PSYCHIATRIC NURSING
Contemporary Practice

SECOND EDITION

PSYCHIATRIC NURSING
Contemporary Practice

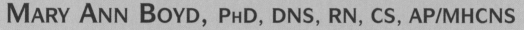

MARY ANN BOYD, PhD, DNS, RN, CS, AP/MHCNS

Professor & Advanced Practice Nurse
Coordinator, Graduate Psychiatric Mental Health Nursing Specialization
School of Nursing
Southern Illinois University Edwardsville
Edwardsville, Illinois

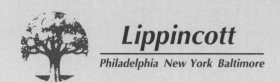
Lippincott
Philadelphia New York Baltimore

Acquisitions Editor: Margaret Zuccarini
Managing Editor/Development: Barclay Cunningham
Developmental Editor: Carol Loyd/Renee Gagliardi
Editorial Assistant: Helen Kogut
Project Editor: Nicole Walz
Senior Production Manager: Helen Ewan
Managing Editor/Production: Barbara Ryalls
Art Director: Carolyn O'Brien
Design: Melissa Olson
Manufacturing Manager: William Alberti
Indexer: Alexandra Nickerson
Compositor: Circle Graphics
Printer: R.R. Donnelley & Sons—Willard

2nd Edition

9 8 7 6 5 4 3 2 1

Library of Congress Cataloging-in-Publication Data

Psychiatric nursing : contemporary practice / [edited by] Mary Ann Boyd.—2nd ed.
    p. ; cm.
  Includes bibliographical references and index.
  ISBN 0-7817-2846-0 (alk. paper)
   1. Psychiatric nursing. I. Boyd, M. (Mary Ann)
  [DNLM: 1. Mental Disorders—nursing. 2. Psychiatric Nursing. WY 160 P9726 2001]
  RC440 .P749 2001
  610.73′68—dc21
                                                            2001041287

This text is dedicated to the development of professionally competent
psychiatric mental health nurses who
balance the art and science of nursing

To Edward & Emma Long, whose life's journey is an inspiration for all.
Mary Ann Boyd

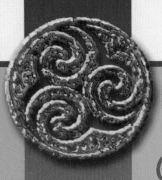

Contributors

Marjorie Baier, RN, PhD, CS
Assistant Professor
Southern Illinois University Edwardsville
Edwardsville, Illinois

Catharine P. Bailey, MSN
Assistant Professor, Psychiatric-Mental Health Specialty
University, School of Nursing
Haven, Connecticut

...ell, PhD, RN, CS

Illinois University Edwardsville
...e, Illinois

...trom, PhD, RN, CS
...fessor and
...an of Academic Programs
...of Nursing
...te University
...and Rapids, Michigan

...hD, RN
..., College of Nursing
...nistration and Clinical Nursing
...arolina
...lina

...er, PhD, RN, FAAN
...e Health Sciences &
...dation Distinguished

...of Nursing

...N, MSN
...s Program
...ion Health Care System

...RN, CS

...y

Barbara G. Faltz, RN, MS
Clinical Nurse Specialist, Addiction Treatment Services
Palo Alto Veterans Administration Health Care System
Palo Alto, California

Linda Garand, PhD, RN, CS
Post Doctoral Fellow,
Western Psychiatric Institute and Clinic
Assistant Professor, University of
    Pittsburgh School of Nursing
Pittsburgh, Pennsylvania

Linda A. Gerdner, PhD, RN
Assistant Professor
College of Nursing
University of Minnesota
Minneapolis, Minnesota

Denise M. Gibson, RN, CS, MSN
Director of Nursing
Alton Mental Health Center
Alton, Illinois

Vanya Hamrin, RN, MS, CS
Program Instructor, Department of
    Psychiatric Nursing
Yale University
New Haven, Connecticut

Sandy Harper-Jaques, MN
Coordinator, Psychiatric Assessment Service
Calgary Regional Health Authority
Calgary, Alberta, Canada

Emily J. Hauenstein, PhD, LCP, RN, CS
Associate Professor
School of Nursing
University of Virginia
Charlottesville, Virginia

Nancy Anne Hilliker, MA, RN, ANP, CS
Nurse Practitioner
Washington University School of Medicine
St. Louis, Missouri

Gail L. Kongable-Beckman, RN, MSN, FNP
Associate Professor
Neurology and Neurological Surgery
University of Virginia Health Systems
Charlottesville, Virginia

Ronna E. Krozy, EdD, RN
Associate Professor of Nursing
Boston College, School of Nursing
Chestnut Hill, Massachusetts

Kathy Lee, MS, RN, CS
Clinical Nurse Specialist
Memorial Behavioral Health Group
Memorial Medical Center
Springfield, Illinois

Barbara J. Limandri, DNSc, RN, CS
Associate Professor
Department of Primary Care, Mental Health Division
Oregon Health Sciences University
Portland, Oregon

Kimberly H. Littrell, MS, ARNP, CS
President and CEO
The Promedica Research Center
Tucker, Georgia
Adjunct Professor
Georgia State University College of Health Sciences

Lyn Marshall, MSN, RN, CS
Director of Psychiatric Nursing
San Mateo County General Hospital
San Mateo, California

Susan McCabe, EdD, RN, CS
Associate Professor, College of Nursing
East Tennessee State University
Johnson City, Tennessee

Mark J. Muehlbach, PhD
Diplomate of the American Board of Sleep Medicine
Associate Director
Sleep Disorders and Research Center
Forest Park Hospital
St. Louis, Missouri
And
Adjunct Faculty
Webster University
Webster Groves, Missouri

Ruth Beckmann Murray, EdD,
  MSN, RN, CS, N-NAP
Professor, Coordinator of Psychiatric-Mental
  Health Nursing
Graduate Specialty
School of Nursing, Saint Louis University
St. Louis, Missouri

Robert B. Noud, RN, MS
Adult Psychiatric Nurse
Illinois Department of Human Services
Alton Mental Health Center
Edwardsville, Illinois

Carol D. Peabody, MS, CCRC
Vice President
The Promedica Research Center
Tucker, Georgia

Marlene Reimer, RN, PhD, CNN(C)
Associate Professor and Associate Dean,
  Research and Graduate Programs,
Faculty of Nursing
University of Calgary
Calgary, Alberta, Canada

Nan Roberts, RN, CS, AP/MHCNS
Advanced Practice Nurse
Private Practice
St. Louis, Missouri

Lawrence Scahill, MSN, PhD
Associate Professor of Nursing and Child Psychiatry
Yale School of Nursing and Yale School of Medicine
New Haven, Connecticut

Mary K. Skinner, RN, MSN, CNS
Clinical Nurse Specialist
Telemedicine Coordinator
Palo Alto Veterans Administration Health Care System
Palo Alto, California

Mickey Stanley, PhD, RN, CS
Associate Professor
School of Nursing
Southern Illinois University Edwardsville
Edwardsville, Illinois

Toni Tripp-Reimer, PhD, RN, FAAN
Professor and Associate Dean for Research
College of Nursing
The University of Iowa
Iowa City, Iowa

Bonnie J. Wakefield, PhD, RN
Research Scientist
Iowa City VA Medical Center
Clinical Associate Professor
College of Nursing
University of Iowa
Iowa City, Iowa

Jane H. White, DNSc, RN, CS
Professor
The Catholic University of America
School of Nursing
Washington, DC
And
Private Practice
Washington, DC

REVIEWERS

Barbara F. Bell, RN, MSEd, MSN
Professor of Nursing
New Mexico Junior College
Hobbs, New Mexico

Linda M. Bulger, MSEd, RNCS, LPC
Faculty
Riverside School of Professional Nursing
Newport News, Virginia

Howard Karl Butcher, RN, PhD, CS
Assistant Professor
The University of Iowa
College of Nursing
Iowa City, Iowa

Nancy L. Cowan, RN, BSN, MSN, EdD
Director of Nursing Program
Chabot College
Hayward, California

Maria deMontigny-Korb, BS, MS, PhD
Assistant Professor
University of Northern Colorado
Greeley, Colorado

Susan Dewey-Hammer, MN, RN, CS
Associate Professor
Suffolk County Community College
Ammerman Campus
Selden, New York

Karen Espeland, MSN, RN, CARN
Associate Professor
Med Center One College of Nursing
Bismarck, North Dakota

Sarah P. Farrell, PhD, RN, CS
Assistant Professor
University of Virginia
Charlottesville, Virginia

Mary Fenimore, AAS, BS, MA, EdD
Professor
Pasco-Hernando Community College
New Port Richey, Florida

Anne H. Fishel, PhD, RN, CS
Professor
University of North Carolina at Chapel Hill
Chapel Hill, North Carolina

Bonnie Gnadt, MSN
Associate Professor
Southwestern Adventist University
Department of Nursing
Keene, Texas

Ella Hunter, PhD, RN
Professor of Nursing
Eastern Kentucky University
Richmond, Kentucky

Katherine Jorgensen, RN, MA, MSN
Assistant Professor
University of South Dakota, Department of Nursing
Vermillion, South Dakota

Merrie J. Kaas, DNSc, RN, CS
Associate Professor
University of Minnesota
School of Nursing
Minneapolis, Minnesota

Eileen W. Keefe, MS, RN, C
Assistant Professor of Clinical Nursing
School of Nursing
Louisiana State University Health Sciences Center
New Orleans, Louisiana

Joanne Lavin, RN, EdD, CS
Professor
Kingsborough Community College
Brooklyn, New York

Jennifer L. Lewis, RN, MS
Associate Professor
Front Range Community College
Westminster, Colorado

Wanda K. Mohr, PhD, RN, FAAN
Associate Professor
Rutgers, The State University of New Jersey
Newark, New Jersey

Elaine Mordoch, RN, BN, MN
Lecturer
University of Manitoba
Winnipeg, Manitoba
Canada

Marianne Hattar Pollara, RN, DNSc
Professor
Azusa Pacific University
Azusa, California

Charlotte Spade, MS, RN, CS, CNS
Professor
Community College of Denver
Health & Human Services Division
Denver, Colorado

Pamela Phillips White, RN, MSN
Assistant Professor
Spalding University
Louisville, Kentucky

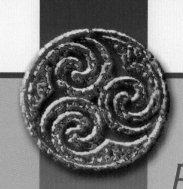

Preface

It is with much excitement that we introduce the second edition of *Psychiatric Nursing: Contemporary Practice*. As we enter the 21st century, psychiatric nursing is facing new challenges in the care and treatment of people with mental illness. Knowledge about mental disorders exploded during the 1990s, the "Decade of the Brain." We are pleased to greet this opportunity by incorporating new scientific findings into this text. We now have scientific knowledge to understand our patients as complex human beings. The biopsychosocial paradigm is alive and well. It provides a solid organizing framework for education, research and practice. *Psychiatric Nursing: Contemporary Practice* is written by seasoned expert faculty and practitioners who are at the cutting edge of both the science and art of psychiatric nursing. As recognized leaders in their field, they are able to provide a comprehensive perspective of mental health and disorders in clear, easily understood terms.

This second edition presents the most current advances in psychiatric care, psychiatric nursing care, and nursing education including current research into the biologic basis of mental illness, psychopharmacologic treatment of mental disorders, the increasing professional demands of delivering care in a continuum of settings, and wide curriculum changes in nursing education. These and other advances make it even more important for nursing students to develop critical thinking skills. With this in mind, the text has been developed to provide the theoretical and informational knowledge base to assist students in sharpening their critical thinking skills as well as their ability to make sound clinical judgments. This edition is in full color with a dynamic new design to attract and sustain the learner's interest.

This text is solidly grounded in the biopsychosocial paradigm as the foundation for teaching and practicing psychiatric mental health nursing. Using the *Diagnostic and Statistical Manual of Psychiatric Disorders Text Revision* (DSM-IV-TR) as a guide, specific disorders have been selected to be highlighted and addressed in depth in the text. These highlighted disorders are the more typical examples that the beginning nurse will encounter. Based upon student and faculty feedback, this edition has been expanded to include separate assessment chapters of adults, children, the elderly, and the family. Psychiatric nursing assessment instruments are included for each group. Group interventions are also found in a separate chapter. Because of the complexity of the mental disorders, students asked for help in matching interventions with assessment data. To this end, in those chapters presenting significant major mental disorders, assessment data, nursing diagnosis, and interventions are presented within the context of each domain. This level of detail enables the student to develop a thorough understanding of the biologic, psychological, and social domains of each disorder before being expected to integrate these concepts in the real world of clinical practice.

It is the goal of this text, however, to help prepare a well-rounded graduate nurse who can apply the knowledge and understanding of human behavior and psychiatric disorders gained from using this text to caring for any human being, whether in a professional or personal capacity. To address this goal, this text is based on the following beliefs:

- A textbook should provide the student with a bridge, connecting theory with clinical application.
- Beginning nurses need to gain competence in assessing human behavior, developing therapeutic communication skills, and understanding how to diagnose, identify outcomes, and plan and evaluate basic interventions for psychiatric patients.
- Appropriate assessment tools are necessary to provide a structured approach for gathering meaningful patient data.
- A textbook should provide knowledge that is easily transferred from the classroom to the clinical setting.
- A psychiatric nursing textbook should focus on teaching the fundamentals of nursing care of patients with commonly occurring *DSM-IV-TR* psychiatric disorders.
- It is important to impart theoretical, research-based knowledge and skills that reflect contemporary

practice, to enhance the capacity of nursing professionals to practice in any health care delivery environment.

- It is imperative to prepare culturally diverse nurses who can provide culturally competent care in culturally diverse environments.

Chapter authors for this textbook were carefully selected based on their psychiatric nursing expertise. Mastery of their respective areas is readily evident. Although the material is complex, content is explained in a language that is easily understood by the undergraduate student. We have incorporated Canadian nursing practice considerations when possible.

TEXT ORGANIZATION

Each of the chapters that focus on patient care highlights a carefully selected number of the more frequently occurring disorders or patient situations that require some degree of psychiatric nursing care. This approach permits a more in-depth exploration of the current knowledge related to etiology, risk factors, assessment, and treatment that is appropriate in the contemporary psychiatric health care delivery setting. In this way, students can assimilate the key principles that are important for providing effective psychiatric nursing care within the constraints of our fast-changing health care environment. Less frequently occurring disorders are summarized in text and tables, provide students with the basis for developing appropriate nursing care for patients with a variety of diagnoses in any setting.

PEDAGOGICAL FEATURES

Psychiatric Nursing: Contemporary Practice incorporates a multitude of pedagogical features to focus and direct student learning, including:

- Chapter Opener pedagogy
- The Chapter Outline presents an overview of content to be studied, providing a frame within which to organize information.
- Learning Objectives provide a road map for student learning.
- The Key Terms list identifies new terms used and defined in the chapter context.
- The Key Concepts list identifies concepts that are critical to fully understanding the chapter content.
- Other text pedagogy
- The Summary of Key Points encapsulates important chapter content to focus chapter study and encourage content assimilation.
- The Critical Thinking Challenges use aspects of chapter content to stimulate independent thinking and encourage the development of higher cognitive function.

- The Glossary offers easily accessible definitions of important terms.

NEW PEDAGOGICAL FEATURES

- Movies: Each chapter has at least one entertainment video that can be rented to depict an important concept in the chapter. Students are encouraged to view the video and use it as a basis of discussion in class. "Viewing points" are provided so that students can focus their attention to certain aspects of the film.
- Web Links: Each chapter has several web links for the student to use for supplemental information.

SPECIAL FEATURES

- Highlighted Disorders Approach provides an in-depth study of the more commonly occurring major psychiatric disorders.
- Case Study-Based Nursing Care Plans present actual clinical examples of patients with the highlighted diagnosis and demonstrate plans of care that follow patients through various diagnostic stages and care-delivery settings. These care plans help students understand the dynamic nature of the nursing process: the ongoing need to constantly assess, develop nursing diagnoses and interventions, identify outcomes, and evaluate patient outcomes.
- Interdisciplinary treatment plans (ITPs) are linked with their respective nursing care plans in three disorders chapters. ITPs are used extensively in the real world of practice.
- Therapeutic Dialogue Boxes contrast therapeutic with nontherapeutic dialogue to encourage by example the development of therapeutic communication.
- Psychoeducation Checklists identify content areas for patient and family education related to a specific disorder and its treatment, which supports critical thinking by encouraging students to develop a patient-specific teaching plan based on chapter content.
- Clinical Vignettes present a vivid clinical portrait of patients exhibiting the symptoms described within the text discussion.
- Family focus is identified throughout the text with a family icon. The emphasis on the family indicates that assessment and interventions apply to the care of the family.
- Research Utilization Boxes present current research and its application to practice and underscore the importance of reading, evaluating, and applying research in clinical practice when appropriate.

- Key Diagnostic Characteristics Tables present DSM-IV-TR diagnostic criteria, target symptoms, and related findings for highlighted disorders, and help identify behavior, treatment, and physical and lab assessment parameters, thereby expanding the student's understanding of the clinical picture.
- Summary of Diagnostic Characteristics Tables present *DSM-IV-TR* diagnostic criteria for other disorders within the chapter's diagnostic category.
- Biologic art provides visual explanation of complex neurophysiology.
- Biopsychosocial three-ring art highlights the biopsychosocial aspects of patient outcomes, disorder etiologies, and nursing interventions, providing a succinct and visual summary of these key dimensions for highlighted disorders.
- A variety of scans illustrate the biologic nature of the etiology of many *DSM-IV-TR disorders and show the effects of biologic intervention.*

TEACHING-LEARNING PACKAGE

The teaching-learning package that accompanies this edition includes a student study guide, a computerized testbank, a printed testbank, an instructor's manual, and overhead transparency masters.

- The Study Guide, based on the text, is clinically focused and dedicated to helping the student use critical thinking skills to make the transition from the classroom to the clinical setting. A wide variety of approaches are offered to meet a range of learning needs. Examples of features and learning activities include: summarized chapter highlights and key points, critical thinking exercises, communication exercises, self-exploration situations, short-answer questions, case study-based nursing care plans, nursing diagnoses tables for specified disorders, and other learning activities such as crossword puzzles and word scrambles, matching, sentence completion, and biologic art labeling exercises.
- The Testbank on CD-ROM, consists of 1,000 NCLEX-style test items. It is available free to instructors upon adoption of the text.

- The Instructor's Manual on 'connection' website [connection.lww.com/go/boyd] is designed to provide the instructor with concrete support in designing meaningful student in-class activities, whether a traditional lecture or a case study—based approach to teaching and learning. The Instructor's Manual includes material that supports faculty understanding of the biologic basis of psychiatric disorders, and integrates the textbook contents with Study Guide activities to encourage full use of every aspect of this psychiatric nursing material in the student curriculum.
- Image Bank on CD-ROM provides line art, schematics, graphs and tables from the textbook electronically that can be imported to PowerPoint slides or printed out and prepared as overhead transparencies.
- PowerPoint slides on CD-ROM provide ready-made lecture outlines that can be used as part of any electronic presentation program.

I hope that this text will more firmly establish psychiatric nursing as a substantive health care specialty with a well-defined knowledge base. I believe that the biopsychosocial paradigm provides a strong research-based foundation for integrating these multiple diverse human dimensions into psychiatric nursing practice. I hope that through the teaching of the biologic basis of psychiatric disorders, the stigma of mental illness will eventually be ameliorated and that psychiatric disorders will be viewed as any other health care problem.

Care has been taken to present psychiatric nursing as an exciting and challenging specialty that presents opportunities to make a difference in the lives of patients and their families. The ultimate aim is to help improve the care of our patients and their quality of life. I firmly believe that this thoroughly contemporary and clinically relevant text will effectively nurture students in their quest to become competent nursing professionals who are capable of providing theoretically sound and culturally competent care to patients in any setting.

Mary Ann Boyd, PhD, DNS, RN, CS, AP/MHCNS
Professor & Advanced Practice Nurse

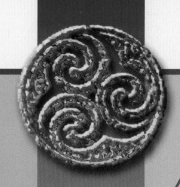

Acknowledgments

The publication of this second edition was an exciting journey. The contributors and I were challenged to re-examine our previous work within the context of new research findings and thinking. Ideas shift rapidly. New research quickly invalidates previous beliefs. We continued to be challenged to re-synthesize current scientific knowledge, then re-conceptualize and re-explain the world of psychiatric nursing in a way that is meaningful to the undergraduate student. The second edition is seen as a work in progress. Editorial guidance and resources were in constant demand from the Lippincott Williams & Wilkins staff, who enthusiastically and tirelessly responded to our many questions.

I wish to express my sincere appreciation to the contributors, who spent many hours writing and revising the numerous drafts of their manuscripts, and to the reviewers, whose expertise was invaluable in the development of this text. Recognition is due to Mary Ann Nihart, whose suggestion it was to adopt the biopsychosocial model as a way of organizing the content. I especially want to acknowledge Dr. Jeanne Fox and Dr. Catherine Kane for their guidance in the first edition. I wish to extend my warmest thanks to Mary E. Johnson and the library staff of the Missouri Institute of Mental Health for their support and professionalism as they responded to my infinite number of requests. To the students from Southern Illinois University Edwardsville, I thank you for your careful critiques and for helping me to understand the student's perspective. I want to extend my very deepest appreciation to the staff at Lippincott Williams & Wilkins, especially Margaret Zuccarini, Helen Kogut, Carol Loyd, Barclay Cunningham, Renee Gagliardi, and Nicole Walz, who worked tirelessly in making this book a reality.

Finally, I want to thank my husband, James, for his patience, support, and understanding throughout this project.

Mary Ann Boyd, PhD, DNS, RN, CS, AP/MHCNS

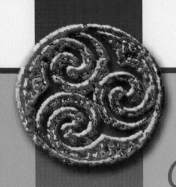

Contents

PSYCHIATRIC NURSING
Contemporary Practice

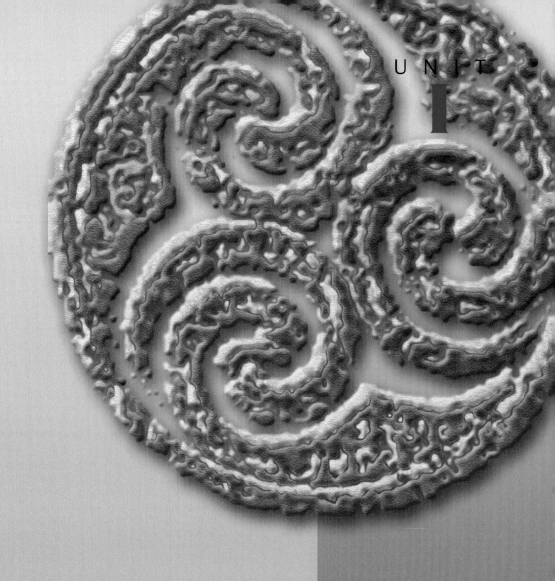

The Nature of Mental Health and Mental Illness

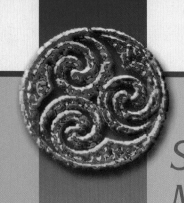

Social Change and Mental Health

Mary Ann Boyd

**LEARNING
OBJECTIVES**

After studying this chapter, you will be able to:

➤ Identify agents of social change that affect the delivery of mental health care.

➤ Relate the concept of social change to the history of psychiatric–mental health care.

➤ Discuss the history of psychiatric–mental health nursing and its place within nursing history.

➤ Analyze the theoretic arguments that shaped the development of contemporary scientific thought.

➤ Summarize the impact of the current economic and political forces on the delivery of mental health services.

Throughout history, mental disorders were believed to have been caused by an interplay of biologic, spiritual, and environmental factors. Acceptable methods of treatment reflected the underlying popular beliefs of the times. In periods when the causes of mental disorders were believed to be primarily biologic, individuals were treated with the latest biologic therapy. Prehistoric healers practiced an ancient surgical technique of removing a disk of bone from the skull to let out the evil spirits. In the early Christian period (1 to 100 AD), when mental disorders were believed to be caused by sin or demonic possession, clergymen treated patients, often through prescribed exorcisms. If such measures did not succeed, patients were excluded from the community and sometimes even put to death. Later in the Medieval era (1000–1300), disorders were often believed to be products of dysfunctional environments, and individuals were removed from their "sick" environments and placed in protected asylums.

The differences in treatment of mentally ill patients may depend on the community's perceived notions and fears of those with mental disorders. History reflects that generally, in periods of relative social stability, there is less fear and more tolerance for deviant behavior, and it is easier for individuals with mental disorders to live safely within their communities. During periods of rapid social change and instability, there is more general anxiety and fear regarding people with mental disorders

and subsequently more intolerance and ill treatment of them. See Table 1-1 for a summary of historical events and correlating perspectives on mental health during the Pre–Moral Treatment Era (800 BC to the Colonial Period).

A REVOLUTIONARY IDEA: HUMANE TREATMENT

The emergence of enlightened political ideas and an increasing availability of economic resources in the late 18th century led to the advent of **moral treatment** in mental health care, characterized by kindness, compassion, and a pleasant environment for patients. Publicly and privately supported asylums for individuals with mental disorders were built during this time, and patients were routinely removed from their home environments, which were believed to be causing the illnesses. It was the first humane treatment period since the Greek and Roman eras.

By the height of the French Revolution in 1792, moral treatment had become a standard practice. It was during this time that Philippe Pinel (1745–1826) was appointed physician to Bicetre, a hospital for men that had the unfortunate distinction of being touted as the worst asylum in the world. Pinel believed that the insane were sick patients who needed special treatment, and once installed in his position, he ordered the removal of the chains, stopped the abuses of drugging and bloodletting,

TABLE 1.1   Social Change in the Pre–Moral Treatment Era

Period	Socioeconomic and Political Events and People	Changing Attitudes and Practice in Mental Health Care
Ancient Times to 800 BC	Sickness was an indication of the displeasure of deities for sins. Viewed as supernatural.	Persons with psychiatric symptoms were driven from homes and ostracized by relatives. When behavioral manifestations were viewed as supernatural powers, the persons who exhibited them were revered.
Greek and Roman: 800 BC to 1 AD	Egypt and Greek periods of inquiry. Physical and mental health viewed as interrelated. Hippocrates argued abnormal behaviors were due to brain disturbances. Aristotle related mental to physical disorders.	Counseling, work, music were provided in temples by priests to relieve the distress of those with mental disorders. Observation and documentation were a part of the care. The mental disorders were treated as diseases. The aim of treatment was to correct imbalances.
Early Christian and Early Medieval: 1–1000 AD	Power of Christian church grew. St. Augustine pronounced all diseases ascribed to demons.	Persons with psychiatric symptoms were incarcerated in dungeons, beaten, and starved.
Later Medieval: 1000–1300 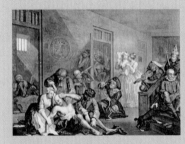	In Western Europe, spirit of inquiry dead. Healing by theologians and witchdoctors. Persons with psychiatric symptoms were incarcerated in dungeons, beaten, and starved. In Mideast, Avicenna said mental disorders are illnesses.	First asylums built by Moslems. Persons with psychiatric symptoms were treated as being sick.
Renaissance: 1300–1600 Interior of Bethlehem Hospital, London *Colonial: 1700–1790*	In England, differentiated insane from criminal. In colonies, mental illness believed caused by demonic possession. Witch hunts were common.	Persons with psychiatric symptoms who presented a threat to society were apprehended and locked up. There were no public provisions for persons with mental disorders except jail. Private hospitalization for the wealthy who could pay. Bethlehem Asylum was used as a private institution.
	1751: Benjamin Franklin established Pennsylvania Hospital (in Philadelphia)—the first institution in United States to receive those with mental disorder for treatment and cure. 1773: First public, free-standing asylum at Williamsburg, Virginia. 1783: Benjamin Rush categorized mental illnesses and began to treat mental disorders with medical interventions such as bloodletting, mechanical devices.	The beginnings of mental diseases viewed as illness to be treated.

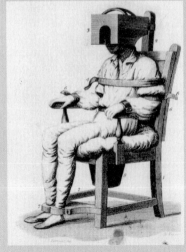

The Tranquilizer Chair of Benjamin Rush. A patient is sitting in a chair, his body immobilized, a bucket attached beneath the seat. U.S. National Library of Medicine, *Images from the History of Medicine*, National Institutes of Health, Department of Health and Human Services.

and placed the patients under the care of physicians. Three years later, the same standards were extended to Salpetriere, the asylum for female patients. At about the same time in England, William Tuke (1732–1822), a member of the Society of Friends, raised funds for a retreat for members who had mental disorders. The York Retreat was opened in 1796; restraints were abandoned, and sympathetic care in quiet, pleasant surroundings with some form of industrial occupation, such as weaving or farming, was provided (Fig. 1-1).

While Tuke was influential in England, the Quakers also exercised their influence in the United States, where they were instrumental in stopping the practice of bloodletting and placed great emphasis on providing a proper religious atmosphere (Deutsch, 1949). The Quaker Friends Asylum was proposed in 1811 and opened 6 years later in Frankford, Pennsylvania, to become the second asylum in the United States. The humane and supportive rehabilitative attitude of the Quakers was seen as an extremely important influence in changing management techniques toward the mentally disordered. As states were founded, new hospitals were opened that were dedicated to the care of patients with mental disorders. By the end of the first quarter of the 19th century, institutions were established in Kentucky, South Carolina, Maryland, Massachusetts, Ohio, Connecticut, New York, and Pennsylvania. Virginia established its second state hospital during this period in Staunton.

Even with these hospitals, only a small fraction of people with mental disorders received treatment. Those who were judged dangerous were hospitalized; those deemed harmless or mildly insane were treated the same as other indigents and given no public support. In farm communities, as was the custom during the first half of the 19th century, the poor and indigent were often auctioned and bought by landowners to provide cheap labor. Landowners eagerly sought them out for their strong backs and weak minds. The arrangement had its own economic usefulness because it provided the community with a low-cost way to care for its mentally ill. Some states used almshouses (poorhouses) for housing the mentally ill.

THE 19TH AND EARLY 20TH CENTURIES

Horace Mann and the Beginning of Public Responsibility

Horace Mann was a representative in the Massachusetts state legislature whose plea that the "insane are wards of the state" became a reality in 1828. State governments were expected to assume financial responsibility for the care of people with mental illnesses. This is an important milestone because it set a precedent for tax-supported mental health funding. Canada also embraced mental health care as a public responsibility. By the time the British North America Act was passed in 1867, which created the Dominion of Canada, the care of the mentally ill was the responsibility of provinces.

A Social Reformer: Dorothea Lynde Dix

Dorothea Lynde Dix (1802–1887), a militant crusader for the humane treatment of patients with mental illness, was responsible for much of the reform of the mental health care system in the 19th century. At nearly 40 years of age, Dix, a retired school teacher living in Massachusetts, was solicited by a young theology student to help in preparing a Sunday School class for women inmates at the East Cambridge jail. Dix led the class herself and was shocked by the filth and dirt in the jail. She was particularly struck by the treatment of inmates with mental disorders. It was the dead of winter, and no heat was provided. When she questioned the jailer about the lack of heat, his answer was that "the insane need no heat." The prevailing myth was that the insane were insensible to extremes of temperature. Her outrage initiated a long struggle in the reform of care.

An early feminist, Dix disregarded the New England role of a Puritan woman and diligently investigated the conditions of jails and the plight of the mentally ill. Her solution was state hospitals. She first influenced the Massachusetts legislature to expand the Massachusetts State Hospital. Then, through public awareness campaigns and lobbying efforts, she managed to convince state after state to build hospitals. Dorothea Dix also turned her attention to the plight of the mentally ill in Canada, where she was instrumental in creating mental hospitals in Halifax, Nova Scotia and St. John, Newfoundland (Fig. 1-2).

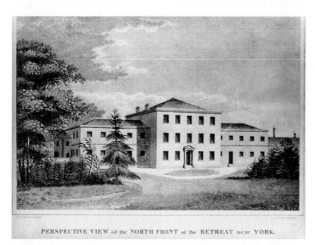

PERSPECTIVE VIEW of the NORTH FRONT of the RETREAT near YORK.

FIGURE 1.1 The perspective view of the north front of the retreat near York. U.S. National Library of Medicine, *Images from the History of Medicine*. National Institutes of Health, Department of Health and Human Services.

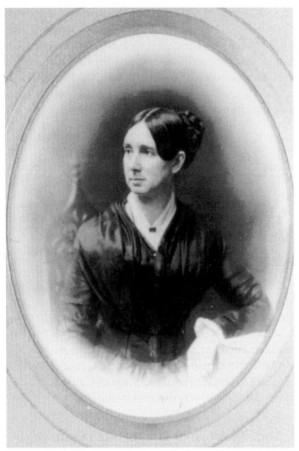

FIGURE 1.2 Dorothea Lynde Dix. U.S. National Library of Medicine, *Images from the History of Medicine*. National Institutes of Health, Department of Health and Human Services.

At the end of her long career, 20 states had responded directly to her appeals by establishing or enlarging state hospitals. Dix played an important role in the establishment of the Government Hospital for the Insane in Washington, DC (which later became St. Elizabeth's Hospital). In addition to Canada, she extended her work into Great Britain and other parts of Europe. During the Civil War, Dix was appointed to the post of Superintendent of Women Nurses, the highest position held by a woman during the war.

Life Within Early Institutions

The approach inside the institution was one of practical management, not treatment. The patients did not possess the interpersonal and social skills to live within a family setting, let alone in the complex group-living environment of a state hospital, with others who were equally ill. The major concern was the management of a large number of people with bizarre thoughts and behaviors who lived in close quarters.

Women had a particularly difficult time and were often institutionalized at the convenience of their fathers or husbands. Because a woman's role in the late 1800s was to function as a domestic extension of her husband, any behavior or beliefs that did not conform to male expectations could be used to justify the claim of insanity. These women were literally held prisoner for years (Geller & Harris, 1994). In the asylums, women were psychologically degraded, used as servants, and physically tortured by male physicians and female attendants. First-hand accounts of women's experiences dating from 1840 to 1945 are described in the book *Women of the Asylum: Voices From Behind the Walls, 1840–1945*, by Jeffrey L. Geller and Maxine Harris.

For male patients, these institutions had little more to offer than food, clothing, pleasant surroundings, and perhaps some means of employment and exercise. Because the scientific hypotheses linking mental disorders to brain dysfunction were generally ignored, the emphasis in the institutions was on humane custodial care within an efficient organization. Many people believed that this custodial care was the highest possible level of treatment that could be provided.

People with mental disorders who were warehoused in state mental institutions had little hope of reentering society. In 1908, Clifford Beers (1876–1943) published an autobiography, *A Mind That Found Itself*, depicting his 3-year experience in three different types of hospitals, a private for-profit hospital, a private nonprofit hospital, and a state institution. In all of these facilities, he was beaten, choked, imprisoned for long periods in dark, dank, padded cells, and confined many days in a straightjacket. At the end of his book, he recommended that a national society be established for the purpose of reforming care and treatment, disseminating information, and encouraging and conducting research. Beers' cause was supported by a prominent Swiss neuropathologist, Adolf Meyer (1866–1950), who suggested the term "mental hygiene" to denote mental health. By 1909, Beers formed a National Committee for Mental Hygiene. Through the committee's efforts, child guidance clinics, prison clinics, and industrial mental health approaches were developed.

Early institutions eventually evolved into self-contained communities that produced their own food and made their own clothing. A medical superintendent, who was usually more adept in executive and business ability than in treatment, managed the closed mental health community. Attendants, many of whom were untrained, staffed these institutions. Nursing care was not introduced until the very late 1800s.

Development of Psychiatric–Mental Health Nursing Thought

Early Views

The roots of contemporary psychiatric–mental health nursing thought can be traced back to Florence Nightingale's seminal work, *Notes on Nursing*, originally published in 1839 (Nightingale, 1859; Barker, 1990). The holistic view of the patient, with the body and soul seen as inseparable and the patient viewed as a member of a family and community, was central to Nightingale's view of nursing. Even though she did not address the care of patients in asylums, Nightingale was sensitive to human emotion and recommended interactions that would be classified as therapeutic communication today (see Chap. 9). This early nursing leader advocated promotion of health and development of independence by encouraging patients to perform their own health care. She believed that this, in turn, would reduce their anxiety in the face of illness.

The need for specialized psychiatric–mental health nursing was recognized when the humane care that characterized the Moral Treatment Era was emerging as a model for practice. Dr. Edward Cowles, director of the McLean Asylum in Massachusetts, firmly believed that patients in mental hospitals should receive nursing care. His attempts to employ nurses to meet the particular needs of asylum patients, however, proved fruitless for two reasons. First, the nurses received no formal education in mental diseases; in addition, many of them were resistant to being associated with the asylum because of the stigma attached to mental disorders. Cowles sought to remedy both shortcomings by assisting Linda Richards, the United States' first trained nurse, to open a training school for psychiatric–mental health nurses that

was based on Florence Nightingale's principles and training practices (Cowles, 1887). The Boston City Hospital Training School for Nurses, which was established in 1882 at McLean Hospital, answered those specific needs.

Although there was still much social resistance toward the education of women, especially for the care of the insane, the first candidates for admission to the McLean training school were both male and female attendants who worked at the McLean Asylum (Campinha, 1987). McLean was noteworthy for more than just providing nurses with the rudiments of caring for the mentally ill. It was the first institution in the United States to provide men the opportunity to become trained nurses (Mericle, 1983) (Text Box 1-1).

Although nurses were trained in the care of patients in psychiatric institutions, their training was financially and academically dependent on the institution's organizational structure and was outside of mainstream nursing education. In 1913, Effie Taylor initiated the first nursing program of study organized by nurses for psychiatric training at Johns Hopkins' Phipps Clinic. Taylor sought to integrate the concepts from general and mental health nursing to establish a more comprehensive knowledge base for all nursing care. She was committed to the concept of wholeness and warned that mental health nursing and general nursing could not and should not exist independently of each other. In Taylor's classes at Johns Hopkins, the psychobiologic

TEXT BOX 1.1

History of Psychiatric Mental Health Nursing

1882 First training school for psychiatric nursing at McLean Asylum by E. Cowles; first nursing program to admit men.

1913 First nurse-organized program of study for psychiatric training by Euphemia (Effie) Jane Taylor at Johns Hopkins Phipps Clinic.

1914 Mary Adelaide Nutting emphasized nursing role development.

1920 First psychiatric nursing text published, *Nursing Mental Disease,* by Harriet Bailey.

1950 Accredited schools required to offer a psychiatric nursing experience.

1952 Publication of Hildegarde E. Peplau's *Interpersonal Relations in Nursing.*

1954 First graduate program in psychiatric nursing established at Rutgers University by Hildegarde E. Peplau.

1963 *Perspectives in Psychiatric Care* and *Journal of Psychiatric Nursing* published.

1967 *Standards of Psychiatric–Mental Health Nursing Practice* published. American Nurses Association (ANA) initiated the certification of generalists in psychiatric mental health nursing.

1979 *Issues in Mental Health Nursing* published. ANA initiated the certification of specialists in psychiatric mental health nursing.

1980 *Nursing: A Social Policy Statement* published by the ANA.

1982 *Revised Standards of Psychiatric and Mental Health Nursing Practice* issued by the ANA.

1985 *Standards of Child and Adolescent Psychiatric and Mental Health Nursing Practice* published by the ANA.

1987 *Archives of Psychiatric Nursing* and *Journal of Child and Adolescent Psychiatric and Mental Health Nursing* published.

1994 *Statement on Psychiatric–Mental Health Clinical Nursing Practice and Standards of Psychiatric–Mental Health Clinical Nursing Practice* written by ANA, American Psychiatric Nurses Association, Association of Child and Adolescent Psychiatric Nurses, Inc., and Society for Education and Research in Psychiatric–Mental Health Nursing (SERPN).

1996 Guidelines specifying course content and competencies published by *SERPN.*

2000 *Statement on Psychiatric Mental Health Nursing Practice.*

orientation was basic to all patients, not just to those labeled mentally ill. Taylor, like Nightingale before her, encouraged nurses to avoid the false dichotomy of mind and body (Church, 1987). She believed that the integrated whole was the focus of nursing. In 1914, distinguished nursing leader and educator Mary Adelaide Nutting (1858–1948) addressed a conference at the new Psychopathic Hospital in Boston on the role of the psychopathic nurse. Her unique message was that nursing care should be based on scientific study and conceptualized in terms of diagnosis, care, and treatment.

Social Influences

The development of nursing thought has been significantly influenced by the larger social climate in which women in the profession operated. During Cowles' era, women could neither vote nor own property, and nursing training reflected the societal view of women as helpmates of men (physicians). In the early 1900s, nurses were expected to stay subservient to physicians and administrators and quietly play out the maternal role outside the home (Church, 1987). Although this may have been an acceptable social policy, it effectively barred nurses from obtaining full access to information they needed to treat their patients properly. For example, in 1920, Effie Taylor complained bitterly to Adolf Meyer that nurses were not allowed to view medical records, whereas medical students (men) were.

Despite the oppressive social climate for psychiatric nurses, nursing thought continued to develop. The first psychiatric nursing textbook, *Nursing Mental Disease*, was written by Harriet Bailey in 1920. The content of the book reflected an understanding of mental disorders of the times and set forth nursing care in terms of procedures.

MODERN THINKING

Evolution of Scientific Thought

As psychiatric–mental health nursing continued to develop as a profession in the early part of the 20th century, modern perspectives on mental illness were emerging in research, and these new theories would profoundly shape the future of mental health care for all practitioners. Further examination of the underlying ideologies is discussed in Chapter 6, but it is important to understand their development within the social and historical context to appreciate fully their impact on treatment approaches.

In the early 1900s, two opposing views were held regarding mental illnesses: the belief that mental disorders had biologic origins and the belief that the problems were attributed to environmental and social stresses. The **psychosocial theory** proposed that mental disorders resulted from environmental and social deprivation. Moral management (nonrestraint, kindness, and hygiene) in an asylum was the answer. However, by the 1900s, it was realized that moral treatment alone would not cure mental disorders. The **biologic view** held that mental illnesses had a biologic cause and could be treated with physical interventions. Biologic science was not far enough advanced to offer reasonable treatment approaches, however, and existing primitive physical treatments (venesections [bloodletting] and gyrations [strapping patients to a rotating board]) were either painful or considered barbaric. What ensued was a complete and bitter split between the two groups.

Meyer and Psychiatric Pluralism

Adolf Meyer attempted to bridge the ideologic gap between the two groups by introducing the concept of **psychiatric pluralism,** an integration of human biologic functions with the environment. Meyer became interested in psychiatry after he received an appointment at Kankakee, Illinois State Hospital in 1892. Although he had no clinical training in psychiatry, he eventually became a professor of psychiatry at Johns Hopkins University and chief of the Phipps Psychiatric Clinic. His approach focused on investigating how the organs related to the person and how the person, constituted of these organs, related to the environment (Neill, 1980). However, the biologic explanations were so far removed from later scientific evidence that Meyer's concept of psychiatric pluralism won little support. The times were right for a new approach.

Freud and the Psychoanalytic Theory

Sigmund Freud (1856–1939) and the **psychoanalytic movement** of the early 1900s promised an even more radical approach to psychiatric–mental health care. Freud, trained as a neuropathologist, developed a personality theory based on unconscious motivations for behavior, or drives. Using a new technique, psychoanalysis, he delved into the patient's feelings and emotions regarding past experiences, particularly early childhood and adolescent memories, to explain the basis of aberrant behavior. He showed that symptoms of hysteria could be produced and made to disappear while patients were in a subconscious state of hypnosis.

As psychoanalytic theory gained in popularity, ideas of the mind–body relationship were lost. According to the freudian model, normal development occurred in stages, with the first three being the most important: oral, anal, and genital. The infant progressed through the oral stage, experiencing the world through symbolic oral ingestion; through the anal stage, in which the toddler developed a sense of autonomy through withholding; and on to the genital stage, in which a beginning sense of sexuality emerged within the framework of the oedipal relationship. If there was any interference in normal development, such as psychological trauma, psychosis or neurosis would develop.

Primary causes of mental illnesses were now viewed as psychological, and any physical manifestations or social influences were considered secondary (Malamud, 1944). It was generally believed within the psychiatric community that mental illnesses were a result of disturbed personality development and faulty parenting. Mental illnesses were categorized either as a psychosis (severe) or neurosis (less severe). A psychosis impaired daily functioning because of breaks in contact with reality. A neurosis was less severe, but individuals were often distressed about their problems. The terms *psychosis* and *neurosis* entered common, everyday language and added credibility to Freud's conceptualization of mental disorders. Soon, Freud's ideas represented the forefront of psychiatric thought and began to shape society's view of mental health care. Freudian ideology dominated psychiatric thought well into the 1970s.

Intensive psychoanalysis, which focused on repairing the trauma of the original psychological injury, was the treatment of choice. Psychoanalysis was costly, was time-consuming, and required lengthy training. Few could perform it. It thus became the treatment of choice for a select clientele: the idle wealthy who had access to a trained psychoanalyst. People who could engage in a lengthy therapeutic relationship and had the economic resources to pay for frequent visits were treated for many years. Thousands of patients in state institutions with severe mental illnesses were essentially ignored. Because Freud's ideas about mental illnesses were so widely accepted, however, there was little interest or support for pursuing any other explanation or treatment for mental disorders.

Diagnostic Classifications

The ideologic struggles of the biologic, psychosocial, and psychoanalytic groups are apparent in the changes that have occurred in diagnosing mental disorders. In the early 1900s, Emil Kraepelin introduced a diagnostic classification framework based on descriptive symptomatology. Before that time, mental disorders were divided into mania, melancholia, and dementia. Although Kraepelin's classification was based on symptoms rather than causes, it did account for the whole course of diseases. He recognized manic-depressive illness (bipolar) as a distinct disorder and developed the concept of dementia praecox (schizophrenia). This classification was quickly adopted.

Kraepelin's classification system was inconsistent with Freud's conceptualization of psychological drives. Freudian psychoanalysts were diagnosing and treating disorders that were not identified in the kraepelinian

classification. A standardized classification system was needed to provide a common framework. In 1952, the American Psychiatric Association (APA) Committee on Nomenclature and Statistics developed the first edition of the *Diagnostic and Statistical Manual of Mental Disorders* (*DSM-I*). This first standardized diagnostic classification system categorized mental disorders according to the freudian model, using the categories of psychosis and neurosis. Other disorders, such as hysteria, which Freud and his followers discovered, were included in the taxonomy. Freudian thought clearly dominated psychiatry. The *DSM-I* was followed by a similar *DSM-II* (APA, 1968).

Even though the freudian conceptualization of mental illness initially received considerable political support from the psychiatric community, its heavy reliance on subjective assessment and the lack of research support caused the model to be rejected as a classification for mental illness. In the 1960s, a "neo-kraepelinian" movement began at Washington University in St. Louis. After years of systematically investigating psychiatric symptomatology, a change in direction took place in 1980. No longer were the categories of psychosis and neurosis used. Instead, the *Diagnostic and Statistical Manual of Mental Disorders* (*DSM-III* and *DSM-IV* (APA, 1980, 1994) returned to a taxonomy based on descriptive symptomatology.

Integration of Biologic Theories Into Psychosocial Treatment

Up until the 1940s, the biologic understanding of mental illness was fairly unsophisticated and often misguided. Biologic treatments in this century were often unsuccessful because of the lack of understanding and knowledge of the biologic basis of mental disorders. For example, the use of hydrotherapy, or baths, was an established procedure in mental institutions. The use of warm baths and in some instances, ice cold baths, produced calming effects for patients with mental disorders. However, the treatment's success was ascribed to its effectiveness as a form of restraint because the physiologic responses that hydrotherapy produced were not understood. Baths were applied indiscriminately and used as a form of restraint, rather than a therapeutic practice. Other examples of biologic procedures applied either indiscriminately or inappropriately include psychosurgery and electroconvulsive therapy (see Chap. 8). Thanks to modern technology, neurosurgical techniques and electroconvulsive therapy can be humanely applied with positive therapeutic outcomes for some psychiatric disorders.

Support for the biologic approaches increased as successful symptom management with psychopharmacologic agents was reported. When a pharmacologic agent made a difference in care, a biologic hypothesis was considered. Modern psychopharmacology began in the 1930s, when barbiturates, particularly amobarbital sodium (Amytal Sodium), were tried for the treatment of mental diseases (Malamud, 1944). Psychopharmacology revolutionized the treatment of mental illness and led to an increased number of patients discharged into the community and the eventual focus on the brain as the key to understanding psychiatric disorders.

Increased Government Involvement in Mental Health Care

As scientific advances led to an increased intellectual understanding of the biologic foundations of mental illness, social change and historical events fostered a new level of empathy on an emotional level. During World War II, mental illness was beginning to be seen as a problem that could happen to anyone. Many "normal" people who volunteered for the armed services were disqualified on the grounds that they were psychologically unfit to serve. Others who had already served a tour of duty were diagnosed with psychiatric and emotional problems believed to be caused by the war. Consequently, in 1946, President Truman signed into law the National Mental Health Act, which supported research, training, and the establishment of clinics and treatment centers. This act created a six-member National Mental Health Advisory Council that established the National Institute of Mental Health (NIMH), which was responsible for overseeing and coordinating research and training.

The Hill-Burton Act of 1946 provided substantial federal support for hospital construction, which facilitated the expansion of psychiatric units in general hospitals. With the passage of the National Mental Health Act, the federal government became more involved in financing and controlling the delivery of care. Under its provisions, the federal government provided grants to states to support existing outpatient facilities and programs to establish new ones. Before 1948, more than half of all states had no clinics; by 1949, all but five had one or more. Six years later, there were about 1,234 outpatient clinics.

Continued Evolution of Psychiatric– Mental Health Nursing

Another consequence of the passing of the National Mental Health Act of 1946 was the provision of training grants to institutions for stipends and fellowships to prepare specialty nurses in advanced practice (Chamberlain, 1983). The first graduate nursing program, developed by Hildegarde E. Peplau in 1954 at Rutgers University, was in the specialty of psychiatric nursing (Donahue, 1985). Subspecialties began to emerge focusing on children, adolescents, or elderly people. Today in the

United States, nearly 100 master's degree programs offer specializations in psychiatric–mental health.

In 1952, Peplau published a landmark work titled *Interpersonal Relations in Nursing*. It introduced psychiatric–mental health nursing practice to the concepts of interpersonal relations and the importance of the therapeutic relationship. In fact, the nurse–patient relationship was defined as the very essence of psychiatric–mental health nursing (see Chaps. 6 and 9). This was a significant switch in perspective from the neurobiologic approach that had characterized the discipline before that time. Peplau's perspective was also important in its conceptualization of nursing care as truly independent of physicians. The nurse's use of self as a nursing tool was outside the dominance of both hospital administrators and physicians.

Gradually, nursing education programs in specialized hospitals were phased into generalized programs in nursing (Peplau, 1989). Nursing programs offered in psychiatric hospitals closed. This mainstreaming of psychiatric–mental health nursing education into the general nursing curriculum obviated the need for specialized hospitals.

THE LATE 20TH CENTURY
Community Health Movement and Deinstitutionalization

In 1955, the Joint Commission on Mental Illness and Health was formed to study the problems of mental health care delivery. During its 6-year existence, the commission sponsored several scholarly studies and created an atmosphere conducive to the discussion of new federal policy initiatives that would eventually undermine the traditional emphasis on institutional care. In 1961, the commission transmitted its final report, "Action for Mental Health." The report called for larger investments in basic research; national personnel recruitment and training programs; one full-time clinic for every 50,000 individuals, supplemented by general hospital units and state-run regional intensive psychiatric treatment centers; and access to emergency care and treatment in general, both in mental hospitals and community clinics. It was recommended that planning and implementation of the system would include the consumers and that funding for the construction and operation of the community mental health system would be shared by federal, state, and local governments.

"Action for Mental Health" was presented at a time that was politically ripe for the new ideas. The 1960 presidential election of John F. Kennedy brought a new type of leadership to the United States. The ideas expressed in the report clearly shifted authority for mental health programming to the federal government. This report was the basis of the federal legislation, the Mental Retardation Facilities and Community Mental Health Centers Construction Act, which President Kennedy signed into law in 1963.

In reality, this act included only some of the ideas proposed by the commission and did not encompass state-run regional intensive psychiatric centers. Supporters of the legislation believed that the new community-oriented policy would provide better care and eliminate the need for institutions providing custodial care. The supporters of this 1963 legislation believed the exact opposite of what the supporters of Dorothea Dix believed during the previous century. That is, instead of viewing custodial care as the treatment of mental disorders, institutionalization was viewed as contributing to the illness. The predominant view was that many of the problems of mental disorders were caused by the deplorable conditions of the state mental institutions and that, if patients were moved into a "normal" community-living setting, the symptoms of mental disorders could easily be treated and would eventually disappear. Thus, **deinstitutionalization,** the discharge of the institutionalized people into the community, became a national objective. The inpatient population fell by about 15% between 1955 and 1965 and by about 59% during the succeeding decade.

The goal of the Community Mental Health Centers Construction Act was to expand community mental health services and diminish society's sole reliance on mental hospitals. Guidelines for implementing the act were somewhat vague, and administering the program became the responsibility of NIMH. Each community mental health center (CMHC) was mandated to have five basic services:

1. Inpatient services
2. Outpatient services
3. Partial hospitalization services (including day care, at the minimum)
4. Twenty-four-hour emergency services
5. Consultation and educational services for community agencies and profession personnel

Only centers providing all of these services were eligible for funding. The regulations were also designed to encourage states to offer diagnostic, rehabilitative, pre-care and after-care services, training, research, and evaluation. In this act, a community was defined as a population range of 75,000 to 200,000. Any mention of the role for or linkages to state hospitals was absent.

The Community Mental Health Construction Act, originally a construction grant, was amended in 1965 to strengthen the funding for staffing new facilities. Even so, the number of CMHCs grew slowly. There were a limited number of communities with large enough populations to support the centers and a shortage of trained personnel, even in urban areas. In smaller and rural communities, there was often no one (or no mental health provider) prepared for the new role. By the spring of 1967, only 173 funded projects existed.

There was no evidence that deinstitutionalized patients constituted a significant population of those receiving services at the new CMHCs. One problem was that the treatment of choice in most of the centers, individual psychotherapy, had not been shown to be effective for patients with long-term mental disorders. Many urban CMHC clients, as compared with former state hospital patients, tended to be younger and poorer and were disproportionately drawn from minority backgrounds. Also, many centers focused on the treatment of alcoholism and drug addiction.

Sanctioning of Holistic Nursing Care

By 1963, two nursing journals focused on psychiatric nursing: the *Journal of Psychiatric Nursing* (now the *Journal of Psychosocial Nursing and Mental Health Services*) and *Perspectives in Psychiatric Care*. In 1967, the Division of Psychiatric and Mental Health Nursing Practice of the American Nurses Association (ANA) published the *Statement on Psychiatric Nursing Practice*. For the first time, there was official sanction of a holistic approach to nursing care, with psychiatric–mental health nurses practicing in a variety of settings with a variety of clientele. The emphasis was on activities ranging from health promotion to health restoration. Since 1967, there have been three more updates of the psychiatric–mental health nursing practice statement that continue to expand the role of the psychiatric nurse and delineate practice functions and roles. Today in the United States, nearly 100 master's degree programs offer specializations in psychiatric–mental health.

Contemporary Issues

Changing Demographics

The social changes of the 1980s set the stage for the continuing evolution of mental health care. The population was rapidly aging. Family structure was diversifying through divorce, cohabitation, and a variety of other family configurations. Women entered the work force in record numbers. Rapid growth of cities, or urbanization, was the single most characteristic phenomenon in the United States (Aldrich, 1986). The population in the United States was shifting toward the southwest. (In 1983, Los Angeles replaced Chicago as the second largest city.) Many of the new residents had migrated to the southwest from Mexico and Asian countries and not simply relocated from other areas of the country.

By the 1990s, wrinkles in the social fabric had begun to show. The deinstitutionalization movement, so long hailed as an efficient, cost-effective means of reabsorbing the mentally ill into society, was considered a failure. People with mental disorders were discharged into communities that were unprepared to offer them little in the way of treatment, housing, or vocational opportunities; these communities were also sometimes vastly different from the ones they had left behind at the time of their hospitalization. In addition, fewer community-based facilities were in place to serve the growing population of people with mental disorders.

The 2,000 projected CMHCs that should have been in place by 1980 never materialized. By 1990, about 1,300 programs provided various types of psychosocial rehabilitation services, such as vocation, educational, or social-recreational services (International Association of Psychosocial Rehabilitation, 1990). The CMHCs, by and large, ignored people with serious mental illnesses, who had become legion. Today it is estimated that within a 12-month period, 16.7 million adults (10% of the U.S. population) have a mental-emotional problem. The reported prevalence rate of mental-emotional problems that seriously interfere with the ability to work, attend school, or manage day-to-day activities is 8.2 million (4.9%). The rate in children is even higher. It is estimated that 9% to 13% of children between the ages of 9 and 17 years have serious emotional disturbances (Friedman et al., 1998).

The Age of Managed Care

Both public and private expenditures for health care services have increased in the United States. Financial barriers account for the different resource allocation rules for financing mental health services compared with general health care services, leading to less overall funding for mental health. To control costs, privately "insured" mental health care has been "carved out" from the rest of health care and is managed separately. Privately owned behavioral health care firms not only manage care but also provide services through directly owned or contracted networks of providers. In theory, people with psychiatric problems have direct access to the specialists who provide the best care. In reality, services are still limited and sometimes withheld. Once care is limited or denied, individuals once again turn to public funds, which may or may not be available.

States are also reducing mental health expenditures by securing federal waivers to permit managed care of the Medicaid population (publicly funded health care). Now, large networks of public and private organizations share responsibility for mental health care, with the state remaining as the major decision maker for resource allocation. That is, private organizations are contracting with the states to coordinate and deliver cost-effective care. Emphasis is on reducing expensive institutional care and increasing the resources devoted to communities of individuals with mental disorders. This managed care approach raises several issues, including the legal ramifications of admission denial and confidentiality of patient information.

The mental health work force is shifting from providing care in traditional health care institutions to community settings: clinics, homes, schools, and treatment centers. New skills are need in these settings. There is a closer relationship with family and community support networks. It is a time of change and uncertainty about the new wave of community practice.

National Mental Health Objectives

Mental Health: A Report of the Surgeon General, was submitted by Dr. David Sachter to Secretary of Health and Human Services Donna E. Shalala in 1999 (U.S. Department of Health and Human Services, 1999). This informative report was the first report by the Office of the Surgeon General and supported two main findings:

1. The efficacy of mental health treatments is well documented.
2. A range of treatments exits for most mental disorders.

Two major reports were published in 2000.

Another landmark report by the Office of the Surgeon General is the *Report of the Surgeon General's Conference on Children's Mental Health: A National Action Agenda*. This report highlights consensus recommendations for identifying, recognizing, and referring children to services, increasing access to services for families, and identifying the evidence in treatments services, systems of care and financing (U.S. Public Health Service, 2000).

One of the most important documents for the advancement of a mental health agenda is *Healthy People 2010: National Health Promotion and Disease Prevention Objectives*, which was submitted and accepted by the Secretary Donna E. Shalala (U.S. Department of Health and Human Services, 2000). Many of the health care goals pertain specifically to mental health objectives (Text Box 1-2). The challenge before nurses is to strive to meet these goals while obeying marketplace demands to provide the most cost-effective care possible. This translates into an emphasis on preventing the symptoms of mental disorders and using hospitalization as a treatment of last resort. Devising and implementing a continuum of mental health services that provides access for all is an integral part of the strategy for accomplishing these goals.

TEXT BOX 1.2

Mental Health and Mental Disorders Objectives for the Year 2010

Mental Health Status Improvement
- Reduce the suicide rate to no more than 6.0 per 100,000 (baseline, 10.8/1,000 in 1998)
- Reduce the suicide attempts by adolescents to no more than 1% (baseline, 2.6% in 1997)
- Reduce the proportion of homeless adults who have serious mental illness (SMI)
- Increase the proportion of persons with serious mental illnesses who are employed

Treatment Expansion
- Reduce the relapse rates for persons with eating disorders, including anorexia nervosa and bulimia nervosa.
- Increase the number of persons seen in primary health care who receive mental health screening and assessment.
- Increase the proportion of children with mental health problems who receive treatment.
- Increase the proportion of juvenile justice facilities that screen new admissions for mental health problems.

- Increase the proportion of adults with mental disorders who receive treatment.
- Increase the proportion of persons with co-occurring substance abuse and mental disorders who receive treatment for both disorders.
- Increase the proportion of local governments with community-based jail diversion programs for adults with serious mental illness.

State Activities
- Increase the number of states and the District of Columbia that track consumers' satisfaction with the mental health services they receive.
- Increase the number of states, territories, and the District of Columbia with an operational mental health plan that addresses cultural competence.
- Increase the number of states, territories, and the District of Columbia with an operational mental health plan that addresses mental health crisis interventions, ongoing screening, and treatment services for elderly persons.

Summary of Key Points

- ➤ Throughout history, attitudes and treatment toward those with mental disorders have drastically changed as a result of the changing socioeconomic backdrop of our society and the development of new theories and study by key individuals and groups.
- ➤ During periods of economic and political instability, uncertainty, or narrow-minded thinking, attitudes and treatment of the mentally disordered were often characterized by intolerance and cruelty.
- ➤ During the 1800s, as mental illness began to be viewed as an illness, more humane and moral treatments began to develop.
- ➤ Key individuals throughout modern history have been instrumental in changing attitudes through research and revolutionary ideas in helping to establish mental disorders as an illness. True social reformers, such as Dorothea Dix, Horace Mann, and Clifford Beers, dedicated their efforts to raising society's awareness and advocating public responsibility for proper treatment of patients with mental disorders.
- ➤ Although the need for psychiatric–mental health nursing was recognized near the end of the 19th century, there was much resistance to training women for the care of the insane. Dr. Edward Cowles, director of the McLean Asylum in Massachusetts, assisted Linda Richards to open Boston City Hospital Training School for Nurses in 1882.

- ➤ Although nurses were receiving mental health training in these institutions, it was still outside the mainstream of nursing education. In 1913, Effie Taylor initiated the first nurse-organized program of study for psychiatric training at the Johns Hopkins Phipps Clinic. Gradually, all psychiatric nursing education in the United States and Canada was phased into generalist nursing education, and nursing programs offered in psychiatric hospitals closed.
- ➤ Psychiatric–mental health nursing content was eventually incorporated into all diploma and baccalaureate nursing programs. The first graduate program in psychiatric–mental health nursing was initiated in 1954 by Hildegarde Peplau at Rutgers University.
- ➤ Through key legislation and state and local organizations in the 20th century, community mental health centers developed and now offer a wider variety of services, treatment, and follow-up care.
- ➤ Theoretic arguments characterized the evolution of scientific thought and psychiatric practice. Gradually, the importance of the biologic aspect of mental disorders has been recognized.
- ➤ Economic and political factors influence the availability of mental health services.

Critical Thinking Challenges

1. Compare the ideas of psychiatric care during the 1800s with those of the 1980s and identify the

major political and economic forces that influenced care.

2. Analyze the social, political, and economic changes that influenced the community mental health movement.

3. Present an argument for the moral treatment of people with mental disorders.

4. Trace the history of the development of biologic psychiatry and highlight the major ideas and treatments.

 WEB LINKS

www.health.gov/healthypeople   This is the Healthy People 2010 website.

www.surgeongeneral.com   This website of the U.S. Surgeon General contains major mental health reports.

www.nlm.nih.gov   The National Library of Medicine site offers excellent access to PUBMED for nursing articles and mental health information. It provides links to the History in Medicine Library.

www.mentalhealth.com   This site is an excellent resource on disorders and diagnoses and provides links to other sites.

www.cmhc.com   This site provides access to the Mental Health Net, self-help groups, professional resources, and discussions.

www.samhsa.gov/oas/oasftp.htm   This Substance Abuse and Mental Health Statistics site provides national statistics on alcohol, tobacco, and illegal drug use, substance abuse treatment, and mental health.

www.who.org/aboutwho/en/preventingmental.htm
This site of the World Health Organization has information on mental health disability and programs.

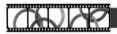 **MOVIES**

One Flew Over the Cuckoo's Nest.   1975. This classic film stars Jack Nicholson as Randle P. McMurphy, who takes on the state hospital establishment. This picture won all five of the top Oscars, including Best Picture, Best Actor, Best Actress, Best Director, and Best Screenplay. The film depicts the life of an inpatient psychiatric ward of the late 1960s and increased public awareness of the potential human rights violations inherent in a large, public mental system. However, the portrayal of electroconvulsive therapy is stereotyped and inaccurate, and the suicide of Billy appears to be simplistically linked to his domineering mother. Overall, this film probably contributes to the stigma of mental illness.

Viewing Points: This film should be viewed from several different perspectives: What is the basis of McMurphy's admission? How does Nurse Ratchet interact with the patients? What is missing? What is different today in public mental health systems?

An Angel at My Table.   1990, New Zealand. This thought-provoking trilogy was based on Janet Frame's autobiography that traces her life from being a shy, socially inept little girl to New Zealand's most famous novelist-poet. Produced by Jane Champion and starring Kerry Fox, the story is told within a trilogy of three stages—childhood, young adulthood, and adulthood. During the second period, Janet Frame was misdiagnosed with schizophrenia and hospitalized for 8 years. She barely avoided a leukotomy.

Viewing Points: Observe how the role of the woman in society influenced Janet's admission to the hospital. Would Janet be considered "mentally ill and needing hospitalization" by today's standard?

Beautiful Dreamers.   1992, Canada. This film is based on a true story about poet Walt Whitman's visit to an asylum in London, Ontario. Whitman, played by Rip Torn, is shocked by what he sees and persuades the hospital director to offer humane treatment. Eventually, the patients wind up playing the townspeople in a game of cricket.

Viewing Points: Observe the stigma that is associated with having a mental illness.

REFERENCES

Aldrich, R. (1986). The social context of change. *Psychiatric Annals, 16*(10), 613–618.

American Psychiatric Association. (1968). *Diagnostic and statistical manual of mental disorders* (2nd ed.). Washington, DC: Author.

American Psychiatric Association. (1980). *Diagnostic and statistical manual of mental disorders* (3rd ed.). Washington, DC: Author.

American Psychiatric Association. (1994). *Diagnostic and statistical manual of mental disorders* (4th ed.). Washington, DC: Author.

Bailey, H. (1920). *Nursing mental diseases.* New York: Macmillan.

Barker, P. (1990). The conceptual basis of mental health nursing. *Nurse Education Today, 10*(5), 339–348.

Beers, C. (1908). *A mind that found itself.* New York: Longmans, Green, & Co.

Campinha, J. (1987). The training of a "Mental Nurse": An historical look at McLean Training School for Nurses. *Virginia Nurse, 55*(1), 18–20.

Chamberlain, J. (1983). The role of the federal government in the development of psychiatric nursing. *Journal of Psychosocial Nursing and Mental Health Services, 21*(4), 11–18.

Church, O. (1987). From custody to community in psychiatric nursing. *Nursing Research, 36*(10), 48–55.

Cowles, E. (1887, October). Nursing reform for the insane. *American Journal of Insanity, 44,* 176, 191.

Deutsch, S. (1949). *The mentally ill in America*. London: Oxford University Press.

Donahue, M. (1985). *Nursing, the finest art*. St. Louis: Mosby.

Friedman, R., Katz-Leavy, J., Manderscheid, R., & Sondheimer, D. (1998). Prevalence of serious emotional disturbance: An update. In R. Manderscheid, & M. Henderson (Eds.), *Mental health, United States, 1998*. (DHHS Publication No. SMA99-3285, pp. 110–123). Washington, DC: U.S. Government Printing Office.

Geller, J., & Harris, M. (1994). *Women of the asylum: Voices from behind the walls, 1840–1945*. New York: Anchor Books.

International Association of Psychosocial Rehabilitation Services (IAPRS). (1990). *A national directory: Organizations providing psychosocial rehabilitation and related community support services in the United States*. Boston: Center for Psychiatric Rehabilitation, Boston University.

Malamud, W. (1944). The history of psychiatric therapies. In J. K. Hall, G. Zilboorg, & H. Bunker (Eds.), *One hundred years of American psychiatry*. New York: Columbia University Press.

Mericle, B. (1983). The male as a psychiatric nurse. *Journal of Psychosocial Nursing, 21*(11), 30.

Neill, J. (1980). Adolf Meyer and American psychiatry today. *American Journal of Psychiatry, 137*(4), 460–464.

Nightingale, F. (1859). *Notes on nursing: What it is and what it is not*. London: Harrison & Son.

Peplau, H. (1952). *Interpersonal relations in nursing*. New York: Putnam.

Peplau, H. (1989). Future directions in psychiatric nursing from the perspective of history. *Journal of Psychosocial Nursing and Mental Health Services, 27*(2), 18–21.

U.S. Public Health Service. (2000). *Report of the Surgeon General's conference on children's mental health: A national action agenda*. Washington, DC: Department of Health and Human Services.

U.S. Department of Health and Human Services. (1999). *Mental health: A report of the Surgeon General*. Washington, DC: U.S. Department of Health and Human Services, Substance Abuse and Mental Health Services Administration, Center for Mental Health Services, National Institutes of Health, National Institute of Mental Health.

U.S. Department of Health and Human Services. (2000). *Healthy people 2010* (2nd ed.) With: Understanding and improving health and objectives for improving health. Washington, DC: U.S. Government Printing Office.

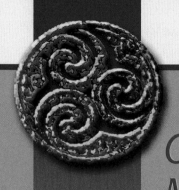

Cultural Issues Related to Mental Health Care

Mary Ann Boyd

IMPORTANCE OF CULTURE TO PSYCHIATRIC NURSING

CULTURAL TERMS AND ISSUES
Acculturation
Segregation Versus Integration
Prejudice, Discrimination, and Stereotyping
Stigmatization
Gender and Culture

VARIOUS CULTURAL AND RELIGIOUS VIEWS OF MENTAL ILLNESS
Religion and Mental Illness
Cultural Groups

African Americans
Latino Americans
Asian Americans, Polynesians, and Pacific Islanders
Native Americans

SOCIOECONOMIC INFLUENCES ON MENTAL HEALTH CARE
Poverty and Mental Illness
Geographic Location and Access to Mental Health Care
Changing Family Structure
Family Size
Changing Roles
Mobility and Relocation
Unmarried Couples

Single-Parent Families
Stepfamilies
Childless Families
Same-Gender Families

STIGMA AND MENTAL ILLNESS
Effects of Stigma on Individuals With Mental Illness
Stigmatization and Stress for Family Members

CHANGING PUBLIC ATTITUDE: NATIONAL ALLIANCE FOR THE MENTALLY ILL

LEARNING OBJECTIVES

After studying this chapter, you will be able to:

➤ Identify various cultural and ethnic groups in the United States and Canada.
➤ Compare the concepts of prejudice, discrimination, and stereotyping and their relationship to stigmatization.
➤ Define the process of stigmatization as an influence in mental health care delivery.
➤ Describe the beliefs about mental health and illness in different cultural groups.
➤ Trace the changing view of families from causing mental illness to collaborating in the care.
➤ Discuss the changing family structure and the mental health implications.
➤ Describe the important role of consumer groups in developing awareness of the special problems of patients with mental disorders.

CHAPTER 2

(Fig. 2-1).

KEY TERMS

acculturation   integration
cultural competence   prejudice
discrimination   segregation
homophobia   stereotyping

KEY CONCEPTS

culture
stigmatization

All cultural groups have sets of values, beliefs, and patterns of accepted behavior, and it is often difficult for those of one cultural background to understand those of another. This fact is especially true in regard to how people view mental illness—some cultures view it as a condition for which they must be punished and ostracized from society, whereas other cultures are more tolerant of mental illness and believe that family and community members are crucial to their care and treatment.

In this chapter, we examine the definitions of prejudice, stereotyping, and stigma and the various minority groups or cultures that have traditionally been victims of stereotyping and stigma in the United States. We examine the differences in cultural and social mores of these groups and the overall changing profile of the traditional American family structure today. Our hope is that when nurses understand these different cultures, people, and groups, they will be better prepared to understand each individual's feelings and motivations, which are so crucial in treating patients with mental disorders, and will be better able to adapt treatment to all those of different backgrounds and lifestyles whom they encounter in mental health practice.

KEY CONCEPT **Culture.** **Culture** is a way of life for people who identify or associate with one another on the basis of some common purpose, need, or similarity of background and is the totality of learned, socially transmitted beliefs, values, and behaviors that emerge from its members' interpersonal transactions.

IMPORTANCE OF CULTURE TO PSYCHIATRIC NURSING

Nursing care of people with mental disorders and emotional problems can often be more complex because of cultural differences. Nurses' and patients' backgrounds and cultural heritages may be different; hence, it is important for nurses to understand clearly the thinking and perspectives of other cultures and groups. Because treating mental disorders deals so heavily with peoples' attitudes about themselves, their beliefs, values, and ways of interacting with families and their communities, it is critical that psychiatric nurses be culturally competent in their practice. **Cultural competence** is a process in which the "nurse continuously strives to achieve the ability to effectively work within the cultural context of an individual or community from a diverse cultural or ethnic background" (Campinha-Bacote, 1995, p. 1). It is developed through cultural awareness, acquisition of cultural knowledge, development of cultural skills, and engagement of numerous cultural encounters (Fig. 2-1).

CULTURAL TERMS AND ISSUES

Acculturation

When a minority group succeeds in melding into the predominant culture and assumes not only the language but also the beliefs, values, and practices of the predominant culture, the members are said to be **acculturated.**

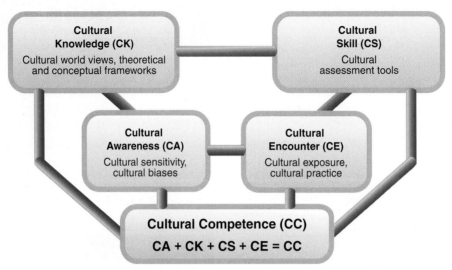

FIGURE 2.1 Culturally competent model of care. (Adapted from Campinha-Bacote J. [1994]. Cultural competence in psychiatric mental health nursing. *Nursing Clinics of North America, 29* [1], 2.)

Many of the masses of minority populations that immigrated from Europe during the late 1800s and throughout the 20th century have succeeded in acculturating to American culture, such as the Irish Americans, Polish Americans, and Italian Americans. For these groups, English is their primary language, and they have accepted the customs and practices of the American culture. Many of their descendants have intermarried with those of other cultural heritages, and these groups are no longer viewed as minority or ethnic groups. They have become acculturated into the larger, predominant society.

Segregation Versus Integration

As cultural groups enter a new society, they may have difficulties becoming a part of the larger dominant society. Often, minority groups are separated from the majority culture through legally sanctioned societal practices, or **segregation.** For example, before the *Brown v. Board of Education* decision in 1954, it was legally sanctioned in some states that African American children attend separate (but poorer) schools. Through segregation, individuals are prevented from having the same opportunities as other society members. Incorporation of disparate ethnic or religious elements of the population into a unified society, or **integration,** provides equality of opportunity for all members of that society's culture, and although the process may be difficult, it is usually a desired goal of the disenfranchised minority group. Segregation, or staying separate and apart as a group, may serve desired short-term advantages by providing support and protection by the group members and reducing their exposure to direct prejudice, but ultimately, integration offers minorities more economic

stability, more even-quality services within the dominant society, and eventually the reduction of prejudice.

Curiously, countries that have encouraged the "melting pot" policy, one of integrating minority cultures into the larger society, such as the United States and Australia, also report high rates of psychiatric admissions among immigrant groups. Those countries in which groups have maintained their own independent identities, such as Canada, have reported lower rates (Murphy, 1965). Halpern (1993) argues that it is not important that everyone in the neighborhood be of one's group, but that there be a critical mass, perhaps 30% to 40%, of the local population, for there to be social support through a local network.

Prejudice, Discrimination, and Stereotyping

The concepts of prejudice, discrimination, and stereotyping are important in understanding the life of people with mental disorders. **Prejudice** is a hostile attitude toward others simply because they belong to a particular group that is considered to have objectionable characteristics. **Discrimination** is the differential treatment of others because they are members of a particular group. It can include ignoring, derogatory name calling, denying services, and threatening. **Stereotyping** is expecting individuals to act in a characteristic manner that conforms to a negative perception of their cultural group. Individual characteristics are not considered. Stereotyping occurs because of lack of exposure to enough people in a particular group. Prejudice, discrimination, and stereotyping lead to a lack of understanding and appreciation of differences among people.

Stigmatization

People with mental illnesses or emotional problems are often stigmatized by the society in which they live.

KEY CONCEPT Stigmatization. **Stigmatization** is the process of assigning negative characteristics and identity to one person or group and causing that person or group to feel unaccepted, devalued, ostracized, and isolated from the larger society (Jones et al., 1984).

Through prejudice, discrimination, and stereotyping, stigmatization occurs. Although individuals can be victims of stigmatization, even large groups within a society can become victims of stigma, such as those of certain ethnic or cultural groups, those of certain socioeconomic status, and certainly those with a mental handicap or illness.

Gender and Culture

Women within minority groups may experience more conflicting feelings and psychological stressors than men in trying to adjust to both their defined role in the minority culture and a different role in the larger predominant society. For men, who are often earning a living and working within the cultural neighborhood, their socioeconomic status and social position remain the same. But for women, who are often forced to find employment outside of the cultural neighborhood, they must often cope with disparity between their status and role within their minority group and that defined by their workplace or the larger society (Cho, 1985). In cultures in which the traditional role of the woman is subservient to her husband, such as in most Asian American groups, it is difficult for a woman to assume the assertive stance that is needed in her work world (see Research Box 2-1).

In African American cultures, in which women with high career aspirations are often head of the household, the role conflict is different. In a study of nine African American women, all reported role conflict when they were immersed in a work world that discriminated against members of their cultural group. Their work was scrutinized, and they were excluded from professional interactions. They also experienced negative attitudes from coworkers, even from other African Americans they supervised (Sims & Napholz, 1996). These experiences produced conflicting feelings and confusion regarding their social role and caused additional stressors. These experiences and their resulting conflict may explain the higher rates of psychiatric admissions and psychopathology for women in minority subcultures (Halpern, 1993).

RESEARCH BOX 2.1

Depression in Korean Immigrant Wives

Korean immigrant wives volunteered to participate in a research study that looked at their coping strategies and the development of depression. The study group consisted of 282 women ranging in age from 25 to 55 years (mean age, 41.7 years). Most of these women (92%) arrived in the United States with at least a high school education. Most (86%) had children. All of the women were employed outside the home and worked from 20 to 84 hours per week. The researchers found that depression was positively correlated to the management of stress by working harder at cleaning the house. Depression was negatively correlated to negotiation (discussion with husband).

Um, C., & Dancy, B. (1999). Relationship between coping strategies and depression among employed Korean immigrant wives. *Issues in Mental Health Nursing, 20,* 485–494.

VARIOUS CULTURAL AND RELIGIOUS VIEWS OF MENTAL ILLNESS

Religion and Mental Illness

Religious beliefs often define an individual's relationship within a family and community. Many different religions are practiced throughout the world. Judeo-Christian thinking tends to dominate Western societies. Other religions, such as Islam, Hinduism, and Buddhism, dominate Eastern and Middle Eastern cultures (Table 2-1). Because religious beliefs often influence approaches to mental health, it is important to understand the basis of various religions that appear to be growing in the United States and Canada.

Cultural Groups

African Americans

Lives of African Americans Today. The African American population is expected to reach 40 million by the year 2010 (U.S. Bureau of the Census, 1998). Although African Americans share many common beliefs, attitudes, values, and behaviors, there are also many subcultural and individual differences based on social class, country of origin, occupation, religion, educational level, and geographic location. Many have extensive family networks in which members can be relied on for moral support, help with childrearing, provide financial aid, and help in crises. In most African American families, elderly members are treated with great respect.

(text continues on page 22)

TABLE 2.1   World's Major Religions or Belief Forms

Source of Power or Force (Deity)	Historical Sacred Texts or Beliefs	Key Beliefs or Ethical Life Philosophy
Christianity		
God, a unity in tripersonality; Father, Son, and Holy Ghost	Bible Teachings of Jesus through the Apostles and the Church Fathers	God's love for all creatures is a basic belief. Salvation is gained by those who have faith and show humility toward God. Brotherly love is emphasized in acts of charity, kindness, and forgiveness.
Islam		

Allah (the only God)
Has two major sects:
  Sunni (orthodox), traditional and simple practices are followed, human will is determined by outside forces
  Shiite, practices are rapturous and trance-like; human beings have free will.
	Koran (the words of God delivered to Mohammed by the angel Gabriel)
	Hadith (commentaries by Mohammed)
	Five Pillars of Islam (religious conduct)
	Islam was built on Christianity and Judaism
		God is just and merciful; humans are limited and sinful. God rewards the good and punishes the sinful. Mohammed, through the Koran, guides and teaches people truth. Peace is gained through submission to Allah. The sinless go to Paradise, and the evil go to Hell. A "good" Muslim obeys the Five Pillars of Islam.

Hinduism		

Brahma (the Infinite Being and Creator that pervades all reality)
Other gods:
  Vishnu (preserver)
  Shiva (destroyer)
  Krishna (love)
	Vedas (doctrine and commentaries)	All people are assigned to castes (permanent hereditary orders, each having different privileges in society; each was created from different parts of Brahma):
		1. *Brahmans:* includes priests and intellectuals.
		2. *Kshatriyas:* includes rulers and soldiers.
		3. *Vaisya:* includes farmers, skilled workers, and merchants.
		4. *Sudras:* includes those who serve the other three castes (servants, laborers, peasants).
		5. *Untouchables:* the outcasts, those not included in the other castes.

Buddhism		

Buddha
Individual responsibility and logical or intuitive thinking
Buddhist subjects include:
  Lamaism (Tibet) where Buddhism is blended with spirit worship.
  Mantrayana (Himalayan area, Mongolia, Japan) where intimate relationship with a guru and reciting secret mantras is emphasized; the belief in sexual symbolism and demons is also practiced.
  Ch'an (China) *Zen* (Japan) where self-reliance and awareness through intuitive understanding are stressed.
  Satori (enlightenment) may come from "sudden insight" or through self-discipline, meditation, and instruction.
	Tripitaka (scripture)
	Middle Path (way of life)
	The Four Noble Truths
	Eightfold Path (guides for life)
	The Texts of Taoism (include the Tao Te Ching of Lao Tzŭ and The Writings of Chuang Tzŭ)
	Sutras (Buddhist commentaries)
	Sangha (Buddhist Community)
		Buddhism attempts to deal with problems of human existence such as suffering and death.
		Life is misery, unhappiness, and suffering with no ultimate reality in the world or behind it.
		The cause of all human suffering and misery is desire.
		The "middle path" of life avoids the personal extremes of self-denial and self-indulgence.
		Visions can be gained through personal meditation and contemplation; good deeds and compassion also facilitate the process toward nirvana, the ultimate mode of existence.
		The end of suffering is the extinction of desire and emotion, and ultimately the unreal self. Present behavior is a result of past deed.

(continued)

TABLE 2.1   World's Major Religions or Belief Forms (Continued)

Source of Power or Force (Deity)	Historical Sacred Texts or Beliefs	Key Beliefs or Ethical Life Philosophy
Confucianism		
No doctrine of a god or gods or life after death Individual responsibility and logical and intuitive thinking	Five Classics (Confucian thought) Analects (conversations and sayings of Confucius)	Considered a philosophy or a system of ethics for living, rather than a religion that teaches how people should act toward one another. People are born "good." Moral character is stressed through sincerity in personal and public behavior. Respect is shown for parents and figures of authority. Improvement is gained through self-responsibility, introspection, and compassion for others.
Shintoism		
Gods of nature, ancestor worship, national heroes	Tradition and custom (the way of the gods) Beliefs were influenced by Confucianism and Buddhism	Reverence for ancestors and traditional Japanese way of life is emphasized. Loyalty to places and locations where one lives or works and purity and balance in physical and mental life are major motivators of personal conduct.
Taoism		
All the forces in nature	Tao-te-Ching ("The Way and the Power")	Quiet and happy harmony with nature is the key belief. Peace and contentment are found in the personal behaviors of optimism, passivity, humility, and internal calmness. Humility is an especially valued virtue. Conformity to the rhythm of nature and the universe leads to a simple, natural, and ideal life.
Judaism		
God	Hebrew Bible (Old Testament) Torah (first five books of Hebrew Bible) Talmud (commentaries on the Torah)	Jews have a special relationship with God: obeying God's law through ethical behavior and ritual obedience earns the mercy and justice of God. God is worshiped through love, not out of fear.
Tribal Beliefs		
Animism: Souls or spirits embodied in all beings and everything in nature (trees, rivers, mountains) Polytheism: Many gods, in the basic powers of nature (sun, moon, earth, water)	Passed on through ceremonies, rituals, myths, and legends. Oral history, rather than written literature, is the common medium.	All living things are related. Respect for powers of nature and pleasing the spirits are fundamental beliefs to meet basic and practical needs for food, fertility, health, and interpersonal relationships and individual development. Harmonious living is comprehension and respect of natural forces.

(continued)

TABLE 2.1   World's Major Religions or Belief Forms (Continued)

Summary of Other Belief Forms

- *Atheism:* the belief that no God exists, as "God" is defined in any current existing culture of society
- *Agnosticism:* the belief that whether there is a God and a spiritual world or any ultimate reality is unknown and probably unknowable
- *Scientism:* the belief that values and guidance for living come from scientific knowledge, principles, and practices; systematic study and analysis of life, rather than superstition, lead to true understanding and practice of life
- *Maoism:* the faith that is centered in the leadership of the Communist Party and all the people; the major belief goal is to move away from individual personal desires and ambitions, toward viewing and serving each other and all people as a whole.

Adapted from *Counseling and Development in a Multicultural Society,* by J. A. Axelson & P. McGrath. Copyright 1998, 1993, 1985 Brooks/Cole Publishing Company, Pacific Grove, CA 93950, a division of International Thomson Publishing Inc. By permission of the publisher.

Beliefs About Mental Illness. African Americans with mental illness suffer from the stresses of double stigmata—not only from within their own culture but also from a long history of racial discrimination. To make matters worse, there has been racial discrimination from within the health community itself, with several studies showing that diagnoses for African Americans are often racially biased (Fisher, 1969; Frumkin, 1954; Lindsey & Paul, 1989). In a classic study, it was shown that in state and county mental hospitals, men of European descent tended to be diagnosed with alcoholism and African American men with schizophrenia (Simon et al., 1973). One more recent study showed that in most situations, African Americans are still more likely to be admitted to psychiatric hospitals and misdiagnosed (Lindsey & Paul, 1989). In general hospitals, African American men and women were more often diagnosed with schizophrenia than men and women of European descent, who were more often diagnosed as having depressive disorders (Capers, 1994; Worthington, 1992). One nursing study investigated racial differences in health status and health behavior of African American and white elderly patients. The researchers found that the African Americans had significantly lower mental health and poorer self-perceived health than did their white counterparts (Kim et al., 1998).

Latino Americans

Lives of Latino Americans Today. The number of Latino Americans living in the United States has been gradually increasing. From 1980 to 1997, there was a 101% increase in population, from 14.6 to 29.3 million. It is estimated that there will be 41 million people of Latino descent by the year 2010 (U.S. Bureau of the Census, 1998). Immigration contributed about half of this growth, and a high fertility rate the other half. Immigrants came from Mexico (64%), Central and South America (14%), Puerto Rico (10%), and Cuba (5%). It

is forecasted that within the next 25 years, the Latino population will become the largest minority group in the United States. Latino populations are largest in urban areas, such as Los Angeles, Dallas–Fort Worth, Boston, San Diego, Miami–Fort Lauderdale, and New York. Despite the diversity within this group, people are united by language, religion, and customs and attitudes toward self, family, and community. Although evidence indicates that second-generation Latino Americans are speaking English as their first language, many cities are becoming increasingly bilingual. For example, television programs and commercials are bound to be more persuasive if they are broadcast in Spanish rather than English (Roslow & Nicholls, 1996).

Access to Mental Health Care. Studies have begun to show that Latino Americans tend to use all other resources before seeking help from mental health professionals. Reasons have been reported for this lack of access to mental health care: (1) many Latino patients believe that mental health facilities do not accommodate their cultural needs (eg, language, beliefs, values); and (2) many still seek help through supportive home care and counseling from the church. If bilingual, bicultural mental health facilities are available, Latino patients will seek care. One study examined the perception of services in an outpatient mental health facility located in a border city in southwest Texas serving Mexican American patients with severe mental illness. Data from 56 patients reported a highly favorable and positive rating of the mental health services (Lantican, 1998).

Asian Americans, Polynesians, and Pacific Islanders

Lives of Asian Americans, Polynesians, and Pacific Islanders Today. In 1997, Asian Americans, Polynesians, and Pacific Islanders numbered more than 10 million in the United States. This large multicultural group includes Chinese, Filipino, Japanese,

Asian Indian, Korean, Vietnamese, Laotian, Cambodian, Hawaiian, Samoan, and Guamanian people. Most Chinese, Japanese, Korean, Asian Indian, and Filipino immigrants have migrated to urban areas, whereas the Vietnamese have settled throughout the United States.

Beliefs About Mental Illness. Generally, Asian cultures have a tradition of denying or disguising the existence of mental illnesses. In many of these cultures, it is an embarrassment to have a family member treated for mental illness. For example, in both China and Japan, to disguise the severity of the illness, schizophrenia is called "neurasthenia." In China, many psychiatrists and general physicians use this term because they believe that it will improve the treatment and establish good communication with patients (Rin & Huang, 1989). In Japan, psychiatrists disguise diagnoses from patients to protect their patients and their families from the loneliness, alienation, powerlessness, and hopelessness they believe will result from the knowledge of their illnesses or the social prejudice against them (Munakata, 1989). Mental disorders, including alcoholism, are kept hidden by family members until the disorder has progressed too far for interventions to be useful (Sharts-Hopko, 1996). In the United States, however, the more acculturated the Asian Americans, the more likely they will seek psychiatric services (Atkinson & Gim, 1989). There is little research regarding specific mental health problems in Asian cultures, but there are data that suggest high rates of suicide related to social isolation, increasing use of alcohol (leading to alcoholism), and increasing somatization (the physical manifestation of psychological disturbances) (Herrick & Brown, 1999).

Traditional Korean beliefs are derived from shamanism, traditional Chinese medicine, and Buddhism or Taoism. Mental illnesses were regarded as a supernatural intervention or as afflictions caused by evil or vengeful spirits. Today, many Koreans believe that mental illnesses are caused by hereditary weakness, character weakness, physical and emotional strain, or imbalance within the body of yin and yang. Many believe that mental illnesses are incurable and that people with mental illnesses may have to spend the rest of their lives in mental hospitals. It is an embarrassment for a family member to be mentally ill (Kim, 1993).

Traditional Philippine folk medicine did not differentiate mental from physical illnesses. Any illness was perceived as a disruption of the harmonious functioning of the individual in interacting with the natural, social, and spiritual environment. Among the westernized group, mental illnesses are believed to be caused by physical and emotional strain or exhaustion, sexual frustration, sexual excess, unreturned love, lack of self-discipline, weakness of character, and inherited defects (Araneta, 1993). There is very little research regarding

the mental health needs of Filipino Americans. The admission and length of stay at psychiatric hospitals for Filipino patients is lower than for other Asian Americans. However, this does not mean there is less need. Instead, it is believed that the stigma of mental illnesses is so great that families are reluctant to acknowledge the existence of mental illness. Also, within the Filipino culture, other available alternative resources, such as churches, family, physicians, and elders, reduce the dependence on mental health facilities (Araneta, 1993).

Although several different cultural groups immigrated to America from Southeast Asia after the Vietnam War (Vietnamese, Cambodians, Laotians, Hmong, and Mien), we will discuss the Vietnamese because they comprise the largest group. These groups may have different languages and customs, but they all share the common factor of being driven from their homeland. Mental illness is stigmatized within the Vietnamese culture. Shame and social ostracism are typical treatments of families with a mentally ill member. Families avoid seeking help until the relative's behavior is unmanageable. Milder mental illnesses may not be recognized because of the tendency to somaticize (experience physical symptoms) the illness. Many Southeast Asian patients with mental disorders seek help for physical problems that are, in reality, a manifestation of psychiatric conditions (Kinzie & Leung, 1993).

Native Americans

Native American cultures have the basic ideology of respect and reverence for the earth and nature, from which comes not only survival, but also the comprehension of life and one's relationships with a separate, higher spiritual being and with other human beings. Shamans, or medicine men, were central to most cultures and were the healers who were believed to possess psychic abilities. Herbal medicines are often used, as well as healing ceremonies and feasts. The self is understood by observing nature, and relationships with others emphasize interdependence and sharing.

Traditional views about mental illnesses varied among the tribes. In some, mental illness is viewed as a supernatural possession, as being out of balance with nature. In certain Native American groups, people with mental illnesses are stigmatized. The degree of stigmatization, however, is not the same for all disorders. In tribal groups that make little distinction between physical and mental illnesses, there is little stigma. In other groups, a particular event is stigmatized, such as suicide. Clinical evidence suggests that different illnesses may be encountered in different Native American cultures and gene pools. For example, panic disorder is often seen in people from the Plains group and not in those from other groups (Neligh, 1988).

SOCIOECONOMIC INFLUENCES ON MENTAL HEALTH CARE

Not only are cultural and ethnic groups victims of stigma, but also these groups are sometimes denied access to mental health care because of where and how they live. Those who are without economic resources to afford treatment and those who are unemployed and not eligible for public assistance are often denied access to mental health care. Mental health care facilities and programs are also limited for those in certain geographic areas of the United States, such as rural or sparsely populated areas.

The deinstitutionalization of the mentally ill, which followed the passage of the 1963 Mental Retardation Facilities and Community Mental Health Centers Construction Act, released thousands of people from state psychiatric institutions into the communities of the United States and Canada (see Chap. 1). The health care system was not prepared for such a mass transition from institutionalized care to focus on community programs, and social service programs needed to help integrate these patients back into work, school, and family and social relationships. Public and private funding sources were not equipped to deal with the tremendous costs of providing these community mental health care services for the mentally ill. Consequently, both the level of services and reimbursement for those services have remained somewhat limited, particularly for certain segments of the population.

Although many employers are now providing working people with private health insurance that covers mental illness, and other people receive some public assistance for mental health care through Medicare and Medicaid, often reimbursement for outpatient services is limited. In addition, an estimated 44 million people are not covered by any of the public and private health care plans and cannot afford treatment at all.

Poverty and Mental Illness

The "culture of poverty" is a term used to describe the norms and behavior of people living in poverty. Poverty affects all cultural groups and other groups, including elderly, disabled, and psychiatrically impaired people and single-parent families. In the United States, one third of people living below the poverty line are single mothers and their children. Elderly people comprise a large percentage of poverty-stricken individuals—27% of African Americans older than 65 years of age live below the poverty level, as do 23% of Latino Americans and 10% of Americans of European descent.

Families living in poverty are under tremendous financial and emotional stress, which can often trigger or exacerbate mental problems. Not only must they face the daily stressors of trying to provide food and shelter for themselves and their families, but also they have neither the time, energy, nor money to attend to psychological needs. Often, these families become trapped in a downward economic spiral, and tension and stress mount. The inability to gain employment and the lack of financial independence only contribute to the feeling of powerlessness and low self-esteem. Being self-supporting gives one a feeling of control over life and bolsters self-esteem. Dependence on others or the government causes frustration, anger, apathy, and feelings of depression and meaninglessness (Axelson, 1999). Alcoholism, depression, and child and spouse abuse may seem to be the only means of coping with such hopelessness and despair. The homeless population is the group most at risk for being unable to escape this spiral of poverty.

Geographic Location and Access to Mental Health Care

Most mental health services are located in urban areas because most people live near cities. All age groups in rural areas have limited access to health care. The lack of resources is particularly problematic for children and elderly people, who have specialized needs. Rural areas are diverse in both geography and culture. The mental health needs of those in the deep South are different than those with the same problems in the Northwest. Treatment approaches may be effective in one part of the country, but not in another. There is a void of consumer and family-focused treatment and leadership in mental health services in rural areas. Hopefully, through information technology and increasing behavioral health managed care contractors, mental health care will improve (Beeson et al., 1998).

Changing Family Structure

Even though families may be defined differently within various cultures, they all play an important role in the life of the individual and influence who and what we are. Traditionally, families have been a source of guidance, security, love, and understanding. This is also true for people who have mental illnesses and emotional problems. It is often the family who assumes primary care for the person with mental illness and supports that individual throughout treatment. For patients, the family unit provides the only constant support throughout their lives. Although the nuclear family remains the basic unit of social organization, its structure and size have changed drastically since the 1950s, and so have the functions and roles of family members.

Family Size

Family size in the United States has decreased. In 1790, about one third of all households, including servants, slaves, and other people not related to the head, consisted of seven people or more. By 1960, only 1 household in 20 was this size. Few households contained members not related to the head (Taeuber, 1968). The average family household in 1995 was 2.65 people (U.S. Bureau of the Census, 1998).

Changing Roles

Women's role in the family structure has changed drastically during the past 35 years. Today, most women, including those who are mothers, work, both in dual-income families and single-parent families. Women make up 45% of the American civilian work force. More than half the female work force is made up of married women. Half the single, never-married women have children under the age of 18 years. More than 75% of divorced, widowed, or separated women have children, and more than 70% of married women have children (U.S. Bureau of the Census, 1998). Although the traditional roles for men and women have changed somewhat by women entering the workforce, working women still bear the bulk of responsibility for child care and household duties and often feel guilty and stressed from trying to be everything—a good parent and a success at a demanding job. Women often become emotionally exhausted, particularly during periods of personal conflict, and are at high risk for depression (Leiter & Durup, 1996).

Mobility and Relocation

Families are more mobile and may often change residences. Such relocations are stressful to families because they must leave familiar environments and readjust to new surroundings and lifestyles. These moves often cause separation from extended family, who have traditionally been a stabilizing force and have provided a much-needed support system to core families.

Unmarried Couples

More unmarried couples are cohabiting before or instead of marrying. Some elderly couples, most often widowed, are finding it more economically practical to cohabitate without marrying. The number of unmarried couples among the total U.S. population about tripled between 1970 and 1980, to an estimated 1.56 million households shared by two unrelated adults (with or without children) of opposite sex; by 1995, the number exceeded 3.5 million. Of the nation's 99 million households in 1995, married couples (with or without children) accounted for 53.8 million; there were 24.7 million single-person households, a significant increase since 1970 (U.S. Bureau of the Census, 1998). Unfortunately, the lifestyles chosen as an alternative to the traditional two-parent nuclear families are often stigmatized.

Single-Parent Families

It is estimated that 50% to 60% of all American children will reside at some point in a single-parent home. In the past, one-parent families were usually the result of the death of a spouse. Now, one-parent families are mostly the result of divorce. The divorce rate has been steadily rising in the United States since the 1960s; by 1997, more than one of four children lived with only one parent. Of all children in one-parent homes, 84% live with their mother. Because women maintaining families tend to have considerably lower incomes than their male counterparts, they now make up a disproportionate share of the poor population in the United States. More than 50% of single women with children under the age of 18 years live below the poverty level (U.S. Bureau of the Census, 1998).

Stepfamilies

Remarried families or stepfamilies have a unique set of problems that are not yet completely understood. Many parents find that stepparenting is much more difficult than parenting a biologic child. The bonding that occurs with biologic children rarely occurs with the stepchildren, whose natural bond is with a parent not living with them. However, it is the stepparent who often assumes a measure of financial and parental responsibility. The care and management of children often become the primary stressor to the marital partners. Additionally, the children are faced with multiple sets of parents whose expectations may be different from each other. They may also compete for the children's attention. It is not unusual for second marriages to fail because of the stressors inherent in a remarried family.

Childless Families

Couples often elect not to have children or to postpone having them until their careers are well established. Because many people consider having children as an expected adult behavior, families who do not have children are often stigmatized by society. For many years, the proportion of couples who were childless declined steadily as venereal and other diseases that caused infertility were conquered. In the 1970s, however, the changes in the status of women reversed this trend. Many people chose not to have children. Couples who voluntarily chose not to have children were more stigmatized than those who were infertile (Lampman & Dowling-Guyer, 1995).

Same-Gender Families

Among the most stigmatized groups are those who live a homosexual lifestyle. It is estimated that half the lesbian and gay male populations have encountered some form of verbal harassment or violence in their lives (Comstock, 1991). **Homophobia** is prejudice that leads to discrimination and stereotyping and ultimately stigmatization.

It is estimated that 1 in every 10 people has a homosexual orientation. Many argue that this estimate is probably low because of the stigmatization of homosexual people by Western society (Dworkin & Gutierrez, 1989). Even today, many religions condemn homosexuality. Although at one time people believed that being gay or lesbian was a result of faulty parenting or personal choice, it is generally accepted that sexual orientation is determined early in a child's development by a combination of factors, including genetic predisposition, biologic development, and environmental events. In the past, it was also believed that sexual preference could be changed through counseling by making a concerted effort to establish new relationships. There is no evidence that supports the hypothesis that change in sexual orientation is possible.

STIGMA AND MENTAL ILLNESS

As discussed in the historical account of mental illness and mental health practice in Chapter 1, patients with mental disorders have always been victims of stigma. Even within the past 20 years, with a more enlightened view of mental illness, a stigma still remains attached to those with mental disorders or those who seek help for mental illness. In 1999, the U.S. Surgeon General's Report on Mental Health described the negative attitude that continues to persist in the United States. Individuals with these illnesses are often still characterized in today's society as "crazy." Hollywood's portrayal of people with mental illness still seems to stereotype characters as clowns, buffoons, or frightening, possessed serial killers. These negative labels, misconceptions, and stigmata regarding mental illness persist for the same reasons that racial and ethnic stigmata persist—they are rooted in misunderstanding and fear.

Effects of Stigma on Individuals With Mental Illness

Stigmatization is a powerful force in influencing the treatment and rehabilitation of the person with a mental disorder. It is estimated that nearly two thirds of people with mental disorders do not seek treatment. Stigma surrounding mental health treatment is one of the many barriers that discourages people from seeking help (U.S. Surgeon General's Report, 1999). Its effects

are not easily overcome. Stigmatization is very real to those with mental illnesses, especially for those who exhibit bizarre, mysterious, or irrational behaviors. When people are subjected to stigmatization over long periods of time, they often try to conceal their disorders and worry that others may discover the presence of an illness. They become discouraged, hurt, and angry and develop low self-esteem (Wahl, 1999).

Stigmatization and Stress for Family Members

Families are often responsible for a lifetime of coordinating care for relatives with mental illnesses. Unlike many medical illnesses, psychiatric illnesses usually are chronic, with periods of exacerbation and remission. Stigma affects relatives of patients with mental illness. Family members cite that the effects of stigmatization of mentally ill family members damage their self-esteem and make it difficult to make friends or find a job. Denial of mental illness is therefore common among family members. The psychiatric nurse needs to be aware of the effects of stigma on patients and families and to support efforts to change the social view of mental disorders.

CHANGING PUBLIC ATTITUDE: NATIONAL ALLIANCE FOR THE MENTALLY ILL

During most of the 1900s, before the complexity of mental illnesses and the impact of the environment on symptom manifestations were recognized, family members were often blamed as "causing" mental illnesses. They were placed in the position of seeking treatment for family members and then being excluded from the treatment process because they were seen as the culprit. Family members were disrespected, blamed, or ignored. This negative treatment of the family was frustrating for both the patient and family and did not provide an atmosphere conducive to collaboration.

Once the fallacy of blaming parents was recognized and the stigma toward parents lessened, family members became involved in supporting the delivery of services. Through the formation of self-help groups, parents organized and responded to the inadequacies of the mental health system. In 1973, the first organized family group, Parents of Adult Schizophrenics, was formed in San Mateo County, California. The idea soon spread, and within 6 years, there were seven affiliated groups in California under a new name, Families for the Mentally Disabled. In 1979, groups from across the nation met in Madison, Wisconsin and formed a new organization, the National Alliance for the Mentally Ill (NAMI). The mission of NAMI is to eradicate mental illness and improve the quality of life for patients. One of the driving goals of NAMI is that the general public will understand that mental illnesses are no-fault, biologically based, treatable, and eventually curable.

NAMI has local chapters with family support groups operating in cities or counties that are affiliated with state organizations, which in turn are affiliated with the national office in Washington, DC. The organization has more than 70,000 member households. At the national level, NAMI promotes federal legislation to improve the delivery of care. It also rates the care delivered by the state departments of mental health. Statewide offices emphasize legislative contacts and advocacy for specific treatment programs. The state office distributes educational materials produced by the national office and other mental health agencies. NAMI members are often active at the local level in surveying the quality of community mental health services and fighting the stigmatization of their ill relatives.

Summary of Key Points

➤ The United States and Canada consist of a variety of cultural groups with unique values, beliefs, and health care practices. The term culture is defined as a way of life that manifests the learned beliefs, values, and accepted behaviors that are transmitted socially within a specific group.

➤ Cultural competence consists of cultural awareness, cultural knowledge, cultural skills, and cultural encounters. Developing cultural competence in psychiatric nursing practice is an ongoing process in caring for patients within the context of their culture.

➤ Many Americans of European descent have been acculturated into mainstream American culture. Some groups have been segregated from the predominant society, such as African Americans.

➤ Stigmatization occurs as a result of prejudice, discrimination, and stereotyping. Cultural groups and people with mental illness are stigmatized.

➤ Stigmatization involves the negative valuation of a characteristic or trait by society. The people who have the traits not only are ostracized by society but also view themselves in a negative, demoralizing way.

➤ Religious beliefs are closely intertwined with beliefs about health and mental illness.

➤ Mental illnesses are stigmatized in most cultural groups. A variety of cultural and religious beliefs underlie the stigmatization.

➤ Access to mental health treatment is particularly limited for those living in rural areas or those within the culture of poverty.

➤ The family is an important societal unit that is often responsible for the care and coordination of treatment of members with mental disorders. The family structure, size, and roles of members are rapidly changing. The traditional health care services will have to adapt to meet the mental health care needs of these families.

➤ In the past, families have been stigmatized, but they now serve as advocates and are often in the forefront of positive legislative changes. The National Institute of Mental Health has initiated campaigns to improve the understanding of mental disorders that should reduce the stigmatization of mental illness.

Critical Thinking Challenges

1. Identify a group that you know in your area that has been stigmatized and analyze the process of stigmatization of that group.
2. Compare the stigma of patients with physical illnesses to that of those with mental illnesses.
3. Differentiate the concepts of prejudice, discrimination, and stereotyping and their relationship to stigmatization.
4. Compare the access to mental health services in your state or county in rural areas to urban areas.
5. Define the culture of poverty and discuss how powerlessness affects the life of people living in poverty.
6. Trace the structure of the changing family through the 1900s.
7. Discuss how changing lifestyles, such as single-parent, stepfamilies, and single-sex families, are stigmatized by society.
8. Describe the role of consumer and government groups in the development of awareness of the problems of people with mental illnesses.
9. Visit a consumer group such as a branch of the National Alliance for the Mentally Ill and survey how it advocates for people with mental disorders.

REFERENCES

Araneta, E. (1993). Psychiatric care of Philipino Americans. In A. Gaw (Ed.), *Culture, ethnicity, and mental illness* (pp. 377–411). Washington, DC: American Psychiatric Association.

Atkinson, D., & Gim, R. (1989). Asian-American cultural identity and attitudes toward mental health services. *Journal of Counseling Psychology, 36*(2), 209–212.

Axelson, J. (1999). *Counseling and development in a multicultural society.* Belmont, CA: Wadsworth: Brooks/Cole.

Beeson, P. G., Britain, C., Howell, M. L., et al. (1998). Rural mental health at the millennium. In R. Manderscheid & M. Henderson (Eds.), *Mental Health, United States, 1998.* (DHHS Publication No. SMA 99-3285, pp. 82–97). Washington, DC: U.S. Government Printing Office.

Campinha-Bacote, J. (1994). Cultural competence in psychiatric mental health nursing: A conceptual model. *Nursing Clinics of North America, 29*(1), 1–8.

Capers, C. (1994). Mental health issues and African-Americans. *Nursing Clinics of North America, 29*(1), 57–64.

Cho, S. (1985). The labour process and capital mobility: The limits of the new international division of labour. *Politics in Society, 14*, 185–222.

Comstock, G. (1991). *Violence against lesbians and gay men.* New York: Columbia University Press.

Dworkin, S., & Gutierrez, F. (1989). Counselors be aware clients come in every size, shape, color, and sexual orientation. *Journal of Counseling and Development, 68*(1), 6–10.

Fischer, J. (1969). Negro and white rates of mental illness: Reconstruction of a myth. *Psychiatry, 32*(4), 428–466.

Frumkin, R. (1954). Race and major mental disorders. *Journal of Negro Education, 23*(1), 97–98.

Halpern, D. (1993). Minorities and mental health. *Social Science and Medicine, 36*(5), 597–607.

Hershberger, S., & D'Augelli, R. (1995). The impact of victimization on the mental health and suicidality of lesbian, gay, and bisexual youths. *Developmental Psychology, 31*(1), 65–74.

Herrick, C., & Brown, H. (1999). Mental disorders and syndromes found among Asians residing in the United States. *Issues in Mental Health Nursing, 20*, 275–296.

Jones, I., Farina, A., Hastorf, A., et al. (1984). *Social stigma: The psychology of marked relationships.* New York: Freeman.

Kim, L. (1993). Psychiatric care of Korean Americans. In A. Gaw (Ed.), *Culture, ethnicity, and mental illness* (pp. 347–375). Washington, DC: American Psychiatric Association.

Kim, J., Bramlett, M. H., Wright, L. K., & Poon, L. W. (1998). Racial differences in health status and health behaviors of older adults. *Nursing Research, 47*(4), 243–250.

Kinzie, J., & Leung, P. (1993). Psychiatric care of Indochinese Americans. In A. Gaw (Ed.), *Culture, ethnicity, and mental illness* (pp. 281–304). Washington, DC: American Psychiatric Association.

Lampman, C., & Dowling-Guyer, S. (1995). *Basic and applied social psychology, 17*(1–2), 213–222.

Lantican, L. S. (1998). Mexican American clients' perceptions of services in an outpatient mental health facility in a border city. *Issues in Mental Health Nursing, 19*, 125–137.

Leiter, M., & Durup, M. (1996). Work, home, and in-between: A longitudinal study of spillover. *Journal of Applied Behavioral Science, 32*(1), 29–47.

Lindsey, K., & Paul, G. (1989). Involuntary commitments to public mental institutions: Issues involving the overrepresentation of blacks and assessment of relevant functioning. *Psychological Bulletin, 106*(2), 171–183.

Munakata, R. (1989). The socio-cultural significance of the diagnostic label "neurasthenia" in Japan's mental health care system. Special issue: Neurasthenia in Asian cultures. *Culture, Medicine, and Psychiatry, 13*(2), 203–213.

Murphy, H. (1965). Migration and the major mental disorders: A reappraisal. In M. Kantor (Ed.), *Mobility and mental health* (pp. 5–29). Springfield, IL: Charles C. Thomas.

Neligh, G. (1988). Major mental disorders and behavior among American Indians and Alaska Natives. *American Indians and Alaska Native Mental Health Research, 1*(Monograph 1), 116–150.

Rin, H., & Huang, M. (1989). Neurasthenia as nosological dilemma. Special issue: Neurasthenia in Asian cultures. *Culture, Medicine, and Psychiatry, 13*(2), 215–226.

Roslow, P., & Nicholls, J. (1996). Targeting the Hispanic market: Comparative percussion of TV commercials in Spanish and English. *Journal of Advertising Research, 36*(3), 67–77.

Sharts-Hopko, N. (1996). Health and illness concepts for cultural competence with Japanese clients. *Journal of Cultural Diversity, 3*(3), 74–79.

Simon, R., Fleiss, J., Gurland, B., et al. (1973). Depression and schizophrenia in black and white mental patients. *Archives of General Psychiatry, 28*(4), 509–512.

Sims, O., & Napholz, L. (1996). What are some African American working women's expressed experiences of role conflict? *Journal of Cultural Diversity, 3*(4), 116–122.

Taeuber, C. (1968). Population trends. In E. Sheldon & W. Moore (Eds.), *Indication of social change* (pp. 27–74). New York: Russell Sage Foundation.

Um, C., & Dancy, B. (1999). Relationship between coping strategies and depression among employed Korean immigrant wives. *Issues in Mental Health Nursing, 20*, 485–494.

U.S. Bureau of the Census. (1998). *Statistical abstract of the United States: 1998* (118th ed.). Washington, DC: U.S. Government Printing Office.

U.S. Department of Health and Human Services. (1999). *Mental health: A report of the Surgeon General.* Washington, DC: U.S. Department of Health and Human Services Substance Abuse and Mental Health Administration, Center for Mental Health Services, National Institutes of Health, National Institute of Mental Health.

Wahl, O. F. (1999). Mental health consumers' experience of stigma. *Schizophrenia Bulletin, 25*(3), 467–478.

Worthington, C. (1992). An examination of factors influencing the diagnosis and treatment of black patients in the mental health system. *Archives of Psychiatric Nursing, 6*(3), 195–204.

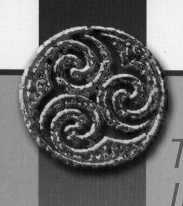

The Mental Health–Mental Illness Continuum

Mary Ann Boyd

EPIDEMIOLOGY OF MENTAL DISORDERS
Epidemiologic Terms
Barriers to Psychiatric Epidemiology
Risk Factors Related to Mental Disorders

DIAGNOSES IN MENTAL HEALTH
Categoric Versus Dimensional Diagnoses
Labeling and Its Consequences

Psychiatric Diagnosis: *The Diagnostic and Statistical Manual of Mental Disorders* (DSM-IV)

INTERVENTIONS IN PSYCHIATRIC MENTAL HEALTH
Caplan's Model: Primary, Secondary, and Tertiary Prevention
Intervention Spectrum: Prevention, Treatment, Maintenance

CLINICAL DECISION MAKING

INTERDISCIPLINARY APPROACH AND THE NURSE'S ROLE
Nursing Care Plans
Critical Pathways
Treatment Guidelines in Psychiatric Mental Health Care
Nurse as Coordinator

LEARNING OBJECTIVES

After studying the chapter, you will be able to:

➤ Differentiate the concepts of mental health, mental illness, mental disorder, and mental health problem.

➤ Define the epidemiologic terms *rate*, *prevalence*, and *incidence*.

➤ Identify categoric and dimensional diagnoses and their relevance to psychiatric nursing.

➤ Differentiate the five axes used in the *Diagnostic and Statistical Manual for Mental Disorders* (DSM-IV).

➤ Compare Caplan's conceptualization of prevention with the newer *intervention spectrum* recommended by the Committee on Prevention of Mental Disorders.

➤ Discuss discipline relationships and the use of nursing care plans and critical pathways.

CHAPTER 3

KEY TERMS

axes
categoric diagnoses
clinical decision making
critical pathways
dimensional diagnoses
epidemiology
incidence
indicated preventive
   interventions
interdisciplinary
   approach
interdisciplinary
   treatment plan
maintenance
   interventions
mental disorder
mental health

mental health problem
mental illness
multiaxial diagnostic
   system
multidisciplinary
   approach
point prevalence
prevalence
prevention
rate
risk factors
selective preventive
   interventions
treatment interventions
universal preventive
   interventions

KEY CONCEPT

mental disorders

Mental health *and mental illness are not polar opposites but instead can be viewed as points on a continuum. A person who is mentally healthy is able to deal with normal human emotion, is productive, has successful relationships with others, can adapt to change, and can cope with adversity. Mental health is the basis for thinking, mood, and communication.* *Mental illness* *is a term that is used to mean all diagnosable mental disorders.*

KEY CONCEPT **Mental disorders. Mental disorders** are health conditions that are characterized by alterations in thinking, mood, or behavior and are associated with distress or impaired functioning.

Mental disorders are unexpected, culturally sanctioned responses to events, such as the normal sadness, grief, and mild depression associated with the death of a spouse. Unit

IV will explain the various mental disorders and their nursing care.

Mental health problem *is a term that is used when signs and symptoms of mental illnesses occur but do not meet specified criteria for a disorder. These problems cause distress to the individual, who feels as if a mental disorder is present. In reality, most people behave in bizarre or strange ways at one time or another, especially during stressful times, such as after a natural disaster, after loss of a loved one, or during a serious illness. Mental health interventions are useful during these periods.*

EPIDEMIOLOGY OF MENTAL DISORDERS

The occurrence of mental disorders is studied just like any other disorder. **Epidemiology** is the study of patterns of disease distribution in time and space. It focuses on the health status of population groups, or aggregates, rather than individuals, and it involves quantitative analysis of the occurrence of illnesses in population groups. Epidemiologic approaches are useful in understanding the occurrences of mental disorders. Throughout this book, mental disorders are described using epidemiologic data. The following discussion defines the epidemiologic terms that are used.

Epidemiologic Terms

In epidemiology, certain terms have specific meanings relative to what they measure. When expressing the number of cases of a disorder, population rates, rather than raw numbers, are used. A **rate** is a proportion of the cases in the population when compared with the total population. It is expressed as a fraction, in which the numerator is the number of cases and the denominator is the total number in the population, including the cases and noncases. The term *average rate* is used for measures that involve rates over specified time periods:

$$\text{Rate} = \frac{\text{Cases in the population}}{\text{Total Population}}$$
$$\text{(includes cases and noncases)}$$

Prevalence refers to the total number of people who have the disorder within a given population at a specified time, regardless of how long ago the disorder started. **Point prevalence** is the basic measure that refers to the proportion of individuals in the population who have the disorder at a specified point in time. For example, the point prevalence of schizophrenia is estimated at 3.2 people per 1,000 (Bromet et al., 1995). This point can be a day on the calendar, such as April 1, 2010, or a point defined in relation to the study assessment, such as the day of the interview. This is also expressed as a fraction:

$$\text{Point prevalence rate} = \frac{\text{Cases at } t}{\text{Population at } t}$$

Incidence refers to a rate that includes only *new* cases that have occurred within a clearly defined time period. For example, the incidence of schizophrenia is estimated at 0.2 per 1,000, much less than the prevalence rate (Bromet et al., 1995). The most common time period evaluated is 1 year. The study of incidence cases is more difficult than a study of prevalent cases because a study of incidence cases requires at least two measurements to be taken, one at the start of the prescribed time period and another at the end of it (Regier & Burke, 2000).

Barriers to Psychiatric Epidemiology

The major obstacle to psychiatric epidemiologic studies has been establishing specific criteria for diagnosis.

Because epidemiologic studies may take many years to complete, it is important that the diagnostic criteria be the same at the beginning and at the end of the study. It is also important that the same diagnosis be reached by different people. With the emergence of the American Psychiatric Association's (APA) diagnostic and statistical manuals, reliable diagnostic criteria became available. These diagnoses are expected to be stable over time.

Risk Factors Related to Mental Disorders

An important epidemiologic concept is **risk factors**, characteristics that increase the likelihood of developing a disorder. They do not cause the disorder or problem and are not symptoms of the illness, but are factors that influence the likelihood that the symptoms will appear. The existence of a risk factor does not always mean the person will get the disorder or disease, it just increases the chances. Risk factors are determined by research evidence of a relationship between a variety of factors and a specific problem. There are many different kinds of risk factors, including genetic, biologic, environmental, cultural, and occupational. Even gender is a risk factor for some disorders (eg, more women suffer from depression than men).

Some risk factors can be controlled or changed, others cannot. Genetic risk factors cannot be changed because individuals cannot change the genetic makeup with which they are born. In some types of dementia, in schizophrenia, and in mood disorders, genetic factors increase the likelihood of the manifestation of the illness. Modern health care has no way of changing these genetic risk factors.

Risk factors that can be changed include those related to lifestyle behaviors or environment. For someone who is genetically at high risk for bipolar disorder (ie, family members have the disorder), this individual can modify lifestyle and environment to decrease the impact of these factors. Selecting a job with less stress can reduce the likelihood of manifestations related to some of the anxiety disorders. However, even if it is possible to change behaviors, occupations, and environmental conditions, the actual change can be difficult. Many of the risky behaviors are physically, psychologically, or socially rewarding and pleasurable, such as eating a high-calorie meal, engaging in unprotected sexual intercourse, or sustaining an interpersonal relationship with someone who is abusive. One of the challenges of nursing is helping people identify and monitor their own risk factors.

DIAGNOSES IN MENTAL HEALTH
Categoric Versus Dimensional Diagnoses

Through the use of standardized classification systems, it is possible to communicate with other health professionals a large amount of information about a patient in a shorthand phrase or system. Assessment data are commonly classified according to categories or dimensions. **Categoric diagnoses** include or exclude data for the purposes of giving a name to a set of symptoms. For example, diabetes mellitus, schizophrenia, or ulcerative colitis are categoric diagnoses that communicate a common set of signs and symptoms. The International Classification of Diseases (ICD) and DSM-IV (discussed in the next section) are two examples of categoric diagnostic systems. However, this type of diagnosis is limited because not all people respond to an illness in exactly the same way. Although two individuals may acquire the same flu virus, one may develop a high fever, an upset stomach, and a dry, harsh cough, and the other may have only a mild fever, a slight cough, and no nausea.

Dimensional diagnoses are descriptions of individuals' responses and behaviors to illnesses. Human dimensions, such as anxiety, aggression, depression, or self-destruction, are experienced on a continuum that ranges from normal to abnormal. These responses and behaviors are viewed in terms of degree or level of severity. For example, the dimension of aggression can be seen on a continuum from verbal anger to physical assault. There can be many dimensional continua (eg, anxiety from mild to panic, self-destruction from indirect to direct, or depression from grief to major depression). Dimensional diagnoses specify human responses to illness and provide direction for treatment. The North American Nursing Diagnosis Association (NANDA) taxonomy is dimensional (see Chap. 13).

Labeling and Its Consequences

A diagnosis becomes a way of labeling a particular patient problem. In mental health, there can be a negative impact caused by labeling. Studies have shown that once individuals are labeled with certain diagnoses, they may be socially rejected and stigmatized (see Chap. 2). For example, Link and colleagues (1997) studied the enduring effects on well-being of 84 men diagnosed with the dual diagnoses of mental disorder and substance abuse. The researchers found a strong and enduring effect of stigma on these individuals' well-being.

The labeling process is an important clinical tool, but the potential negative impact must be considered. Just as a person with diabetes mellitus should not be referred to as a "diabetic," but rather as a "person with diabetes," a person with a mental disorder should never be referred to as a "schizophrenic" or "bipolar," but rather as a "person with schizophrenia" or a "person with bipolar disorder." This method of labeling allows the nurse to view the individual as a whole person who happens to have a disorder, rather than defining the whole person in terms of the disorder or disability. Nurses and health professionals must be careful to avoid the pitfalls of negative labeling and stigmatization of patients.

Psychiatric Diagnosis: *The Diagnostic and Statistical Manual of Mental Disorders (DSM-IV)*

The diagnosis of mental disorders is based on the classification system of the fourth edition of the *Diagnostic and Statistical Manual of Mental Disorders* (DSM-IV) (American Psychiatric Association, 2000). The DSM-IV system contains subtypes and other specifiers to describe further the characteristics of the diagnosis as exhibited in a given individual. This classification system is designed to be useful in research and educational settings, but the primary purpose of the DSM-IV is to provide a commonly understood diagnostic taxonomy for clinical practice.

The diagnosis of mental disorders is based on groups of symptoms that tend to appear together and not on etiology alone. As such, they are useful for the development of a common language, but they do not give specific direction for treatment, which may tend to be symptom or problem based. There is also the issue of its applicability across all cultures. Some disorders are influenced by cultural factors and others are *culture-bound syndromes* that are present in only a particular setting Text Box 3-1). Although the DSM-IV provides criteria for diagnosing mental disorders, there are no absolute boundaries separating one disorder from another, and similar disorders may have different manifestations at different points in time.

TEXT BOX 3.1

Selected Culture-Bound Syndromes

Definition: Behaviors limited to specific cultures that have meaning within that culture

Name	Description
Amok	A dissociative experience of brooding followed by violent outbursts; reported in Malaysia, Laos, Philippines, and Polynesia
Ghost sickness	Preoccupation with death, including bad dreams, weakness, feelings of danger, loss of appetite; observed among Native American tribes
Shin-byung	Initially anxiety and somatic complaints (weakness, dizziness, anorexia, etc.), followed by dissociation and possession of ancestral spirits; part of the Korean folk heritage

Adapted from American Psychiatric Association. (2000). *Diagnostic and statistical manual of mental disorders* (4th ed.) (pp. 898–903). Washington, DC: Author.

The DSM-IV is a **multiaxial diagnostic system** and includes five **axes**, or domains of information. Axis I includes most *clinical disorders* and other conditions that may be the focus of clinical attention, and Axis II contains *personality disorders and mental retardation.* Axis III includes the *general medical conditions*, which must be considered in the diagnosis and treatment of the primary psychiatric disorders. Each of the first three axes is essential to the complete understanding and treatment of an individual with psychiatric concerns. For example, a person with a major depression (Axis I) may meet the criteria for having a dependent personality disorder (Axis II) and also have diabetes (Axis III). See Table 3-1 for a listing of disorders and conditions that might be considered under each axis and Text Box 3-2 for a clinical example.

Although the first three axes appear to contain all of the diagnostic information, a truly accurate picture of the individual is incomplete without considering other factors, such as life stressors and current level of functioning. Axis IV concerns any *psychosocial or environmental problems* that may produce added stress, confound the diagnosis, or must be considered in the treatment of the primary psychiatric problem. These problems may be conceptualized in terms of life stressors, which may be negative or positive. For example, a negative life event, such as a death of a spouse, a recent divorce, or job discrimination, may exacerbate symptoms of depression. On the other hand, positive stressors, such as starting a new job, getting married, or having a baby, may also prompt the appearance of symptoms. Although the DSM-IV suggests a number of problem areas to be considered, the clinician making the diagnosis should write out the individual's specific problems on this axis.

Ratings given on Axis V provide an estimate of *overall functioning* in psychological, social, and occupational spheres of life. These data are useful in planning treatment and measuring its impact. The global assessment functioning (GAF) scale is usually used and is scored from low functioning of 0 to 10, to high functioning of 91 to 100 (see Table 3-1). This rating may be made at the beginning of treatment, at discharge from the hospital, or at any point thereafter. When including this rating, the point of time should also be indicated, such as "current," or "at discharge from the hospital."

INTERVENTIONS IN PSYCHIATRIC MENTAL HEALTH

Caplan's Model: Primary, Secondary, and Tertiary Prevention

In the 1960s, mental health embraced the ideas of primary, secondary, and tertiary prevention from the public health field in an attempt to understand how to lower the statistical rates of a disorder within a population (Caplan, 1964). Through the pioneering works of Gerald Caplan, the field of preventive psychiatry was born. Using Caplan's model, preventive programs are organized to achieve three different goals. Primary prevention seeks to reduce the incidence (rate of occurrence of new cases) of mental disorders within a population over time. For example, primary prevention interventions targeted at suicide have focused on preventing the development of suicidal tendencies in individuals. These interventions have included restricting access to suicide methods (gun control), establishing community-based services, and educating the public and health care professionals. Secondary prevention seeks to lower the prevalence (rate of new and old cases at a point in time). Secondary prevention interventions would include hotlines and short-term hospitalizations targeted for those on the verge of suicide. Tertiary prevention seeks to lower the rate of residual disability, such as by the reduction of occupational and role dysfunctioning (Caplan, 1993). Tertiary prevention interventions also focus on the prevention of recurring suicide attempts (Lester, 1994; Spirito & Overholser, 1993). In Caplan's model, community prevention programs are organized around either *global* risk factors, such as poverty, prejudice, and inadequate living situations, or *target* risk factors, such as biopsychosocial stressors associated with the risk for a mental disorder.

Even though the conceptualization of mental health care in terms of primary, secondary, and tertiary prevention is still being used, there have been consistent difficulties in applying this model to mental disorders. One problem is that this model implies a cause and effect. In mental health, multiple factors influence the manifestation of a disorder, not just one factor. Also, Caplan's use of the term prevention encompasses preventing the illness (primary) as well as treating it. Thus, the ambiguous meaning of the term prevention led to considerable confusion about exactly what prevention activities are.

Intervention Spectrum: Prevention, Treatment, Maintenance

In 1992, the Institute of Medicine (an advisory group to the federal government) established a Committee on Prevention of Mental Disorders to work with the National Institute of Mental Health (NIMH) in identifying current prevention knowledge and recommending future research directions. The committee quickly recognized the conceptual problems of the traditional approach of the primary, secondary, and tertiary prevention model. A new definition of the term prevention was agreed on by this committee. **Prevention** was redefined

TABLE 3.1 DSM-IV Multiaxial Diagnoses for Persons With Mental Disorders

Diagnostic Axes and Their Disorders and Conditions

*Axis I: Clinical Disorders and Other Conditions
That May Be a Focus of Clinical Attention*

Disorders Usually First Diagnosed During Infancy,
  Childhood, or Adolescence
Delirium, Dementia, Amnestic, and Other Cognitive
  Disorders
Mental Disorders Due to General Medical Conditions
Substance-Related Disorders
Schizophrenia and Other Psychotic Disorders
Mood Disorders
Somatoform Disorders
Factitious Disorders
Dissociative Disorders
Sexual and Gender Identity Disorders
Eating Disorders
Sleep Disorders
Impulse Control Disorders (Not Elsewhere Classified)
Adjustment Disorders
Other Conditions That May Be a Focus of Clinical Attention

Axis II: Personality Disorders and Mental Retardation

Personality Disorders:
  Paranoid Personality Disorder
  Schizoid Personality Disorder
  Schizotypal Personality Disorder
  Antisocial Personality Disorder
  Borderline Personality Disorder
  Histrionic Personality Disorder
  Narcissistic Personality Disorder
  Avoidant Personality Disorder
  Dependent Personality Disorder
  Obsessive-Compulsive Personality Disorder
  Personality Disorder Not Otherwise Specified
Mental Retardation

Axis III: General Medical Conditions

Infectious and Parasitic Diseases
Neoplasms
Endocrine, Nutritional, and Metabolic Diseases and
  Immunity Disorders
Diseases of the Blood and Blood-Forming Organs
Diseases of the Nervous and Sense Organs
Diseases of the Respiratory System
Diseases of the Digestive System
Diseases of the Genitourinary System
Complications of Pregnancy, Childbirth, and
  the Puerperium
Diseases of the Skin and Subcutaneous Tissue
Diseases of the Musculoskeletal System and
  Connective Tissue
Congenital Anomalies
Certain Conditions Originating in the Perinatal Period
Symptoms, Signs, and Ill-Defined Conditions
Injury and Poisoning

Axis IV: Psychosocial and Environmental Problems

Problems with primary support group
Problems related to the social environment
Educational problems
Occupational problems
Housing problems
Economic problems
Problems with access to health care services
Problems related to interaction with the legal system/crime
Other psychosocial and environmental problems

Axis V: Global Assessment of Functioning:

  Current =

  Potential =

Psychologic, social, and occupational functioning on a
  hypothetical continuum of mental health–illness.

Scores

91–100	Superior functioning, no symptoms
81–90	Absent or minimal symptoms, good functioning in all areas
71–80	If symptoms are present, they are transient and expectable reactions to psychosocial stressors; no more than slight impairment in social, occupational, or school functioning
61–70	Some mild symptoms or some difficulty in social, occupational, or school functioning, but generally functioning well; has some meaningful interpersonal relationships
51–60	Moderate symptoms or moderate difficulty in social, occupational, or school functioning
41–50	Serious symptoms or any serious impairment in social, occupational, or school functioning
31–40	Some impairment in reality testing or communication or major impairment in several areas, such as work or school, family relations, judgment, thinking, or mood
21–30	Behavior is considerably influenced by delusions or hallucinations or serious impairment in communication or judgment or inability to function in almost all areas
11–20	Some danger of hurting self or others or occasionally fails to maintain minimal personal hygiene or gross impairment in communication
1–10	Persistent danger of severely hurting self or others or persistent inability to maintain minimal personal hygiene or serious suicidal act with clear expectation of death

TEXT BOX 3.2

*Diagnostic Axes and Their Disorders
and Conditions*

Clinical Example

Axis I: 296.2a* Major Depressive Disorder, single
          episode, severe w/o psychotic features
          305.00 Alcohol abuse

Axis II: 301.83 Borderline Personality Disorder

Axis III: 250.00† Diabetes mellitus

Axis IV: Occupational problems: Interpersonal conflict
          at work

Axis V: Global Assessment of Function
          GAF = 55 (current)
                90 (potential)

---

*In this example, code numbers are used and can be found in the *Diagnostic and Statistical Manual of Mental Disorders, 4th ed. (DSM-IV)*. To improve readability, these code numbers are not used when discussing the various disorders. The student will see them used in the clinical setting. †The medical conditions in Axis III are coded according to the *International Classification of Diseases (ICD)*.

as only those interventions used before the initial onset of a disorder and became distinct from treatment. The committee recommended that the mental health intervention spectrum for mental disorders be used as the standard intervention system (Fig. 3-1) (Mrazek & Haggerty, 1994). In this model, prevention interventions are classified according to the following:

- **Universal preventive interventions:** targeted to everyone within a general public or whole population group
- **Selective preventive interventions:** targeted to an individual or a subgroup of the population whose risk for developing a disorder is higher than average

- **Indicated preventive interventions:** targeted to high-risk individuals who are identified as having minimal, but detectable, signs or symptoms foreshadowing a disorder or biologic markers indicating a predisposition, but who do not have the disorder (Mrazek & Haggerty, 1994)

Treatment interventions include case identification and standard treatment for all known disorders. Treatment aims to reduce the likelihood of future co-occurring disorders and the length of stay as well as to halt the progression of severity of the illness. **Maintenance interventions**, in turn, are those supportive, educational, or pharmacologic interventions that are provided on a long-term basis to individuals who have been diagnosed with a disorder. They aim to decrease the disability associated with the disorder. Maintenance components include the patient's compliance with long-term treatment to reduce relapse and recurrence and the provision of after-care services to the patient, including rehabilitation.

CLINICAL DECISION MAKING

The development and implementation of efficacious interventions involves critical analysis of patient, family, and community data and making decisions about care. Although nurses are often leaders in the implementation of prevention programs to designated populations, most nurses focus on the delivery of care to individuals. Treatment decisions for individual patients with psychiatric mental health problems are multifaceted. There are a variety of theoretic perspectives from which the patient can be viewed, and each has a treatment component. Nurses are responsible for familiarizing themselves with the many treatment possibilities and for determining which approach fits a particular patient.

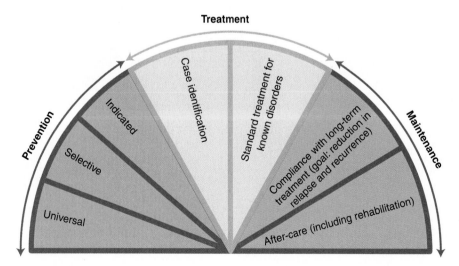

FIGURE 3.1 The mental health intervention spectrum for mental disorders. (Adapted from Mrazek, P., & Haggerty, R. [Eds.]. [1994]. *Reducing risks for mental disorders: Frontiers for preventive intervention research* [p. 23]. Committee on Prevention of Mental Disorders, Institute of Medicine. Washington, DC: National Academy Press.

Decision making is a type of critical thinking and is at the core of clinical practice. Job satisfaction is directly related to involvement in decision making. One survey of 230 critical care nurses showed that their level of work satisfaction was directly related to the level of involvement in decision making. Thus, the nurses who were autonomous in their decision making were the most satisfied (Bucknall & Thomas, 1996). In addition to the complex decisions, such as collecting, processing, and organizing information, and formulating nursing approaches, many moment-to-moment decisions are made, such as deciding whether a patient can leave a unit or whether a patient should receive a medication. Clinical decision making is a specific type of critical thinking that focuses on the choices made in clinical settings.

INTERDISCIPLINARY APPROACH AND THE NURSE'S ROLE

Several other professionals besides nurses and physicians provide mental health services to people with emotional problems and mental disorders. These professionals come from a variety of discipline backgrounds and provide services based on their training and licensure, which may vary from state to state. Psychiatric mental health care has a long tradition of using a **multidisciplinary approach**, with several disciplines providing service to a patient at one time. Table 3-2 describes other health professionals with whom the nurse will come in contact. In the hospital, a patient may be seeing a psychiatrist for

management of the disorder symptoms and the prescribing of medication; a psychiatric social worker for individual psychotherapy; a psychiatric nurse for management of responses related to the mental disorder, administration of medication, and monitoring side effects; and an occupational therapist for transition into the workplace. In the community clinic, the patient may be meeting weekly with a therapist, monthly with a mental health provider who prescribes medication, and twice a week with a group leader in a day treatment program. All of these professionals bring a specialized skill to the patient.

A multidisciplinary approach, however, is not quite the ideal for patient care because the care can be fragmented when approaches are independent of each other. An **interdisciplinary approach**, in which interventions from the different disciplines are integrated into delivery of patient care, is ideal. In this model, a nurse and a psychologist may simultaneously intervene with a patient on changing a behavior related to medication compliance. An interdisciplinary approach differs from a multidisciplinary one because it requires a close working relationship among personnel from the different disciplines who no longer provide services independently from each other.

Whether a multidisciplinary or interdisciplinary approach is used, the psychiatric mental health nurse can expect to collaborate with other professionals in all settings, including hospital and community. However, it is usually the nurse who coordinates the delivery of the

TABLE 3.2   The Interdisciplinary Mental Health Team Involved in the Multidisciplinary Approach

Discipline	Education	Focus of Treatment
Psychiatrist	MD/DO + psychiatric residency	Diagnosis and treatment of mental disorders
Psychologist	MS or PhD	Diagnosis of mental disorders, psychological testing, psychological treatments such as psychotherapy
Social worker	MS	Diagnosis of mental disorders, psychosocial therapies such as family, couple; also linked with community resources
Counselor	MS or PhD	Counseling
Occupational therapist	BS	Functional independence in tasks of daily living
Recreational therapist	BS	Leisure-related activities
Speech therapist	MS	Communication disorders
Art therapist	MA	Expressive therapy through art
Music or dance therapist	BA	Expressive therapy through music or dance
Dietitian	MS	Nutritional therapy, education, maintaining balanced diet
Chaplain or pastoral counselor	Masters in Theology (or equivalent) Ecclesiastical endorsement by faith group	Ascertain the spiritual and faith assets of each patient in the healing process

care of these different disciplines. In the hospital and in the community, the nurses oversee the completion of the **interdisciplinary treatment plan**, a plan of care that identifies the patient's problems, outcomes, interventions, members of different disciplines assigned to implement interventions, and evaluation criteria. In this text, interdisciplinary treatment plans will be presented in Chapters 18, 20, and 21.

Nursing Care Plans

Clinical decision making is the cornerstone of the development of nursing care plans. Just like patients in medical surgical settings, the person receiving psychiatric mental health services has a written plan of care. If only nursing care is being provided, such as in home care, then a nursing care plan may be used. If other disciplines are providing services to the same patient, which often occurs in a hospital, then an individual treatment plan may be used with or instead of a traditional nursing care plan. When a interdisciplinary plan is used, components of the nursing care plan should always be easily identified. The nurse provides the care that is judged to be within the scope of practice of the psychiatric mental health nurse (see Chap. 5). Thus, the traditional nursing care plan may or may not be used, depending on institutional policies. Whether a nursing care plan or an individual treatment plan is used, these plans are important because they are individualized to a patient's needs. They are sometimes approved by third-party payers who cover the cost of the service. In this text, the emphasis will be on developing nursing care plans because they serve as a basis of practice even if the interventions are included in a multidisciplinary or interdisciplinary individual treatment plan.

Critical Pathways

Many psychiatric institutions use **critical pathways** to ensure a quality level of care in a cost-effective way. These care paths are similar to individual treatment plans in that all the discipline interventions are included on one plan. They are different in that critical pathways are designed for a hypothetical patient with typical symptoms who follows an expected course of treatment. Care paths are not developed for each patient. Instead, each facility or agency has only a few psychiatric mental health care paths that are used to guide care. Also, critical pathways are used in determining appropriate length of treatment within a particular setting, hospital, clinic, or home. Each problem has an expected length of stay within each type of setting. If a patient is not improving according to the time designated on the care

path, the patient and caregivers are evaluated by others in the system.

The use of critical pathways in mental health has met with some resistance. Proponents of the use of care paths argue that consumers are protected because up-to-date research-based care is guaranteed and care is not solely directed by physicians, who may use out-of-date approaches. It is viewed as a cost-effective approach to delivering mental health care. Those opposed to the use of critical pathways respond that individuality of patient treatment is jeopardized by a standard treatment for everyone. The efficacy of critical pathways is still being studied. In this text, examples of critical pathways can be found in the appendices.

Treatment Guidelines in Psychiatric Mental Health Care

There is general agreement in the psychiatric community that treatment guidelines are useful. These guidelines usually include algorithms (or decision trees) that can be used in making treatment decisions. The best guidelines are evidenced based and can be uniformly applied to people with a particular disorder. Most of the disorders discussed in this book have several treatment guidelines.

Nurse as Coordinator

In the inpatient setting, it is the nurse who coordinates the delivery of care. The nurse interfaces with other disciplines in planning and implementing the care. In the outpatient setting, the nurse can serve as the coordinator of care as well as the primary provider. Critical thinking skills are crucial. A patient with a psychiatric disorder will have a diagnosis that may have at least five problem areas (axes) that need to be considered. Each axis focuses on an aspect of the person. One of the axes is the medical condition, which has its own set of interventions and interacts with the problems inherent in the other axes. The nurse must synthesize all of the information and approach the patient from a holistic perspective.

Summary of Key Points

➤ Mentally healthy people are able to deal with normal human emotions. Mental disorders are health conditions characterized by alterations in thinking, mood, or behavior and are associated with distress or impaired functioning. Mental health problems may need intervention but do not meet criteria for a mental disorder.

➤ Epidemiology is important in understanding the distribution of mental illness within a given population. The rate of occurrence refers to the proportion of the population that has the disorder. The incidence is the rate of new cases within a specified time. The prevalence is the rate of occurrence of all cases at a particular point in time.

➤ Risk factors include factors that can and cannot be changed. Genetic predisposition cannot be changed, but lifestyle and behavior can.

➤ Categoric and dimensional diagnoses are used in nursing. The use of diagnosis in mental health can be problematic because of the negative association of the label *mental illness*. The categoric diagnoses outlined in the DSM-IV are the standardized, accepted language in the mental health field. There are five diagnostic axes: clinical disorders; personality disorders and mental retardation; general medical problems; psychosocial or environmental problems; and overall functioning.

➤ Mental health interventions can be viewed along a spectrum of prevention, treatment, and maintenance strategies. They can target an individual or a whole population.

➤ Within the intervention spectrum, prevention is categorized according to universal, selective, and indicated preventive interventions. Prevention is defined as only those interventions used before the onset of the disorder.

➤ Clinical decision making is an important aspect of developing nursing care plans, critical pathways, and algorithms.

➤ The psychiatric mental health nurse interacts with other disciplines and many times acts as a coordinator in the delivery of care. There is always a plan of care for a patient, but it may be either a nursing care plan or an individualized treatment plan that includes other disciplines. Critical pathways, different from individualized care plans, are used throughout the care continuum to ensure quality care and cost-effectiveness.

Critical Thinking Challenges

1. Define the terms *mental health*, *mental disorder*, and *mental health problem*. How can they be differentiated?
2. Define the epidemiologic terms *prevalence*, *incidence*, and *rate*.
3. Define risk factors and identify the different types of risk factors in psychiatric mental health.

4. Discuss the negative impact of labeling someone with a psychiatric diagnosis.
5. Explain the difference between a categoric and a dimensional diagnosis. Give examples.
6. Explain the purposes of the five axes of the DSM-IV.
7. Compare the spectrum of interventions advocated by the Committee on Prevention of Mental Disorders with the traditional view of prevention.
8. Contrast multidisciplinary and interdisciplinary practice. Describe how and when nursing care plans and integrated care paths should be used.

 WEB LINKS

www.mentalhealth.com   This useful site examines many aspects of mental health and mental illness, including psychiatric diagnosis.

www.ahcpr.gov   This website of the Agency for Healthcare Research and Quality has a repository of practice guidelines.

www.nursingnet.com   This nursing student website includes nursing care plans.

www.nurseintraining.8m.com/nursing/careplans. htm   This site includes care plans, a chat room, and Internet hot sites.

REFERENCES

American Psychiatric Association. (2000). *Diagnostic and statistical manual of mental disorders* (4th ed., Text revision). Washington, DC: Author.

Bromet, E., Dew, M., & Eaton, W. (1995). Epidemiology of psychosis with special reference to schizophrenia. In M. Tsuang, M. Tohen, & G. Zahner (Eds.), *Textbook in psychiatric epidemiology* (pp. 283–300). New York: Wiley-Liss.

Bucknall, T., & Thomas, S. (1996). Critical care nurse satisfaction with levels of involvement in the clinical decisions. *Journal of Advanced Nursing, 23*(3), 571–577.

Caplan, G. (1964). *Principles of preventive psychiatry.* New York: Basic Books.

Caplan, G. (1993). Organization of preventive psychiatry programs. *Community Mental Health Journal, 29*(4), 367–395.

Lester, D. (1994). Challenges in preventing suicide. *Death Studies, 18*(6), 623–639.

Link, B. G., Struening, E. L., Rahav, M., et al. (1997). On stigma and its consequences: Evidence from a longitudinal study of men with dial diagnoses of mental illness and substance abuse. *Journal of Health & Social Behavior, 38*(2), 177–190.

Mrazek, P., & Haggerty, R. (Eds.). (1994). *Reducing risks for mental disorders: Frontiers for preventive intervention research.* Committee on Prevention of Mental Disorders, Institute of Medicine. Washington, DC: National Academy Press.

Regier, D., & Burke, J. (2000). Epidemiology. In B. Sadock & V. Sadock (Eds.), *Comprehensive textbook of psychiatry* (vol. VII) (pp. 500–522). Philadelphia: Lippincott Williams & Wilkins.

Spirito, A., & Overholser, J. (1993). Primary and secondary prevention strategies for reducing suicide among youth. Special issue: Family treatment. *Child and Adolescent Mental Healthcare, 3*(3), 205–217.

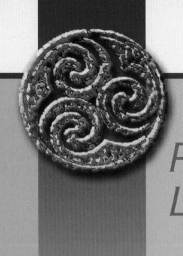

Patient Rights and Legal Issues

Mary Ann Boyd

PATIENT RIGHTS
Bill of Rights
The Americans With Disabilities
   Act and Job Discrimination

ISSUES OF CONSENT
Self-Determinism
   Self-Determination Act
   Advance Care Directives
      in Mental Health
Competency
Informed Consent
Voluntary and Involuntary
   Treatment

**RIGHT TO TREATMENT IN
THE LEAST RESTRICTIVE
ENVIRONMENT**

ISSUES OF CONFIDENTIALITY
Privacy Versus Confidentiality
Mandates to Inform

**DOCUMENTATION
AND LEGAL ISSUES**

**CRIMINAL LAW
AND PSYCHIATRY**
Not Guilty by Reason
   of Insanity (NGRI)

Guilty But Mentally Ill (GBMI)
Forensic Commitment
Misconceptions Regarding
   the Insanity Plea
Public Safety

**LAWS AND SYSTEMS THAT
PROTECT HUMAN RIGHTS**
Internal Rights Protection System
External Advocacy Systems
Accreditation of Mental Health
   Care Delivery Systems

**LEARNING
OBJECTIVES**

After studying this chapter, you will be able to:

➤ Discuss the role of informed consent in the delivery of psychiatric–mental health care.

➤ Use the concepts of self-determinism and competence in discussing patient treatment choices.

➤ Delineate the differences between voluntary and involuntary treatment.

➤ Explain the rationale for providing the least restrictive treatment environment.

➤ Discuss the issues of confidentiality and mandates to inform and their implications in psychiatric–mental health care.

➤ Identify the importance of accurate, descriptive documentation of the biopsychosocial areas.

➤ Discuss the issues underlying the insanity plea.

accreditation
advance care directives
breach of confidentiality
competence
confidentiality
external advocacy
  systems
forensic commitment
incompetent

informed consent
internal rights
  protection system
involuntary commitment
least restrictive
  environment
privacy
voluntary admission
voluntary commitment

self-determinism

In the past, people with mental disorders often received in-adequate treatment and were punished because their disorder was misunderstood. It was difficult to protect human rights and maintain ethical practice standards. In the first three chapters, you learned how society's misunderstanding and sociocultural beliefs and events often led to maltreatment of those with mental disorders. Today, legal rights of those with mental disorders and ethical health care practices of mental health providers are ongoing concerns for psychiatric–mental health nurses. For example, who decides the care plan for a person with a mental disorder? Can a person be forced into a hospital if his or her behavior is bizarre but harmless? What human rights can be denied to a person who has a mental disorder and under what circumstances? These questions are not easily answered. This chapter summarizes some of the key patient rights and legal issues that underlie psychiatric–mental health nursing practice across the continuum of care.

PATIENT RIGHTS

Bill of Rights

People with psychiatric problems are vulnerable to mistreatment and abuse; consequently, laws have been passed that guarantee them legal protection. The spe-cific laws and regulations are discussed later in the chap-ter. In some instances, people with mental disorders are unable to make sound decisions regarding their treat-ment and care. Fortunately, certain laws protect them from their own poor decision-making abilities. The following is a discussion of certain important patients' rights outlined in the Universal Bill of Rights for Mental Health Patients (Text Box 4-1), first established by the President's Commission on Mental Health and later made into law by the Mental Health Systems Act of 1980.

The Americans With Disabilities Act and Job Discrimination

The Americans With Disabilities Act of 1990 (ADA) makes it unlawful to discriminate in employment against a qualified individual with a disability. The ADA also outlaws discrimination against individuals with dis-abilities in state and local government services, public accommodations, transportation, and telecommuni-cation. The ADA defines an *individual with a disability* as a person who has a physical or mental impairment that substantially limits one or more major life activities, has a record of such an impairment, or is regarded as having such an impairment (U.S. Equal Employment

TEXT BOX 4.1

Universal Bill of Rights for Mental Health Patients

1. The right to appropriate treatment and related services in a setting and under conditions that are the most supportive of such person's personal liberty, and restrict such liberty only to the extent necessary consistent with such person's treatment needs, applicable requirement of law, and applicable judicial orders.

2. The right to an individualized, written treatment or service plan (such plan to be developed promptly after admission of such person), the right to treatment based on such plan, the right to periodic review and reassessment of treatment and related service needs, and the right to appropriate revision of such plan, including any revision necessary to provide a description of mental health services that may be needed after such person is discharged from such program or facility.

3. The right to ongoing participation, in a manner appropriate to a person's capabilities, in the planning of mental health services to be provided (including the right to participate in the development and periodic revision of the plan).

4. The right to be provided with a reasonable explanation, in terms and language appropriate to a person's condition and ability to understand the person's general mental and physical (if appropriate) condition, the objectives of treatment, the nature and significant possible adverse effects of recommended treatment, the reasons why a particular treatment is considered, the reasons why access to certain visitors may not be appropriate, and any appropriate and available alternative treatments, services, and types of providers of mental health services.

5. The right not to receive a mode or course of treatment in the absence of informed, voluntary, written consent to treatment except during an emergency situation.

6. The right not to participate in experimentation in the absence of informed, voluntary, written consent (includes human subject protection).

7. The right to freedom from restraint or seclusion, other than as a mode or course of treatment or restraint or seclusion during an emergency situation with a written order by a responsible mental health professional.

8. The right to a humane treatment environment that affords reasonable protection from harm and appropriate privacy with regard to personal needs.

9. The right to access, on request, to such person's mental health care records.

10. The right, in the case of a person admitted on a residential or inpatient care basis, to converse with others privately, to have convenient and reasonable access to the telephone and mails, and to see visitors during regularly scheduled hours. (For treatment purposes, specific individuals may be excluded.)

11. The right to be informed promptly and in writing at the time of admission of these rights.

12. The right to assert grievances with respect to infringement of these rights.

13. The right to exercise these rights without reprisal.

14. The right of referral to other providers.

Title II, Public Law 99-319, *Restatement of Bill of Rights for Mental Health Patients*, Title II—Restatement of Bill of Rights for Mental Health Patients established by Mental Health Systems Act of 1980.

Opportunity Commission, 1991). An employer is free to select the most qualified applicant available, but if the most qualified person has a mental disorder, this law mandates that reasonable accommodations need to be made for that individual. Accommodations are any adjustments to a job or work environment, such as restructuring a job, modifying work schedules, and acquiring or modifying equipment.

ISSUES OF CONSENT

Self-Determinism

KEY CONCEPT **Self-Determinism.** In general, **self-determinism** can be defined as being empowered or having the free will to make moral judgments.

A self-determined individual chooses a course of action without being restrained by others' expectations. Personal autonomy and avoidance of dependency on others are key values. A self-determined individual has *intrinsic* motivation to make choices based on personal goals, not to please others or to be rewarded. That is, a person engages in activities that are interesting, challenging, pleasing, exciting, or fun, requiring no reward other than the positive feelings that accompany them (Deci, 1987). Researchers believe that self-determinism is a basic and fundamental psychological need.

In mental health care, self-determinism is the right to choose one's own health-related behaviors, which, at times, differ from those recommended by health professionals. A patient's right to refuse treatment, to choose the second or third best health care recommendation rather than the first, and to seek a second opinion are all self-deterministic acts. In mental health care, compliance to treatment regimes may be at odds with the self-deterministic views of an individual. Supporting an individual's ability to choose treatment becomes complex because of related issues of competency, informed consent, voluntary and involuntary commitment, and public safety.

Self-Determination Act

A competent individual can make a decision about a treatment that can be honored if that person becomes incompetent. The Patient Self-Determination Act (PSDA) was implemented on December 1, 1991 as a part of the Omnibus Budget Reconciliation Act of 1990 and requires hospitals, health maintenance organizations, skilled nursing facilities, home health agencies, and hospices receiving Medicare and Medicaid reimbursement to inform patients at the time of admission of their right to be a central part of any and all health care decisions made about them or for them. These rights include the following:

- Developing written policies on advance care documents and providing patients information on the policies
- Asking patients at admission or enrollment whether they have an advance care document and recording this fact in the medical record
- Providing patients information on their rights to complete advance care documents and refuse medical care
- Educating health care personnel and the local community about advance care planning (Omnibus Budget Reconciliation Act, 1990)

Advance Care Directives in Mental Health

Advance care directives include treatment directives, often referred to as *living wills*, and appointment directives, often referred to as *power of attorney* or *health proxies*. A living will states what treatment should be omitted or refused in the event that a person is unable to make those decisions. A durable power of attorney for health care appoints a proxy, usually a relative or trusted friend, to make health care decisions on that individual's behalf if that person is incapacitated. An advance directive does not need to be written, reviewed, or signed by an attorney. It must be witnessed by two people and notarized and applies only if the individual is unable to make his or her own decisions as a result of being incapacitated or if, in the opinion of two physicians, the person is otherwise unable to make decisions for himself or herself.

States have started to legislate separate statutes for advance care directives in mental health. Minnesota has enacted a living will act for mental health (SB 187, Chapter 148, 1991 Laws) that allows a competent adult to make a declaration of preference or instruction regarding intrusive mental health treatment. This declaration must be made in advance and signed by the patient and two witnesses. Although a physician can override this declaration during times when the patient's decision-making capacity is clearly distorted because of the mental illness, the patient must be informed first and the order made by the court.

Competency

In psychiatric–mental health care, individuals may make poor treatment decisions because they are experiencing symptoms of their illness. These individuals would most likely make different choices if they did not have symptoms. One of the most important concepts underlying the legal rights of individuals is competency to consent to or to refuse treatment. Even though competency is a legal determination, it is not clearly defined across the states. It is generally agreed that **competence**, or the degree to which the patient is able to understand and appreciate the information given during the consent process, refers to a patient's cognitive ability to process information at a specific time (Culver, 1991). A patient may be competent to make a treatment decision at one time and not be competent at another time. Competence is also decision specific, so that a patient may be competent to decide on a simple treatment with a relatively clear consequence, but may not be competent to decide about a treatment with a complex set of outcomes. A competent patient can refuse any aspect of the treatment plan, except in the case of an emergency (Trudeau, 1993).

Competence is different from rationality, which is a characteristic of a patient's decision, not of the patient's ability to make a decision. An irrational decision is one that involves hurting oneself pointlessly, such as stopping recommended treatment even though symptoms return (Culver, 1991). A person who is competent may make what appears to be an irrational decision, and it cannot be overruled by health care providers; however, if a person is judged **incompetent** (ie, unable to understand and appreciate the information given during the consent process), it is possible to force treatment on the individual. There are strong arguments, however, against forced treatment under these circumstances. Forced treatment denigrates individuals, and according to self-determinism theory, individuals are not as likely to experience treatment success if it is externally imposed. For example, some clinicians report that medications are less effective when they are imposed on an unwilling person (Parrish, 1993; Winick, 1994).

Informed Consent

Individuals seeking mental health care must provide **informed consent**, the right to determine what shall be done with their own body and mind. To provide informed consent, the patient must be given adequate information on which to base decisions about care and is thus an active participant and ultimately decides the course of treatment. Informed consent is not an option, but is mandated by state or provincial laws. In most states or provinces, the law mandates that a mental health provider must inform a patient in such a way that an average, reasonable person would be able to make an educated decision about the interventions.

Informed consent is complicated in mental health treatment. A patient must be competent to give consent, but the individual's decision-making ability is often compromised by the mental illness. This dilemma might be illustrated by the case in which a person who is informed of the medication side effects refuses treatment, not because of the potential negative impact of the medication, but because he or she denies the illness outright. The health care provider knows that once the person begins taking the medication, the symptoms of the illness will subside, and the decision-making ability will return. Thus, an adequate mental status of the patient is the basis of the informed consent dilemma (Trudeau, 1993).

How is it determined that a patient is competent to give informed consent? Mental health legal experts generally agree that four areas should be directly assessed (Galen, 1993; Applebaum & Grisso, 1988). The patient who is competent to give informed consent should be able to achieve the following:

1. Communicate choices
2. Understand relevant information
3. Appreciate the situation and its consequence
4. Use a logical thought process to compare the risks and benefits of treatment options

These areas are further explained in Table 4-1. In mental health care, informed consent is important because of the potential side effects of many of the treatments, including medications and electroconvulsive therapy. Once consent is given, nursing and medical personnel are absolved from legal liability for actions they take provided they practice according to discipline standards (see Chap. 5). Most institutions have policies that outline the nursing responsibilities within the informed consent process. The nurse has a key role in the process of informed consent, from structuring the written informed consent document to educating the patient about a particular procedure. The nurse makes sure that consent has been obtained before any treatment is given. Informed consent is especially important in research projects involving experimental drugs or therapies.

Voluntary and Involuntary Treatment

Patients seeking mental health treatment gain access to the delivery system by seeking out the care of a mental health provider. The process is similar to that of seeking any other type of medical care. Treatment is recommended and agreed on by both the provider and the individual, and the individual then complies with the treatment. If hospitalization is required, the person enters the facility, participates in the treatment planning process, and then follows through with the treatment. This individual maintains all civil rights and is free to leave at any time, even if it is against medical advice. In most settings, this type of admission is called a **voluntary admission.** If an individual is admitted to a public facility, the state statute may refer to the process as **voluntary commitment**, rather than admission; however, in both instances, full legal rights are retained.

Involuntary commitment is the confined hospitalization of a person without the person's consent, but with a court order. There are also legal provisions for people to be involuntarily committed to outpatient mental health facilities through state civil laws. Because involuntary commitment to mental health agencies is a province of state laws, each state and the District of

TABLE 4.1 Determination of Competency		
Assessment Area	**Definition**	**Patient Attributes**
Communicate choices	Ability to express choices	Patient should be able to repeat what he or she has heard.
Understand relevant information	Capacity to comprehend the meaning of the information given about treatment	Patient should be able to paraphrase understanding of treatment.
Appreciate the situation and its consequence	Capacity to grasp what the information means specifically to the patient	Patient should be able to discuss the disorder, the need for treatment, the likely outcomes, and the reason the treatment is being suggested.
Use a logical thought process to compare the risks and benefits of treatment options	Capacity to reach a logical conclusion consistent with the starting premise	Patient should be able to discuss logical reasons for the choice of treatment.

Columbia has separate commitment statutes; however, three common elements are found in most of these statutes. The individual must be (1) mentally disordered, (2) dangerous to self or others, or (3) unable to provide for basic needs (ie, "gravely disabled"). Involuntary commitment is a fairly common occurrence. One study conducted in an urban emergency department found that during a 1-month period, 8.5% of the patients (*n* = 3,637) required involuntary treatment orders (Lavoie, 1992). About one of every four admissions to inpatient mental health programs is involuntary (L. M. Sayre, personal communication, Center for Mental Health Services, October 3, 1996).

Commitment procedures vary considerably among the states and provinces. Most have provisions for an emergency short-term hospitalization of 48 to 92 hours authorized by a certified mental health provider without court approval. At the end of that period, the individual either agrees to voluntary treatment, or extended commitment procedures are begun that can be renewed for periods of 90 days or 6 months. The judge must order the commitment, and the individual is afforded several legal rights, including notice of the proceedings, a full hearing (jury trial if requested) in which the government must prove the grounds for commitment, and the right to legal counsel at state expense.

RIGHT TO TREATMENT IN THE LEAST RESTRICTIVE ENVIRONMENT

Not only do people who are involuntarily committed have the right to receive treatment, they also may have the right to refuse it. Arguments over the rights of civilly committed patients to refuse treatment first surfaced in 1975, when a federal district court judge issued a temporary restraining order prohibiting the use of psychotropic medication against the patient's will at a state hospital in Boston. Half the states and one third of the Canadian provinces have recognized the right of involuntary patients to refuse medication (Hermann, 1990). The state trend is to grant patients the right to refuse treatment.

The right to refuse treatment is related to a larger concept, the right to be treated in the **least restrictive environment**, which means that an individual cannot be restricted to an institution when he or she can be successfully treated in the community. In 1975, the courts ruled that a person committed to psychiatric treatment had a right to be treated in the least restrictive environment (Dixon v. Weinberger, 1975). Medication cannot be given unnecessarily. An individual cannot be restrained or locked in a room unless all other "less restrictive" interventions are tried first.

ISSUES OF CONFIDENTIALITY

Communication between patient and health care provider is protected by law. Psychiatric–mental health care requires an intense level of communication in which extremely personal information is shared. Often, the information relates to other people; for example, information regarding a married woman's sexual fantasy about her coworker is confidential and cannot be shared with her husband. Under certain circumstances, however, confidential information needs to be shared with others, for example, when a patient relates an intention to harm someone else. Although laws have been enacted to protect patients' privacy, maintain confidentiality, and protect human rights, laws have also been enacted to protect society from actions of people with symptoms that may endanger others. The following section discusses the issues related to privacy and confidentiality.

Privacy Versus Confidentiality

Privacy refers to that part of an individual's personal life that is not governed by society's laws and government intrusion. Protecting an individual from intrusion is a responsibility of health care providers. **Confidentiality** can be defined as an ethical duty of nondisclosure. The provider who receives confidential information must protect that information from being accessed by others and resist disclosing it. Confidentiality involves two people: the individual who discloses and the person with whom the information is shared. If confidentiality is broken, a person's privacy is also violated; however, a person's privacy can be violated but confidentiality maintained. For example, if a nurse observes an adult patient reading pornography alone in his or her room, the patient's privacy has been violated. If the patient asks the nurse not to tell anyone and the request is honored, confidentiality is maintained.

Maintaining a person's privacy and protecting confidentiality involve legal and ethical considerations. A **breach of confidentiality** is the release of patient information without the patient's consent in the absence of legal compulsion or authorization to release information (Wettstein, 1994). For example, discussing a patient's problem with one of his or her relatives without the patient's consent is a breach of confidentiality. Even sharing patient information with another professional who is not involved in the care is a breach of confidentiality because the individual has not given permission for the information to be shared. Maintaining confidentiality is not as easy as it first appears. Because of confidentiality laws, family members are legally excluded from receiving any information about an adult member without consent, even if that member is receiving care from the family. Ideally, a patient gives consent for information to be shared with the family.

Mandates to Inform

At certain times, a professional is legally obligated to breach confidentiality. When there is a judgment that the patient has harmed any person or is about to injure someone, the professional is mandated by law to report it to authorities. The legal "duty to warn" was a result of the 1976 decision of *Tarasoff v. Regents of the University of California*. In this case, a 26-year-old graduate student told university psychologists about his obsession with another student, Tatiana Tarasoff, whom he subsequently killed. Tatiana Tarasoff's parents initiated a separate civil action and brought suit against the therapist, the university, and the campus police, claiming that her death was a result of negligence on the part of the defendants. The plaintiffs claimed that the therapists should have warned Ms. Tarasoff that the graduate student presented a danger to her and that he should have been confined to a hospital. Both claims were originally dismissed in the lower courts, but in 1974, the California Supreme Court reversed the lower courts' decisions and said that Ms. Tarasoff should have been warned. The high court said that psychotherapists have a duty to warn the foreseeable victims of their patients' violent actions. Because of the outcry from professional mental health organizations, the court agreed to review the case, and in 1976, the original decision was revised by the ruling that psychotherapists have a duty to exercise reasonable care in protecting the foreseeable victims of their patients' violent actions.

The results of this case have had far-reaching consequences and have influenced many decisions in other jurisdictions (Pettis, 1992). For example, the duty to warn has been extended to instances of intentions to abuse others, alcohol abuse and driver safety, and damage of property (Felthous, 1993; Helminski, 1993; Pettis, 1992; Pettis & Gutheil, 1993; Zellman, 1992). Although many lawsuits have been based on the Tarasoff case, most have failed. Usually, if there are clear threats of violence toward others, then the therapist is mandated to warn potential victims.

The Tarasoff case has generated debate in Canada regarding the duty to warn (Emson, 1993; Kleinman, 1993). Canadian courts have not been faced with an identical case, but the reasoning of the Tarasoff decision played a role in Wenden v. Trikha, Royal Alexandra Hospital and Yaltho (1991). Mr. Trikha, a voluntarily admitted psychiatric patient, left the psychiatric unit without authorization and drove a car at high speed through numerous traffic lights and crashed into Ms. Wenden's car. Wenden had numerous residual medical problems and eventually lost custody of her three children because of her inability to care for them. The court concluded that the psychiatrist has a duty to take reasonable steps to protect such people if a patient posed a serious danger to the well-being of a third party. In this instance, however, there was no way to foresee that Trikha would pose a threat to himself or others, and the court concluded that there was no basis for the psychiatrist to impose greater restraints on him.

DOCUMENTATION AND LEGAL ISSUES

Documentation is a portrayal of the patient, nursing care, and responses to nursing care. It can be hand written or computer generated. Patient records contain the data for evidenced-based care. It is very common in psychiatric care that all disciplines record on one progress note. Patients also have access to their records. Nursing documentation is based on nursing standards (see Chap. 5) and the policies of the particular facility. There are several different documentation styles that are used. Many are problem focused. That is, documentation is organized around specific problems that are identified on the Nursing Care Plan or interdisciplinary treatment plan. No matter the setting or structure of the documentation, nurses are responsible for documenting the following:

- Observations of patients' subjective and objective physical, psychological, and social responses to mental disorders and emotional problems
- Interventions implemented
- Evaluation of outcomes of interventions

Particular attention should be paid to the reason the patient is admitted for care. Nurses are always responsible for monitoring therapeutic actions and side effects of medications that are administered. If the person's initial problem was suicide or homicidal ideation, the patient should routinely be assessed for suicidality and homicidal thoughts, even if the treatment plan does not specifically identify suicide and homicide as potential problems. Careful documentation is always needed for patients who are suicidal, homicidal, aggressive, or restrained in any way. PRN medication also requires a separate entry, including reason for administration, dosage, route, and response to the agent.

Patient records are legal documents and can be used in courts of law. The records are often the only written evidence of a patient's problems at the time of care. It is the only documentation that care has been provided. The entries should always be written in pen, with no erasures. If an entry is corrected, it should be initialed by the person making the correction. Any entry should be clear, well written, and void of jargon. Judgmental statements, such as "patient is manipulating staff," have no place in patients' records. Only meaningful, accurate, objective descriptions of the behavior should be used. General, stereotypic statements, such as "had a good night," or "no complaints" are meaningless and should be avoided.

CRIMINAL LAW AND PSYCHIATRY

Not Guilty by Reason of Insanity (NGRI)

The beginning of the relationship between law and psychiatry can be traced to 1843, when Daniel M'Naghten was tried for the murder of a public official and acquitted on the grounds of insanity. M'Naghten suffered from a paranoid delusion that the Tories in England were conspiring to destroy him. He attempted to assassinate the prime minister, who was the Tory leader. Truly believing that he was acting in self-defense, M'Naghten mistakenly shot and killed the prime minister's secretary. M'Naghten was judged to be criminally insane and acquitted of the crime. There was such a public outcry that the House of Lords convened a special session of the judges to give an advisory opinion as to the law of England governing the insanity defense. They set forth what has come to be known as the M'Naghten rule. To be considered criminally insane, the accused with a mental disorder either does not know the nature and quality of the act or whether it is right or wrong. When the M'Naghten rule is applied, the underlying issue in the insanity defense is responsibility—is the individual responsible for his or her actions? The individual is not responsible for the act only when he or she is unaware of the nature and quality of the act or does not know that the act is wrong. The M'Naghten rule is a narrow and rigid test that relates only to the individual's cognitive ability.

The American Law Institute's (ALI's) legal definition of insanity includes the phrases "substantial appreciation of his or her behavior" or "capacity to conform to the requirements of the law." This definition focuses not just on proving the individual knew whether an act is right or wrong but also on whether one "appreciates" or understands the actions and has the ability to control one's actions (Palermo & Knudten, 1994).

Since the 1950s, the ALI test has been adopted in all federal jurisdictions, but wide variations exist in the state jurisdictions. In about half the states, the ALI test is applied, and in about one third of the states, some variation of the M'Naghten rule is used. Montana and Idaho have abolished the insanity defense altogether (Palermo & Knudten, 1994).

Guilty But Mentally Ill (GBMI)

Another insanity defense is GBMI. Different from the NGRI disposition, in which "not guilty" individuals are committed to the mental health system, GBMI people are convicted of the crime and are typically remanded to the correctional system. Both individuals with NGRI and GBMI are treated for their mental disorders, but the conditions of release are different. GBMI individuals are subject to the correction system's parole decisions, whereas the NGRIs are released through the courts on recommendations of the forensic mental health providers.

Forensic Commitment

A **forensic commitment** is a special type of involuntary commitment of people with a mental disorder who are charged with a crime and are criminally committed to a mental hospital. There are five different groups who may be committed in this way, and each is treated somewhat differently:

1. People charged with a crime who are found incompetent to stand trial because of a mental disorder are treated in a mental hospital until competency is restored. When competency is restored, they are returned to stand trial.
2. People NGRI are treated in a mental hospital until competency is restored.
3. For mentally disordered sex offenders, states usually have special statutes for hospitalization and discharge (such as registration and community notification).
4. People found GBMI are treated in a hospital and then released according to the specific state laws.
5. Prisoners who develop mental illness are transferred to a mental hospital, treated, and returned to prison to complete their sentences.

Misconceptions Regarding the Insanity Plea

Many people in our society believe that the court systems have failed and the NGRI defense is often applied to keep criminals from being sent to prison. One of the most prevalent concerns is that the insanity defense provides a loophole through which criminals can escape punishment for illegal acts. In a large-scale study of insanity pleas ($n = 8,953$), an analysis showed that the public overestimates the use and success of the insanity defense and underestimates the extent to which insanity acquittees are confined on acquittal (Silver et al., 1994). In reality, very few insanity pleas are successful. In examining insanity pleas and acquittals across eight states over a 5-year period, the insanity defense was used in about 1% of all felony cases. Most of the people who used this defense ($n = 8,979$) were seriously mentally ill, and only the most seriously disturbed defendants were successful in their plea ($n = 2,500$) (Callahan et al., 1991). It is estimated that less than 2% of all patients admitted to an inpatient psychiatric facility and only 7% of all involuntary commitments are criminally committed (L. M. Sayre, personal communication, Center for Mental Health Services, October 3, 1996).

Some of the insanity defense cases have been highly publicized, which could contribute to the misconceptions that the NGRI defense is overused. One such case was that of John Hinkley, who attempted to assassinate President Ronald Reagan in 1981 and was found NGRI. On psychiatric examination, Hinkley was found to be living in a "fantasy world with magical and grandiose expectations of impressing and winning over his secret lover, actress Jodie Foster" (Goldstein, 1995, p. 309). Hinkley attempted to commit a historic deed that would make him famous and unite him with his delusional love object. His acquittal stimulated public cries for reform of the insanity defense. Within 2½ years after John Hinkley's acquittal, 34 states changed their insanity defense statutes to limit its use or to prevent the premature release of dangerous people.

A famous case in which the insanity defense was unsuccessful was the State of Wisconsin v. Jeffrey Dahmer. In 1991, Dahmer was charged with first-degree murder of 15 young boys whom he sexually seduced, tortured, and eventually killed by stabbing or strangling. He disposed of the bodies by crushing bones, cutting, dismembering, disemboweling, or boiling the flesh. He made sexual fetishes from the body parts. On psychiatric examination, it was found that he had calmly calculated and prearranged each murder, including obtaining all the necessary equipment and securing his apartment with a high-quality security system. He pled NGRI, but the jury found him legally sane at the time of each and every crime (Palermo & Knudten, 1994).

The key factors in these cases appear to focus on the standards of whether the person has a "substantial appreciation" or understanding of the criminality (wrongfulness) of his conduct or ability to conform with the requirements of the law. In Dahmer's case, his behavior indicated that he meticulously planned and premeditated 15 murders and took extreme precautions to hide his actions by having a security system installed in his apartment and carefully disposing of the bodies. It was clear to the jury that he understood the wrongfulness of his actions and had enough control over his behavior to formulate and implement actions to hide his crimes.

Public Safety

The issue of public safety is often raised around the care and discharge of patients with psychiatric disorders. The reality is that patients with psychiatric problems are more likely victims than perpetrators of criminal activity. For patients who are admitted because they have

committed a crime, the development of sound conditional release programs is one approach many states use. In conditional release, patients are discharged provided that they are monitored by the court.

LAWS AND SYSTEMS THAT PROTECT HUMAN RIGHTS

Internal Rights Protection System

The rights of people with mental disorders, emotional problems, and mental retardation are of special concern because of the vulnerability of this population to stigmatization and societal abuse. Title II of Public Law 99-319, Restatement of Bill of Rights for Mental Health Patients, reaffirms the Bill of Rights for Mental Health Patients originally recommended by the President's Commission on Mental Health and part of the Mental Health Systems Act of 1980. These rights are guaranteed by federal law to each person admitted to a program or facility for the purpose of receiving mental health services.

To help combat any violation of rights, mental health care systems in the United States have developed protective mechanisms that exist within their organizations and make up the **internal rights protection system.** This system was set up by Public Law 99-319, the Protection and Advocacy for Mentally Ill Individuals Act of 1986, which requires each state mental health provider to establish and operate a system that protects and advocates the rights of individuals with mental illnesses and investigates any incidents of abuse and neglect. As states authorized the formation of their respective advocacy and protection systems, they developed their own Bill of Rights based on the federal Bill of Rights. Although there may be variation among states, all states incorporate the rights listed in Text Box 4-1.

In Canada, the 1982 Canadian Charter of Rights and Freedoms specified the rights of Canadian citizens and is used in a number of jurisdictions. All medical patients must give consent for treatment and have the right to refuse treatment with the exception of an emergency in which it is impossible to obtain permission or if a patient is not competent; however, in mental health care, it is different. In seven Canadian provinces, legislation authorizes routine treatment without consent to individuals who have been committed involuntarily (Verdun-Jones, 1988). Nova Scotia, Ontario, Saskatchewan, and the Northwest Territories make it illegal for a competent patient who is involuntarily committed to receive compulsory treatment. In these provinces, a competent person can refuse treatment, even if the individual is committed involuntarily.

External Advocacy Systems

Organizations that operate outside these mental health agencies and serve as advocates for the rights and treatment of mental health patients are part of an **external advocacy system.** Some of these organizations include the American Hospital Association, American Healthcare Association, the American Public Health Association, and the United Nations. They are financially and administratively independent from the state agencies. These groups advocate through negotiation and recommendations but have no legal authority. In instances in which agencies believe their advocacy attempts are unsuccessful, they can resort to litigation that leads to lawsuits and consent decrees (legal mandates that are monitored by the Department of Justice) or, in some instances, a denial of being accredited by their certifying body.

Accreditation of Mental Health Care Delivery Systems

Mental health care is regulated by many different agencies, and nursing is integrally involved with meeting the agency accreditation standards. **Accreditation** is the process by which any mental health agency is judged by established standards to be providing acceptable quality of care. Accreditation is important to the consumer because accreditation not only ensures that the institution meets the acceptable standards of quality of care but also is necessary for third-party payers (managed care companies, Medicare) to reimburse facilities.

Mental health agencies are accredited by a variety of organizations. One of the most influential organizations in the total health care system is the Joint Commission on Accreditation of Healthcare Organizations (JCAHO), the body that accredits hospitals in the United States. One of JCAHO's survey areas is patient's rights. Thus, all institutions seeking accreditation from this organization must also meet its patients' rights standards. The Healthcare Finance Administration (HCFA) sets accreditation standards for institutions seeking Medicare and Medicaid funding. Community mental health centers are not accredited by either JCAHO or HCFA, but by another accrediting agency, the Commission on Accreditation of Rehabilitation Facilities.

Summary of Key Points

➤ The right of self-determination entitles all patients to refuse treatment, to obtain other opinions, and to choose other forms of treatment. It is one of the basic patients' rights established by Title II, Public Law 99-139, outlining the Universal Bill of Rights for Mental Health Patients.

➤ Informed consent is another protective right that helps patients decide what can be done to their bodies and minds. It must be obtained from a competent individual before any treatment is begun to ensure that the information is not only received but understood. A competent person can refuse any treatment. Incompetence is determined by the court when the patient cannot understand the information. Nurses play a key role in informed consent by making sure that the patient is competent and understands the risks and interventions.

➤ The right to the least restrictive environment entitles patients to be treated in the least restrictive setting and by the least restrictive interventions, and protects patients from unnecessary confinement and medication.

➤ There are special legal terms and considerations for individuals who have mental disorders and commit crimes. Those determined to be not guilty by reason of insanity are those who demonstrate they had no understanding of their actions and no control over them. These patients are committed to a mental health facility for treatment and then discharged after treatment. Guilty but mentally ill applies to those who demonstrate they knew the wrongfulness of their actions and had the ability to act otherwise. These patients enter the correctional system and receive treatment for their disorder but are returned after treatment to serve their sentences.

➤ Laws and systems are established to protect the rights of the mentally disordered. The internal rights protection system operates from within the state mental health system and consists of special departments or agencies that monitor the treatment of patients in the system according to the Universal Patient Bill of Rights and state regulations and laws.

➤ The external advocacy system comprises organizations working outside the state and federal systems to protect the rights of the mentally disordered or handicapped and includes the American Hospital Association, American Healthcare Association, American Public Health Association, and the United Nations—all of which are involved in setting standards and licensing procedures.

Critical Thinking Challenges

1. Explain the relationship between self-determinism and motivation.
2. Consider the relationship of self-determinism to competence by differentiating patients who are competent to give consent and those who are incompetent. Discuss the steps in determining whether a patient is competent to provide informed consent for a treatment.

3. Contrast the rights of individuals with voluntary admissions and involuntary commitments.

4. Define competency to consent or refuse treatment and relate the definition to the Self-Determination Act.

5. Justify the patient's right to treatment in the least restrictive environment.

6. Discuss the purposes of living wills and health proxies. Discuss their use in psychiatric–mental health care.

7. Identify the legal and ethical issues underlying the Tarasoff case and mandates to inform.

8. Compare the definitions of insanity in the M'Naghten rule and the American Law Institute. What are the major differences?

9. Compare the authority and responsibilities of the internal rights protection system with those of the external advocacy system.

 WEB LINKS

www.nami.org The National Alliance for the Mentally Ill is a grassroots, self-help support and advocacy organization.

www.cnps.ca The Canadian Nurses Protective Society (CNPS) is a nonprofit society, owned and operated by nurses for nurses, offering legal liability protection related to nursing practice to registered nurses by providing information on education.

www.nursingnet.org This site provides information on nurses as legal consultants.

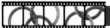 **MOVIES**

Nuts: 1987. Starring Barbara Streisand, Richard Dreyfuss, Maureen Stapleton, Eli Wallach, Robert Webber. A strong-willed, high-class prostitute has committed murder, and her family and attorney want her to plead guilty by reason of insanity. The movie centers around her family's attempt to have her declared incompetent to stand trial, which would commit her to a mental health center without ever going to trial for the murder. She insists on holding on to her sanity, and her lawyer must battle his own prejudice and her inexplicable belligerence to discover the truth. *Viewing Point:* Watch how the family members attempt to use the competency hearings for maintaining family secrets.

REFERENCES

Applebaum, P., & Grisso, T. (1988). Assessing patients' capacities to consent to treatment. *New England Journal of Medicine, 319*(25), 1635–1638.

Callahan, L., Steadman, H., McGreevy, J., & Robbins, P. (1991). The volume and characteristics of insanity defense pleas: An eight state study. *Bulletin of the American Academy of Psychiatry and the Law, 19*(4), 331–338.

Culver, C. (1991). Healthcare ethics and mental health law. In S. A. Shah & B. D. Sales (Eds.), *Law and mental health* (DHHS Publication No. ASD 91-1875, pp. 25–47). Washington, DC: National Institute of Mental Health.

Deci, E. (1987). Theories and paradigms, constructs and operations: Intrinsic motivation research is already exciting. *Journal of Social Behavior and Personality, 2*(2, Part 1), 177–185.

Dixon v. Weinberger, 405 F. Supp. 974 (D.D.C.), (1975).

Emson, H. (1993). The duty to warn in the Canadian context. *Canadian Medical Association Journal, 149*(12), 1781–1782.

Felthous, A. (1993). Substance abuse and the duty to protect. *Bulletin of the American Academy of Psychiatry and the Law, 21*(4), 419–426.

Galen, K. (1993). Assessing psychiatric patients' competency to agree to treatment plans. *Hospital and Community Psychiatry, 44*(4), 362–364.

Goldstein, R. (1995). Paranoids in the legal system: The litigious paranoid and the paranoid criminal. *Psychiatric Clinics of North America, 18*(2), 303–315.

Helminski, F. (1993). Near the conflagration: The wide duty to warn. *Mayo Clinic Proceedings, 68*(7), 709–710.

Hermann, D. (1990). Autonomy, self-determination, the right of involuntarily committed persons to refuse treatment, and the use of substituted judgment in medication decisions involving incompetent persons. *International Journal of Law and Psychiatry, 13*(4), 361–385.

Kleinman, I. (1993). Confidentiality and the duty to warn. *Canadian Medical Association Journal, 149*(12), 1783–1785.

Lavoie, R. (1992). Consent, involuntary treatment and the use of force in an urban emergency department. *Annals of Emergency Medicine, 21*(1), 25–32.

Omnibus Budget Reconciliation Act of 1990. Public Law No. 101–158, Paragraph 4206, 4751.

Palermo, G., & Knudten, R. (1994). The insanity plea in the case of a serial killer. *International Journal of Offender Therapy and Comparative Criminology, 38*(1), 3–16.

Parrish, J. (1993). Involuntary use of interventions: Pros and cons. *Innovations and Research in Clinical Services, Community Support, and Rehabilitation, 2*(1), 15–22.

Pettis, R. (1992). Tarasoff and the dangerous driver: A look at the driving cases. *Bulletin of the American Academy of Psychiatry and the Law, 20*(4), 427–437.

Pettis, R., & Gutheil, T. (1993). Misapplication of the Tarasoff duty to driving cases: A call for a reframing of theory. *Bulletin of the American Academy of Psychiatry and the Law, 21*(3), 263–275.

Silver, E., Cirincione, C., & Steadman, H. (1994). Demythologizing inaccurate perceptions of the insanity defense. *Law and Human Behavior, 18*(1), 63–70.

Tarasoff v. Regents of the University of California, 551P. 2d 334 (Cal. 1976).

Trudeau, M. (1993). Informed consent: The patient's right to decide. *Journal of Psychosocial Nursing, 31*(6), 9–12.

U.S. Equal Employment Opportunity Commission, Office of the Americans With Disabilities Act. (1991). *The Americans With Disabilities Act: Questions and answers.* Washington, DC: U. S. Government Printing Office.

Verdun-Jones, S. (1988). The right to refuse treatment: Recent developments in Canadian jurisprudence. *International Journal of Law and Psychiatry, 11*(1), 51–60.

Wenden v. Trikha, Royal Alexandra Hospital and Yaltho. 116 AR (2d) 81, 1991.

Wettstein, R. (1994). Confidentiality. In J. Oldham & M. Riba (Eds.), *Review of Psychiatry* (Vol. 13, pp. 343–364). Washington, DC: American Psychiatric Press.

Winick, B. (1994). The right to refuse mental health treatment: A therapeutic jurisprudence analysis. *International Journal of Law and Psychiatry, 17*(1), 99–117.

Zellman, G. (1992). The impact of case characteristics on child abuse reporting decision. *Child Abuse and Neglect, 16*(1), 57–74.

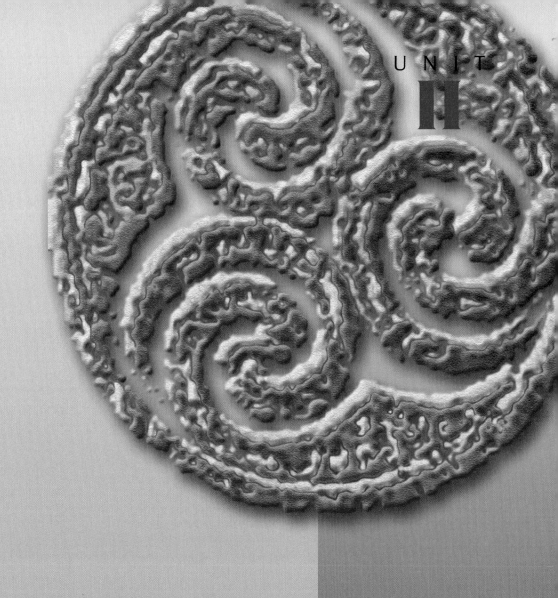

Principles of Psychiatric Nursing

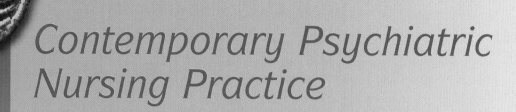

Contemporary Psychiatric Nursing Practice

Mary Ann Boyd

THE BIOPSYCHOSOCIAL MODEL IN PSYCHIATRIC–MENTAL HEALTH NURSING
Biologic Domain
Psychological Domain
Social Domain

STANDARDS OF CARE AND PROFESSIONAL PRACTICE
Scope of Psychiatric–Mental Health Nursing Areas of Concern

Standards of Care
Standards of Professional Performance
Basic and Advanced Practice Levels
  Basic Level
  Advanced Level

CHALLENGES OF PSYCHIATRIC NURSING
Knowledge Development, Dissemination, and Application

Overcoming the Stigma
Health Care Delivery
  System Challenges
Impact of Technology

ETHICAL FRAMEWORKS

PSYCHIATRIC–MENTAL HEALTH NURSING ORGANIZATIONS

LEARNING OBJECTIVES

After studying the chapter, you will be able to:

➤ Explain the biopsychosocial model as a conceptual framework for understanding and treating mental health problems.

➤ Delineate the scope and standards of psychiatric–mental health nursing practice.

➤ Discuss selected challenges of psychiatric–mental health nursing.

➤ Identify ethical framework and principles used in the practice of psychiatric nursing.

➤ Discuss the impact of psychiatric–mental health nursing professional organizations on practice.

CHAPTER 5

KEY TERMS

advanced practice
  psychiatric–mental
  health nurse
autonomy

basic level of practice
beneficence
standards of care

KEY CONCEPTS

biopsychosocial model
nursing process

*T*his chapter introduces the biopsychosocial model as the organizational thread for the rest of the book. The scope of practice of the psychiatric nurse is then explained, followed by a discussion of the standards of care that serve as a basis of practice. These standards are integral to the understanding of the day-to-day practice of psychiatric–mental health nursing and should be familiar to any student involved in mental health nursing practice. The discussion of the challenges of psychiatric nursing sets the stage for the rest of the text through an overview of the dynamic nature of this specialty.

THE BIOPSYCHOSOCIAL MODEL IN PSYCHIATRIC–MENTAL HEALTH NURSING

Contemporary psychiatric nursing uses theories from the biologic, psychological and social sciences as a basis of practice. This holistic approach, referred to as the biopsychosocial model, is necessary to truly understand the individual who has a mental disorder or emotional problems. The model is ideal for organizing nursing care and is used throughout this text for organizing theoretic knowledge and the nursing process.

KEY CONCEPT Biopsychosocial Model. The **biopsychosocial model** consists of three separate but interdependent domains: biologic, psychological, and social (Abraham et al., 1992). Each domain has an independent knowledge and treatment focus but can interact and be mutually interdependent with the other dimensions (Fig. 5-1).

Biologic Domain

The *biologic* domain consists of the theories that explain neurobiologic changes related to mental disorders (see Chaps. 6 and 7.) This domain has gained increasing importance in the understanding of mental disorders and is grounded primarily in the biologic sciences. Today, there is evidence of neurobiologic changes in most psychiatric disorders. Even in normal emotional reactions, such as happiness and sadness, there are neurobiologic changes. This domain is associated with the brain and the processing of information as well as *all* of the biologic activity related to other health problems. For example, patients with schizophrenia may also have other health-threatening disorders, such as diabetes mellitus or cardiac disease. In addition, the neurobiologic theories also serve as a basis for understanding and administering pharmacologic agents (see Chap. 8.)

Within the biologic domain, there are also theories and concepts used as a basis of interventions focusing on the patient's physical functioning. These theories are generated in the "bench" sciences, such as biology or chemistry, and also within other sciences, such as nursing. Exercise, sleep, and adequate nutrition are all important in psychiatric nursing.

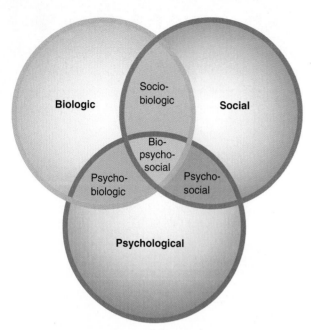

FIGURE 5.1 Biopsychosocial model. (Adapted from Abraham, I., Fox, J., & Cohen, B. [1992]. Integrating the bio into the biopsychosocial: Understanding and treating biological phenomena in psychiatric mental health nursing. *Archives of Psychiatric Nursing, 6*[5], 298.)

Psychological Domain

The *psychological* domain contains the theoretic basis related to the psychological processes of thoughts, feelings, and behavior (intrapersonal dynamics) that influence one's emotion, cognition, and behavior. The psychological and nursing sciences generate theories and research that are critical in understanding the patient symptoms and responses to mental disorders. Even though mental disorders have a biologic component, they are often manifested in psychological symptoms as well as physical changes. The person with a thought disorder may have bizarre behavior that needs to be interpreted within the context of the neurobiologic dysfunction of the mental disorder.

Many psychiatric nursing interventions are based on knowledge generated within this domain. Cognitive approaches, behavior therapy, and patient education are all based on the use of theories from the psychological domain. These interventions are explained in Unit III. Psychiatric–mental health interventions are also based on the use of interpersonal communication techniques, which require nurses to develop awareness of their own, as well as their patients', internal feelings and behavior. For mental health nurses, understanding their own and their patients' intrapersonal dynamics and motivation is critical in developing a therapeutic relationship and motivating patients to learn and understand their disorders and participate in their management. Motivating patients to engage in learning activities best occurs within the context of a therapeutic relationship (see Chap. 9).

Social Domain

The *social* domain includes theories that account for the influence of social forces encompassing the patient, family, and community within cultural settings. This knowledge base is generated from social and nursing sciences and explains the connections within the family and communities that affect the mental health and treatment of mental disorders. Psychiatric disorders are not caused by social factors, but their manifestations and treatment can be significantly affected by the society in which they live. Family support can actually improve treatment outcomes. Family factors, including origin, extended family, and other significant relationships, contribute to the total understanding and treatment of patients. Community forces, including cultural and ethnic groups within larger communities, shape patients' manifestation of disorders, response to treatment, and overall view of mental illness.

STANDARDS OF CARE AND PROFESSIONAL PRACTICE

The practice of psychiatric nursing is regulated by law but guided by standards of care. Legal authority to practice nursing is granted by the states and provinces, but professional **standards of care** or professional nursing activities are set by professional nursing organizations. The American Nurses Association (ANA) and the psychiatric nursing organizations (discussed later in this chapter) collaborate in specifying the health problems that match the skills of psychiatric nurses and set standards of care and professional practice.

Scope of Psychiatric–Mental Health Nursing Areas of Concern

The areas of concern for the psychiatric–mental health nurse include a wide range of actual or potential mental health problems, such as emotional stress or crisis, self-concept changes, developmental issues, physical symptoms that occur with psychological changes, and symptom management of patients with mental disorders. To understand the problem and select an appropriate intervention, integration of knowledge from the biologic, psychological, and social domain is necessary. Text Box 5-1 presents details on the actual and potential mental health problems of patients to whom psychiatric nurses attend.

Standards of Care

The standards of care are organized around the nursing process and include six components: assessment, diagnosis, outcome identification, planning, implementation, and evaluation (Text Box 5-2).

Text Box 5.1

Psychiatric Mental Health Nursing's Phenomena of Concern

Actual or potential mental health problems of patients pertaining to:

- The maintenance of optimal health and well-being and the prevention of psychobiologic illness
- Self-care limitations or impaired functioning related to mental, emotional, and physiologic distress
- Deficits in the functioning of significant biologic, emotional, and cognitive systems
- Emotional stress or crisis related to illness, pain, disability, and loss
- Self-concept and body image changes, developmental issues, life process changes, and end-of-life issues
- Problems related to emotions such as anxiety, anger, powerlessness, confusion, fear, sadness, loneliness, and grief
- Physical symptoms that occur along with altered psychological functioning
- Psychological symptoms that occur along with altered physiologic functioning
- Alterations in thinking, perceiving, symbolizing, communicating, and decision making
- Difficulties in relating to others
- Behaviors and mental states that indicate the patient is a danger to self or others or has a severe disability
- Symptom management, side effects, and toxicities associated with psychopharmacologic intervention and other aspects of the treatment regimen
- Interpersonal, organizational, sociocultural, spiritual, or environmental circumstances or events that have an affect on the mental and emotional well-being of the individual, family, or community

From American Nurses Association, American Psychiatric Nurses Association, International Society of Psychiatric–Mental Health Nurses. (2000). *Scope and Standards of Psychiatric–Mental Health Nursing Practice* (28-41). Washington, D.C.: American Nurses Publishers.

KEY CONCEPT **The Nursing Process.** The **nursing process** is the basis of clinical decision making and nursing actions (ANA et al., 2000).

Each standard has a rationale and measurement criteria that are indicators for meeting the standard. The fifth standard, implementation, has several subcategories that specify standards for each intervention. These standards of care represent the nursing profession's commitment to the general public. It is important that nurses know their practice standards and are able to practice at this level. Nurses ultimately are held accountable for practicing according to their standards. The Canadian Nursing standards are organized into themes (Text Box-5-3).

Standards of Professional Performance

Developing and maintaining competency is the responsibility of a professional psychiatric–mental health nurse.

All nurses are expected to achieve competency in psychiatric nursing practice as specified by the standards of professional performance within the *Scope and Standards of Psychiatric–Mental Health Nursing* in the areas of quality of care, performance appraisal, education, collegiality, ethics, collaboration, research, and resource utilization (ANA et al., 2000) (Table 5-1).

Basic and Advanced Practice Levels

There are two levels of practice in psychiatric–mental health nursing: basic and advanced. These levels are differentiated by educational preparation, complexity of practice, and performance of nursing function (Text Box 5-4).

Basic Level

According to the *Scope and Standards of Psychiatric–Mental Health Nursing*, the **basic level of practice** includes two groups of nurses. The first group consists of registered nurses who practice in psychiatric settings as staff nurses, case managers, or nurse managers or in other nursing roles. The second is the psychiatric–mental health nurse (RN-PMH) who has a baccalaureate degree in nursing and has worked in the field for at least 2 years. Both groups of nurses are expected to adhere to the scope and standards of practice (ANA et al., 2000). Nursing practice at this level is "characterized by interventions that promote and foster health, assess dysfunction, assist patients to regain or improve their coping abilities, maximize strength, and prevent further disability" (ANA et al., 2000, p. 13). The nurse performs a wide range of interventions, including health promotion and health maintenance strategies, intake screening and evaluation, case management, milieu therapy, promotion of self-care activities, psychobiologic interventions, complementary interventions, health teaching, counseling, crisis care, and psychiatric rehabilitation (Table 5-2). An overview of psychiatric nursing interventions is presented in Chapter 14.

Advanced Level

The **advanced practice psychiatric–mental health nurse** (APRN-PMH) is also a licensed registered nurse but is educationally prepared at the master's level and is nationally certified as a specialist by the American Nurses Credentialing Center (ANCC). The APRN-PMH is either a clinical nurse specialist or a nurse practitioner in psychiatric nursing. The advanced level also includes nurses with doctoral preparation who have earned a Doctor in Nursing Science (DNS, DNSc) or a Doctor of Philosophy (PhD). The APRN-PMH's responsibilities include the complete delivery of direct primary mental health services, including, but not limited to, formulating differential diagnoses; ordering, conducting, and interpreting pertinent laboratory and

TEXT BOX 5.2

Standards of Care

Standard I. Assessment
The psychiatric–mental health nurse collects patient health data.

Rationale:
The assessment interview—which requires linguistically and culturally effective communication skills, interviewing, behavioral observation, database record review, and comprehensive assessment of the patient and relevant systems—enables the psychiatric–mental health nurse to make sound clinical judgments and plan appropriate interventions with the client.

Standard II. Diagnosis
The psychiatric–mental health nurse analyzes the assessment data in determining diagnoses.

Rationale:
The basis for providing psychiatric–mental health nursing care is the recognition and identification of patterns of response to actual or potential psychiatric illnesses, mental health problems, and potential morbid physical illness.

Standard III. Outcome Identification
The psychiatric–mental health nurse identifies expected outcomes individualized to the patient.

Rationale:
Within the context of providing nursing care, the ultimate goal is to influence health outcomes and improve the patient's health status.

Standard IV. Planning
The psychiatric–mental health nurse develops a plan of care that is negotiated among the patient, nurse, family, and health care team and prescribes evidence-based interventions to attain expected outcomes.

Rationale:
A plan of care is used to guide therapeutic intervention systematically, document progress, and achieve the expected patient outcomes.

Standard V. Implementation
The psychiatric–mental health nurse implements the interventions identified in the plan of care.

Rationale:
In implementing the plan of care, psychiatric–mental health nurses use a wide range of interventions designed to prevent mental and physical illness and promote, maintain, and restore mental and physical health. Psychiatric–mental health nurses select interventions according to their level of practice.
[Note: Va–Vg are basic level interventions. Vh–Vj are advanced practice interventions.]

Standard Va. Counseling
The psychiatric–mental health nurse uses counseling interventions to assist patients in improving or regaining their previous coping abilities, fostering mental health, and preventing mental illness and disability.

Standard Vb. Milieu Therapy
The psychiatric–mental health nurse provides, structures, and maintains a therapeutic environment in collaboration with the patient and other health care clinicians.

Standard Vc. Self-Care Activities
The psychiatric–mental health nurse structures interventions around the patient's activities of daily living to foster self-care and mental and physical well-being.

Standard Vd. Psychobiologic interventions
The psychiatric–mental health nurse uses knowledge of psychobiologic interventions and applies clinical skills to restore the patient's health and prevent further disability.

Standard Ve. Health Teaching
The psychiatric–mental health nurse, through health teaching, assists patients in achieving satisfying, productive, and healthy patterns of living.

Standard Vf. Case Management
The psychiatric–mental health nurse provides case management to coordinate comprehensive health services and ensure continuity of care.

Standard Vg. Health Promotion and Health Maintenance
The psychiatric–mental health nurse employs strategies and interventions to promote and maintain mental health and prevent mental illness.

Standard Vh. Psychotherapy
The APRN-PMH uses individual, group, and family psychotherapy, and other therapeutic treatments to assist patient in preventing mental illness and disability, treating mental health disorders, and improving mental health status and functional abilities.

Standard VI. Prescription Authority and Treatment Agents
The APRN-PMH uses prescriptive authority, procedures, and treatments in accordance with state and federal laws and regulations, to treat symptoms of psychiatric illness and to improve functional health status.

Standard VI. Consultation
The APRN-PMH provides consultation to enhance the abilities of other clinicians to provide services for patients and effect change in systems.

Standard VI. Evaluation
The psychiatric–mental health nurse evaluates the patient's progress in attaining expected outcomes.

Rationale:
Nursing care is a dynamic process involving change in the patient's health status over time, giving rise to the need for new data, different diagnoses, and modifications in the plan of care. Therefore, evaluation is a continuous process of appraising the effect of nursing and the treatment regimen on the patient's health status and expected health outcomes.

From American Nurses Association, American Psychiatric Nurses Association, International Society of Psychiatric–Mental Health Nurses. (2000). *Scope and Standards of Psychiatric–Mental Health Nursing Practice* (28-41). Washington, D.C.: American Nurses Publishers.

TABLE 5.1 Standards of Professional Performance

Standard I	Quality of care	Systematically evaluates the quality of care and effectiveness of psychiatric–mental health nursing practice
Standard II	Performance appraisal	Evaluates own psychiatric–mental health nursing practice in relation to professional practice standards and relevant statutes and regulations
Standard III	Education	Acquires and maintains current knowledge in nursing practice
Standard IV	Collegiality	Interacts and contributes to the professional development of peers, health care clinicians, and others
Standard V	Ethics	Determines and implements assessments, actions, and recommendations on behalf of patients in an ethical manner
Standard VI	Collaboration	Collaborates with the patient, significant others, and health care clinicians in providing care
Standard VII	Research	Contributes to nursing and mental health through the use of research methods and findings
Standard VIII	Resource utilization	Considers factors related to safety, effectiveness, and cost in planning and delivering patient care

From American Nurses Association, American Psychiatric Nurses Association, International Society of Psychiatric–Mental Health Nurses. (2000). *Scope and Standards of Psychiatric–Mental Health Nursing Practice* (28-41). Washington, D.C.: American Nurses Publishers.

diagnostic studies and procedures; conducting individual, family group, and network psychotherapy; and prescribing, monitoring managing, and evaluating psychopharmacologic and related medication.

CHALLENGES OF PSYCHIATRIC NURSING

The challenges of psychiatric nursing are increasing in the 21st century. New knowledge is being generated, technology is shaping health care into new dimensions, and nursing practice is becoming more specialized and autonomous. This section discusses a few of the challenges in psychiatric nursing.

TEXT BOX 5.3

Canadian Standards of Psychiatric and Mental Health Nursing Practice (2nd ed.)

Standards Theme

  I. Provides competent professional care through the helping role.
 II. Perform/refines client assessments through the diagnostic and monitoring function.
III. Administers and monitors therapeutic interventions.
IV. Effectively manages rapidly changing situations.
 V. Intervenes through the teaching-coaching function.
VI. Monitors and ensures the quality of health care practices.
VII. Practices within organizational and work-role structures.

Standards Committee (1998). *The Canadian standards of psychiatric and mental health nursing practice* (2nd ed.). The Canadian Federation of the Mental Health Nurses.

TEXT BOX 5.4

Functions of Psychiatric–Mental Health Nurses

Basic Level Functions
Health promotion and health maintenance
Intake screening and evaluation
Case management
Milieu therapy
Promotion of self-care activities
Psychobiologic interventions
Complementary interventions
Health teaching
Counseling
Crisis care
Psychiatric rehabilitation
Advanced Level Functions
Psychopharmacology interventions
Psychotherapy interventions
Community interventions
Case management activities
Clinical supervisory activities

TABLE 5.2	Basic Psychiatric Nursing Interventions
Area	**Interventions**
Health promotion and maintenance	Conducts health assessment and targets high-risk situations and potential complications of disorder and treatment. Interventions include, but are not limited to, assertiveness training, stress management, parenting classes, and health teaching.
Intake screening and evaluation	Conducts intake assessment, makes triage decisions. Facilitates patient moving into appropriate service. Interventions include, but are not limited to, data collection guided by principles of human behavior and the interviewing process. Refers patient for additional assessment when needed.
Case management	Supports the patient's highest level of functioning, self-efficacy, and optimal health. Interventions include risk assessment, supportive counseling problem solving, teaching medication and health status monitoring, comprehensive care planning, and coordination of other health services.
Milieu therapy	Assesses and develops the therapeutic potential of a particular environment. Interventions focus on the physical environment, social structure interaction processes, and culture of the setting.
Promotion of self-care activities	Supports independence in self-care activities of daily living. Interventions include, but are not limited to, teaching medication regimen and symptom management, fostering recreational activities, and facilitating development of practical skills for community life.
Psychobiologic interventions	Assess holistically and treat patients' responses to actual and potential health problems. Interventions include, but are not limited to, administering, monitoring, and overseeing pharmacotherapeutic treatment, relaxation techniques, nutrition and diet regulation, exercise and rest schedules, preoperative and postoperative care of patient receiving electroconvulsive therapy, and medication education.
Complementary interventions	Wide range of interventions included diet and nutrition regulation, relaxation techniques, therapeutic touch, mindfulness meditation, and guided imagery.
Health teaching	Identifies learning needs related to biologic, pharmacologic, physical, sociocultural, or psychological aspects of care. Interventions include formal and informal approaches, developing real-life experiences, and role modeling.
Counseling	Supports problem solving of an immediate difficulty and constructive personal change. Interventions include time-limited sessions with patient, family, or group.
Crisis care	Supports the resolution of an immediate crisis or emergency. Interventions include crisis intervention, stabilization, and direct counseling services using supportive problem solving and mobilization of resources.
Psychiatric rehabilitation	Facilitates symptom management and relapse prevention within a rehabilitation and recovery context. Interventions include developing a collaborative partnership with patient, supporting the development of life skills, and identifying and using environmental support.

Adapted from American Nurses Association, American Psychiatric Nurses Association, and International Society of Psychiatric–Mental Health Nurses. (2000). *Scope and standards of psychiatric–mental health nursing* (pp. 13–17). Washington, DC: American Nurses Publishing.

Knowledge Development, Dissemination, and Application

Results of new research efforts continually redefine our knowledge base relative to mental disorders and their treatment. For example, in the 1900s, the explanation for schizophrenia was hypothesized to be overactivity of dopamine. Later, it was discovered that overactivity of dopamine was involved in some of the pathophysiology of schizophrenia but other transmitters seemed to play a role in this elusive syndrome. As a result, new medications with various side-effect profiles became available, which in turn meant that nurses needed to redefine their

monitoring and interventions related to medication administration.

The presence of comorbid medical disorders is gaining increasing importance in the treatment of mental disorders. Psychiatric nurses are challenged to continue to stay abreast of new advances in total health care in order to provide safe, competent care to individuals with mental disorders. Hypertension, hypothyroidism, hyperthyroidism, and diabetes mellitus all affect the treatment of psychiatric disorders.

Psychiatric nurses are challenged to stay current in their knowledge in order to apply the results of studies in the care of patients. Accessing new information through journals, electronic databases, and continuing education programs requires vigilance but provides a sound basis for application of new knowledge. Nurse have to evaluate the usefulness of the results of research studies. One research study supporting a particular treatment approach may not be as meaningful as several statistically significant studies. On the other hand, results of a small study can sometimes have useful clinical application, even though findings are not reported in terms of statistical significance. Psychiatric nurses are challenged to improve patient treatment by integrating knowledge into a biopsychosocial model that includes all human responses to potential or actual health problems.

Overcoming the Stigma

Nurses can play an important role in dispelling myths of mental illnesses. Stigma often prevents individuals from seeking help for mental health problems (see Chap. 2). The issue of stigma, identified as a major problem in the 1999 *Report of the Surgeon General*, should be addressed by every nurse, whether or not practicing psychiatric nursing. To reduce the burden of mental illness and improve access to care, nurses can educate all of their patients about etiology, symptoms, and treatment of mental illnesses.

Health Care Delivery System Challenges

Psychiatric nurses continue to be challenged to provide nursing care within integrated community-based services. Culturally sensitive and high-quality nursing care will need to meet the emerging mental health care needs of our patients. Nurses will be caring for patients who require support from the social welfare system in the form of housing, job opportunities, welfare, and transportation (*Report of the Surgeon General*, 1999) and need to be knowledgeable about these systems. In some settings, the nurse may be the only one who has a background in medical disorders, such as HIV, AIDS, and other somatic health problems.

Nursing roles are expanding and include not only hospital-based but also community-based care. Assertive community treatment (ACT) reduces inpatient service use, promotes continuity of outpatient care, and increases stability of people with serious mental illnesses (see Chap. 17). The nurse is involved in moving the current fragmented health care system toward one focusing on consumer needs.

Nurses have an opportunity to participate in development of a health care system that calls for *parity*, that is, equality between mental health and other health coverage. In 1998, the Federal Mental Health Parity Act went into effect. Under this law, group health plans providing mental health benefits may not impose a lower lifetime or annual dollar limit on mental health benefits than exists for medical-surgical benefits. Financial barriers that have prevented many people from accessing services are slowly being removed. As people access services, it is important that nurses step forward to provide quality, evidenced-based care to individuals and their families.

Impact of Technology

The impact of technologic advances on the delivery of psychiatric nursing care is unprecedented. Nurses are challenged to continue to develop their technologic and computer skills and to use this technology in the improvement of care. *Telemedicine* is a reality and takes many forms, from communication to remote sites to completion of education programs of study. It is important that patients have the opportunity to use technology to learn about their disorders and treatment. Because many of the disorders can affect cognitive functioning, it is also important that software programs be developed that can be used by these individuals to facilitate cognitive functioning.

New technology also challenges nurses in maintaining patient confidentiality. Patient records, once stored in remote areas and rarely viewed, are now readily available and easily accessed. Nurses need to be more vigilant in maintaining privacy and confidentiality. Nursing documentation skills need to be updated continually to reflect quality patient care within a changing health care environment.

ETHICAL FRAMEWORKS

Ethical issues are clearly inherent in mental health care. The interests of the patients, nurses, health care team, and society may be in conflict and may manifest in any number of psychiatric–mental health care delivery settings. Ethical conflicts can occur when the patient is being guided by the principle of autonomy and the nurse by the principle of beneficence. The fundamental ethical principles of autonomy and beneficence are in conflict in many clinical situations. According to the principle of **autonomy,** each person has the fundamental right of self-determination. According to the principle of **beneficence**, the health care provider uses knowledge of science and incorporates the art of caring to develop an environment in which individuals achieve their maximal health care potential.

For nurses to provide patient care within ethical frameworks, they need knowledge of basic rights and ethical principles, conceptual models as ways of thinking about ethical dilemmas, and opportunities to explore and resolve clinical dilemmas. Knowledge of the legal issues and patients' rights that have been discussed in this chap-

TEXT BOX 5.5

Code for Nurses

1. The nurse provides services with respect for human dignity and the uniqueness of the patients, unrestricted by considerations of social or economic status, personal attributes, or the nature of health problem.

2. The nurse safeguards the patient's right to privacy by judiciously protecting information of a confidential nature.

3. The nurse acts to safeguard the patient and the public when health care and safety are affected by the incompetent, unethical, or illegal practice of any person.

4. The nurse assumes responsibility and accountability for individual nursing judgments and actions.

5. The nurse maintains competence in nursing.

6. The nurse participates in activities that contribute to the ongoing development of the profession's body of knowledge.

7. The nurse participates in the profession's efforts to implement and improve standards of nursing.

8. The nurse participates in the profession's effort to protect the public from misinformation and misrepresentation and to maintain the integrity of nursing.

9. The nurse collaborates with members of the health professions and other citizens in promoting community and national efforts to meet the health needs of the public.

American Nurses Association. (1985). *Code for nurses with interpretive statements* (p. 1). Washington, DC: Author.

ter should be used in making clinical decisions. Nursing actions are guided by the *Code for Nurses With Interpretive Statements*, adopted by the ANA in 1950, which serves to inform both the nurse and society of the profession's expectations and requirements in ethical matters (ANA, 1985) (Text Box 5-5.) In the United States, nurses are guided by this code for nurses, which is a framework within which nurses can make ethical decisions. This document is currently being revised as a "code of ethics" for nurses. In Canada, the Canadian Nurses Association Code of Ethics (1985) is accepted as the standard.

PSYCHIATRIC–MENTAL HEALTH NURSING ORGANIZATIONS

Whereas the establishment and reinforcement of standards go a long way toward legitimizing psychiatric–mental health nursing, it is professional organizations that provide leadership in shaping mental health care. They do so by providing a strong voice for meaningful legislation that promotes quality patient care and advocates for maximal utilization of nursing skills.

The ANA is one such organization. Although its focus is on addressing the emergent needs of nursing in general, the ANA supports psychiatric–mental health nursing practice through liaison activities, such as advocating for psychiatric–mental health nursing at the national and state levels and working closely with psychiatric–mental health nursing organizations. The American Psychiatric Nurses Association (APNA) and the International Society of Psychiatric–Mental Health Nurses (ISPN) are two organizations for psychiatric nurses that focus on mental health care.

The APNA is the largest psychiatric–mental health nursing organization with the primary mission of advancing psychiatric–mental health nursing practice; improving mental health care for culturally diverse individuals, families, groups, and communities; and shaping health policy for the delivery of mental health services. The APNA envisions that all people will have accessible, effective, and efficient psychiatric–mental health care in delivery systems that fully use the skills and expertise of psychiatric nurses.

The ISPN consists of three specialist divisions: the Association of Child and Adolescent Psychiatric Nurses, the International Society of Psychiatric Consultation Liaison Nurses, and the Society for Education and Research in Psychiatric–Mental Health Nursing. The purpose of ISPN is to unite and strengthen the presence and the voice of psychiatric–mental health nurses and to promote quality care for individuals and families with mental health problems. The goals of ISPN are to promote equitable quality care for individuals and families with mental health problems, enhance the ability of psychiatric–mental health nurses to work collaboratively on major issues facing the nursing profession, provide expanded opportunities for networking and leadership development, and affect health care policy to facilitate more effective use of available human and financial resources.

Both organizations serve important functions in promoting quality mental health care and furthering the specialty of psychiatric–mental health nurses. Both organizations have annual meetings at which new research is presented. Student memberships are available.

Summary of Key Points

➤ The biopsychosocial model focuses on the three separate but interdependent dimensions of biologic, psychological, and social factors in the assessment and treatment of mental disorders. This comprehensive and holistic approach to mental disorders is the foundation for effective psychiatric–mental health nursing practice and is used as the basic organizational framework for this book.

➤ The *Scope and Standards of Psychiatric–Mental Health Nursing* published in 2000 established the areas of concern, standards of care according to the nursing process, and standards of nursing performance and differentiates between the functions of the basic and advanced practice nurse.

➤ New challenges facing psychiatric nurses are emerging. Interpretation of research findings will assume new importance in the care of individuals with psychiatric disorders. The roles of nurses are expanding as nursing care becomes an established part of the community-based delivery system.

➤ Several professional nursing organizations provided leadership in shaping mental health care, including the American Nurses Association, the American Psychiatric Nurses Association, and the International Society of Psychiatric–Mental Health Nurses.

➤ Psychiatric nurses will practice within ethical frameworks, including the ethical code established by the American Nurses Association.

Critical Thinking Challenges

1. Explain the biopsychosocial model, and apply it to the following three clinical examples:
   a. An adult man with hypertension is extremely distraught at the death of his wife.
   b. A child is unable to sleep at night because of terrifying nightmares.
   c. A young mother is extremely depressed after the birth of her child, who is perfectly healthy.
2. Compare the variety of patients for whom psychiatric–mental health nurses care. Factors to be considered are age, health problems, and social aspects.
3. Compare the basic level functions of a psychiatric nurse to the advanced practice psychiatric nurse.
4. Discuss the purposes of the following organizations in promoting quality mental health care and supporting nursing practice.
   a. American Nurses Association
   b. American Psychiatric Nurses Association

   c. International Society of Psychiatric–Mental Health Nurses
5. Compare the difference between the ethical concepts of autonomy and beneficence.

 WEB LINKS

www.nursingworld.org   This is the American Nurses Association website.

www.ispn-psych.org   This is the site of the International Society of Psychiatric–Mental Health Nurses.

www.apna.org   This is the American Psychiatric Nurses Association website.

www.surgeongeneral.com   At the Surgeon General's website, one can obtain a copy of *Mental Health: Report of the Surgeon General*.

www.cna-nurses.ca   The Canadian Nurses Association.

www.cfmhn.org   The Canadian Federation of Mental Health Nurses website which has the Canadian standards of psychiatric nursing practice.

References

Abraham, I., Fox, J., & Cohen, B. (1992). Integrating the bio into the biopsychosocial: Understanding and treating biological phenomena in psychiatric–mental health nursing. *Archives of Psychiatric Nursing, 6*(5), 296–305.

American Nurses Association, American Psychiatric Nurses Association, & International Society of Psychiatric–Mental Health Nurses. (2000). *Scope and standards of psychiatric–mental health nursing practice.* Washington, DC: American Nurses Publishing.

American Nurses Association. (1985). *Code for nurses with interpretive statements.* Washington, DC: Author.

Canadian Nurses Association Code for Nurses. (1985). *Code of ethics.* Ottawa: Author.

Standards Committee (1998). *The Canadian standards of psychiatric and mental health nursing* (2nd ed.). The Canadian Federation of the Mental Health Nurses.

U.S. Department of Health and Human Services (1999). Mental health: A report of the Surgeon General. Rockville, MD: Author.

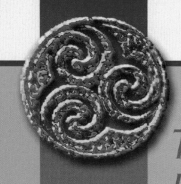

Theoretic Basis of Psychiatric Nursing

Mary Ann Boyd

BIOLOGIC THEORIES
General Adaptation Syndrome
Diathesis-Stress Model

PSYCHOLOGICAL THEORIES
Psychodynamic Theories
  Psychoanalytic Theory
  Neo-Freudian Models
  Humanistic Theories
  Applicability of Psychodynamic
    Theories to Psychiatric–Mental
    Health Nursing
Behavioral Theories
  Early Stimulus-Response Theories
  Reinforcement Theories
  Cognitive Theories
  Applicability of Behavioral
    Theories to Psychiatric–Mental
    Health Nursing
Developmental Theories
  Erik Erikson: Psychosocial
    Development
  Jean Piaget: Learning in Children
  Carol Gilligan: Gender
    Differentiation

Jean Baker Miller: A Sense
  of Connection
Applicability of Developmental
  Theories to Psychiatric–Mental
  Health Nursing

SOCIAL THEORIES
Family Dynamics
  Interactional View
  Problem-Solving Approach
  Multigenerational System
  Structural Family Theory
  Applicability of Family Theories
    to Psychiatric–Mental
    Health Nursing
Social Distance
  Balance Theory
  Applicability of Balance Theory
    to Psychiatric–Mental
    Health Nursing
Role Theories
  Role Theory Perspectives
  Applicability of Role Theories
    to Psychiatric–Mental
    Health Nursing

Sociocultural Perspectives
  Margaret Mead: Culture
    and Gender
  Madeleine Leininger:
    Transcultural Health Care
  Applicability of Sociocultural
    Theories to Psychiatric–
    Mental Health Nursing

NURSING THEORIES
Interpersonal Relations Models
  Hildegarde Peplau: The Power
    of Empathy
  Ida Jean Orlando
Existential and Humanistic
  Theoretic Perspectives
  Joyce Travelbee
  Jean Watson
Systems Models
  Imogene M. King
  Betty Neuman
  Dorothea Orem
Other Nursing Theories

LEARNING OBJECTIVES

After studying this chapter, you will be able to:

➤ Discuss the need for a theory-based practice and supporting research.
➤ Identify the underlying theories that contribute to the understanding of human beings and behavior.
➤ Compare the key elements of each theory that provides a basis for psychiatric–mental health nursing practice.
➤ Identify common nursing theoretic models used in psychiatric–mental health nursing.

This chapter presents an overview of the biologic, psychological, and social theories that serve as the knowledge base for psychiatric–mental health nursing practice. Many of the theories underlying psychiatric nursing practice are evolving and have limited research support. Lack of research does not necessarily mean that theories are useless, but researchers must acknowledge the limitations of existing experimentation and knowledge. In this chapter, published research support for the theories and their applicability in psychiatric nursing practice are discussed.

BIOLOGIC THEORIES

Biologic theories are clearly important in understanding the manifestations of mental disorders and caring for people with these illnesses. Chapter 7 explains many of the important neurobiologic theories, and Chapter 8 focuses on psychopharmacology. Many of the biologically focused interventions explained in Chapter 14 have their theoretic roots in basic nursing knowledge. This chapter describes two well-known biologic theoretic approaches that are used to understand the expression of mental disorders.

General Adaptation Syndrome

Hans Selye's landmark studies on stress described the interaction of environmental events and biologic response (Selye, 1956). Selye looked for a link between illness and stressful events and identified the *general adaptation syndrome* (GAS), describing a three-stage process: *alarm reaction*, *resistance*, and *exhaustion*. He hypothesized that during the alarm stage, patients exhibit an adrenocortical response associated with "fight-or-flight" behavior. During the resistance phase, the body adapts to stress but functions at a lower than optimal level. If the adaptive mechanisms fail or become worn out, the individual enters the third stage of exhaustion. At this point, the negative effects of the stressor spread to the entire organism, and Selye believed that ensuing illnesses could ultimately lead to death.

In this decade, research supports the relationship between illness and stressful events but has raised questions about some of Selye's basic ideas (see Chap. 35). Although there is support for biologic responses to stress, Selye's ideas of a general physical reaction to diverse environmental stimuli are being questioned. Many responses, such as those within the neuroendocrine system, are not general at all, but very specific.

Diathesis-Stress Model

Another perspective related to biology is the diathesis-stress model, an integration of the concepts of genetic vulnerability and environmental stressors. According to the model, certain genes or genetic combinations produce a **diathesis**, or constitutional predisposition to a disorder. When diathesis is combined with environmental stressors, abnormal behavior results. The diathesis-stress model suggests that for a mental disorder to develop, both the diathesis and stress must interact, that is, an individual with a predisposition toward a disorder must be "challenged" by a stressor. This model is supported by several research studies. One recent study found that living with chronic pain (stress) is related to elevated rates of depression (Dohrenwend et al., 1999). Another study that examined college students also found a relationship between the stress of holding especially high academic standards and the development of depressive symptoms (Carver, 1998).

PSYCHOLOGICAL THEORIES

Psychodynamic Theories

Psychodynamic theories explain the mental or emotional forces or developing processes, especially in early childhood, and their effects on behavior and mental states. The study of the unconscious is part of psychodynamic theory, and many of the models that are important in psychiatric nursing began with the Austrian physician Sigmund Freud (1856–1939). Since his time, Freud's theories have been enhanced by so-called interpersonal and humanist models. Psychodynamic theories initially attempted to explain the cause of mental disorders, but etiologic explanations were not supported by controlled research. These theories, however, proved to be especially important in the development of therapeutic relationships, techniques, and interventions (Table 6-1).

Psychoanalytic Theory

Study of the Unconscious. In Freud's psychoanalytic model, the human mind was conceptualized in terms of consciousness (an awareness of events, thoughts, and feelings with the ability to recall them) and unconscious mental processes (thoughts and feelings that are outside awareness and are not remembered). The unconscious was considered a repository for material that had never been subject to conscious awareness, or was part of consciousness and later repressed. The laws of logic did not apply to the unconscious. That is, thoughts and feelings that normally belonged together could be shifted or displaced out of context. Disparate ideas or images could be condensed into one, and objects could have symbolic representations. Freud believed that the unconscious part of the human mind is only rarely recognized by the conscious, as in remembered dreams (see Movies at the end of this chapter). The term *preconscious* was used to describe unconscious material that is capable of entering consciousness.

Personality and Its Development. Freud's personality structure consisted of three parts: the id, ego, and superego (Freud, 1927). The *id* was formed by unconscious desires, primitive instincts, and unstructured drives, including sexual and aggressive tendencies that arose from the body. Freud proposed that at birth, a neonate is endowed with an id with instinctual drives seeking gratification. The energy or psychic drive associated with the sexual instinct, called the libido, literally translated from Latin to mean "pleasure" or "lust," resided in the id. These inherent drives claimed immediate satisfaction, which were experienced as pleasurable. Thus, the pleasure principle dominated the id but was rarely experienced directly because any expressions of thoughts or feelings were filtered through the ego, the part responsible for resolving intrapsychic conflict.

Freud believed the *ego* consisted of the sum of certain mental mechanisms, such as perception, memory, and motor control, as well as specific defense mechanisms. The ego controlled movement, perception, and contact with reality. The capacity to form mutually satisfying relationships was a fundamental function of the ego, which is not present at birth but is formed throughout the child's development. Freud believed that as the ego was formed, it gradually replaced the domination of the pleasure principle with the reality principle, which only strengthens ego functioning. The ego assessed external conditions while the desires of the id adapted to the environment. The ego, in turn, was responsible for testing reality and postponing satisfaction of the instinctual impulses originating in the id.

The *superego* was that part of the personality structure associated with ethics, standards, and self-criticism. A child's identification with important and esteemed people in early life, particularly parents, helped form the superego; the supposed or actual wishes of significant people were taken over as part of the child's own standards to develop a conscience. In Freudian theory, the

TABLE 6.1 Psychodynamic Models

Theorist	Overview	Major Concepts	Applicability
Psychoanalytic Models			
Sigmund Freud (1856–1939)	Founder of psychoanalysis. Believed that the unconscious could be accessed through dreams and free association. Developed a personality theory and theory of infantile sexuality.	Id, ego, superego Consciousness Unconscious mental processes Libido Object relations Anxiety and defense mechanisms Free associations, transference, and countertransference	Individual therapy approach used for enhancement of personal maturity and personal growth
Anna Freud (1895–1982)	Application of ego psychology to psychoanalytic treatment and child analysis with emphasis on the adaptive function of defense mechanisms.	Refinement of concepts of anxiety, defense mechanisms	Individual therapy, childhood psychoanalysis
Neo-Freudian Models			
Alfred Adler (1870–1937)	First defected from Freud. Founded the school of individual psychology.	Inferiority	Added to the understanding of human motivation
Carl Gustav Jung (1875–1961)	After separating from Freud, founded the school of psychoanalytic psychology. Developed new therapeutic approaches.	Redefined libido Introversion Extroversion Persona	Personalities are often assessed on the introversion and extroversion dimensions
Otto Rank (1884–1939)	Introduced idea of primary trauma of birth. Active technique of therapy including more nurturing than Freud. Emphasized feeling aspect of analytic process.	Birth trauma Will	Recognized the importance of feelings within psychoanalysis
Erich Fromm (1900–1980)	Emphasized the relationship of the individual to society.	Society and individual are not separate	Individual desires are formed by society
Melanie Klein (1882–1960)	Devised play therapy techniques. Believed that complex unconscious fantasies existed in children younger than 6 months of age. Principal source of anxiety arose from the threat to existence posed by the death instinct.	Pioneer in object relations Identification	Developed different ways of applying psychoanalysis to children; influenced present-day English and American schools of child psychiatry
Karen Horney (1885–1952)	Opposed Freud's theory of castration complex in women and his emphasis on the oedipal complex. Argued that neurosis was influenced by the society in which one lived.	Situational neurosis Character	Beginning of feminist analysis of psychoanalytic thought
Interpersonal Relations			
Harry Stack Sullivan (1892–1949)	Impulses and striving need to be understood in terms of interpersonal situations.	Participant observer Parataxic distortion Consensual validation	Provided the framework for the introduction of the interpersonal theories in nursing
Humanist Theories			
Abraham Maslow (1921–1970)	Concerned himself with healthy rather than sick people. Approached individuals from a holistic-dynamic viewpoint.	Needs Motivation	Used as a model to understand how people are motivated and needs that should be met
Frederick S. Perls (1893–1970)	Awareness of emotion, physical state, and repressed needs would enhance the ability to deal with emotional problems.	Reality Here-and-now	Used as a therapeutic approach to resolve current life problems that are influenced by old, unresolved emotional problems
Carl Rogers (1902–1987)	Based theory on the view of human potential for goodness. Used the term *client* rather than *patient*. Stressed the relationship between therapist and client.	Empathy Positive regard	Individual therapy approach that involves never giving advice and always clarifying client's feelings

superego originated in the struggle to overcome the oedipal conflict and consequently had the power of an instinctual drive. In part unconscious, the superego gave rise to feelings of guilt not justified by any conscious transgression.

Freud believed that when sexual desire was controlled and not expressed, tension resulted and was transformed into anxiety (Freud, 1905). For Freud, anxiety was a specific state of unpleasantness accompanied by motor discharge along definite pathways, the reaction to danger of object loss. His conviction that sexuality was an essential force led to his development of a theory of infantile sexuality, which was criticized by many of his colleagues and the Victorian society in which he lived. Freud believed that adult sexuality was an end product of a complex process of development that began in early childhood and involved a variety of body functions or areas (oral, anal, and genital zones) that corresponded to stages of relationships, especially with parents.

Psychoanalysis. Freud developed psychoanalysis, a therapeutic process of accessing the unconscious and resolving the conflicts that originated in childhood with a mature adult mind. As a system of psychotherapy, psychoanalysis attempted to reconstruct the personality by examining free associations (spontaneous, uncensored verbalizations of whatever comes to mind) and the interpretation of dreams. Therapeutic relationships had their beginnings within the psychoanalytic framework. As Freud initiated psychoanalysis, a therapeutic relationship evolved with the patient, and Freud identified many concepts, including defense mechanisms, object relations, transference, and countertransference, all of which are discussed later in this chapter.

The process of psychoanalysis required a large investment of time (several individual sessions a week for several years) and was not a practical approach for delivering mental health care on a widespread basis. Psychoanalysis was also not effective for people with mental disorders, but it continues to be a respected therapeutic approach for those seeking to enhance personal maturity and growth. Many of the techniques and concepts have been incorporated into other psychodynamic models.

Neo-Freudian Models

Freud had many followers who were either in analysis with him or were colleagues treating people with emotional problems. Many of Freud's followers ultimately broke away, establishing their own form of psychoanalysis. Freud did not receive criticism well. The rejection of some of his basic beliefs often cost his friendship as well. Various psychoanalytic schools have adopted other names because their doctrines deviated from Freudian theory.

Adler's Foundation for Individual Psychology. Alfred Adler (1870–1937), a Viennese psychiatrist and founder of the school of individual psychology, was a student of Freud who believed that the motivating force in human life is a sense of inferiority. Avoiding feelings of inferiority leads the individual to adopt a life goal that is often unrealistic and frequently expressed as an unreasoning will to power and dominance. Because inferiority is intolerable, the compensatory mechanisms set up by the mind may get out of hand, resulting in self-centered neurotic attitudes, overcompensation, and a retreat from the real world and its problems.

Adler's contributions included identifying the importance of birth order. According to his model, the first-born child is generally given much attention until the second child is born. The first-born child is then "dethroned" and often placed in a position of responsibility for the new sibling. Consequently, when the oldest child grows up, he or she usually protects others and is concerned with issues of power and authority. The second-born child is in a different position because he or she is always sharing attention with another child. Therefore, the second child more easily learns to cooperate with others. Adler believed that second children tended to compete with their older sibling and in adulthood rejected the strict leadership of others. The youngest child, as the baby of the family, could never be "dethroned." The youngest may also excel, but many times ended up being spoiled and, as a result, the problem child of the family (Adler, 1931).

The effects of birth order on personality development have been studied with conflicting results. Early studies support the idea that birth order is related to criminal activities. In an investigation of the birth order of 249 inmates in jail for felony, drunkenness, and miscellaneous crimes between 1977 and 1986, it was determined that more first- and last-born people were in jail for these crimes than were middle-born children (Weinstein & Sackhoff, 1987). However, a later study failed to support any significant influence of birth order on aggression (Claxton, 1999). In studies of the effects of birth order on personality achievements using four diverse data sets, first-borns were nominated as most achieving and most conscientious and later-borns were nominated as most rebellious, liberal, and aggressive (Paulhus et al., 1999). These results may be related not only to birth order but also to other variables, such as ethnicity, family environment, and family size (Marjoribanks, 1999; Salmon & Daly, 1998; Parker, 1998).

Today, Adler's theories and principles have been adapted and applied to both psychotherapy and education. Adlerian theory is based on principles of mutual respect, choice, responsibility, consequences, and belonging. This theory provides a framework for nurses working with children to react concretely to misbehavior, give encouragement, implement natural and logical consequences, and handle special need children with sensitivity (Pryor & Tollerud, 1999). The Adlerian approach was a basis of a parent education and evaluation program for abusive parents. Through participation in this education program, parents improved their perceptions of their children and were less potentially abusive (Fennell & Fishel, 1998).

Jung's Analytical Psychology: The Existence of Archetypes. One of Freud's earliest students, Carl Gustav Jung (1875–1961), a Swiss psychoanalyst, created a model called analytical psychology. Jung believed in the existence of two basically different types of personalities: extroverted and introverted. Extroverted people tend to be generally interested in other people and objects of the external world, whereas introverted people tend to be interested in themselves and their internal environment. Even though he argued that both tendencies exist in the normal individual, the libido usually channels itself mainly in one direction or the other. Jung rejected Freud's distinction between the ego and superego. Instead, he developed the concept of persona (what a person appears to be to others, in contrast with what he or she actually is) that was similar to the superego (Jung, 1966).

Horney's Feminine Psychology. Karen Horney (1885–1952), a German American psychiatrist, challenged many of Freud's basic concepts and introduced principles of feminine psychology. Recognizing early on the male bias in psychoanalysis, Horney was the first to challenge the traditional psychoanalytic belief that women felt disadvantaged because of their genital organs. Freud believed that women felt inferior to men because their bodies were less completely equipped, a theory he described as "penis envy." Horney rejected this concept, as well as the oedipal complex, arguing that there are significant cultural reasons why women may strive to obtain qualities or privileges that are defined by a society as being masculine. For example, university education, the ability to vote, and economic independence have only been recently available to women. She argued that women truly were at a disadvantage because of the authoritarian culture in which they lived (Horney, 1939).

Other Neo-Freudian Theories: Birth Trauma and Child's Play. Otto Rank (1884–1939), an Austrian psychologist and psychotherapist, was also a student of Freud. Introducing a theory of neurosis that attributed all neurotic disturbances to the primary trauma of birth, he described individual development as a progression from complete dependence on the mother and family to physical independence coupled with intellectual dependence on society, and finally to complete intellec-

tual and psychological emancipation. Rank believed in the importance of will, a positive guiding organization in the integration of self.

Other psychoanalytic theorists include Erich Fromm and Melanie Klein. Erich Fromm (1900–1980), an American psychoanalyst, focused on the relationship of society and the individual. He argued that individual and societal needs are not separate and opposing forces; their relationship with each other is determined by the historic background of the culture. Fromm also believed that the needs and desires of individuals are largely formed by their society. For Fromm, the fundamental problem of psychoanalysis and psychology was to bring about harmony and understanding of the relationship between the individual and society.

Melanie Klein (1882–1960), an Austrian psychoanalyst, devised play therapy techniques to demonstrate how a child's interaction with toys revealed earlier infantile fantasies and anxieties. She believed that complex unconscious fantasies existed in children younger than 6 months of age. She is generally acknowledged as a pioneer in presenting an object relations viewpoint to the psychodynamic field, introducing the idea of early identification, a defense mechanism by which one patterns oneself after another person, such as a parent. Her theoretic inferences were based on her clinical observations.

Departure From Freudianism: Sullivan's Interpersonal Forces. Interpersonal theories were developed as an alternative explanation of human development and behavior. Although there are similarities between psychoanalytic and interpersonal theories, the major difference is that interpersonal theories acknowledge the importance of individual relationships in personality development. Instincts and drives are less important. Childhood relationships with parenting figures are especially significant and are believed to influence important adult relationships, such as the choice of a mate.

Harry Stack Sullivan (1892–1949), an American psychiatrist, extended the concept of **interpersonal relations** to include characteristic interaction patterns. Sullivan studied personality characteristics that could be directly observed, heard, and felt. He believed that the health or sickness of one's personality was determined by the characteristic ways in which he or she dealt with other people. Health also depended on the constantly changing physical, social, and interpersonal environment as well as past and current life experiences (Sullivan, 1953).

Humanistic Theories

Humanistic theories were generated as a reaction against psychoanalytic premises of instinctual drives. Humanistic therapies are based on the views of human potential for goodness. Instead of focusing on instinctual drives, humanist therapists focus on a person's ability to learn about himself or herself, acceptance of self, and exploration of personal capabilities. Within the therapeutic relationship, the patient begins to view himself or herself as a person of worth. A positive attitude is developed. The focus is not on investigation of repressed memories, but on learning to experience the world in a different way.

Rogers' Client-Centered Therapy. Carl Rogers (1902–1987), an American psychologist, developed new methods of client-centered therapy. Rogers defined **empathy** as the capacity to assume the internal reference of the client in order to perceive the world in the same way as the client. To use empathy in the therapeutic process, the counselor must be nondirect, but not passive. Thus, the counselor's attitude and nonverbal communication are crucial. He also advocated that the therapist develop *unconditional positive regard*, a nonjudgmental caring for the client (Rogers, 1980). *Genuineness* is also important in a therapist, in contrast with the passivity of the psychoanalytic therapist. Rogers believed that the therapist's emotional investment (ie, true caring) in the client is essential in the therapeutic process.

Gestalt Therapy. Another humanistic approach created as a response to the psychoanalytic model was Gestalt therapy, developed by Frederick S. (Fritz) Perls (1893–1970), a German-born former psychoanalyst who immigrated to the United States. Perls believed that modern civilization inevitably produces neurosis because it forces people to repress natural desires and frustrates an inherent human tendency to adjust biologically and psychologically to the environment. Neurotic anxiety results. For a person to be cured, unmet needs must be brought back to awareness. He did not believe that the intellectual insight gained through psychoanalysis enabled people to change. Instead, he devised individual and group exercises that enhanced the person's awareness of emotions, physical state, and repressed needs as well as physical and psychological stimuli in the environment (Perls, 1969).

Abraham Maslow's Hierarchy of Needs. Abraham Maslow (1921–1970) developed a humanistic theory that is used in psychiatric–mental health nursing today. His major contributions were to the area of needs and motivation (Maslow, 1970). Maslow advocated viewing human behavior from a perspective of needs. Human beings have a hierarchy of needs that range from basic food, shelter, and warmth to a high-level requirement for self-actualization (Fig. 6-1). This model is used in understanding individual needs. For example, the need for food and shelter must be met before caring for the symptoms of a mental illness.

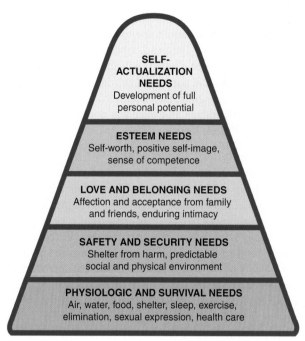

FIGURE 6.1 Maslow's hierarchy of needs.

Applicability of Psychodynamic Theories to Psychiatric–Mental Health Nursing

Several concepts that are traced to the psychodynamic theories are important in the practice of psychiatric–mental health nursing. They include interpersonal relationships, defense mechanisms, transference, countertransference, empathy, levels of consciousness, and internal objects (Wheeler & Lord, 1999; Ens, 1998). In particular, a therapeutic interpersonal relationship is a core of psychiatric–mental health nursing. Through the strength and support of the therapeutic relationship, patients can examine and solve mental health problems (see Chap. 14 for nursing interventions).

Defense Mechanisms. Even though they are defined differently than in Freud's day, defense mechanisms still play an explanatory role in contemporary psychiatric–mental health practice.

KEY CONCEPT   **Defense Mechanism.** The fourth edition of the *Diagnostic and Statistical Manual of Mental Disorders* (DSM-IV) published by the American Psychiatric Association (1994) defines **defense mechanisms** (or coping styles) as the automatic psychological process protecting the individual against anxiety and from the awareness of internal or external dangers or stressors. Individuals are often unaware of these processes even though they mediate their reaction to emotional conflicts and to internal and external stressors.

Table 6-2 lists defense mechanisms. Some defense mechanisms (eg, projection, splitting, and acting out) are almost invariably maladaptive. Others, such as suppres-

TABLE 6.2   Specific Defense Mechanisms and Coping Styles*

Defense Mechanism	Definition	Example
Acting out	Using actions rather than reflections or feelings during periods of emotional conflict	A teenager gets mad at parents and begins staying out late at night.
Affiliation	Turning to others for help or support (sharing problems with others without implying that someone else is responsible for them)	An individual has a fight with spouse and turns to best friend for emotional support.
Altruism	Dedicating life to meeting the needs of others (receives gratification either vicariously or from the response of others)	After being rejected by boyfriend, a young girl joins the Peace Corps.
Anticipation	Experiencing emotional reactions in advance or anticipating consequences of possible future events and considering realistic, alternative responses or solutions	A parent cries for 3 weeks before the last child leaves for college. On the day of the separation, the parent spends the day with friends.
Autistic fantasy	Excessive daydreaming as a substitute for human relationships, more effective action, or problem solving	A young man sits in his room all day and dreams about being a rock star instead of attending a baseball game with a friend.
Denial	Refusing to acknowledge some painful aspect of external reality or subjective experience that would be apparent to others (*psychotic denial* used when there is gross impairment in reality testing)	A teenager's best friend moves away, but the adolescent says he does not feel sad.
Devaluation	Attributing exaggerated negative qualities to self or others	A boy has been rejected by his long time girlfriend. He tells his friends that he realizes that she is stupid and ugly.
Displacement	Transferring a feeling about, or a response to, one object onto another (usually less threatening), substitute object	A child is mad at her mother for leaving for the day, but says she is really mad at the sitter for serving her food she does not like.
Dissociation	Experiencing a breakdown in the usually integrated functions of consciousness, memory, perception of self or the environment, or sensory and motor behavior	An adult relates severe sexual abuse experienced as a child, but does it without feeling. She says that the experience was as if she were outside her body watching the abuse.
Help-rejecting complaining	Complaining or making repetitious requests for help that disguise covert feelings of hostility or reproach toward others, which are then expressed by rejecting the suggestions, advice, or help that others offer (complaints or requests may involve physical or psychological symptoms or life problems)	A college student asks a teacher for help after receiving a bad grade on a test. Every suggestion the teacher has is rejected by the student.
Humor	Emphasizing the amusing or ironic aspects of the conflict or stressor	A person makes a joke right after experiencing an embarrassing situation.
Idealization	Attributing exaggerated positive qualities to others	An adult falls in love and fails to see the negative qualities in the other person.
Intellectualization	Excessive use of abstract thinking or the making of generalizations to control or minimize disturbing feelings	After rejection in a love relationship, the rejected explains about the relationship dynamics to a friend.
Isolation of affect	Separation of ideas from the feelings originally associated with them	The individual loses touch with the feelings associated with a rape while remaining aware of the details.
Omnipotence	Feeling or acting as if one possesses special powers or abilities and is superior to others	An individual tells a friend about personal expertise in the stock market and the ability to predict the best stocks.
Passive aggression	Indirectly and unassertively expressing aggression toward others. There is a facade of overt compliance masking covert resistance, resentment, or hostility.	Passive aggression often occurs in response to demands for independent action or performance or the lack of gratification of dependent wishes but may be adaptive for individuals in subordinate positions who have no other way to express assertiveness more overtly.

(continued)

TABLE 6.2   Specific Defense Mechanisms and Coping Styles* (Continued)

Defense Mechanism	Definition	Example
Projection	Falsely attributing to another one's own unacceptable feelings, impulses, or thoughts	A child is very angry at a parent, but accuses the parent of being angry.
Projective identification	Falsely attributing to another one's own unacceptable feelings, impulses, or thoughts. Unlike simple projection, the individual does not fully disavow what is projected. Instead, the individual remains aware of his or her own affect or impulses but misattributes them as justifiable reactions to the other person. Not infrequently, the individual induces the very feelings in others that were first mistakenly believed to be there, making it difficult to clarify who did what to whom first.	A child is mad at a parent, who in turn becomes angry at the child, but may be unsure of why. The child then feels justified at being angry with the parent.
Rationalization	Concealing the true motivations for one's own thoughts, actions, or feelings through the elaboration of reassuring or self-serving but incorrect explanations	A man is rejected by his girlfriend, but explains to his friends that her leaving was best because she was beneath him socially and would not be liked by his family.
Reaction formation	Substituting behavior, thoughts, or feelings that are diametrically opposed to one's own unacceptable thoughts or feelings (this usually occurs in conjunction with their repression)	A wife finds out about her husband's extramarital affairs and tells her friends that she thinks his affairs are perfectly appropriate. She truly does not feel, on a conscious level, any anger or hurt.
Repression	Expelling disturbing wishes, thoughts, or experiences from conscious awareness (the feeling component may remain conscious, detached from its associated ideas)	A woman does not remember the experience of being raped in the basement, but does feel anxious when going into that house.
Self-assertion	Expressing feelings and thoughts directly in a way that is not coercive or manipulative	An individual reaffirms to another that going to a ball game is not what he or she wants to do.
Self-observation	Reflecting feelings, thoughts, motivation, and behavior and responding to them appropriately	An individual notices an irritation at his friend's late arrival and decides to tell the friend of the irritation.
Splitting	Compartmentalizing opposite affect states and failing to integrate the positive and negative qualities of the self or others into cohesive images.	Self and object images tend to alternate between polar opposites: exclusively loving, powerful, worthy, nurturant, and kind—or exclusively bad, hateful, angry, destructive, rejecting, or worthless. One friend is wonderful and another former friend, who was at one time viewed as being perfect, is now believed to be an evil person.
Sublimation	Channeling potentially maladaptive feelings or impulses into socially acceptable behavior	An adolescent boy is very angry with his parents. On the football field, he tackles someone very forcefully.
Suppression	Intentionally avoiding thinking about disturbing problems, wishes, feelings, or experiences	A student is anxiously waiting test results, but goes to a movie to stop thinking about it.
Undoing	Words or behavior designed to negate or to make amends symbolically for unacceptable thoughts, feelings, or actions	A man has sexual fantasies about his wife's sister. He takes his wife away for a romantic weekend.

* The following defense mechanisms and coping styles are identified in the *DSM-IV* as being used when the individual deals with emotional conflict or stressors (either internal or external).
Adapted from the American Psychiatric Association. (2000). *Diagnostic and statistical manual of mental disorders* (4th ed., Text revision, pp. 811–814). Washington, DC: Author.

sion and denial, may be either maladaptive or adaptive, depending on the severity and the context in which they occur. Defense mechanisms are divided into seven related groups called **defense levels** (Table 6-3). These groups identify and categorize mechanisms, or coping styles, that individuals use.

Transference and Countertransference. **Transference** is defined as the displacement of thoughts, feelings, and behaviors originally associated with significant others from childhood onto a person in a current therapeutic relationship (Moore & Fine, 1990). For example, a woman's feelings toward her parents as a child may be directed toward the therapist. If a woman were unconsciously angry with her parents, she may feel unexplainable anger and hostility toward her therapist. In psychoanalysis, the therapist used transference as a therapeutic tool to help the patient understand emotional problems and their origin. **Countertransference**, on the other hand, is defined as the direction of all of the therapist's feelings and attitudes toward the patient. Feelings and perceptions caused by countertransference may interfere with the therapist's ability to understand the patient.

Object Relations and Identification. Freud introduced the concept of **object relations**, the psychological attachment to an another person or object. He believed that the choice of a love object in adulthood and the nature of the relationship would depend on the nature and quality of the child's object relationships during the early formative years. The child's first love object was the mother, who is the source of nourishment and the provider of pleasure. Gradually, as the child

TABLE 6.3 Defense Levels

Defense Levels	Definition	Examples
High adaptive level	This level of defensive functioning results in optimal adaptation in the handling of stressors. These defenses usually maximize gratification and allow the conscious awareness of feelings, ideas, and their consequences. They also promote an optimum balance among conflicting motives.	Anticipation Affiliation Altruism Humor Self-assertion Self-observation Sublimation Suppression
Mental inhibitions (compromise formation) level	Defensive functioning at this level keeps potentially threatening ideas, feelings, memories, wishes, or fears out of awareness.	Displacement Dissociation Intellectualization Isolation of affect Reaction formation Repression Undoing
Minor image-distorting level	This level is characterized by distortions in the image of the self, body, or others that may be used to regulate self-esteem.	Devaluation Idealization Omnipotence
Disavowal level	This level is characterized by keeping unpleasant or unacceptable stressors, impulses, ideas, affects, or responsibility out of awareness with or without a misattribution of these to external causes.	Denial Projection Rationalization
Major image-distorting level	This level is characterized by gross distortion or misattribution of the image of self or others.	Autistic fantasy Projective identification Splitting of self-image or image of others
Action level	This level is characterized by defensive functioning that deals with internal or external stressors by action or withdrawal.	Acting out Apathetic withdrawal Help-rejecting complaining Passive aggression
Level of defensive dysregulation	This level is characterized by failure of defensive regulation to contain the individual's reaction to stressors, leading to a pronounced break with objective reality.	Delusional projection Psychotic denial Psychotic distortion

Adapted from the American Psychiatric Association. (2000). *Diagnostic and statistical manual of mental disorders* (4th ed., Text revision, pp. 807–810). Washington, DC: Author.

separated from the mother, the nature of this initial attachment influenced any future relationships. The development of the child's capacity for relationships with others progressed from a state of narcissism to social relationships, first within the family and then within the larger community. Although the concept of object relations is fairly abstract, it can be understood in terms of a child who is imitating her mother and then becomes like her mother in adulthood. This child has incorporated her mother as a love object, identifies with her, and becomes like her as an adult. This process becomes especially important in understanding an abused child who, under certain circumstances, becomes the adult abuser.

Empathy. Because nursing relies on interpersonal interactions, the concept of empathy is important in all areas of nursing and has been studied by many nursing experts (Peplau, 1992; Reynolds & Scott, 2000; Evans et al., 1998). Empathy can be defined as one person voluntarily experiencing another person's emotions of situation (Greiner, 1989). The empathic person has not actually had this experience, but feels the other person's emotion generated within the situation. This experience is based on cues consciously taken in while observing another. A special bond is established with the other person, who may have no knowledge of the empathy. Empathy is an internal state and cannot be measured by observable actions or behavior. However, being empathic is observable and is associated with active listening behavior, such as maintaining eye contact. The development of empathy is discussed in Chapter 9.

Behavioral Theories

One important group of theories that serves as a knowledge base for the practice of psychiatric–mental health nursing is the behavioral theories, which have their roots in the discipline of psychology. Behavioral theories attempt to explain how people learn and act. Behavioral theories never attempt to explain the cause of mental disorders but instead focus on normal human behavior. Research results are then applied to the clinical situation (Table 6-4).

Early Stimulus-Response Theories

Pavlov's Dog. One of the earliest behavioral theorists was Ivan P. Pavlov (1849–1936), a Russian physiologist, who won the Nobel Prize in physiology and medicine in 1904 for his work on digestion. Pavlov noticed that stomach secretions of dogs were stimulated by other triggers besides food reaching the stomach. He found that the sight and smell of food triggered stomach secretions, and he became interested in this anticipatory secretion. Through his experiments, he was able to stimulate secretions with a variety of other laboratory non-

physiologic stimuli. Thus, a clear connection was made between thought processes and physiologic responses.

In Pavlov's model, there is an *unconditioned stimulus* (not dependent on previous training) that elicits an *unconditioned* (ie, specific) *response.* In his experiments, meat was the unconditioned stimulus, and salivation was the unconditioned response. Pavlov would then select other stimuli, such as a bell, a ticking metronome, and a triangle drawn on a large cue card, presenting this conditioned stimulus just before the meat, the unconditioned response. If the conditioned stimulus was repeatedly presented before the meat, eventually salivation was elicited only by the conditioned stimulus. This phenomenon was called **classical** (pavlovian) **conditioning.**

John B. Watson and the Behaviorist Revolution. At about the same time as Pavlov was working in Russia, John B. Watson (1878–1958) initiated the psychological revolution known as **behaviorism** in the United States. Watson received the first doctorate in psychology granted from the University of Chicago. The psychological revolution known as behaviorism had begun. He developed two principles: *frequency* and *recency.* The principle of frequency states that the more often a given response is made to a given stimulus, the more likely the response to that stimulus will be repeated. The principle of recency states that the more recently a given response to a particular stimulus is made, the more likely it will be repeated. Watson's major contribution was the rejection of the distinction between body and mind and his emphasis on the study of objective behavior.

Reinforcement Theories

Edward L. Thorndike. A pioneer in experimental animal psychology, Edwin L. Thorndike (1874–1949) studied the problem-solving behavior of cats to determine whether animals solved problems by reasoning or instinct. He found that neither choice was completely correct; animals gradually learn the correct response by "stamping in" the stimulus-response connection. The major difference between Thorndike and behaviorists like Watson was that Thorndike believed in the importance of the effects that followed the response or the reinforcement of the behavior. He was the first reinforcement theorist, and his view of learning became the dominant view in American learning theory.

B. F. Skinner. One of the most influential behaviorists, B. F. Skinner (1904–1990) recognized two different kinds of learning, each involving a separate kind of behavior. Respondent behavior, or the end result of classical conditioning, is elicited by specific stimuli. Given the stimulus, the response occurs automatically. The other kind of learning is referred to as **operant behav-**

TABLE 6.4 Behavioral Theorists

Theorist	Overview	Major Concepts	Applicability
Stimulus-Response			
Edwin R. Guthrie (1886–1959)	Continued with understanding conditioning as being important in learning	Recurrence of responses tends to follow a specific stimulus	Important in analyzing habitual behavior
Ivan P. Pavlov (1849–1936)	Classical conditioning	Unconditioned stimuli Unconditioned response Conditioned stimuli	Important in understanding learning of automatic responses such as habitual behaviors
John B. Watson (1878–1958)	Introduced behaviorism, believed that learning was classical conditioning called reflexes; rejected distinction between mind and body	Principle of frequency Principle of recency	Focuses on the relationship between the mind and body
Reinforcement Theories			
B. F. Skinner (1904–1990)	Developed an understanding of the importance of reinforcement and differentiated types and schedules	Operant behavior Respondent behavior Continuous reinforcement Intermittent reinforcement	Important in behavior modification
Edward L. Thorndike (1874–1949)	Believed in the importance of effects that followed behavior	Reinforcement	Important in behavior modification programs
Cognitive Theories			
Albert Bandura (b. 1925)	Developed social cognitive theory, a model for understanding how behavior is learned from others	Modeling Disinhibition Elicitation Self-efficacy	Important in helping patients learn appropriate behaviors
Aaron Beck (b. 1921)	Conceptualized distorted cognitions as a basis for depression	Cognitions Beliefs	Important in cognitive therapy
Kurt Lewin (1890–1947)	Developed field theory, a system for understanding learning, motivation, personality and social behavior	Life space Positive valences Negative valences	Important in understanding motivation for changing behavior
Edward Chace Tolman (1886–1959)	Introduced the concept of cognitions; believed that human beings act on beliefs and attitudes and strive toward goals	Cognition	Important in identifying person's beliefs

ior. In this type of learning, the distinctive characteristic is the consequence of a particular behavioral response, not a specific stimulus. The learning of operant behavior is also known as conditioning, but it is different from the conditioning of reflexes. If a behavior occurs and is followed by reinforcement, it is probable that the behavior will recur. For example, if a child climbs on a chair, reaches the faucet, and is able to get a drink of water successfully, it is more likely that the child will repeat the behavior.

Reinforcers can be set up on a variable schedule. The simplest schedule is continuous reinforcement, in which the reinforcement is given for every response. This schedule is generally used when training is begun. After the response is learned, the schedule can be shifted to *intermittent reinforcement*, in which only some of the responses are reinforced.

Even though he was mostly concerned with positive reinforcers, Skinner recognized that negative reinforcers also exist. These include aversive stimuli, ones that the individual seeks to avoid. According to Skinner, negative reinforcers are different from punishment. Negative reinforcement results from the removal of an aversive stimuli, whereas punishment involves the presentation of a negative reinforcer. This is an important distinction because negative reinforcers may sometimes be used in a clinical situation when in reality they are actually punishment. For example, if a new patient is restricted to a unit for suicide precautions, this becomes a negative reinforcer when the restriction is removed once the individual's risk to self is reduced. However, if a patient regularly watches television at 10:00 PM, and the television is removed suddenly because the patient violated a smoking policy, this is punishment. Skinner points out that punishment is not a reliable way of preventing responses from occurring. Negative reinforcement increases the probability of a response, but punishment does not necessarily reduce it. Punishment is also likely to have negative emotional effects.

Skinner also developed the concept of shaping behavior, which has been used in the process of learning how to perform complex tasks. **Shaping** is a technique by which trained animals perform complex acts that are outside their normal range of behavior. The behavior is shaped through a series of reinforcements for successive approximations to the desired behavior. For example, if a pigeon is to be taught how to bowl, the first step would be establishing an initial positive reinforcer, such as a sound that indicates the availability of food. Once the positive reinforcer is well established, any movement close to the ball would be reinforced by the sound and food. Gradually, the reinforcer is used less and only as the activity becomes more specific and approximates rolling the ball down the alley.

Cognitive Theories

The initial behavioral studies focused attention on human actions without much attention to the internal thinking process. As complex behavior was examined and could not be accounted for by strictly behavioral explanations, thought processes became new subjects for study. Cognitive theories, an outgrowth of different theoretic perspectives, including the behavioral and the psychodynamic, attempted to link the internal thought processes with human behavior.

Albert Bandura's Social Cognitive Theory. Acquiring behaviors by learning from other people is the basis of social cognitive theory developed by Albert Bandura (b. 1925). Bandura developed his ideas after being concerned about violence on television contributing to aggression in children. He believes that important behaviors are learned by internalizing behaviors of others. His initial contribution was identifying the process of **modeling**: pervasive imitation, or one person trying to be like another. According to Bandura, the model may not need to be a real person, but could be a character in history or generalized to an ideal person (Bandura, 1977).

The concept of **disinhibition** is important to Bandura's model and refers to the situation in which someone has learned not to make a response; then, in a given situation, when another is making the inhibited response, the individual becomes disinhibited and also makes the response. Thus, the response that was "inhibited" now becomes disinhibited through a process of imitation. For example, during severe dieting, an individual may have learned to resist eating large amounts of food. However, when at a party with a friend who eagerly fills a plate at a buffet, the person also eats large amounts of food.

In the instance of disinhibition, the desire to eat is already there, and the individual indulges that desire. However, in another instance, called *elicitation*, there is no desire present, but when one person starts an activity, others want to do the same. An example of this occurs when a child is playing with a toy, and the other children also want to play with the same toy even though they showed no interest in it before that time.

An important concept of Bandura's is **self-efficacy**, a person's sense of his or her ability to deal effectively with the environment (Bandura, 1993). Efficacy beliefs influence how people feel, think, motivate themselves, and behave. The stronger the self-efficacy, the higher the goals people set for themselves and the firmer their commitment to them.

Aaron Beck: Thinking and Feeling. American psychiatrist Aaron T. Beck (b. 1921) of the University of Pennsylvania devoted his career to understanding the relationship between **cognition** and mental health. For Beck, cognitions are verbal or pictorial events in the stream of consciousness. He realized the importance of cognitions when treating people with depression, finding that the depression improved when patients began thinking differently.

He believed that people with depression had faulty information—processing systems that led to biased cognitions. These faulty beliefs cause errors in judgment that become habitual errors in thinking. These individuals incorrectly interpret life situations, judge themselves too harshly, and jump to inaccurate conclusions. A person may truly believe that he or she has no friends and therefore no one cares. On examination, the evidence for the beliefs is based on the fact that there has been no contact with anyone because of moving from one city to another. Thus, a distorted belief is the basis of the cognition. Beck and his colleagues developed cognitive therapy, a successful approach for the treatment of depression (see Research Box 6-1) (see Chap. 20).

Applicability of Behavioral Theories to Psychiatric–Mental Health Nursing

Basing interventions on behavioral theories is widespread in psychiatric nursing. For example, patient education interventions are usually based on learning principles derived from any number of the behavioral theories. Teaching patients new coping skills for their symptoms of mental illnesses is usually based on behavioral theories. Changing an entrenched habit involves helping patients identify what motivates them and how these new lifestyle habits can become permanent. In psychiatric units, behavioral interventions include the privilege systems and token economies (see Chap. 14).

RESEARCH BOX 6.1

Depression and Psychosocial Functioning

This nursing research study tests Beck's cognitive theory, which suggests that depressive cognitions (negative views of self-world and future) affect psychosocial functioning. There were three groups in this study: hospitalized patients with depression, outpatients who were depressed, and those who were not depressed. In the two groups that were depressed, the individuals' views of themselves and the world had a greater impact on psychosocial functioning than did the view of the future.

Nursing Utilization. Interventions that build self-esteem and enhance self-control may be most effective in improving psychosocial functioning of depressed adults.

Zauszniewski, J. A., & Rong, J. R. (1999). Depressive cognitions and psychosocial functioning: A test of Beck's cognitive theory. *Archives of Psychiatric Nursing, 13*(6), 286–293.

Developmental Theories

The developmental theories explain normal human growth and development, focusing on change over time. Many developmental theories are presented in terms of *stages* based on the assumption that normal development proceeds longitudinally from the beginning to the ending stage. Although this approach is useful, unless a stage model has been truly supported by research, the model may not represent reality. Trying to fit a patient into a particular stage without support for the existence of the stages would be inappropriate without acknowledging the lack of research support for the model. In addition, there has been criticism that time-tables do not reflect the reality of today's world.

Erik Erikson: Psychosocial Development

Freud and Sullivan both published treatises on stages of human development, but Erik Erikson (1902–1994) outlined the psychosocial developmental model that is most often used in nursing. Erikson's model was an expansion of Freud's psychosexual development theory. Whereas Freud emphasized intrapsychic experiences, Erikson recognized the importance of culture. Erikson followed Freud in recognizing that certain physical zones dominate different phases of development: in the early phase, the mouth; later, the anus; and finally, the genital area. He believed that similar events may be experienced differently depending on a person's reaction, family background, and cultural situation. To Erikson, viewing the person in the historical-cultural situation is the all-encompassing concern.

Each of Erikson's eight stages is associated with a specific task that can be successfully or unsuccessfully resolved. The model is organized into the following developmental conflicts according to age: basic trust versus mistrust, autonomy versus shame and doubt, initiative versus guilt, industry versus inferiority, identity versus role diffusion, intimacy versus isolation, generativity versus stagnation, and ego integrity versus despair (Table 6-5). Implicit is a focus on dichotomous personality characteristics that typically dominate a specific age, such as the development of trust for the infant, autonomy for the toddler, and identity for the adolescent. Successful resolution of a crisis leads to essential strength and virtues. For example, a positive outcome of the first crisis (basic trust versus mistrust) is the development of trust that can be maintained for a lifetime. If the crisis is unsuccessfully resolved, the infant develops mistrust

TABLE 6.5	**Erikson's Eight Ages of Man**	
Approximate Chronologic Age	Developmental Conflict*	Long-Term Outcome of Successful Resolution
Infant	Basic trust vs. mistrust	Drive and hope
Toddler	Autonomy vs. shame and doubt	Self-control and willpower
Preschool-aged child	Initiative vs. guilt	Direction and purpose
School-aged child	Industry vs. inferiority	Method and competence
Adolescence	Identity vs. role diffusion	Devotion and fidelity
Young adult	Intimacy vs. isolation	Affiliation and love
Adulthood	Generativity vs. stagnation	Production and care
Maturity	Ego integrity vs. despair	Renunciation and wisdom

* Successful outcome is evidenced by the development of the characteristic listed first.
Adapted from Erikson, E. (1963). *Childhood and society* (pp. 273–274). New York: Norton.

and moves into the next stage with the lack of social trust. According to this model, a child who is mistrustful will be unable to complete the next crisis successfully and, instead of developing a sense of autonomy, will develop shame and doubt.

Identity and Adolescents. One of Erikson's major contributions, however, was the recognition of the complexity and turbulence of adolescent development. Erikson (1968) wrote extensively about adolescence, youth, and identity formation. Throughout childhood, the ego is formed by successive identifications. Children are always losing their love objects; the child and mother of today are not the same as the child and mother of yesterday. These lost objects are taken into the ego and become its building blocks. When adolescence begins, childhood ways must be given up, and body changes must be reconciled with the individual's social position, previous history, and identifications. What is formed is an identity, which is something more than the sum of identifications. During this time, there must be reasonable congruence between how young people see themselves and how society perceives them. This task can become overwhelming and lead to role confusion, which carries the possibility of role alienation. He believed that the virtue of fidelity, the ability to sustain loyalties freely pledged despite the inevitable contradictions of value systems, would guide young people through this time and make it possible for adolescents to assume their place in society. He also pointed out that adolescence was a time when past and future history of the community take on new significance (Erikson, 1968).

Research Support for Erikson's Models. Erikson's developmental concepts of identity, intimacy, and generativity have been studied. Favorable resolution of the intimacy-isolation crisis (the capacity to commit to a sexual partnership rather than avoidance of intimate relationships) has been associated with successful resolution of the identity crisis (Orlofsky et al., 1973). In this study, 53 male college students' identity and intimacy states were correlated with measures of intimacy, isolation, social desirability, autonomy, affiliation, and heterosexuality. Those who scored lowest on the identity measures (determined by standard interview) also scored lowest on intimacy status. The researchers concluded that these findings supported the hypothesis that favorable resolution of the intimacy-isolation crisis is related to successful resolution of the identity crisis. However, the subjects were all men and were most likely predominantly white, middle-class students. Thus, conclusions of the researchers can only be generalized to a similar population.

A later study questioned the applicability of Erikson's sequencing of stages to women and other cultural groups.

In a South African study, Ochse and Plug (1986) developed a self-report personality inventory that measured Erikson's dichotomous personality components of adults that would be suitable for cross-cultural studies. When adult men and women from white and black cultures were tested, researchers found that Erikson's concepts of identity, intimacy, and generativity (productivity, creativity) were extremely important. However, sequential formation at the times Erikson suggested was not supported. They found that white women resolved the crisis of identity at a younger age than did white men. They also found evidence that the formation of identity occurs when intimacy and generativity have already started to develop. Additionally, other gender and cultural differences were discovered. White women develop intimacy before their male counterparts and already have a sense of intimacy in adolescence. In this study, it appeared that both men and women gained identity through experiencing intimacy. However, somewhat different results were reported for black men and women. In a South African cultural group, the black men demonstrated higher intimacy scores than women.

Because Erikson's model has its roots in Freudian psychoanalytic theory, it is not surprising that his model is criticized for male bias. Researchers who study female development argue that Erikson could not account for gender differences in personality development. For men, separation and individuation are critical to the development of masculine identity. For women, identity does not depend on separation but instead relies on attachment and relationships. Male identity may be threatened by intimacy, and female identity is threatened by separation. Men tend to have problems with relationships, and women tend to have problems with separation. If Erikson's model is applied to women, their failure to separate then becomes defined as a developmental failure (Gilligan, 1982). Currently, there is considerable debate whether or not Erikson's developmental model is applicable to women.

Recent research on the Erikson model supports the idea that *generativity* (defined as the need or drive to produce, create, or effect a change) is associated with well-being in both males and females. In males, generativity may be related to the urge for self-protection, self-assertion, self-expansion, and mastery; in women, the antecedents may be the desire for contact, connection, and union (Ackerman et al., 2000). This study is consistent with the idea that the development of women is not identical to that of men. In another study of fathers with young children, the fathers' level of generativity was associated with a paternal identity, psychosocial identity, and psychosocial intimacy. Fathers who had a religious identification also had higher generativity scores than did others (Christiansen & Palkovitz, 1998).

Jean Piaget: Learning in Children

One of the most influential people in child psychology was Jean Piaget (1896–1980), who easily contributed over 40 books and more than 100 articles on child psychology alone. Piaget viewed intelligence as an adaptation to the environment. He proposed that cognitive growth is like embryologic growth: an organized structure becomes more and more differentiated over time. Piaget developed a system that explains how knowledge is developed and changed. Each stage of cognitive development represents a particular structure with major characteristics (Table 6-6). Piaget's theory was developed through observation of his own children and therefore never really received any formalized testing. The major strength of his model was its recognition of the central role of cognition in development and the discovery of surprising features of young children's thinking. For psychiatric–mental health nursing, Piaget's model provides a framework on which to define different levels of thinking and use the data in the assessment and intervention processes. For example, the assessment of concrete thinking would be typical of people with schizophrenia who are unable to perform abstract thinking.

Carol Gilligan: Gender Differentiation

Carol Gilligan (b. 1936), showed how most development models have been male centered and therefore inappropriate to girls and women. In 1982, she compared male and female personality development and highlighted the differences (Gilligan, 1982). For Gilligan, attachment within relationships is the important factor in successful female development. She argued that because the first primary relationship of both boys and girls is with the mother, the boys need to focus on separating to achieve masculine identity. Female identity occurs within the ongoing relationship with the mother, and girls experience themselves like their mother. Thus, girls learn to value relationships and become interdependent at an earlier age. They learn to value the ideal of care, begin to respond to human need, and want to take care of the world by sustaining attachments so no one is left alone. Female development does not necessarily follow a progression of stages, but it can be determined from experiences within relationships. However, some researchers suggest that relationships may also be equally important for boys in their development of a strong sense of self (Nelson, 1996).

TABLE 6.6 Piaget's Periods of Intellectual Development

Age (years)	Period	Cognitive Developmental Characteristics	Description
Birth to 2	Sensorimotor	Divided into six stages, characterized by (1) inborn motor and sensory reflexes, (2) primary circular reaction and first habit, (3) secondary circular reaction, (4) use of familiar means to obtain ends, (5) tertiary circular reaction and discovery through active experimentation, and (6) insight and object permanence	The infant understands the world in terms of overt, physical action on that world. The infant moves from simple reflexes through several steps to an organized set of schemes. Significant concepts are developed, including space, time, and causality. Above all, during this period, the child develops the scheme of the permanent object.
2–7	Preoperational	Deferred imitation; symbolic play, graphic imagery (drawing); mental imagery; and language. Egocentrism, rigidity of thought, semilogical reasoning, and limited social cognition	Child no longer only makes perceptual and motor adjustment to objects and events. Child can now use symbols (mental images, words, gestures) to represent these objects and events; uses these symbols in an increasingly organized and logical fashion.
7–11	Concrete operations	Conservation of quantity, weight, volume, length, and time based on reversibility by inversion or reciprocity; operations: class inclusion and seriation	Conservation is the understanding of what values remain the same. For example, if liquid is poured from a short, wide glass into a tall, narrow one, the preoperational child thinks that the quantity has changed. For the concrete operation child, the amount stays the same.
11 through end of adolescence	Formal operations	Combination system, whereby variables are isolated and all possible combinations are examined; hypothetical-deductive thinking	Mental operations are applied to objects and events. The child classifies, orders, and reverses them. Hypotheses can be generated from these concrete operations.

Gilligan's conclusion that female development depends on relationships has implications for everyone who provides care to women. Traditional models that advocate separation as the primary goal of human development immediately place women at a disadvantage. By negating the value and importance of attachments within relationships, the natural development of women is impaired.

Jean Baker Miller: A Sense of Connection

Jean Baker Miller (b. 1927) conceptualizes women's development completely differently from either Erikson or Freud. Consistent with the thinking of Carol Gilligan, Miller argues for the importance of experience and relationships. The Miller relational model rejects forcing observations into specific, predetermined categories or stages, arguing instead that the central organizing feature of women's development is a sense of connection to others. Consequently, women make and maintain relationships to feel important and worthwhile. "Most women find a sense of value and effectiveness if they experience all of their life activity as arising from a context of relationships and as leading into a greater sense of connection rather than a sense of separation" (Miller, 1994, p. 81).

One of the assumptions of the model is that positive interactions foster development. For example, failure-to-thrive syndrome, well documented in the pediatric literature, is caused by a lack of human contact. Active participation in the development of other people is important to women, but the ideal relationship is one that promotes a concept of mutuality—development not only of the other person but also of the woman.

The psychological development of women depends on their **connections** (mutually responsive and enhancing relationships) and **disconnections** (lack of mutually responsive and enhancing relationships). Miller advocates viewing the goal of development as "the increasing ability to build and enlarge mutually enhancing relationships" (Miller, 1994, p. 83). Connections lead to mutual engagement (attention), empathy, and empowerment. In those relationships in which everyone interacts beneficially, mutual psychological development can occur. Miller believes that many formative relationships have not have been based on mutuality, but have been directed in one way. Women foster the growth of others. Traditionally, psychological theories have not valued these relationships and, in many instances, have focused on separation from others. Explanations as to how children would learn to engage in these types of relationships are missing from the parenting literature (Miller & Stiver, 1997).

Disconnections occur when a child or adult expresses a feeling or explains an experience and does not receive any response from others. For example, if a child is hurt and crying and is told not to cry or is ignored by her parents, she may feel startled and angry at her parents' reaction. Then, she has to deal with more complex feelings than the original hurt. However, if the parents are responsive, then she feels an increase in her ability to have an effect on the relationship between her parents and herself. The most serious types of disconnection arise from the lack of response that occurs after abuse or attacks. Violation occurs when a girl or woman is sexually abused. In this instance, she is violated physically and psychologically. Both violation and disconnection can occur when one person has more power in the relationship than the other.

The theory is currently evolving. Research is ongoing, but there is support for the importance of relationships in female development (Gilligan, 1994; Miller & Stiver, 1997). Further development of the underlying processes of mutual engagement, empathy, and empowerment are being initiated.

Applicability of Developmental Theories to Psychiatric–Mental Health Nursing

Developmental theories are used in understanding childhood and adolescent experiences and their manifestations as adult problems. When working with children, nurses can use developmental models to help gauge development and mood. However, because most of the models are based on the assumptions of the linear progression of stages and have not been adequately tested, applicability has limitations. Additionally, these models were based on a relatively small number of children who typically were raised in a Western middle-class environment; most do not account for gender differences and diversity in lifestyles and cultures. The new research on female development is a paradigm shift in the field of human development. Evidence suggests that girls do not follow a staged developmental path. The new female development paradigm needs to be included in any developmental assessment performed. Interventions should account for the differences in male and female development. Miller's relational model may be especially useful in dealing with female patients who experience periods of disconnection. There is a report of one psychiatric unit organized around this model in which the emphasis is on changing the responses of individuals to remain connected to others rather than trying to change their fundamental personality (Riggs & Bright, 1997).

SOCIAL THEORIES

Numerous social theories underlie psychiatric–mental health nursing practice. In Chapter 2, some of the sociocultural issues and various social groups were identified. The nursing profession serves a specific societal function (caregivers and families). This section represents a sampling of important social theories that nurses may use. The selected theories explain family functioning from an interpersonal and societal perspective, present an overview of role theory, and discuss the application of transcultural theory. This discussion is not exhaustive and should be viewed by the student as including some of the theoretic perspectives that may be applicable.

Family Dynamics

Family dynamics are the patterned interpersonal and social interactions that occur within the family structure over the life of a family. Family dynamics models are based on systems theory describing a phenomenon in terms of a set of interrelated parts, in which the change of one part affects the total functioning of the system. A system can be "open" and interacting in the environment or "closed," completely self-contained and not influenced by the environment. In family theories, the family is viewed organizationally as an open system in which one member's actions influence the functioning of the total system. Family theories important in psychiatric–mental health nursing are based on systems models but have rarely been tested for wide-range validity. Most of the theoretic explanations have emerged from case studies involved in treatment instead of systematic development of theory based on large samplings. Consequently, the limitation of available research should be considered when these models are used to understand family interactions and plan patient care.

The understanding of family dynamics comes from the development of family therapy, which had its beginning in the early 1950s and emerged within the psychodynamic climate. An important team of psychiatrists and social scientists at the Mental Research Institute in Palo Alto, California, including Gregory Bateson, Don Jackson, Jay Haley, and Virginia Satir, developed models of family communication derived from the study of animal play. They emphasized pathologic communication. At about the same time at Yale University, another group, including Murray Bowen, studied marital relationships. It is from these initial works that family theories have developed.

Interactional View

The Bateson group studied family interactions in the context of communication and the etiology of schizophrenia (Bateson et al., 1956). The group consisted of respected psychotherapists who were mental health providers. This model introduced the revolutionary idea that rules, not roles, determined human behavior. This paradigm shift from individual and didactic units to family units as a rule-governed, hemostatic system was revolutionary thinking for the time (Jackson, 1981).

The model, an alternative to the accepted sex-role theory of marriage and family, emphasized the importance of behavioral rules as well as verbal interactions.

The interactionist model has been criticized for several reasons. The initial research attempted to show faulty communication as a cause of schizophrenia (Bateson et al., 1956). Bateson argued that in families with a member with schizophrenia, communication is characterized by a "double-bind." That is, schizophrenia developed in circumstances where an individual is given two contradictory messages—I love you, go away. Although that seems like an absurd idea today, during the 1960s, that explanation won widespread acceptance. Parents, translated as mothers, were viewed as causing schizophrenia because of their faulty interaction patterns with their children. This view had detrimental effects on the treatment of individuals with long-term psychiatric illnesses, on their families, and on families' relationships with mental health systems.

Today, the interaction pattern of families who have a member with schizophrenia continues to be investigated. The concept **expressed emotion** describes family members' responses that include one or more of the following dynamics: critical comments, hostility, or emotional overinvolvement. It is assessed by the Camberwell Family Interview (CFI), a semistructured interview that is usually administered to "key" relatives of people with schizophrenia. The CFI is believed to provide an effective measure of the emotional climate in a household that, in turn, can correctly identify family members' responses toward a relative with schizophrenia. It is hypothesized that individuals who live in households in which one or more family members are either highly critical, hostile, or emotionally overinvolved have a higher risk for symptom development and relapse (King & Dixon, 1996). The research regarding expressed emotion and its relationship to symptom management is contradictory. Some studies show that expressed emotion is related to low social functioning (Mavreas et al., 1992), but in another study of 69 patients ranging in age from 19 to 36 years, emotional overinvolvement of relatives was associated with a better social outcome (Stirling, 1994). In the future, family dynamics will continue to be studied in an attempt to better understand the impact of different interactional patterns on people with mental disorders.

Problem-Solving Approach

Jay Haley (b. 1923), a communication analyst, was concerned with building a model of therapeutic change rather than a theory of family. However, he added two important dimensions to Jackson's ideas. Emphasizing the importance of viewing the family and problem formation from a life cycle perspective, he believed that families undergo a developmental process over time; human distress and psychiatric symptoms appear when this process is disrupted. Haley also recognized that families are hierarchically organized and introduced the idea of inequality of power among family members (Haley, 1976). Most of his discussion was limited to inequality of power across generations and between parents, grandparents, and children. He did not address power relationships between men and women within families, an omission that was roundly criticized by contemporary feminists (Walsh & Scheinkman, 1991).

Virginia Satir (1916–1988), a respected and gifted psychiatric social worker, had two basic assumptions: (1) human beings have all the resources they need and (2) every human can grow. A well-known family therapist, Satir believed that dysfunctional families were systems in disharmony. The role of the therapist was to help the families improve their self-esteem and communication. She assumed that everyone could grow and change and that human beings had the skills they needed. Although she viewed families from a system perspective, her theoretic roots were in humanism. She believed that therapy was a process of interaction, communication, and mutual growth (Satir et al., 1991).

Multigenerational System

Murray Bowen (1913–1990) viewed the family within a multigenerational context. Bowen believed that emotional experiences were carried from one generation to another. Focusing on the impact of the parent on family members' mental health, Bowen emphasized collecting information about the family-of-origin relationship patterns and unresolved conflicts or losses. The goal in collecting the data is to change one's perspectives and current relationships with key family members. Bowen advocated a healthy differentiation of self in relation to one's family. The goal of therapy is to differentiate self from others and involves being a separate person as well as a connected family member. Bowen has been criticized for disproportionately focusing on the mother and not including the importance of the father's role. This model is discussed in more depth in Chapter 16.

Structural Family Theory

Structural family models emphasize the importance of organization to the functioning of the family unit and the well-being of its members. Salvador Minuchin (b. 1921) proposed a conceptual schema of family functioning to guide therapy, especially for families with children with eating disorders. He viewed the family structure as an open social system functioning within a certain cultural context and believed that the family progresses through successive stages of development, with each transition requiring restructuring. The family must adapt to changed environmental circumstances in ways that allow individual members to maintain continuity and adaptive re-

structuring. Autonomy and interdependence are key concepts, important both to individual growth and family system maintenance. Family structure is the invisible set of functional demands organizing interactions, whereas transactional patterns define relationships and regulate behavior. These relationship patterns are maintained by universal rules governing family organization (especially power hierarchy) and mutual behavioral expectations. In the well-functioning family, boundaries are clear, and a hierarchy exists with a strong parental subsystem (see Chap. 16.)

Problems result when there is a malfunctioning of the hierarchical arrangement or boundaries or a maladaptive reaction to changing developmental or environmental requirements. The family structure then needs to be reorganized to shift the malfunctioning pattern and strengthen parental hierarchy. Minuchin believes in clear, flexible boundaries by which all family members can live comfortably.

Applicability of Family Theories to Psychiatric–Mental Health Nursing

Family theories are especially useful to nurses who are assessing family dynamics and planning interventions. Family systems models are used to help nurses form collaborative relationships with patients and families dealing with health problems. Generalist psychiatric–mental health nurses will not be engaged in family therapy. However, they will be caring for individuals and families. Understanding family dynamics is important in every nurse's practice. Many family interventions are consistent with these theories (see Chap. 16). Many of the symptoms of mental disorders, such as hallucinations or delusions, have implications for the total family and affect interactions.

Social Distance

Balance Theory

A useful theory for understanding caregiving activities within a community is balance theory, proposed in 1966 by sociologist Eugene Litwak (b. 1925). This theory explains the importance of informal and formal support systems in the delivery of health care. **Formal support systems** are large organizations, such as hospitals and nursing homes, which provide care to individuals. **Informal support systems** are family, friends, and neighbors. Litwak found that individuals with strong informal support networks actually live longer than those without this type of support. In addition, those without informal support have significantly higher mortality rates when the causes of death are accidents (eg, smoking in bed) or suicides (Litwak, 1985). He argues that large-scale organizations work best when they include informal groups or are cooperating with them—a healthy balance develops between the formal and informal systems. The formal systems manage tasks that require technical knowledge; the informal groups provide help for those unpredictable, but necessary tasks. For example, a home health nursing agency (the formal system) provides nursing care twice a week and housekeeping services three times a week. The informal system, primary groups such as family and friends, checks on the person daily, makes emergency loans of items or finances, stores clothing and valuables, and keeps other family members informed.

A key concept in balance theory is **social distance**, the degree to which the values of the formal organization and primary group members differ. The formal and informal groups are considered to be balanced when they are at a midpoint of social distance, that is, close enough to communicate, but not so close to destroy each other, neither enmeshment nor isolation (Litwak et al., 1990; Messeri et al., 1993). If the primary groups and the formal care system begin performing similar caregiving services, the formal system increases the social distance by developing linkages with the primary group. Thus, a balance is maintained between the two systems. For example, if a patient relies only on the health care provider for care and support (eg, calls the nurse every day, visits the doctor weekly, refuses any help from family), the individual will be linked with an informal support system for help with some of the caregiving tasks. If the individual refuses any health promotion interventions from providers, the patient will be directly approached by the health care team.

Applicability of Balance Theory to Psychiatric–Mental Health Nursing

Balance theory is a practical model for conceptualizing delivery of mental health care in the community, particularly in rural areas where resources are limited. By using the framework of formal and informal support systems and social distance, mental health services can be developed and evaluated from this perspective. Nurse researchers at the Southeastern Rural Mental Health Research Center at the University of Virginia, Charlottesville, developed a model for establishing linkages of formal and informal caregivers for mental health service for those with serious mental illnesses in rural areas (Fox et al., 1994). In this model, case managers adjust the social distance between the formal and informal systems by identifying communication barriers and helping the two groups work together. For example, a patient misses an appointment because of lack of transportation. The case manager helps the patient communicate the problem to the system to obtain another appointment. Informal caregivers are valued by the case manager, who recognizes the important services performed by family and friends. Thus, linkages between mental health providers (formal support) and the consumer network (informal support) are reinforced.

Role Theories

Role Theory Perspectives

A **role** describes an individual's social position and function within an environment. Anthropologic theories explain members' roles that relate to a specific society. For example, the universal roles of healer may be assumed by a nurse in one culture and a spiritual leader in another. Societal expectations, social status, and rights are attached to these roles. Psychological theories, which are concerned about roles from a different perspective, focus on the relationship of an individual's role—the self. The responsibilities of a parent are often in conflict with the personal needs for time alone. All of the neo-Freudian and humanist models that have been discussed focus on reciprocal social relationships or interactions that determine how the mind develops.

Applicability of Role Theories to Psychiatric–Mental Health Nursing

Role theories emphasize the importance of social interaction in either the individual's choice of a particular role or society's recognition of it. Psychiatric–mental health nursing uses role concepts in understanding group interaction and the role of the patient in the family and community (see Chap. 16). Additionally, milieu therapy approaches discussed in later chapters are based on the patient's assumption of a role within the psychiatric environment.

Sociocultural Perspectives

Margaret Mead: Culture and Gender

American anthropologist Margaret Mead (1901–1978) is widely known for her studies of primitive societies and her contributions to social anthropology. She conducted studies in New Guinea, Samoa, and Bali and devoted much of her studies to the patterns of childrearing in various cultures. She was particularly interested in the cultural influences determining male and female behavior (Mead, 1970). Although her research was often criticized as not having scientific rigor and being filled with misinterpretations, it became accepted as a classic in the field of anthropology (Torrey, 1992). The importance of culture in determining human behavior was acknowledged.

Madeleine Leininger: Transcultural Health Care

Concern about the impact of culture on the treatment of children with psychiatric and emotional problems led Madeleine Leininger (b. 1924) to develop a new field, transcultural nursing, directed toward holistic, congruent, and beneficial care. Leininger developed the theory of culture care diversity and universality, which focused on diverse and universal dimensions of human caring. Thus, nursing care in one culture is different from that in another because definitions are different. Because caring is an integral part of being human, as well as a learned behavior, caring is culturally based (Leininger, 1999). Leininger developed a model to depict her theory that symbolically portrayed the rising sun. According to Leininger, the model depicts the "world view, religion, kinship, cultural values, economics, technology, language, ethnohistory, and environmental factors that are predicted to explain and influence culture care" (1993, p. 27) (Fig. 6-2).

Applicability of Sociocultural Theories to Psychiatric–Mental Health Nursing

The use of sociocultural theories is especially important for psychiatric–mental health nurses. In any individual or family assessment, the sociocultural aspect is analyzed and related to the individual's biopsychosocial problem. It would be impossible to complete an adequate assessment without considering the role of the individual within the family and society. Interventions are designed based on the understanding and signifi-

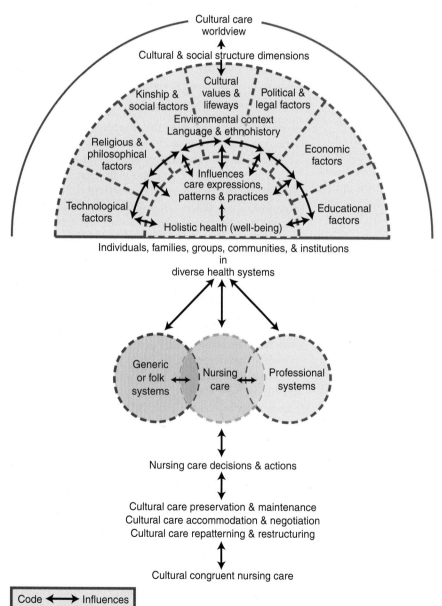

FIGURE 6.2 Leininger's sunrise model to depict theory of cultural care diversity and universality. (Adapted from Leininger, M. [Ed.]. [1991]. *Culture care diversity and universality: A theory of nursing.* New York: National League for Nursing.)

cance of family and cultural norms. It would be impossible to interact with the family in a meaningful way without the understanding of the family's cultural values. In the inpatient setting, the nurse is responsible for designing the social environment of the unit as well as ensuring that the patient is safe from self and others. To accomplish this complex task, an understanding of the unit as a small social community helps the nurse use the environment in patient treatment (see Chap. 14). Additionally, many group interventions are based on sociocultural theories (see Chap. 15).

NURSING THEORIES

A number of nursing theories are applicable to psychiatric–mental health nursing. Nursing theories are useful in conceptualizing the individual, family, or community and in planning nursing interventions. Chapter 14 explains the actual implementation of the interventions. The use of theories depends on the patients and their problems. For example, in people with schizophrenia who have problems related to maintenance of self-care, Dorothea Orem's theory of self-care may be useful. By contrast, Hildegarde Peplau's theories may be appropriate when the nurse is developing a relationship with the patient. Because of the wide range of possible problems requiring different approaches, familiarity with a variety of nursing theories is essential. The following discussion includes nursing models typically used in psychiatric–mental health nursing.

Interpersonal Relations Models

Hildegarde Peplau: The Power of Empathy

Hildegarde Peplau's (1909–1999) theoretic perspectives continue to be an important base for the practice of psychiatric–mental health nursing. Influenced by Harry Stack Sullivan, she introduced the first systematic theoretic framework for psychiatric nursing and focused on the nurse–patient relationship in her book *Interpersonal Relations in Nursing* in 1952. Although her work continues to stimulate debate, she has led psychiatric–mental health nursing out of the confinement of custodial care into a theory-driven professional practice. One of her major contributions was the introduction of the nurse–patient relationship (see Chap. 9).

Peplau believed in the importance of the environment, defined as those external factors considered essential to human development (Peplau, 1992): cultural forces, presence of adults, secure economic status of the family, and a healthy prenatal environment. She believed in the importance of the "interpersonal environment," which included interactions between person

and family, parent and child, or patient and nurse. The nurse–patient relationship is discussed more fully in Chapter 9.

Peplau also emphasized the importance of **empathic linkage**, the ability to feel in oneself the feelings experienced by another person or people. The interpersonal transmission of anxiety or panic is the most common empathic linkage. However, according to Peplau, other feelings, such as anger, disgust, and envy, can also be communicated nonverbally by way of empathic transmission to others. Although the process is not yet understood, she explains that empathic communication occurs. She believes that if nurses pay attention to what they feel during a relationship with a patient, they can gain invaluable observations of feelings a patient is experiencing and has not yet noticed or talked about.

The **self-system** is an important concept in Peplau's model. Drawn from Sullivan, she defined the self as an "anti-anxiety system" and a product of socialization. The self proceeds through personal development that is always open to revision but tends toward a certain stability. For example, in parent–child relationships, patterns of approval, disapproval, and indifference are used by children to define themselves. If the verbal and nonverbal messages have been derogatory, children incorporate these messages and also view themselves negatively. The concept of need is important to Peplau's model. Needs are primarily of biologic origin but need to be met within a sociocultural environment. When a biologic need is present, it gives rise to tension that is reduced and relieved by behaviors meeting that need. According to Peplau, nurses are not concerned about needs *per se*, but recognize the patient's patterns and style of meeting their needs in relation to their health status. Nurses interact with the patient to identify available resources, such as the quantity of food, availability of interpersonal support, and support for interaction patterns that help patients obtain what is needed.

Anxiety is a key concept for Peplau, who argues that professional practice is unsafe if this concept is not understood.

> **KEY CONCEPT** Anxiety. **Anxiety** is defined as an energy that arises when expectations that are present are not met.

If anxiety is not recognized, it continues to rise and escalates toward panic. There are various levels of anxiety, each having its observable behavioral cues (see Text Box 6-1). These cues are sometimes called defensive, but Peplau argues that they are often "relief behavior." For example, some people may relieve their anxiety by yelling and swearing, whereas others seek relief by withdrawing. In both instances, anxiety was generated by an unmet self-system security need.

Ida Jean Orlando

In 1954, Ida Jean Orlando (b. 1926) studied the factors that enhanced or impeded the integration of mental health principles in the basic nursing curriculum. From this study, she published, *The Dynamic Nurse–Patient Relationship*, which was intended to offer the nursing student a theory of effective nursing practice. She studied nursing care of patients on medical-surgical units, not people with psychiatric problems in mental hospitals. Orlando identified three areas of nursing concern: the nurse–patient relationship, the nurse's professional role, and the identity and development of knowledge that is distinctly nursing (Orlando, 1961). A nursing situation involves the behavior of the patient, the reaction of the nurse, and anything that does not relieve the distress of the patient. Patient distress is related to the inability of the individual to meet or communicate his or her own needs (Orlando, 1961; 1972).

Orlando's contribution to nursing practice helped nurses focus on the whole patient rather than on the disease or institutional demands. Her ideas continue to be useful today, and current research supports her model (Olson & Hanchett, 1997). A small nursing study investigated whether Orlando's nursing theory–based practice had a measurable impact on patients' immediate distress ($n = 19$) when compared with nonspecified nursing interventions ($n = 11$) (Potter & Bockenhauer, 2000). Orlando's approach consisted of the nurse validating the patient's distress before taking any action to reduce it. Those patients being cared for by the Orlando group experienced significantly less stress than those being cared for with traditional nursing care.

Existential and Humanistic Theoretic Perspectives

Joyce Travelbee

Influenced not only by Peplau and Orlando, Joyce Travelbee provided an existential perspective to nursing based on the works of Victor Frankl, an existential philosopher who was a survivor of Nazi concentration camps. Existentialists believe that humans seek meaning in their life and experiences. Suffering is defined as a feeling of displeasure ranging from simple and transitory mental, physical, or spiritual discomfort to extreme anguish, and to those phases beyond anguish, namely, the malignant phase of despair. Despair can be experienced as "not caring"; the terminal phase that follows is apathetic indifference (Travelbee, 1971). Travelbee also applied the concept of hope and defined it as a mental state characterized by the desire to gain an end or accomplish a goal combined with some degree of expectation that what is desired or sought is attainable.

Travelbee expanded the area of concern of psychiatric–mental health illness to include long-term physical illnesses. Focusing her attention on individuals who must learn to live with chronic illness, she believed that the nurse's spiritual values and philosophical beliefs about suffering would determine the extent to which she could help ill people find meaning in these situations.

Travelbee's model was never subjected to empiric testing, and because of the philosophical underpinnings, it is unlikely that scientific research will be useful. However, her use of the interpersonal process as a nursing intervention and her focus on suffering and illness helped to define areas of concern and psychiatric nursing practice.

Jean Watson

The science of caring was initiated by Jean Watson (b. 1940). Watson believes that caring is the foundation of nursing and recommends that specific theories of caring be developed in relation to specific human conditions and health and illness experiences (Watson, 1990). She distinguishes between caring and curing, the work of medicine. The science of caring is based on 7 assumptions and 10 carative factors (see Text Box 6-2).

Watson's theory is especially applicable to the care of those who seek help for mental illness. This model emphasizes the importance of sensitivity to self and others, the development of helping and trusting relations, the promotion of interpersonal teaching and learning, and provision for a supportive, protective, and corrective mental, physical, sociocultural, and spiritual environment. Research studies supporting the model use qualitative approaches.

Systems Models

Imogene M. King

The theory of goal attainment developed by Imogene King (b. 1923) is based on a systems model that includes three interacting systems: personal, interpersonal, and

TEXT BOX 6.2

Nursing: Human Science and Human Care Assumptions and Factors in Care

Assumptions

1. Caring can be effectively demonstrated and practiced only interpersonally.

2. Caring consists of factors that result in the satisfaction of certain human needs.

3. Effective caring promotes health and individual or family growth.

4. Caring responses accept a person not only as he or she is now but also as what he or she may become.

5. A caring environment offers the development of potential while allowing the person to choose the best action for himself or herself at a given point in time.

6. Caring is more "healthogenic" than is curing. It integrates biophysical knowledge with knowledge of human behavior to generate or promote health and provide ministrations to those who are ill. A science of caring is complementary to the science of curing.

7. The practice of caring is central to nursing.

Carative Factors

1. Formation of a humanistic-altruistic system of values

2. Instillation of faith or hope

3. Cultivation of sensitivity to one's self and to others

4. Development of a helping, trusting relationship

5. Promotion and acceptance of the expression of positive and negative feelings

6. Systematic use of the scientific problem solving method for decision making

7. Promotion of interpersonal teaching and learning

8. Provision for a supportive, protective, and corrective mental, physical, sociocultural, and spiritual environment

9. Assistance with the gratification of human needs

10. Allowance for existential-phenomenologic force

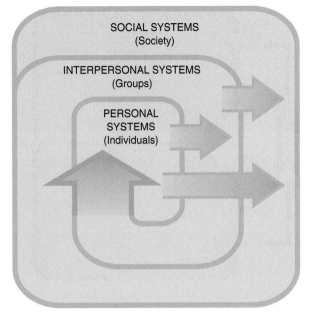

FIGURE 6.3 Imogene King's conceptual framework for nursing: dynamic interacting systems. (Adapted from King, I. [1981]. *A theory for nursing: Systems, concepts, process.* New York: Wiley.)

social. She believes that human beings interact with the environment and that the individual's perceptions influence reactions and interactions (Fig. 6-3). For King, nursing involves caring for the human being with the goal of health defined as adjusting to the stressors in both internal and external environments. She defines nursing as a "process of human interactions between nurse and patient whereby each perceives the other and the situation; and through communication, they set goals, explore means, and agree on means to achieve goals" (King, 1981, p. 144). This model focuses on the process that occurs between a nurse and a patient, which is initiated to help the patient cope with a health problem that compromises his or her ability to maintain social roles, functions, and activities of daily living (King, 1992).

In this model, the person is goal oriented and purposeful, reacting to stressors and viewed as an open system interacting with the environment. The variables in nursing situations are as follows:

- Geographic place of the transacting system, such as the hospital
- Perceptions of nurse and patient
- Communications of nurse and patient
- Expectations of nurse and patient
- Mutual goals of nurse and patient
- Nurse and patient as a system of interdependent roles in a nursing situation (King, 1981, p. 88)

The quality of nurse–patient interactions may have positive or negative influences on the promotion of health in any nursing situation. It is within this interpersonal system of nurse and patient that the healing process is performed. Interaction is depicted in which the outcome is a **transaction**, defined as the transfer of value between two or more people. This behavior is unique, based on experience, and is goal directed (Fig. 6-4).

King's work reflects her understanding of the systematic process of theory development. As a contemporary nursing theorist, her model continues to be developed and applied in different settings, including psychiatric–mental health care. The King model was applied in group therapy for inpatient juvenile offenders, maximum security state offenders, and community parolees (Laben et al., 1991). This model has also been used as a nursing framework for individual psychotherapy (DeHowitt, 1992).

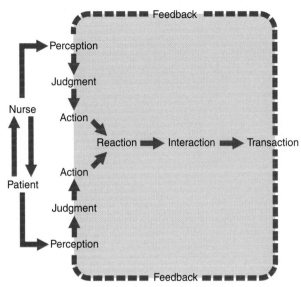

FIGURE 6.4 Imogene King's model of transaction. (Adapted from King, I. [1981]. A theory for nursing: Systems, concepts, process. New York: Wiley.)

Betty Neuman

Betty Neuman (b. 1924) also used a systems approach as a model of nursing care. Neuman wanted to extend care beyond an illness model, incorporating concepts of problem finding and prevention and the newer behavioral science concepts and environmental approaches to wellness. Neuman developed her framework in the late 1960s as chairwoman of the University of California at Los Angeles graduate nursing program. Although the original model was published in 1972, it has continued to be developed into the 1990s (Neuman, 1989). The purpose of the model is to guide the actions of the professional caregiver through the assessment and intervention processes (Fig. 6-5).

The Neuman systems model focuses on two major components: the nature of the relationship between the nurse and patient, and the patient's response to stressors. The patient may be an individual, group (eg, a family), or a community. The nurse is an "intervener" who attempts to reduce an individual's encounter with stress and to strengthen the person's ability to deal with stressors. The patient is viewed as a collaborator in setting health care goals and determining interventions. Neuman was one of the first psychiatric nurses to include the concept of stressors in understanding nursing care.

The model continues to be developed and applied. The latest edition of the Neuman systems model, for example, is applied to a diversity of settings, including community health, family therapy, renal nursing, perinatal nursing, and mental health nursing of older adults (Moore & Munro, 1990; Neuman, 1989). The model has also been applied to nursing care of patients with

multiple sclerosis (Knight, 1990) and quality-of-life indicators defined as a perception of good physical health, being comfortable with socioeconomic status, and developing a psychospiritual self (Hinds, 1990). The Neuman Systems Model Trustee Group, Inc. was established in 1988 to preserve, protect, and perpetuate the integrity of the model for the future of nursing.

Dorothea Orem

Self-care is the focus of the general theory of nursing initiated by Dorothea Orem in the early 1960s. The theory consists of three separate parts: a theory of self-care, theory of self-care deficit, and theory of nursing systems (Orem, 1991). The theory of self-care defines the term as those activities performed independently by an individual to promote and maintain personal well-being throughout life. The central focus of Orem's theory is the self-care deficit theory, which describes how people can be helped by nursing. Nurses can help meet self-care requisites through five approaches: acting or doing for; guiding; teaching; supporting; and providing an environment to promote the patient's ability to meet current or future demands. The nursing systems theory refers to a series of actions a nurse takes to meet the patient's self-care requisites. This system varies from the patient being totally dependent on the nurse for care, to needing only some education and support.

Orem's model is used extensively in psychiatric–mental health nursing because of its emphasis on promoting independence of the individual and on self-care activities (Campbell & Soeken, 1999). Although many psychiatric disorders have an underlying problem, such as motivation, these problems are generally manifested as difficulties conducting ordinary self-care activities (eg, personal hygiene) or developing independent thinking skills.

Other Nursing Theories

Other nursing models are applied in psychiatric settings. Martha Rogers' model of unitary human beings and Calista Roy's adaptation model have been the basis of many psychiatric nursing approaches.

Summary of Key Points

➤ The biologic framework forms a new basis for nursing considerations based on such models as diathesis-stress and imbalances in brain chemistry.
➤ The traditional psychodynamic framework helped form the basis of early nursing interpersonal interventions, including the development of therapeutic relationships and use of such concepts as transference and countertransference, empathy, and object relations.
➤ The behavioral theories are often used in strategies that help patients change behavior and thinking.

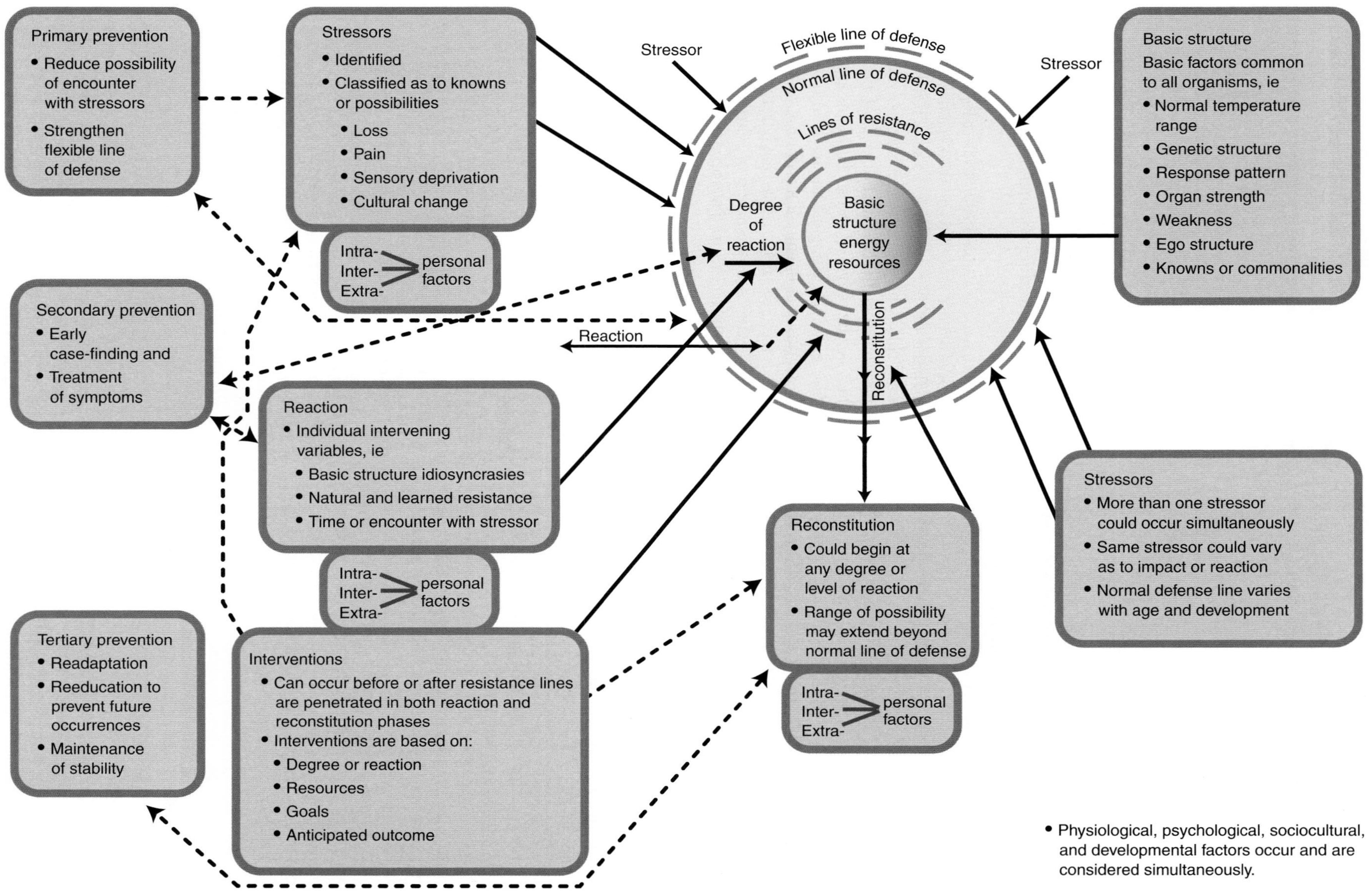

Primary prevention
• Reduce possibility of encounter with stressors
• Strengthen flexible line of defense
Stressors
• Identified
• Classified as to knowns or possibilities
• Loss
• Pain
• Sensory deprivation
• Cultural change
Intra- Inter- Extra- personal factors
Stressor
Flexible line of defense
Normal line of defense
Lines of resistance
Degree of reaction
Basic structure energy resources
Stressor
Basic structure
Basic factors common to all organisms, ie
• Normal temperature range
• Genetic structure
• Response pattern
• Organ strength
• Weakness
• Ego structure
• Knowns or commonalities
Secondary prevention
• Early case-finding and
• Treatment of symptoms
Reaction
Reconstitution
Reaction
• Individual intervening variables, ie
• Basic structure idiosyncrasies
• Natural and learned resistance
• Time or encounter with stressor
Intra- Inter- Extra- personal factors
Stressors
• More than one stressor could occur simultaneously
• Same stressor could vary as to impact or reaction
• Normal defense line varies with age and development
Reconstitution
• Could begin at any degree or level of reaction
• Range of possibility may extend beyond normal line of defense
Intra- Inter- Extra- personal factors
Tertiary prevention
• Readaptation
• Reeducation to prevent future occurrences
• Maintenance of stability
Interventions
• Can occur before or after resistance lines are penetrated in both reaction and reconstitution phases
• Interventions are based on:
• Degree or reaction
• Resources
• Goals
• Anticipated outcome
• Physiological, psychological, sociocultural, and developmental factors occur and are considered simultaneously.

FIGURE 6-5. The Betty Neumann model: A total person approach to viewing patient problems. (Adapted from Neuman, B., & Yound, R. J. [1972]. A model for teaching total person approach to patient problems. *Nursing Research, 21*, 264–269.)

➤ Sociocultural theories remain important in understanding and interacting with patients as members of families and cultures.

➤ Nursing theories form the conceptual basis for nursing practice and are useful in a variety of psychiatric–mental health settings.

Critical Thinking Challenges

1. Discuss the importance of the biologic theories in mental health practice. Compare Selye's model with the diathesis-stress model.

2. Discuss the similarities and differences between Freud's ideas and the neo-Freudians including Jung, Adler, Horney, and Sullivan.

3. Compare and contrast the basic ideas of psychodynamic and behavioral theories.

4. Define the following terms and discuss their applicability in psychiatric–mental health nursing: defense mechanisms, transference and countertransference, object relations, identification, empathy, and level of consciousness.

5. Compare and differentiate classic conditioning from operant behavior.

6. Define the following terms and discuss their applicability to psychiatric–mental health nursing: classical conditioning, operant conditioning, positive reinforcement, and negative reinforcement.

7. List the major developmental theorists and their main ideas.

8. Discuss the cognitive therapy approaches to mental disorders and how they can be used in psychiatric–mental health nursing practice.

9. Compare the focus of the interactional, problem-solving, and multigenerational approaches with family theory. How are they alike? How are they different?

10. Define formal and informal support systems. How does the concept of social distance relate to these two systems?

11. Compare and contrast the basic ideas of the nursing theorists.

   WEB LINKS

www.ualberta.ca/~jrnorris/nt/theory.html   This site provides a nursing theory page.

www.healthsci.clayton.edu/eichelberger/nursing.htm   This site provides a nursing theory link page.

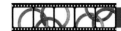   **MOVIES**

Freud: 1962. This video depicts Sigmund Freud as a young doctor, focusing on his early psychiatric theories and treatments. His struggles for acceptance of his ideas among the Viennese medical community are depicted. This fascinating film is well done and gives an interesting overview of the impact of psychoanalysis.
Viewing Points: Watch for the impact of the political thinking on the gradual acceptance of Freud's ideas. Discuss the "dream sequence" and its impact on the development of psychoanalysis as a therapeutic technique.

An Angel at My Table: 1990. This trilogy tells the story of Novelist Janet Frame who is a novelist and poet. Based on her autobiography, Janet is a shy, awkward child who experiences a family tragedy that alienates her socially. She studies in England to be a teacher, but her shyness and social ineptness causes extreme anxiety. Seeking out mental health care, she is misdiagnosed as having schizophrenia and spends 8 years in a mental institution. She barely escapes a lobotomy when she is notified of a literary award. She then again begins to develop friendships and a new life.
Viewing Points: Observe Janet Frame's childhood development. Does she "fit" any of the models that are discussed in this chapter? Consider her life in light of Gilligan and Miller's theories that it is important for women to have a sense of connection.

REFERENCES

Ackerman, S., Zuroff, D. C., Moskowitz, D. S. (2000). Generativity in midlife and young adults: Links to agency, communion, and subjective well-being. *International Journal of Aging and Human Development, 5*(1), 17–41.

Adler, A. (1931). Birth-order position. In H. Ansbacher & R. Ansbacher (Eds.). (1956). *The individual psychology of Alfred Adler* (pp. 376–383). New York: Basic Books.

American Psychiatric Association. (1994). *Diagnostic and statistical manual of mental disorders* (4th ed.). Washington, DC: Author.

Bandura, A. (1977). *Social learning theory.* Englewood Cliffs, NJ: Prentice-Hall.

Bandura, A. (1993). Perceived self-efficacy in cognitive development and function. American Educational Research Association Annual Meeting. *Educational Psychologist, 28*(2), 117–148.

Bateson, G., Jackson, D., Haley, J., & Weakland, J. (1956). Toward a theory of schizophrenia. *Behavioral Science, 1,* 251–264.

Campbell, J. C., & Soeken, K. L. (1999). Women's responses to battering: A test of the model. *Research in Nursing and Health, 22*(1), 49–58.

Carver, C. S. (1998). Generalization, adverse events, and development of repressive symptoms. *Journal of Personality, 66*(4), 607–619.

Christiansen, S. L., & Palkovitz, R. (1998). Exploring Erikson's psychosocial theory and development: Gernactivity and its relationship to paternal identity, intimacy, and involvement in childcare. *The Journal of Men's Studies, 7*(1), 133–156.

Claxton, R. P. (1999). Birth order and two marketing-related measures of aggression. *Psychological Reports, 84*(1), 236–238.

DeHowitt, M. (1992). King's conceptual model and individual psychotherapy. *Perspectives in Psychiatric Care, 28*(4), 11–14.

Dohrenwend, B. P., Raphael, K. G., Marbach, J. J., & Gallagher, R. M. (1999). Why is depression comorbid with chronic myofascial face pain? A family study test of alternative hypotheses. *Pain, 83*(2), 183–192.

Ens, I. C. (1998). An analysis of the concept of countertransference. *Archives of Psychiatric Nursing, 12*(5), 273–281.

Erikson, E. (1963). *Childhood and society* (2nd ed.). New York: Norton.

Erikson, E. (1968). *Identity: Youth and crisis.* New York: Norton.

Evans, G. W., Wilt, D. L., Alligood, M. R., & O'Neil, M. (1998). Empathy: A study of two types. *Issues in Mental Health Nursing, 19*(5), 453–479.

Fennell, D., & Fishel, A. (1998). Parent education: An evaluation of STEP on abusive parents? Perceptions and abuse potential. *Journal of Child and Adolescent Psychiatric Nursing, 11*(3), 107–120.

Freud, S. (1905). Three essays on the theory of sexuality. In J. Strachey, A. Freud, A. Strachey, & A. Tyson, (Eds.). (1953). *The standard edition of the complete psychological works of Sigmund Freud* (pp. 135–248). London: Hogarth Press.

Freud, S. (1927). The ego and the id. In E. Jones (Ed.). (1957). *The international psycho-analytical library* (No. 12). London: Hogarth Press.

Fox, J., Blank, M., & Kane, C. (1994). Balance theory as a model for coordinating delivery of rural mental health services. *Applied and Preventive Psychology, 3*(2), 121–129.

Gilligan, C. (1982). *In a different voice.* Cambridge, MA: Harvard University Press.

Gilligan, C. (1994). Joining the resistance: Psychology, politics, girls and women. In M. Berger (Ed.), *Women beyond Freud: New concepts of feminine psychology* (pp. 99–145). New York: Brunner Mazel.

Greiner, P. (1989). *The ideas of empathy in nursing: A conceptual analysis.* Dissertation. University of Pennsylvania, Philadelphia.

Haley, J. (1976). *Problem-solving therapy.* New York: Harper & Row.

Hinds, C. (1990). Personal and contextual factors predicting patients' reported quality of life: Exploring congruency with Betty Neuman's assumptions. *Journal of Advanced Nursing, 15,* 456–462.

Horney, K. (1939). *New ways in psychoanalysis.* New York: Norton.

Jackson, D. (1981). The question of family homeostasis. *International Journal of Family Therapy, 3*(1), 5–15.

Jung, C. (1966). On the psychology of the unconscious. V. The personal and the collective unconscious. In Jung, C. (Ed.), *Collected works of C. G. Jung* (2nd ed., Vol. 7, pp. 64–79). Princeton, NJ: Princeton University Press.

King, I. (1981). *A theory for nursing: Systems, concepts, process.* New York: Wiley.

King, I. (1992). King's theory of goal attainment. *Nursing Science Quarterly, 5*(1), 19–26.

King, S., & Dixon, M. (1996). The influence of expressed emotion, family dynamics and symptom type on the social adjustment of schizophrenic young adults. *Archives of General Psychiatry, 53*(12), 1098–1104.

Knight, J. (1990). The Betty Neuman systems model applied to practice: A client with multiple sclerosis. *Journal of Advanced Nursing, 15,* 447–455.

Laben, J., Dodd, D., & Snead, L. (1991). King's theory of goal attainment applied in group therapy for inpatient juvenile sexual offenders, maximum security state offenders, and community parolees, using visual aids. *Issues in Mental Health Nursing, 12*(1), 51–64.

Leininger, M. (1993). Assumptive premises of the theory. In C. Reynolds & M. Leininger (Eds.), *Madeleine Leininger: Cultural care diversity and universality theory. Notes on nursing theories* (Vol. 8, pp. 15–30). Newbury Park, CA: Sage.

Leininger, M. (1999). What is transcultural nursing and culturally competent care? *Journal of Transcultural Nursing, 10*(1), 9.

Litwak, E. (1985). Complementary roles for formal and informal support groups: A study of nursing homes and mortality rates. *Journal of Applied Behavioral Science, 21*(4), 407–425.

Litwak, E., Messeri, P., & Silverstein, M. (1990). The role of formal and informal groups in providing help to older people. *Marriage and Family Review, 15*(1–2), 171–193.

Marjoribanks, D. (1999). Ethnicity, birth order and family environment. *Psychological Reports, 84*(3, Pt. 1), 758–760.

Maslow, A. (1970). *Motivation and personality* (Rev. ed.). New York: Harper & Brothers.

Mavreas, V., Tomaras, V., Karydi, V., et al. (1992). Expressed emotion in families of chronic schizophrenics and its association with clinical measures. *Social Psychiatry and Psychiatric Epidemiology, 27*(1), 4–9.

Mead, M. (1970). *Culture and commitment: A study of the generation gap.* Garden City, NY: Natural History Press/Doubleday & Co.

Messeri, P., Silverstein, M., & Litwak, E. (1993). Choosing optimal support groups: A review and reformulation. *Journal of Health and Social Behavior, 34*(6), 122–137.

Miller, J. (1994). Women's psychological development. Connections, disconnections, and violations. In M. Berger (Ed.), *Women beyond Freud: New concepts of feminine psychology* (pp. 79–97). New York: Brunner Mazel.

Miller, J., & Stiver, P. (1997). *The healing connection: How women form relationships in therapy and life.* Boston: Beacon Press.

Moore, B., & Fine, B. (Eds.). (1990). *Psychoanalytic terms and concepts.* New Haven, CT: The American Psychoanalytic Association and Yale University Press.

Moore, S., & Munro, M. (1990). The Neuman system model applied to mental health nursing of older adults. *Journal of Advanced Nursing, 15*(3), 293–299.

Nelson, M. (1996). Separation versus connection, the gender controversy: Implications for counseling women. *Journal of Counseling and Development, 74*(4), 339–344.

Neuman, B. (1989). *The Neuman systems model* (2nd. ed.). East Norwalk, CT: Appleton & Lange.

Ochse, R., & Plug, C. (1986). Cross-cultural investigation of the validity of Erikson's theory of personality development. *Journal of Personality and Social Psychology, 50*(6), 1240–1252.

Olson, J., & Hanchett, E. (1997). Nurse-expressed empathy, patient outcomes, and the development of a middle-range theory. *Image: The Journal of Nursing Scholarship, 29*(1), 71–76.

Orem, D. (1991). *Nursing concepts of practice.* St. Louis: Mosby–Year Book.

Orlando, I. J. (1961). *The dynamic nurse–patient relationship.* New York: G. P. Putnam's Sons.

Orlando, I. J. (1972). *The discipline and teaching of nursing process.* New York: G. P. Putnam's Sons.

Orlofsky, J., Marcia, J., & Lesser, I. (1973). Ego identity status and the intimacy versus isolation crisis of young adulthood. *Journal of Personality and Social Psychology, 27*(2), 211–219.

Parker, W. (1998). Birth order effects in the academically talented. *Gifted Child Quarterly, 42*(1), 29–38.

Paulhus, D. L., Trapnell, P. D., & Chen, D. (1999). Birth order effects on personality and achievement within families. *Psychological Science, 10*(6), 482–488.

Peplau, H. (1992). Interpersonal relations: A theoretical framework for application in nursing practice. *Nursing Science Quarterly, 5*(1), 13–18.

Perls, F. (1969). *In and out of the garbage pail.* Lafayette, CA: Real People Press.

Piaget, J. (1952). Autobiography. In E. G. Boring & W. Bingham (Eds.), *A history of psychology in autobiography* (Vol. IV). Worcester, MA: Clark University Press.

Potter, M. L., & Bockenhauer, B. J. (2000). Implementing Orlando's nursing theory. *Journal of Psychosocial Nursing and Mental Health Services, 3813,* 14–21.

Pryor, D. B., & Tollerud, T. R. (1999). Applications of Alderian principles in school settings. *Professional School Counseling, 2*(4), 299–304.

Reynolds, W. J., & Scott, B. (2000). Do nurses and other professional helpers normally display much empathy? *Journal of Advanced Nursing, 31*(1), 226–234.

Riggs, S. R., & Bright, M. S. (1997). Dissociative identity disorder: A feminist approach to inpatient treatment using Jean Baker Miller's relational model. *Archives of Psychiatric Nursing, 11*(4), 218–224.

Rogers, C. (1980). *A way of being.* Boston: Houghton Mifflin.

Salmon, C. & Daly, M. (1998). Birth order and familial sentiment: Middleborns are different. *Evolution and Human Behavior, 19*(5), 299–312.

Satir, V., Banmen, J., Gerber, J., & Gamori, M. (1991). *The Satir model: Family therapy and beyond.* Palo Alto, CA: Science and Behavior Books.

Selye, H. (1956). *The stress of life.* New York: McGraw-Hill.

Stirling, J. (1994). Schizophrenia and expressed emotion. *Perspectives in Psychiatric Care, 30*(2), 20–25.

Sullivan, H. (1953). *The interpersonal theory of psychiatry.* New York: Norton.

Torrey, E. (1992). *Freudian fraud.* New York: Harper Collins.

Travelbee, J. (1971). *Interpersonal aspects of nursing* (2nd ed.). Philadelphia: F. A. Davis.

Watson, J. (1990). Caring knowledge and informed moral passion. *Advances in Nursing Sciences, 13*(1), 15–24.

Weinstein, L., & Sackhoff, J. (1987). Adler is right. *Bulletin of the Psychonomic Society, 25*(3), 201.

Wheeler, S., & Lord, L., (1999). Denial: A conceptual analysis. *Archives of Psychiatric Nursing, 13*(6), 311–320.

Zauszniewski, J. A., & Rong, J. R. (1999). Depressive cognitions and psychosocial functioning: A test of Beck's cognitive theory. *Archives of Psychiatric Nursing, 13*(6), 286–293.

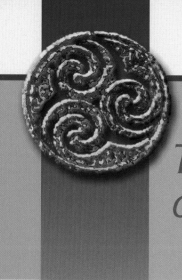

The Biologic Foundations of Psychiatric Nursing

Susan McCabe

CURRENT APPROACHES AND TECHNOLOGIC ADVANCES
Structural Neuroimaging
  Computed Tomography
  Magnetic Resonance Imaging
Functional Neuroimaging
  Positron Emission Tomography
  Single Photon Emission
    Computed Tomography
Bridging the Gap

NEUROANATOMY OF THE CENTRAL NERVOUS SYSTEM
Cerebrum
Left and Right Hemispheres
Lobes of the Brain
  Frontal Lobes
  Parietal Lobes
  Temporal Lobes

  Occipital Lobes
  Association Cortex
Subcortical Structures
  Basal Ganglia
  Limbic System
  Hippocampus
  Thalamus
  Hypothalamus
  Amygdala
  Limbic Midbrain Nuclei
Other Important Central Nervous
  System Structures

NEUROPHYSIOLOGY OF THE CENTRAL NERVOUS SYSTEM
Neurons and Nerve Impulses
Synaptic Transmission
Changing Receptor Sensitivity
Receptor Subtypes

Neurotransmitters
  Cholinergic
  Biogenic Amines
  Amino Acids
  Neuropeptides

NEW FIELDS OF STUDY
Psychoendocrinology
Psychoimmunology
Chronobiology
Diagnostic Approaches
  Laboratory Tests
  Neurophysiologic Procedures
Genetics
  Transmission
  Risk Factors

INTEGRATION OF THE BIOLOGIC, PSYCHOLOGICAL, AND SOCIAL DIMENSIONS

LEARNING OBJECTIVES

After studying this chapter, you will be able to:

➤ Identify the location of brain structures primarily involved in mental disorders; describe the primary functions of these structures in the brain.

➤ Describe the various approaches researchers have used to study the central nervous system and the significance of each approach.

➤ Describe the mechanisms of neuronal transmission.

➤ Identify the location and function of neurotransmitters significant to hypotheses regarding major mental disorders.

➤ Discuss the basic purpose of new fields of study in psychiatry, including psychoendocrinology, psychoimmunology, and chronobiology.

➤ Compare the application and use of various research methods in biologic psychiatry.

➤ Discuss the methods of study related to genetics.

CHAPTER 7

KEY TERMS

amino acids
autonomic nervous
   system
basal ganglia
biogenic amines
biologic markers
circadian cycle
chronobiology
cortex
frontal, temporal,
   parietal, and
   occipital lobes

hippocampus
limbic system
neurohormones
neuropeptides
neurotransmitters
plasticity
psychoendocrinology
psychoimmunology
receptors
risk factors
synapse
zeitgebers

The brain, or encephalon, is perhaps the most complex organ within the human body, weighing between 1,200 and 1,400 g in adults. All behavior recognized as human results from actions originating in the brain and its amazing interconnection of neural networks. Modern research has increased understanding of how the complex circuitry of the brain interacts with external environment, memories, and experiences. Through the spinal column and peripheral nerves, along with other systems, such as the endocrine and immune systems, the brain constantly receives and processes information that leads to action, allowing each person to behave in entirely unique ways.

This chapter reviews the information necessary for a basic understanding of neuroscience as it relates to the role of the psychiatric–mental health nurse, including basic central nervous system (CNS) structures and functions; basic mechanisms of neurotransmission; general functions of the major neurotransmitters; basic structure and function of the endocrine system; genetic research; circadian rhythms; neuroimaging techniques; and biologic tests. The chapter assumes that the reader has a basic knowledge of human biology, anatomy, and pathophysiology and is not intended as a full presentation of neuroanatomy and physiology, but rather as an overview of the structures and functions most critical to understanding the role of the psychiatric–mental health nurse.

CURRENT APPROACHES AND TECHNOLOGIC ADVANCES

Before reviewing the structures within the CNS and each of their related functions, it is important to remember that neuroscience researchers have used several approaches to the study of neuroanatomy. These approaches are highlighted in Table 7-1 and include the following:

- Comparative
- Developmental

This chapter is based on the chapter in the first edition, written by Mary Ann Nihart, MA, RN, CS, Clinical Nurse Specialist, Turning Point Center, San Francisco, California; Partner and Consultant, Professional Growth Facilitators, San Clemente, California.

	TABLE 7.1	Approaches to the Study of Neuroanatomy

Approach	Purpose	Potential Limitations
Comparative	Explores and compares behavior across animal nervous systems from a simple primitive cordlike structure in some species to the large complex of the human brain	Difficult to correlate animal behavior to human, especially emotional New brain structures do not necessarily correlate to new behavior
Developmental	Studies nervous system structure within an individual or species of animal across different stages of development	Impossible to follow one human being's neuronal development Individual variation in development complicates comparisons of individuals across a specific point of time in development
Chemoarchitecture	Identifies differences in location of neurochemicals, such as neurotransmitters, throughout the brain	Boundaries between regional changes are subtle and may vary across individuals
Cytoarchitecture	Identifies differences or variations in cell type, structure, and density throughout the brain, mapping these variations by location	Boundaries between regional changes are subtle and may vary across individuals
Functional	Identifies location of predominant control over various behavioral functions within the brain Studies often conducted on the basis of dysfunction from a localized injury to the brain	Several regions or structures within the brain may contribute to one behavior, making predominant control difficult to assign Controversy exists in correlating normal brain function to damaged brain tissue

- Chemoarchitecture
- Cytoarchitecture
- Functional

These different approaches to studying the CNS have led to significant findings that have increased understanding of how changes in the normal CNS contribute to the development of mental illness. It is now understood that areas of the brain or groups of nerve cells often work together in functional units. A hierarchy of function exists in which primary sensory input is used in an increasingly more complex and integrated manner across areas of the brain. In addition, some areas of the brain, such as those that control basic levels of alertness and attention, must be present before information can be received and understood or used to organize a response. It is important to recognize the limitations of theories implying that specific structures of the brain control specific functions. The results of recent research clearly indicate that the brain must be viewed in functional units that predominantly work together to control or contribute to specific behaviors or emotions, sometimes referred to as the *integrated approach* to brain development and function.

Neuroscientists also now recognize the importance of the concept of plasticity in describing brain function. **Plasticity** is the ability of the brain to change in various ways to compensate for loss of function in specific areas. Nerve signals may be rerouted, cells may learn new functions, or some nerve tissue may be regener-

ated in a limited way. All of these methods and more may explain how function may be restored over time after brain tissue has been damaged.

The technologic advances made in neuroimaging techniques that have been developed primarily since the 1980s have been a major aid to current research and understanding of how the human brain functions. There are two basic types of neuroimaging methods: structural and functional neuroimaging.

Structural Neuroimaging

Structural neuroimaging techniques allow for visualization of the structures of the brain. These images have identified what the normal structures of the brain look like and allow clinicians to identify any tissue changes, damage, or tissue that does not belong. Commonly used structural neuroimaging techniques include computed tomography (CT) scanning and magnetic resonance imaging (MRI). Whereas these techniques are useful in identifying what the brain looks like, the structural imaging procedures do not reveal anything about how the brain works.

Computed Tomography

Sometimes referred to as computerized axial tomography (CAT), CT first allowed scientists and clinicians to visualize the structures inside the brain without more invasive and potentially dangerous methods. A CT scan still uses an x-ray beam passed through the head in serial slices. High-speed computers measure the attenuation or decrease in the x-ray beam that results from absorption. The computer assigns a shade of gray that reflects the degree of attenuation. The degree of energy absorbed by a tissue is proportional to its density. Cerebrospinal fluid (CSF) attenuates the least, so it appears the darkest, whereas bone absorbs the most and appears light. White matter and gray matter are more difficult to discriminate.

A CT examination can be done without any invasion of the patient's body or CNS; however, iodinated contrast materials may be administered intravenously to enhance the image. Although these contrast materials help the radiologist to differentiate particular types of tumors, cerebrovascular disease, or infections, they may have some adverse effects. Patients receiving contrast materials frequently complain of a metallic taste in the mouth. Some experience mild nausea, rashes, or joint pain. In rare instances, severe allergic responses, including anaphylaxis, may develop. CT scanning is a relatively safe, noninvasive measure, but patients should be educated about the procedure. The equipment itself may be frightening to the unprepared psychiatric patient. Some patients may need to be accompanied during the procedure for ongoing reassurance. After the examination, nurses must be aware of potential untoward effects and closely monitor patients who have received contrast media.

In psychiatry, a CT scan may be required to rule out neurologic conditions that present with psychiatric symptoms. In addition, CT examination is frequently used in psychiatric research to assess pathologic changes in brain tissue that may develop in some mental disorders, such as schizophrenia.

Magnetic Resonance Imaging

An MRI scan looks like a CT scan, although the image is produced in an entirely different way. First introduced into clinical practice in 1983, an MRI is performed by placing a patient into a long tube that contains powerful magnets. This magnetic field causes hydrogen-containing molecules (primarily water) to line up and move in symmetric ways around their axes. The magnetic field is then interrupted in pulses, causing the molecules to turn 90 or 180 degrees. When the molecules return to their original position, electromagnetic energy is released, which can be detected by the device that measures the density of tissue. Although a CT scan is limited to one plane, the MRI can reconstruct three-dimensional images. The image produced by an MRI is extremely clear, much clearer than that from a CT scan, allowing for discrimination of white and gray matter along with other subtle changes in tissue. An MRI offers many different imaging options. Seemingly minor adjustments by the technician can substantially change the appearance of the image. Specific areas of tissue may be highlighted. Given the right information to know what to look for, the radiologist can make adjustments to the scan that may aid in making determinations about the quality of the tissue itself.

Based on this information alone, it may appear that the MRI should replace the CT. However, at this point, MRI scans remain somewhat more complicated and more costly than CT. In addition, the scan is not without potential complications. First of all, because the patient is entering a magnetic field, individuals with pacemakers, metal plates, bone replacements, aneurysm clips, or other metal in their body cannot undergo the procedure, nor can pregnant women. In addition, the long tube in which the patient must lie still for a considerable period of time causes some individuals to feel claustrophobic. Adequate preparation of the patient by the nurse should eliminate any surprises. Assistance with shallow breathing techniques or mental distractions may also help. Many MRI facilities are equipped with music to mask the whirring of the equipment, which some patients find distressing or frightening, and to provide a distraction through the long testing period, during which the patient must lay completely still. The nurse should investigate this feature; it may be possible to bring a favorite cassette of the patient's to the examination. Nonetheless, the individual may need to be accompanied to the procedure for the added reassurance of a familiar person. Some patients feel nauseated after the experience, but other complications are minimal.

Functional Neuroimaging

Functional neuroimaging techniques provide measurement of physiologic activities, providing insight into how the brain is working. These methods allow researchers to study such activities as cerebral blood flow, neuroreceptor location and function, and distribution patterns of specific chemicals within the brain. Single photon emission computed tomography (SPECT) and positron emission tomography (PET) are the two primary methods used to observe metabolic functioning. These two imaging procedures require the administration of radioactive compounds that emit charged particles, which can be measured by scanning equipment when they are released.

Positron Emission Tomography

The PET scanning method was developed in the late 1970s. Initially, the isotopes that emit positrons (positively charged electrons) were used to measure glucose consumption in various regions of the brain. Because cells use glucose as fuel for cellular action, the higher the rate of glucose utilization detected by the PET scan, the higher the rate of metabolic activity occurring in different areas of the brain. Abnormalities in glucose consumption, indicating more or less cellular activity, have been found in Alzheimer's disease, seizures, stroke, tumor, and a number of psychiatric disorders. Scanning may be performed at rest or while the individual is performing a cognitive task. PET scans have also been used to measure regional cerebral blood flow and in the rapidly developing study of neurotransmitter systems.

Single Photon Emission Computed Tomography

In SPECT, the radioactive isotopes emit a single photon. SPECT has an advantage over PET in that the isotopes are more stable, so that they may be commercially made and stored for use (Nahas et al., 1998). This makes the cost of each scan considerably less than for PET. These isotopes are made of molecules that are foreign to the human body. They are also difficult to attach to compounds used by the brain. Therefore, SPECT scans are used primarily to measure regional cerebral blood flow. Evidence has already accumulated to document the use of SPECT scans in the differentiation of depression and dementia. Decreased cerebral blood flow in specific areas of the brain has been well documented in Alzheimer's disease. This decrease has not been found in depression. SPECT scans have also been used to confirm changes in cerebral blood flow caused by certain drugs. For example, caffeine and nicotine cause a generalized decrease in cerebral blood flow. New compounds have been developed recently to visualize the numbers or density of receptors in various areas of the brain. This information may be useful in understanding treatment effects of psychopharmacologic medications.

Because these procedures identify function, the patient is often asked to perform a specific neuropsychological task during the imaging. The Wisconsin Card Sorting Test (WCST) is commonly used; it requires the individual to sort cards with different numbers, colors, and shapes into piles based on specified rules. This task requires considerable use of the frontal lobe of the brain, an important area for concept formation and decision making. Figure 7-1 illustrates the differences between the frontal lobe activity of a pair of twins, one who has the mental disorder of schizophrenia and the one who does not have the disorder.

Bridging the Gap

As structural and functional neuroimaging techniques have advanced, attempts have been made to develop imaging procedures that give detailed information on

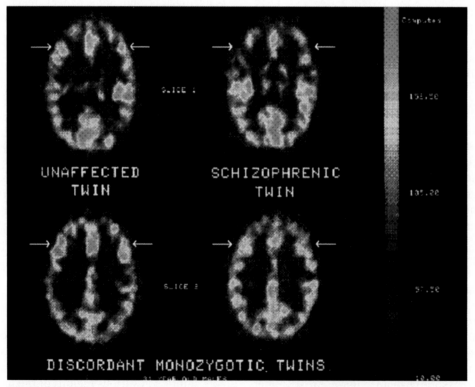

FIGURE 7.1 Differences in the frontal lobe activity of a pair of twins, one with the mental disorder of schizophrenia, and one who does not have the disorder. Figure courtesy of Drs. K. F. Berman and D. R. Weinberger, Clinical Brain Disorders Branch, National Institute of Mental Health.

both structure and function. Magnetic resonance spectroscopy (MRS) and functional magnetic resonance imaging (fMRI) are examples of attempts to combine imaging techniques. The fMRI is most useful in showing structure while localizing functioning and providing high-resolution, clear images. Like other forms of neuroimaging, the fMRI is noninvasive, but it requires no radioactive agent, making it both cheaper and safer than the PET and SPECT images (McIntosh, 1998). The MRS utilizes the same machinery as the fMRI and provides precise and clear imaging of neuron membranes as well as metabolic cellular functioning (Lorberbaum et al., 1998). In addition to these new imaging procedures, electromagnetoencephalography (EEG/MEG) is increasingly being used. This procedure combines traditional EEG measurement (discussed later in this chapter) with imaging and allows for the visualization of cellular electrical activity in the brain. Table 7-2 summarizes these neuroimaging methods.

Although these neuroimaging procedures are used primarily as research tools, it is reasonable to assume that they will increasingly move from research to clinical practice, becoming commonplace procedures in the near future.

NEUROANATOMY OF THE CENTRAL NERVOUS SYSTEM

The symptoms that constitute mental illness are most commonly manifested as abnormalities of behavior. As advances have occurred in brain science, understanding of the biochemical basis of these symptoms has grown. Psychiatric nurses increasingly need to be aware of the anatomic intricacy of the CNS, which forms the basis of modern psychiatric nursing assessments and interventions presented in later chapters of this textbook.

This section discusses each functioning area of the brain separately, but it must be remembered that these areas are intricately connected and function interactively. The CNS contains the brain, brain stem, and spinal cord. Although this section focuses on the CNS, remember that the total human nervous system contains the peripheral nervous system (PNS) as well as the CNS. The PNS consists of those neurons that connect the CNS to the muscles, organs, and other systems in the periphery of the body. Whatever affects the CNS may also affect the PNS, and vice versa.

Cerebrum

The largest part of the human brain is the cerebrum, which fills the entire upper portion of the cranium. The **cortex**, or outermost surface of the cerebrum, makes up about 80% of the human brain. The cortex is four to six cellular layers thick, and each layer is composed of cell bodies mixed with capillary blood vessels. This mixture gives the cortex a gray-brown color, and the tissue is called *gray matter*. The cortex contains a number of bumps and grooves in a fully developed adult brain, as shown in Figure 7-2. This "wrinkling" allows for a large amount of surface area to be confined in the limited space of the skull. The increased surface area allows for more potential connections between cells within the cortex. The grooves are called *fissures* if they extend deep into the brain and *sulci* if they are shallower. The bumps or convolutions are called *gyri*. Together, they provide many of the landmarks for the subdivisions of the cortex. The longest and deepest groove, the longitudinal fissure, separates the cerebrum into left and right hemispheres. Although these two divisions are nearly symmetric, there is some variation in the location and size of the sulci and gyri in each hemisphere. Substantial variation in these convolutions may be found when examining the cortex of different individuals.

Left and Right Hemispheres

The cerebrum can be roughly divided into two halves, or hemispheres. For most people, one hemisphere is dominant, whereas about 5% of individuals have mixed dominance. Each hemisphere controls functioning mainly on the opposite side of the body. For example, the left hemisphere, dominant in about 95% of people, controls functions mainly the right side of the body. The right hemisphere provides input into receptive nonverbal communication, spatial orientation and recognition; intonation of speech and aspects of music; facial recognition and facial expression of emotion; and nonverbal learning and memory. In general, the left hemisphere is more involved with verbal language function, including areas for both receptive and expressive speech control. In addition, the left hemisphere provides strong contributions to temporal order and sequencing, numeric symbols, and verbal learning and memory. The two hemispheres are connected by the corpus coliseum, a bundle of neuronal tissue that allows information to be exchanged quickly between the right and left hemispheres. An intact corpus coliseum is required for the hemispheres to function in a smooth and coordinated manner.

Lobes of the Brain

The lateral surface of each hemisphere is further divided into four lobes: the **frontal, parietal, temporal, and occipital lobes** (Fig. 7-2). While working in coordinated ways, each lobe is responsible for specific functions. An understanding of these unique functions is helpful in understanding how damage to these areas produces the symptoms of mental illness and how

TABLE 7.2   Methods of Neuroimaging

Method	Description	Considerations
Structural Imaging		
Computed tomography (CT), also called computerized axial tomography (CAT)	Uses x-ray technology to measure tissue density; is readily available, can be completed quickly, and less costly; may be used for screening, but many disease states are not clearly seen; use of contrast medium improves resolution	Contrast medium may produce allergic reactions; individuals with increased risk for contrast media complications include those with: History of previous reactions Cardiac disease Hypertension Diabetes Sickle cell disease Contraindications for use of contrast: Iodine/shellfish allergies Renal disease Pregnancy
Magnetic resonance imaging (MRI)	Uses a magnetic field to magnetize hydrogen atoms in soft tissue, changing their alignment—this creates a tiny electric signal, which can be received to produce an image; produces greater resolution than a CT, diagnosing more subtle pathologic changes	Patients may experience headaches, dizziness, and nausea; symptoms of anxiety, claustrophobia, or psychosis can increase; contraindicated when patients have: Aneurysm clips Internal electrical, magnetic, or mechanical devices, such as pacemakers Metallic surgical clips, sutures; and dental work distort the image Claustrophobia
Functional Neuroimaging		
Positron emission tomography (PET)	Uses positron emitting isotopes (very short-lived radioactive entities such as oxygen-15) to image brain functioning; isotopes are incorporated into specific molecules to study cerebral metabolism, cerebral blood flow, and specific neurochemicals	Images appear blurry, lacking anatomic detail, but have been extremely useful in research to study distribution of neuroreceptors and the action of pharmacologic agents; invasive procedure; use of radioactivity limits the number of scans done with a single individual
Single photon emission computed tomography (SPECT)	Like PET, SPECT uses radioisotopes that produce only one photon; these isotopes are readily available from commercial sources and are accessible in many clinical centers	Less resolution than the PET, but inhalation methods may be used, allowing for some repeated studies
Functional magnetic resonance imaging (fMRI)	Combines spatial resolution of MRI with the ability to image neural activity; methods are still very early in development	Requires no radiation and can be completely noninvasive; individual can be imaged many times, in different clinical states, before or after treatments; removes many of the ethical constraints when studying children and adolescents with psychiatric disorders.
Magnetic resonance spectroscopy (MRS)	Uses the same imaging equipment of the fMRI; by altering scanning parameters, signals represent specific chemicals in the brain	Noninvasive, repeatable, may be ideal for longitudinal studies, but has limited spatial resolution, especially with molecules that occur in low concentrations

medications that affect the functioning of these lobes can produce certain effects.

Frontal Lobes

The right and left frontal lobes make up about one fourth of the entire cerebral cortex and are proportionately larger in humans than in any other mammal. The precentral gyrus, the gyrus immediately anterior to the central sulcus, contains the primary motor area, or homunculi. Damage to this gyrus, or to the anterior neighboring gyri, causes spastic paralysis in the opposite side of the body. The frontal lobe also contains Broca's

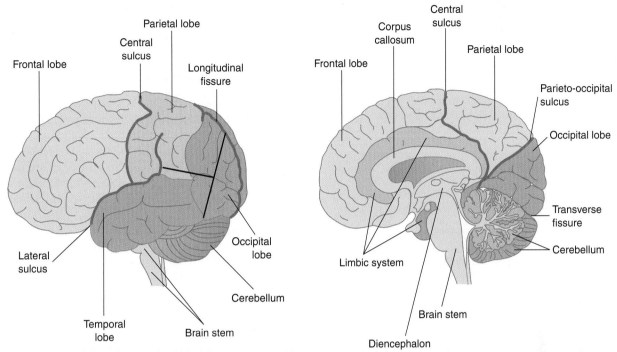

Figure 7.2 Lateral and medial surfaces of the brain. *Left*, the left lateral surface of the brain. *Right*, the medial surface of the right half of a sagittally hemisected brain.

area, which controls the motor function of speech. Damage to Broca's area produces expressive aphasia, or difficulty with the motor movements of speech. The frontal lobes are also thought to contain the highest or most complex aspects of cortical functioning, which collectively make up a large part of what we call personality. Working memory is an important aspect of frontal lobe function, including the ability to plan and initiate activity with future goals in mind. Insight, judgment, reasoning, concept formation, problem-solving skills, abstraction, and self-evaluation are all abilities that are modulated and affected by the action of the frontal lobes. These skills are often referred to as *executive functions* because they modulate more primitive impulses through numerous connections to other areas of the cerebrum. When normal frontal lobe functioning is altered, executive functioning is decreased, and modulation of impulses can be lost, leading to changes in mood and personality. Text Box 7-1 describes how altered frontal lobe functioning can affect mood and personality.

Parietal Lobes

The postcentral gyrus, immediately behind the central sulcus, contains the primary somatosensory area (Fig. 7-3). Damage to this area and neighboring gyri results in deficits in discriminative sensory function, but not in the ability to perceive sensory input. The posterior areas of the parietal lobe appear to coordinate visual and somatosensory information. Damage to this area produces complex sensory deficits, including neglect of contralateral sensory stimuli and spatial relationships. The parietal lobes contribute to the ability to recognize objects by touch, calculate, write, recognize fingers of the opposite hands, draw, and organize spatial directions, such as how to travel to familiar places.

Temporal Lobes

The temporal lobes contain the primary auditory and olfactory areas. Wernicke's area, located at the posterior aspect of the superior temporal gyrus, is primarily responsible for receptive speech. The temporal lobes also integrate sensory and visual information involved in control of written and verbal language skills as well as visual recognition. The hippocampus, an important structure discussed later, lies in the internal aspects of each temporal lobe and contributes to memory. Other internal structures of this lobe are involved in the modulation of mood and emotion.

Occipital Lobes

The primary visual area is located in the most posterior aspect of the occipital lobes. Damage to this area results in a condition called *cortical blindness*. In other words, the retina and optic nerve remain intact, but the individual is unable to see. The occipital lobes are involved in many aspects of visual integration of information, including color vision, object and facial recognition, and the ability to perceive objects in motion.

TEXT BOX 7.1

Frontal Lobe Syndrome

In the 1860s, Phineas Gage became a famous example of frontal lobe dysfunction. Mr. Gage was a New England railroad worker who had a thick iron-tamping rod propelled through his frontal lobes by an explosion. He survived, but suffered significant changes in his personality. Mr. Gage, who had previously been a capable and calm supervisor, began to show impatience, labile mood, disrespect for others, and frequent use of profanity after his injury (Harlow, 1868).

Similar conditions are often called *frontal lobe syndrome*. Symptoms vary widely from individual to individual. In general, after damage to the dorsolateral (upper and outer) areas of the frontal lobes, the symptoms include a lack of drive and spontaneity. With damage to the most anterior aspects of the frontal lobes, the symptoms tend to involve more changes in mood and affect, such as impulsive and inappropriate behavior.

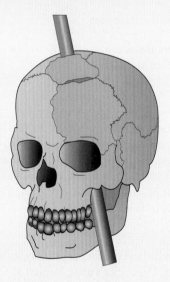

The skull of Phineas Gage, showing the route the tamping rod took through his skull. The angle of entry of the rod shot it behind the left eye and through the front part of the brain, sparing regions that are directly concerned with vital functions like breathing and heartbeat.

Association Cortex

Although not a lobe, the association cortex is an important area that allows the lobes to work in an integrated manner. Areas of one lobe of the cortex often share functions with an area of the adjacent lobe. When these neighboring nerve fibers are related to the same sensory modality, they are often referred to as *association areas*. For example, an area in the inferior parietal, posterior temporal, and anterior occipital lobes integrates visual, somatosensory, and auditory information to provide the abilities required for basic academic skills. These areas,

along with numerous connections beneath the cortex, are part of the mechanisms that allow for the human brain to work as an integrated whole.

Subcortical Structures

Beneath the cortex are layers of tissue composed of the axons of cell bodies. The axon tissue forms pathways that are surrounded by glia, a fatty or lipid substance, which have a white appearance and give these layers of neuron axons their name—*white matter*. Structures inside the hemispheres, beneath the cortex, are considered subcortical. Many of these structures, essential in the regulation of emotions and behaviors, play important roles in our understanding of mental disorders. Figure 7-4 provides a coronal section view of the gray matter, white matter, and important subcortical structures.

Basal Ganglia

The **basal ganglia** are subcortical gray-matter areas in both the right and the left hemisphere that contain many cell bodies or nuclei. The basal ganglia are involved with motor functions and association in both the learning and the programming of behavior or activities that are repetitive and, done over time, become automatic. The basal ganglia have many connections with the cerebral cortex, thalamus, midbrain structures, and spinal cord. Damage to portions of these nuclei may produce changes in posture or muscle tone. In addition, damage may produce abnormal movements, such as twitches or tremors. The primary subdivisions of the basal ganglia are the putamen, globus pallidus, and caudate.

Limbic System

The **limbic system** is essential to understanding the many hypotheses related to psychiatric disorders and emotional behavior in general. Basic emotions, needs, drives, and instinct begin and are modulated in the limbic system. Hate, love, anger, aggression, and caring are basic emotions that originate within the limbic system. Not only does the limbic system function as the seat of emotions, but also, because emotions are often generated based on our personal experiences, the limbic system is involved with aspects of memory. Hypothesized changes in the limbic system play a significant role in many theories of major mental disorders, including schizophrenia, depression, and anxiety disorders (discussed in later chapters). The limbic system is called a "system" because it comprises several small structures that work in a highly organized way. These structures include the hippocampus, thalamus, hypothalamus, amygdala, and limbic midbrain nuclei. See Figure 7-5 for identification and location of the structures within the limbic system and their relationship to other common CNS structures.

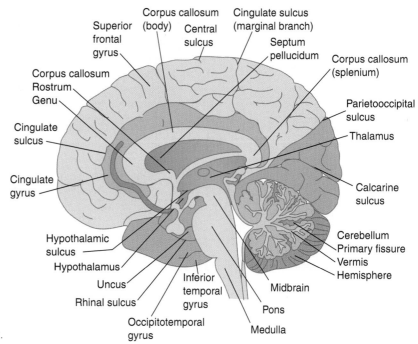

FIGURE 7.3 Gyri and Sulci of the cortex.

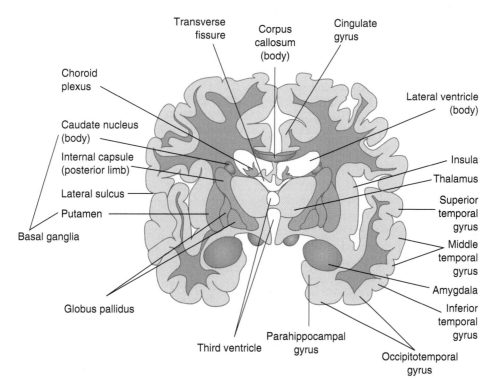

FIGURE 7.4 Coronal section of the brain illustrating the corpus callosum, basal ganglia, and lateral ventricles.

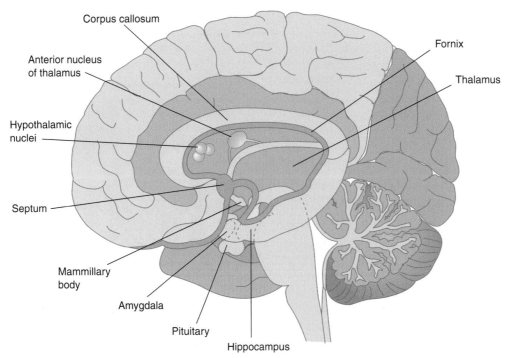

FIGURE 7.5 The structures of the limbic system are integrally involved in memory and emotional behavior. Theories link changes in the limbic system to many major mental disorders, including schizophrenia, depression, and anxiety disorders.

Hippocampus

The **hippocampus** is involved in storing information, especially the emotions attached to a memory. Our emotional response to memories and our association with other related memories are functions of how information is stored within the hippocampus. Although memory storage is not limited to one area of the brain, destruction of the left hippocampus impairs verbal memory, and damage to the right hippocampus results in difficulty with recognition and recall of complex visual and auditory patterns. Deterioration of the nerves of the hippocampus and other related temporal lobe structures found in Alzheimer's disease produces the disorder's hallmark symptoms of memory dysfunction.

Thalamus

The thalamus can be considered the relay-switching center of the brain. It functions as a regulatory structure to relay all sensory information, except smell, that is sent to the CNS from the PNS. From the thalamus, the sensory information is then relayed mostly to the cerebral cortex. The thalamus accomplishes its relay and regulatory function by filtering incoming information and determining what to pass on or not pass on to the cortex. In this fashion, the thalamus prevents the cortex from becoming overloaded with too much sensory stim-

ulus. The thalamus is thought to play a part in controlling electrical activity in the cortex. Because of its primary relay function, damage to a very small area of the thalamus may produce deficits in a large number of cortical functions, producing abnormalities of behaviors.

Hypothalamus

Basic human activities, such as sleep–rest patterns, body temperature, and physical drives like hunger and sex, are regulated by another part of the limbic system that rests deep within the brain and is called the hypothalamus. Dysfunction of this structure, whether from disorders or as a consequence of the adverse effect of drugs used to treat mental illness, produces common psychiatric symptoms such as appetite and sleep problems. Nerve cells within the hypothalamus secrete hormones such as antidiuretic hormone, which when sent to the kidneys, accelerates the reabsorption of water, and oxytocin, which acts on smooth muscles to promote contractions, particularly within the walls of the uterus. Because cells within the nervous system produce these hormones, they are often referred to as **neurohormones** and form a communication mechanism through the bloodstream to control organs that are not directly connected to nervous system structures. The pituitary gland, often called the *master gland*, is directly connected by thousands of neurons that attach it to the ventral aspects of the hypothalamus. Together with the pituitary gland, the hypothalamus functions as one of the primary regulators of many aspects of the endocrine system. Its functions are involved in control of visceral activities, such as body temperature, arterial blood pressure, hunger, thirst, fluid balance, gastric motility, and gastric secretions.

Amygdala

The amygdala is directly connected to more primitive centers of the brain involving the sense of smell. It has numerous connections to the hypothalamus and lies adjacent to the hippocampus. The amygdala provides an emotional component to memory and is involved in modulation of aggression and sexuality. Impulsive acts of aggression and violence have been linked to dysregulation of the amygdala, and erratic firing of the nerve cells in the amygdala has become a focus of investigation in bipolar affective disorders (see Chap. 20).

Limbic Midbrain Nuclei

The limbic midbrain nuclei are a collection of neurons, including the ventral tegmental area and the locus ceruleus, that appears to play a role in the biologic basis of addiction. Sometimes referred to as the pleasure center or reward center of the brain, the limbic midbrain nuclei function to reinforce chemically certain behaviors, ensuring their repetition. Emotions such as feeling satisfied with good food, the pleasure of nurturing young, and the enjoyment of sexual activity originate in the limbic midbrain nuclei. The reinforcement of activities such as nutrition, procreation, and nurturing young are all primitive aspects of ensuring the survival of a species. When functioning in abnormal ways, the limbic midbrain nuclei can begin to reinforce unhealthy or risky behaviors, such as drug abuse. Exploration of this area of the brain is in its infancy but offers promising potential new insights into the treatment of addictions.

Other Important Central Nervous System Structures

The extrapyramidal motor system is a bundle of nerve fibers connecting the thalamus to the basal ganglia and cerebral cortex. Muscle tone, common reflexes, and automatic voluntary motor functioning, such as walking, are controlled by this nerve track. Dysfunction of this motor track can produce hypertonicity in muscle groups. In Parkinson's disease, the cells that compose the extrapyramidal motor system are severely affected, producing many involuntary motor movements. A number of medications, which will be discussed in Chapter 8, affect this system as well.

The pineal body is located above and medial to the thalamus. Because the pineal gland easily calcifies, it can be visualized in neuroimaging scans and often is a medial landmark. Its functions remain somewhat of a mystery, despite long knowledge of its existence. It contains secretory cells that emit the neurohormone melatonin as well as other substances. These hormones are thought to have a number of regulatory functions within the endocrine system. Information received from light–dark sources control release of melatonin, which has been associated with sleep and emotional disorders (see Chap. 26). In addition, a modulation of immune function has been postulated for melatonin from the pineal gland.

The locus ceruleus is a tiny cluster of neurons whose fan out and innervate almost every part of the brain, including most of the cortex, the thalamus and hypothalamus, cerebellum, and the spinal cord. Just one neuron from cus ceruleus can connect to more than a quarter-million other neurons. Although it is very small, because of its wide-ranging neuronal connections, this tiny ure has influence in the regulation of attention, time perception, sleep–rest cycles, arousal, learning, pain, and mood and seems most involved with information processing of new, unexpected, and novel experiences. It has been hypothesized to explain part of the mystery of why individuals become addicted to substances and seek out risky behaviors, despite awareness of negative consequences.

The brain stem can be found beneath the thalamus and is composed of the midbrain, pons, and medulla. In addition to many important life-sustaining functions, nuclei of numerous neural pathways to the cerebrum are located in the brain stem. They are significantly involved in the mediation of symptoms of emotional dysfunction. These nuclei are also the primary source of production of several neurochemicals, such as serotonin, commonly associated with psychiatric disorders. Table 7-3 summarizes some of the key related nuclei.

The cerebellum can be found in the posterior aspect of the skull, beneath the cerebral hemispheres. This large structure is an important center for control of movements and postural adjustments. To regulate postural balance and positioning, the cerebellum receives information from all parts of the body, including muscles, joints, skin, and visceral organs, as well as from many parts of the CNS.

Closely associated with the spinal cord, but not lying entirely within its column, is the **autonomic nervous system**, a subdivision of the PNS. It was originally given this name for being independent of conscious thought, that is, automatic. However, it does not necessarily function as autonomously as the name indicates. This system contains efferent (nerves moving away from the CNS), or motor system neurons, which affect target organs such as cardiac muscle, smooth muscle, and the glands.

TABLE 7.3   Classic and Putative Neurotransmitters, Their Distribution and Proposed Functions

Neurotransmitter	Cell Bodies	Projections	Proposed Function
Acetylcholine			
Dietary precursor: choline	Basal forebrain Pons Other areas	Diffuse throughout the cortex, hippocampus Peripheral nervous system	Important role in learning and memory Some role in wakefulness, and basic attention Peripherally activates muscles and is the major neuro-chemical in the autonomic system
Monoamines			
Dopamine Dietary precursor: tyrosine	Substantia nigra Ventral tegmental area Arcuate nucleus Retina, olfactory bulb	Striatum (basal ganglia) Limbic system and cerebral cortex Pituitary	Involved in involuntary motor movements Some role in mood states, pleasure components in reward systems, and complex behavior such as judgment, reasoning, and insight
Norepinephrine Dietary precursor: tyrosine	Locus ceruleus Lateral tegmental area and others throughout the pons and medulla	Very widespread throughout the cortex, thalamus, cerebellum, brain stem, and spinal cord Basal forebrain, thalamus, hypothalamus, brain stem, and spinal cord	Proposed role in learning and memory, attributing value in reward systems, fluctuates in sleep and wakefulness Major component of the sympathetic nervous system responses, including "fight or flight"
Serotonin Dietary precursor: tryptophan	Raphe nuclei Others in the pons and medulla	Very widespread throughout the cortex, thalamus, cerebellum, brain stem, and spinal cord	Proposed role in the control of appetite, sleep, mood states, hallucinations, pain perception, and vomiting
Histamine Precursor: histidine	Hypothalamus	Cerebral cortex Limbic system Hypothalamus Found in all mast cells	Control of gastric secretions, smooth muscle control, cardiac stimulation, stimulation of sensory nerve endings, and alertness
Amino acids			
GABA	Derived from glutamate without localized cell bodies	Found in cells and projections throughout the central nervous system (CNS), especially in intrinsic feedback loops and interneurons of the cerebrum Also in the extrapyramidal motor system and cerebellum	Fast inhibitory response post-synaptically, inhibits the excitability of the neurons and therefore contributes to seizure, agitation, and anxiety control
Glycine	Primarily the spinal cord and brain stem	Limited projection, but especially in the auditory system and olfactory bulb Also found in the spinal cord, medulla, midbrain, cerebellum, and cortex	Inhibitory Decreases the excitability of spinal motor neurons but not cortical
Glutamate	Diffuse	Diffuse, but especially in the sensory organs	Excitatory Responsible for the bulk of information flow

TABLE 7.3 **Classic and Putative Neurotransmitters, Their Distribution and Proposed Functions** (Continued)

Neurotransmitter	Cell Bodies	Projections	Proposed Function
Neuropeptides			
Endogenous opioids, (ie, endorphins, enkephalins)	A large family of neuropeptides, which has three distinct subgroups, all of which are manufactured widely throughout the CNS	Widely distributed within and outside of the CNS	Suppresses pain, modulates mood and stress Likely involvement in reward systems and addiction Also may regulate pituitary hormone release Implicated in the pathophysiology of diseases of the basal ganglia
Melatonin One of its precursors: serotonin	Pineal body	Widely distributed within and outside of the CNS	Secreted in dark and suppressed in light, helps regulate the sleep–wake cycle as well as other biologic rhythms
Substance P	Widespread; significant in the raphe system and spinal cord	Spinal cord, cortex, brain stem and especially sensory neurons associated with pain perception	Involved in pain transmission, movement, and mood regulation
Cholecystokinin	Predominates in the ventral tegmental area of the midbrain	Frontal cortex where it is often colocalized with dopamine Widely distributed within and outside of the CNS	Primary intestinal hormone involved in satiety, also has some involvement in the control of anxiety and panic

Compiled from Cooper, J. R., Bloom, F. E., & Roth, R. H. (1991). *The biochemical basis of neuropharmacology* (6th ed.). New York: Oxford University Press; Kaplan, H. I., & Sadock, B. J. (Eds.). (1995). *Comprehensive textbook of psychiatry/VI* (6th ed.). Baltimore: Williams & Wilkins; and Rang, H. P., & Dale, M. M. (1991). *Pharmacology* (2nd ed.). New York: Churchill Livingstone.

It also contains afferent nerves, which are sensory and function to conduct information from these organs back into the CNS. The autonomic nervous system is further divided into the sympathetic and parasympathetic nervous systems. These systems, although peripheral, are included here because they are involved in the emergency, or "fight-or-flight," response as well as the peripheral actions of many medications (see Chap. 8). Figure 7-6 illustrates the innervations of various target organs by the autonomic nervous system. Table 7-4 identifies the actions of the sympathetic and parasympathetic nervous systems on various target organs.

NEUROPHYSIOLOGY OF THE CENTRAL NERVOUS SYSTEM

Neurons and Nerve Impulses

At their most basic level, the human brain and connecting nervous system are composed of billions of cells (Fig. 7-7). Most are connective and supportive glial cells with ancillary functions in the nervous system. About 10 billion cells are nerve cells, or neurons, responsible for receiving, organizing, and transmitting information. Each neuron has a cell body, or soma, which holds the nucleus containing most of the cell's genetic information. The soma also includes other organelles, such as ribosomes and endoplasmic reticulum, both of which carry out protein synthesis; the Golgi apparatus, which contains enzymes to modify the proteins for specific functions; vesicles, which transport and store proteins; and lysosomes, responsible for degradation of these proteins. Located throughout the neuron, mitochondria, containing enzymes and often called the "cell's engine," are the site of many energy-producing chemical reactions. These cell structures provide the basis for numerous secretions by which neurons communicate.

It is not just the sheer number of neurons that accounts for the complexities of the brain, but rather the enormous number of neurochemical interconnections and interactions between neurons. A single motor neuron in the spinal cord may receive signals from more than 10,000 sources of interconnections with other nerves. Although most neurons have only one axon, which varies in length and conducts impulses away from the soma, each

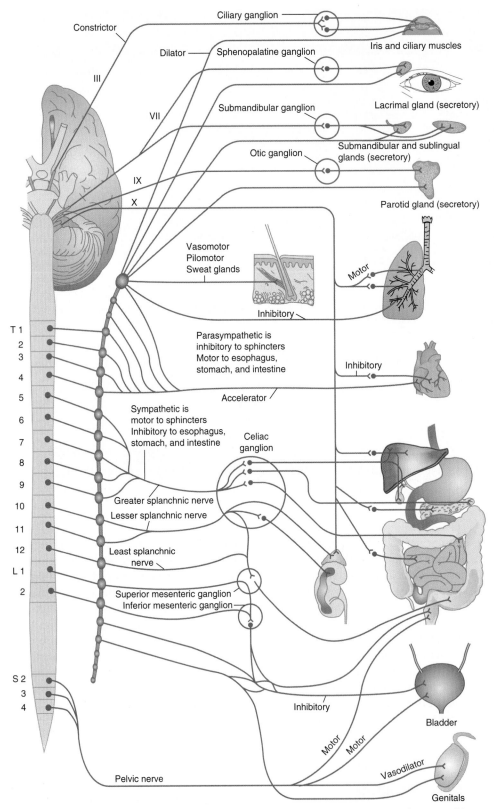

FIGURE 7.6 Diagram of the autonomic nervous system. Note that many organs are innervated by both sympathetic and parasympathetic nerves. (Adapted from Schaffe, E. E., & Lytle, I. M. [1980]. *Basic physiology and anatomy*. Philadelphia: J. B. Lippincott).

TABLE 7.4   Peripheral Organ Response in the Autonomic Nervous System

Effector Organ	Sympathetic Response (Mostly Norepinephrine)	Parasympathetic Response (Acetylcholine)
Eye		
• Iris sphincter muscle	Dilation	Constriction
• Ciliary muscle	Relaxation	Accommodation for near vision
Heart		
• Sinoatrial node	Increased rate	Decrease in rate
• Atria	Increased contractility	Decrease in contractility
• Atrioventricular node	Increased contractility	Decrease in conduction velocity
Blood vessels	Constriction	Dilation
Lungs		
• Bronchial muscles	Relaxation	Bronchoconstriction
• Bronchial glands		Secretion
Gastrointestinal tract		
• Motility and tone	Relaxation	Increased
• Sphincters	Contraction	Relaxation
• Secretion		Stimulation
Urinary bladder		
• Detrusor muscle	Relaxation	Contraction
• Trigone and sphincter	Contraction	Relaxation
Uterus	Contraction (pregnant) Relaxation (nonpregnant)	Variable
Skin		
• Pilomotor muscles	Contraction	No effect
• Sweat glands	Increased secretion	No effect
Glands		
• Salivary, lachrymal		Increased secretion
• Sweat		Increased secretion

has numerous dendrites, receiving signals from other neurons. Because axons may branch as they terminate, they have multiple contacts with other neurons as well.

Nerve signals are prompted to fire by a variety of chemical or physical stimuli. This firing produces an electrical impulse. The cell's membrane is a double layer of phospholipid molecules with embedded proteins. Some of these proteins provide water-filled channels through which inorganic ions may pass (Fig. 7-8). Each of the common ions—sodium, potassium, calcium, and chloride—has its own specific molecular channel. These channels are voltage gated and thus open or close in response to changes in the electrical potential across the membrane. At rest, the cell membrane is polarized with a positive charge on the outside and about a 270-millivolt charge on the inside, owing to the resting distribution of sodium and potassium ions. As potassium passively diffuses across the membrane, the sodium pump uses energy to move sodium from the inside of the cell against a concentration gradient to maintain this distribution. An action potential, or nerve impulse, is generated as the membrane is depolarized and a threshold value is reached, which triggers the opening of the voltage-gated sodium channels, allowing sodium to

surge into the cell. The inside of the cell briefly becomes positively charged and the outside negatively charged. Once initiated, the action potential becomes self-propagating, opening nearby sodium channels. This electrical communication moves into the soma from the dendrites or down the axon by this mechanism.

Synaptic Transmission

For one neuron to communicate with another, the electrical process described thus far must change to a chemical communication. The synaptic cleft, a junction between one nerve and another, is the space where the electrical intracellular signal becomes a chemical extracellular signal. Various substances are recognized as the chemical messengers between neurons. **Neurotransmitters** are small molecules that directly and indirectly control the opening or closing of ion channels. Neuromodulators are chemical messengers that make the target cell membrane or postsynaptic membrane more or less susceptible to the effects of the primary neurotransmitter. Some of these neurochemicals are synthesized quickly from dietary precursors, such as tyrosine or tryptophan, by enzymes inside the cytoplasm of the

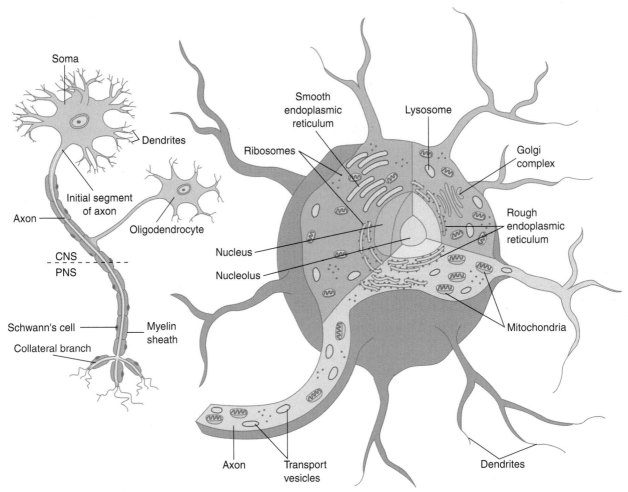

FIGURE 7.7 Cell body and organelles of an axon.

neuron, but most synthesis occurs in the terminals or the neuron itself. Some neurochemicals can reduce the membrane potential and enhance the transmission of the signal between neurons. These chemicals are called *excitatory neurotransmitters*. Other neurochemicals have the opposite effect, slowing down nerve impulses, and these substances are called *inhibitory neurotransmitters*.

As the electrical action potential reaches the ends of the axon, called *terminals*, calcium ion channels are opened, causing an influx of Ca^{++} ions into the neuron. This increase in calcium stimulates the release of neurotransmitters into the **synapse**. Rapid signaling between neurons requires a ready supply of neurotransmitter. These neurotransmitters are stored in small vesicles

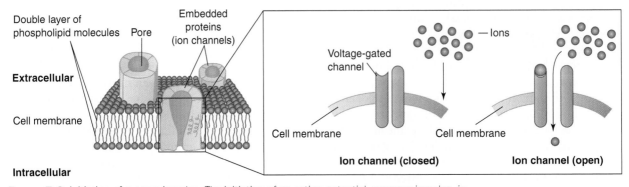

FIGURE 7.8 Initiation of a nerve impulse. The initiation of an action potential, or nerve impulse, involves the opening and closing of the voltage-gated channels on the cell membrane and the passage of ions into the cell. The resulting electrical activity sends communication impulses from the dendrites or axon into the body.

grouped near the cell membrane at the end of the axon. Because nerve terminals do not have the ability to manufacture proteins, the transmitters that fill these vesicles are small molecules, such as the bioamines (dopamine and norepinephrine) or the amino acids (glutamate or γ-aminobutyric acid [GABA]). The actions of these small molecules are discussed later in this chapter. When stimulated, the vesicles containing the neurotransmitter fuse with the cell membrane, and the neurotransmitter is released into the synapse (Fig. 7-9). The neurotransmitter then crosses the synaptic cleft to a receptor site on the postsynaptic neuron and stimulates adjacent neurons. This is the process of neuronal communication.

Embedded in the postsynaptic membrane are a number of proteins that act as **receptors** for the released neurotransmitters. The "lock-and-key" analogy has often been used to describe the fit of a given neurotransmitter to its receptor site. Each neurotransmitter has a specific receptor, or protein, for which it and only it will fit. The target cell, when stimulated by the

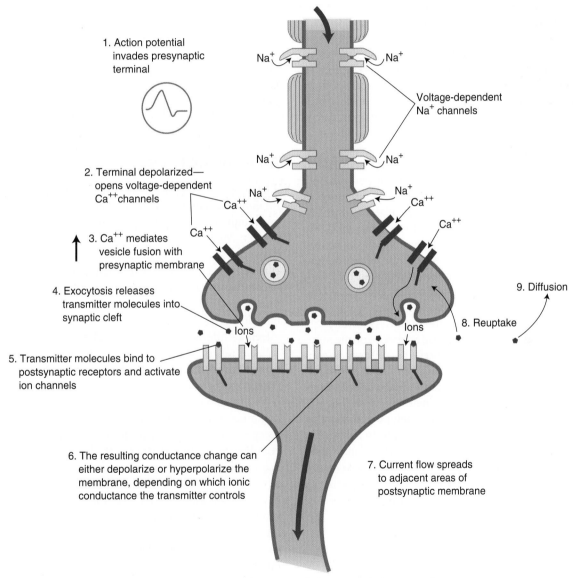

FIGURE 7.9 Synaptic transmission. The most significant events that occur during synaptic transmission: (1) the action potential reaches the presynaptic terminal; (2) membrane depolarization causes Ca++ terminals to open; (3) Ca++ mediates fusion of the vesicles with the presynaptic membrane; (4) transmitter molecules are released into the synaptic cleft, by exocytosis; (5) transmitter molecules bind to postsynaptic receptors and activate ion channels; (6) conductance changes cause an excitatory or inhibitory postsynaptic potential, depending on the specific transmitter; (7) current flow spreads along the postsynaptic membrane; (8) transmitter remaining in the synaptic cleft returns to the presynaptic terminal by reuptake; or (9) diffuses into the extracellular fluid. (Adapted and reproduced with permission from Schauf, C., Moffett, D., & Moffett, S. [1990]. *Human physiology*. St. Louis: Times Mirror/Mosby.)

neurotransmitter, will then respond by evoking its own action potential and either producing some action common to that cell or acting as a relay to keep the message moving throughout the CNS. This pattern of the electrical signal from one neuron, converted to chemical signal at the synaptic cleft, picked up by an adjacent neuron, again converted to an electrical action potential, and then to a chemical signal, occurs billions of times a day in billions of different brain cells. It is this electrical-chemical communication process that allows the structures of the brain to function together in a coordinated and organized manner.

When the neurotransmitter has completed its interaction with the postsynaptic receptor and stimulated that cell, its work is done, and it needs to be removed. It can be removed by natural diffusion away from the area of high neurotransmitter concentration at the receptors by being broken down by enzymes in the synaptic cleft, or through reuptake through highly specific mechanisms into the presynaptic terminal. Many psychopharmacologic agents, particularly antidepressants, act by blocking the reuptake of the neurotransmitters, thereby increasing the available amount of chemical messenger. Presynaptic binding sites for neurotransmitters not only may serve as reuptake mechanisms but also may act as autoreceptors to perform various regulatory functions on the flow of neurotransmitter into the synapse. When these presynaptic autoreceptors are saturated, the neuron knows it is time to slow down or stop the release of neurotransmitter. The neurotransmitters taken back into the presynaptic neuron may be stored in vesicles for later re-release, or they may be broken down by enzymes, such as monoamine oxidase, and removed entirely.

The primary steps in synaptic transmission are summarized in Figure 7-10. The preceding discussion contains only the basic mechanisms of neuronal communication. Many other factors that modulate or contribute to the communication between neurons are only beginning to be discovered. Examples include peptides that are released into the synapse and thought to behave like neurotransmitters or that also can appear in combination with another neurotransmitter. These peptides, known as *co-transmitters*, are believed to have a modulatory effect on the primary neurotransmitter.

Changing Receptor Sensitivity

Both presynaptic and postsynaptic receptors have the capacity to change, developing either a greater-than-usual response to the neurotransmitter, known as *supersensitivity*, or a less-than-usual response, called *subsensitivity*. These changes in sensitivity of the receptor are most commonly caused by the impact of a drug on a receptor site or by disease that affects the normal functioning of a receptor site. Drugs can affect the sensitivity of the receptor by altering the strength of attraction or affinity of a receptor for the neurotransmitter, by changing the efficiency with which the receptor activity translates the message inside the receiving cell, or by decreasing over time the number of receptors. These mechanisms may account for the long-term, sometimes severely adverse, effects of psychopharmacologic drugs, the loss of effectiveness of a given medication, or the loss of effectiveness of a medication after repeated use in treating recurring episodes of a psychiatric disorder. Disease may cause a change in the normal number or function of receptors, thereby altering their sensitivity (Friedman, 2000). It has been hypothesized that depression is caused by a reduction in the normal number of certain receptors, leading to an abnormality in their sensitivity to neurotransmitters such as serotonin and norepinephrine. A decreased response to continued stimulation of these receptors is usually referred to as *desensitization* or *refractoriness*. This suspected subsensitivity, referred to as *down-regulation* of the receptors.

Receptor Subtypes

The nervous system uses many different neurochemicals for communication, and each specific chemical messenger requires a specific receptor on which the chemical can act. More than 100 different chemical messengers have been identified, with new ones being frequently uncovered as research on the functioning of the brain becomes more and more precise. In addition to the sheer number of receptors needed to accommodate these chemicals, the neurotransmitters may produce different effects at different synaptic sites. The ability of a neurotransmitter to produce different actions is, in part, because of the specialization of its receptors. The different receptors for each neurochemical messenger are referred to as receptor subtypes for the chemical. Each major neurotransmitter has several different subtypes of receptors, allowing the neurotransmitter to have different effects in different areas of the brain. For example, dopamine, a common neurotransmitter discussed in the next section, has five different subtypes of receptors that have been identified so far. Numbers usually name the receptor subtypes. In the example of dopamine, the various subtypes of receptors are called D1, D2, D3, and so on. Understanding the different subtypes helps in understanding both the effects and side effects of medications used to treat mental disorders.

Neurotransmitters

Many substances have been identified as possible chemical messengers, but not all chemical messengers are neurotransmitters. Classic neurotransmitters are those

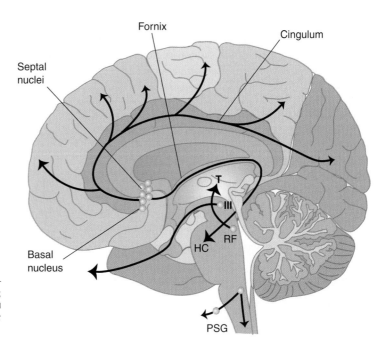

FIGURE 7.10 Cholinergic pathways. HC, hippocampal formation; PSG, parasympathetic ganglion cell; RF, reticular formation; T, thalamus. (Adapted from Nolte, J., & Angevine, J. [1995]. *The human brain: In photographs and diagrams*. St. Louis: Mosby.)

that meet certain criteria agreed on by neuroscientists. The traditional criteria include the following:

1. The chemical is synthesized inside the neuron.
2. The chemical is present in the presynaptic terminals.
3. The chemical is released into the synaptic cleft and causes a particular effect on the postsynaptic receptors.
4. An exogenous form of the chemical administered as a drug causes identical action.
5. The chemical is removed from the synaptic cleft by a specific mechanism.

Neurotransmitters can be classified into categories that reflect chemical similarities of the neurotransmitter. Common practice classifies certain chemicals as neurotransmitters even though their ability to meet the strict traditional definition may be incomplete. For the purposes of this section, the classification of neurotransmitters will use this common system of classifying neurotransmitters. Common categories of neurotransmitters include cholinergic neurotransmitters, biogenic amine neurotransmitters (sometimes called *monoamines* or *bioamines*), amino acid neurotransmitters, and neuropeptide neurotransmitters.

Neurotransmitters are also classified by whether their action causes physiologic activity to occur or to stop occurring. All of the neurotransmitters commonly involved in the development of mental illness or that are affected by the drugs used to treat these illnesses are excitatory except one, GABA, which is inhibitory. The significance of this concept will be

discussed in more detail as each neurotransmitter is described in the following section.

Neurotransmitters are found wherever there are neurons. Whereas neurons are contained in both the CNS and the PNS, psychiatric mental disorders occur in the CNS, and therefore, neurotransmitters will be discussed from the perspective of the CNS.

Cholinergic

Acetylcholine (ACh) is the primary cholinergic neurotransmitter. Found in the greatest concentration in the PNS, ACh provides the basic synaptic communication for the parasympathetic neurons and part of the sympathetic neurons, which send information to the CNS. Understanding both the action of Ach and the receptor subtypes for this neurotransmitter assists psychiatric mental health nurses in understanding the complex side effects of common medications used to treat mental disorders.

Cholinergic neurons, so named because they contain ACh, follow diffuse projections throughout the cerebral cortex and limbic system, arising primarily from cell bodies in the base of the frontal lobes. Pathways from this region also project throughout the hippocampus (Fig. 7-10). These connections suggest that ACh is involved in higher intellectual functioning and memory. Individuals who have Alzheimer's disease or Down's syndrome often exhibit patterns of cholinergic neuron loss in regions innervated by these pathways (such as the hippocampus), which may contribute to their memory difficulties and other cognitive deficits. Some cholinergic neurons are afferent to these areas bringing information from the limbic system, highlighting the role that ACh plays in communicating emotional state to the cerebral cortex. Ach is an excitatory neurotransmitter, meaning that when released into a synapse, it causes the postsynaptic neuron to initiate some action.

The subtypes of ACh receptors are divided into two groups: the muscarinic receptors and the nicotinic receptors. Many psychiatric medications are anticholinergic agents, which block the effects of the muscarinic ACh receptors. This blocking effect of Ach causes common side effects such as dry mouth, blurred vision, constipation, urinary retention, and tachycardia, which are seen in many psychotropic medications. Excessive blockade of ACh can cause confusion and delirium, especially in elderly patients, as discussed in Chapter 31.

Biogenic Amines

The **biogenic amines** (bioamines) consist of small molecules manufactured in the neuron that contain an amine group, hence the name. These include dopamine, norepinephrine, and epinephrine, which are all synthesized from the amino acid tyrosine; serotonin, which is synthesized from tryptophan; and histamine, manufactured from histidine. Of all the neurotransmitters, the biogenic amines are most central to current hypotheses of psychiatric disorders and are therefore described individually in more detail.

Dopamine. Dopamine is an excitatory neurotransmitter found in distinct regions of the CNS and is involved in cognition, motor, and neuroendocrine functions. Dopamine levels are decreased in Parkinson's disease, and abnormally high levels of production of dopamine have been associated with the illness of schizophrenia, discussed in more detail in Chapter 18.

Dopamine pathways are distinct neuronal areas within the CNS in which the neurotransmitter dopamine predominates. Three major dopaminergic pathway have been identified.

The first, the mesocortical or mesolimbic pathway, originates in the ventral tegmental area and projects into the medial aspects of the cortex and the medial aspects of the limbic system inside the temporal lobes, including the hippocampus and amygdala. This pathway has major effects on cognition, including such functions as judgment, reasoning, insight, social conscience, motivation, the ability to generalize learning, and reward systems in the human brain. It contributes to some of the highest seats of cortical functioning. It also strongly influences emotions and has projections that affect memory and auditory reception. Abnormalities in this pathway have been associated with the illness schizophrenia.

The second major dopaminergic pathway begins in the substantia nigra and projects into the basal ganglia, parts of which are known as the *striatum*. Therefore, this pathway is called the *nigrostriatal pathway*. This influences the extrapyramidal motor system, which serves the voluntary motor system and allows involuntary motor movements. Destruction of dopaminergic neurons in this pathway has been associated with Parkinson's disease.

The third dopamine pathway originates from projections of the mesolimbic pathway and continues into the hypothalamus, which then projects into the pituitary gland. Therefore, this pathway, called the *tuberoinfundibular pathway*, has an impact on endocrine function and other functions such as metabolism, hunger, thirst, sexual function, circadian rhythms, digestion, and temperature control. Figure 7-11 illustrates the dopaminergic pathways.

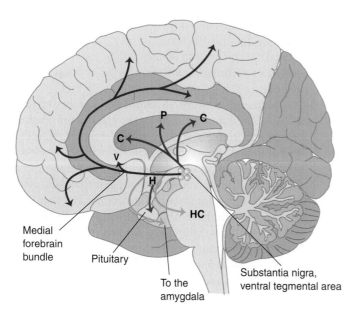

Medial forebrain bundle

Pituitary

To the amygdala

Substantia nigra, ventral tegmental area

FIGURE 7.11 Dopaminergic pathways. C, caudate nucleus; H, hypothalamus; HC, hippocampal formation; P, putamen; S, striatum; V, ventral striatum. (Adapted from Nolte, J., & Angevine, J. [1995]. *The human brain: In photographs and diagrams.* St. Louis: Mosby.)

Scientists have identified at least five subtypes of dopamine receptors in the CNS. These subtypes are distributed differently throughout the brain. For example, the D1 subtype receptor, and its related receptor subtype, D5, predominate in areas that affect memory and emotions such as the cortex, hippocampus, and amygdala. They have not been detected in the substantia nigra. D2 receptors are richly distributed throughout neurons in the extrapyramidal motor system, whereas D4 receptors are richly distributed in the frontal cortex, with few in the nigrostriatal system. Antipsychotic medications, discussed in Chapter 8, act by blocking the effects of dopamine at the receptor sites. Many of the medications that are most effective on the acute symptoms of psychosis have a strong attraction or affinity for D2 receptors and a weaker but modest correlation with D1 receptors. Because D2 receptors predominate in the nigrostriatal pathway, medications that have a weaker blockade of D2 will have fewer extrapyramidal motor system effects. Side effects and adverse effects from the involuntary motor system are at times extremely debilitating to individuals. Based on the assumption that these dopamine receptor subtypes have different functions in the CNS, new medications are being designed to affect more predominantly one subtype than another, presumably avoiding effects on systems containing other subtypes and thus avoiding potential side effects of the medication. Researchers are attempting to develop new antipsychotic medications that avoid or minimize the effects on D2 and, therefore, diminish the occurrence of extrapyramidal effects.

Norepinephrine. Norepinephrine was first demonstrated to be the primary neurotransmitter of the peripheral sympathetic nervous system in 1946. Whereas it is commonly found in the PNS, norepinephrine is critical to CNS functioning as well. Norepinephrine is an excitatory neurochemical that plays a major role in the generation and maintenance of mood states. Decreased norepinephrine has been associated with depression, and excessive norepinephrine has been associated with manic symptoms (Montgomery, 2000). Because norepinephrine is so heavily concentrated in the terminal sites of sympathetic nerves, it can be released quickly to ready the individual for a fight-or-flight response to threats in the environment. For this reason, norepinephrine is thought to play a role in the development of the physical symptoms of anxiety. Nerve tracts and pathways containing predominantly norepinephrine are called noradrenergic and are less clearly delineated than the dopamine pathways. In the CNS, noradrenergic neurons originate in the locus ceruleus, where more than half of the noradrenergic cell bodies are located. Because the locus ceruleus is one of the major timekeepers of the human body, norepinephrine is involved in sleep and

wakefulness. From the locus ceruleus, noradrenergic pathways ascend into the neocortex, spread diffusely (Fig. 7-12), and enhance the ability of neurons to respond to whatever input they may be receiving. Also, norepinephrine appears to be involved in the process of reinforcement, which facilitates learning. Noradrenergic pathways innervate the hypothalamus and as such are involved to some degree in endocrine function. Anxiety disorders and depression are examples of psychiatric illnesses in which dysfunction of the noradrenergic neurons may be involved. Table 7-4 lists the effects of ACh on various organs in the parasympathetic system.

Serotonin. Serotonin (also called 5-hydroxytryptamine, or 5-HT) is primarily an excitatory neurotransmitter that is diffusely distributed within the cerebral cortex, limbic system, and basal ganglia of the CNS. Serotonergic neurons also project into the hypothalamus and cerebellum. Figure 7-13 illustrates serotonergic pathways. Serotonin plays a role in emotions, cognition, sensory perceptions, and essential biologic functions, such as sleep and appetite. During the rapid-eye-movement (REM) phase of sleep, the dream state, serotonin concentrations decrease, and muscles subsequently relax. Serotonin is also involved in the control of food intake, hormone secretion, sexual behavior, thermoregulation, and cardiovascular regulation. Some serotonergic fibers reach the cranial blood vessels within the brain and the pia mater, where they have a vasoconstricting effect. The potency of some new migraine medications is related to

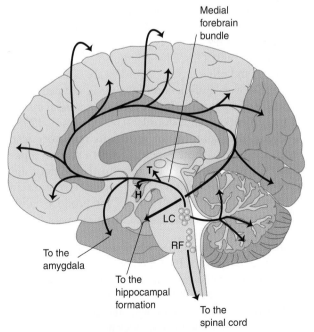

FIGURE 7.12 Noradrenergic pathways. H, hypothalamus; LC, locus ceruleus; RF, reticular formation; T, thalamus. (Adapted from Nolte, J., & Angevine, J. [1995]. *The human brain: In photographs and diagrams.* St. Louis: Mosby.)

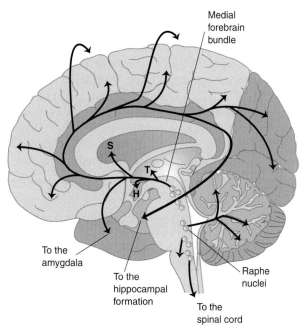

Medial
forebrain
bundle

S

T

H

To the
amygdala

To the
hippocampal
formation

Raphe
nuclei

To the
spinal cord

FIGURE 7.13 Serotonergic pathways. H, hypothalamus; S, septal nuclei; T, thalamus. (Adapted from Nolte, J., & Angevine, J. [1995]. *The human brain: In photographs and diagrams*. St. Louis: Mosby.)

their ability to block serotonin transmission in the cranial blood vessels. Descending serotonergic pathways are important in central pain control. Depression and insomnia have been associated with decreased levels of 5-HT, whereas mania has been associated with increased 5-HT. Some of the most well-known antidepressant medications, such as Prozac and Zoloft, which are discussed in more depth in Chapter 8, function by raising serotonin levels within certain areas of the CNS (Keck & Arnold, 2000). Obsessive-compulsive disorder, panic disorder, and other anxiety disorders are believed to be associated with dysfunction of the serotonin pathways, explaining why these antidepressants have several uses in the treatment of mental disorders (Battaglia et al., 1998).

Numerous subtypes of serotonin receptors also exist, and each of these appears to have a distinct function. 5-HT1a is involved in the control of anxiety, aggression, and depression. Drugs such as lysergic acid diethylamide (LSD) affect 5-HT2 and produce hallucinatory effects.

Histamine. Histamine has only recently been identified as a neurotransmitter. Its cell bodies originate predominantly in the hypothalamus and project to all major structures in the cerebrum, brain stem, and spinal cord. Its functions are not well known, but it appears to have a role in autonomic and neuroendocrine regulation. Many psychiatric medications can block the effects of histamine postsynaptically and produce side effects such as sedation, weight gain, and hypotension.

Amino Acids

Amino acids are the building blocks of proteins and have many roles in intraneuronal metabolism. In addition, amino acids can function as neurotransmitters in as many as 60% to 70% of the synaptic sites in the brain. Amino acids are the most prevalent neurotransmitters. Virtually all of the neurons in the CNS are activated by excitatory amino acids, such as glutamate, and inhibited by inhibitory amino acids, such as GABA and glycine. Many of these amino acids coexist with other neurotransmitters.

γ-Aminobutyric Acid. GABA is the primary inhibitory neurotransmitter for the CNS. The pathways of GABA exist almost exclusively in the CNS, with the largest GABA concentrations in the hypothalamus, hippocampus, basal ganglia, spinal cord, and cerebellum. GABA functions in an inhibitory role in control of spinal reflexes and cerebellar reflexes. It has a major role in the control of neuronal excitability through the brain. In addition, GABA has an inhibitory influence on the activity of the dopaminergic nigrostriatal projections. GABA also has interconnections with other neurotransmitters. For example, dopamine inhibits cholinergic neurons, and GABA provides feedback and balance. Dysregulation of GABA and GABA receptors has been associated with anxiety disorders, and decreased GABA activity is involved in the development of seizure disorders.

Two specific subtype receptors have been identified for GABA: A and B. Two classes of medication, benzodiazepine antianxiety drugs and sedative-hypnotic barbiturate drugs, work because of their affinity for GABA receptor sites. Interest in the beneficial effects of these drugs has lead to increased interest in GABA receptor sites. Researchers are finding endogenous chemicals that bind to the same receptor sites as benzodiazepines and serve as natural inhibitory regulators (Little et al., 1998).

Glutamate. Glutamate is the most widely distributed excitatory neurotransmitter. It is the main transmitter in the associational areas of the cortex. Glutamate occurs in a number of pathways from the cortex to the thalamus, pons, striatum, and spinal cord. In addition, glutamate pathways have a number of connections with the hippocampus. It has been hypothesized that some glutamate receptors may play a role in the long-lasting enhancement of synaptic activity. In turn, in the hippocampus, this enhancement may have a role in learning and memory. Too much glutamate is harmful to neurons, and considerable interest has emerged regarding its neurotoxic effects. Degeneration of glutamate neurons has been implicated in the development of Huntington's disease and schizophrenia.

Neuropeptides

Peptides are short chains of amino acids. **Neuropeptides** exist in the CNS and have a number of important roles as neurotransmitters, neuromodulators, or neurohormones. Neuropeptides were first thought to be pituitary hormones, such as adrenocorticotropin, oxytocin, and vasopressin, or hypothalamic-releasing hormones (eg, corticotropin-releasing hormone and thyrotropin-releasing hormone [TRH]). However, when an endogenous morphine-like substance was discovered in the 1970s, the term *endorphin*, or endogenous morphine, was introduced. Although the amino acids and monoamine neurotransmitters can be produced directly from dietary precursors in any part of the neuron, neuropeptides are, almost without exception, synthesized from messenger RNA in the cell body. Currently two, types of neuropeptides have been identified. Opioid neuropeptides, such as endorphins, enkephalins, and dynorphins, function in endocrine functioning and pain suppression. The nonopioid neuropeptides, such as substance P and somatostatin, play roles in pain transmission as well as in endocrine functioning.

There are considerable variations in the distribution of individual neuropeptides, but some areas are especially rich in cell bodies containing neuropeptides. These areas include the amygdala, striatum, hypothalamus, raphe nuclei, brain stem, and spinal cord. Many of the interneurons of the cerebral cortex contain neuropeptides, but there are considerably fewer in the thalamus and almost none in the cerebellum.

By now, it should be obvious that the complexities of neuronal transmission are enormous. Psychiatric nurses have a significant role in the assessment of symptoms and in the administering and monitoring of medications, and knowledge of this system is essential. Even a single dose of a drug affecting this system may cause relief of symptoms or have adverse effects. The actions of psychopharmacologic agents and related nursing responsibilities are discussed more fully in Chapter 8. In addition, many nursing interventions designed to effect changes in such functions as sleep, diet, stress management, exercise, and mood modulation affect these neurotransmitters and neuropeptides, directly or indirectly. More research is clearly needed to understand the biopsychosocial aspects of nursing care.

NEW FIELDS OF STUDY

As the complexity of the nervous system and its interrelationship with other body systems and the environment have become more fully understood, new fields of study have emerged. From the discussion of neuroanatomy and neurotransmitters, it is logical to deduce that understanding the endocrine system and its interrelationship with the nervous system is essential. Although it has long been observed that individuals under stress have compromised immune systems and are more likely to acquire common diseases, only recently have changes in the immune system been noted as endemic to some psychiatric illnesses. In addition, as biologic rhythms have become more fully understood and defined, new information suggests that dysfunction of these rhythms may not only result from a psychiatric illness but also contribute to its development. Therefore, the following sections provide a brief overview of psychoendocrinology, psychoimmunology, and chronobiology.

Psychoendocrinology

Psychoendocrinology examines the relationships among the nervous system, endocrine system, and behavior. Messages are conveyed within the endocrine system primarily by hormones, and neurohormones are those substances excreted by special neurons within the nervous system. Neurohormones are cellular substances secreted into the bloodstream and transported to a site where they exert their effect. There are several types of hormones, but peptides are by far the most common hormones within the CNS.

The hypothalamus sends and receives information through the pituitary, which then communicates with structures in the peripheral aspects of the body. Figure 7-14 presents an example of the communication of the anterior pituitary with a number of organs and structures. Axes, the structures within which the neurohormones are providing messages, are the most often studied aspect of the neuroendocrine system. These axes always involve a feedback mechanism. For example, the hypothalamus–pituitary–thyroid axis regulates the release of thyroid hormone by the thyroid gland using TRH hormone from the hypothalamus to the pituitary and thyroid-stimulating hormone (TSH) from the pituitary to the thyroid. Figure 7-15 illustrates the hypothalamic–pituitary–thyroid axis. The hypothalamic–pituitary–gonadal axis regulates estrogen and testosterone secretion through luteinizing hormone and follicle-stimulating hormone.

Interest in the study of psychoendocrinology is heightened by a number of endocrine disorders that produce psychiatric symptoms. Addison's disease (hypoadrenalism) produces depression, apathy, fatigue, and occasionally psychosis. Hypothyroidism produces depression and some anxiety. Administration of steroids can cause depression, hypomania, irritability, and in some cases, psychosis. Some psychiatric disorders have been associated with endocrine system dysfunction. For example, some individuals with mood disorders show evidence of dysregulation in adrenal, thyroid, and growth hormone axes.

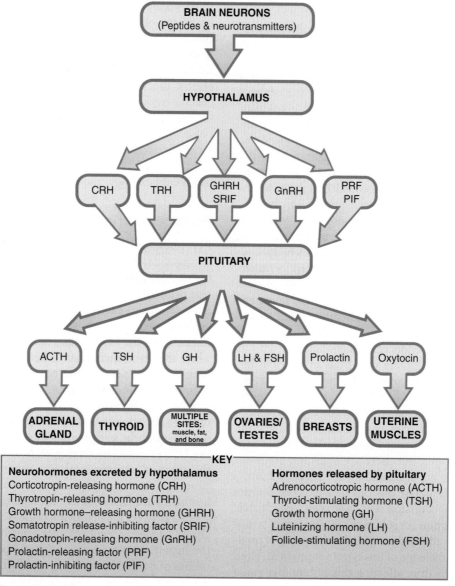

FIGURE 7.14 Hypothalamic and pituitary communication system. The neurohormonal communication system between the hypothalamus and the pituitary exerts effects on many organs and systems.

Psychoimmunology

Psychoimmunology involves the study of immunology as it relates to emotions and behavior. The immune system protects the body from foreign pathogens. Overactivity of the immune system can occur in autoimmune diseases such as systemic lupus erythematous (SLE), allergies, or anaphylaxis. Underactivity may result from cancer and serious infections, such as is the case with AIDS. Evidence suggests that the nervous system regulates many aspects of immune function. Specific immune system dysfunctions may result from damage to the hypothalamus, hippocampus, or pituitary and may produce symptoms of psychiatric disorders. Figure 7-16 illustrates the interaction between stress and the immune system. This figure also demonstrates the true biopsychosocial nature of the complex interrelationship of the nervous system, the endocrine system, the immune system, and environmental or emotional stress.

Immune dysregulation may also be involved in the development of psychiatric disorders. This can occur by allowing neurotoxins to affect the brain, by damaging neuroendocrine tissue, or by damaging tissues in the brain at locations such as the receptor sites. Some antidepressants have been thought to have antiviral effects. Symptoms of diseases such as depression may follow an occurrence of serious infection, and prenatal exposure to infectious organisms has been associated with the development of schizophrenia. Stress and conditioning also have specific effects on suppression

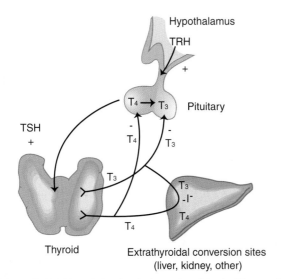

Hypothalamus

TRH

+

T₄ → T₃   Pituitary

TSH
+

−   −
T₄   T₃

T₃

T₃
-I⁻

T₄

T₄

Thyroid   Extrathyroidal conversion sites
(liver, kidney, other)

FIGURE 7.15 Hypothalamic–pituitary–thyroid axis. The regulation of thyroid-stimulating hormone (TSH or thyrotropin) secretion by the anterior pituitary. Positive effects of thyrotropin-releasing hormone (TRH) from the hypothalamus and negative effects of circulating triiodothyronine (T_3) and T_3 from intrapituitary conversion of thyroxine (T_4).

of immune function (Friedman, 2000). Individuals with SLE often experience symptoms of depression, insomnia, nervousness, and confusion. Although there is still much to learn about the relationship of psychiatric disorders and the immune system, it is clear that psychiatric–mental health nurses must develop and implement interventions designed to enhance immune function in psychiatric patients.

Chronobiology

Chronobiology involves the study and measure of time structures or biologic rhythms. Some rhythms have a **circadian cycle**, or 24-hour cycle, whereas others, such as the menstrual cycle, operate in different time frames. Rhythms exist in the human body to control endocrine secretions, sleep–wake, body temperature, neurotransmitter synthesis, and more. These cycles may become deregulated and may begin earlier than usual, known as a *phase advance*, or later than usual, known as a *phase delay*. **Zeitgebers** are specific events that function as time givers or synchronizers and that result in the setting of biologic rhythms. Light is the most common example of an external zeitgeber. The suprachiasmatic nucleus of the hypothalamus is an example of an internal zeitgeber. Figure 7-17 provides a schematic representation of the far-reaching influence and interrelationships of the suprachiasmatic nucleus as well as the involvement of another internal zeitgeber, the pineal body. Some theorists believe that psychiatric disorders may be the result of one or more biologic rhythm dysfunctions. For example, depression may be, in part, a phase ad-

vance disorder, including early morning awakening and decreased time of onset of REM sleep. Seasonal affective disorder may be the result of shortened exposure to light during the winter months. Exposure to specific artificial light often improves symptoms of fatigue, overeating, hypersomnia, and depression. More of this information is discussed in Chapter 20.

Diagnostic Approaches

In recent years, a great deal of attention has turned to the study of the biologic basis of psychiatric disorders. Although this research has provided greatly increased understanding of neural transmission and psychopharmacology, an additional focus has been to find biologic markers for many of the disorders previously thought to have only a functional component. **Biologic markers** may include laboratory test results, neuropathologic changes, or other diagnostic tests that occur only in the presence of the psychiatric disorder. These markers serve to increase diagnostic certainty and may have predictive value, whereby preventive interventions might forestall or avoid the onset of symptoms. In addition, biologic markers could provide indications of the most effective treatments and information about prognosis that could be used in treatment planning. The psychiatric–mental health nurse should be aware of the most common avenues of study so that information, limitations, and results can be knowledgeably discussed with the patient.

Laboratory Tests

For many years, laboratory tests have attempted to measure levels of neurotransmitters and other CNS substances in the bloodstream. Many of the metabolites of neurotransmitters can be found in the urine and CSF as well. These measures, however, have had only limited utility in understanding what is happening in the brain. Levels of neurotransmitters and metabolites in the bloodstream or urine do not necessarily equate with levels in the CNS. In addition, availability of the neurotransmitter or metabolite does not predict the availability of the neurotransmitter in the synapse where it must act, or directly relate to the receptor sensitivity. Nonetheless, numerous research studies have focused on changes in neurotransmitters and metabolites in blood, urine, and CSF. These studies have provided clues but remain without conclusive predictive value and are therefore not routinely used.

Another laboratory approach to the study of some of the psychiatric disorders is the challenge test. A challenge test has been most often used in the study of panic disorders. These tests are usually conducted by intravenously administering a chemical known to produce a specific set of psychiatric symptoms. For example,

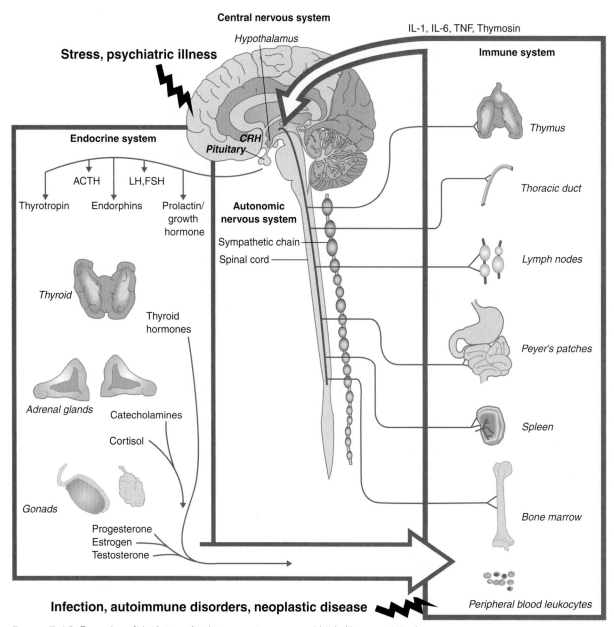

Central nervous system

Hypothalamus

IL-1, IL-6, TNF, Thymosin

Stress, psychiatric illness

Immune system

Thymus

Endocrine system

CRH
Pituitary

ACTH   LH,FSH

Thyrotropin   Endorphins   Prolactin/
growth
hormone

Thoracic duct

**Autonomic
nervous system**

Sympathetic chain

Spinal cord

Lymph nodes

Thyroid

Thyroid
hormones

Peyer's patches

Adrenal glands   Catecholamines

Cortisol

Spleen

Gonads

Progesterone
Estrogen
Testosterone

Bone marrow

Infection, autoimmune disorders, neoplastic disease

Peripheral blood leukocytes

FIGURE 7.16 Examples of the interaction between stress or psychiatric illness and the immune system through the endocrine system. CRH, corticotropin-releasing hormone; IL, interleukin; TNF, tumor necrosis factor; ACTH, adrenocorticotropic hormone; LH, luteinizing hormone; FSH, follicle-stimulating hormone.

lactate or caffeine may be used to induce the symptoms of panic in a person who has panic disorder. The biologic response of the individual is then monitored. These tests have been developed primarily for research purposes. However, endocrine stimulation tests, such as the TRH stimulation test and the dexamethasone suppression test, have found some limited clinical utility.

In the TRH stimulation test, an individual is given TRH and the TSH blood level is measured over time, usually at intervals over 3 to 4 hours. The hypothyroid patient has an elevation of TSH. A blunted TRH stim-

ulation test has been proposed as a biologic marker for major depression; however, only about 30% of individuals with major depression show the response. In addition, the blunted TRH stimulation test result has been found in a number of other psychiatric disorders.

The dexamethasone suppression test involves the administration of 1 mg dexamethasone at 11 PM. Cortisol blood levels are then measured. In the healthy individual, dexamethasone suppresses cortisol levels, but numerous studies have suggested that there is nonsuppression in certain types of depression. Typically, the

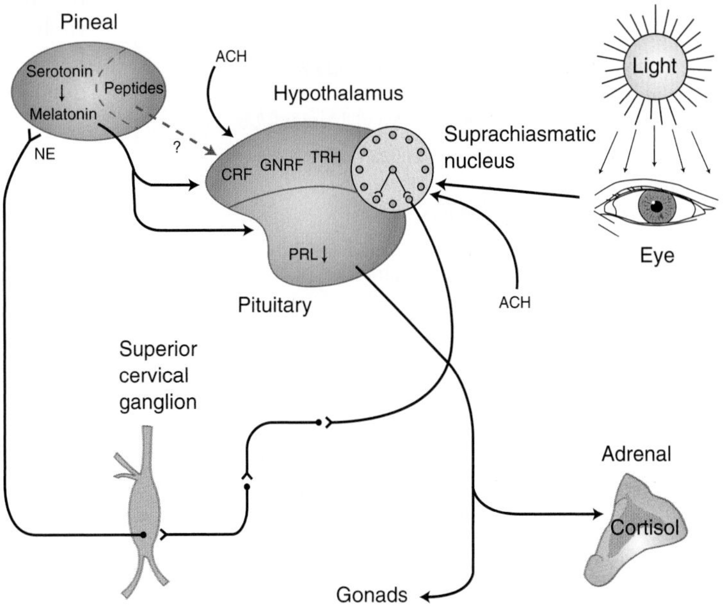

FIGURE 7.17 The far-reaching influence of the suprachiasmatic nucleus (SCN). The SCN is drawn as a clock, indicating its function as an internal time-keeper. It receives information through a neuronal pathway from the retina of the eye to the hypo-thalamus (the retinohypothalamic pathway) where the SCN is located. The hypothalamus also receives feedback from another internal timekeeper, the pineal body, through a complex pathway that regulates secretion of melatonin. This information influences the hypothalamus-releasing hormones and the pituitary hormones, which regulate the go-nads, adrenals, and other endocrine glands. ACH, acetylcholine; CRH, corticotropin-releasing hor-mone; GNRF, gonadotropin-releasing factor; TRH thyrofropin-releasing hormone; NE, norepinephrine.

cortisol levels are drawn before administration of the dexamethasone and then again at 8 AM, 4 PM, and 11 PM on the following day. Many medical conditions, such as diabetes mellitus, obesity, infection, pregnancy, recent surgery, and medications such as carbamazepine or high doses of estrogen, may alter the test results, producing false-positive results. Overall, a positive result, or abnor-mal nonsuppression, appears to indicate major depres-sion, but a negative result does not rule out depression. Considerable controversy continues over the clinical usefulness of this test.

Although no commonly used laboratory tests exist that directly confirm the presence of a mental disorder, laboratory tests are still an active part of the overall care and assessment of psychiatric patients. Many physical conditions mimic the symptoms of mental illness, and many of the medications used to treat psychiatric illness can produce health problems. For these reasons, the routine care of psychiatric patients includes the use of laboratory tests such as complete blood counts, thyroid studies, electrolytes, hepatic enzymes, and other evalu-ative tests. Psychiatric–mental health nurses need to be familiar with these procedures and assist patients in un-derstanding the use and implications of such tests.

Neurophysiologic Procedures

Electroencephalography. EEG is the oldest of the currently used methods for understanding what is hap-pening inside the living human brain. Developed in the 1920s by Hans Berger, an EEG measures electrical ac-tivity in the uppermost nerve layers of the cortex. Usu-ally, 16 electrodes are placed on the patient's scalp, and recording pens draw the waves measured from each elec-

trode on paper. Until the use of CT in the 1970s, the EEG was the only method for identifying brain abnor-malities. It remains the simplest and most noninvasive method for identifying some disorders.

An EEG may be used in psychiatry to differentiate possible causes of the patient's symptoms. For example, some types of seizure disorders, such as temporal lobe epilepsy, head injuries, or tumors, may present with pre-dominantly psychiatric symptoms. In addition, meta-bolic dysfunction, delirium, dementia, altered levels of consciousness, hallucinations, and dissociative states may require EEG evaluation.

Amplitude, frequency, and distribution of waveforms are among the many important aspects of an EEG recording. For example, frequency is measured in cy-cles per second, or hertz (Hz). These frequencies are typically divided into four categories: alpha activity (8 to 12 Hz), beta activity (13 to 20 Hz or more), theta ac-tivity (4 to 8 Hz), and delta activity (less than 4 Hz). Normal awake adults have mostly alpha activity when their eyes are closed. With their eyes open, beta activity begins to occur. In sleep, theta and delta activity develop. A normal awake adult does not have theta or delta activ-ity. Figure 7-18 demonstrates the variation of frequen-cies in a single-channel EEG across the stages of sleep.

Spikes and wave-pattern changes are indications of brain abnormalities. Spikes may be the focal point from which a seizure occurs. However, abnormal activity is often not discovered on a routine EEG while the indi-vidual is awake. For this reason, additional methods are sometimes used. Nasopharyngeal leads may be used to get physically closer to the limbic regions. The patient may be exposed to a flashing strobe light while the

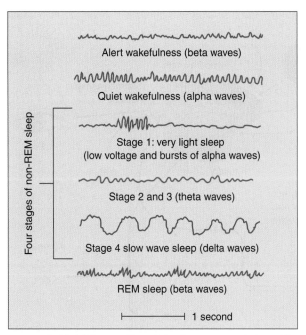

Four stages of non-REM sleep

Alert wakefulness (beta waves)

Quiet wakefulness (alpha waves)

Stage 1: very light sleep
(low voltage and bursts of alpha waves)

Stage 2 and 3 (theta waves)

Stage 4 slow wave sleep (delta waves)

REM sleep (beta waves)

1 second

FIGURE 7.18 EEG recording of the four stages of sleep. The beta waves of REM sleep, commonly referred to as *dream sleep*, resemble the beta waves of alert wakefulness on the EEG.

examiner looks for activity that is not in phase with the flashing light or may be asked to hyperventilate for 3 minutes to induce abnormal activity if it exists. Sleep deprivation may also be used. This involves keeping the patient awake throughout the night before the EEG evaluation. The patient may then be drowsy and fall asleep during the procedure. Abnormalities are more likely to occur when the patient is asleep. Sleep may also be induced using medication; however, many medications change wave patterns on an EEG. For example, the benzodiazepine class of drugs increases the rapid and fast beta activity. Many other prescribed and illicit drugs, such as lithium, which increases theta activity, can cause EEG alterations. In addition to reassuring, preparing, and educating the patient for the examination, the nurse should carefully assess the history of substance use and report this information to the examiner. If a sleep deprivation EEG is to be done, caffeine or other stimulants that might assist the patient in staying awake should be withheld because they may change the EEG patterns.

Polysomnography. Polysomnography is a special procedure that involves recording of the EEG throughout a night of sleep. This test is usually conducted in a sleep laboratory. Other information is usually collected at the same time, including an electrocardiogram and an electromyogram. Blood oxygenation, body movement, body temperature, and other information may be collected as well, especially in research settings. This procedure is

usually conducted for the evaluation of sleep disorders, such as sleep apnea, enuresis, or somnambulism (see Chap. 26). However, sleep pattern changes are frequently researched in mental disorders as well.

In the normal sleep of an adult, there are two major divisions of sleep patterns: REM sleep and non-REM sleep. During non-REM sleep, an individual passes through four stages as alpha activity on the EEG is gradually replaced by theta and slow delta activity. In REM sleep, commonly referred to as dream sleep, the EEG resembles that of an awake and alert person. On falling asleep, a healthy adult gradually descends through stages 1 through 4 and enters the first episode of REM sleep about 90 minutes after falling asleep. This cycle repeats about five times during the night, with gradually increasing amounts of time spent in REM sleep. See Chapter 26 for a more complete discussion of normal and abnormal sleep.

Research has found that normal sleep divisions and stages are affected by many factors, including drugs, alcohol, general medical conditions, and psychiatric disorders. For example, REM latency, the length of time it takes an individual to enter the first REM episode, is shortened in depression. Reduced delta sleep is also observed. These findings have been replicated so frequently that some researchers consider them to be biologic markers for depression.

Other Neurophysiologic Methods. Evoked potentials (EPs), also called event-related potentials, use the same basic principles as an EEG. They measure changes in electrical activity of the brain in specific regions as a response to a given stimulus. Electrodes placed on the scalp measure a large waveform that stands out after the administration of repetitive stimuli, such as a click or flash of light. There are several different types of EPs to be measured, depending on the sensory area affected by the stimulus, the cognitive task required, or the region monitored, any of which can change the length of time until the wave occurrence. EPs are used extensively in psychiatric research. In clinical practice, EPs are used primarily in the assessment of demyelinating disorders, such as multiple sclerosis.

Various computer programs have been developed to translate EEG and EP information by calculating the amount of voltage present in each area of the brain and representing this information on gray-scale or color-scale maps, indicating areas of more or less activity for a given frequency. One example is brain electrical activity mapping (BEAM), which involves a 20-electrode EEG that generates computerized maps of the brain's electrical activity. Using these techniques, some studies have found a slowing of electrical activity in the frontal lobes of individuals who have schizophrenia. These findings are consistent with other findings that suggest a "hypofrontality" in schizophrenia (see Chap. 18). Although these procedures are limited primarily to research, some investigators believe that clinical applications are close at hand.

Overall, neurophysiologic methods provide only rough approximations compared with current structural and functional neuroimaging techniques. Yet they provide a snapshot measured in milliseconds rather than the minutes and even hours of other methods. Today, they remain the most noninvasive, inexpensive, and accessible examinations of brain activity.

Genetics

It has long been noted that family members of individuals who have one of the major mental disorders, such as schizophrenia, mania, or panic disorder, have an increased risk for developing the same disorder. For this reason, the study of genetics has been of great interest in psychiatry. This endeavor is also a source of great controversy. Embedded in this controversy are the arguments of nature versus nurture. In other words, is there a gene that passes on the disorder, or is it the family interactions and environment that induce the disorder? An overview of how genetics are studied may be helpful in addressing this issue.

On a molecular level, DNA is known to be the basic carrier of genetic information. A gene, in its classic sense, is actually a segment of the DNA. There are estimated to be 100,000 genes in the human genome, but the brain accounts for only about 1% of the body's DNA. The nucleus of every cell contains the same basic genetic information, but not all genes are expressed within that cell. Simply consider the vast number of different cell types within the nervous system alone. Then consider all of the possible cell types in the human body. Finally, consider that each cell must produce a number of different proteins that make up unique cell features such as the vesicles, neuromodulators, and neuroreceptors. The idea that one gene encodes information for the amino acid sequence of only one protein is a dramatic and inaccurate oversimplification. In addition, gene expression is not a static condition, fixed at some point in neuronal development. Individual nerve cells may respond to neurochemical changes outside of the cell, producing different proteins for adaptation to the new environment. Obviously, gene expression is extremely complex.

Transmission

The study of molecular genetics in psychiatric disorders is in its infancy. Most genetic studies in psychiatry involve tracing a given disorder within groups of people. This falls under the rubric of population genetics, which involves the analysis of genetic transmission of a trait within families and populations to determine risk and pattern of transmission. Risk for the occurrence of a given disorder in the general population is often compared with risk within families and between groups of relatives. These studies rely on the initial identification of an individual who has the disorder under investigation and include the following principal methods:

- Family studies analyze the occurrence of a disorder in first-degree relatives (biologic parents, siblings, and children), second-degree relatives (grandparents, uncles, aunts, nieces, nephews, and grandchildren), and so on.
- Twin studies analyze the presence or absence of the disorder in pairs of twins. The measure of similarity of occurrence is called the *concordance rate*.
- Adoption studies compare the risk for developing the illness in offspring raised in different environments. The strongest inferences may be drawn from studies that involve children separated from their parents at birth.

Few traits are completely heritable. Color blindness and blood type are examples of traits that exist as a result of heredity alone. Monozygotic twins have identical genetic contributions; therefore, both would have color blindness or the same blood type if they expressed that gene. This is 100% concordance. If a disorder is completely unrelated to genetics, then monozygotic twins would have the same concordance rates as dizygotic (fraternal) twins, who share roughly the same proportion of genes that ordinary siblings do—50%. If there is a genetic contribution with environmental influence, the concordance rates would be less than 100% for monozygotic twins but significantly greater than for dizygotic twins. Such is the case with several psychiatric disorders.

When considering information regarding risks for genetic transmission of psychiatric disorders, it is important to remember several key points:

- Psychiatric disorders may have been described and labeled quite differently across generations. Errors in diagnosis may also have occurred.
- Similar psychiatric symptoms may have considerably different causes.
- Genes that are present in an individual may not always cause the appearance of the trait.
- Several genes may need to be present in an individual to produce a given trait or disorder.
- A biologic cause is not necessarily solely genetic in origin, and an environmental influence is not solely psychological.

Although no conclusive evidence exists for a genetic cause of most psychiatric disorders, significant evidence exists to suggest a strong genetic contribution for some

(Trippitelli et al., 1998). It is likely that more than one gene produces a psychiatric disorder and that development of the disorder results from an interaction of the genetic contributions with environmental influences. The environmental factors may include such experiences as stress, infections, poor nutrition, catastrophic loss, complications during pregnancy, and exposure to toxins.

As evidence accumulates and is reported to the public, it is likely that a psychiatric–mental health nurse will be confronted with patients or family members requesting information regarding the likelihood that they too are at risk for a psychiatric disorder. As a result, more psychiatric professionals are considering the need for skills in genetic counseling.

Risk Factors

The concept of genetic susceptibility suggests that an individual may be at increased risk for developing a psychiatric disorder. Research into **risk factors** is an important avenue of study. Some of the environmental influences listed previously may be examples of risk factors. These are events, circumstances, or demographic information that is more likely to have occurred in individuals who develop a particular psychiatric disorder. In the absence of a specific gene for the major psychiatric disorders, risk factor assessment may be a logical alternative for predicting who is more likely to develop psychiatric disorders or certain conditions, such as aggression or suicidality.

INTEGRATION OF THE BIOLOGIC, PSYCHOLOGICAL, AND SOCIAL DIMENSIONS

Basic knowledge in the neurosciences has become essential information for the practicing psychiatric nurse. In a truly holistic biopsychosocial model, all psychological and social influences interact with a complex biologic system. For example, treatment of generalized anxiety disorder would involve addressing etiologies in each of these areas (see Fig. 7-19). As research continues to increase our understanding of the biologic dimension of psychiatric disorders and mental health, nursing care will focus on human biology in increasingly sophisticated ways. Psychiatric nurses must integrate this information into all aspects of nursing management, including:

- Assessment—physical factors and environmental stressors that may contribute to the symptoms of the disorder; biologic rhythm changes; cognitive abilities that may effect or complicate interventions; and risk factors that may predict development of psychiatric symptoms or disorders
- Diagnosis—difficulties related to diet, exercise, or sleep that may change the individual's biology; quality-of-life difficulties based on biologic changes; knowledge deficits concerning the biologic basis of psychiatric disorders or treatment
- Interventions—designed to modify biologic changes and physical functioning; designed to

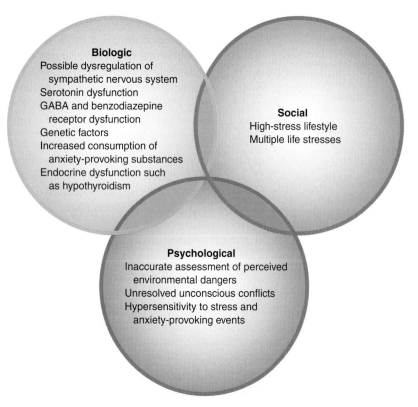

FIGURE 7.19 Biopsychosocial etiologies for patients with generalized anxiety disorders. GABA, γ-aminobutyric acid.

enhance biologic treatments; or modified to consider cognitive dysfunction related to psychiatric disorders

Summary of Key Points

➤ Neuroscientists now view behavior and cognitive function as a result of complex interactions within the central nervous system and its plasticity (ability to adapt and change).

➤ Each hemisphere of the brain is divided into four lobes: the frontal lobe, which controls motor speech function, personality, and working memory—often called the executive functions that govern one's ability to plan and initiate action; the parietal lobe, which controls the sensory functions; the temporal lobe, which contains the primary auditory and olfactory areas; and the occipital lobe, which controls visual integration of information.

➤ The structures of the limbic system are integrally involved in memory and emotional behavior. Dysfunction of the limbic system has been linked with major mental disorders, including schizophrenia, depression, and anxiety disorders.

➤ Neurons communicate with each other through synaptic transmission. Neurotransmitters excite or inhibit a response at the receptor sites and have been linked to certain mental disorders. These neurotransmitters include acetylcholine, dopamine, norepinephrine, serotonin, γ-aminobutyric acid, and glutamate.

➤ Psychoendocrinology examines the relationship between the nervous system and endocrine system and the effects of neurohormones excreted by special neurons to communicate with the endocrine system in effecting behavior. Psychoimmunology focuses on the nervous system as regulating immune function, which may play a significant role in effecting psychological states and psychiatric disorders. Chronobiology focuses on the study and measure of time structures or biologic rhythms occurring in the body and associates dysregulation of these cycles as contributing factors to the development of psychiatric disorders.

➤ Biologic markers are physical indicators of disturbances within the central nervous system that differentiate one disease process from another, such as biochemical changes or neuropathologic changes. These biologic markers can be measured by several methods of testing, including challenge tests, electroencephalography, polysomnography, evoked potentials, computed tomography scanning, magnetic resonance imaging, positron emission tomography, and single photon emission computed tomography—all of which the psychiatric nurse must be familiar with.

➤ Although no one gene has been found to produce any psychiatric disorder, for several disorders, significant evidence indicates there is genetic predisposition or susceptibility in certain individuals. For individuals who have such genetic susceptibility, the identification of risk factors is crucial in helping to plan interventions to prevent development of that disorder or to prevent certain behavior patterns, such as aggression or suicide.

Critical Thinking Challenges

1. A patient who is scheduled for magnetic resonance imaging asks how this test can possibly help explain why he is "all nerved up." He states that his friend had a "CAT scan" and he wants that instead. Think about what the nurse might do to assist this patient at this time.
2. Five different approaches to the study of neuroanatomy are discussed in this chapter. Do you believe that one of these approaches is better or more practical than another? Why or why not?
3. An individual who has experienced a small cerebrovascular accident continues to regain lost cognitive function months after the stroke. How would this be explained if the stroke did damage to her brain?
4. A patient is described as having impaired executive functioning. Consider if it would be reasonable to schedule this patient for counseling sessions at 1:00 PM weekly? Would we expect the patient to be able to keep to this schedule? Why or why not?
5. A patient who has had a right sided stroke and now cannot move their left leg. Explain why this is happening.
6. Describe what behavioral problems may be present in a patient with dysfunction of the following and analyze how dysfunction in these areas might relate to psychiatric symptoms:
   a. Basal ganglia
   b. Hippocampus
   c. Limbic system
   d. Thalamus
   e. Hypothalamus
7. Compare and contrast the functions of the sympathetic and parasympathetic nervous systems.
8. Explain the steps in synaptic transmission beginning with the action potential and ending with how the neurotransmitter no longer communicates its message to the receiving neuron.
9. Examine how a receptor's usual response to a neurotransmitter might change.
10. Analyze the significance of the discovery of receptor subtypes.

11. Explain how dopamine, norepinephrine, and serotonin all contribute to endocrine system regulation. Suggest some other transmitters that may affect endocrine function.

12. Based on the information in this chapter, examine how stress may affect emotional functions from a biologic perspective.

13. Suggest how the fields of psychoendocrinology, psychoimmunology, and chronobiology might overlap.

14. Compare the methods used to find biologic markers of psychiatric disorders reviewed in this chapter. Consider the potential risks and benefits to the patient.

15. Determine the actions you would take in preparing a patient for an MRI.

16. Explain the role of genetics within the biopsychosocial model.

REFERENCES

Battaglia, M., Bertella, S., Bajo, S., et al. (1998). Anticipation of age at onset in panic disorder. *American Journal of Psychiatry, 155*(5), 590–594.

Friedman, M. J. (2000). What might the psychobiology of post traumatic stress disorder teach us about the future approaches to pharmacotherapy. *Journal of Clinical Psychiatry, 61*(7), 44–51.

Harlow, J. M. (1868). Recovery after severe injury to the head. *Publication of the Massachusetts Medical Society, 2*, 327.

Keck, P. E., & Arnold, L. A. (2000). The serotonin syndrome. *Psychiatric Annals, 30*(5), 333–346.

Little, K. Y., McLaughlin, D. P., Zhang, L., et al. (1998) Cocaine, ethanol, and genotype effect on human midbrain serotonin transporter binding sites and mRNA levels. *American Journal of Psychiatry, 155*(2), 207–213.

Lorberbaum, J. P., Bohning, D. E., Shastri, A., et al. (1998). Functional magnetic resonance imaging (fMRI) for the psychiatrist. *Primary Psychiatry, 5*(3), 60–71.

McIntosh, K. (1998). Neuroimaging tools offer new ways to study Autism. *APA Monitor, 29*(11), 1–2.

Montgomery, S. A. (2000). Understanding depression and its treatment: Restoration of chemical balance or creation of conditions promoting recovery. *Journal of Clinical Psychiatry, 61*(6), 3–6.

Nahas, Z., George, M. S., Lorberbaum, J. P., et al. (1998). SPECT and PET in neuropsychiatry. *Primary Psychiatry, 5*(3), 52–59.

Trippitelli, C. L., Jamison, K. R., Folstein, M. F., et al. (1998). Pilot study on patient's and spouses' attitudes towards potential genetic testing for bipolar disorder. *American Journal of Psychiatry, 155*(7), 899–904.

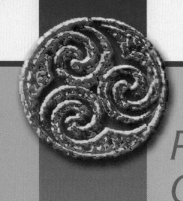

Psychopharmacology and Other Biologic Treatments

Susan McCabe

PHARMACODYNAMICS
Targets of Drug Action:
 Where Drugs Act
 Receptors
 Ion Channels
 Enzymes
 Carrier Proteins:
  Uptake Receptors
Efficacy and Potency:
 How Drugs Act
 Loss of Effect:
  Biologic Adaptation
 Target Symptoms and
  Side Effects
 Drug Toxicity

**PHARMACOKINETICS:
HOW THE BODY ACTS
ON THE DRUGS**
Absorption and Routes
 of Administration
Bioavailability
Distribution
Metabolism
Elimination
Individual Variations in
 Drug Effects

**PHASES OF
DRUG TREATMENT**
Initiation
Stabilization
Maintenance
Discontinuation

**ANTIPSYCHOTIC
MEDICATIONS**
Target Symptoms and Mechanism
 of Action
Pharmacokinetics
Depot Preparations
Side Effects, Adverse Reactions,
 and Toxicity
 Cardiovascular Side Effects
 Anticholinergic Side Effects
 Weight Gain
 Endocrine and Sexual
  Side Effects
 Blood Disorders
 Miscellaneous Side Effects
 Medication-Related
  Movement Disorders

**MOOD STABILIZERS
(ANTIMANIA MEDICATIONS)**
Lithium
 Indications and Mechanisms
  of Action
 Pharmacokinetics
 Side Effects, Adverse Reactions,
  and Toxicity
Anticonvulsants
 Indications and Mechanisms
  of Action
 Pharmacokinetics
 Side Effects, Adverse Reactions,
  and Toxicity

**ANTIDEPRESSANT
MEDICATIONS**

Indications
Pharmacokinetics and
 Mechanism of Action
Side Effects, Adverse Reactions,
 and Toxicity

**ANTIANXIETY AND SEDATIVE-
HYPNOTIC MEDICATIONS**
Benzodiazepines
 Indications and Mechanisms
  of Action
 Pharmacokinetics
 Side Effects, Adverse Reactions,
  and Toxicity
Nonbenzodiazepines

STIMULANTS
Indications and Mechanisms
 of Action
Pharmacokinetics
Side Effects, Adverse Reactions,
 and Toxicity

**DEVELOPMENT OF
NEW MEDICATIONS**

**OTHER BIOLOGIC
TREATMENTS**
Electroconvulsive Therapy
Light Therapy (Phototherapy)
Nutritional Therapies
Psychosocial Issues in the Use of
 Biologic Treatments

LEARNING OBJECTIVES

After studying this chapter, you will be able to:

➤ Explain the key role of neurotransmitter chemicals and their receptor sites in the action of psychopharmacologic medications.

➤ Explain the four action sites where current psychotropic medications work: receptors, ion channels, enzymes, and carrier proteins.

➤ Define the three properties that determine the strength and effectiveness of a medication.

➤ Describe the hypothesized mechanism of action for each class of psychopharmacologic medication.

➤ Describe the target symptoms and major side effects of various classes of psychotropic medications.

➤ Suggest appropriate nursing methods to administer medications that facilitate efficacy.

➤ Implement interventions to minimize side effects of psychopharmacologic medications.

➤ Differentiate acute and chronic medication-induced movement disorders.

➤ Identify aspects of patient teaching that nurses must implement for successful maintenance of patients using psychotropic medications.

➤ Analyze the potential benefits of other forms of somatic treatments, including electroconvulsive therapy, light therapy, and nutrition therapy.

➤ Evaluate potential causes of noncompliance and implement interventions to improve compliance with treatment regimens.

KEY TERMS

adverse reactions
affinity
agonists
akathisia
antagonists
compliance
desensitization
dystonia
efficacy
intrinsic activity
phototherapy

pseudoparkinsonism
psychopharmacology
receptor
selectivity
side effects
tardive dyskinesia
target symptoms
therapeutic index
tolerance
toxicity

The treatment of mental disorders has always been linked to assumptions about the etiology of these illnesses. In the early 1900s, Emil Kraeplin classified mental disorders on the basis of clusters of observed symptoms, providing the basic tenets of the contemporary biologic approach to understanding and treating psychiatric disorders. However, this approach fell out of favor as psychoanalytic, psychodynamic, interpersonal, and other therapies flourished, and mental disorders were assumed to have primarily a psychological etiology. In the 1950s, when it was discovered that the phenothiazine medications, such as chlorpromazine (Thorazine), relieved many of the symptoms of psychosis and iproniazid, a medication for the treatment of tuberculosis, improved depression, there was renewed interest in biologic treatments. Recent scientific and technologic developments have once again renewed awareness of the biologic basis of mental disorders, leading to a proliferation of new medications that, while acting at the cellular level, produce major behavioral and psychological change. These medications provide relief from debilitating symptoms in millions of individuals suffering from psychiatric disorders. They have become the dominant form of treatment for mental disorders and form the cornerstones of psychiatric treatment.

Most psychiatric–mental health nurses work with individuals who are receiving psychopharmacologic agents as at least part of their treatment, making knowledge of these treatments essential for effective clinical practice. As awareness of the prevalence of mental disorders increases, these medications are increasingly prescribed in primary care settings, and even nurses working in nonpsychiatric settings now need an in-depth knowledge of these medications to be able to care for their patients. Because these medications form the cornerstone of treatment for mental disorders, the American Nurses Association (ANA) formed a task force to study what nurses need to know about psychopharmacology. The task force (Scahill & Laraia, 1994) produced a report, the Psychopharmacology Guidelines for Psychiatric Mental Health Nurses, which states the following:

> The psychiatric mental health nurse involved in the care of patients who have been prescribed psychopharmacologic agents demonstrates knowledge of psychopharmacologic principles, including pharmacokinetics, pharmacodynamics, drug classification, intended and unintended effects, and related nursing implications. (American Nurses Association, 1994, p. 42)

As an integral part of the treatment team, nurses, particularly psychiatric–mental health nurses, must retain current knowledge of developing biologic or somatic treatments.

This chapter is based on the chapter in the first edition, written by Mary Ann Nihart, MA, RN, CS, Clinical Nurse Specialist, Turning Point Center, San Francisco, California; and Partner and Consultant, Professional Growth Facilitators, San Clemente, California.

*This chapter provides the reader with an understanding of the pharmacodynamics of drugs used to treat mental disorders. Pharmacodynamics is the study of the biologic actions of drugs by examining the mechanisms of action of the drug, or where and how the drugs work. Pharmacokinetics is the study of how the human body processes the drug, including absorption, distribution, metabolism, and elimination. The first part of this chapter reviews general principles of pharmacodynamics and pharmacokinetics of medications used for psychiatric reasons. This chapter assumes that the reader has a basic knowledge of organic chemistry and pharmacology. **Psychopharmacology** is the subspecialty of pharmacology that includes medications affecting the brain and behaviors used to treat psychiatric disorders. This chapter reviews the major classes of psychopharmacologic drugs used in the treatment of mental disorders, including antipsychotics, mood stabilizers, antidepressants, antianxiety medications, and stimulants, and provides a basis for understanding the specific biologic treatments of psychiatric disorders that are described more fully in this text within later chapters related to each disorder.*

Medications used to treat mental disorders all affect the central nervous system (CNS) at the synaptic level. For this reason, this chapter focuses on a basic understanding of synaptic physiology as it relates to the actions of psychotropic medications. This basic understanding allows the psychiatric–mental health nurse to accept the role and responsibilities of administering medications, monitoring and treating side effects, and educating the patient and family, which is crucial to successful psychopharmacologic therapy. Because the primary focus of all biologic therapy is improvement in the quality of life for individuals experiencing psychiatric disorders, other biologic treatments (sometimes referred to as somatic treatments) are used. These include electroconvulsive therapy, light therapy, and nutritional therapy and are further discussed in this chapter.

PHARMACODYNAMICS

A comparatively small amount of medication can have a significantly large impact on cells, their function, and resulting behavior. When tiny molecules of medication are compared with the vast amount of cell surface in the human body, the fraction seems disproportionate. And yet the drugs used to treat mental disorders often have profound effects on behavior. To understand how this occurs, one needs to understand both where and how drugs work.

Targets of Drug Action: Where Drugs Act

There are four action sites where psychopharmacologic drugs act: receptors, ion channels, enzymes, and carrier proteins. Drug molecules do not act on the entire cell surface, but rather at a specific receptor site. In 1900, a German chemist, Paul Erhlich, suggested that a receptive substance exists within the cell membrane. His work, along with that of Langley, an English physiologist, provided the basis for the concept of a receptor region or area on which a specific chemical may act (see Chap. 7). The biologic action of a drug depends on how its structure interacts with a specific receptor. The importance of receptor sites has now been firmly established and is critical in understanding how drugs work in the body.

Several different types of proteins exist in the cell membrane, both presynaptically and postsynaptically. These proteins serve as receptors for both chemicals found normally in the body and administered drugs. Normally occurring chemicals involved in neurotransmission, such as dopamine and serotonin, adhere to a specific group of receptors. Administered drugs may compete with neurotransmitters for these receptor sites, attempting to mimic or block the action of the normally occurring neurotransmitter. Some authors use the term receptor to mean any target protein with which a drug molecule can combine, but this interpretation may cause considerable confusion because there are many types of regulatory proteins in the nervous system that serve as targets for drugs. These include receptors, ion channels, carrier molecules, and enzymes. Drugs also bind to a few other types of proteins in the nervous system as well as in the bloodstream. However, current medications used in psychiatry primarily produce their actions at these four sites. Therefore, in this chapter, **receptor** refers only to those sites to which a neurotransmitter can specifically adhere to produce a change in the cell membrane, serving a physiologic regulatory function (such as those discussed in Chap. 7). These include the ligand-gated ion channel or the G-protein–linked receptor.

Receptors

Many drugs have been developed to act specifically at the receptor sites. Their chemical structure is similar to the neurotransmitter substance for that receptor. When attached, these drugs act as **agonists**—chemicals producing the same biologic action as the neurotransmitter itself, or as **antagonists**—chemicals blocking the biologic response at a given receptor. Figure 8-1 illustrates the action of an agonist and an antagonist drug at a receptor site.

A drug's ability to interact with a given receptor type may be judged on the basis of three properties. The first property, called **selectivity,** is the ability of the drug to be specific for a particular receptor. If a drug is highly selective, it will interact only with its specific receptors in the areas of the body where these receptors occur and, therefore, not affect tissues and organs where its receptors do not occur. Using a "lock-and-key" analogy, only a specific (or highly selective) key will fit a given lock. The more selective or structurally specific a drug is, the more likely it will affect only the specific receptors for which it is meant, and not the receptors for other neurochemicals that would produce unintended effects, or **side effects.** Selectivity is important to understand because it helps explain the concept of side effects from medications, a major cause of concern in medication treatment, that is discussed more completely later in the chapter.

The second property is that of **affinity,** which is the degree of attraction or strength of the bond between the drug and its receptor. Normally, these bonds are relatively weak chemical bonds. When a drug has more than one type of chemical bond with a receptor, its affinity may be increased. A drug's affinity may also be increased by the number of specific receptors on the cell membrane to which it might adhere. However, these types of weak chemical bonds with a receptor allow a

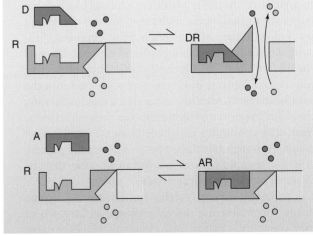

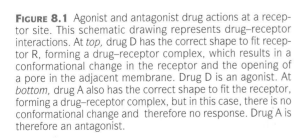

FIGURE 8.1 Agonist and antagonist drug actions at a receptor site. This schematic drawing represents drug–receptor interactions. At *top,* drug D has the correct shape to fit receptor R, forming a drug–receptor complex, which results in a conformational change in the receptor and the opening of a pore in the adjacent membrane. Drug D is an agonist. At *bottom,* drug A also has the correct shape to fit the receptor, forming a drug–receptor complex, but in this case, there is no conformational change and therefore no response. Drug A is therefore an antagonist.

drug's effects to be easily reversible when the drug is discontinued. Whereas most drugs used in psychiatry adhere to receptors through weak chemical bonds, some drugs, specifically the monoamine oxidase inhibitors (discussed later), have a different type of bond, called a *covalent bond.* A covalent bond is formed when two atoms share a pair of electrons. This type of bond is stronger and irreversible at normal temperatures. The effects of the drugs that form covalent bonds are often called "irreversible" because they are long-lasting, taking several weeks to resolve.

The final property of a drug's ability to interact with a given receptor is that of **intrinsic activity,** or the ability of the drug to produce a biologic response once it becomes attached to the receptor. Some drugs have selectivity and affinity, but produce no biologic response; therefore, an important measure of a drug is whether it produces a change in the cell containing the receptor. Drugs that act as agonists have all three properties: selectivity, affinity, and intrinsic activity. However, antagonists have only selectivity and affinity because they produce no biologic response by attaching to the receptor.

Some drugs are referred to as *partial agonists.* When a stronger agonist with high intrinsic activity is combined with a weaker agonist (low intrinsic activity) that has high affinity for a given receptor, the net effect is that the weaker agonist will act as an antagonist to the stronger agonist. Because it has some intrinsic activity (although weak), it is referred to as a partial agonist. Because there are no "pure" drugs, affecting only one neurotransmitter, most drugs have multiple effects. A drug may act as an agonist for one neurotransmitter and an antagonist for another. Medications that have both agonist and antagonist effects are called *mixed agonist–antagonists.*

Ion Channels

Some drugs directly block the ion channels of the nerve cell membrane. For example, local anesthetics block the entry of sodium into the cell, preventing a nerve impulse. In psychiatry, the utility of calcium-channel blockers has been investigated for use with the symptoms of mania, a psychological state of increased activity, euphoria, difficulty sleeping, racing thoughts, and rapid and forced speech (see Chap. 20). Operating on the hypothesis that too much neurotransmitter is being released into the synapse in mania, researchers suggested that modulating the influx of calcium (which stimulates the vesicles to release neurotransmitter) might decrease the symptoms of mania. Although this theory has not been fully proved, it is an example of how neurotransmission may be changed by different drug actions.

Frequently used in psychiatry, the benzodiazepine drugs, which decrease the symptoms of anxiety, are an example of drugs that affect the ion channels of the nerve

cell membrane. The benzodiazepine molecule, in such drugs as diazepam (Valium), works by binding to a region of the γ-aminobutyric acid (GABA)-receptor chloride channel complex. They facilitate GABA in opening the chloride ion channel, rather than replacing GABA, and have a modulatory effect in opening the ion channel.

Enzymes

Enzymes are complex proteins that catalyze specific biochemical reactions within cells and are the targets for some drugs used to treat mental disorders. For example, monoamine oxidase, the enzyme required to break down most bioamine neurotransmitters, such as norepinephrine, serotonin, and dopamine, can be inhibited by medications from a group of antidepressants called monoamine oxidase inhibitors (MAOIs). Strong covalent bonds are formed between the medication and the enzyme, which inhibit the ability of the enzyme to inactivate the bioamine neurotransmitters after they have been used, resulting in increased amounts of these neurotransmitters ready for release in the nerve terminals. The inhibitory effect is greater for norepinephrine and serotonin than it is for dopamine. This increase in available norepinephrine and serotonin is thought to be the primary mechanism by which MAOIs relieve the symptoms of depression.

Carrier Proteins: Uptake Receptors

Neurotransmitters are small organic molecules, and a carrier protein is usually required for these molecules to cross cell membranes. In much the same way as receptors, these carrier proteins (also referred to as *uptake receptors*) have recognition sites specific for the type of molecule to be transported. When a neurotransmitter such as serotonin needs to be removed from the synapse, specific carrier molecules transport the serotonin back into the presynaptic nerve, where most of it is stored to be used again. Medications specific for this site may block or inhibit this transport and, therefore, increase the amount of the neurotransmitter in the synaptic space available for action on the receptors.

A primary action of most of the antidepressants is to increase the amount of neurotransmitters in the synapse by blocking their reuptake. Older antidepressants block the reuptake of more than one neurotransmitter. The newer antidepressants, such as fluoxetine (Prozac) and sertraline (Zoloft), are more selective for serotonin, the primary neurotransmitter thought to be involved in the development of depression. For this reason, these newer medications have been called selective serotonin reuptake inhibitors (SSRIs). By more selectively acting on serotonin reuptake rather than norepinephrine, acetylcholine, and others, these medications have reduced the number of side effects or untoward effects experienced by the individuals who need this type of medication. Figure 8-2 illustrates the reuptake blockade of serotonin by an SSRI.

Efficacy and Potency: How Drugs Act

Efficacy is another characteristic of medications that must be considered when selecting a drug for treatment of a particular set of symptoms. **Efficacy** is the ability of a drug to produce a response as a result of the receptor or receptors being occupied. It is important to remember that the degree of receptor occupancy contributes to efficacy, yet it is not the only variable. A drug may occupy a large number of receptors, but not produce a response. Potency is also important when comparing drug actions. This factor considers the dose required to produce the desired biologic response. One drug may be able to achieve the same clinical effect as another drug but at a lower dose, making it more potent. Although the drug given at the lower dose is more potent, because both drugs achieve similar effects, they may be considered to have equal efficacy.

Loss of Effect: Biologic Adaptation

In some instances, the effects of medications diminish over time, especially when they are given repeatedly, as in the treatment of chronic psychiatric disorders. This loss of effect is most often a form of physiologic adaptation that may develop as the cell attempts to regain homeostatic control to counteract the effects of the drug. **Desensitization** is a rapid decrease in drug effects that may develop in a few minutes of exposure to a drug. This reaction is rare with most psychiatric medications, but can occur with some medications used to treat serious side effects (eg, physostigmine, sometimes used to relieve severe anticholinergic side effects). **Tolerance** is a gradual decrease in the action of a drug at a given dose or concentration in the blood. This decrease may take days or weeks to develop and results in loss of therapeutic effect of a drug. This loss of effect is sometimes referred to as *treatment refractoriness.*

There are many reasons for decrease in drug effectiveness (Text Box 8-1). A rapid decrease can occur with some drugs because of immediate transformation of the receptor when the drug molecule binds to the receptor. Other drugs cause a decrease in the number of receptors. It is hypothesized that the receptors are taken into the cell in a self-regulatory effort. In part, this may explain the development of some long-term side effects, such as **tardive dyskinesia,** a neuromuscular condition resulting from long-term use of some medications used in the treatment of psychosis.

Some drugs may exhaust the mediators of neurotransmission. For example, amphetamines deplete the supplies of norepinephrine stored in the vesicles at the terminals of the nerve cell. Drug tolerance can also be caused by an increase in the metabolism of the medication, such as with barbiturates, which trigger an increase in some hepatic enzymes that increase their own metabolism. This may add to the tolerance that develops to a given dose of barbiturate or may cause a precipitant drop in the blood level of the anticonvulsant carbamazepine (Tegretol).

Other forms of physiologic adaptation result in a gradual tolerance that may be helpful when affecting unpleasant side effects such as drowsiness or nausea. This information is important for the nurse to communicate to patients experiencing such side effects, so that they can be reassured that the effects will subside. The psychiatric nurse must also know when tolerance will not occur and when a lack of tolerance to a significant side effect warrants discontinuation of the medication.

Target Symptoms and Side Effects

Psychiatric medications are prescribed for specific symptoms, referred to as **target symptoms.** The target

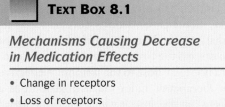

FIGURE 8.2 Reuptake blockade of a carrier molecule for serotonin by a selective serotonin reuptake inhibitor.

■ **TEXT BOX 8.1**

Mechanisms Causing Decrease in Medication Effects

- Change in receptors
- Loss of receptors
- Exhaustion of neurotransmitter supply
- Increased metabolism of the drug
- Physiologic adaptation

symptoms for each class of medication are discussed more fully in later sections of this chapter. As yet, no drug has been developed to be so specific as to attack only its target symptoms; instead, drugs act on target symptoms as well as a number of other organs and sites within the body. Because most neurotransmitters have a number of functions, even drugs with a high affinity and selectivity for a specific neurotransmitter, such as serotonin, will cause some responses in the body that are not related to the target symptoms. These unwanted effects of medications are referred to as side effects or untoward effects. Some of these unwanted effects may have serious physiologic consequences and are referred to as **adverse reactions.** These three terms are often used interchangeably in the literature.

Knowledge of medication's affinity for receptors and subtypes of receptors may give some indication of the likelihood that specific target symptoms might improve and what side effects might be predicted. Table 8-1 provides a brief summation of possible side effects from drug actions on specific neurotransmitters. For example, medications with a high affinity for acetylcholine receptors of the muscarinic subtype, producing antagonism or blockage at the receptor site, will be more likely to cause anticholinergic side effects, including dry mouth, blurred vision, constipation, urinary hesitancy or retention, and nasal congestion. This information should serve only as a guide in predicting side effects because many physical outcomes or behaviors resulting from neural transmission are controlled by multiple receptors and neurotransmitters. A psychiatric–mental health nurse should use this information to focus assessment on these areas. If the symptoms are mild, simple nursing interventions suggested in Table 8-2 may then be implemented. If symptoms persist or are severe, the prescriber should be notified immediately.

Drug Toxicity

All drugs have the capacity to be harmful as well as helpful. **Toxicity** generally refers to the point at which concentrations of the drug in the bloodstream become harmful or poisonous to the body. However, what is considered harmful? Side effects can be harmful, but not toxic, and individuals vary widely in their responses to medications. Some patients suffer adverse reactions more easily than others. **Therapeutic index,** a concept often used to discuss the toxicity of a drug, is a ratio of the maximum nontoxic dose to the minimum effective dose. A high therapeutic index means that there is a large range between the dose at which the drug begins to take effect and a dose that would be toxic to the body. Drugs with a low therapeutic index have a narrow range. This concept has some limitations. The concept of toxicity is only vaguely defined. The range can also be

affected by drug tolerance. For example, accidental suicides have been caused by individuals increasing their dosages of barbiturates as they became increasingly more tolerant to the effects and required larger doses to make them sleep. The therapeutic index of a medication may be also greatly changed by the coadministration of other medications or drugs. For example, alcohol consumed with most CNS depressant drugs will have added depressant effects, greatly increasing the likelihood of toxicity or death.

Despite the limitations of the therapeutic index, it is a helpful guide for nurses, particularly when working with potentially suicidal individuals. Psychiatric–mental health nurses must be aware of the potential for overdose and closely monitor availability of drugs for these patients. In some cases, prescriptions may have to be dispensed every few days or each week until a suicidal crisis has passed to ensure that patients do not have a lethal dose available to them. The SSRIs, such as fluoxetine, have a relatively high therapeutic index. Therefore, they are frequently considered the preferred antidepressants for treatment of acutely suicidal individuals.

PHARMACOKINETICS: HOW THE BODY ACTS ON THE DRUGS

The field of pharmacokinetics describes, often in mathematic models, how biologic functions within the living organism act on a drug. The processes of absorption, distribution, metabolism, and excretion are of central importance. Overall, the goal in pharmacokinetics is to describe and predict the time course of drug concentrations throughout the body and factors that may interfere with these processes. Together with the principles of pharmacodynamics, this information can be helpful to the psychiatric nurse in such ways as facilitating or inhibiting drug effects and predicting behavioral response.

Absorption and Routes of Administration

The first phase of drug disposition in the human body is absorption, defined as the movement of the drug from the site of administration into the plasma. It is important to first consider the routes by which a drug is administered. Not all potential routes of administration are available for medications used to treat psychiatric disorders. The primary routes available include oral (both tablet and liquid), intramuscular (short- and long-acting agents), and intravenous (rarely used for treatment of the primary psychiatric disorder, but instead for rapid treatment of adverse reactions). The psychiatric–mental health nurse must be knowledgeable of the advantages and disadvantages of each route and the subsequent effects on absorption (Table 8-3).

TABLE 8.1 Drug Affinity for Specific Neurotransmitters and Receptors and Subsequent Effects

Neurotransmitter/ Receptor Action	Physiologic Effects	Example of Drugs That Exhibit High Affinity
Receptor Blockade		
Norepinephrine reuptake inhibition	Antidepressant action Potentiation of pressor effects of norepinephrine Interaction with guanethidine Side effects: tachycardia, tremors, insomnia, erectile and ejaculation dysfunction	Desipramine Venlafaxine
Serotonin reuptake inhibition	Antidepressant action Antiobsessional effect Increase or decrease in anxiety, dose dependent Side effects: gastrointestinal distress, nausea, headache, nervousness, motor restlessness and sexual side effects, including anorgasmia	Fluoxetine Fluvoxamine
Dopamine reuptake inhibition	Antidepressant action Antiparkinsonian effect Side effects: increase in psychomotor activity, aggravation of psychosis	Buproprion
Reuptake Inhibition		
Histamine receptor blockade (H$_1$)	Side effects: sedation, drowsiness, hypotension, and weight gain	Quetiapine Imipramine Clozapine Olanzapine
Acetylcholine receptor blockade (muscarinic)	Side effects: anticholinergic (dry mouth, blurred vision, constipation, urinary hesitancy and retention, memory dysfunction) and sinus tachycardia	Imipramine Amitriptyline Thioridazine Clozapine
Norepinephrine receptor blockade (α_1 receptor)	Potentiation of antihypertensive effect of prazosin and terazosin Side effects: postural hypotension, dizziness, reflex tachycardia, sedation	Amitriptyline Clomipramine Clozapine
Norepinephrine receptor blockade (α_2 receptor)	Increased sexual desire (yohimbine) Interactions with antihypertensive medications, blockade of the antihypertensive effects of clonidine Side effect: priapism	Amitriptyline Clomipramine Clozapine Trazodone Yohimbine
Norepinephrine receptor blockade (β_1 receptor)	Antihypertensive action (propranolol) Side effects: orthostatic hypotension, sedation, depression, sexual dysfunction (including impotence and decreased ejaculation)	Propranolol
Serotonin receptor blockade (5-HT$_{1a}$)	Antidepressant action Antianxiety effect Possible control of aggression	Trazodone Risperidone Ziprasidone
Serotonin receptor blockade (5-HT$_2$)	Antipsychotic action Some antimigraine effect Decreased rhinitis Side effects: hypotension, ejaculatory problems	Risperidone Clozapine Olanzapine Ziprasidone
Dopamine receptor blockade (D$_2$)	Antipsychotic action Side effects: extrapyramidal symptoms, such as tremor, rigidity (especially acute dystonia and parkinsonism); endocrine changes, including elevated prolactin levels	Haloperidol Ziprasidone

Drugs taken orally are usually the most convenient for the patient; however, this route is also the most variable because absorption may be slowed or enhanced by a number of factors. Taking certain drugs orally with food or antacids may slow the rate of absorption or change the amount of the drug absorbed. For example, the β-receptor antagonist, propranolol, a cardiac medication used in psychiatry for control of the physical symptoms of anxiety, exhibits increased blood levels when given with food. Antacids containing aluminum

TABLE 8.2 Interventions for the Management of Common Side Effects of Psychiatric Medications

Assessment (Side Effect or Discomfort)	Intervention
Blurred vision	Reassurance (generally subsides in 2–6 wk) Warn ophthalmologist, no eye exam for new glasses for at least 3 wk after a stable dose
Dry eyes	Artificial tears may be required, or increase use of wetting solutions for those wearing contact lens
Dry mouth and lips	Frequent rinsing of mouth, good oral hygiene, sucking sugarless candies, lozenges, lip balm, lemon juice, and glycerin mouth swabs
Constipation	High-fiber diet, encourage bran, fresh fruits and vegetables, Metamucil (must consume at least 16 oz of fluid with dose) Increase hydration Exercise, increase fluids Mild laxative
Urinary hesitancy or retention	Monitor frequently for difficulty with urination, changes in starting or stopping stream Notify prescriber if difficulty develops A cholinergic agonist such as bethanechol may be required
Nasal congestion	Nose drops, moisturizer, ***not*** nasal spray Assess for infections
Sinus tachycardia	Monitor pulse for rate and irregularities Withhold medication and notify prescriber if resting rate is faster than 120
Decreased libido and inhibition of ejaculation	Reassurance (reversible) Consider change to less antiadrenergic drug
Postural hypotension	Frequent monitoring of lying to standing blood pressure during dosage adjustment period, immediate changes and accommodation, measure pulse in both positions Advise patient to get up slowly, sit for at least 1 min before standing (dangling legs over side of bed) and stand for 1 min before walking or until light-headedness subsides Increase hydration, avoid caffeine Elastic stockings if necessary Notify prescriber if symptoms persist or significant blood pressure changes are present, medication may have to be changed if patient does not have impulse control to get up slowly
Photosensitivity	Protective clothing Dark glasses Use of sun block, remember to cover ***all*** exposed areas
Dermatitis	Stop medication Consider medication change, may require a systemic antihistamine Initiate comfort measures to decrease itching
Impaired psychomotor functions	Advise patient to avoid dangerous tasks, such as driving Avoid alcohol, which increases this impairment
Drowsiness	Encourage activity during the day to increase accommodation Avoid tasks that require mental alertness, such as driving May need to adjust dosing schedule or, if possible, give single daily dose at bedtime
Weight gain	Exercise and diet teaching Caloric control Check fluid retention
Edema	Reassurance May need a diuretic
Irregular menstruation	Reassurance (reversible) May need to change class of drug
Amenorrhea	Reassurance and counseling (does not indicate lack of ovulation) Instruct patient to continue birth control
Vaginal dryness	Instruct in use of lubricants May need a cholinergic medication
Sedation	Instruct not to drive or operate potentially dangerous equipment May need change to less sedating medication Provide quiet and decreased stimulation when sedation is the desired effect

TABLE 8.3 **Preparation and Route of Administration for Medications Used in the Treatment of Psychiatric Disorders**

Preparation and Route	Examples	Advantages	Disadvantages
Oral tablet	Basic preparation for most psychopharmacologic agents, including antidepressants, antipsychotics, mood stabilizers, anxiolytics, etc.	Usually most convenient	Variable rate and extent of absorption, depending on the drug May be affected by the contents of the gut May show first pass metabolism effects May not be easily swallowed by some individuals
Oral liquid	Also known as concentrates Many antipsychotics, such as haloperidol, chlorpromazine, thioridazine, risperidone The antidepressant, fluoxetine Antihistamines, such as diphenhydramine Mood stabilizers, such as lithium citrate	Ease of incremental dosing Easily swallowed In some cases, more quickly absorbed	More difficult to measure accurately Depending on drug: 1. Possible interactions with other liquids such as juice, forming precipitants 2. Possible irritation to mucosal lining of mouth if not properly diluted
Intramuscular	Some antipsychotics, such as haloperidol and chlorpromazine Anxiolytics, such as lorazepam Anticholinergics, such as diphenhydramine and benztropine mesylate No antidepressants No mood stabilizers	More rapid acting than oral preparations No first-pass metabolism	Injection-site pain and irritation Some medications may have erratic absorption if heavy muscle tissue at the site of injection is not in use High-potency antipsychotics in this form may be more prone to adverse reactions such as neuroleptic malignant syndrome
Intramuscular depot or long-acting	Haloperidol decanoate Fluphenazine decanoate	May be more convenient for some individuals who have difficulty following medication regimens	Significant pain at injection site
Intravenous	Anticholinergics, such as diphenhydramine, benztropine mesylate Anxiolytics, such as diazepam, lorazepam, and chlordiazepoxide The antipsychotic, haloperidol (unlabeled use)	Rapid and complete availability to systemic circulation	Inflammation of tissue surrounding site Often inconvenient for patient and uncomfortable Continuous dosage requires use of a constant-rate IV infusion

salts decrease the absorption of most antipsychotic drugs; thus, antacids must be given at least 1 hour before administration or 2 hours after.

Oral preparations absorbed from the gastrointestinal tract into the bloodstream first go to the liver through the portal vein. There, they may be metabolized in such a way that most of the drug is inactivated before it reaches the rest of the body. Some drugs are also subjected to metabolism in the gastrointestinal wall, resulting in loss of available drug in the gastrointestinal system or the liver, called the *first-pass effect*.

Tacrine (see Chap. 31) and propranolol undergo significant first-pass effect, and yet enough of each drug reaches the rest of the body to be effective. However, the absorption of tacrine is also reduced 30% to 40% by the concurrent presence of food. If improved absorption is needed, tacrine should be given without food. It is extremely important for psychiatric–mental health nurses to attend conscientiously to drug administration times that meet the individual patient's needs, rather than adhere to all standardized administration schedules.

C = Generally compatible together
X = Incompatible: DO NOT MIX
Blank = No information available—
    choose "C" liquid to dilute

	Oral Liquid Neuroleptics										
	Chlorpromazine (generics, Thorazine)	Fluphenazine (Permitil)	Haloperidol (Haldol)	Lithium citrate (generic)	Loxapine (Loxitane)	Mesoridazine (Serentil)	Perphenazine (Trilafon)	Thioridazine 30 mg/ml (Mellaril)	Thioridazine 100 mg/ml (Mellaril)	Thiothixene (Navane)	Trifluoperazine (generic, Stelazine)
Liquids											
Water	C	C	C	C			C	X	X	C	C
Saline	C	C	X	C			C	X	X	C	
Milk	C	C	C	C			C	X	X	C	C
Coffee	C*	X	X	C			X	X	X		C
Tea	C*	X	X	C			X	X	X		C
Fruit Juices											
Apple juice or cider		X	C	C			X	X	X	X	
Apricot		C		C			C	X		C	
Cranberry	X			C		C		C	C	C	
Grape juice or drink				C		C		X	X		
Grapefruit	C	C		C	C	C	C	C	C‡	C	C
Lemonade, reconst. frozen				C				C	C		
Orange juice	C	C	C	C	C	C	C	C†	C**	C	C

Pineapple	C	C	C	C	C	X	C
Prune	X	C	C	X	X	X	C
Tang	X	C	C				
Tomato	C	C	C	X	X	C	C
V-8	C	C	C	X	X	C	C
Carbonated Liquids							
Cola (Coke, Pepsi, etc.)	X	C	C	X	X	X	C
Mellow-Yellow	C	C	C	C	C	C	C
Orange	C	C	C	C	C	C	C
7-Up, Sprite	C	C	C	C	C	C	C
Soups, Pudding	C	C		C			C
Oral Liquid Neuroleptics							
Chlorpromazine	X						
Haloperidol	X						
Lithium citrate	X	X	X	X	X	X	X
Thioridazine	X						
Trifluoperazine	X						

*Data differs with brand—avoid if using generics.
†Incompatible with orange "drink."
‡Canned only, not frozen concentrate.
**Canned orange juice only.
From Kerr, L. E. (1986). Oral liquid neuroleptics: Administer with care. *Journal of Psychosocial Nursing, 24*(3), 33–35.

Gastric motility also affects how the drug is absorbed. Increasing age, many disease states, and concurrent medications can reduce motility and slow absorption. Other factors, such as blood flow in the gastrointestinal system, drug formulation, and chemical factors, may also interfere with absorption. Nurses must be aware of a patient's physical condition and use of medications or other substances that can interfere with drug absorption.

Absorption of liquid preparations is usually more stable. However, some drugs continue to exhibit first-pass effects. Many liquid preparations, especially antipsychotics, are irritating in full strength to the mucosal lining of the mouth, esophagus, and stomach and must be adequately diluted. Nurses must be careful when diluting liquid medications because some liquid concentrate preparations are incompatible with certain juices or other liquids. If a drug is mixed with an incompatible liquid, a white or grainy precipitant usually forms, indicating that some of the drug has bound to the liquid and inactivated. Thus, the patient actually receives a lower dose of the medication than intended. Precipitants can also form from combining two liquid medications in one diluent, such as juice. Sometimes, precipitants may be difficult to see, such as in orange juice, so nurses must be aware of the compatibilities of liquid preparations. If the precipitant of these liquids forms in the cup, it will also form when mixed in the stomach, causing further inactivation of the drugs. Therefore, some medications should be given at least an hour apart, depending on gastric emptying. For more information regarding compatibilities of liquid preparations, see Table 8-4.

Bioavailability

Bioavailability describes the amount of the drug that actually reaches systemic circulation unchanged. The route by which a drug is administered significantly affects bioavailability. Given orally, many drugs undergo first-pass metabolism, which decreases the amount of drug that gets into the bloodstream. Drugs that experience this effect have a lower bioavailability than drugs that do not undergo first-pass effects.

Bioavailability is a concept often used to compare one drug to another, obviously implying that increased bioavailability makes one drug "better" than another. When generic forms of a drug are developed, the U.S. Food and Drug Administration (FDA) uses bioavailability as one measure for comparing the equivalency of the drugs. Although increased bioavailability of a drug may sound impressive, it is important to remember that this is not a characteristic solely of the drug preparation. It may be low if absorption is incomplete. Wide individual variations in the enzyme activity of the gut or liver, gastric pH, and intestinal motility will all affect it. In practice, bioavailability is difficult to quantify. Psychiatric–mental health nurses must keep in mind that many factors on any particular occasion may affect the absorption and bioavailability of the drug for an individual patient.

Distribution

Even after a drug has entered the bloodstream, several factors affect how it is distributed in the body. Distribution of a drug is defined as the amount of the drug found in various tissues, particularly the target organ at the site of drug action for which it is intended. Factors that affect medication distribution to specific organs in the body include the size of the organ, amount of blood flow or perfusion within the organ, solubility of the drug, plasma protein binding, and anatomic barriers, such as the blood–brain barrier, that the drug must cross. A drug may have rapid absorption and high bioavailability, but if it does not cross the blood–brain barrier to reach the CNS, it is of little use in psychiatry. Table 8-5 provides a summary of how some significant factors affect distribution.

TABLE 8.5 Factors Affecting Distribution of a Drug

Factor	Effect on Drug Distribution
Size of the organ	Larger organs require more drug to reach a concentration level equivalent to other organs and tissues.
Blood flow to the organ	The more blood flow to and within an organ (perfusion), the greater the drug concentration. The brain has high perfusion.
Solubility of the drug	The greater the solubility of a drug within a tissue, the greater its concentration.
Plasma protein binding	If a drug binds well to plasma proteins, particularly to albumin, it will stay in the body longer, but have a slower distribution.
Anatomic barriers	Both the gastrointestinal tract and the brain are surrounded by layers of cells that control the passage or uptake of substances. Lipid-soluble substances are usually readily absorbed and pass the blood–brain barrier.

Two of these factors, solubility and protein binding, warrant further discussion as they relate to psychiatric medications.

Substances may cross a membrane in a number of ways, but passive diffusion is by far the simplest. To do this, the drug must dissolve in the structure of the cell membrane. Therefore, solubility of a drug is an important characteristic. Drugs may be soluble in a number of substances, but being lipid soluble allows a drug to cross most of the membranes in the body. The degree to which a drug is lipid soluble varies somewhat depending on the chemical structure of the drug and may affect how readily the medication reaches its primary site of action. The tissues of the CNS are less permeable to water-soluble drugs than other areas of the body. Most psychopharmacologic agents are lipid soluble to easily cross the blood–brain barrier. However, this characteristic also means that psychopharmacologic agents cross the placenta as well.

Lipid-soluble drugs will also bind to other large molecules in the body. Of considerable importance is the degree to which the drug binds to plasma proteins. Only unbound or "free" drugs will be able to act at the receptor sites because drug–protein complexes are too large to cross cell membranes. High protein binding reduces the concentration of the drug at the receptor sites. However, because the binding is reversible, as the unbound drug is metabolized, more drug is released from the protein bonds. This process can prolong the duration of action of the drug. In addition, highly lipid-soluble drugs bind to other sites in the body as well, particularly fat cells. As the concentration of unbound drug decreases, more drug is released from fat depots. This concept is important for medications such as chlorpromazine, an antipsychotic medication, which are highly lipid soluble. Often, patients who discontinue their medication do not experience an immediate return of symptoms. This is because they are continuing to receive the drug as it is released from sites of storage in their body. Medications such as chlorpromazine may be found in the bloodstream and urine for several weeks or months after discontinuation. With this knowledge, nurses can help patients to understand why their symptoms did not return, even though they have not been taking their medication for several days or weeks.

Metabolism

The extent of drug action depends to a large part on the body's ability to change or alter a drug chemically so that it can be rendered inactive and removed from the body. Metabolism, or biotransformation, is the process by which the drug is altered and broken down into smaller substances, known as *metabolites*. In most cases, metabolites are pharmacologically inactive substances. Through the processes of metabolism, lipid-soluble drugs become more water soluble, so that they may be more readily excreted.

Most metabolism occurs in the liver, but it can also occur in the kidneys, lungs, and intestine. The outcome of this process is most often an inactive metabolite. However, metabolism can also change a drug to an active metabolite with potentially similar action as the parent compound. For instance, the antidepressant imipramine is metabolized to a pharmacologically active substance, desipramine, which also has antidepressant effects. This becomes important when measuring the therapeutic blood level of imipramine. It is more clinically relevant and accurate to obtain both imipramine and desipramine levels, even though the patient may only be taking the drug imipramine. Metabolism may also change an inactive drug to an active one or an active drug to a toxic metabolite. For example, with an overdose of acetaminophen, N-hydroxyacetaminophen is formed, which is further oxidized to a chemical that can destroy liver cells. Pharmacology textbooks provide a more complete review of drug metabolism.

Many of the processes of drug metabolism are carried out by the hepatic microsomal drug-metabolizing enzymes that exist in the smooth endoplasmic reticulum. The popularity of the SSRIs has renewed attention to these enzymes and the potential harmful effects of drug–drug interactions.

Cytochrome P-450 is the major member of one class of enzymes that is localized in the liver and has a high affinity for lipid-soluble drugs. This class of enzyme is involved in the metabolism of most medications used in psychiatric treatment. Each human P-450 enzyme is an expression of a unique gene. Most medications in psychiatry are metabolized by three distinct gene families (coded 1, 2, or 3) of enzymes within the cytochrome P-450 class, each of which may or may not be involved in the metabolism of a specific drug. Further research has delineated and coded for identification of subfamilies of enzymes within each of these gene families. Each subfamily can be induced, as well as inhibited, by a variety of drugs. For example, the SSRIs are inhibitors of the P-4502D6 subfamily. When the enzymes are inhibited, they decrease the clearance of the drugs they metabolize and elevate the plasma levels of other coadministered drugs metabolized by this same enzyme subfamily. Adverse reactions may occur from the coadministration of such drugs as propranolol (Inderal), codeine, carbamazepine, diphenhydramine (Benadryl), and dextromethorphan (found in many nonprescription cough remedies). Not all SSRIs are equal in their potency to inhibit P-4502D6. Paroxetine (Paxil) is the most potent, producing more than 90% inhibition of this enzyme subfamily (Olin, 1996), whereas sertraline exhibits mild effects, with only 20% to 50% inhibition (Preskorn, 1996).

The P-4502D6 subfamily is also notorious because it is genetically defective in about 9% of white patients (Glod, 1996), rendering these individuals "slow metabolizers" of a number of drugs, including the SSRIs, other common antidepressants, β-blockers, and analgesics. Because of the significance of this genetic defect, a laboratory test may be used to determine its presence in patients. A urinalysis measuring the ratio of metabolites from a test substance, debrisoquin (an antihypertensive), administered in an oral dose of 10 mg can identify individuals as "slow metabolizers" of P-4502D6.

Because knowledge of the P-450 enzymatic pathway is relatively new, and the technology that detects such effects was not available when many drugs were developed, not all drugs are currently classified by which of these hepatic enzyme subfamilies act in their metabolism. This information is available for only about 20% of commonly prescribed medications (Preskorn, 1996). Research is continuing, and more information is constantly emerging. For now, it is important to note that common substances such as cigarette smoke, chronic alcohol consumption, coal tar in charcoal-broiled foods, and estrogens induce the P-450 enzyme system. Acute alcohol ingestion and the antiulcer medication cimetidine inhibit these enzymes. Until more information is available, nurses should remain alert to the possibilities of drug–drug interactions wherever patients are receiving more than one medication. In addition, if an individual receiving a medication experiences an unusual reaction or suddenly loses effect from a medication that had previously been working, the nurse should carefully assess other substances that the person has recently consumed, including prescription medications, nonprescription remedies, dietary supplements or changes, and substances of abuse.

Elimination

Clearance refers to the total amount of blood, serum, or plasma from which a drug is completely removed per unit of time. The half-life of a drug provides a measure of the expected rate of clearance. *Half-life* refers to the time required for plasma concentrations of the drug to be reduced by 50%. For most drugs, the rate of elimination slows while the half-life remains unchanged. It usually takes four half-lives or more of a drug in total time for more than 90% of the drug to be eliminated.

Only a few medications used in psychiatry are removed predominantly by renal excretion. Most notably, lithium, a mood stabilizer, is eliminated primarily by the kidneys. Any impairment in renal function or renal disease may lead to severe toxic symptoms. Drugs bound to plasma proteins do not cross the glomerular filter freely. These lipid-soluble drugs are passively reabsorbed by diffusion across the renal tubule and are therefore not rapidly excreted in the urine. Because many psychiatric medications are protein bound and lipid soluble, most of their elimination occurs through the liver, where they are excreted in the bile and delivered into the intestine. This is the process by which active metabolites may be reabsorbed in the intestine. In fact, as much as 20% of the drug may "recirculate," which tends to prolong the duration of action. The half-life of these metabolites may also be calculated. Sometimes, the "mean" half-life is provided to represent an average measure of the elimination half-lives of both the parent drug and its metabolites.

Dosing refers to the administration of medication over time, so that therapeutic levels may be achieved or maintained without reaching toxic levels. In general, it is necessary to give a drug at intervals no greater than the half-life of the medication to avoid excessive fluctuation of concentration in the plasma between doses. With repeated dosing, a certain amount of the drug is accumulated in the body. This accumulation slows as the dosing continues and plateaus when absorption equals elimination. This is called *steady-state plasma concentration* or simply *steady state*. The rate of accumulation is determined by the half-life of the drug. Drugs generally reach steady state in about five times the elimination half-life. However, because elimination rates may vary significantly in any individual, fluctuations may still occur, and dose schedules may need to be modified. The psychiatric–mental health nurse should remember that these measures are subject to physiologic processes and individual variation. They are guidelines; accurate assessment for indicators of treatment response or unwanted effects may be the better tool for individualizing care.

Individual Variations in Drug Effects

Many factors affect drug absorption, distribution, metabolism, and elimination. These factors may vary among individuals depending on their age, genetics, and ethnicity. Nurses must be aware of and consider these individual variations in the effects of medications.

Pharmacokinetics are significantly altered at the extremes of the life cycle. Gastric absorption changes as individuals age because of increased gastric pH, decreased gastric emptying, slowed gastric motility, and reduced splanchnic circulation. Normally, these changes do not significantly impair oral absorption of a medication, but addition of common conditions, such as diarrhea, may significantly alter and reduce absorption.

Renal function is also altered in both very young and elderly patients. Infants who are exposed in utero to medications that are excreted through the kidneys may develop toxic reactions to these medications because renal function in the newborn is only about 20% that of an adult. In less than a week, renal function develops to adult levels, but in premature infants, the process may take longer. Renal function also declines with age. Creatinine clearance in a young adult is normally 100 to 120 mL/min, but after 40 years of age, this rate declines by about 10% per decade. Medical illnesses, such as diabetes and hypertension, may further the loss of renal function. When creatinine clearance falls below 30 mL/min, the excretion of drugs by the kidneys is significantly impaired, and potentially toxic levels may accumulate.

Metabolism of medications changes across the life span. In newborns, many of the liver enzymes take as long as 8 weeks to become fully functional. Drugs metabolized by these enzymes will accumulate, exhibiting very long half-lives. With age, blood flow to the liver and the mass of liver tissue both decrease. The activity of hepatic enzymes also slows with age. As a result, the ability of the liver to metabolize medications may show as much as a fourfold decrease between the ages of 20 and 70 years.

Most psychiatric medications are bound to proteins. Albumin is one of the primary circulating proteins to which drugs bind. Production of albumin by the liver generally declines with age. In addition, a number of medical conditions change the ability of medications to bind to albumin. Malnutrition, cancer, and liver disease decrease the production of albumin, which means that more free drug is acting in the system, producing higher blood levels of the medication and potentially toxic effects.

Less information is known about pharmacodynamic changes with age, but changes in the sites of medication actions may make older individuals more sensitive to certain side effects. Changes in the parasympathetic nervous system produce a greater sensitivity in elderly patients to anticholinergic side effects, which are more severe with this age group.

Although only a small amount of information is available at this time, it is clear that genetics play a significant role in the metabolism of medications. Studies of identical and nonidentical twins have documented that much of the individual variability in elimination half-life of a given drug is genetically determined. Individuals of Asian descent may metabolize ethanol to produce higher concentrations of acetaldehyde than white individuals, resulting in a higher incidence of symptoms such as flushing and palpitations. Asian research subjects have been found to be more susceptible to the cardiovascular effects of propranolol than whites, whereas individuals of African descent were less sensitive (Schatzberg et al., 1997). Early indications are that differences in rates of side effects and therapeutic effects may also exist with other medications used in psychiatry. Several reports indicate that Asians require one half to one third the dose of antipsychotic medications that whites require and that they may be more sensitive to side effects because of higher blood levels (Yamamoto & Lin, 1995). Lower doses of antidepressant medications are also often required for individuals of Asian descent. More research is needed to understand fully the underlying mechanisms and to identify groups that may require different approaches to medication treatment.

Concurrent medication use is the most common factor for individual variations in drug response. Both prescription and nonprescription medications may alter other drugs when they are present in the body. Medications may compete for the same sites of action in target organs or at the sites of unwanted effects. Drugs may compete for the same mechanisms of metabolism or alter another drug's route of metabolism. Each of these factors must be carefully explored when considering individual responses and side effects to all medications as well as psychopharmacologic agents. Working closely with individuals receiving these medications and their families, psychiatric–mental health nurses may be instrumental in uncovering the source of individual variations in medication response and in planning for optimizing response to psychopharmacologic drugs.

PHASES OF DRUG TREATMENT

The psychiatric–mental health nurse is involved in all of the phases of medication treatment. Considerations in terms of assessment, treatment issues such as adherence, predominance of side effects, and expected symptom relief vary across the phases of treatment, but all involve potential nursing actions. These phases include initiation, stabilization, maintenance, and discontinuation of the medication. In the ANA Psychopharmacology Guidelines for Psychiatric Mental Health Nurses, special considerations for treatment are organized within each of these phases, as listed in Table 8-6. Although the advanced practice psychiatric–mental health nurse may prescribe medications or operate in other, more independent roles, generalist level psychiatric–mental health nurses must still be concerned with the phases of treatment as a guide for what may be expected as they administer medications or monitor individuals receiving medications across each of these phases. The following subsections discuss some of the knowledge required

	TABLE 8.6 Clinical Considerations in the Phases of Treatment With Psychopharmacological Medications	

Phase of Treatment	Clinical Considerations
Initiation	• Pharmacokinetics/pharmacodynamics • Patient education about medication and alternative treatments • Informed consent • Identification of target symptoms and rating scales for assessment • Alternative treatments • Development of treatment plans • Implications of information obtained in assessment
Stabilization	• Continued assessment of target symptoms • Expected timing of medication effects • Therapeutic drug monitoring • When and how to change medication strategies • Ongoing patient education • Transition between treatment settings
Maintenance	• Education regarding relapse and recognition of stressors • Monitoring efficacy, side effects, and laboratory values • Consider long-term side-effect potential • Address compliance issues • When and how to discontinue medication treatment • Patient education for relapse prevention
Discontinuation (medication free)	• Duration of treatment for a given disorder • Tapering methods/schedules • Symptom recognition • Relapse prevention

From Nihart, M. A., & Laraia, M. T. (1994). Clinical psychopharmacology: Considerations for nursing practice. *American Nurses Association: Psychiatric Mental Health Nursing Psychopharmacology Project* (p. 27). Washington, DC: American Nurses Publishing.

and the assessments and interventions to be performed by the generalist-level psychiatric–mental health nurse within each phase.

Initiation

Before beginning medications, patients must undergo several assessments. A psychiatric evaluation, including past history and previous medication treatment response, will clarify diagnosis and determine target symptoms for the medication. Physical examination and indicated laboratory tests, most likely a complete blood count (CBC), liver and kidney function tests, electrolytes, and urinalysis, and possibly also thyroid function tests and electrocardiogram (ECG), will help determine whether a physical condition may be causing the symptoms. In addition, the individual's liver and kidney functions may identify potential problems with metabolism of the medications. Nurses must be aware of the outcomes of these evaluations and determine what aspects of treatment may need to be more closely monitored.

Psychiatric–mental health nurses should perform their own premedication evaluations, including physical assessments that focus on pre-existing symptoms, such as gastrointestinal distress, or restrictions in range of motion that may later be confused with side effects. Side effects are difficult to assess if baseline status has not been evaluated. A pharmacologic history must be obtained to determine prescription, nonprescription, and substances of abuse that the individual may be taking concurrently with psychiatric medications. An assessment of cognitive functioning will assist the nurse in assessing whether memory aids or other supports are necessary to assist the individual in accurately completing the medication regimen. Psychosocial factors, such as support networks, financial health resources, occupation, family history of psychiatric disorders, and beliefs about psychiatric disorders, should also be addressed, with special attention to factors that may interfere with treatment. This information should be reviewed in consultation with the prescriber and other members of the multidisciplinary team to develop a plan that is acceptable to the patient and that will improve the individual's functioning, minimize side effects, improve quality of life, and maximize the ability to follow the medication regimen successfully.

In all situations, recommendations and treatment alternatives should be developed and reviewed with input from the individual seeking treatment. Doing so will allow the patient to ask questions, receive complete information, and give informed consent to the selected approach. Patients are often overwhelmed during the initial phases of treatment and may have symptoms that make it difficult for them to participate fully in treatment planning. Information is forgotten or may often need to be repeated. Nurses must be fully knowledgeable of the indications, target symptoms, actions, pharmacokinetics, and side effects of each medication to be able to answer questions and provide ongoing education.

When the medication is actually initiated, psychiatric–mental health nurses should treat the first dose as if it were a "test" dose. They should observe closely for sensitivity to the medication, such as changes in blood pressure, pulse, or temperature; changes in mental status; allergic reactions; dizziness; ataxia; or gastric distress. Other common side effects that may occur with even one dose of medication should also be closely monitored. If any of these symptoms develop, they should be reported to the prescriber.

Stabilization

During stabilization, the medication dosage is often being adjusted and increased to achieve the maximum amount of improvement with a minimum number of side effects. This process is sometimes referred to as *titration*. Psychiatric–mental health nurses must continue to assess target symptoms, looking for change or improvement and side effects that may develop. If medications are being increased rapidly, such as in a hospital setting, nurses must closely monitor temperature, blood pressure, pulse, mental status, common side effects, and unusual adverse reactions. On an outpatient basis, nurses must educate individuals who are receiving the medication as to the expected outcome and potential side effects. This education should include factors that may influence the effectiveness of the medication, such as whether to take the medication with food, common interventions that may minimize side effects if they develop, and what side effects require immediate attention. A plan should be developed for patients and their families that clearly identifies what to do if adverse reactions develop. The plan should include emergency telephone numbers or available emergency treatment and should be reviewed frequently with the individual.

Therapeutic drug monitoring is also an important aspect of this phase of treatment. Many medications used in psychiatry improve target symptoms only when a therapeutic level of medication has been obtained in the individual's blood. Some medications, such as lithium, have a narrow therapeutic range and must be monitored frequently and accurately. Nurses must be aware of when and how these levels are to be determined and assist patients in learning these procedures. Because of protein binding and lipid solubility, most medications do not have obtainable plasma levels that are clinically relevant. However, plasma levels of these medications may still be requested to evaluate further such issues as absorption and adverse reactions.

Sometimes, the first medication chosen does not improve the patient's target symptoms. This medication will be discontinued and a new medication started. Medications may also be changed when adverse reactions or seriously uncomfortable side effects occur, or these effects substantially interfere with the individual's quality of life. Nurses should be familiar with the pharmacokinetics of both drugs to be able to monitor side effects and possible drug–drug interactions during this change.

At times, an individual may show only partial improvement from a medication, and the prescriber may wish to try an augmentation strategy. Augmentation adds another medication to enhance or potentiate the effects of the first medication. For example, a prescriber may add a mood stabilizer, such as lithium, to an antidepressant to improve the effects of the antidepressant. These strategies are often used with so-called treatment-resistant situations. Treatment resistance has various definitions, but most often it means that after several medication trials, the individual has received at best only partial improvement. Polypharmacy, using more than one group from a class of medications, is usually not recommended and is avoided with most psychopharmacologic agents. Nonetheless, treatment-resistant symptoms may require combinations of medications to affect more than one neurotransmitter group. Nurses must be familiar with the potential effects, side effects, drug interactions, and rationale for each approach.

Maintenance

Once the individual's target symptoms have improved, medications may be continued to prevent relapse. Relapse means that the symptoms of the disorder return. In some cases, this may occur despite the patient's continued use of the medication. Some medications lose their efficacy over time. Other medications activate or speed up their own metabolism, causing a precipitant drop in the therapeutic blood level of the drug. Other factors, such as medical illness, psychosocial stressors, or concurrent use of prescription or nonprescription medication, may cause the medications to lose their effect. Whatever the reason, patients must be educated about their target symptoms and have a plan of action if the symptoms return. The psychiatric–mental health nurse has a central role in assisting individuals to monitor their own symptoms, manage psychosocial stressors, and avoid other factors that may cause the medications to lose effect.

Some side effects or adverse reactions emerge only after the individual has been receiving the medication for an extended period of time. Psychiatric–mental health nurses must be familiar with standardized assessment tools to monitor the development of these unwanted effects. Some of these tools are discussed more fully in Chapter 10. In addition, medications may alter the function of other body organs, such as the liver or thyroid, or result in the development of blood dyscrasias, such as leukopenia or agranulocytosis. Nurses should be familiar with the appropriate laboratory tests required to ensure that patients receive these tests at appropriate intervals as well as monitoring for symptoms of these adverse events.

Discontinuation

Most medications require a tapered discontinuation. Tapering involves the slow reduction in dosage of the medication, monitoring closely for re-emergence of the symptoms being treated. Some psychiatric disorders, such as depression, often respond to several months of treatment and do not recur. Other disorders, such as schizophrenia, usually require continued medication treatment throughout the person's life. Some medications have withdrawal symptoms; others do not. Nurses must be aware of the potential for these symptoms, monitor them closely, and implement measures to minimize their effects. Psychiatric–mental health nurses should support individuals throughout this process, whether they can successfully stop the medication or must continue. Even if patients can successfully discontinue the medication without return of symptoms, nurses may help implement preventive measures to avoid recurrence of the psychiatric disorder. In the roles of advocate, patient educator, and provider of interpersonal support, psychiatric–mental health nurses often have a central role in relapse prevention.

ANTIPSYCHOTIC MEDICATIONS

First synthesized by Paul Charpentier in 1950, chlorpromazine became the interest of Henri Lorit, a French surgeon, who was attempting to develop medications that controlled preoperative anxiety. Administered in intravenous doses of 50 to 100 mg, it produced drowsiness and indifference to surgical procedures. At Lorit's suggestion, a number of psychiatrists began to administer chlorpromazine to agitated psychotic patients. In 1952, Jean Delay and Pierre Deniker, two French psychiatrists, published the first report of chlorpromazine's calming effects with psychiatric patients. They soon discovered it was especially effective in relieving hallucinations and delusions associated with schizophrenia. As more psychiatrists began to prescribe the medication, the use of restraints and seclusion in psychiatric hospitals dropped sharply, ushering in a revolution in psychiatric treatment.

Since that time, a number of antipsychotic medications have been developed. Older, typical antipsychotic medications, available since 1954, are considered to be equally effective, varying only in the degree to which they caused certain groups of side effects. Table 8-7 provides a list of selected antipsychotics grouped by the nature of their chemical structure and indicating the likelihood of certain side effects. These medications treat the symptoms of psychosis, such as hallucinations, delusions, bizarre behavior, disorganized thinking, and agitation.

Initially, the term *major tranquilizer* was used to describe this group of medications, but it has since been deemed a misnomer because mentally healthy individuals have reported that these medications produce a somewhat unpleasant state of indifference. The term major tranquilizer has been replaced more recently by the term *neuroleptic* to describe the action of drugs like chlorpromazine. Literally translated, neuroleptic means "to clasp the neuron," and reflected the often significant neurologic side effects that these types of drugs are known to produce. The development of newer antipsychotic drugs that have less significant neurologic side effects has reduced the use of this term, making it less appropriate, and antipsychotic is a more accurate descriptor of these medications. The term *typical antipsychotic* is used to identify the older antipsychotic drugs, and *atypical antipsychotic* is used to identify the newer generation of antipsychotic drugs.

The typical, older antipsychotics have a range of dosage options, including intramuscular injection, but have many adverse side effects leading to poor patient compliance and poor symptom relief. The atypical antipsychotic drugs have less adverse events associated with them, but are available only in oral form.

Target Symptoms and Mechanism of Action

Antipsychotic medications are generally indicated for the treatment of psychosis. Possible target symptoms for the antipsychotics include hallucinations, delusions, paranoia, agitation, assaultive behavior, bizarre ideation, disorientation, social withdrawal, catatonia, blunted affect, thought blocking, insomnia, and anorexia, when these symptoms are the result of a psychotic process. (These symptoms are described more fully in later chapters.) In general, the older, typical antipsychotics, such as haloperidol (Haldol), chlorpromazine, and thioridazine (Mellaril) are equally effective in relieving hallucina-

TABLE 8.7   Side-Effect Comparison of Selected Antipsychotic Medications

Drug Category Drug Name	Sedation	Extrapyramidal	Anticholinergic	Orthostatic Hypotension
Standard (Typical) Antipsychotics				
PHENOTHIAZINES				
ALIPHATICS				
Chlorpromazine (Thorazine)	+4	+2	+3	+4
PIPERIDINES				
Thioridazine (Mellaril)	+3	+1	+4	+4
Mesoridazine (Serentil)	+3	+1	+4	+3
PIPERAZINES				
Fluphenazine (Prolixin)	+1	+4	+1	+1
Perphenazine (Trilafon)	+2	+3	+2	+2
Trifluoperazine (Stelazine)	+1	+3	+1	+1
THIOXANTHENES				
Thiothixene (Navane)	+1	+4	+1	+1
DIBENZOXAZEPINES				
Loxapine (Loxitane)	+2	+3	+2	+3
BUTYROPHENONES				
Haloperidol (Haldol)	+1	+4	+1	+1
DIHYDROINDOLONES				
Molindone (Moban)	+2	+3	+2	+1
Atypical Antipsychotics				
DIBENZODIAZEPINES				
Clozapine (Clozaril)	+4	+/0	+4	+4
BENZISOXAZOLE				
Risperidone (Risperdal)	+1	+/0	+/0	+2
THIENOBENZODIAZEPINE				
Olanzapine (Zyprexa)	+4	+/0	+2	+1
DIBENZOTHIAZEPINE				
Quetiapine fumarate (Seroquel)	+4	+/0	+/0	+3
MONOHYDROCHLORIDE				
Ziprasidone HCL (Geodon)	+1	+/0	+1	+2

+/0 = lowest likelihood
+4 = highest likelihood
From Maxmen, J. S., & Ward, N. G. (1995). *Psychotropic drugs: Fast facts* (2nd ed., p. 21). New York: Norton.

tions, delusions, and bizarre ideation, considered to be the "positive" symptoms of schizophrenia. The "negative" symptoms—blunted affect, social withdrawal, lack of interest in usual activities, lack of motivation, poverty of speech, thought blocking, and inattention—respond less well to the typical antipsychotics and in some cases may even worsen these symptoms. Newer atypical antipsychotics, such as clozapine, risperidone, olanzapine (Zyprexa), quetiapine (Seroquel), and the newest drug, ziprasidone, are more effective at improving negative symptoms. Therefore, these additional symptoms may be considered some of the target symptoms for atypical antipsychotic drugs.

Although antipsychotic medications are the primary treatment for schizophrenia and related illnesses such as schizoaffective disorder, schizophreniform disorder, and brief psychotic disorder, they have also been used to treat other psychiatric and medical illnesses. Psychotic symptoms that occur during a major depressive episode or bipolar affective disorder are frequently treated with antipsychotics, primarily on a short-term basis. These medications reduce agitation, aggressiveness, and inappropriate behavior in pervasive developmental disorders, such as autism, or severe mental retardation. Haloperidol and pimozide have been approved for the treatment of Tourette's syndrome, reducing the frequency and severity of vocal tics. Some of these drugs, particularly chlorpromazine, are used as antiemetics or for postsurgical intractable hiccoughs.

Uses not in the FDA labeling of the drug have also been found to be effective. Chlorpromazine and haloperidol are both effective in the treatment of drug-related psychosis, such as that caused by phencyclidine. Antipsychotics have been effective in the control of behavioral disturbances in elderly patients who have dementia, reducing symptoms of agitation, hyperactivity, hallucinations, suspiciousness, and hostility. Antipsychotic medications also have potential uses in the treatment of migraines, Huntington's chorea, and some other neurologic disorders (Olin, 1996).

The typical antipsychotic drugs are generally effective in decreasing target symptoms because they are potent postsynaptic dopamine antagonists. Chapter 18 discusses the link between dopamine and disorders like schizophrenia and provides further detail about how lowering dopamine assists in the reduction of target symptoms. The atypical antipsychotic medications differ from the typical antipsychotics in that they block serotonin receptors as well as dopamine receptors. These differences between the mechanism of action of the typical and atypical antipsychotic helps to explain their differences in terms of effect on target symptoms and in the degree of side effects they produce. It also helps to explain why the atypical antipsychotic drugs are, in general, more effective than the typical in addressing the negative target symptoms of disorders such as schizophrenia.

Pharmacokinetics

Antipsychotic medications administered orally have a variable rate of absorption complicated by the presence of food, antacids, smoking, and even the coadministration of anticholinergics, which slow gastric motility. Clinical effects begin to appear in about 30 to 60 minutes. Intramuscular administration is less variable because this method avoids the first-pass effects to which many of these drugs are subjected. Therefore, intramuscular administration produces greater bioavailability. It is important to remember that intramuscular medications are absorbed more slowly when patients are immobile because erratic absorption may occur when muscles are not in use. This knowledge becomes important when administering intramuscular antipsychotic medication to patients who are restrained. For example, the patient's arm may be more mobile than the buttocks. The deltoid has better blood perfusion, and the medication will be more readily absorbed, especially with use. The nurse must also remember that plastic syringes may absorb some medications. This is true of the antipsychotics, and injectable medications should never be allowed to sit in the syringe longer than 15 minutes.

Metabolism of these drugs occurs almost entirely in the liver, where hepatic microsomal enzymes convert these highly lipid-soluble substances into water-soluble metabolites that can be excreted through the kidneys. Therefore, these medications are subjected to the effects of other drugs that induce or inhibit the cytochrome P-450 system described earlier. Table 8-8 summarizes many of the possible medication interactions with antipsychotics, including those resulting from changes in hepatic enzymes. Careful observance of concurrent medication use, including prescribed, over-the-counter, and substances of abuse, is required to avoid drug–drug interactions.

Excretion of these substances tends to be slow. As highly lipid-soluble drugs, antipsychotics easily pass the blood–brain barrier but accumulate in the fatty tissues of the body. Most antipsychotics have a half-life of 24 hours or longer, but many also have active metabolites with longer half-lives. These two effects make it difficult to predict elimination time, and metabolites of some of these agents may be found in the urine months later. Psychiatric nurses must remember that just because a medication was discontinued today, it does not mean that the effects of the drug will be gone tomorrow. If a patient experiences side effects from a medication severe enough to discontinue the drug and start a new one, the adverse effects of the first drug may not necessarily immediately disappear. The patient may continue to experience and sometimes need treatment for the adverse effects of the first drug for several days. In a similar fashion, patients who have discontinued antipsychotic drugs may still derive therapeutic benefit for several days to weeks after discontinuation, leading some patients to believe falsely that they no longer need medication treatment.

Although, initially, antipsychotics are best administered in divided doses to minimize side effects, the long elimination time does allow the medication to be given in once-daily dosing. This schedule increases adherence and reduces the impact of the peak occurrence of some side effects, such as sedation during the day.

High lipid solubility, accumulation in the body, and other factors have also made it difficult to correlate blood levels with therapeutic effects. Dose–response curves have not been established, and the dose required for an individual to experience treatment effects varies widely. Plasma levels of these medications are only partially helpful. Although these can be measured for a number of antipsychotics, their correlation with therapeutic response has been inconsistent. Haloperidol and clozapine correlate well and may be helpful in determining whether an adequate blood level has been reached and maintained during a trial of medication. Table 8-9 provides the therapeutic ranges available for some of the antipsychotic medications. Plasma levels may also be helpful in identifying absorption problems, determining whether the patient is taking the medication as prescribed, and identifying adverse reactions due to drug–drug interactions.

Potency of the antipsychotics also varies widely. As Table 8-9 indicates, 100 mg chlorpromazine is roughly equivalent to 2 mg haloperidol and 5 mg trifluoperazine. Although more potent drugs are not inherently better than less potent drugs, differentiating

TABLE 8.8 Chemical Interactions With Antipsychotic Medications

Agent	Effect
Alcohol	Phenothiazines potentiate CNS depressant effects. Extrapyramidal reactions may occur.
Barbiturates	Speed action of liver microsomal enzymes so antipsychotic is metabolized more quickly, reducing phenothiazine and haloperidol plasma levels; barbiturate levels may also be reduced by phenothiazines; potentiate CNS depressant effect.
Tricyclic antidepressants	Can lead to severe anticholinergic side effects; some antipsychotics (especially phenothiazines or haloperidol) can raise the plasma level of the antidepressant, probably by inhibiting metabolism of the antidepressant.
Hydrochlorothiazide and hydralazine	Can produce severe hypotension.
Guanethidine	Antihypertensive effect is blocked by phenothiazines, haloperidol, and possibly thiothixene.
Aluminum salts (antacids)	Impair gastrointestinal absorption of the phenothiazines, possibly reducing therapeutic effect. Administer antacid at least 1 h before or 2 h after the phenothiazine.
Nicotine	Heavy consumption requires larger doses of antipsychotic due to hepatic microsomal enzyme induction.
Charcoal (and char-broiled food)	Decreases absorption of phenothiazines.
Anticholinergics	May reduce the therapeutic actions of the phenothiazines, increase anticholinergic side effects, lower serum haloperidol levels, worsen symptoms of schizophrenia, increase symptoms of tardive dyskinesia.
Meperidine	May result in excessive sedation and hypotension when coadministered with phenothiazines.
Fluoxetine	Case report of serious extrapyramidal symptoms when used in combination with haloperidol.
Lithium	May induce disorientation, unconsciousness, extrapyramidal symptoms, or possibly the risk for neuroleptic malignant syndrome when combined with phenothiazines or haloperidol.
Carbamazepine	Decreases haloperidol serum levels, decreasing its therapeutic effects.
Phenytoin	Increase or decrease in phenytoin serum levels; thioridazine and haloperidol serum levels may be decreased.
Methyldopa	May potentiate the antipsychotic effects of haloperidol or may produce psychosis. Serious elevations in blood pressure may occur with methyldopa and trifluoperazine.
General anesthesia (barbiturates)	Antipsychotic may potentiate effect of anesthetic; may increase the neuromuscular excitation or hypotension.

low-potency versus high-potency antipsychotics may be somewhat helpful in predicting side effects. Roughly speaking, high-potency medications, such as haloperidol and fluphenazine, produce a greater frequency of extrapyramidal symptoms, and low-potency antipsychotics, such as chlorpromazine and thioridazine, produce more sedation and hypotension. This distinction is often discussed in the literature and is helpful to understand; however, it is not exact and should be only a general guide.

Except for the new atypical drugs, all of the antipsychotics are relatively similar in their effectiveness and action, so that there are limited reasons to prescribe more than one antipsychotic at a time. Polypharmacy also adds to treatment confusion. If the symptoms improve, which drug caused the improvement?

This is also true with the development of side effects. Ultimately, selection of medication from the group of typical antipsychotics depends predominately on predicted side effects, prior history of treatment response, whether or not a depot preparation will be needed during maintenance, concurrent medications, and the presence of other medical conditions.

Depot Preparations

Haloperidol and fluphenazine are available in long-acting forms. These two antipsychotics may be administered by injection once every 2 to 4 weeks. After administration, the drug is slowly released from the injection site; therefore, these forms of the drugs are re-

TABLE 8.9 Antipsychotic Medications				
Generic (Trade) Drug Name	Usual Dosage Range (mg/d)	Half-Life (h)	Therapeutic Blood Level	Approximate Equivalent Dosage (mg)
Standard (Typical) Antipsychotics				
PHENOTHIAZINES				
ALIPHATICS				
Chlorpromazine (Thorazine)	50–1200	2–30	30–100 mg/mL	100
PIPERIDINES				
Thioridazine (Mellaril)	50–600	10–20	1–1.5 ng/mL	100
Mesoridazine (Serentil)	50–400	24–48	Not available	50
PIPERAZINES				
Fluphenazine (Prolixin)	2–20	4.5–15.3	0.2–0.3 ng/mL	2
Perphenazine (Trilafon)	12–64	Unknown	0.8–12.0 ng/mL	10
Trifluoperazine (Stelazine)	5–40	47–100	1–2.3 ng/mL	5
THIOXANTHENES				
Thiothixene (Navane)	5–60	34	2–20 ng/mL	4
DIBENZOXAZEPINES				
Loxapine (Loxitane)	20–250	19	Not available	15
BUTYROPHENONES				
Haloperidol (Haldol)	2–60	21–24	5–15 ng/mL	2
DIHYDROINDOLONES				
Molindone (Moban)	50–400	1.5	Not available	10
Atypical Antipsychotics				
DIBENZODIAZEPINES				
Clozapine (Clozaril)	300–900	4–12	141–204 ng/mL	50
BENZISOXAZOLE				
Risperidone (Risperdal)	2–8	20	Not available	1
THIENOBENZODIAZEPINE				
Olanzapine (Zyprexa)	5–10	21–54	Not available	Not available
DIBENZOTHIAZEPINE				
Quetiapine fumarate (Seroquel)	150–750	7	Not available	Not available
MONOHYDROCHLORIDE				
Ziprasidone HCL (Geodon)	40–160	7	Not available	Not available

ferred to as *depot preparations.* Long-acting injectable medications maintain a fairly constant blood level between injections. Because they bypass problems with gastrointestinal absorption and first-pass metabolism, this method may enhance therapeutic outcomes for the patient. Lower rates of relapse have been reported for patients receiving long-acting injectable medication compared with those taking oral medications. Most often, depot preparations are used when individuals have difficulty remembering to take their oral medications but are able to keep appointments reliably or attend a program regularly where the injection may be administered.

Long-acting forms of fluphenazine are available as fluphenazine decanoate and fluphenazine enanthate. The latter has a markedly increased risk for extrapyramidal side effects and is rarely used. Fluphenazine decanoate and haloperidol decanoate are equally effective in treating the symptoms of psychosis. A change to depot preparation from oral antipsychotic is done on a gradual basis after the patient is fully informed and consents.

Nurses should be aware that the injection site may become sore and inflamed if certain precautions are not taken. The liquids are viscous, and a large-gauge needle (at least 21 gauge) should be used. Because the medication is meant to remain in the injection site, the needle should be dry, and a deep intramuscular injection should be given by the Z-track method. The medication may be given subcutaneously if seepage is difficult to control and the patient does not respond to intramuscular injection. Do not massage the injection site. Rotate sites and document in the patient's record. Do not allow the medication to remain in a plastic syringe longer than 15 minutes. If the patient refuses the injection, assess whether it is the site and related pain rather than the medication that the patient is refusing. Some patients prefer the thigh or deltoid when administration in the buttocks is too painful.

Side Effects, Adverse Reactions, and Toxicity

Cardiovascular Side Effects

Various side effects and interactions can occur with antipsychotics (see Tables 8-7 and 8-8). These side effects vary to a great extent based on their degree of attraction to different neurotransmitter receptors and their subtypes. Cardiovascular side effects, such as orthostatic hypotension, depend on the degree of blockade of α-adrenergic receptors. Low-potency antipsychotics, such as chlorpromazine and thioridazine, and the atypical antipsychotic, clozapine, have a high degree of affinity for α-adrenergic receptors and therefore produce considerable orthostatic hypotension. Other cardiovascular side effects from typical antipsychotics have been rare, but occasionally they cause ECG changes that have a benign or undetermined clinical effect. Both of the low-potency antipsychotics and the new atypical drug, ziprasidone, should be used cautiously in patients who have increased Q-T intervals (Viskin, 1999). High-potency antipsychotics are less likely to cause cardiovascular side effects.

Anticholinergic Side Effects

Anticholinergic side effects resulting from blockade of acetylcholine are another common concern with typical antipsychotics and with some of the atypical drugs such as olanzapine. Dry mouth, slowed gastric motility, constipation, urinary hesitancy or retention, vaginal dryness, blurred vision, dry eyes, nasal congestion, and confusion or decreased memory are examples of these side effects. Interventions for decreasing the impact of these side effects are outlined in Table 8-2. This group of side effects occurs with many of the medications used in psychiatry. Sometimes, a cholinergic medication, such as bethanechol, may reduce the peripheral effects but not the CNS effects. Using more than one medication with anticholinergic effects often increases the symptoms. Elderly patients are often most susceptible to a potential toxicity that results from high blockade of acetylcholine. This toxicity is called an *anticholinergic crisis* and is described more fully, along with its treatment, in Chapter 18. The likelihood of occurrence of anticholinergic side effects, along with sedation and extrapyramidal side effects, from antipsychotics is explored in Table 8-7.

Weight Gain

Other side effects of clinical importance also occur with the antipsychotic medications. Weight gain due to increased appetite is common with the low-potency antipsychotics but occurs in highest proportion with clozapine and olanzapine. Weight gain has been known to be associated with antipsychotic drugs since chlorpromazine was developed. It has become an issue of increasing concern with the increased use of atypical drugs such as clozapine and has been linked to increase risk for diabetes and hyperlipidemia, known risk factors for cardiovascular illness (Allison et al., 1999). This increased awareness of the link between weight gain and antipsychotic drug use emphasizes the need for early, preventive intervention with diet and exercise. The chronic health problems of diabetes and cardiovascular illness occur much more often in individuals with mental illness than in the general population (Harris & Barraclough, 1998), making it essential for nurses to assist patients in dealing effectively with issues of weight gain. Ziprasidone is the first atypical antipsychotic to be associated with little to no weight gain during clinical trials (Allison et al., 1999). Because this is a new drug, research data regarding ziprasidone will need to be collected to determine the drug's effects once it is used in wider patient groups.

Endocrine and Sexual Side Effects

Endocrine and sexual side effects result primarily from the blockade of dopamine in the tuberoinfundibular pathways of the hypothalamus (see Chap. 7). As a result, increased blood levels of prolactin may occur with all of the antipsychotics except clozapine. Increased prolactin causes breast enlargement and rare but potential galactorrhea (milk production and flow), decreased sexual drive, amenorrhea, menstrual irregularities, and increased risk for growth in pre-existing breast cancers. Bromocriptine, a dopamine agonist, may be helpful, but more likely these symptoms will necessitate a change in medication. The prescriber should be notified immediately. Retrograde ejaculation (backward flow of semen) is rare, but it may be painful and can occur with all of the antipsychotics. A more common side effect is erectile dysfunction, including difficulty achieving and maintaining an erection. Anorgasmia, or the inability to achieve orgasm, may develop in women.

Blood Disorders

Blood dyscrasias (disorders) are rare but have received renewed attention since the introduction of clozapine. Agranulocytosis is an acute reaction that causes the individual's white blood cell count to drop to very low levels, and concurrent neutropenia, a drop in neutrophils in the blood, develops. In the case of the antipsychotics, the medication suppresses the bone marrow precursors to blood factors. The exact mechanism by which the drugs produce this effect is unknown. The most notable symptoms of this disorder include high fever, sore throat, and mouth sores. Although benign elevations in temperature have been reported in individuals taking clozapine, no fever should go uninvestigated. Agranulocytosis can be life-threatening if untreated.

Although agranulocytosis can occur with any of the antipsychotics, the risk with clozapine is 10 to 20 times greater than with the other antipsychotics (Schatzberg et al., 1997). Therefore, prescription of clozapine requires weekly blood samples to assess white blood cells and neutrophils. Drawing of these samples must continue for 4 weeks after clozapine has been discontinued. Weekly samples are required because the onset of symptoms can be gradual or quite rapid, occurring in 8 days or less. If sore throat or fever develops, medications should be withheld until a leukocyte count can be obtained. Hospitalization, including reverse isolation to prevent infections, is usually required. Agranulocytosis is more likely to develop in the first 18 weeks of treatment. Some research indicates that it is more common in women.

Miscellaneous Side Effects

Photosensitivity reactions to antipsychotics, including severe sunburns or rash, most commonly develop with the use of low-potency medications. Sun block must be worn on all areas of exposed skin. In addition, sun exposure may cause pigmentary deposits to develop, resulting in discoloration of exposed areas, especially the neck and face. This discoloration may progress from a deep orange color to a blue gray. Skin exposure should be limited and skin tone changes reported to the prescriber. Pigmentary deposits may also develop on the retina of the eye, especially with high doses of thioridazine, even for a few days. This condition is called *retinitis pigmentosa* and can lead to significant visual impairment. Therefore, thioridazine should never be administered in doses over 800 mg/d.

Antipsychotics may also lower the seizure threshold. Patients with an undetected seizure disorder may develop seizures early in treatment. Those who have a preexisting condition should be monitored closely.

Neuroleptic malignant syndrome and water intoxication are two serious complications that may occur with the use of antipsychotic medications. Neuroleptic malignant syndrome, characterized by rigidity and high fever, is a rare condition that may occur abruptly with even one dose of medication. Temperature must always be monitored when administering antipsychotics, especially high-potency medications. Water intoxication may develop gradually over a period of long-term use. This condition is characterized by the patient's consumption of large quantities of fluid (polydipsia) and the resulting effects of sodium depletion (hyponatremia). Both of these conditions are discussed more fully in Chapter 18.

Medication-Related Movement Disorders

Medication-related movement disorders are a group of side effects or adverse reactions that are most commonly caused by typical antipsychotic medications, but they have been identified less commonly with atypical antipsychotic drugs as well. These disorders of abnormal motor movements can be divided into two groups: acute extrapyramidal syndromes, which are acute abnormal movements developing early in the course of treatment (sometimes after just one dose); and chronic syndromes, which develop from longer exposure to antipsychotic drugs. The atypical antipsychotic drugs are most likely to cause movement disorders.

Acute Extrapyramidal Syndromes. Acute extrapyramidal syndromes occur in as many as 90% (Glazer, 2000) of all patients receiving antipsychotic medications. These syndromes develop early in the course of treatment, sometimes from as little as one dose. Although these acute abnormal movements are more easily treatable, they are at times dramatic and frightening, causing physical and emotional impairments that often result in patients discontinuing their own medication. Some milder forms may occur with other classes of medication, including the SSRIs.

The acute extrapyramidal syndromes, including dystonia, parkinsonism, and akathisia, occur early in treatment, but with slightly variable time frames. In addition, each responds somewhat differently to interventions for relief. Nurses play a vital role in the early recognition and treatment of these syndromes. Early recognition can save the patient considerable discomfort, fear, and impairment. All nurses must be aware of these symptoms, notifying the prescriber as soon as possible and implementing selected medication changes and other interventions. A number of medications can control these acute extrapyramidal symptoms (Table 8-10).

Dystonia, sometimes referred to as an *acute dystonic reaction*, is an impairment in muscle tone that is generally the first extrapyramidal symptom to occur, usually within a few days of initiating an antipsychotic. Dystonia is characterized by involuntary muscle spasms, especially of the head and neck muscles. Patients will often first complain of a thick tongue, tight jaw, or stiff neck. The syndrome can progress to include a protruding tongue, oculogyric crisis (eyes rolled up in the head), torticollis (muscle stiffness in the neck, which draws the head to one side with chin pointing to the other), and laryngopharyngeal constriction. Abnormal postures of the upper limbs and torso may be briefly held or sustained. In severe cases, the spasms may progress to the intercostal muscles, producing more significant breathing difficulty for patients who already have respiratory impairment from asthma or emphysema, for example.

Drug-induced parkinsonism is sometimes referred to as **pseudoparkinsonism** because its presentation is identical to Parkinson's disease without the same destruction of dopaminergic cells. These symptoms in-

TABLE 8.10 Common Treatments for Acute Medication-Related Movement Disorders

Agents	Typical Dosage Ranges	Routes Available	Common Side Effects
Anticholinergics			
Benztropine (Cogentin)	2–6 mg/d	PO, IM, IV	Dry mouth, blurred vision, slowed gastric motility causing constipation, urinary retention, increased intraocular pressure, overdose produces toxic psychosis
Trihexyphenidyl (Artane)	4–15 mg/d	PO	Same as benztropine, plus gastrointestinal distress Elderly people are most prone to mental confusion and delirium
Biperiden (Akineton)	2–8 mg/d	PO	Fewer peripheral anticholinergic effects Euphoria and increased tremor may occur
Antihistamines			
Diphenhydramine (Benadryl)	25–50 mg qid to 400 mg daily	PO, IM, IV	Sedation and confusion, especially in elderly people
Dopamine Agonists			
Amantadine (Symmetrel)	100–400 mg daily	PO	Indigestion, decreased concentration, dizziness, anxiety, ataxia, insomnia, lethargy, tremors, and slurred speech may occur on higher doses Tolerance may develop on fixed dose
β-Blockers			
Propranolol (Inderal)	10 mg tid to 120 mg daily	PO	Hypotension and bradycardia Must monitor pulse and blood pressure Do not stop abruptly as may cause rebound tachycardia
Benzodiazepines			
Lorazepam (Ativan)	1–2 mg IM 0.5–2 mg PO	PO, IM	All may cause drowsiness, lethargy, and general sedation or paradoxical agitation Confusion and disorientation in elderly people
Diazepam (Valium)	2–5 mg tid	PO, IV	Most side effects are rare and will disappear if dose is decreased
Clonazepam (Klonopin)	1–4 mg/d	PO	Tolerance and withdrawal are potential problems

From Nihart, M. A. (1995). *Managing the symptoms of schizophrenia: A nursing perspective.* American Psychiatric Nursing Association, Slide Kit, p. 29. Belle Mead, NJ: Excerpta Medica.

clude the classic triad of rigidity, slowed movements (akinesia), and tremor. The rigid muscle stiffness is usually most easily identified in the arms. Akinesia can be observed by the loss of spontaneous movements, such as the absence of the usual relaxed swing of the arms while walking. In addition, masklike facies or loss of facial expression and a decrease in the ability to initiate movements are also present. Usually, the tremor is more pronounced at rest, but it can also be observed with in-

tentional movements, such as while eating. If this tremor becomes severe, it may interfere with the patient's ability to eat or maintain adequate fluid intake. Hypersalivation is possible as well. Pseudoparkinsonism symptoms may occur on one or both sides of the body and develop abruptly or in a subtle manner, usually within the first 30 days of treatment.

Akathisia, another involuntary movement disorder, is characterized by the inability to sit still. The person will frequently be observed pacing, rocking while sitting or standing, marching in place, or crossing and uncrossing the legs. All of these repetitive motions have an intensity that is frequently beyond the explanation of the individual. In addition, akathisia may be present as a primarily subjective experience without obvious motor behavior. This subjective experience includes feelings of anxiety, jitteriness, or the inability to relax, which the individual may or may not be able to communicate. It is extremely uncomfortable for a person experiencing akathisia to be forced to sit still or be confined. These symptoms are sometimes misdiagnosed as agitation or an increase in psychotic symptoms, but if the nurse administers a PRN of an antipsychotic medication, the symptoms will not abate and will often worsen. Differentiating akathisia from agitation may be aided by knowing the person's symptoms before the introduction of medication. Psychotic agitation does not usually begin abruptly after antipsychotic medication has been started, whereas akathisia may occur after administration. In addition, the nurse may ask the patient if the experience is felt primarily in the muscles (akathisia) or in the mind or emotions (agitation).

Akathisia is the most difficult acute medication-related movement disorder to relieve. It does not usually respond well to anticholinergic medications; therefore, it is hypothesized that the still unknown source of pathology may involve more than just the extrapyramidal motor system (Baldassano et al., 1996). A number of medications have been tried to reduce the symptoms of akathisia, including β-adrenergic blockers, anticholinergics, antihistamines, and low-dose antianxiety agents (Sajatovic, 2000). The usual approach to treatment begins with a reduction in dose of antipsychotic medication. During this time, psychiatric–mental health nurses must closely assess for signs of increased psychosis. Then, β-adrenergic blockers, such as propranolol (Inderal), given in doses of 30 to 120 mg/d, have been most successful. Nurses must monitor the patient's pulse and blood pressure because propranolol can cause hypotension and bradycardia. If the individual's pulse is below 60, propranolol should be withheld and the prescriber notified. Normal signs of hypoglycemia may be blocked by propranolol; therefore, patients with diabetes must monitor their blood or urine glucose carefully, especially because they are under physical stress from the disorder. Also, propranolol should be taken with food to facilitate absorption.

A number of nursing interventions may reduce the impact of these syndromes. Individuals with acute extrapyramidal symptoms need frequent reassurance that this is not a worsening of their psychiatric condition, but instead is a treatable side effect of the medication. They also need validation that what they are experiencing is real and that the nurse is concerned and will be responsive to changes in these symptoms. Physical and psychological stress appear to increase the symptoms

and further frighten the patient; therefore, decreasing stressful situations becomes important. These symptoms are often exhausting for the patient, and nurses should ensure that the patient receives adequate rest. Because tremors, muscle rigidity, and motor restlessness may interfere with the individual's ability to eat, the nurse may need to assist the patient with eating and drinking fluids to maintain nutrition and hydration.

Risk factors for the development of acute syndromes include previous presence of extrapyramidal symptoms. Listen closely when patients say they are "allergic" to antipsychotic medications. Often, they are describing one of the medication-related movement disorders, particularly dystonia, rather than a rash or other allergic symptoms. About 90% of the individuals who have experienced extrapyramidal symptoms in the past will again have these symptoms if antipsychotic medications are restarted (Arana, 2000). High-potency medications, such as haloperidol and fluphenazine, are more likely to cause extrapyramidal symptoms. Age and gender appear to be risk factors for specific syndromes. Acute dystonia occurs most often in young men, adolescents, and children; akathisia is more common in middle-aged women. Elderly patients are at the greatest risk for developing pseudoparkinsonism (Madhusoodanan et al., 2000). Risk factors may be helpful in identifying individuals who need closer assessment of acute extrapyramidal syndromes.

Chronic Syndromes. Chronic syndromes develop from long-term use of antipsychotics. They are serious and afflict about 20% of the patients who receive antipsychotics for an extended period of time. These conditions are often irreversible and cause significant impairment in self-image, social interactions, and occupational functioning. Early symptoms and mild forms may go unnoticed by the person experiencing them because they frequently remain beyond the individual's awareness. Therefore, psychiatric–mental health nurses in contact with individuals who are taking antipsychotic medications for months or years must be vigilant to the early symptoms of these chronic conditions.

First identified in 1957, tardive dyskinesia is the most well-known of the chronic syndromes. It involves irregular, repetitive involuntary movements of the mouth, face, and tongue, including chewing, tongue protrusion, lip smacking, puckering of the lips, and rapid eye blinking. Abnormal finger movements are common as well. In some individuals, the trunk and extremities are also involved, and in rare cases, irregular breathing and swallowing lead to belching and grunting noises. These symptoms usually begin no earlier than after 6 months of treatment or when the medication is reduced or withdrawn. Once thought to be irreversible, considerable controversy now exists as to whether or not this is true.

Part of the difficulty in determining the irreversibility of tardive dyskinesia is that any movement disorder that persists after discontinuation of antipsychotic medication has been described as tardive dyskinesia. Atypical forms are now receiving more attention because some researchers believe they may have different underlying mechanisms of causation. Some of these forms of the disorder appear to remit spontaneously. Symptoms of what is now called *withdrawal tardive dyskinesia* appear when an antipsychotic medication is reduced or discontinued and remit spontaneously in 1 to 3 months. Tardive dystonia and tardive akathisia have also been described. Both appear in a manner similar to the acute syndromes but continue after the antipsychotic medication has been withdrawn. More research is needed to determine whether these syndromes are distinctly different in origin and outcome.

The risk for developing tardive dyskinesia increases with age. Although the prevalence of tardive dyskinesia averages 15% to 20%, the rate rises to 50% to 70% in elderly patients receiving antipsychotic medications (Yeung et al., 2000). Cumulative incidence of tardive dyskinesia appears to increase 5% per year of continued exposure to antipsychotic medications (Sajatovic, 2000). Women are at higher risk than men. Individuals with affective disorders, particularly depression, are at higher risk than those who have schizophrenia. Any individual receiving antipsychotic medication may develop tardive dyskinesia; therefore, nurses must be particularly alert to individuals at higher risk. Risk factors are summarized in Text Box 8-2.

The exact cause of tardive dyskinesia remains unclear. Neuroimaging and postmortem studies have failed to provide direct evidence of pathology in the CNS. The most commonly held theory proposes that chronic dopamine suppression in the extrapyramidal motor system causes an overactivation of that system as a possible counterbalance. Increases in antipsychotic medication suppress the symptoms. Reduction in the dose of antipsychotic medication or administration of dopamine agonists frequently increases the symptoms. Therefore, the dopamine receptors have been thought to be hypersensitive, possibly by developing increased numbers, but again, this has not been supported by direct evidence. No other hypotheses concerning other neurotransmitters have produced consistent results.

Lack of a consistent theory of etiology for the chronic medication-related movement disorder syndromes has led to inconsistent and disappointing treatment approaches. No one medication relieves the symptoms. Dopamine agonists, such as bromocriptine, and many other drugs have been tried. Even dietary precursors of acetylcholine, such as lethicin, and nutritional therapies, such as vitamin E supplements, provided initial positive results, but since have been of variable or no benefit.

The best approach to treatment remains avoiding the development of the chronic syndromes. Preventive measures include using the lowest possible dose of medication, minimizing use of PRN medication, and closely monitoring individuals in high-risk groups for development of the symptoms of tardive dyskinesia. All mental health treatment team members who have contact with individuals taking antipsychotics for longer than 3 months must be alert to the risk factors and earliest possible signs of chronic medication-related movement disorders. Monitoring tools, such as the Abnormal Involuntary Movement Scale, should be used routinely to standardize assessment and provide the earliest possible recognition of the symptoms. Standardized assessments should be preformed at no more than 3- to 6-month intervals. The earlier the symptoms are recognized, the more likely they will resolve if the medication can be changed or discontinued. Newer, atypical antipsychotic medications have a much lower risk of causing tardive dyskinesia and are increasingly being considered the first approach to the treatment of schizophrenia. Other medications are under development to provide alternatives that limit the risk for tardive dyskinesia.

MOOD STABILIZERS (ANTIMANIA MEDICATIONS)

Mood stabilizers, or antimania medications, are psychopharmacologic agents used for stabilizing mood swings, particularly those of mania in bipolar affective disorders. For a number of years, lithium was the only drug known to relieve the symptoms of mania. Although it remains the primary treatment for acute mania and maintenance of bipolar affective disorders, not all individuals respond to lithium alone, and increasingly, other drugs are being used as first-line agents. In the 1970s, carbamazepine and later valproate, both anticonvulsants approved for the treatment of epilepsy, were found to have mood-stabilizing effects (see Table 16-4 in Chap. 20). Other medications, such as calcium-channel blockers, have been used to treat the symptoms of mania,

TEXT BOX 8.2

Risk Factors for Tardive Dyskinesia

- Age more than 50 y
- Female
- Affective disorders, particularly depression
- Brain damage or dysfunction
- Increased duration of treatment
- Standard antipsychotic medication
- Possible—higher doses of antipsychotic medication

From Kane, J. M., & Lieberman, J. (1992). Tardive dyskinesia. In J. M. Kane & J. A. Lieberman (Eds.), *Adverse effects of psychotropic drugs* (pp. 235–245). New York: Guilford.

but at this point, they remain experimental. Benzodiazepines, such as clonazepam and lorazepam, have also been used to control some acute symptoms, but have not been proved to have mood-stabilizing effects. Therefore, this section focuses on lithium and the anticonvulsants in current use.

Lithium

Lithium, an element, was first discovered in the early 1800s. It has been in medical use in a variety of forms, including tonics and elixirs, since that time. As a salt substitute, lithium produced a number of cases of toxicity and, as a result, lost favor in the 1940s. Rediscovered in 1949 by the Australian John Cade, lithium was found to reduce agitation in some patients experiencing psychosis, and in the 1950s, Schou published reports that lithium controlled and prevented the symptoms of mania. In 1970, the FDA approved lithium for use in the treatment of manic episodes in bipolar affective disorder. Since then, it has become a mainstay in psychopharmacology. About 70% to 80% of the individuals receiving lithium alone have at least a partial improvement of symptoms, if not total relief (Tondo et al., 2000). Although not a perfect drug, it has restored stability to the lives of thousands of people.

Indications and Mechanisms of Action

The only FDA-approved indication for the use of lithium is treating the symptoms of mania and preventing recurrence of these symptoms. At the very least, it diminishes the intensity and severity of manic episodes. Therefore, its target symptoms are those of mania, such as rapid speech, jumping from topic to topic (flight of ideas), irritability, grandiose thinking, impulsiveness, and agitation. (See Chap. 20 for a further description of the symptoms of mania.) Other psychiatric indications include some antidepressant effects, especially in depression associated with bipolar affective disorder. More recently, lithium has been proved to be an effective addition to antidepressants in the treatment of major depression that has only partially responded to antidepressants alone. Therefore, lithium has been used in augmentation as a potentiator (enhancing the effects) of antidepressant medications. It has also been investigated in the treatment of a number of other psychiatric disorders, but results have either been unconvincing or need further study.

With nonpsychiatric disorders, lithium has been effective in the treatment of cluster headaches. Because lithium stimulates leukocytosis, it often improves the neutrophil counts of patients receiving chemotherapy or who have other conditions that cause neutropenia. In addition, lithium has been investigated as an antiviral agent because it appears to inhibit the replication of several DNA viruses, including herpesvirus. Further research is needed to understand the mechanisms of these effects.

The exact action by which lithium improves the symptoms of mania is unknown. Lithium is actively transported across cell membranes, altering sodium transport in both nerve and muscle cells. It replaces sodium in the sodium–potassium pump and is retained more readily than sodium inside the cell. Conditions that alter sodium content in the body, such as vomiting, diuresis, and diaphoresis, also alter lithium retention. The results of lithium influx into the nerve cell lead to increased storage of catecholamines within the cell, reduced dopamine neurotransmission, increased norepinephrine reuptake, increased GABA activity, and increased serotonin receptor sensitivity (Solomon et al., 2000). Lithium also alters the distribution of calcium and magnesium ions and inhibits second messenger systems within the neuron. Most likely, the mechanisms by which lithium improves the symptoms of mania are complex, involving the sum of all or part of these actions and more. Molecular research in the next decade may provide the answers.

Pharmacokinetics

Lithium carbonate is available orally in capsule, tablet, and liquid forms. Slow-release preparations are also available. Lithium is readily absorbed in the gastric system and may be taken with food, which does not impair absorption. Peak blood levels are reached in 1 to 4 hours, and the medication is usually completely absorbed in 8 hours. Slow-release preparations are absorbed at a slower, more variable rate.

Lithium is not protein bound, and its distribution into the CNS across the blood–brain barrier is slow. The onset of action is usually 5 to 7 days and may take up to 2 weeks. The elimination half-life is 8 to 12 hours, and 18 to 36 hours in individuals whose blood levels have reached steady state and whose symptoms are stable. Lithium is almost entirely excreted by the kidneys but is present in all body fluids. Conditions of renal impairment or decreased renal function in elderly patients decrease lithium clearance and may lead to toxicity. Several medications affect renal function and therefore change lithium clearance. See Chapter 20 for a list of these and other medication interactions with lithium. Eighty percent of lithium is reabsorbed in the proximal tubule of the kidney along with water and sodium. In conditions that cause sodium depletion, such as dehydration due to fever, strenuous exercise, hot weather, increased perspiration, and vomiting, the kidney attempts to conserve sodium. It retains lithium as well, leading to increased blood levels and potential toxicity. Significantly increasing sodium intake causes lithium levels to decrease.

Lithium is usually administered in doses of 300 mg two to three times daily. Blood levels are monitored frequently during acute mania, while the dosage is increased every 3 to 5 days. These increases may be slower in elderly patients or patients who experience uncomfortable side effects. Blood levels should be drawn about 12 hours after the last dose of medication. In the hospital setting, nurses should withhold the morning dose of lithium until the serum sample is drawn to avoid falsely elevated levels. Individuals who are at home should be instructed to have their blood drawn in the morning about 12 hours after their last dose and before they take their first dose of medication. During the acute phases of mania, blood levels of 0.8 to 1.4 mEq/L are usually attained and maintained until symptoms are under control. The therapeutic range for lithium is narrow, and patients in the higher end of that range usually experience more uncomfortable side effects. During maintenance, the dosage is reduced, and blood levels are lowered to 0.4 to 1 mEq/L.

Lithium clears the body relatively quickly after discontinuation. Withdrawal symptoms are rare, but occasional anxiety and emotional lability have been reported. It is important to remember that almost half of the individuals who discontinue lithium treatment abruptly experience a relapse of symptoms within a few weeks (Goodwin & Ghaemi, 2000). Some research suggests that discontinuation of lithium for individuals whose symptoms have been stable may lead to lithium losing its effectiveness when the medication is restarted. Patients should be warned of the risks in abruptly discontinuing their medication. They should be advised to consider the options carefully in consultation with their prescriber.

Side Effects, Adverse Reactions, and Toxicity

At lower therapeutic blood levels, side effects from lithium are relatively mild. These reactions correspond with peaks in plasma concentrations of the medication after administration, and most subside during the first few weeks of therapy. Frequently, individuals taking lithium complain of excessive thirst and a metallic taste. Sugarless throat lozenges may be useful in minimizing this side effect. Other common side effects include increased frequency of urination, fine head tremor, drowsiness, and mild diarrhea. Weight gain occurs in about 20% of the individuals taking lithium. Nausea may be minimized by taking the medication with food or by use of a slow-release preparation. However, slow-release forms of lithium increase diarrhea. Muscle weakness, restlessness, headache, acne, rashes, and exacerbation of psoriasis have also been reported. See Table 16-8 in Chapter 20 for a summary of selected nursing interventions to minimize the impact of common side effects associated with lithium treatment. Patients most frequently discontinued their own medication because of concerns with mental slowness, poor concentration, and memory problems. However, these symptoms have not been well documented in objective psychological testing.

As blood levels of lithium increase, the side effects of lithium become more numerous and severe. Early signs of lithium toxicity include severe diarrhea, vomiting, drowsiness, muscular weakness, and lack of coordination. Lithium should be withheld and the prescriber consulted if these symptoms develop. Lithium toxicity can easily be resolved in 24 to 48 hours by discontinuing the medication, but hemodialysis may be required in severe situations. See Chapter 20 for a summary of the side effects and symptoms of toxicity associated with various blood levels of lithium.

Monitoring of creatinine concentration, thyroid hormones, and CBCs every 6 months during maintenance therapy helps to assess the occurrence of other potential adverse reactions. Although controversial, kidney damage is still considered a potential risk in long-term lithium treatment. This damage is usually reversible after discontinuation of the lithium. A gradual rise in serum creatinine and decline in creatinine clearance indicate the development of renal dysfunction. Individuals with preexisting kidney dysfunction are susceptible to lithium toxicity.

Lithium may alter thyroid function, usually after 6 to 18 months of treatment. About 30% of the individuals taking lithium exhibit elevations in thyroid-stimulating hormone, but most do not show suppression of circulating thyroid hormone. Thyroid dysfunction from lithium treatment is more common in women. Some individuals require the addition of thyroxine. During maintenance, thyroid-stimulating hormone levels may be monitored. Nurses should observe for dry skin, constipation, bradycardia, hair loss, cold intolerance, and other symptoms of hypothyroidism. Other endocrine system effects result from hypoparathyroidism, which increases parathyroid hormone levels and calcium. Clinically, this change is not significant, but elevated calcium levels may cause mood changes, anxiety, lethargy, and sleep disturbances. These symptoms may erroneously be attributed to depression if hypercalcemia is not investigated.

Lithium use should be avoided during pregnancy because it has been associated with birth defects, especially when administered during the first trimester. If lithium is given in the third trimester, toxicity may develop in a newborn, producing signs of hypotonia, cyanosis, bradykinesia, cardiac changes, gastrointestinal bleeding, and shock. Diabetes insipidus may persist for months. Lithium is also present in breast milk, and new mothers should not breast-feed while taking lithium. Women expecting to become pregnant should be advised to consult with their physician before discontinuing birth control methods.

Anticonvulsants

Although lithium alone has provided tremendous relief to thousands of individuals experiencing bipolar affective disorder, 20% to 40% of those affected by the disorder do not respond, most often those with rapid cycling episodes. The psychopharmacologic properties of some anticonvulsant medications have been reported since the 1960s, but it was not until the 1970s in Japan that carbamazepine was found to have mood-stabilizing effects in bipolar affective disorders. Concern about blood dyscrasias delayed its release in the United States. The increased risks for aplastic anemia and agranulocytosis still require close monitoring of CBCs during treatment, and carbamazepine provides a reasonable alternative. Valproate and its derivatives have a similar course of development. Divalproex sodium (Depakote), an enteric-coated valproate derivative, was first marketed in the United States in 1983 and has more recently received FDA approval for treatment of mania in bipolar affective disorder. Recently, gabapentin (Neurontin), lamotrigine (Lamictal), and topiramate (Topamax) are anticonvulsant that are being used as well for control of manic symptoms.

Indications and Mechanisms of Action

Anticonvulsant medications in general are indicated for the treatment of seizure disorders. Specifically, carbamazepine is indicated for treatment of partial seizures with complex motor movements as well as for trigeminal neuralgia. Divalproex sodium is indicated for both simple and complex seizures. Both carbamazepine and divalproex sodium have received FDA approval for treatment of mania and are used widely for this purpose in other countries.

Target symptoms for the use of anticonvulsants with bipolar affective disorder include all of the symptoms of mania discussed earlier. However, anticonvulsants are often used for individuals who have not responded to lithium. Studies have shown some common traits in these individuals. Lithium nonresponders are most often those who have a dysphoric or mixed mania. These individuals experience the increase in physical activity of mania without the elevation in mood. They are often referred to as mixed states because they have elements of both depression and mania. These individuals exhibit symptoms of high anxiety, agitation, and irritability, which are then target symptoms for the use of anticonvulsants. See Chapter 20 for further information regarding subgroups of symptoms in bipolar affective disorder.

Rapid cycling is another subtype of bipolar affective disorder in which individuals experience four or more episodes of either depression or mania during a 12-month period. This occurs more often in women than in men and comprises another group of individuals who respond poorly to lithium treatment. Mood stability is also a target symptom of anticonvulsant medications. The theory of the mechanism of action of the anticonvulsants involves the concept of kindling as it applies to mood disorders. *Kindling* refers to the repeated electrical stimulation of selected brain regions, such as the amygdala, that apparently sensitizes the nerve cells in that region. This stimulation may be subthreshold and may work cumulatively to produce seizure activity. Once these regions are sensitized, it takes considerably less stimulation to initiate a seizure. In the case of mood disorders, the stimulation of these regions, possibly by external stressors or other emotional factors, produces a mood swing instead of a seizure.

Anticonvulsants are thought to have "antikindling" properties and decrease the sensitization of affected cells. Carbamazepine has many actions, but its effects on ion channels reduce repetitive firing of action potentials in the nerves. In addition, carbamazepine affects the release and reuptake of several neurotransmitters, including norepinephrine, GABA, dopamine, and glutamate. It also changes several second messenger systems. No one action has successfully accounted for its ability to stabilize mood. Divalproex sodium also has numerous neurotransmission effects. The most widely held theory of how it stabilizes mood swings relates to its effects on GABA. As the major inhibitory neurotransmitter in the CNS, increased levels of GABA and improved responsiveness of the neurons to GABA lead to control of epileptic activity. Divalproex sodium increases levels of GABA in the CNS by activating its synthesis, inhibiting the catabolism (destructive metabolism) of GABA, increasing its release, and increasing receptor density (Solomon et al., 2000). Although the exact mechanisms of action for the anticonvulsants remain unknown, these theories related to kindling and the enhanced functioning of GABA hold promise for the future of new developments in treatment.

Pharmacokinetics

Carbamazepine is absorbed in a somewhat variable manner. The liquid suspension is absorbed more quickly than the tablet form, but food does not appear to interfere with absorption. Peak plasma levels occur in 2 to 6 hours. Because high doses influence peak plasma levels and increase the risk for side effects, carbamazepine should be given in divided doses two or three times a day. The suspension, which has higher peak plasma levels and lower trough levels, must be given more frequently than the tablet form.

Valproic acid is more rapidly absorbed, but the enteric coating of divalproex sodium adds a delay of up to 1 hour. Peak serum levels occur in about 1 to 4 hours. The liquid form (sodium valproate) is absorbed more rapidly and peaks in 15 minutes to 2 hours (Olin, 1996). Food appears to slow absorption, but does not lower bioavailability of the drug. Absorption of both carbamazepine and valproic acid is decreased by charcoal, which will reduce their effectiveness.

Carbamazepine and valproic acid are highly protein bound; therefore, patients who are medically ill or malnourished may experience the effects of increased unbound levels of both drugs. When given with other drugs that are competing for the same protein-binding sites, higher levels of unbound drug may occur. In both cases, these individuals will experience more side effects and fluctuations in medication plasma levels. Newer agents for treatment of bipolar affective disorder, such as gabapentin, have little protein binding and are therefore not subject to some of these effects. Both drugs also cross easily into the CNS and move into the placenta as well. Both are associated with an increased risk for birth defects, including spina bifida, and carbamazepine does accumulate in fetal tissue.

Carbamazepine and valproic acid are metabolized by the cytochrome P-450 system of microsomal hepatic enzymes. However, one of the metabolites of carbamazepine is potentially toxic. If other concurrent medications inhibit the enzymes that break down this toxic metabolite, severe adverse reactions are often the result. Medications that inhibit this breakdown include erythromycin, verapamil, and cimetidine (now available in nonprescription form). See Chapter 20 for a list of these and other drugs that interact with carbamazepine. Nurses should educate patients as to the potential drug interactions, especially with nonprescription medications, and should inform other health care practitioners who may be prescribing medication that these patients are taking carbamazepine. It is also important to note that oral contraceptives may become ineffective, and female patients should be advised to use other methods of birth control.

Carbamazepine activates its own metabolism through induction of the P-450 microsomal hepatic enzymes. As long as 2 to 3 months after steady state has been achieved, patients receiving carbamazepine may experience a precipitant drop in therapeutic blood levels and a relapse in symptoms if the dosage of medication is not increased. Although valproic acid is also affected by other medications that stimulate the P-450 system, it does not enhance its own metabolism. Gabapentin has no active metabolites and is eliminated by renal excretion primarily as unchanged drug. Recently, both carbamazepine and valproic acid have been available in slow release, extended action forms, allowing for decreased daily dosing and improved compliance.

Side Effects, Adverse Reactions, and Toxicity

The most common side effects of carbamazepine are dizziness, drowsiness, tremor, visual disturbance, nausea, and vomiting. These side effects may be minimized by initiating treatment in low doses. Patients should be advised that these symptoms will diminish, but care should be taken when changing positions or performing tasks that require visual alertness. Nausea may be diminished by giving the drug with food. Valproic acid also causes gastrointestinal disturbances, tremor, and lethargy. In addition, it is more likely to produce weight gain and alopecia (hair loss). These symptoms are transient and should diminish over the course of treatment. Dietary supplements of zinc and selenium may be helpful to patients experiencing hair loss. Constipation and urinary retention occur in some individuals. Nurses should monitor urinary output and assist patients to increase fluid consumption to decrease constipation.

Transient elevations in liver enzymes occur with both carbamazepine and valproic acid. Rarely do symptoms of hepatic injury occur. If the patient reports abnormal pain or shows signs of jaundice, the prescriber should be notified immediately. Several blood dyscrasias may occur with carbamazepine, including aplastic anemia, agranulocytosis, and leukopenia. Patients should be advised to report fever, sore throat, rash, petechiae, or bruising immediately. In addition, advise patients of the importance of completing routine blood tests throughout treatment.

Both valproic acid and carbamazepine may be lethal if high doses are ingested. Toxic symptoms appear in 1 to 3 hours and include neuromuscular disturbances, dizziness, stupor, agitation, disorientation, nystagmus, urinary retention, nausea and vomiting, tachycardia, hypotension or hypertension, cardiovascular shock, coma, and respiratory depression. Carbamazepine appears to be more lethal at lower doses, but valproic acid is absorbed rapidly, and gastric lavage may be ineffective, depending on time from ingestion. Of the newer anticonvulsant drugs, gabapentin has relatively few side effects, whereas lamictal has been associated with ataxia, dizziness, and Stevens-Johnson syndrome.

ANTIDEPRESSANT MEDICATIONS

Researchers in the 1950s who were investigating other drugs related to the phenothiazines for treatment of psychosis discovered that imipramine, a somewhat related compound, relieved the symptoms of depression. Imipramine was the first of a number of medications that contained a three-ring structure in their chemical make up and produced improvement in depression. These medications became known as the *tricyclic antidepressants* (TCAs). Table 8-11 lists other related TCAs still in use today.

Concurrent with the discovery of TCAs, an antibiotic, iproniazid, used in the treatment of tuberculosis, was also found to alleviate the symptoms of depression. Iproniazid increased the bioamine neurotransmitters by inhibiting monoamine oxidase, the enzyme that breaks down these neurotransmitters inside the nerve cell. Iproniazid is no longer used, but related, more effective drugs, phenelzine and tranylcypromine, make up the subgroup of antidepressants called MAOIs.

TABLE 8.11   Antidepressant Medications

Generic (Trade) Drug Name	Usual Dosage Range (mg/d)	Half-Life (h)	Therapeutic Blood Level (ng/mL)
Tricyclic—Tertiary Amines			
Amitriptyline (Elavil)	50–300	31–46	110–250
Clomipramine (Anafranil)	25–250	19–37	80–100
Doxepin (Sinequan)	25–300	8–24	100–200
Imipramine (Tofranil)	30–300	11–25	200–350
Tricyclics—Secondary Amines			
Amoxapine (Asendin)	50–600	8	200–500
Desipramine (Norpramin)	25–300	12–24	125–300
Nortriptyline (Aventyl, Pamelor)	30–100	18–44	50–150
Protriptyline (Vivactil)	15–60	67–89	100–200
Serotonin Selective Reuptake Inhibitors			
Fluoxetine (Prozac)	20–80	2–9 days	72–300
Sertraline (Zoloft)	50–200	24	Not available
Paroxetine (Paxil)	10–50	10–24	Not available
Fluvoxamine (Luvox)	50–300	17–22	Not available
Citalopram (Celexa)	20–50	35	Not available
Other Antidepressant Medications			
PHENETHYLAMINE			
Venlafaxine (Effexor)	75–375	5–11	100–500
TETRACYCLIC			
Maprotiline (Ludiomil)	50–225	21–25	200–300
TRIAZOLOPYRIDINE			
Trazodone (Desyrel)	150–600	4–9	650–1,600
PHENYLPIPERAZINE			
Nefazodone (Serzone)	100–600	2–4	Not available
AMINOKETONE			
Bupropion (Wellbutrin)	200–450	8–24	10–29
PIPERAZINOAZEPINES			
Mirtazapine (Remeron)	15–45	20–40	Not available
Monoamine Oxidase Inhibitors			
Phenelzine (Nardil)	15–90	24 (effect lasts 3–4 d)	Not available
Tranylcypromine (Parnate)	10–60	24 (effect lasts 3–10 d)	Not available

Throughout the 1960s and 1970s, the TCAs and MAOIs were the primary treatment of depression. Research continued to develop new agents with increased effectiveness, while decreasing the side effects and potential lethal effects. In the 1980s, several medications of significantly different chemical structure were introduced. Bupropion (Wellbutrin), introduced in 1987, had actions that were significantly different from those of previous antidepressants, but concern about the risk for seizures and other side effects limited excitement about its use. In 1988, the release of fluoxetine received much public attention and resulted in increased awareness of depression and its treatment. Fluoxetine was the first of a class of drugs that acted "selectively" on one group of neurotransmitters: serotonin. Other similarly selective medications, sertraline, paroxetine, and fluvoxamine, soon followed and together make up the SSRIs.

Indications

The primary indication for the use of antidepressant medications is depression, hence the name *antidepressant*. Symptoms such as loss of interest in the person's usual activities, depressed mood, lethargy or decreased energy, insomnia, decreased concentration, loss of appetite, and suicidal ideation usually respond well (about 70% of individuals who have depression) to antidepressant medications. (See Chap. 20 for a more complete discussion of the symptoms of depression.) Antidepressants are also used to treat a number of other symptoms and disorders. The name antidepressant is therefore somewhat misleading.

Some antidepressants are used to treat anxiety disorders, including panic attacks (see Chap. 21). Others relieve the ruminations and repetitive behaviors of eating disorders (see Chap. 24) and obsessive-compulsive disorders. Antidepressants are also used to treat the symptoms of social phobia, depression in bipolar affective disorders, dysthymia, chronic pain disorders, and premenstrual syndrome. More sedating antidepressants are sometimes used in small doses to improve sleep disturbance. Trazodone in particular but also amitriptyline and other agents have been used alone or as adjunctive interventions for sleep disturbance. Antidepressants are used for other sleep disorders, such as sleep apnea (see Chap. 26) as well. Symptoms of some psychiatric disorders of childhood (see Chap. 29), such as attention deficit hyperactivity disorder (ADHD), enuresis (bed wetting), and school phobia, respond to antidepressant medication.

At times, the symptoms of depression present themselves in a somewhat "atypical" manner, and the entity is therefore sometimes referred to as *atypical depression*. These individuals have a mixture of anxiety and depression, hypersomnia, mood swings, worsening of the symptoms in the evening, and oversensitivity to such interpersonal feelings as rejection. These target symptoms of atypical depression often respond better to the MAOIs, such as phenelzine (Nardil).

Pharmacokinetics and Mechanism of Action

All of the antidepressant medications are well absorbed from the gastrointestinal system; however, some individual variations exist. For example, food delays the absorption of nefazodone and decreases its bioavailability by as much as 20% (Olin, 1996). Food slightly increases the amount of trazodone absorbed but decreases its maximum blood concentrations and lengthens the time to peak effects from 1 hour on an empty stomach to 2 hours with food. Food also increases the maximum concentrations of sertraline in the bloodstream and decreases the time to peak plasma levels, whereas fluoxetine and fluvoxamine are unaffected, although food may delay the absorption of fluoxetine. Food has little effect on the TCAs. Psychiatric–mental health nurses should review this information as it applies to each individual medication. They must consider how this information will affect the patient's use of the medication given the target symptoms for which the drug is intended. For example, if trazodone is being used on a continuous dose schedule for its antidepressant effect, the effects of food probably matter very little. However, if trazodone is being used in a small dose at bedtime to assist a patient to sleep, an empty stomach becomes important because food would lengthen the time of onset of clinical effects, in this case, sleep.

The TCAs undergo considerable first-pass metabolism, but reach peak plasma concentrations in 2 to 4 hours. The TCAs are highly bound to plasma proteins, which makes the association between blood levels and therapeutic clinical effects difficult. However, some plasma ranges have been established. Table 8-11 includes the available ranges for therapeutic blood levels of the TCAs. In addition, times to steady-state plasma levels have wide variations, and the effective dose of medication must be individualized. Other antidepressants are also highly protein bound, which means that drugs that compete for these binding sites may cause fluctuations in blood levels of the antidepressants. Venlafaxine has the lowest protein binding; therefore, drug interactions of this type are not expected with this medication. Blood level changes caused by the presence of other drugs competing with binding sites are not expected.

Onset of action varies considerably as well and appears to depend on factors outside of steady-state plasma levels. Initial improvement with some antidepressants, such as fluoxetine, may appear within 7 days, but complete relief of symptoms may take several weeks. Full enzyme inhibition with the MAOIs may take as long as 2 weeks, but the energizing effects may be seen within a few days. Overcoming issues such as social stigma, viewing depression as a personal failing, fear about taking a medication, and the decreased energy and motivation associated with depression have made deciding to seek treatment a major hurdle. For this and a host of other reasons, some individuals expect rapid and significant relief. The variable onset of action may discourage some patients. Psychiatric–mental health nurses are often involved in providing encouragement and other supportive interventions to assist the patient in "getting through" this period of time.

Antidepressants are primarily excreted in the kidneys; however, their routes of metabolism vary. Most of the TCAs have active metabolites that act in much the same manner as the parent drug. Therefore, determining the rate of elimination must consider the half-lives of these metabolites. Most of these antidepressants may be given in a once-daily single dose. If the medication causes sedation, this dose should be given at bedtime. The SSRIs frequently cause more activation of energy and are often given in the morning. Venlafaxine, nefazodone, and bupropion are examples of antidepressants whose shorter half-life periods and other factors require administration twice or three times per day. Fluoxetine and its active metabolite have particularly long half-lives, remaining present for as long as 5 to 6 weeks. This may affect a number of decisions. For example, women who wish to have children and are taking fluoxetine must discontinue its use at least 6 weeks before attempting to conceive. They should be advised to consult their prescriber before making this decision. Table 8-11 provides information about the average elimination half-lives of most of the antidepressants.

Most of the antidepressants are metabolized by the P-450 enzyme system, so that drugs that activate this system will tend to decrease blood levels of the antidepressants, and inhibitors of this system will increase antidepressant blood levels. This effect varies according to the subfamily that is activated. For example, fluvoxamine (Luvox) substantially inhibits the P-450CYP1A2 subsystem; thus, other drugs that are metabolized by the system will experience slower metabolism. These include such medications as amitriptyline, clomipramine, imipramine, clozapine, propranolol, theophylline, and caffeine (Preskorn, 1996). Fluoxetine inhibits most of the enzymes in the P-450 system, although some are not clinically significant at lower doses of fluoxetine. At higher doses, effects may be significant. Abrupt discontinuation of some of the antidepressants produces uncomfortable symptoms that begin within a few days. For patients who have been taking the TCAs for several weeks or months, abrupt discontinuation often causes headache, anxiety, insomnia, nausea, chills, muscle soreness, and generalized discomfort. These medications require a slow taper, decreasing the medication by 25 to 50 mg each week, to avoid these symptoms. The SSRIs with shorter half-lives, such as paroxetine, also produce flu-like symptoms of nausea, headache, dizziness, and irritability if abruptly discontinued. Individuals taking these medications should be advised not to stop them abruptly without consulting their prescriber. Arrangements or reminders should be implemented to have prescriptions refilled in a timely manner so that these symptoms may be avoided. Fluoxetine, which has a very long half-life, rarely produces a withdrawal syndrome.

Side Effects, Adverse Reactions, and Toxicity

Side effects of the antidepressant medications vary considerably. Because the TCAs act on several neurotransmitters in addition to serotonin and norepinephrine, these drugs have many unwanted effects. Conversely, the SSRIs are more selective for serotonin and have comparatively fewer and better tolerated side effects. As for all medications, uncomfortable side effects are the primary reason for many patients discontinuing treatment. With the TCAs, sedation, orthostatic hypotension, and anticholinergic side effects are the most common sources of discomfort for patients receiving these medications. See Chapter 20 for a comparison of side effects of antidepressant medications.

Receptor affinities may be helpful in predicting which side effects are most likely to occur with a given medication. Table 8-12 provides a relative weighting of the degree of affinity most of the antidepressants have for each of the major neurotransmitters. This is provided for reuptake blockade of serotonin, norepinephrine, and dopamine and for postsynaptic blockade of some of the subtypes of neurotransmitter receptors. Using this table

in conjunction with Chapter 20, nurses may be able to predict which side effects will be most common with each medication. Interventions to assist in minimizing these side effects are listed in Table 8-2.

Tolerance develops gradually to sedation and anticholinergic side effects caused by TCAs, but these may be minimized when the prescriber begins with a low dose and increases gradually. This is the approach used most often when a patient is not in a closely monitored setting, such as a hospital. Other side effects of the TCAs include tremors, restlessness, insomnia, nausea and vomiting, confusion, pedal edema, headache, and seizures. Blood dyscrasias may also occur, and any fever, sore throat, malaise, or rash should be reported to the prescriber.

Sexual dysfunction is a relatively common side effect with most antidepressants. Erectile and ejaculation disturbances occur in men and anorgasmia in women. This side effect is often difficult to assess if the nurse has not obtained a sexual history before initiation of the medication. Anorgasmia is particularly common with the SSRIs and often goes unreported, frequently because nurses and other health care providers do not ask. Bupropion and nefazodone (Serzone) appear to be least likely to cause sexual disturbance. In addition, when sexual dysfunction has been determined to be related to the medication, several options are available for treatment. These include the use of other medications or a change in medications. The patient should be encouraged to discuss these options with the prescriber because this side effect may precipitate self-discontinuation of the medication.

The TCAs have the potential for cardiotoxicity. Symptoms include prolongation of cardiac conduction that may worsen pre-existing cardiac conduction problems. TCAs are contraindicated with second-degree atrioventricular block and should be used cautiously in patients who have other cardiac problems. Occasionally, they may precipitate congestive heart failure, myocardial infarction, arrhythmias, and stroke. The newer antidepressants, such as the SSRIs and bupropion, are less cardiotoxic, and nefazodone currently exhibits no evidence of cardiotoxicity.

Antidepressants that block the dopamine (D_2) receptor, such as amoxapine, have produced symptoms of neuroleptic malignant syndrome. Mild forms of extrapyramidal symptoms and endocrine changes, including galactorrhea and amenorrhea, may develop. Amoxapine should be avoided in elderly patients because it may be associated with the development of tardive dyskinesia with this age group. Rare occurrences and only mild forms of extrapyramidal symptoms, such as tightness in the jaw and muscle spasms, may occur with any of the TCAs or SSRIs (Schatzberg et al., 1997).

The most common side effects of the SSRIs include headache, anxiety, insomnia, transient nausea, vomiting, and diarrhea. Sedation may also occur, especially

TABLE 8.12 Relative Reuptake Inhibition Activity of Antidepressant Medications

Although all of these antidepressant medications have reuptake inhibition activity, serotonin selective reuptake inhibitors (SSRIs) have more selective reuptake activity than older tricyclics.

	Reuptake Blockade Effect		
Generic (Trade) Drug Name	*Norepinephrine*	*Serotonin (5-HT)*	*Dopamine*
Tricyclics: Tertiary Amines			
Amitriptyline (Elavil)	+2	+2	+1
Clomipramine (Anafranil)	+2	+4	+2
Doxepin (Sinequan)	+2	+1	+1
Imipramine (Tofranil)	+2	+3	+1
Trimipramine (Surmontil)	+1	+1	+1
Tricyclics: Secondary Amines			
Amoxapine (Asendin)	+3	+1	+2
Desipramine (Norpramin)	+4	+1	+1
Nortriptyline (Aventyl, Pamelor)	+3	+1	+2
Protriptyline (Vivactil)	+4	+1	+2
SSRIs			
Fluoxetine (Prozac)	+1	+3	+1
Fluvoxamime (Luvox)	+1/−	+3	+1
Sertraline (Zoloft)	+1/−	+4	+2
Paroxetine (Paxil)	+1	+4	+1
Others			
Mirtazapine (Remeron)	+3	+3	+2
Maprotiline (Ludiomil)	+3	+1	+1
Trazodone (Desyrel)	+1	+1	−
Venlafaxine (Effexor)	+3	+3	+1
Bupropion (Wellbutrin)	+1	−	+3

+1 = low affinity
+4 = high affinity
Adapted from Bezchlibnyk-Butler, K. Z., & Jeffries, J. J. (1995). *Clinical handbook of psychotropic drugs* (5th ed.). Seattle: Hogrefe & Huber.

for paroxetine. Most often, these medications are given in the morning, but if daytime sedation occurs, they may be given in the evening. Higher doses, especially of fluoxetine, are more likely to produce sedation.

Venlafaxine (Effexor) has little effect on acetylcholine and histamine; thus, it creates only mild sedation and anticholinergic symptoms. Tolerance develops to the common side effects of nausea and dizziness. These symptoms, along with sexual dysfunction, sedation, diastolic hypertension, and increased perspiration, tend to be dose dependent, occurring more frequently at higher doses. Elevations in blood pressure have been described, and nurses should monitor blood pressure, especially in patients who have a preexisting history of hypertension. Other common side effects include insomnia, constipation, dry mouth, tremors, blurred vision, and asthenia or muscle weakness.

Nefazodone is structurally similar to trazodone. Its most common side effects include dry mouth, nausea, dizziness, muscle weakness, constipation, and tremor.

These effects occur much less often than with the TCAs. Orthostatic hypotension is rare, but resting pulse and blood pressure may be somewhat lower.

Bupropion has a chemical structure unlike any of the other antidepressants. It somewhat resembles a few of the psychostimulants; therefore, its side effects are different from the TCAs. Bupropion's activating effects may be experienced as agitation or anxiety by some patients. Others also experience insomnia and appetite suppression. For a few individuals, bupropion has produced psychosis, including hallucinations and delusions. Most likely, this is secondary to overstimulation of the dopamine system. This effect accounts for the increasingly common use of bupropion, under the trade name of Zyban, as a smoking cessation agent. The slightly increased risk for developing seizures from bupropion has received the most attention. It has been found that if the total daily dose of bupropion is no more than 450 mg and no individual dose is greater than 150 mg, the risk for seizures for bupropion is no greater than the risk with the TCAs (Schatzberg et al., 1997). Most important, bupropion has not caused sexual dysfunction and is often used alone or in conjunction with other antidepressants in individuals who are experiencing these side effects.

The MAOIs frequently produce dizziness, headache, insomnia, dry mouth, blurred vision, constipation, nausea, peripheral edema, urinary hesitancy, muscle weakness, forgetfulness, and weight gain. Elderly patients are especially sensitive to the side effect of orthostatic hypotension and require frequent assessment of lying and standing blood pressures. They may be at risk for falls and subsequent bone fractures and require assistance in changing position. Sexual dysfunction, including decreased libido, impotence, and anorgasmia, is also common with MAOIs.

The most serious side effect of the MAOIs is its interaction with food and certain medications. The food interaction occurs because MAOIs block the breakdown of tyramine. This action increases the level of tyramine in the nerve cells. Tyramine has a pressor action that induces hypertension. If the individual also ingests food that contains high levels of tyramine while taking MAOIs, severe headaches and hypertension, stroke, and in rare instances, death may result. Patients who are taking MAOIs are placed on a low-tyramine diet. This diet has been difficult for some individuals to follow, and concerns about the risk for severe hypertension have led many clinicians to rarely use the MAOIs. Gardener and colleagues (1996) suggest a more practical approach to tyramine restrictions. They suggest that simpler dietary restrictions are easier to follow for most patients. In addition, they found that many of the past reports of food interactions were related to spoiled foods, which have increased levels of tyramine. If these same foods are fresh, they are safe to consume. Their MAOI diet is contained in Table 8-13. They maintain that all food must be fresh. Proper storage or freezing is paramount, and patients are informed that if they do not know that the food was properly stored, they should not consume it. Individuals should be advised to remain on this diet while they are taking MAOIs and continue the diet for at least 2 weeks after drug discontinuation. Because there is some controversy concerning the degree of restriction of some foods, nurses should avoid giving the patient any conflicting information by checking with the prescriber before recommending any dietary restrictions.

Efforts at developing new MAOIs with fewer or no dietary restrictions are ongoing. MAOIs in current use in the United States include phenelzine and tranylcypromine (Parnate). These are considered irreversible MAOIs because they form strong covalent bonds to block the enzyme monoamine oxidase. This inhibition increases with repeated administration of these med-

---

TABLE 8.13   Example of a Tyramine-Restricted Diet

Category of Food	Food to Avoid	Food Allowed
Cheese	All matured or aged cheeses All casseroles made with these cheeses, pizza, lasagna, etc. *Note:* All cheeses are considered matured or aged except those listed under "foods allowed"	Fresh cottage cheese, cream cheese, ricotta cheese, and processed cheese slices. All fresh milk products that have been stored properly (eg, sour cream, yogurt, ice cream)
Meat, fish, and poultry	Fermented/dry sausage: pepperoni, salami, mortadella, summer sausage, etc. Improperly stored meat, fish, or poultry Improperly stored pickled herring	All fresh packaged or processed meat (eg, chicken loaf, hot dogs), fish, or poultry Store in refrigerator immediately and eat as soon as possible
Fruits and vegetables	Fava or broad bean pods (not beans) Banana peel	Banana pulp All others except those listed in "food to avoid"
Alcoholic beverages	All tap beers	Alcohol: No more than two domestic bottled or canned beers or 4-fluid-oz glasses of red or white wine per day; this applies to non-alcoholic beer also; please note that red wine may produce a headache unrelated to a rise in blood pressure
Miscellaneous foods	Marmite concentrated yeast extract Sauerkraut Soy sauce and other soybean condiments	Other yeast extracts (eg, brewer's yeast) Soy milk

Adapted from Gardener, D. M., Shulman, K. I., Walker, S. E., & Tailor, S. A. N. (1996). The making of a user friendly MAOI diet. *Journal of Clinical Psychiatry, 57,* 99–104.

ications and takes at least 2 weeks to resolve after discontinuation of the medication. Moclobemide is an example of a reversible MAOI that is available in Europe and Canada. Although it acts in the same way as the irreversible MAOIs, moclobemide forms weaker bonds that are short-lasting. Its inhibition does not increase with repeated administration of the drug, and it is easily displaced by tyramine in the diet. Therefore, a less restrictive diet may be used with moclobemide. Similar drugs are under investigation in the United States.

In addition to food restrictions, many prescription and nonprescription medications that stimulate the sympathetic nervous system (sympathomimetic) produce the same risk for hypertensive crisis as foods containing tyramine. The nonprescription medication interactions involve primarily diet pills and cold remedies. Patients should be advised to check the labels of any nonprescription drugs carefully for a warning against use with antidepressants, especially the MAOIs, and then consult their prescriber before consuming these medications. Also, symptoms of other serious drug–drug interactions may develop, such as coma, hypertension, and fever, which may occur when patients receive meperidine (Demerol) while taking an MAOI. Patients should notify other health care providers, including dentists, that they are taking an MAOI before being prescribed or given any other medication.

Suicide is a major concern when working with individuals who are depressed. Nurses should closely assess suicide risk (see Chap. 10) when indicated, especially with any individual who is receiving an antidepressant. Some of these medications are more lethal than others. For example, the TCAs pose a significant risk for overdose and are more lethal in children. Symptoms of overdose and treatment are discussed more fully in Chapter 20, but for now, it is important to remember that this potential exists. Sometimes, the prescriber will provide the patient with only small amounts of the medication, requiring more frequent visits, and will closely monitor use. In general, newer antidepressant medications, such as the SSRIs, have less risk for toxicity and lethality in overdose.

ANTIANXIETY AND SEDATIVE-HYPNOTIC MEDICATIONS

Antianxiety medications, sometimes referred to as *anxiolytics*, include medications from a number of pharmacologic classifications, including barbiturates, benzodiazepines, nonbenzodiazepines (eg, buspirone), and nonbarbiturate sedative-hypnotics, such as chloral hydrate. These drugs represent some of the most widely prescribed medications today. Their uses include induction of sleep, maintenance of sleep, reduction of anxiety, and control of the symptoms of panic. Within each pharmacologic classification, some medications

are used more often for sleep, whereas others are used to control anxiety and panic. Some are primarily used for other indications, such as phenobarbital as an anticonvulsant.

Barbiturates were found to be highly addictive and to exhibit a low therapeutic index, which resulted in a number of "accidental" suicides when only these drugs were available for use. For this reason, barbiturates, except for phenobarbital, are rarely prescribed in current practice. Benzodiazepines provided a safer alternative, but tolerance and addiction may develop to these medications, and they should be used cautiously only for short-term, symptomatic relief. This section focuses on the benzodiazepines and newer nonbenzodiazepine anxiolytics most often used with psychiatric disorders. The student should be aware that other medications offer control of some of these symptoms and are sometimes prescribed instead. For example, propranolol and other β-blockers control the physical symptoms of anxiety, such as shakiness, increased perspiration, and tremor. Although use of propranolol has not been approved for this indication by the FDA, some prescribers use these medications for this purpose. Antihistamines, such as diphenhydramine (Benadryl) or hydroxyzine (Vistaril), are sometimes used as well for sedation and relief of anxiety.

Benzodiazepines

Developed in the late 1950s, chlordiazepoxide (Librium) was the first benzodiazepine to provide a sedative and muscle relaxant alternative to the barbiturates. Diazepam was introduced shortly after chlordiazepoxide in the early 1960s and was found to be 3 to 10 times more potent. Since that time, other benzodiazepines have been developed (Table 8-14) as antianxiety medications or for sleep. In 1992, alprazolam (Xanax) received the first FDA approval for treatment of panic disorders.

Indications and Mechanisms of Action

In psychiatry, benzodiazepines are used primarily for the treatment of generalized anxiety disorder (see Chap. 21); for anxiety as it occurs as part of other disorders, such as depression, or withdrawal from alcohol (see Chaps. 20 and 25); and for some sleep disorders (see Chap. 26). Target symptoms for the benzodiazepines are the symptoms of anxiety and related symptoms, such as difficulty concentrating, restlessness, muscle tension, disturbed sleep, irritability, and fatigue. Other target symptoms relate to the specific disorders for which the medication is given, such as the symptoms of withdrawal associated with alcohol and the symptoms of sleep disturbance. Alprazolam has been proved to control the symptoms of panic, such as shortness of breath, chest pain, lighthead-

TABLE 8.14 Anxiety and Sedative-Hypnotic Medications

Generic (Trade) Drug Name	Usual Dosage Range (mg/d)	Half-Life (h)	Speed of Onset After Single Dose
Benzodiazepines			
Diazepam (Valium)	4–40	30–100	Very fast
Chlordiazepoxide (Librium)	15–100	50–100	Intermediate
Clorazepate (Tranxene)	15–60	30–200	Fast
Prazepam (Centrax)	20–60	30–200	Very slow
Flurazepam (Dalmane)	15–30	47–100	Fast
Lorazepam (Ativan)	2–8	10–20	Slow-intermediate
Oxazepam (Serax)	30–120	3–21	Slow-intermediate
Temazepam (Restoril)	15–30	9.5–20	Moderately fast
Triazolam (Halcion)	0.25–0.5	2–4	Fast
Alprazolam (Xanax)	0.5–10	12–15	Intermediate
Halazepam (Paxipam)	80–160	30–200	Slow-intermediate
Clonazepam (Klonopin)	1.5–20	18–50	Intermediate
Nonbenzodiazepines			
Buspirone (BuSpar)	15–30	3–11	Very slow
Zolpidem (Ambien)	5–10	2.6	Fast

Adapted from Maxmen, J. S., & Ward, N. G. (1995). *Psychotropic drugs: Fast facts* (2nd ed.). New York: Norton.

edness, feelings of impending doom, choking, nausea, fear of losing control, chills, or hot flashes. (See Chap. 21 for a complete description of panic attacks.) Some benzodiazepines, such as flurazepam (Dalmane), temazepam (Restoril), and triazolam (Halcion), are used primarily for induction and maintenance of sleep. Benzodiazepines act by potentiating the effect of GABA in opening the chloride ion channel, leading directly to an anxiolytic effect in the limbic system and cortex, ataxia in the cerebellum, and anticonvulsant effects in the brain stem. The muscle relaxant effect of the benzodiazepines occurs in the peripheral nervous system. All of these medications have sedative, muscle relaxant, and anticonvulsant effects, but they vary considerably in their ability to produce each of these effects, depending partly on their individual pharmacokinetic properties.

Pharmacokinetics

All of the benzodiazepines are readily absorbed from the gastrointestinal tract after oral administration. However, the somewhat variable rate of absorption determines the speed of onset. Table 8-14 provides relative indications of the speed of onset, from very fast to slow, for some of the commonly prescribed benzodiazepines. Chlordiazepoxide and diazepam are slow, erratic, and sometimes incompletely absorbed when given intramuscularly, whereas lorazepam (Ativan) is rapidly and completely absorbed when given intramuscularly. Intravenous benzodiazepines often cause phlebitis and thrombosis at the intravenous sites,

which should be monitored closely and changed if any redness or swelling develops.

All of the benzodiazepines are highly lipid soluble and highly protein bound. They are distributed throughout the body and enter the CNS quickly. Other drugs that compete for protein-binding sites may produce drug–drug interactions. The degree to which each of these drugs is lipid soluble affects its duration of action. Most of these drugs have active metabolites, but the degree of activity of each metabolite affects duration of action and elimination half-life. Most of these drugs vary markedly in length of half-life. Oxazepam (Serax) and lorazepam have no active metabolites and therefore have shorter half-lives. These drugs are often preferred for patients with liver disease and for elderly patients. Elderly patients receiving repeated doses of medications such as flurazepam at bedtime often experience paradoxical confusion, agitation, and delirium, sometimes after the first dose. Elimination half-lives may also be sustained for obese patients when using diazepam, chlordiazepoxide, and halazepam.

Side Effects, Adverse Reactions, and Toxicity

The most commonly reported side effects result from the sedative and CNS depression effects of these medications. Drowsiness, impairment of intellectual function, impairment of memory, ataxia, and reduced motor coordination are frequent complications. If used for sleep, many of these medications, especially long-acting benzodiazepines, produce significant "hangover" effects on awakening. In addition, daytime fatigue, drowsiness, and cognitive impairments may continue while the person is awake. For most patients, these side effects subside as tolerance develops; however, alcohol increases all of these symptoms and potentiates the CNS depression. Individuals using these medications should be warned to be cautious driving or performing other tasks that require mental alertness. If these tasks are part of the person's work requirements, another medication may be chosen.

Because tolerance develops to most of the CNS depressant effects, individuals who wish to experience the feeling of "intoxication" from these medications may be tempted to increase their own dosage. Psychological dependence is more likely to occur when using these medications for a longer period of time. Abrupt discontinuation of the benzodiazepines may result in a recurrence of the target symptoms, such as rebound insomnia or anxiety. Other withdrawal symptoms appear rapidly, including tremors, increased perspiration, palpitations, increased sensitivity to light, abdominal discomfort or pain, and elevations in systolic blood pressure. These symptoms may be more pronounced with the short-acting benzodiazepines, such as lorazepam. A gradual taper is recommended for discontinuing all benzodiazepines that have been used for long-term treatment. When tapering short-acting medications, the prescriber may switch the patient to a long-acting benzodiazepine before initiating the taper.

Individual reactions to the benzodiazepines appear to be associated with sensitivity to their effects. Some patients feel apathy, fatigue, tearfulness, emotional lability, irritability, and nervousness. Symptoms of depression may worsen. The psychiatric–mental health nurse should closely monitor these symptoms when individuals are receiving benzodiazepines as adjunctive treatment for anxiety that coexists with depression. Gastrointestinal disturbances, including nausea, vomiting, anorexia, dry mouth, and constipation, may also develop. These medications may be taken with food to ease the gastrointestinal distress.

Elderly patients are particularly susceptible to incontinence, memory disturbances, dizziness, and increased risk for falls when using benzodiazepines. All of these medications cross the placenta and have been associated with increased risk for some birth defects, such as cleft palate, mental retardation, and pyloric stenosis. Infants born addicted to benzodiazepines often exhibit flaccid muscle tone, lethargy, and difficulties sucking. All of the benzodiazepines are excreted in breast milk, and nursing mothers should avoid using these medications. Infants and children metabolize these medications more slowly; therefore, more benzodiazepine accumulates in their bodies.

Toxicity develops in overdose or accumulation of the drug in the body from liver dysfunction or disease. Symptoms include worsening of the CNS depression, ataxia, confusion, delirium, agitation, hypotension, di-minished reflexes, and lethargy. Rarely do the benzodiazepines cause respiratory depression or death. In overdose, these medications have a high therapeutic index and rarely result in death unless combined with another CNS depressant drug, such as alcohol.

Nonbenzodiazepines

Buspirone was first synthesized in 1968 by Michael Eison while searching for an improved antipsychotic medication. Later, it was found that buspirone was effective in controlling the symptoms of anxiety but had no effect on panic disorders. The hope for this drug has been to develop a new class of medications effective in the treatment of anxiety disorders, but without the CNS depressant effects or the potential for abuse and withdrawal syndromes.

Buspirone (BuSpar) has no effect on the benzodiazepine–GABA complex, but instead appears to control anxiety by blocking the serotonin subtype of receptor, 5-HT1a, at both presynaptic reuptake and postsynaptic receptor sites. It has no sedative, muscle relaxant, or anticonvulsant effects. It also lacks potential for abuse. Buspirone is indicated in the treatment of generalized anxiety disorder; therefore, its target symptoms include anxiety and such related symptoms as difficulty concentrating, tension, insomnia, restlessness, irritability, and fatigue. Because buspirone does not add to the symptoms of depression, it has been tried in the treatment of anxiety that coexists with depression. In some instances, it is thought to potentiate the antidepressant actions of other medications. Buspirone does not appear to be effective in treating other anxiety disorders, such as panic disorder or obsessive-compulsive disorder (see Chap. 21).

Buspirone is rapidly absorbed but undergoes extensive first-pass metabolism. Food slows absorption but appears to reduce first-pass effects, increasing the bioavailability of the medication. Buspirone is given on a continual dosing schedule of three times per day because of its short half-life of 2 to 3 hours. Clinical action depends on reaching steady-state concentrations; taking this medication with food may facilitate this process.

Buspirone is highly protein bound but does not displace most other medications. It does, however, displace digoxin and may increase digoxin levels to the point of toxicity. It is metabolized in the liver and excreted predominantly by the kidneys but also in the gastrointestinal tract. Patients with liver or kidney impairment should be given this medication with caution.

Buspirone should not be used as a PRN agent, and it takes 2 to 4 weeks of continual use for symptom relief to occur. It is more effective in reducing anxiety in patients who have never been on a benzodiazepine agent. There is no indication that physical or psychological dependence develops with buspirone. It does not block the withdrawal of other benzodiazepines. Therefore, a switch to buspirone must be done gradually to avoid withdrawal symptoms from the benzodiaze-pines. Nurses should closely monitor patients who are undergoing this change of medication for emergence of withdrawal symptoms from the benzodiazepines and report such symptoms to the prescriber.

Common side effects from buspirone include dizziness, drowsiness, nausea, excitement, and headache. Most other side effects occur at an incidence of less than 1%. There have been no reports of death from an overdose of buspirone alone. Elderly patients, pregnant women, and children have not been adequately studied. For now, buspirone can be assumed to cross the placenta and is present in breast milk; therefore, it should be avoided in pregnant women, and women who are taking this medication should not breast-feed.

Zolpidem (Ambien) is a nonbenzodiazepine medication for sleep that acts on the benzodiazepine–GABA receptor complex. It has a short half-life of 3 hours. It appears to increase slow-wave (deep) sleep, and rebound effects such as insomnia and anxiety are minimal. There are minimal effects on respiratory function and little potential for abuse, but because it acts on GABA, some of the same side effects are possible. Sonota, the newest of the short half-life sleep agents, is also beginning to be used more commonly. The short half-life allows for sleep induction without a hangover feeling upon waking. More research is needed to determine whether these and similar medications offer a substantial improvement over the benzodiazepines.

STIMULANTS

Amphetamines were first synthesized in the late 1800s but were not used for psychiatric reasons until the 1930s. Initially, amphetamines were prescribed for a variety of symptoms and disorders, but their high abuse potential soon became obvious. Medical use of these drugs is now restricted to a few disorders, including narcolepsy, ADHD (particularly in children), and obesity unresponsive to other treatments.

Indications and Mechanisms of Action

Amphetamines indirectly stimulate the sympathetic nervous system, producing alertness, wakefulness, vaso-constriction, suppressed appetite, and hypothermia. Tolerance develops to some of these effects, such as suppression of appetite, but the CNS stimulation continues. Although the exact mechanism of action is not completely understood, stimulants cause a release of catecholamines, particularly norepinephrine and dopamine, into the synapse from the presynaptic nerve cell. They also block reuptake of these catecholamines. Methylphenidate is structurally similar to the amphetamines but produces a milder CNS stimulation. Pemoline is structurally dissimilar from the amphetamines but produces the same pharmacologic actions. Pemoline

predominantly affects the dopamine system and therefore has less effect on the sympathetic nervous system.

Although the stimulant effects of these medications may seem logically indicated for narcolepsy, a disorder in which the individual frequently and abruptly falls asleep, the indications for ADHD in children may seem somewhat less obvious. The etiology and neurobiology of ADHD remain unclear, but psychostimulants produce a paradoxic calming of the increased motor activity related to ADHD. Studies have also shown a decrease in disruptive activity during school hours, decreased noise and verbal activity, improved attention span and short-term memory, improved ability to follow directions, decreased distractibility, and decreased impulsivity. Although these improvements have been well documented in the literature, the diagnosis of ADHD and subsequent use of psychostimulants with children remain controversial (see Chap. 29).

Psychostimulants have also been used for a number of other disorders in psychiatry. Nurses must be aware that these medications may be prescribed for other disorders, but these uses are outside of the FDA-approved indications for the medications. When used alone, stimulants are not indicated for the treatment of depression. However, research has found that these medications may be beneficial as adjunctive medications for treatment-resistant depression. All appetite depressants are stimulants, but most are not related to the amphetamines and have a low potential for abuse. However, psychostimulants have been used for the treatment of obesity when other treatments have failed. In addition, these medications have improved lethargy, increased mood, and reduced cognitive deficits associated with chronic medically debilitating conditions, such as chronic fatigue syndrome, AIDS, and some types of cancer, but more research is needed. Finally, psychostimulants may improve the residual symptoms of attention deficit disorder in adults, such as inattention, impulsivity, decreased concentration, anxiety, and irritability. A childhood history of ADHD must be present. This use remains controversial, and psychostimulants should not be used with individuals who have a history of substance abuse.

Pharmacokinetics

Psychostimulants are rapidly absorbed from the gastrointestinal tract and reach peak plasma levels in 1 to 3 hours. Considerable individual variations occur between the drugs in terms of bioavailability, plasma levels, and half-life. Table 8-15 compares the primary psychostimulants used in psychiatry. Some of these differences are age dependent because children metabolize these medications more rapidly, producing shorter elimination half-lives. Methylphenidate (Ritalin) is available in a sustained-release form for slower absorption and should not be chewed or crushed.

TABLE 8.15 Psychostimulant Medications

Generic (Trade) Drug Name	Usual Dosage Range (mg/d)	Half-Life (h)	Side Effects
Dextroamphetamine (Dexedrine)	5–40	6–7	• Overstimulation • Restlessness • Dry mouth • Palpitations • Cardiomyopathy (with prolonged use or high dosage) • Possible growth retardation (greatest risk); risk reduced with drug holidays
Methylphenidate (Ritalin)	10–60	2–4	• Nervousness • Insomnia • Anorexia • Tachycardia • Impaired cognition (with high doses) • Moderate risk for growth suppression
Pemoline (Cylert)	37.5–112.5	12 (mean)	• Insomnia • Anorexia with weight loss • Elevated liver function tests (ALT, AST, LDH) • Jaundice • Least risk for growth suppression

ALT, alanine aminotransferase; AST, aspartate aminotransferase; LDH, lactic dehydrogenase
Compiled from Olin, B. R. (Ed.). (1996). *Drug facts and comparisons* (1996 Ed.). St. Louis: Facts and Comparisons.

The psychostimulants do not appear to be affected by the presence of food in the stomach and should be given after meals to reduce the appetite-suppressant effects when indicated. However, changes in urine pH may affect the rates of elimination. Excessive sodium bicarbonate alkalizes the urine and reduces amphetamine secretion. Increased vitamin C or citric acid intake may acidify the urine and increase its elimination. Starvation from appetite suppression may have a similar effect.

All of these drugs are highly lipid soluble, crossing easily into the CNS and the placenta. Pemoline has higher protein binding and lower bioavailability than the others but also exhibits less potential for abuse. Psychostimulants undergo metabolic changes in the liver, where they may affect, or be affected by, other drugs. They are primarily excreted through the kidneys; therefore, renal dysfunction may interfere with elimination.

Psychostimulants are usually begun at a low dose and increased weekly, depending on improvement of symptoms and occurrence of side effects. Initially, children with ADHD are frequently given a morning dose so that their school performance may be compared from morning to afternoon. Rebound symptoms of excitability and overtalkativeness may occur when the medication is withdrawn or after dose reduction. These symptoms also begin about 5 hours after the last dose of medication, which may affect the dosing regimen for some individuals. The return of symptoms in the afternoon for children with ADHD may require that a second dose be given at school. Prescribers should work with parents to implement other interventions after school and on weekends when the psychostimulants are not used. Severity of symptoms may require that the medications be continued during these times, but this dosing schedule should be determined after careful evaluation on an individual basis. These medications should not be stopped abruptly, especially when taking higher doses, because the rebound effects may last for several days.

Side Effects, Adverse Reactions, and Toxicity

Side effects from psychostimulants typically arise within 2 to 3 weeks after starting the medication. From most to least common, these side effects include appetite suppression, insomnia, irritability, weight loss, nausea, headache, palpitations, blurred vision, dry mouth, constipation, and dizziness. Because of the effects on the sympathetic nervous system, some individuals experience blood pressure changes (both hypertension and hypotension), tachycardia, tremors, and irregular heart rates. Blood pressure and pulse should be monitored initially and after each dosage change. Pemoline has elevated liver enzymes and produced hepatotoxicity in 1% to 3% of children taking the medication; therefore, liver function tests should be obtained at least every 6 months. Liver function returns to normal when the medication is discontinued.

In relatively rare instances, psychostimulants have suppressed growth and development in children. These effects are controversial, and research has produced conflicting results. Although suppression of height seems unlikely to some researchers, others have indicated that psychostimulants may have an effect on cartilage metabolism. More reports of suppressed growth have occurred with dextroamphetamine than methylphenidate, and both of these drugs have greater growth suppression than pemoline. Height and weight should be monitored several times annually for children taking these medications and compared with prior history of growth. Weight should be monitored especially closely during the initial phases of treatment. These effects may also be minimized by drug "holidays," such as during school vacations.

In rare instances, individuals may develop mild dysphoria, social withdrawal, or mild to moderate depression. These symptoms are more common at higher doses and may require a discontinuation of the medication. Abnormal movements and motor tics may also increase in individuals who have a history of Tourette's syndrome. It is recommended that psychostimulants be avoided in the presence of Tourette's symptoms or a positive family history of the disorder. In addition, dextroamphetamine has been associated with an increased risk for congenital abnormalities. Because there is no compelling reason for a pregnant woman to continue these medications, patients should be informed and should advise their prescriber immediately if they plan to become pregnant or if pregnancy is a possibility.

Death is rare from overdose or toxicity of the psychostimulants, but a 10-day supply may be lethal, especially in children. Symptoms of overdose include agitation, chest pain, hallucinations, paranoia, confusion, and dysphoria. Seizures may develop, along with fever, tremor, hypertension or hypotension, aggression, headache, palpitations, rashes, difficulty breathing, leg pain, and abdominal pain. More data exist concerning dextroamphetamine, placing toxic doses above 20 mg and potential mortality at 400 mg. Parents should be warned regarding the potential lethality of these medications and take preventive measures by keeping the medication in a safe place.

DEVELOPMENT OF NEW MEDICATIONS

Each country has its own approval process for new medications. In the United States, this process is controlled by the FDA. A new drug must be determined to have therapeutic benefit based on theoretic considerations, animal testing, and laboratory models of human disease and its potential toxicity predicted at doses likely to produce clinical improvement in humans. Then, an Investigational New Drug (IND) application is filed by the pharmaceutical company to begin research with human volunteers. Phase I research is the period of testing that defines the range of dosages tolerated in healthy individuals. Phase II begins studies with a limited number of individuals who have the target disorder for the drug. This phase defines the range of clinically effective dosage. Phase III research involves extensive clinical trials at multiple sites throughout the country and larger numbers of patients. These efforts are focused on corroborating the efficacy found in phase II research. A New Drug Application (NDA) is submitted to the FDA at the end of phase III research. Throughout these phases, side effects and adverse reactions are monitored closely. However, it is important for nurses to be aware that these studies are tightly controlled. Strict regulations are enforced at each step. Yet, to prove efficacy, diagnoses are very accurate and follow strict guidelines, and subjects are usually not receiving other medications, nor do they have complicating illnesses. When a new drug is approved by the FDA, it is approved only for the indications for which it has been tested. After a new drug is released on the market, it is usually not prescribed under such strict conditions. Therefore, phase IV research continues after a drug is released to discover new or rare adverse reactions and potentially new indications. During this period, the FDA has a communication mechanism in place for prescribers to report adverse reactions from these medications. Many new psychiatric medications, particularly the atypical antipsychotics, are in various phases of clinical testing and are expected to be released in the coming years. Keeping the phases of new drug development in mind will assist the psychiatric–mental health nurse in understanding what to expect from drugs newly released to the market.

Obviously, new drug development is a long and expensive process, requiring years of animal and human testing and millions of dollars. Less than 1 of every 8,000 chemicals tested is ever approved for use in humans. Although academicians develop basic knowledge, most new drugs come from the research sector of the pharmaceutical industry. This means that the process is often driven by economic rewards as well as clinical gaps in treatment. For this reason, the federal government has a system to award orphan status to some disorders that affect only a small population. This status allows certain tax deductions for pharmaceutical companies to subsidize development of drugs for disorders that would otherwise not be profitable. In recent years, depression, which afflicts as many as 11 million people each year, has received considerable attention, and several new antidepressant medications have been released. Other, much rarer disorders, such as Tourette's syndrome, have received little attention.

As advocates for individuals experiencing psychiatric disorders, nurses may serve as liaisons for patients with the pharmaceutical industry. Most companies have information services or hotlines through which nurses may obtain the latest information concerning a new drug. Because new medications are often expensive, most companies have programs that subsidize the cost of medications for low-income, uninsured patients. As patient advocates, nurses may obtain this information directly from the involved pharmaceutical company. The patient's prescriber usually must complete some forms, but nurses may act to facilitate this process. In addition, many educational tools, including patient monitoring programs, pamphlets, flip charts, and videotapes, are made available by pharmaceutical companies.

OTHER BIOLOGIC TREATMENTS

Throughout the history of psychiatry, numerous treatments have been developed and used to change the biologic basis of what was hypothesized, at the time, to cause psychiatric disorders. Insulin coma, atropine coma, hemodialysis, hyperbaric oxygen therapy, continuous sleep therapy, and ether and carbon dioxide inhalation therapies are just examples of some of those treatments that seemed to produce improvement in symptoms, but results were either unable to be replicated or potential negative effects proved too great a risk. Although the primary biologic interventions remain in the field of psychopharmacology, some other somatic treatments have gained acceptance, remain under investigation, or show promise for the future. This section provides a brief overview of three interventions that have shown consistently effective results or are gaining support for their potential use. These are electroconvulsive therapy (ECT), light therapy, and the use of vitamins and nutrition.

Electroconvulsive Therapy

For hundreds of years, seizures have been known to produce improvement in some psychiatric symptoms. Camphor-induced seizures were used in the 16th century to reduce psychosis and mania. Over time, other substances, such as inhalants, were tried, but most were difficult to control or produced adverse reactions, sometimes even fatalities. ECT was formally introduced in

Italy in 1938. It is one of the oldest medical treatments available and remains safely in use today. It is one of the most effective treatments for severe depression but has been used for other disorders, including mania and schizophrenia, when other treatments have failed.

With ECT, a brief electrical current is passed through the brain to produce generalized seizures lasting 25 to 150 seconds. The patient does not feel the stimulus or recall the procedure. A short-acting anesthetic and a muscle relaxant are given before induction of the current. A brief pulse stimulus, administered unilaterally on the nondominant side of the head, is associated with less confusion after ECT. However, some individuals require bilateral treatment for effective resolution of depressive symptoms. Induction of a seizure is necessary to produce positive treatment outcomes. Because individual seizure thresholds vary, the electrical impulse and treatment method may vary also. In general, the lowest possible electrical stimulus necessary to produce seizure activity should be used. Blood pressure and the ECG are monitored during the procedure. This procedure is repeated twice or three times a week, usually for a total of 6 to 12 treatments. Because there is no particular difference in treatment efficacy and a twice-weekly regimen produces less accumulative memory loss, this treatment course is often chosen. After symptoms have improved, antidepressant medication may be used to prevent relapse. Some patients who cannot take, or do not respond to, antidepressant treatment may be continued on ECT treatment. Usually, once-weekly treatments are gradually decreased in frequency to once monthly. The number and frequency vary depending on the individual's response.

Although ECT produces rapid improvement in depressive symptoms, its exact mechanism of antidepressant action remains unclear. It is known to down-regulate β-adrenergic receptors in much the same way as antidepressant medications. However, unlike antidepressants, it produces an up-regulation in serotonin, especially 5-HT2. ECT also has a number of other known actions on neurochemistry, including increased influx of Ca^{++} and effects on second messenger systems. Any number of possibilities exist as the potential source of relief for depressive symptoms.

Adverse effects may occur with ECT, as with any medical procedure. Brief episodes of hypotension or hypertension, bradycardia or tachycardia, and minor arrhythmias may occur during and immediately after the procedure, but usually resolve quickly. Common aftereffects from ECT include headache, nausea, and muscle pain. Memory loss occurs as the most troublesome long-term effect of ECT. Many patients do not experience amnesia, whereas others complain of loss of some memories for months or even years (Olfson et al., 1998). Most memory loss is for the short period before and during treatments. Evidence is conflicting on the effects of

ECT on the formation of memories after the treatments and on learning, but most patients experience no noticeable change. Memory loss occurring as part of the symptoms of untreated depression presents a confounding factor in determining the exact nature of the memory deficits from ECT. It is important to remember that, despite much negative stigma and publicity regarding ECT, patient surveys are positive. Those surveys report that most individuals felt they were helped by ECT and would not be reluctant to have it again (Salzman, 1998).

The use of ECT is contraindicated in the presence of increased intracranial pressure. Increased risk also is present in patients with recent myocardial infarction, recent cerebrovascular accident, retinal detachment, or pheochromocytoma (a tumor on the adrenal cortex) and in those at high risk for complications from anesthesia. Although ECT should be considered cautiously because of its specific side effects, added risks of general anesthesia, possible contraindications, and substantial social stigma, it is a safe and effective treatment (Salzman, 1998). Even if ECT proves effective, preventive use of antidepressant medication or some form of maintenance treatment is usually necessary.

Psychiatric–mental health nurses are involved in many aspects of care for individuals undergoing ECT. Informed consent is required, and all treating professionals have a responsibility to ensure that the patient's and family's questions are answered completely; available treatment options, risks, and consequences must be fully discussed. Sometimes, memory difficulties associated with severe depression make it difficult for patients to retain information or ask questions. Nurses should be prepared to restate or explain the procedure as often as necessary. Whenever possible, the individual's family or other support systems should be educated and involved in the consent process. Videotapes are available, but they should not replace direct discussions. Language should be in terms the patient and family members can understand. Other nursing interventions involve preparation of the patient before treatment, monitoring immediately after treatment, and follow-up. Many of these considerations are listed in Text Box 8-3.

Light Therapy (Phototherapy)

Human circadian rhythms are set by time clues (zeitgebers) inside and outside the body. One of the most powerful regulators of these body patterns is the cycle of daylight and darkness. Research findings have indicated that some individuals with certain types of depression may experience disturbance in these normal body patterns or of circadian rhythms, particularly those who experience a seasonal variation in their depression. These individuals experience more depressive symptoms during the winter months, when there is less light, and improve spontaneously in the spring.

TEXT BOX 8.3

Interventions for the Patient Receiving Electroconvulsive Therapy

- Informed consent is necessary, including discussion of treatment alternatives, procedures, risks, and benefits.
- Initial and ongoing patient and family education must be provided.
- Patient must be assisted and monitored to remain NPO after the midnight before the procedure.
- The patient must wear loose, comfortable, non-restrictive clothing to the procedure.
- If the procedure is outpatient, the patient must not attempt to drive home. Someone should accompany the patient and stay with him or her after the procedure.
- Ensure that pretreatment laboratory tests are complete, including CBC, serum electrolytes, urinalysis, ECG, chest radiograph, and physical examination.
- Teach patient to use memory aids such as lists and notepads prior to the ECT.
- No foreign or loose objects must be in patient's mouth, such as dentures. A bite block may be inserted during the procedure.
- An intravenous line is inserted, and the patient is oxygenated, usually with a nasal cannula, at 5 L/min of 100% oxygen. Emergency equipment should be checked and ready before the procedure.
- Vital signs are monitored frequently immediately after the procedure as in every postanesthesia recovery period.
- When patient is fully conscious and vital signs are stable, assist to get up slowly, sitting for some time before standing.
- Monitor confusion closely; patient may need to be reoriented to the bathroom and other areas.
- Close supervision should be maintained for at least 12 hours and continued observation for 48 hours after treatment. Family members should observe how patient manages activities at home, assisting when necessary and reporting any problems.
- Assistance, such as reminder telephone calls, may be needed to remind the patient of follow-up appointments or other scheduled treatments.

CBC, complete blood count; ECG, electrocardiogram; ECT, electroconvulsive therapy.

(Refer to Chap. 20 for a complete description of depression and mood disorders.) Usually, these individuals have symptoms that are somewhat different from classic depression, including fatigue, increased need to sleep, increased appetite and weight gain, irritability, and carbohydrate craving. Sometimes, the symptoms appear in the summer, and some individuals have only subtle changes without developing the full pattern. These depressive symptoms have been reduced by administering artificial light to these patients during winter months.

Light therapy, sometimes referred to as **phototherapy,** involves exposing the patient to an artificial light source during winter months to relieve seasonal depression. It is believed the artificial light triggers a shift in the patient's circadian rhythm to an earlier time. Research remains ongoing. The light source must be very bright, full-spectrum light, usually 2,500 lux, which is about 200 times brighter than normal indoor lighting. Harmful ultraviolet light is filtered out. Exposure to this light source has produced improvement and relief of depressive symptoms for significant numbers of seasonally depressed individuals. It produces no change for individuals who are not seasonally depressed. Studies have shown that morning phototherapy produces a better response than either evening or morning and evening timing of the phototherapy session. Light banks with full-spectrum light may be put together by the individual or obtained from various companies now producing these light sources. Light visors, visors containing small, full-spectrum light bulbs that shine on the eyelids, have also been developed. The patient is instructed to sit in front of the lights at a distance of about 3 feet, engaging in a variety of other activities, but glancing directly into the light every few minutes. This should be done immediately on arising and is most effective before 8 AM. The duration of administration may begin with as little as 30 minutes and increase to 2 to 5 hours. One to 2 hours is usually sufficient, and the antidepressant response begins in 1 to 4 days, with the full effect usually complete after 2 weeks. Full antidepressant effect is usually maintained with daily sessions of 30 minutes.

Side effects of phototherapy are rare, but eye strain, headache, and insomnia are possible. Consultation with an ophthalmologist should be consulted if the patient has a pre-existing eye disorder. In rare instances, phototherapy has been reported to produce an episode of mania. Irritability has been a more common complaint. Follow-up visits with the prescriber or therapist are necessary to assist in managing the side effects and assessing positive results. Phototherapy should not be implemented without the assistance of a provider knowledgeable in its use.

Nutritional Therapies

The neurotransmitters necessary for normal healthy functioning are produced from chemical building blocks taken in with the foods we eat. Many nutritional deficiencies may produce symptoms of psychiatric disorders. Fatigue, apathy, and depression are caused by deficiencies in iron, folic acid, pantothenic acid, magnesium, vitamin C, or biotin. Logically, treating these deficiencies with nutritional supplements should improve the psychiatric symptoms. The question becomes: Can nutritional supplements improve psychiatric symptoms that are not the result of such deficiencies?

In 1967, Linus Pauling espoused the theory that ascorbic acid deficiency produced many psychiatric disorders. He implemented a treatment for schizophrenia that included large doses of ascorbic acid and other vitamins. This treatment was referred to as *megavitamin therapy* or *orthomolecular therapy.* Many psychiatrists showed interest in Pauling's proposal, but his research and claims could never be substantiated, and most researchers and clinicians became highly skeptical of this hypothesis. Nonetheless, a small group remains committed to the orthomolecular approach.

Older theories and related diets based on the belief that food controls behavior. High sugar intake was once thought to produce hyperactivity in children, and Benjamin Feingold developed a diet to eliminate food additives that he believed increased hyperactivity. Neither claim was substantiated, but further research has determined that yellow dye no. 5 (tartrazine), sodium benzoate, milk, chocolate, eggs, wheat, corn, oats, and fish may produce behavioral problems for some children. An elimination diet was implemented for some children but was difficult and tedious to follow.

More recently, advances in technology have led research to new investigations regarding dietary precursors for the bioamines. For example, tryptophan, the dietary precursor for serotonin, has been most extensively investigated as it relates to low serotonin levels and increased aggression. Individuals who have low tryptophan levels are prone to have lower levels of serotonin in the brain, resulting in depressed mood and aggressive behavior (Little et al, 1998). However, simply adding tryptophan does not increase brain serotonin.

Many individuals are turning to dietary herbal preparations to address psychiatric symptoms. More than 17% of the adult population has used herbal preparations to address their mood or emotions. From St. John's wort to treat depression, to ginkgo for cognitive impairment, to kava for anxiety, these preparations are increasingly being used. Nurses need to include an assessment of these agents into their overall patient assessment to understand the needs of the patient.

Medications may also influence the development of nutritional deficiencies that may worsen psychiatric symptoms. For example, drugs with strong anticholinergic activity often produce impaired or enhanced gastric motility, which may lead to generalized malabsorption of vitamins and minerals. In addition, many nutritional supplements have toxicities of their own when given in excess. For example, daily ingestion of more than 100 mg pyridoxine (vitamin B_6) can produce neurotoxic symptoms, photosensitivity, and ataxia. More research is needed to identify the underlying mechanisms and relationships of dietary supplements and dietary precursors of the bioamines to mood and behavior and psychopharmacologic medications. For now, it is important for the psychiatric–mental health nurse to recognize that these issues may be potential factors in improvement of the patient's mental status and target symptoms.

Psychosocial Issues in the Use of Biologic Treatments

Many factors influence an individual's successful treatment with medications and other biologic therapies. Of particular importance are issues related to compliance or adherence. **Compliance** refers to the individual's ability to self-administer medications as prescribed, keep appointments, and follow other treatment suggestions. Although individuals often seek treatment and complain of distressing psychiatric symptoms, many are unable or unwilling to continue treatment even after the symptoms have improved. Recent estimates indicate that on the average, 50% or more of the individuals taking antipsychotic medications for the treatment of schizophrenia stop the medications or do not take them as prescribed. This is despite the fact that the symptoms of schizophrenia usually return when the medication is discontinued. Text Box 8-4 provides a list of some of the common reasons for noncompliance. Psychiatric–mental health nurses should be aware that a number of factors influence individuals to stop taking their medication.

The most often sited reasons for noncompliance are side effects related to the medication. Improvement in functioning may be observed by the treating professionals but not felt by the patient. Side effects may interfere with work performance or other important aspects of the individual's life. For example, a construction worker cannot afford to be drowsy and sedated while operating a crane at a construction site, or a woman in a relatively new, intimate relationship may find anorgasmia intolerable. Nurses need to be sensitive to the patient's ability to tolerate side effects and to the impact of those side effects on the individual's life. Medication choice, dosing schedules, and prompt side-effect treatment may be crucial factors for these individuals to continue their treat-

ment, even if the symptoms for which they initially sought help have improved.

Recent studies suggest that denial of the illness may also be important. Taking a medication every day reminds some individuals that they are "sick." Denial may be psychologically protective against the impact of losses or stigma associated with such disorders as schizophrenia. Nurses must support and assist patients as they adjust to changes in their beliefs about psychiatric disorders and about themselves.

Cognitive deficits associated with some psychiatric disorders may make it difficult for the individual to self-monitor, develop insight, make choices, remember to fill prescriptions, or keep appointments. Forgetfulness, cost, and confusion over dosage or timing may also contribute to noncompliance.

Family members may have similar difficulties that influence the individual not to take the medication. They may misunderstand or deny the illness; for example, "My wife's better, so she doesn't need that medicine anymore." Family members may become distressed over the appearance of side effects. Akinesia, which has been linked to suicidal thoughts as a way to relieve the subjective discomfort, may be the most distressing side effect for family members of individuals who have schizophrenia (Meltzer, 2000).

Compliance concerns must not be dismissed as the patient's or family's problem. Psychiatric nurses should actively address this issue. A positive therapeutic relationship between the nurse, patient, and family must provide a strong sense of trust that side effects and other difficulties in treatment will be addressed and minimized. When individuals report experiencing distressing side effects, the nurse should immediately respond with assessment and interventions to reduce these effects. It is important to assess compliance often, asking questions in a nonthreatening manner. It also may be helpful to seek information from others who are involved with the patient.

Denial of the illness may be addressed through psychoeducation. This approach is most helpful if it addresses the individual's specific symptoms and concerns. For example, if the patient is having difficulty with the purpose of the medication, it may be helpful to link taking it to reduction of specific unwanted symptoms or improved functioning, such as continuing to work. Family members should also be included in these discussions.

Other factors that interfere with compliance should also be assessed and plans developed to minimize their effect. For example, an individual who is being considered for clozapine therapy may have missed a number of appointments in the past. On assessment, the nurse may discover that it takes the individual 2 hours on three different buses each way to reach the clinic. The nurse can then assist with arranging for a home health

TEXT BOX 8.4

Common Reasons for Medication Noncompliance

- Uncomfortable side effects
- Side effects that interfere with quality of life, such as work performance or intimate relationships
- Lack of awareness of or denial of illness
- Stigma
- Feeling better
- Confusion about dosage or timing
- Difficulties in access to treatment
- Substance abuse

nurse to visit the patient's apartment, draw blood samples, and assess side effects, thus decreasing the number of trips the patient must make to the clinic.

Summary of Key Points

➤ Psychopharmacology is the study of medications used to affect the brain and behavior in the treatment of psychiatric disorders, including the drug categories of antipsychotics, mood stabilizers, antidepressants, antianxiety medications, and psychostimulants.

➤ Pharmacodynamics involves the study of actions of drugs on living tissue and the human body and primarily has been focused on specific actions at receptor sites, ion channel sites, enzyme actions, and carrier proteins (reuptake receptors).

➤ The importance of receptors is recognized in current psychopharmacology, and it is understood that the biologic action of each drug depends on how its structure interacts with a specific receptor, functioning either as an agonist, reproducing the same biologic action as the neurotransmitter, or as an antagonist, blocking the response.

➤ A drug's ability to interact with a given receptor type may be judged on three qualities: selectivity—ability to interact with specific receptors while not affecting other tissues and organs; affinity—degree of strength of the bond between drug and receptor; and intrinsic activity—ability to produce a certain biologic response.

➤ Many characteristics of specific drugs greatly affect how well they act and how they affect patients. Psychiatric–mental health nurses must be familiar with characteristics, adverse reactions, and toxicity of certain drugs to administer psychotropic medications safely, educate patients regarding their safe use, and encourage compliance.

➤ Pharmacokinetics is the study of how the human body processes the drug, including absorption, distribution, metabolism, and elimination. Bioavailability describes the amount of the drug that actually reaches circulation throughout the body. The wide variations in the way each individual processes any medication are often related to physiologic differences caused by age, genetic makeup, other disease processes, and chemical interactions.

➤ Antipsychotic medications are drugs used in the treatment of psychotic disorders, such as schizophrenia. They primarily act by blocking dopamine or serotonin postsynaptically. In addition, they have a number of actions on other neurotransmitters. For this reason, these medications produce many side effects.

➤ Medication-related movement disorders are a particularly serious group of side effects that principally occur with the antipsychotic medications and that may be acute syndromes, such as dystonia, pseudoparkinsonism, and akathisia, or chronic syndromes, such as tardive dyskinesia.

➤ The mood stabilizers, or antimania medications, are drugs used for the control of wide variations in mood related to mania, but these agents may also be used to treat other disorders. Lithium and the anticonvulsants are chemically unrelated and act in different ways to stabilize mood.

➤ Antidepressant medications are drugs used primarily for the treatment of symptoms of depression and act by blocking reuptake of one or more of the bioamines, especially serotonin and norepinephrine. These medications vary considerably in their structure and action. Newer antidepressants, such as the selective serotonin reuptake inhibitors, have fewer side effects and are less lethal in overdose than the older tricyclic antidepressants.

➤ Antianxiety medications also include several subgroups of medications, but benzodiazepines and nonbenzodiazepines are those principally used in psychiatry. Benzodiazepines act by enhancing the effects of GABA, whereas the nonbenzodiazepine buspirone acts on serotonin.

➤ Psychostimulants enhance neurotransmitter activity, acting at a number of sites in the nerve. These medications are most often used for the treatment of symptoms related to attention deficit hyperactivity disorder and narcolepsy.

➤ Electroconvulsive therapy uses the application of an electrical pulse stimulus to induce seizures in the brain. These seizures produce a number of effects on neurotransmission that result in the rapid relief of the symptoms of depression.

➤ Phototherapy involves the application of full-spectrum light in the morning hours, which appears to reset circadian rhythm delays related to seasonal affective disorder and other forms of depression. Nutritional therapies are in various stages of investigation, but though promising, most remain unsubstantiated at this time.

➤ Compliance refers to the ability of an individual to self-administer medications as prescribed and to follow other instructions related to medication treatment. Noncompliance is related to a number of factors, such as side effects of medications, denial of illness, stigma, and family influences. Nurses play a crucial role in educating patients and helping them to improve compliance.

Critical Thinking Challenges

1. Define the following terms: neurotransmitter, receptor, agonist, and antagonist.

2. Discuss how the concepts of affinity with selectivity and intrinsic activity have meaning for nurses.

3. Discuss the usefulness of the concept of bioavailability for nurses. What does it mean to nurses, and how would nursing actions change if it were considered?

4. Delineate nursing management activities associated with each phase of drug treatment: initiation, stabilization, maintenance, and discontinuation.

5. Discuss how you would go about identifying the target symptoms for the following medications: antipsychotic, antidepressant, and antianxiety drugs.

6. Discuss the ways in which you might explain to a patient the differences between typical and atypical antipsychotic medications.

7. Explain the problems associated with anticholinergic side effects of the antipsychotic medications.

8. Compare the type of movements that characterize tardive dyskinesia with akathisia and dystopia and explore which one is easier for a patient to experience.

9. Explain how your nursing care would be different for a male patient on lithium carbonate than for a female patient.

10. Discuss why the antidepressant class of medications has become so commonly prescribed and explain whether nurses should advocate the use of these drugs.

11. Discuss the efficacy of anticonvulsive therapy and its mechanism of action.

12. Compare different approaches that you might use with a schizophrenic patient who has decided to stop taking his or her typical antipsychotic medication because of intolerance to side effects.

REFERENCES

Allison, D. B., Mentore, J. L., & Heo, M. (1999). Antipsychotic-induced weight gain: A comprehensive research synthesis. *American Journal of Psychiatry, 156,* 1686–1696.

American Nurses Association. (1994). Psychopharmacology guidelines for psychiatric mental health nurses. In ANA (Ed.), *Psychiatric mental health nursing psychopharmacology project* (pp. 41–45). Washington, DC: Author.

Arana, G. W. (2000). An overview of side effects caused by typical antipsychotics. *Journal of Clinical Psychiatry, 61*(Suppl. 8), 5–13.

Baldassano, C. F., Truman, C. J., Nierenberg, A., et al. (1996). Akathisia: A review and case report following paroxetine treatment. *Comprehensive Psychiatry, 37,* 122–124.

Gardener, D. M., Shulman, K. I., Walker, S. E., & Tailor, S. A. N. (1996). The making of a user friendly MAOI diet. *Journal of Clinical Psychiatry, 57,* 99–104.

Glazer, W. M. (2000). Extrapyramidal side effects, tardive dyskinesia, and the concept of atypicality. *Journal of Clinical Psychiatry, 61,* 16–21.

Glod, C. A. (1996). Antidepressants and the cytochrome P-450 enzymes. *Journal of the American Psychiatric Nurses Association, 2*(6), 216–218.

Goodwin, F. K., & Ghaemi, S. N. (2000). The impact of mood stabilizers on suicide in bipolar disorder: A comparative analysis. *CNS Spectrums, 5*(2), 12–19.

Harris, E. C., & Barraclough, B. Schizophrenia: Natural causes of death. *British Journal of Psychiatry, 173,* 11–53.

Little, K. Y., McLaughlin, D., Zhang, L., et al. (1998). Cocaine, ethanol, and genotyping effects on human midbrain serotonin transporter binding sites and mRNA levels. *American Journal of Psychiatry, 155*(2), 207–213.

Madhusoodanan, S., Brenner, R., & Cohen, C. I. (2000). Risperidone for elderly patients with schizophrenia or schizoaffective disorder. *Psychiatric Annals, 30*(3), 175–180.

Meltzer, H. Y. (2000). Introduction. Side effects of antipsychotic medications: Physician's choice of medication and patient compliance. *Journal of Clinical Psychiatry, 61*(Suppl. 8), 3–4.

Olin, B. R. (1996). *Drug facts and comparisons* (1996 ed.). St. Louis: Facts and Comparisons.

Olfson, M., Marcus, S., Sackeim, H. A., et al. (1998). Use of ECT for the inpatient treatment of recurrent major depression. *American Journal of Psychiatry, 155*(1), 22–29.

Preskorn, S. H. (1996). Reducing the risk of drug-drug interactions: A goal of rational drug development. *Journal of Clinical Psychiatry, 57*(Suppl. 1), 3–6.

Sajatovic, M. (2000). Clozapine for elderly patients. *Psychiatric Annals, 30*(3), 170–174.

Salzman, C. (1998). ECT, research, and professional ambivalence. *American Journal of Psychiatry, 155*(1), 1–2.

Scahill, L., & Laraia, M. (1994). Education survey. In American Nurses Association (Ed.), *Psychiatric mental health nursing psychopharmacology project.* Washington, DC: Author.

Schatzberg, A. F., Cole, J. O., & DeBattista, C. (1997). *Manual of clinical psychopharmacology* (3rd. ed.). Washington, DC: American Psychiatric Press, Inc.

Solomon, D. A., Keitner, G. I., Ryan, C. E., et al. (2000). Lithium plus valproate as maintenance polypharmacy for patients with bipolar I disorder: A review. *CNS Spectrums, 5*(2), 19–28.

Tondo, L., Baldessarini, R. J., & Hennen, J. (2000). Lithium and suicide risk in bipolar disorder. *CNS Spectrums, 5*(2), 11.

Viskin, S. (1999). Long QT syndromes and torsade de pointes. *Lancet, 654,* 1625–1633.

Weiden, P. (1994). Neuroleptics and quality of life: The patient's perspective. *Neuropsychopharmacology, 10,* 241–244.

Yamamoto, J., & Lin, K-M. (1995). Psychopharmacology, ethnicity and culture. In J. M. Oldman & M. B. Riba (Eds.), *Review of psychiatry* (Vol. 14, pp. 529–541). Washington, DC: American Psychiatric Press.

Yeung, P. P., Tariot, P. N., Schneider, L. S., et al. (2000). Quetiapine for elderly patients with psychotic disorders. *Psychiatric Annals, 30*(3), 197–201.

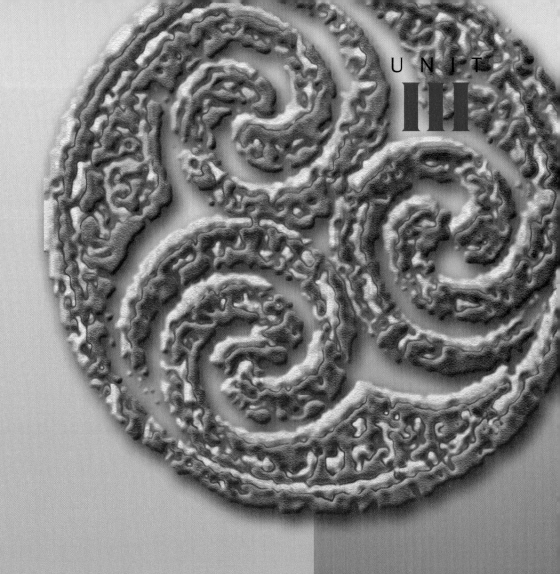

Contemporary Psychiatric Nursing Practice

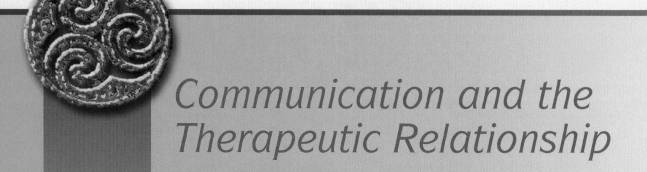

Communication and the Therapeutic Relationship

Mary Ann Boyd

**LEARNING
OBJECTIVES**

After studying this chapter, you will be able to:

➤ Identify the importance of self-awareness in nursing practice.

➤ Develop a repertoire of verbal and nonverbal communication skills.

➤ Develop a process for selecting effective communication techniques.

➤ Explain how the nurse can establish a therapeutic relationship with patients by using rapport and empathy.

➤ Explain the physical, emotional, and social boundaries of the nurse–patient relationship.

➤ Explain what occurs in each of the three phases of the nurse–patient relationship: orientation, working, and resolution.

CHAPTER 9

KEY TERMS

active listening
boundaries
communication blocks
content themes
empathy
nonverbal
  communication
orientation phase

passive listening
process recording
rapport
resolution
self-disclosure
symbolism
verbal communication
working phase

KEY CONCEPTS

nurse–patient relationship
self-awareness
therapeutic communication

Patients with psychiatric disorders have special communication needs that require advanced therapeutic communication skills. In psychiatric nursing, the nurse–patient relationship is an important intervention tool that is used to reach treatment goals. The purpose of this chapter is threefold: (1) to help the nurse develop self-awareness and good communication techniques necessary to establish a therapeutic nurse–patient relationship; (2) to examine the specific stages or steps involved in establishing the relationship; and (3) to explore the specific factors that make a nurse–patient relationship successful and therapeutic.

SELF-AWARENESS

Self-awareness is the process of understanding one's own beliefs, thoughts, motivations, biases, and limitations and recognizing how they affect others. Without being self-aware, recognizing personal and cultural beliefs, and understanding intrapersonal strengths and limitations, attending nurses will find it impossible to establish and maintain therapeutic relationships with patients. "Know thyself" is a basic tenet of psychiatric mental health nursing (see Text Box 9-1).

Nurses can carry out self-examination, which can provoke anxiety and is rarely comfortable, either alone or with help from others. Self-examination without the benefit of another's perspective can lead to a biased view of self. Conducting self-examinations with a trusted individual who can give objective but realistic feedback is best. The development of self-awareness requires a willingness to be introspective and to examine personal beliefs, attitudes, and motivations.

KEY CONCEPT   **Self-awareness.** **Self-awareness** is the process of understanding one's own beliefs, thoughts, motivations, biases, and limitations and recognizing how they affect others.

The Biopsychosocial Self

Each nurse brings his or her biopsychosocial self to nursing practice. The patient perceives the biologic dimension of the nurse in terms of the nurse's physical characteristics: age, sex, body weight, height, and any other observed physical characteristics. The nurse, too, can have a certain genetic composition, chronic illness, or unobservable physical disability that may influence the quality or delivery of nursing care. The nurse's psychological state also influences how he or she analyzes patient information and selects treatment interventions. An emotional state or behavior can inadvertently

TEXT BOX 9.1

"Know Thyself"

- Do you have any physical problems or illnesses?
- Have you had significant traumatic life events (eg, divorce, death of significant person, abuse, disaster)?
- Did your family or significant others have prejudiced or embarrassing beliefs and attitudes about groups different than yours?
- Would sociocultural factors in your background contribute to being rejected by members of other cultures?
- If you answer "Yes" to any of these questions, how would these experiences affect your ability to care for patients with these characteristics?

influence the therapeutic relationship. For example, if a nurse has just found out that her child is using illegal drugs and a patient has a history of drug use, she may inadvertently project a judgmental attitude toward her patient, which would interfere with the formation of a therapeutic relationship. The nurse needs to examine underlying emotions, motivations, and beliefs and determine how these factors shape behavior. The nurse's social biases can be particularly problematic for the nurse–patient relationship. Although the nurse may not verbalize these values to patients, some are readily evident in the nurse's behavior and appearance, such as how the nurse appears at or conducts work. Other sociocultural values may not be immediately obvious to the patient; for example, the nurse's religious or spiritual beliefs or feelings about divorce, abortion, or homosexuality. These beliefs and thoughts can influence how the nurse interacts with a patient who is dealing with such issues.

Understanding Personal Feelings and Beliefs and Changing Behavior

Nurses must understand their own personal feelings and beliefs and try to avoid projecting them on patients. The development of self-awareness will enhance the nurse's objectivity and allow him or her to adopt a nonjudgmental attitude, which is so important in building and maintaining trust throughout the nurse–patient relationship. Soliciting feedback from colleagues and supervisors about how personal beliefs or thoughts are being projected onto others is a useful self-assessment technique. One of the reasons that ongoing supervision is so important is that the supervisor really knows the nurse and can continually observe for inappropriate communication.

Once a nurse has identified and analyzed personal beliefs and attitudes, he or she may change behavior

that was driven by prejudicial ideas. The change process requires introspective analysis that may result in viewing the world differently. Through self-awareness and conscious effort, the nurse can change learned behaviors to engage effectively in therapeutic relationships with patients who have different beliefs and values. Nevertheless, sometimes nurses realize that their attitudes are too ingrained to be able to engage in a therapeutic relationship with a person with different beliefs. They should then refer the patient to someone who can be therapeutic.

COMMUNICATION

Effective communication skills, including verbal and nonverbal techniques, are the basic building blocks for all successful relationships. The nurse–patient relationship is built on therapeutic communication, the ongoing process of interaction through which meaning emerges (see Text Box 9-2). **Verbal communication,** which is principally achieved by spoken words, includes the underlying emotion, context, and connotation of what is actually said. **Nonverbal communication** includes gestures, expressions, and body language. Both the patient and the nurse use verbal and nonverbal communication. In a nurse–patient relationship, the nurse is responsible for assessing and interpreting patient communication to respond therapeutically.

TEXT BOX 9.2

Principles of Therapeutic Communication

1. The patient should be the primary focus of the interaction.
2. A professional attitude sets the tone of the therapeutic relationship.
3. Use self-disclosure cautiously and only when the disclosure has a therapeutic purpose.
4. Avoid social relationships with patients.
5. Maintain patient confidentiality.
6. Assess the patient's intellectual competence to determine the level of understanding.
7. Implement interventions from a theoretic base.
8. Maintain a nonjudgmental attitude. Avoid making judgments about patient's behavior and giving advice. By the time the patient sees the nurse, he or she has had plenty of advice.
9. Guide the patient to reinterpret his or her experiences rationally.
10. Track the patient's verbal interaction through the use of clarifying statements. Avoid changing the subject unless the content change is in the patient's best interest.

KEY CONCEPT Therapeutic communication. **Therapeutic communication** is the ongoing process of interaction through which meaning emerges.

Therapeutic and social relationships are very different. In a therapeutic relationship, the nurse focuses on the patient and patient-related issues, even when engaging in social activities with that patient. For example, a nurse may take a patient shopping and out for lunch. Even though the nurse is engaged in a social activity, that trip should have a definite purpose, and conversation should focus only on the patient. The nurse must not attempt to meet his or her own social needs during the activity.

Using Verbal Communication

The process of verbal communication involves a sender, message, and receiver. The patient is usually the sender, and the nurse is usually the receiver (Fig. 9-1). The patient formulates an idea, encodes a message (puts ideas into words), and then transmits the message with emotion. The patient's words and their underlying emotional tone and connotation communicate the individual's needs and emotional problems. The nurse receives the message, decodes it (interprets the message, including its feelings, connotation, and context), and then responds to the patient. On the surface, this interaction is deceptively simple; unseen complications lie underneath. For example, is the message the nurse receives consistent with the patient's original idea? Did the nurse interpret the message as the patient intended? Is the verbal message consistent with the nonverbal flourishes that accompany it?

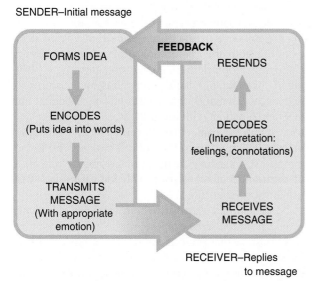

SENDER–Initial message

FORMS IDEA

FEEDBACK

RESENDS

ENCODES
(Puts idea into words)

DECODES
(Interpretation:
feelings, connotations)

TRANSMITS
MESSAGE
(With appropriate
emotion)

RECEIVES
MESSAGE

RECEIVER–Replies
to message

FIGURE 9.1 The communication process. (Adapted from Boyd, M. [1995]. Communication with patients, families, healthcare providers, and diverse cultures. In M. Strader, & P. Decker [Eds.], *Role transition to patient care management* [p. 431]. Norwalk, CT: Appleton & Lange.)

Self-Disclosure

One of the most important principles of therapeutic communication for the nurse to follow is to focus the interaction on the patient's concerns. **Self-disclosure,** telling the patient personal information, is generally not a good idea. The conversation should focus on the patient, not the nurse. If a patient asks the nurse personal questions, the nurse should elicit the underlying reason for the request. The nurse can then determine how much personal information to disclose, if any. If he or she reveals personal information, the self-disclosure should be purposeful with identified therapeutic outcomes. For example, a male patient who was struggling with the implications of marriage and fidelity asked a male nurse if he had ever had an extramarital affair. The nurse interpreted the patient's statement as seeking role-modeling behavior for an adult man and judged self-disclosure in this instance to be therapeutic. He honestly responded that he did not engage in affairs and redirected the discussion back to the patient's concerns.

Nurses sometimes may feel uncomfortable avoiding patients' questions for fear of seeming rude. They sometimes disclose too much personal information because they are trying to be "nice." Being nice, however, is not necessarily therapeutic. When a patient asks a nurse for personal information, the nurse must quickly decide how much to disclose and what purpose such disclosure would serve. Redirecting the patient, giving a neutral or vague answer, or saying, "Let's talk about you" may be all that is necessary to limit self-disclosure. In some instances, nurses may need to tell the patient directly that the nurse will not share personal information (Table 9-1).

Verbal Communication Techniques

Psychiatric nurses use many verbal techniques in establishing relationships and helping patients focus on their problems. Asking a question, restating, and reflecting are examples of such techniques. These techniques may at first seem artificial, but with practice, they can be useful in therapeutic communication (Table 9-2). One of the most difficult but often most effective techniques is the use of silence during verbal interactions. By maintaining silence, the nurse allows the patient to gather thoughts and to proceed at his or her own pace.

Listening is another valuable tool. Silence and listening differ in that silence consists of deliberate pauses to encourage the patient to reflect and eventually respond. Listening is an ongoing activity by which the nurse attends to the patient's verbal and nonverbal communication. The art of listening is developed through careful attention to the content and meaning of the patient's speech. There are two types of listening: passive and active. **Passive listening** involves sitting quietly and letting the patient talk. A passive listener allows the patient to ramble and does not focus or guide the thought process.

TABLE 9.1 Self-Disclosure in Therapeutic Versus Social Relationships

Situation	Appropriate Therapeutic Response	Inappropriate Social Response With Rationale
A patient asks the nurse if she had fun over the weekend.	"The weekend was fine. How did you spend your weekend?"	"It was great. My boyfriend and I went to dinner and a movie." *(This self-disclosure has no therapeutic purpose. The response focuses the conversation on the nurse, not the patient.)*
A patient asks a student nurse if she has ever been to a particular bar.	"Many people go there. I'm wondering if you have ever been there?"	"Oh yes—all the time. It's a lot of fun." *(Sharing information about outside activities is inappropriate.)*
A patient asks a nurse if mental illness is in his family.	"Mental illnesses do run in families. I've had a lot of experience caring for people with mental illnesses."	"My sister is being treated for depression." *(This self-disclosure has no purpose, and the nurse is missing the meaning of the question.)*
While shopping with a patient, the nurse sees a friend, who approaches them.	To her friend: "I know it looks like I'm not working, but I really am. I'll see you later."	"Hi, Bob. This is Jane Doe, a patient." *(Introducing the patient to the friend is very inappropriate and violates patient confidentiality.)*

Passive listening does not foster a therapeutic relationship. Body language during passive listening usually communicates boredom, indifference, or hostility (Fig. 9-2).

Through **active listening,** the nurse focuses on what the patient is saying to interpret and respond to the message objectively. While listening, the nurse concentrates only on what the patient says and the underlying meaning. The nurse's verbal and nonverbal behavior indicates active listening. The nurse usually responds indirectly, using techniques such as open-ended statements, reflection (see Table 9-2), and questions that elicit additional responses from the patient. In active listening, the nurse should avoid changing the subject and instead follow the patient's lead; however, at times it is necessary to respond directly to help a patient focus on a specific topic or to clarify thoughts and beliefs.

Some verbal techniques block interactions and inhibit therapeutic communication (Table 9-3). One of the biggest blocks to communication is giving advice, particularly that which others have already given. Giving advice is different from supporting a patient through decision making. As shown in Therapeutic Dialogue: Giving Advice Versus Recommendations, when giving advice, the nurse tells the patient what to do or how to act. In therapeutic communication, the nurse and patient explore alternative ways of viewing the patient's world. The patient then can reach his or her own conclusions about the best approaches to use.

Using Nonverbal Communication

Gestures, facial expressions, and body language actually communicate more than verbal messages. Under the best circumstances, body language mirrors or enhances what is verbally communicated. If, however, verbal and nonverbal messages are conflicting, the listener will receive the nonverbal message. For example, if a patient says that he feels fine, but has a sad facial expression and is slumped in a chair away from others, the message of sadness and depression will be communicated rather than the patient's words. The same is true of a nurse's behavior. If a nurse tells a patient that she is happy to see him, but her facial expression communicates indifference, the patient will receive the message that the nurse is bored.

Because people with psychiatric problems often have difficulty verbally expressing themselves and interpreting the emotions of others, nurses need to assess continually the nonverbal communication needs of patients. Eye contact (or lack thereof), posture, movement (shifting in chair, pacing), facial expressions, and gestures are nonverbal behaviors that communicate thoughts and feelings. A patient with low self-esteem may not be able to maintain eye contact and thus may spend a great deal of time looking toward the floor. A patient who is pacing and restless may be upset or having a reaction to medication. A clinched fist usually indicates that a person is angry or hostile.

Nurses should use positive body language. The nurse should sit at the same eye level as the patient with a relaxed posture that projects interest and attention. Leaning slightly forward helps engage the patient. Generally, the nurse should not cross arms or legs during therapeutic communication because such postures erect barriers to interaction. Uncrossed arms and legs project openness and a willingness to engage in conversation (Fig. 9-3). Any verbal response should be consistent with nonverbal messages.

TABLE 9.2   Techniques of Verbal Communication

Technique	Definition	Example	Use
Acceptance	Encouraging and receiving information in a nonjudgmental and interested manner	*Pt:* I have done something terrible. *Nurse:* I would like to hear about it. It's OK to discuss it with me.	Used in establishing trust and developing empathy
Confrontation	Presenting the patient with a different reality of the situation	*Pt:* My best friend never calls me. She hates me. Nurse: I was in the room yesterday when she called.	Used cautiously to immediately redefine the patient's reality. However, it can alienate the patient if used inappropriately. A nonjudgmental attitude is critical for confrontation to be effective.
Doubt	Expressing or voicing doubt when a patient relates a situation	*Pt:* My best friend hates me. She never calls me. *Nurse:* From what you have told me, that does not sound like her. When did she call you last?	Used carefully and only when the nurse feels confident about the details. It is used when the nurse wants to guide the patient toward other explanations.
Interpretation	Putting into words what the patients is implying or feeling	*Pt:* I could not sleep because someone would come in my room and rape me. *Nurse:* It sounds like you were scared last night.	Used in helping patient identify underlying thoughts or feelings
Observation	Stating to the patient what the nurse is observing	*Nurse:* You are trembling and perspiring. When did this start?	Used when a patient's behaviors (verbal or nonverbal) are obvious and unusual for that patient
Open-ended statements	Introducing an idea and letting the patient respond	*Nurse:* Trust means. . . . *Pt:* That someone will keep you safe.	Used when helping patient explore feelings or gain insight
Reflection	Redirecting the idea back to the patient	*Pt:* Should I go home for the weekend? *Nurse:* Should you go home for the weekend?	Used when patient is asking for the nurse's approval or judgment. Use of reflecting helps nurse maintain a nonjudgmental approach.
Restatement	Repeating the main idea expressed; lets patient know what was heard	*Pt:* I hate this place. I don't belong here. *Nurse:* You don't want to be here.	Used when trying to clarify what patient has said
Silence	Remaining quiet, but nonverbally expressing interest during an interaction	*Pt:* I am angry!! *Nurse:* (Silence) *Pt:* My wife had an affair.	Used when patient needs to express ideas but may not know quite how to do it. With silence, patient can focus on putting thoughts together.
Validation	Clarifying the nurse's understanding of the situation	*Nurse:* Let me see if I understand.	Used when nurse is trying to understand a situation the patient is trying to describe

Selecting Communication Techniques

In therapeutic communication, the nurse chooses the best words to say and uses nonverbal behaviors that are consistent with these words. If a patient is angry and upset, should the nurse (1) invite the patient to sit down and discuss the problem, (2) walk with the patient silently, or (3) simply observe the patient from a distance and not initiate conversation? Choosing the best response begins with assessing the meaning of the patient's communication.

The first step in determining an appropriate response is listening to the patient's verbal and nonverbal messages and interpreting their meaning. Nurses should not necessarily take verbal messages literally, especially when a patient is upset or angry. For example, one nurse walked into the room of a newly admitted patient who accused her of "locking me up and throwing away the key." The nurse could have responded defensively that she had nothing to do with the patient being admitted; however, that response

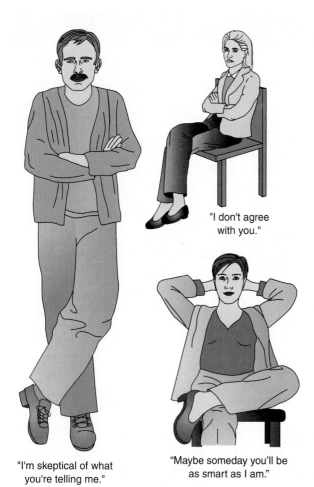

"I don't agree with you."

"I'm skeptical of what you're telling me."

"Maybe someday you'll be as smart as I am."

FIGURE 9.2 Negative body language.

would have ended in an argument, and communication would have been blocked. Fortunately, the nurse recognized that the patient was communicating frustration at being in a locked psychiatric unit and did not take the accusation personally.

The next step is deciding the desired patient outcome. To do so, the nurse should engage the patient with eye contact and quietly try to interpret the patient's feelings. In this example, the desired patient outcome was for the patient to clarify her hospitalization experience. The nurse responded that, "It must be frustrating to feel locked up." The nurse focused on the patient's feelings rather than the accusations and reflected that she understood the patient's feelings. The patient knew that the nurse accepted her feelings, which led to further discussion. It may seem impossible to plan reactions for each situation, but with practice, the nurse will begin to respond automatically in a therapeutic way.

Applying Communication Concepts

When the nurse is interacting with patients, additional considerations can enhance the quality of communication. This section describes the importance of rapport, the development of empathy, and the role of boundaries and body space in nurse–patient interactions.

Rapport

Rapport, interpersonal harmony characterized by understanding and respect, is important in developing a

TABLE 9.3 Techniques That Inhibit Communication

Technique	Definition	Example	Problem
Advice	Telling a patient what to do	*Pt:* I can't sleep. It is too noisy. *Nurse:* Turn off the light and shut your door.	Nurse solves the patient's problem, which may not be the appropriate solution, and encourages dependency on the nurse.
Agreement	Agreeing with a particular viewpoint of a patient	*Pt:* Abortions are sinful. *Nurse:* I agree.	Patient is denied opportunity to change view now that the nurse agrees.
Challenges	Disputing patient's beliefs with arguments, logical thinking, or direct order	*Pt:* I'm a cowboy. *Nurse:* If you are a cowboy, what are you doing in the hospital?	Nurse belittles the patient, and decreases self-esteem. Patient will avoid relating to the nurse who challenges.
Reassurance	Telling a patient that everything will be OK	*Pt:* Everyone thinks I'm bad. *Nurse:* You are a good person.	Nurse makes a statement that may not be true. Patient is blocked from exploring feelings.
Disapproval	Judging patient's situation and behavior	*Pt:* I'm so sorry. I did not mean to kill my mother. *Nurse:* You should be. How could anyone kill their mother?	Nurse belittles the patient. The patient will avoid the nurse.

THERAPEUTIC DIALOGUE | Giving Advice Versus Recommendations

Ms. J has just been diagnosed with phobic disorder and been given a prescription for fluoxetine. She was referred to the home health agency because she does not want to take her medication. She is fearful of becoming suicidal. Two approaches are given below.

Ineffective Communication (Advice)

Nurse: Ms. J, the doctor has ordered the medication because it will help you.

Ms. J: I don't want to take the medication because I am afraid of becoming suicidal. I heard that some of this psychiatric medication does that. I haven't had any attacks for 2 weeks.

Nurse: This medication has rarely had that side effect. You should try it and see if you have any suicidal thoughts.

Ms. J: OK.

(The nurse leaves and Ms. J does not take the medication. Within a week, Ms. J is taken to the emergency room with a panic attack.)

Effective Communication

Nurse: Ms. J, how have you been doing?

Ms. J: So far, so good. I haven't had any attacks for 2 weeks.

Nurse: I understand that the doctor gave you a prescription for medication that may help with the panic attacks.

Ms. J: Yes, but I don't want to take it because I am afraid of becoming suicidal. I heard that some of this psychiatric medication does that.

Nurse: Have you ever had feelings of hurting yourself?

Ms. J: Not really.

Nurse: If you took the medication and had thoughts like that what would you do?

Ms. J: I don't know.

Nurse: I think I see your dilemma. This medication may help your panic attacks, but the suicidal thoughts are a real fear. Is this perception true?

Ms. J: Yeah, that's it.

Nurse: Are there any circumstances under which you would be able to try the medication?

Ms. J: If I knew that I would not have suicidal thoughts.

Nurse: I can't guarantee that, but I would be able to call you every couple of days to determine if you are having any of these thoughts and help you deal with them.

Ms. J: Oh, that will be OK.

(Ms. J successfully took the medication.)

Critical Thinking Challenge

• Contrast the communication in the first scenario with that in the second.

• What therapeutic communication techniques did the second nurse employ that may have contributed to a better outcome?

• Are there any cues in the first scenario that indicate that the patient will not follow the nurse's advice? Explain.

---

trusting, therapeutic relationship. Nurses establish rapport through interpersonal warmth, a nonjudgmental attitude, and a demonstration of understanding. A skilled nurse will establish rapport that will alleviate the patient's anxiety in discussing personal problems.

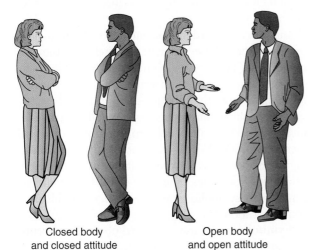

Closed body
and closed attitude

Open body
and open attitude

FIGURE 9.3 Open and closed body language.

People with psychiatric problems often feel alone and isolated from family and friends. Establishing rapport helps lessen feelings of being alone. When rapport develops, a patient feels comfortable with the nurse and finds it easier to self-disclose. The nurse also feels comfortable and recognizes that an interpersonal bond or alliance is developing. All these factors—comfort, sense of sharing, and decreased anxiety—are important in establishing and building the nurse–patient relationship.

Empathy

The use of empathy in a therapeutic relationship is central to psychiatric mental health nursing. **Empathy** is the ability to experience, in the present, a situation as another did at some time in the past. It is the ability to put oneself in another person's circumstances and feelings. The nurse does not actually have to have had the experience, but has to be able to imagine the feelings associated with it. For empathy to develop, there must be a giving of self to the other individual and a reciprocal desire to know each other personally. The process involves the nurse receiving information from the patient with open, nonjudgmental acceptance and communicating this understanding of the experience and feelings so that the patient feels understood.

Biopsychosocial Boundaries and Body Space Zones

Boundaries are the defining limits of individuals, objects, or relationships. Boundaries mark territory or what is "mine" or "not mine." Human beings have many different types of boundaries. Material boundaries, such as fences around property, artificially imposed state lines, and bodies of water, define territory as well as provide security and order. Personal boundaries can be conceptualized within the biopsychosocial model as including physical, psychological, and social dimensions. Physical boundaries are those established in terms of physical closeness to others—whom we allow to touch us or how close we want others to stand near us. Psychological boundaries are established in terms of emotional distance from others—how much of our innermost feelings and thoughts we want to share. Social boundaries, such as norms, customs, and roles, help us establish our closeness and place within the family, culture, and community.

Boundaries are not fixed, but dynamic. When boundaries are involuntarily transgressed, the individual feels threatened and responds to the perceived threat. The nurse must elicit permission before implementing interventions that invade personal space and boundaries.

Every individual is surrounded by four different body zones that provide varying degrees of protection against unwanted physical closeness during interactions with others (Pease, 1992) (Fig. 9-4). The actual sizes of the different zones vary according to culture. Some cultures define the intimate zone narrowly and the personal zones widely. Thus, friends in these cultures stand and sit close while interacting. People of other cultures define the intimate zone widely and are uncomfortable when others stand close to them. The variability of intimate and personal zones has implications for nursing. For a patient to be comfortable with a nurse, the nurse needs to protect the intimate zone of that individual. The patient usually will allow the nurse to enter the personal zone but will express discomfort if the nurse breaches the intimate zone. For the nurse, the difficulty lies in differentiating the personal zone from the intimate zone for each patient.

The nurse's awareness of his or her own need for intimate and personal space is another prerequisite for therapeutic interaction with the patient. It is important that a nurse feels comfortable while interacting with patients. Establishing a comfort zone may well entail fine-tuning the size of body zones. Recognizing this will help nurses understand their occasionally inexplicable reactions to the proximity of patients.

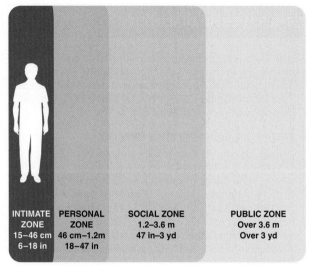

| INTIMATE ZONE 15–46 cm 6–18 in | PERSONAL ZONE 46 cm–1.2m 18–47 in | SOCIAL ZONE 1.2–3.6 m 47 in–3 yd | PUBLIC ZONE Over 3.6 m Over 3 yd |

FIGURE 9.4 Body space zones.

Analyzing Interactions

Many patients with psychiatric disorders have difficulty communicating. For example, perceptual, cognitive, and information-processing deficits, typical of people with schizophrenia, can interfere with the patient's ability to express ideas, understand concepts, and accurately perceive the environment. Because of the complexity of communication, mental health professionals monitor their interactions with patients using various methods, including audio recording, video recording, and **process recording,** which entails writing a verbatim transcript of the interaction. A video or audio recording of an interaction provides the most accurate monitoring but is cumbersome to use. Process recording, one of the easiest methods to use, is adequate in most situations. Nurses should use it when first learning therapeutic communication and during times when communication becomes a problem.

In a process recording, the nurse records, from memory, the verbatim interaction immediately after the communication (Text Box 9-3). The nurse then analyzes the content of the interaction in terms of the words and their meaning for both the patient and the nurse. The analysis is especially important because the ability to communicate verbally is often compromised in people with mental disorders. Words may not have the same meaning for the patient as they do for the nurse. Clarification of meaning becomes especially critical. The analysis can identify symbolic meanings, themes, and blocks in communication.

Symbolism, the use of a word or phrase to represent an object, event, or feeling, is used universally. For example, automobiles are named for wild animals

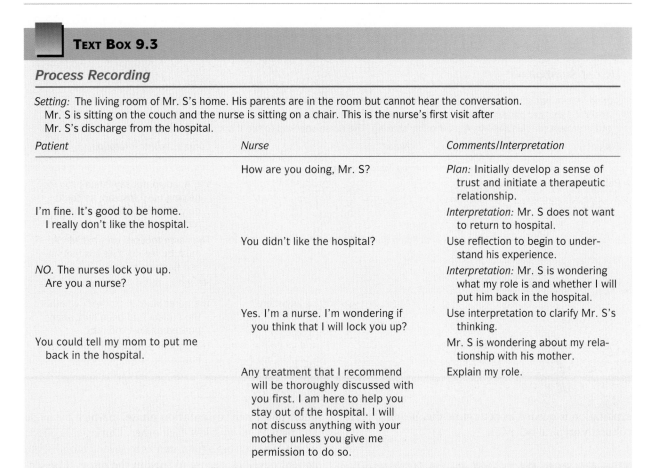

TEXT BOX 9.3

Process Recording

Setting: The living room of Mr. S's home. His parents are in the room but cannot hear the conversation. Mr. S is sitting on the couch and the nurse is sitting on a chair. This is the nurse's first visit after Mr. S's discharge from the hospital.

Patient	Nurse	Comments/Interpretation
	How are you doing, Mr. S?	*Plan:* Initially develop a sense of trust and initiate a therapeutic relationship.
I'm fine. It's good to be home. I really don't like the hospital.		*Interpretation:* Mr. S does not want to return to hospital.
	You didn't like the hospital?	Use reflection to begin to understand his experience.
NO. The nurses lock you up. Are you a nurse?		*Interpretation:* Mr. S is wondering what my role is and whether I will put him back in the hospital.
	Yes. I'm a nurse. I'm wondering if you think that I will lock you up?	Use interpretation to clarify Mr. S's thinking.
You could tell my mom to put me back in the hospital.		Mr. S is wondering about my relationship with his mother.
	Any treatment that I recommend will be thoroughly discussed with you first. I am here to help you stay out of the hospital. I will not discuss anything with your mother unless you give me permission to do so.	Explain my role.

that represent speed, prowess, and beauty. In people with mental disorders, the use of words to symbolize events, objects, or feelings is often idiosyncratic, and they cannot explain their choices. For example, a person who is feeling scared and anxious may tell the nurse that bombs and guns are exploding. It is up to the nurse to make the connection between the bombs and guns and the patient's feelings. Because of the patient's cognitive limitations, the individual can only express feelings symbolically. Another example is found in Text Box 9-4.

Verbal behavior is also interpreted by analyzing **content themes.** Patients often express concerns or feelings repeatedly in several different ways. After a few sessions, a common theme emerges. Themes may emerge symbolically, as in the case with the patient who constantly talks about the "guns and bombs." Alternatively, a theme may simply be identified as a recurrent thread of a story that a patient retells at each session. For example, one patient always explained his early abandonment by his family. This led the nurse to hypothesize that he had an underlying fear of rejection. The nurse was then able to test whether there was an underlying fear and to develop strategies to help the patient explore the fear (Text Box 9-5).

Communication blocks are identified by topic changes that either the nurse or the patient makes. Topics are changed for various reasons. A patient may change the topic from one that does not interest him to one that he finds more meaningful. Usually, however, an individual changes the topic because he or she is uncomfortable with a particular subject. Once a topic change is identified, the nurse hypothesizes the reason for it. If the nurse changes the topic, he or she needs to determine why. The nurse may find that he or she is uncomfortable with the topic or may not be listening to the patient. Beginning mental health nurses who are uncomfortable with silences or trying to elicit specific information from the patient often change topics.

The nurse must also record and interpret the patient's nonverbal behavior in light of the verbal behavior. Is the patient saying one thing verbally and another nonverbally? The nurse must consider the patient's cultural background. Is the behavior consistent with cultural norms? For example, if a patient denies any problems, but is affectionate and physically demonstrative (which is antithetical to her naturally stoic cultural beliefs and behaviors), the nonverbal behavior is inconsistent with what is normal behavior for that person. Further

TEXT BOX 9.4

Use of Symbolism

Setting: Mr. A has schizophrenia and expresses himself through the use of television characters. A nurse observed another patient shoving him against the wall. As the nurse approached the two patients, the other patient ran, leaving Mr. A. noticeably shaking. The nurse checked to see if Mr. A. was all right.

Patient	Nurse	Comments/Interpretation
	Mr. A, are you OK?	
Robin Hood saved the day.		Mr. A. could not say "thank you for helping me." Instead, he could only describe a fictional character's response.
	You feel that you are saved?	The nurse focused on what Mr. A. must be feeling if he felt that he had been rescued.
It's a glorious day in Sherwood forest!		He seems to be happy now.
	Mr. A, are you hurting anywhere?	The nurse wanted to check whether the patient had been hurt when pushed against the wall.
The angel of mercy put out the fire.		The patient is apparently not hurting now.

exploration is needed to determine the meaning of the culturally atypical behavior.

THE NURSE–PATIENT RELATIONSHIP

The nurse–patient relationship is a dynamic process that changes over time. It can be viewed in steps or phases with characteristic behaviors for both patient and nurse. This text uses an adaptation of Hildegarde Peplau's model that she introduced in her seminal work, *Interpersonal Relations in Nursing* (1952, 1992).

The nurse–patient relationship is conceptualized in three overlapping phases that evolve over time: orientation phase, working phase, and resolution phase. The

TEXT BOX 9.5

Use of Themes for Analyzing Interactions

Session I	Patient discusses the death of his mother at a young age.
Session II	Patient explains that his sister is now married and never visits him.
Session III	Patient says that his best friend in the hospital was discharged and he really misses her.
Session IV	Patient cries about a lost kitten.

Interpretation: Theme of loss is pervasive in several sessions.

initial phase is the **orientation phase**, in which the nurse and patient get to know each other. During this phase, which can last from a few minutes to several months, the patient develops a sense of trust in the nurse. The second is the **working phase**, in which the patient uses the relationship to examine specific problems and learn new ways of approaching them. The final stage, **resolution**, is the termination stage of the relationship and lasts from the time the problems are actually resolved to the close of the relationship. The relationship does not evolve as a simple linear relationship. Instead, the relationship may be predominantly in one phase, but reflections of all phases can be seen in each interaction (Table 9-4).

KEY CONCEPT **Nurse–patient relationship.** The **nurse–patient relationship** is a dynamic process that changes over time. It can be viewed in steps or phases with characteristic behaviors for both patient and nurse.

Orientation Phase

The orientation phase begins when the nurse and patient meet and ends when the patient begins to identify problems to examine. During the orientation phase, the nurse discusses the patient's expectations, explains the purpose of the relationship and its boundaries, and facilitates the development of the relationship. It is natural for the nurse to be nervous during the first few sessions. The goal of the orientation phase is to develop trust and security within the nurse–patient relationship.

TABLE 9.4   Phases of the Nurse–Patient Relationship

	Orientation	Working	Resolution
Patient	Seeks assistance Identifies needs Commits to a therapeutic relationship Later part, begins to test relationship	Discusses problems underlying needs Uses emotional safety of relationship to examine personal issues Tests new ways of solving problems Feels comfortable with nurse May use transference	May express ambivalence about the relationship and its termination Uses personal style to say "good-bye"
Nurse	Actively listens Establishes boundaries of the relationship Clarifies expectations Uses empathy Establishes rapport	Supports development of healthy problem solving Identifies countertransference issues	Avoids returning to patient's initial problems Encourages patient to prepare for the future Encourages independence Promotes positive family interactions

During this initial phase, the nurse listens intently to the patient's history and perception of problems and begins to understand the patient and identify themes. The use of empathy facilitates the development of a positive therapeutic relationship.

First Meeting

During the first meeting, outlining both nursing and patient responsibilities is important. The nurse is responsible for providing guidance throughout the therapeutic relationship, protecting confidential information, and maintaining professional boundaries. The patient is responsible for attending agreed-upon sessions, interacting during the sessions, and participating in the nurse–patient relationship. The nurse should also explain clearly to the patient meeting times, handling of missed sessions, and estimated length of the relationship.

Usually, both the nurse and the patient are anxious at the first meeting. The nurse should recognize his or her anxieties and attempt to alleviate them before the meeting. The patient's behavior during this first meeting may indicate to the nurse some of the patient's problems in interpersonal relationships. For example, a patient may talk nonstop for 15 minutes or may brag of sexual conquests. What the patient chooses to tell (or not to tell) is significant. What a patient first does or says may not accurately indicate his or her true feelings or the situation. In the beginning, patients may deny problems or choose not to discuss them as defense mechanisms or to prevent the nurse from getting to know them. The patient is usually nervous and insecure during the first few sessions and may exhibit behavior reflective of these emotions, such as rambling. Usually, by the third session, the patient can focus on a topic.

Confidentiality in Treatment

Ideally, nurses include people who are important to the patient in planning and implementing care. The nurse and patient should discuss the issue of confidentiality in the first session. The nurse should be clear about any information that is to be shared with anyone else. Usually, the nurse shares significant assessment data and patient progress with a supervisor and a physician. Most patients expect the nurse to communicate with other mental health professionals and are comfortable with this arrangement.

Testing the Relationship

This first part of the orientation phase, called the "honeymoon phase," is usually pleasant. Typically, however, the therapeutic team hits rough spots before completing this phase. The patient begins to test the relationship to become convinced that the nurse will really accept him or her. Typical "testing behaviors" include forgetting a scheduled session or being late. Patients may also express anger at something a nurse says or accuse the nurse of breaking confidentiality. The nurse must recognize that these behaviors are designed to test the relationship and establish its parameters, not to express rejection or dissatisfaction with the nurse. The student nurse often feels personally rejected during the patient's testing and may even become angry with the patient. If the nurse simply accepts the behavior and continues to be available to the patient, these behaviors usually subside (see Research Box 9-1).

RESEARCH BOX 9.1

Is A Nurse–Patient Relationship Really Important?

The purpose of this study was to examine the importance of an ongoing therapeutic relationship. Nurse psychotherapists ($n = 6$) and their patients ($n = 8$) were studied to see if they had developed a level of understanding in which they recognized dense meanings and familiar, shorthand communications. The findings were that the nurses and patients could read each other's responses with sensitivity and attunement, which contributed to a sense of comfort and openness during therapy sessions.

Utilization in Clinical Setting: Students can learn the power of relationships. As the relationship develops, it contributes to sensitivity to nuances of meaning and development of an individualized approach.

Raingruber, B. J. (1999). Recognizing, understanding, and responding to familiar responses: The importance of a relationship history for therapeutic effectiveness. *Perspectives in Psychiatric Care, 35*(2), 5–17.

Working Phase

When the patient begins identifying problems to work on, the working phase of the relationship has started. Problem identification can yield a wide range of issues, such as managing symptoms of a mental disorder, coping with chronic pain, examining issues related to sexual abuse, or dealing with problematic interpersonal relationships. Through the relationship, the patient begins to explore the identified problems and develop strategies to resolve them. By the time the working phase is reached, the patient has developed enough trust that he or she can examine the identified problems within the security of the therapeutic relationship. In the working phase, the nurse can use various verbal and nonverbal techniques to help the patient examine problems.

Transference (unconscious assignment to others of the feelings and attitudes that the patient originally associated with important figures) and countertransference (the provider's emotional reaction to the patient based on personal unconscious needs and conflicts) become important issues in the working phase. For example, a patient could be hostile to a nurse because of underlying resentment of authority figures; the nurse, in turn, could respond defensively because of earlier experiences of anger (see Chap. 6). The patient uses transference to examine problems. During this phase, the patient is psychologically vulnerable and emotionally dependent on the nurse. The nurse needs to recognize countertransference and prevent it from eroding professional boundaries.

Resolution Phase

The final stage of the nurse–patient relationship is **resolution**, which begins when the actual problems are resolved and ends with the termination of the relationship. During this phase, the patient is redirected toward a life without a therapeutic relationship. The patient connects with community resources, solidifies a newly found understanding, and practices new behaviors. The patient takes responsibility for follow-up appointments and interacts with significant others in new ways. New problems are not addressed during this phase except in terms of what was learned during the working stage.

Termination begins the first day of the relationship, when the nurse explains that this relationship is time limited and was established to resolve the patient's problems and help him or her handle them. Because a therapeutic relationship is dependent, the nurse must constantly evaluate the patient's level of dependence and continually support the patient's move toward independence. Termination is usually stressful for the patient, who must sever ties with the nurse who has shared thoughts and feelings and given guidance and support over many sessions. Depending on previous experiences with terminating relationships, some patients may not handle their emotions well during termination. Some may not show up for the last session at all to avoid their feelings of sadness and separation. Many patients display anger about the relationship ending. Patients may express anger toward the nurse or displace it onto others. For example, one patient yelled obscenities at another patient after he was told that his therapeutic relationship with the nurse would end in a few weeks. One of the best ways to handle the anger is to help the patient acknowledge it, to explain that anger is a normal emotion when a relationship is ending, and to reassure the patient that it is acceptable to feel angry. The nurse should also reassure the patient that anger subsides once the relationship is over.

Another typical termination behavior is raising old problems that have already been resolved. The nurse may feel frustrated if patients in the termination phase present resolved problems as if they were new. The nurse may feel that the sessions were unsuccessful. In reality, patients are attempting to prolong the relationship and avoid its ending. Nurses should avoid addressing these problems. Instead, they should reassure patients that they already covered those issues and learned methods to control them. They should explain that the patient may be feeling anxious about the relationship ending and redirect the patient to newly found skills and abilities in forming new relationships, including support

THERAPEUTIC DIALOGUE | The Last Meeting

Ineffective Approach

Nurse: Today is my last day.
Patient: I need to talk to you about something important.
Nurse: What is it?
Patient: I have been hearing voices again.
Nurse: Oh, how often?
Patient: Every night. You are the only one I'm going to tell.
Nurse: I think you should tell the new nurse.
Patient: She is too new. She won't understand. I feel so bad about your leaving. Is there anyway you can stay?
Nurse: Well, I could check on you tomorrow?
Patient: Oh, would you? I would really appreciate it if you would give me your new telephone number.
Nurse: I don't know what the number will be, but it will be listed in the telephone book.

Effective Approach

Nurse: Today is my last day.
Patient: I need to talk to you about something important.

Nurse: We talked about that. Anything "Important" needs to be shared with the new nurse.
Patient: But, I want to tell you.
Nurse: Saying goodbye can be very hard.
Patient: I will miss you.
Nurse: Your feelings are very normal when relationships are ending. I will remember you in a very special way.
Patient: Can I please have your telephone number?
Nurse: No, I can't give that to you. It is important that we say good-bye today.
Patient: OK. Good-bye. Good luck.
Nurse: Good-bye.

Critical Thinking Challenge

- What were some of the mistakes the nurse in the first scenario made?

- In the second scenario, how does therapeutic communication in the termination phase differ from effective communication in the working phase?

---

groups and social groups. The final meeting should focus on the future (see Therapeutic Dialogue: The Last Meeting). The nurse can reassure the patient that the nurse will remember him or her, but the nurse should not agree to see the patient outside the relationship.

Summary of Key Points

➤ Before nurses can attempt to deal therapeutically with the emotions, feelings, and problems of patients, they must understand their own cultural values and beliefs and interpersonal strengths and limitations.

➤ The nurse–patient relationship is built on therapeutic communication, including verbal and nonverbal interactions between nurse and patient. Some communication skills include active listening, positive body language, appropriate verbal responses, and ability of the nurse to interpret appropriately and analyze the patient's verbal and nonverbal behaviors.

➤ Two of the most important communication concepts are empathy and rapport.

➤ In the nurse–patient relationship, as in all types of relationships, certain physical, emotional, and social boundaries and limitations need to be observed.

➤ The nurse–patient relationship consists of three major and overlapping stages or phases: the orientation phase, in which the patient and nurse meet and establish the parameters of the relationship; the working phase, in which the patient identifies and explores problems; and the resolution phase, in which the patient learns to manage the problems and the relationship is terminated.

Critical Thinking Challenges

1. Identify three times within the last year that you have "changed your mind" about a group, person, or idea. What did you learn about yourself?

2. Complete the self-assessment in Text Box 9-1. Examine how these views can influence your interaction with patients.

3. Interview a patient for 20 minutes, and complete a process recording. Identify both the therapeutic and nontherapeutic verbal techniques you used. Develop a plan to avoid the nontherapeutic verbal techniques in the future. Select at least two more therapeutic verbal techniques you did not use. Practice using them. At the end of 1 week, evaluate your comfort level in using the new techniques.

4. Compare the concepts of rapport and empathy.

5. Discuss how the following behaviors might mean something different depending on the phase of the relationship:
   a. A patient starts calling the nurse at home.
   b. A patient is late for a session.
   c. A patient reports all new symptoms.
   d. A patient is angry.

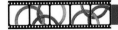 **MOVIES**

Good Will Hunting: 1997. Robin Williams plays a therapist to Will Hunting, a janitor identified as a mathematical genius, played by Matt Damon. Through a strong relationship, Will begins to realize his potential.

Viewing Points: Watch closely how the relationship develops between the characters played by Williams and Damon. How does the relationship change as the characters move through different stages of their relationship?

Ordinary People: 1980. Timothy Hutton plays Conrad Jarrett, a teenager consumed with guilt over his older brother's accidental death, his own subsequent suicide attempt, and his troubled relationship with his mother (Mary Tyler Moore). Therapy sessions with Dr. Berger (Judd Hirsch) and the support of Conrad's concerned father (Donald Sutherland) help Conrad to deal appropriately with his past and present problems and to find hope for the future.

Viewing Points: Dr. Berger uses several communication techniques discussed in this chapter to build a therapeutic relationship with Conrad. Look for examples of acceptance, confrontation, observation, open-ended statements, reflection, and silence. Can you identify others? Also, note the differences in the communication patterns between various people in the film: Conrad and Dr. Berger, Mr. and Mrs. Jarrett, Conrad and Mrs. Jarrett, Conrad and Mr. Jarrett. How does communication change in each relationship throughout the film?

REFERENCES

Boyd, M. (1995). Communication with patients, families, healthcare providers, and diverse cultures. In M. Strader & P. Decker (Eds.), *Role transition to patient care management.* East Norwalk, CT: Appleton & Lange.

Pease, A. (1992). *Body language.* London: Sheldon Press.

Peplau, H. (1952). *Interpersonal relations in nursing.* New York: G. Putnam & Sons.

Peplau, H. (1992). Interpersonal relations: A theoretical framework for application in nursing practice. *Nursing Science Quarterly, 5*(1), 13–18.

Raingruber, B. J. (1999). Recognizing, understanding, and responding to familiar responses: The importance of a relationship history for therapeutic effectiveness. *Perspectives in Psychiatric Care, 35*(2), 5–17.

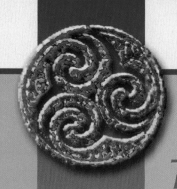

The Assessment Process

Mary Ann Boyd

ASSESSMENT AS A PROCESS
Initial Assessment
Ongoing Assessment

TECHNIQUES OF DATA COLLECTION
Patient Observations
Patient and Family Interviews
Physical and Mental Examinations
Records and Diagnostic Reports
Collaboration With Colleagues

BIOPSYCHOSOCIAL PSYCHIATRIC NURSING ASSESSMENT
Biologic Domain

Present and Past Health Status
Physical Examination
Physical Functions
Pharmacologic Assessment
Psychological Domain
  *Responses to Mental
    Health Problems*
  Mental Status Examination
  Behavior
  Self-Concept
  Stress and Coping Patterns
  Risk Assessment
Social Domain
  Functional Status
  Social Systems

Spiritual Assessment
Occupational Status
Economic Status
Legal Status
Quality of Life

After studying this chapter, you will be able to:

➤ Define the assessment process.

➤ Differentiate an initial assessment from an ongoing assessment.

➤ Discuss the different techniques of data collection.

➤ Discuss the synthesis of the biopsychosocial assessment data.

➤ Delineate important areas of assessment for the biologic domain in completing the psychiatric nursing assessment.

➤ Delineate important areas of assessment for the psychological domain in completing the psychiatric nursing assessment.

➤ Delineate important areas of assessment for the social domain in completing the psychiatric nursing assessment.

Effective nursing interventions are based on accurate and relevant information about the patient receiving assistance. Psychiatric nurses discover such information, used throughout the delivery of patient care, through careful and thorough assessment. In the Scope and Standards of Psychiatric–Mental Health Nursing Practice, *the American Nurses Association (ANA) identifies assessment as the first standard, stating "the psychiatric–mental health nurse collects client health data" (ANA et al., 2000, p. 28). Placing this standard first justly underscores the importance of assessment as the basis for all other aspects of nursing (see Chap. 5). The assessment data will provide the nurse with the foundation for developing an appropriate plan of care.*

The purpose of this chapter is to present an overview of the biopsychosocial nursing assessment for people with actual or potential mental health problems. The biopsychosocial approach to nursing assessment is used throughout this text. Although the biologic, psychological, and social areas of assessment are presented here in somewhat finite divisions, the student should remember that each area overlaps and is interdependent with the others.

ASSESSMENT AS A PROCESS

Assessment is the deliberate and systematic collection and interpretation of biopsychosocial information or data to determine current and past health, functional status, and human responses to mental health problems, both actual and potential. These responses may be biologic, psychological, or social, or they may integrate or encompass all the biopsychosocial dimensions. Assessment is not an isolated activity. It is a systematic process that can occur over several sessions.

KEY CONCEPT Assessment. **Assessment** is the deliberate and systematic collection and interpretation of biopsychosocial information or data to determine current and past health, functional status, and human responses to mental health problems, both actual and potential.

Assessment is integral throughout the nursing process. It may have many purposes. It may be comprehensive or short and focused. Assessment begins with the first contact with the patient and may incorporate several different methods of data collection.

The psychiatric nurse approaches the patient assessment with a solid theoretic background in human social behavior, knowledge about mental disorders, and therapeutic relationship-building skills. All these elements are necessary to determine the patient's response to an emotional problem or mental disorder. The assessment process is based on the establishment of rapport with the patient and the initiation of the nurse–patient relationship (see Chap. 9). The patient must develop a sense of trust within the relationship before he or she comfortably reveals intimate life details to the nurse, who is a stranger. It is of paramount importance that the nurse has a healthy knowledge of self as well (Text Box 10-1). The nurse's own biases and values, which may be different than those of the patient, can influence the nurse's interpretation of assessment data. A careful self-assessment helps the nurse interpret the data objectively.

TEXT BOX 10.1

Self-Concept Awareness

Self-awareness is important in any interaction. To understand a patient's self-concept, the nurse must be aware of his or her own self-concept. By answering these questions, nurses can evaluate self-concept components and increase their self-understanding. The more comfortable the nurse is with himself or herself, the more effective the nurse can be in each and every patient interaction.

Body Image

How do I feel about my body?

How important is my physical appearance?

How does my body measure up to my ideal body? (How would I like to appear?)

What is positive about my body?

What would I like to change about my body?

How does my body image affect my self-esteem?

Self-Esteem

When do I feel confident and good about myself?

When do I feel unimportant?

What do I do when I feel good about myself? (Call friends, socialize?)

What do I do when I have negative feelings about myself? (Withdraw, dress poorly?)

When do I make negative statements?

Am I able to correct my negative self-statements?

Personal Identity

How do I describe myself?

What three adjectives describe who I am?

Do I identify with a particular cultural group, family role, or place of residence?

What would I like to have on my tombstone?

Initial Assessment

The initial assessment can be either a comprehensive or a screening assessment. A **comprehensive assessment** is the collection of all relevant data to identify problems for which a nursing diagnosis is stated. The biopsychosocial nursing assessment discussed later in the chapter represents a comprehensive assessment. Because there are so many areas to cover and it may take time for the nurse–patient relationship to develop, completing the comprehensive assessment at one time may be impossible. Additional sessions with the patient, family, and other health care providers may be necessary to obtain an accurate picture of the patient. Sometimes, the nurse must prioritize problems and address first those that pose imminent danger to the patient's well-being. For example, if a patient is experiencing active suicidal intent, the nurse should choose to forestall further assessment until certain safety measures and crisis intervention strategies are implemented (see Chap. 35). Once the patient's immediate safety is ensured, a more comprehensive assessment may continue later.

A **screening assessment** is the collection of data to identify individuals who may a mental disorder but have not yet recognized its symptoms; who have risk factors for the development of a psychiatric disorder; or who are experiencing emotional difficulties but have not yet formally sought treatment. This type of assessment is usually conducted in a fairly structured and brief format depending on the setting. For example, after a natural disaster such as an earthquake, community mental health services may establish screening clinics in a population to recognize early symptoms of or risks for posttraumatic stress disorder or other psychiatric disorders. These clinics serve as a source of information and referral as well, but usually do not provide on-site treatment.

Screening assessments may also take place when a person requests assistance or comes to a mental health hospital or clinic. In these cases, the screening assessment focuses on determining the most appropriate services or resources for addressing the person's difficulties. Some mental health programs call this form of screening assessment an *intake interview*, designed to determine whether the person's goals or identified problems match the service to which he or she has presented. This brief assessment may result in referral to other services or may develop into a more comprehensive assessment at the place of initial contact.

Ongoing Assessment

Ongoing assessments are made to monitor the progress and outcomes of the interventions implemented. They are shorter and more focused than initial assessments. Ongoing assessments may contain aspects of the initial comprehensive assessment, such as a symptom-monitoring tool or rating scale, discussed later in this chapter. They may involve evaluation of the effectiveness of medications, monitoring for the development of potential side effects, assessment of target symptoms, or evaluation of risks to the patient's safety. Ongoing assessments may focus on specific factors related to knowledge deficits, support resources, or sociocultural status.

TECHNIQUES OF DATA COLLECTION

Psychiatric–mental health nurses collect assessment data through various methods. Such methods include observations of the patient, interviews with the patient and family, analysis of findings from physical and mental examinations, review of records and diagnostic and laboratory reports, and comparisons of data from other providers.

Patient Observations

The psychiatric–mental health nurse begins the assessment from the first moment of observation of the patient. Although verbal communication can be revealing, patients may communicate many signs and symptoms of emotional distress nonverbally. The nurse gathers clues to what the patient may be experiencing by paying attention to nonverbal cues throughout the interview. Dress, manner, facial expression, and gestures are all examples of nonverbal information (see Chap. 9). For example, the patient may wear a winter coat in warm weather, seem agitated, look angry, or gesture wildly. The nurse must note each aspect and how it changes throughout the interview. Nurses must withhold judgment. They may note the patient's nonverbal and verbal cues but must be careful not to make value judgments about them.

Patient and Family Interviews

An interview, especially an assessment interview, is a dynamic process that evolves as the nurse obtains more information and develops more questions to clarify descriptions, perceptions, attitudes, behaviors, beliefs, feelings, or values. The nurse must clearly state the purpose of the interview and, if necessary, modify the interview process so that both patient and nurse agree on its purpose.

An assessment interview usually involves direct questions to obtain facts, clarify perceptions, validate observations, interpret the meanings of groups of facts, or compare information. The specific questions may take on different forms. The nurse may choose to use open-ended questions or closed-ended questions to complete the assessment.

Open-ended questions, such as "How did you come to this clinic today?" allow patients to describe their experience in their own way. Patients may answer this question concretely by saying, "I took a taxi" or "I came by car." Or they may address this question by responding, "My family thought I should come so they brought me" or "Well, I got up this morning . . . I took a shower, got dressed . . . and then, well you know, it is difficult sometimes to decide." Each of these answers helps the nurse assess the patient's thinking process as well as evaluate the content of the response. Open-ended questions are most helpful when beginning the interview because they allow the nurse to observe how the patient is responding verbally and nonverbally. They also convey caring and interest in the person's well-being, which establishes rapport. Using only open-ended questions may cause patients to become sidetracked, however, losing the focus and purpose of the interview for both nurse and patient. Therefore, nurses must use other types of questions as well.

Nurses should use closed-ended questions when they need specific information. For example, "How old are you?" asks for specific information about the patient's age. These types of questions limit the individual's response but often serve as good follow-up questions for clarification of thoughts or feelings expressed. Health professionals commonly rely on closed-ended questions when conducting an initial assessment because such questions feel safe. In fact, patients may appear more relaxed with these types of questions because they clearly indicate what response is expected. However, depending too much on these types of questions tends to block the free flow of information. Nurses may easily miss issues or problems important to the patient when they use only closed-ended questions.

Clarification is extremely important during the assessment process. The nurse must never simply assume that all words have the same meaning to all people. Education, language, culture, history, and experience may influence the meaning of words. Nurses should use as many techniques for clarification as possible. Sometimes, simple and direct questioning provides clarification. In other situations, the nurse may clarify by providing a specific example for a more global thought the patient is trying to express. For example, a patient may say, "Things have been so strange since the children left." The nurse may respond with, "Sometimes, parents feel sad and empty when their children leave home. They do not know what to do with their time." Frequently summarizing what has been said allows the patient the opportunity to correct the nurse's interpretation. For example, verbalizing a sequence of events that the patient has reported may help to identify omissions or inconsistencies. Restating information or reflecting feelings that the patient has described also allows opportunity for clarification. It is essential that nurses understand exactly what patients are attempting to communicate before beginning to intervene. Text Box 10-2

TEXT BOX 10.2

Assessment Interview Behaviors

The following behaviors carried out by the nurse will enhance the effectiveness of the assessment interview:

- Exhibiting empathy—to show empathy to the patient, the nurse uses phrases such as, "That must have been upsetting for you" or "I can understand your hurt feelings."
- Giving recognition—the nurse gives recognition by listening actively: verbally encouraging the patient to continue, and nonverbally presenting an open, interested demeanor.
- Demonstrating acceptance—note that acceptance does not mean agreement or nonagreement with the patient, but is a neutral stance that allows the patient to continue.
- Restating—the nurse tries to clarify what the patient is trying to say by restating it.
- Reflecting—the nurse presents the patient's last statement as a question. This gives the patient a chance to expand on the information.
- Focusing—the nurse attempts to bring the conversation back to the questions at hand when the patient goes off on a tangent.
- Using open-ended questions—general questions give the patient a chance to speak freely.
- Presenting reality—the nurse presents reality when the patient makes unrealistic or exaggerated statements.
- Making observations—the nurse says aloud what patient behaviors are observed, to give the patient a chance to speak to those behaviors. For example, the nurse may say, "I notice you are twisting your fingers; are you nervous about something?"

provides a summary of other behaviors that enhance the effectiveness of an assessment interview.

Many psychiatric symptoms are beyond a patient's awareness. Sometimes, only other people involved with the patient notice the impact of a disorder or that a patient's behavior has changed. With the patient's permission to consult them, family members, friends, and other health care professionals are important sources of information. Confidentiality of information related to the patient is essential. Legally, all rights to release of this information belong to the patient unless these rights have been overridden by legal means discussed in Chapter 4. In almost all cases, state laws strongly protect confidentiality. When seeking information about the patient, the nurse should be careful to obtain permission from the patient. Seeking permission before speaking with relatives or friends also builds the individual's trust in the nurse. The nurse should give a clear explanation to the patient regarding why the information is needed and how it will be used.

Physical and Mental Examinations

The assessment process includes collection of data through physical examinations and mental functioning tests. Usually, the psychiatric nurse does not actually perform the physical examination but collects the information from the provider who does. It is important that the physical examination is recent. The psychiatric nurse will need to learn the results of various mental status and psychological examinations. Other professionals will conduct some of these examinations, and the nurse will use the results in treatment planning.

Records and Diagnostic Reports

The comprehensive assessment includes the review and interpretation of other reports, records, and diagnostic examinations. To access records that are not included in the patient's chart, written permission is required. Because requesting records takes time, the assessment is usually revised after the records are received. Examples of records that are reviewed include past medical records, past psychiatric treatments, psychological evaluations, legal records, and school records.

Because many medical disorders often present with psychiatric symptoms, a general medical workup is also usually completed. This includes a medical history, physical examination, neurologic evaluation, and laboratory work. Although the specific tests ordered vary with the setting, practitioner, and patient's condition, the most common laboratory work obtained includes a complete blood count, urinalysis, serum electrolytes, liver enzymes, serum creatinine, blood urea nitrogen, and sometimes thyroid function tests.

Collaboration With Colleagues

The psychiatric–mental health nurse works in settings with various health care professionals from other disciplines. Many of these professionals are completing assessments at the same time as the nurse. This may prove confusing for the patient if nurses do not clearly convey their roles and relationships to the individual receiving care. The health care team uses psychiatric nursing assessments in developing a comprehensive treatment plan for the patient that includes nursing care. In addition, as part of the multidisciplinary team, nurses must have knowledge and understanding of the assessment data that other health care professionals have obtained. The primary goal of the psychiatric evaluation performed by a psychiatrist, advanced practice nurse, or other primary provider of mental health services is to establish a diagnosis based on the *Diagnostic and Statistical Manual of Mental Health Disorders*, 4th ed. (DSM-IV), published by the American Psychiatric Association (2000). Psychologists are also involved in psychological testing and developing a DSM-IV diagnosis. Although social workers may also be involved in many aspects of assessment, some of their primary concerns are the financial, environmental, and interpersonal well-being of the patient who has a psychiatric disorder. Social workers are often aware of community resources and eligibility requirements for financial assistance. Their assessment involves the individual's social level of functioning and whether his or her current living situation is compromising well-being. Recreational, occupational, art, music, and other therapists have special training in their specific area to assist the patient in recovery. Their assessment focuses on the patient's current abilities and skills to enjoy and function, capitalizing on strengths and interests. Nurses can use this information obtained from these multidisciplinary assessments to learn more about the patient's circumstances and how other disciplines approach patient assessment.

BIOPSYCHOSOCIAL PSYCHIATRIC NURSING ASSESSMENT

The assessment of human responses to emotional difficulties or mental disorders includes the integration of biologic, psychological, and social data. The biopsychosocial model presented in Chapter 5 provides the essential framework for integration of data from all three dimensions. Any single event in the individual's life may produce responses in all of these dimensions. For example, a substance, such as cocaine, produces physiologic responses, such as tachycardia, and changes the actions of neurochemicals, such as dopamine. Although the use of cocaine may be considered basically biologic, it also produces many psychological responses, such as euphoria, hypervigilance, difficulty with judgment, and agitation. In addition, the use of cocaine may change the individual's ability to relate interpersonally and may contribute to legal difficulties, which are considered responses within the social context.

The Biopsychosocial Psychiatric Nursing Assessment (Text Box 10-3) is a basic guide to collecting assessment data using both open- and closed-ended questions. Throughout this book, other assessment tools are presented that are used for specific populations or disorders. All the assessment tools in this book have a biopsychosocial perspective. Even though the following discussion is specific to biologic, psychological, and social areas, nurses should integrate these data within the biopsychosocial context (Fig. 10-1).

Assessment information is entered into the patient's written or computerized record, which may take on several different formats. Forms, checklists, narratives, and problem-oriented notes are examples of such formats. Text Box 10-4 provides a narrative note of the results

from a patient's mental status examination. Regardless of the format used, psychiatric–mental health nurses must be careful to describe behavior exhibited rather than interpret or judge it. They must be careful to eliminate bias, providing a brief, concise, and clear picture of the patient's symptoms, behaviors, strengths, weaknesses, improvements, and concerns. The standard of practice is to complete a psychiatric–mental health nursing assessment and generate nursing diagnoses, identify outcomes, and plan interventions based on the assessment data.

Biologic Domain

Many psychiatric disorders produce physical symptoms, such as the tachycardia, increased perspiration, and tremors associated with anxiety and the lack of appetite and weight loss associated with depression. A person's physical condition may also affect mental health, producing a recurrence or increase in symptoms. Many physical disorders may present first with symptoms considered to be psychiatric. For example, hypothyroidism often presents with feelings of lethargy, decreased concentration, and low mood. For these reasons, biologic information about the patient is always considered.

Present and Past Health Status

Beginning with a history of the patient's general medical condition, the nurse should consider the following:

- Availability of, frequency of, and most recent medical evaluation, including test results
- Past hospitalizations and operations
- Cardiac problems, including cerebrovascular accidents, myocardial infarctions, and childhood illnesses
- Respiratory problems, particularly those that result in a lack of oxygen to the brain
- Neurologic problems, particularly head injuries, seizure disorders, or any periods of loss of consciousness
- Endocrine disorders, particularly unstable diabetes or thyroid or adrenal dysfunction
- Immune disorders, particularly HIV and autoimmune disorders
- Use, exposure, abuse, or dependence on substances, including alcohol, tobacco, prescription drugs, and illegal drugs

Physical Examination

Body Systems Review. Once the nurse has obtained historical information, he or she should examine physiologic systems to evaluate the patient's current physical condition. The nurse should keep in mind that a (*text continues on page 203*)

TEXT BOX 10.3

Biopsychosocial Psychiatric Nursing Assessment

I. Major reason for seeking help _____

II. Initial information

Name _____

Age _____ Marital status _____

Gender _____

Ethnic identification _____

III. Present and past health status

_____

_____

	Normal	Treated	Untreated
Physical functions: System review	☐	☐	☐
Elimination	☐	☐	☐
Activity/exercise	☐	☐	☐
Sleep	☐	☐	☐
Appetite and nutrition	☐	☐	☐
Hydration	☐	☐	☐
Sexuality	☐	☐	☐
Self-Care	☐	☐	☐
Existing physical illnesses	☐	☐	☐

Medications (prescription and over-the-counter)	**Dosage**	**Side effects**	**Frequency**

Significant laboratory tests	**Values**	**Normal range**

IV. Responses to mental health problems

Major concerns regarding mental health problem _____

_____

Major loss/change in past year: No _____ Yes _____

Fear of violence: No _____ Yes _____

Strategies for managing problems/disorder _____

_____

TEXT BOX 10.3 (*Continued*)

V. Mental status examination

    General observations (appearance, psychomotor activity, attitude) _____

    _____

    Orientation (time, place, person) _____

    Mood, affect, emotions _____

    Speech (verbal ability, speed, use of words correctly) _____

    _____

    Thought processes (tangential, logic, repetition, rhyming of words, loose connections, disorganized)

    _____

    Cognition and intellectual performance

      Attention and concentration _____

      Abstract reasoning and comprehension _____

      Memory (recall, short-term, recent, and remote) _____

      _____

      Judgment and insight _____

      MMSE score (optional) _____

VI. Significant behaviors (psychomotor, agitation, aggression, withdrawn) _____

    _____

    _____

VII. Self-concept (body image, self-esteem, personal identity) _____

    _____

    _____

VIII. Stress and coping patterns _____

    _____

    _____

IX. Risk assessment

    Suicide: High _____ Low _____ Assault/homicide: High _____ Low _____

    Suicide thoughts or ideation: No _____ Yes _____

      Current thoughts of harming self _____

      Plan _____

      Means _____

      Means available _____

    Assault/homicide thoughts: No _____ Yes _____

      What do you do when angry with stranger?_____

      What do you do when angry with family or partner?_____

      Have you ever hit or pushed anyone? No _____ Yes _____

      Have you ever been arrested for assault? No _____ Yes _____

      Current thoughts of harming others _____

X. Functional status

    GAF score (see Chap. 3) _____

XI. Social systems

    Cultural assessment

      Cultural group _____

      Cultural group's view of health and mental illness _____

      What cultural rules do you try to live by? _____

      Important cultural foods _____

(continued)

Text Box 10.3 (*Continued*)

Family assessment
   Family members _____
   Members important to patient _____
   Decision makers, family roles, supportive members _____
   _____
   Community resources _____
   _____

XII. Spiritual assessment _____
   _____

XIII. Economic status _____
XIV. Legal status _____
 XV. Quality of life _____

Summary of significant data that can be used in formulating a nursing diagnosis:

SIGNATURE/TITLE _____   Date_____

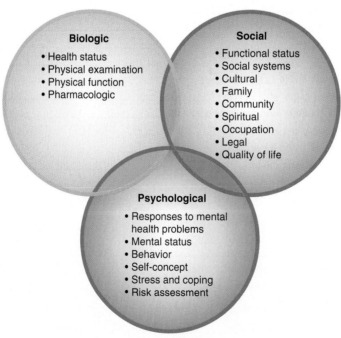

Figure 10.1 Biopsychosocial nursing assessment.

TEXT BOX 10.4

Narrative Mental Status Examination Note

The patient is a 65-year-old widowed man who is slightly disheveled. He is cooperative with the interviewer and judged to be an adequate historian. His mood and affect are depressed and anxious. He becomes tearful throughout the interview when speaking about his wife. His flow of thought is hesitant when speaking about his wife, but coherent. He is oriented to time, place, and person. He shows good recent and remote memory. He is able to recall several items given him by the interviewer. The patient shows poor insight and judgment regarding his sadness since the loss of his wife. He repeatedly says, "Mary wouldn't want me to be sad. She would want me to continue with my life."

physician or nurse practitioner may be conducting a thorough examination. Nevertheless, the psychiatric nurse should pay special attention to various systems that treatment may affect. For example, if a patient is being treated with antihypertensive medication, the dosage may need to be adjusted if an antipsychotic medication is prescribed. If a patient is overweight or has diabetes, some psychiatric medications can affect these conditions.

Neurologic Status. Particular attention is paid to recent head trauma, episodes of hypertension, and changes in personality, speech, or ability to handle activities of daily living. Also noted are any movement disorders.

Laboratory Results. Available laboratory data are reviewed for any abnormalities and documented. Particular attention is paid to any abnormalities of hepatic, renal, or urinary function because these systems metabolize or excrete many psychiatric medications. Also, abnormal white blood cell and electrolyte levels should be noted. Laboratory data are especially important, particularly if the nurse is the only person in the mental health team who has a "medical" background (Table 10-1).

Physical Functions

Elimination. The patient's daily urinary and bowel habits should be questioned and documented. Various medications can affect bladder and bowel functioning; hence, a baseline must be noted. For example, diarrhea and frequency of urination can occur with lithium carbonate. Anticholinergic effects of antipsychotic medication can cause constipation and urinary hesitancy or retention.

Activity and Exercise. The patient's daily methods and levels of activity and exercise must be queried and documented. Activities are important interventions, and baseline information is needed to determine what

the patient already enjoys or dislikes and to determine whether he or she is getting sufficient exercise or adequate recreation. A patient may respond to medication or therapies with a change in activity or exercise. Also, many psychiatric medications cause weight gain, and nurses need to develop interventions that increase activities to counteract the weight gain.

Sleep. Often, changes in sleep patterns reflect changes in a patient's emotions and are symptoms of disorders. If the patient responds positively to a question about changes in sleep patterns, it is important to clarify just what those changes are. For example, "difficulty falling asleep" means different things to different people. For the person who usually falls right to sleep, it could mean that it takes 10 extra minutes to fall asleep. For the person who normally takes 35 minutes to fall asleep, it could mean that it takes 1½ hours to do so.

Appetite and Nutrition. Questions that ascertain changes in the patient's appetite and nutritional intake can uncover how a patient's everyday patterns are changing as mentation changes. For example, a patient who is depressed may not notice hunger or even that he or she does not have the energy to prepare food. Others may handle stressful emotions through eating more than usual. This information also provides valuable clues to possible eating disorders and problems with body image.

Hydration. Gaining perspective on how much fluid patients normally drink and how much they are drinking now provides important data. Some medications can cause retention of fluids, and others can cause diuresis; thus, the patient's current fluid status must be understood.

Sexuality. Questioning a patient on issues involving sexuality requires comfort with one's own sexuality. Changes in sexual activity as well as comfort with sexual orientation are important to assess. Issues involving sexual orientation that are unsettled in a patient or between a patient and family member may cause anxiety, shame, or discomfort. It is necessary to explore how comfortable the patient is with his or her sexuality and sexual functioning. These questions should be asked in a matter-of-fact, but gentle and nonjudgmental, manner. Initiating the topic of sexuality may begin with a question such as "Are you sexually active?"

Self-Care. Often, a patient's ability to care for self or carry out activities of daily living, such as washing and dressing, are indicative of his or her psychological state. For example, a depressed patient may not have the energy to iron a shirt before putting it on. This information may also help the nurse to determine actual or potential obstacles to a patient's compliance with a treatment plan.

(*text continues on page 206*)

TABLE 10.1 Selected Hematologic Measures and Their Relevance to Psychiatric Disorders

Test	Possible Results	Possible Cause or Meaning
Complete Blood Count (CBC)		
Leukocyte count (WBC)	Leukopenia—decrease in leukocytes (white blood cells) Agranulocytosis—decrease in number of granulocytic leukocytes	May be produced by: Phenothiazines Clozapine Carbamazepine
	Leukocytosis—increase in leukocyte count above normal limits	Lithium causes a benign mild-to-moderate increase (11,000–17,000/µL). Neuroleptic malignant syndrome (NMS) can be associated with increases of 15,000 to 30,000/mm³ in about 40% of cases.
WBC differential	"Shift to the left"—from segmented neutrophils to band forms	Shift often suggests a bacterial infection, but has been reported in about 40% of cases of NMS.
Red blood cell count (RBC)	Polycythemia-increased RBCs	Primary form—true polycythemia caused by several disease states Secondary form—compensation for decreased oxygenation, such as in chronic pulmonary disease Blood is more viscous, and the patient should not become dehydrated.
	Decreased RBCs	Decrease may be related to some types of anemia, which requires further evaluation.
Hematocrit (Hct)	Elevations	Elevation may be due to dehydration.
	Decreased Hct	Anemia may be associated with a wide range of mental status changes, including asthenia, depression, and psychosis. 20% of women of childbearing age in the United States have iron-deficiency anemia.
Hemoglobin (Hb)	Decreased	Another indicator of anemia, further evaluation of source requires review of erythrocyte indices.
Erythrocyte indices, such as red cell distribution width (RDW)	Elevated RDW	Finding suggests a combined anemia as in that from chronic alcoholism, resulting from both vitamin B_{12} and folate acid deficiencies and iron deficiency. Oral contraceptives also decrease vitamin B_{12}.
Other Hematologic Measures		
Vitamin B_{12}	Deficiency	Neuropsychiatric symptoms such as psychosis, paranoia, fatigue, agitation, marked personality change, dementia, and delirium may develop.
Folate	Deficiency	The use of alcohol, phenytoin, oral contraceptives, and estrogens, may be responsible.
Platelet count	Thrombocytopenia—decreased platelet count	Some psychiatric medications, such as carbamazepine, phenothiazines, or clozapine, or other non-psychiatric medications, may cause thrombocytopenia. Several medical conditions are other causes.
Serum Electrolytes		
Sodium	Hyponatremia—low serum sodium	Significant mental status changes may ensue. Condition is associated with Addison's disease, the syndrome of inappropriate secretion of antidiuretic hormone (SIADH), and polydipsia (water intoxication) as well as carbamazepine use.

TABLE 10.1 Selected Hematologic Measures and Their Relevance to Psychiatric Disorders (Continued)

Test	Possible Results	Possible Cause or Meaning
Potassium	Hypokalemia—low serum potassium	Produces weakness, fatigue, electrocardiogram (ECG) changes; paralytic ileus and muscle paresis may develop. Common in individuals with bulimic behavior or psychogenic vomiting and use or abuse of diuretics; laxative abuse may contribute; can be life-threatening.
Chloride	Elevation	Chloride tends to increase to compensate for lower bicarbonate.
	Decrease	Binging–purging behavior and repeated vomiting may be causes.
Bicarbonate	Elevation	Causes may be during binging and purging in eating disorders, excessive use of laxatives, or psychogenic vomiting.
	Decrease	Decrease may develop in some patients with hyperventilation syndrome and panic disorder.
Renal Function Tests		
Blood urea nitrogen (BUN)	Elevation	Increase is associated with mental status changes, lethargy, and delirium. Cause may be dehydration. Potential toxicity of medications cleared via the kidney, such as lithium and amantadine, may increase.
Serum creatinine	Elevation	Level usually does not become elevated until about 50% of nephrons in the kidney are damaged.
Serum Enzymes		
Amylase	Elevation	Level appears to increase after binging and purging behavior in eating disorders and declines when these behaviors stop.
Alanine aminotransferase (ALT)—formerly serum glutamic pyruvic transaminase (SGPT)	ALT > AST	Disparity is common in acute forms of viral and drug-induced hepatic dysfunction.
Aspartate aminotransferase (AST)—formerly serum glutamic oxaloacetic transaminase (SGOT)	Elevation AST > ALT	Mild elevations are common with use of sodium valproate. Severe elevations in chronic forms of liver disease and postmyocardial infarction may develop.
Creatine phosphokinase (CPK)	Elevations of the isoenzyme related to muscle tissue	Muscle tissue injury is the cause. Level is elevated in neuroleptic malignant syndrome (NMS). Level is also elevated by repeated intramuscular injections (eg, antipsychotics).
Thyroid Function		
Serum triiodothyronine (T₃)	Decrease	Hypothyroidism and nonthyroid illness cause decrease. Individuals with depression may convert less T_4 to T_3 peripherally, but not out of the normal range. Medications such as lithium and sodium valproate may suppress thyroid function, but clinical significance is unknown.
	Elevations	Hyperthyroidism, T_3 toxicosis, may produce mood changes, anxiety, and symptoms of mania.
Serum thyroxine (T₄)	Elevations	Hyperthyroidism is a cause.
Thyroid stimulating hormone (TSH)—called *thyrotropin*	Elevations	Hypothyroidism—symptoms may appear very much like depression, except for additional physical signs of cold intolerance, dry skin, hair loss, bradycardia, etc. Lithium—may also cause elevations.
	Decrease	Considered nondiagnostic—may be hyperthyroidism, pituitary hypothyroidism, or even euthyroid status.

Pharmacologic Assessment

If the patient is to receive psychopharmacologic treatment, the review of systems will serve as a baseline by which the nurse may judge whether the medication exacerbates symptoms or causes new ones to develop. It is important to determine the current and past medications that the patient is taking. This includes over-the-counter (OTC) or nonprescription medications as well as those prescribed. This assessment is important for reasons other than serving as a baseline. It helps target possible drug interactions, determine whether the patient has already used medications that are being considered, and identify if medications may be causing psychiatric symptoms.

Psychological Domain

Assessment of the psychological domain is the traditional focus of the psychiatric nursing assessment. By definition, psychiatric disorders are manifested through psychological symptoms related to mental status, moods, thoughts, behaviors, and interpersonal relationships. This domain also includes data related to psychological growth and development. Assessing this domain is important in developing a comprehensive picture of the patient.

Responses to Mental Health Problems

Individual concerns regarding the mental health problem or its consequences are included in the mental health assessment. A mental disorder, like any other illness, affects patients and families in many different ways. It is safe to say that a mental illness changes a person's life, and the nurse should identify what the changes are and their meaning to the patient and family members. Many patients develop specific fears such as losing their job, family, or safety. Included in this part of the assessment is identification of current strategies or behaviors in dealing with the disorder. A simple question such as "How do you deal with your voices when you are with other people?" may initiate a discussion about responses to the mental disorder or emotional problem.

Mental Status Examination

The mental status examination involves an organized, systematic approach to the assessment of an individual's current psychiatric condition. It is the basic means of evaluation used by all mental health disciplines. The mental status examination establishes a baseline, provides a snapshot of where the patient is at a particular moment, and creates a written record. It provides information about whether the patient is a reliable historian and sows the beginning seeds of the nurse–patient relationship. Of great importance for the nurse is to

withhold judgment and to allow the patient to explain. The mental status examination may be lengthy and thorough, as in an initial evaluation, or conducted in a shorter form to monitor changes in symptoms. In each case, the primary areas for evaluation remain the same. Unlike a physical examination, in which the nurse asks a systematic series of questions, the nurse draws conclusions throughout the mental health examination as he or she observes and communicates with the patient. General areas of discussion in the mental health examination include general observations, orientation, mood and affect, speech, thought processes, and cognition.

KEY CONCEPT   Mental status examination. The **mental status examination** is an organized systematic approach to assessment of an individual's current psychiatric condition.

General Observations.   At the beginning of the interview, the nurse should record his or her initial impressions of the patient. These general observations include the patient's appearance, affect, psychomotor activity, and overall behavior. How is the patient dressed? Is the dress appropriate for weather and setting? What is the patient's affect? What behaviors is the patient displaying? For example, the same nurse assessed two male patients with depression. At the beginning of the mental status examination, the differences between these two men were very clear. The nurse described the first patient as "a large, well-dressed man who is agitated and appears angry, shifts in his seat, and does not maintain eye contact. He interrupts often in the initial explanation of mental status." The nurse described the other patient as a "small, unshaven, disheveled man with a strong body odor who appears withdrawn. He shuffles as he walks, speaks very softly, appears sad, and avoids direct eye contact."

Orientation.   The nurse can determine the patient's orientation to date, day, time, place, and person by asking the date, time, and current location of the interview setting. If a patient knows the year, but not the exact date, the interviewer can ask the season. A person's orientation tells the nurse the extent of confusion. If a patient does not know the year or the place of the interview, he or she is exhibiting considerable confusion.

Mood and Affect.   **Mood** refers to the prominent, sustained, overall emotions that the person expresses and exhibits. Mood may be sustained for days or weeks, or it may fluctuate during the course of a day. For example, some patients with depression have a diurnal variation in their mood. They experience their lowest mood in the morning, but as the day progresses, their depressed mood lifts and they feel somewhat better in the evening. Terms used to describe mood include **euthymic** (normal), **euphoric** (elated), and **dysphoric** (depressed, disquieted, restless).

Affect refers to the person's capacity to vary emotional expression. Affect fluctuates with thought content. During the assessment, the patient's affect may change as he or she talks about life, expressing happiness concerning some events and sadness about others. The patient may exhibit anger, frustration, irritation, apathy, helplessness, and so on while his or her overall mood remains unchanged. Affect can often be observed in facial expressions, vocal fluctuations, and gestures.

Affect can be described in terms of range, intensity, appropriateness, and stability. Range can be described as full or restricted. An individual who expresses several different emotions consistent with the stated feelings and content being expressed is described as having a full range of affect that is congruent with the situation. An individual who expresses few emotions has a constricted affect. For example, a patient could be describing the recent, tragic death of a loved one in a monotone with little expression. In determining whether this response is normal, the nurse should compare the patient's emotional response with the cultural norm for that particular response. Intensity can be increased, flat, or blunted. For example, a patient may show an extreme reaction to the death of a public figure, as if the celebrity were a personal friend. One patient said that his life stopped when Princess Diana died. He could not eat or sleep for weeks afterward. Stability can be described as mobile (normal) or labile. If a patient reports being happy one minute and reduced to tears the next, the person probably has an unstable mood. During the interview, the nurse should look for rapid mood changes that indicate lability of mood. A patient who exhibits intense, frequently shifting emotional extremes has a labile affect.

Speech. Observation of speech may provide the nurse with clues about the patient's thoughts, emotional patterns, and cognitive organization. The speech may be pressured, fast, slow, or fragmented. Speech patterns may connect to the thought patterns the patient is experiencing. To check the patient's comprehension, the nurse can ask the patient to name objects. During conversation, the nurse assesses the fluency and quality of the patient's speech. The nurse listens for repetition or rhyming of words.

Thought Processes. Patients with mental health problems may exhibit many different difficulties with thought processes. The nurse assesses the patient for rapid movement of ideas; inability or taking a long time to get to the point; loose or no connections among ideas or words; rhyming or repetition of words, questions, or phrases; or use of unheard of words. Any of these observations indicates abnormal thought patterns. The content spoken is also important. What thought is the patient expressing? The nurse listens for unreal stories and fears; for example, "The FBI is tracking me." He or she also listens for phobias, obsessions, and suicidal or homicidal thoughts.

Cognition and Intellectual Performance. To assess the patient's **cognition,** that is, the ability to think and know, the nurse asks the patient to remember, calculate, and reason abstractly. The Mini-Mental State Examination (MMSE) is a helpful, frequently used tool (Text Box 10-5).

Attention and Concentration. To test attention and concentration, the nurse asks the patient, without pencil or paper, to start with 100 and subtract 7 until reaching 65 or to start with 20 and subtract 3. The nurse must decide which is most appropriate for the patient considering education and understanding. Subtracting 3s from 20 is the easier of the two tasks.

Abstract Reasoning and Comprehension. To test abstract reasoning and comprehension, the nurse gives the patient a proverb to interpret. Examples include "People in glass houses shouldn't throw stones," "A rolling stone gathers no moss," and "A penny saved is a penny earned."

Memory: Recall, Short-Term, Recent, and Remote. There are four spheres of memory to check: recall, or immediate, memory; short-term memory; recent memory; and long-term, or remote, memory. To check immediate and short-term memory, the nurse gives the patient three unrelated words to remember and asks him or her to recite them right after telling them, and at 5-minute and 15-minute intervals during the interview. To test recent memory, the nurse may question about a holiday or world event within the past few months. The nurse tests long-term or remote memory by asking about events years ago. If they are personal events and the answers seem incorrect, the nurse may check them with a family member.

Insight and Judgment. Insight and judgment are related concepts that involve the ability to examine thoughts, conceptualize facts, solve problems, think abstractly, and possess self-awareness. **Insight** is a person's awareness of his or her own thoughts and feelings and ability to compare them with the thoughts and feelings of others. It involves an awareness of how others view one's behavior and its meaning. For example, many patients do not believe that they have mental illness. They may have delusions and hallucinations or be hospitalized for bizarre and sometimes dangerous behavior, but they are completely unaware that their behavior is unusual or abnormal. During an interview, a patient may adamantly proclaim that nothing is wrong or that he or she does not have a mental illness.

Judgment is the ability to reach a logical decision about a situation and to choose a course of action after

TEXT BOX 10.5

Mini-Mental State Examination

Orientation
(Score 1 point for correct response)
1. What is the year?
2. What is the season?
3. What is the date?
4. What is the day of the week?
5. What is the month?
6. Where are we? building or hospital?
7. Where are we? floor?
8. Where are we? town or city?
9. Where are we? county?
10. Where are we? state?

Registration
(Score 1 point for each object identified correctly, maximum is 3 points)
11. Name three objects at about one each second. Ask the patient to repeat them. If the patient misses an object, repeat them until all three are learned.

Attention and Calculation
(Score 1 point for each correct answer up to maximum of 5 points)
12. Subtract 7s from 100 until 65 (or, as an alternative, spell "world" backward).

Recall
(Score 1 point for each correct answer, maximum of 3)
13. Ask for names of three objects learned in question 11.

Language
14. Point to a pencil and a watch. Ask the patient to name each object. Score 1 point for each correct answer, maximum of 2 points.

15. Have the patient repeat "No ifs, ands, or buts." Score one point if correct.

16. Have the patient follow a three-stage command: "(1) Take the paper in your right hand. (2) Fold the paper in half. (3) Put the paper on the floor." Score 1 point for each command done correctly, maximum of 3 points.

17. Write the following in large letters: "CLOSE YOUR EYES." Ask the patient to read the command and perform the task. Score 1 point if correct.

18. Ask the patient to write a sentence of his or her own choice. Score 1 point if the sentence has a subject, an object, and a verb.

19. Draw the design printed below. Ask the patient to copy the design. Score 1 point if all sides and angles are preserved and if the intersecting sides form a quadrangle.

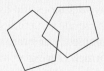

From Folstein, M. F., Folstein, S. E., & McHugh, P. R. Mini-mental state: A practical method for grading the cognitive state of patients for the clinician. *Journal of Psychiatric Research, 12*(189), 1975. Used with permission.

examining and analyzing various possibilities. Throughout the interview, the nurse evaluates the patient's ability to make logical decisions. For example, some patients may continually choose partners who are abusive. The nurse could logically conclude that these patients have poor judgment in selecting partners. Another way to examine a patient's judgment is to give a simple scenario and ask the person to identify the best response. An example of such a scenario is "What would you do if you found a bag of money outside a bank on a busy street?" If the patient responds, "Run with it," his or her judgment is questionable.

Behavior

Throughout the assessment, the nurse observes any behavior that may have significance in understanding the patient's response or symptoms of the mental disorder or emotional problem. For example, a depressed patient may be tearful throughout the session, whereas an anxious patient may twist or pull hair, shift in the chair, or be unable to maintain eye contact. The nurse needs to connect the behavior with the assessment topic. The nurse may find that whenever a particular topic is addressed, the patient's behavior changes. Throughout the assessment, the nurse attempts to identify patterned behaviors to significant events. For example, a patient may change jobs frequently, causing family distress and financial problems. Exploration of the events leading up to job changes may elicit important data regarding the patient's ability to solve problems.

Self-Concept

Self-concept, which develops over a lifetime, represents the total beliefs about three interrelated dimensions of the self: body image, self-esteem, and personal identity. The importance of each of the three dimensions of self-concept varies among individuals. For some, beliefs about themselves are strongly tied to body image; for others, personal identity is most important. Still others develop personal identity from what others have told them over the years. The nurse carrying out an assessment must keep in mind that self-concept and its components are dynamic and variable. For example, a woman may have a consistent self-concept until her first pregnancy. At that time, the many physiologic changes of pregnancy may cause her body image to change. She may be comfortable and enjoy the "glow of pregnancy," or she may feel like a "bloated cow." Suddenly, her body image is the most important part of her self-concept, and how she handles it can increase or decrease her self-esteem or sense of personal identity. Thus, all the components are tied together, and each one affects the others.

Even though self-concept evolves as a dynamic segment of the personality, changing early, ingrained impressions of self is difficult. Because children base their self-concepts on how significant adults view them, verbally or physically abused children are likely to develop poor self-concepts. These early experiences are so powerful that later positive messages from others will not easily alter the entrenched poor self-concept.

Nurses may use various approaches to assess a patient's self-concept, depending on the patient's sex, age, and development; the reason the patient is seeking mental health care; and the purpose of the assessment (ie, screening, comprehensive, ongoing). The assessment criteria also depend on (1) the nurse's own self-concept and (2) how the data will be used (clinical practice or research). The generalist psychiatric nurse usually gathers data through a direct interview or simple questionnaire to plan and implement interventions and then uses these data as a baseline in determining any changes during treatment. The same nurse will find standardized instruments such as the Tennessee Self-Concept scale used in the nursing research literature. The self-concept research instruments are generally too cumbersome to use in a clinical assessment; however, the nurse can use the findings reported in the literature to understand the concept.

Nurses can assess self-concept through understanding and eliciting patients' cognition or patterns of thinking about themselves and their ability to navigate in the world. A patient's self-concept becomes evident during other parts of the assessment. Physical appearance that is disheveled, sloppy, and outside cultural norms is an indication of poor self-concept. Certain statements, such as "I could never do that," "I have no control over my life," and "I'm so stupid" are typical self-diminishing statements. During a comprehensive assessment, the nurse should explore the patient's negative self-statements to understand the patient's underlying self-concept. Moreover, the nurse must be aware of his or her own self-concept and its influence on the patient during the assessment because it can shape the nurse's view of the patient. For example, a nurse who is self-confident and feels inwardly scornful of a patient who lacks such confidence may intimidate the patient through unconscious behaviors or inconsiderate comments.

A useful approach to measuring self-concept for an ongoing assessment is asking the patient to draw a self-portrait. For many patients, drawing is much easier than writing and serves as an excellent technique to monitor changes over time. Interpretation of self-concept from drawings focuses on size, color, level of detail, pressure, line quality, symmetry, and placement. Low self-esteem is expressed by small size, lack of color variation, and sparse details. Powerlessness and feelings of inadequacy are expressed through lack of head, mouth, arms, feet, or eyes. A lack of symmetry (placement of figure parts or

entire drawings off-center) represents feelings of insecurity and inadequacy. As self-esteem builds, size increases, color tends to become more varied and brighter, and more detail appears. Figure 10-2 shows a self-portrait of a patient at the beginning of treatment for depression and another done 3 months later.

Three nursing diagnoses are generated from self-concept assessment:

- Body Image Disturbance
- Self-Esteem Disturbance (Chronic and Low)
- Personal Identity Disturbance

Body Image. **Body image** represents a person's beliefs and attitudes about his or her body and includes such dimensions as size (large or small) and attractiveness (pretty or ugly). People who are satisfied with their body have a more positive body image than those who do not. Body image is more important to some people than it is to others. The patient's sex is a consideration when assessing body image. Generally, women attach more importance to their body image than men and may even define themselves in terms of their body. In psychiatric settings, a patient's delusion or hallucination may represent a body image disturbance.

Patients express body image beliefs through statements about their bodies. Such statements as "I feel so ugly," "I'm so fat," and "No one will want to have sex with me" express negative body images. Nonverbal

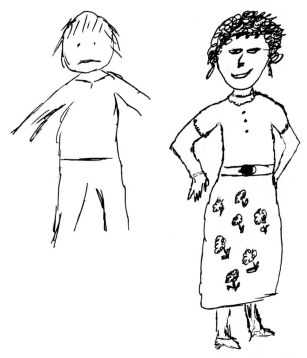

Figure 10.2 *Left:* Self-portrait of a 52-year-old woman at first group session following discharge from hospital for treatment of depression. *Right:* Self-portrait after 3 months of weekly group interventions.

behavior that indicates problems with body image includes avoiding looking at or touching a body part, hiding the body in oversized clothing, or bandaging a particular sensitive area such as a mole on the face. Cultural differences must be considered when evaluating behavior related to body image. For example, some cultures have the expectation for women and girls to keep their bodies completely covered and to wear loose-fitting garments.

Body image is especially important in patients with eating and somatoform disorders. For example, patients with eating disorders are convinced that they are overweight when they are actually emaciated. Patients with somatoform disorders may believe a body part is missing even though evidence does not support the belief. See Chapters 23 and 25 for more information.

Self-Esteem. **Self-esteem** is the person's attitude about the self. Self-esteem differs from body image. It means satisfaction with one's overall self. People who feel good about themselves are more likely to have the confidence to try new health behaviors. They are also less likely to be depressed. Negative self-esteem statements include, "I'm a worthless person" and "I never do anything right." Self-esteem is important in patients who are depressed (see Chap. 20).

Personal Identity. **Personal identity** is knowing "who I am" and is formed through meeting the numerous biologic, psychological, and social challenges and demands throughout the stages of life. Every life experience and interaction contributes to knowing oneself better. Personal identity allows people to establish boundaries and understand personal strengths and limitations. In some psychiatric disorders, individuals cannot separate themselves from others, which shows that their personal identity is not strongly developed. A problem with personal identity is difficult to assess. Statements such as, "I'm just like my mother and she was always in trouble," "I become whatever my current boyfriend wants me to be," and "I can't make a decision unless I check it out first" are all statements that require further exploration into how the person views oneself. Assessment of personal identity is important in patients with personality disorders (see Chap. 22).

Stress and Coping Patterns

Everyone has stress (see Chap. 35). Sometimes, the experience of stress contributes to the development of mental disorders. Identification of major stresses in a patient's life helps the nurse to understand the person as well as to support the use of successful coping behaviors in the future. The nurse should explore with the patient past stresses and coping mechanisms (see Chap. 6). During this aspect of assessment, the nurse

uncovers coping mechanisms that are helpful and can encourage their use. He or she also ascertains coping mechanisms that are not useful, such as use of drugs or alcohol. From this information, the nurse can begin to plan what appropriate coping mechanisms the patient can learn. In addition to the patient's personal behavior patterns, use of family and community resources adds more information.

Risk Assessment

Risk factors are those characteristics, conditions, situations, or events that increase the patient's vulnerability to threats to safety or well-being. Risk factors may be thought of in several ways. Throughout this text, the sections concerning risk factors focus on (1) risks to the patient's safety, (2) risks for developing psychiatric disorders, and (3) risks for increasing, or exacerbating, symptoms and impairment in an individual who already has a psychiatric disorder.

The assessment of risk factors involving patient safety must occur within the first minutes to first hour of the initial assessment as well as ongoing assessments. Examples of these risks include the risk for suicide and violence toward others or the risk for events such as falling, seizures, allergic reactions, or elopement. Nurses must assess some of these risk factors on a priority basis. For example, they must assess the patient's risk for violence or suicide and take measures to prevent injury, such as implementing environmental constraints, before addressing other assessment factors.

Suicidal Ideation. During the assessment, the nurse needs to listen closely to whether the patient describes or mentions thinking about any harm to self. If the patient does not openly express ideas of self-harm, it is necessary to ask in a straightforward and gentle manner, "Have you ever thought about injuring or killing yourself?" If the patient answers, "Yes, I am thinking about it right now," the nurse knows not to leave the patient unobserved and to institute suicide precautions as indicated by the facility protocols. Questions to ask to ascertain suicidal ideation are as follows:

- Have you ever tried to harm or kill yourself?
- Do you have thoughts of suicide at this time? If yes, do you have a plan? If yes, can you tell me the details of the plan?
- Do you have the means to carry out this plan? (If the plan requires a weapon, does the patient have it available?)
- Have you made preparations for your death (eg, writing a note to loved ones, putting finances in order, giving away possessions)?
- Has a significant episode in your life caused you to think this way (eg, recent loss of spouse or job)?

Assaultive or Homicidal Ideation. When assessing a patient, the nurse also needs to listen carefully to any delusions or hallucinations that the patient shares. If the patient gives any indication that he or she must or is being told to harm someone, the nurse must first think of self-safety and institute assaultive precautions as indicated by the facility protocols. Questions to ask to ascertain assaultive or homicidal ideation are as follows:

- Do you intend to harm someone? If yes, who?
- Do you have a plan? If yes, what are the details of the plan?
- Do you have the means to carry out the plan? (If the plan requires a weapon, is it readily available?)

Social Domain

The assessment continues with examination of the patient's social dimensions. During this phase, the nurse inquires about interactions with others in the family and community; the patient's parents and their marital relationship; the patient's place in birth order; names and ages of any siblings; and relationships with spouse, siblings, and children. The nurse also assesses work and education history and community activities. The nurse observes how the patient relates to any family or friends who may be in attendance. This component of the assessment helps the nurse anticipate how the patient may get along with other patients in an inpatient setting. It also allows the nurse to plan for any anticipated difficulties.

Functional Status

Assessment is necessary to understand how the patient functions in a social setting, whether with family or in the community. How the patient copes with strangers and those with whom he or she does not get along is important information. Many nurses use the Global Assessment of Functioning (GAF) scale (discussed in Chap. 3) as a single measure of functioning.

Social Systems

A significant component of the patient's life involves the social systems in which he or she may be enmeshed. The social systems to examine include the family, the culture to which the patient belongs, and the community in which he or she lives.

Family Assessment. How the patient fits in with and relates to his or her family is important to know. See Chapter 16 for discussion of a comprehensive family assessment. General questions to ask include the following:

- Whom do you consider family?
- How important to you is your family?

- How does your family make decisions?
- What are the roles in your family and who fills them?
- Where do you fit in your family?
- With whom in your family do you get along best?
- With whom in your family do you have the most conflict?
- Who in your family is supportive of you?

Cultural Assessment. Culture can profoundly affect a patient's world view. Culture helps a person frame beliefs about life, death, health and illness, and roles and relationships. During cultural assessment, the nurse must consider factors that influence the manifestations of the current mental disorder. For example, a patient mentions "speaking in tongues." The nurse may identify this experience as a hallucination when, in fact, the patient was having a religious experience common within some branches of Christianity. In this instance, knowing and understanding such religious practices will prevent a misinterpretation of the symptoms.

If the patient can respond, the nurse should ask the following questions:

- To what cultural group do you belong?
- Were you raised in an ethnic community?
- How do you define health?
- How do you define illness?
- How do you define good and evil?
- What do you do to get better when you are physically ill? Mentally ill?
- Whom do you see for help when you are physically ill? Mentally ill?
- By what cultural rules or taboos do you try to live?
- Do you eat special foods?

Community Support and Resources. Many patients are connected to community resources, and the nurse needs to assess what they are and the patterns of usage. For example, a homeless patient may know of a church where he or she can sleep but may go there only on cold nights. Or a patient may go to the community center daily for lunch to be with other people.

Spiritual Assessment

Spirituality is defined as "the unifying force of a person; the essence of being that shapes, gives meaning to, and is aware of one's self-becoming. Spirituality permeates all of life and is manifested in one's being, knowing, and doing. It is expressed and experienced uniquely by each individual through and within connection to God, Life Force, the Absolute, the environment, nature, other people, and the self" (Burkhardt & Jacobson, 1997, p. 42). Nurses must be clear about their own spirituality to ensure it does not interfere with assessment of the patient's spirituality. Questions to ask include the following:

- What gives your life meaning?
- What is the purpose of your life?
- What do you do to bring joy into your life?
- What life goals have you set for yourself?
- Do you think that stress in any way has caused your illness?
- Can you forgive others?
- Can you forgive yourself?
- Is your faith helpful to you in stressful situations?
- Is worship important to you?
- Do you participate in any religious activities?
- Do any religious beliefs control your life?
- Do you believe in God or a higher power?
- Do you pray?
- Do you meditate?
- Do you feel connected with the world?

Occupational Status

The nurse should document the occupation the patient is now in as well as a history of jobs. If the patient has changed jobs frequently, the nurse should ask about the reasons. Perhaps the patient has faced such problems as an inability to focus on the job at hand or to get along with others. If so, such issues require further exploration.

Economic Status

Finances are private for many people; thus, the nurse must ask questions about economic status carefully. What the nurse needs to ascertain is not specific dollar amounts, but whether the patient feels stressed by finances and has enough for basic needs.

Legal Status

Because of laws governing mentally ill people, ascertaining the patient's correct age, marital status, and any legal guardianships is important. The nurse may need to check the patient's medical records for this information.

Quality of Life

The patient's perspective on quality of life means how the patient rates his or her life. Does a patient feel his life is poor because he cannot purchase everything he wants? Does another patient feel blessed because the sun is out today? Listening carefully to the patient's discussion of his or her life and how he or she measures the quality of that life provides important information about self-concept, coping skills, wants, and dreams.

Summary of Key Points

- ➤ Assessment is the deliberate and systematic collection of biopsychosocial information or data to determine current and past health and functional status and to evaluate present and past coping patterns.
- ➤ There are different types of assessments. A comprehensive assessment is the collection of all relevant data to identify problems for which a nursing diagnosis is stated. A screening assessment is the collection of data to identify individuals who have not yet recognized the symptoms caused by a psychiatric disorder, who have risk factors for the development of a psychiatric disorder, or who may be experiencing emotional difficulties but have not yet formally sought treatment. Ongoing assessments monitor the progress and outcomes of the interventions implemented.
- ➤ Techniques of data collection include patient observations, patient and family interviews, physical and mental examinations, records and diagnostic reports, and collaboration with colleagues.
- ➤ The biologic assessment includes present and past health status, physical examination with review of body systems, review of physical functions, and pharmacologic assessment.
- ➤ The psychological assessment includes the mental status examination, behavioral responses, and risk factor assessment.
- ➤ The mental status examination includes general observation of appearance, psychomotor activity, and attitude; orientations; mood; affect; emotions; speech; and thought processes.
- ➤ Behavioral responses are assessed, as are self-concept and present and past coping patterns.
- ➤ Risk factor assessment includes ascertaining whether the patient has any suicidal, assaultive, or homicidal ideation.
- ➤ The social assessment includes functional status; social systems; spirituality; occupational, economic, and legal status; and quality of life.

Critical Thinking Challenges

1. A 23-year-old white woman is admitted to an acute psychiatric setting for depression and suicidal gestures. This admission is her first, but she has suffered from bouts of depression since early adolescence. She and her fiancé have just broken their engagement and moved into separate apartments. She has not yet told anyone that she is pregnant. She said that her mother had told her that she was "living in sin" and that she would "pay for it." The patient wants to "end it all!"

From this scenario, develop three assessment questions for each domain: biologic, psychological, and social.

2. Identify normal laboratory values for sodium, blood urea nitrogen (BUN), liver enzymes, leukocyte count and differential, and thyroid functioning. Why are these values important to know?

3. Write a paragraph on your self-concept, including all three components: body image, self-esteem, and personal identity. Explore the type of patient situations in which your self-concept can help your interactions with patients. Explore the types of patient situations in which your self-concept can hinder your interactions with patients.

4. Complete an assessment for an assigned patient, and discuss the findings with your clinical instructor.

WEB LINKS

www.cybernurse.com/books/nursingassessment. html   This bookstore website contains books on nursing assessment and diagnosis.

www.who.int/msa/mnh/ems.primacre/edukit A World Health Organization website that contains checklists useful in primary care and could be useful in screening for specific symptoms.

www.pharmacy.unc.edu/xpharmd/phpr177/ carson/msel.htm   This site contains an online mental status examination, with the classic parts of the history and physical examination used to evaluate patients for general medical conditions.

REFERENCES

American Nurses Association, American Psychiatric Association, & International Society of Psychiatric–Mental Health Nurses. (2000). *Scope and standards of psychiatric–mental health nursing practice.* Washington, DC: American Nurses Publishing.

American Psychiatric Association. (2000). *Diagnostic and statistical manual of mental disorders* (Text revision). Washington, DC: Author.

Burkhardt, M. A., & Jacobson, M. N. (1997). In B. M. Dossey (Ed.), *Core curriculum for holistic nursing.* Gaithersburg, MD: Aspen.

Carpenito, L. (2000). *Nursing diagnosis: Application to clinical practice* (8th ed.). Philadelphia: Lippincott Williams & Wilkins.

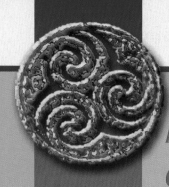

Mental Health Assessment of Children and Adolescents

Vanya Hamrin, Catherine Gray Deering, and Lawrence Scahill

ASSESSMENT PROCESS FOR CHILDREN AND ADOLESCENTS
DATA COLLECTION THROUGH THE CLINICAL INTERVIEW
Treatment Alliance
Child and Parent Observation
Interviewing Techniques
 Discussion With the Child
 Discussion With the Parents
Building Rapport
 Preschool-Aged Children
 School-Aged Children
 Adolescents

BIOPSYCHOSOCIAL PSYCHIATRIC NURSING ASSESSMENT OF CHILDREN AND ADOLESCENTS
Biologic Domain
 Genetic Vulnerability
 Neurologic Examination
Psychological Domain
 Mental Status Examination
 Developmental Assessment
 Attachment
 Temperament and Behavior
 Self-Concept
 Risk Assessment

Social Domain
 Family Relationship
 School and Peer Adjustment
 Community
 Functional Status
 Stresses and Coping Behaviors

LEARNING OBJECTIVES

After studying this chapter, you will be able to:

➤ Define the assessment process for children and adolescents.

➤ Discuss techniques of data collection used with children and adolescents.

➤ Discuss the synthesis of biopsychosocial assessment data for children and adolescents.

➤ Delineate important biopsychosocial areas of assessment for children and adolescents.

214

assortative mating
attachment
attachment disorganization
developmental delays
egocentrism

maturation
temperament (easy,
    difficulty, slow-to-
    warm-up)

ASSESSMENT PROCESS FOR CHILDREN AND ADOLESCENTS

The assessment of children and adolescents is a specialized process that considers their unique problems and responses within the context of their development. The *Standards of Psychiatric-Mental Health Nursing of Children and Adolescents* serves as a guide for this process (American Nurses Association, 2000). The assessment of children and adolescents generally follows the same format as for adults (see Chap. 10), but there are significant differences. Children think in more concrete terms; hence, nurses need to ask more specific and fewer open-ended questions than they would typically ask adults. Nurses should use simple phrasing because children have a narrower vocabulary than adults. Examples include saying "sad" instead of "depressed," or "nervous" instead of "anxious." Nurses need to corroborate information that children offer with more sources (eg, parents, teachers) than they would for adults. Nurses may want to use artistic and play media (eg, puppets, family drawings) to engage children and evaluate their perceptions, inner worlds, fine motor skills, and intellectual functions. Children have a less specific sense of time and a less developed memory than adults. When children are asked about a sequence of events or specific times when events occurred, they may not be able to provide accurate information.

A comprehensive evaluation includes a biopsychosocial history; mental status examination; additional testing (eg, cognitive or neuropsychological), if necessary; records of the child's school performance and medical-physical history; and information from other agencies that may be providing services (eg, department of child and family services [DCF], juvenile court). Nurses may use various assessment tools, including the Child Attention Profile (CAP) and the Devereux Childhood Assessment (DECA).

DATA COLLECTION THROUGH THE CLINICAL INTERVIEW

The clinical interview is the primary assessment tool used in child and adolescent psychiatry. A unique set of skills is necessary for interviewing children and adolescents. How nurses obtain mental health information depends on the developmental level of each child, specifically considering the child's language, cognitive, social, and emotional skills. For example, the nurse should simplify questions for young children or children with developmental delays (eg, mental retardation, Asperger's syndrome pervasive developmental disorder) so that these children can understand and respond appropriately.

The assessment interview may be the initial contact between the child and parent or guardian and the nurse. The first step is to establish a treatment alliance, and the second is to begin assessing the interactions between the child and parent.

Treatment Alliance

The nurse can establish rapport by greeting the child or adolescent in a friendly, polite, open manner and putting him or her at ease. Speaking clearly and at a normal volume and using friendly, reassuring tones are essential measures. The nurse can establish a treatment alliance by recognizing the child's individuality and showing respect and concern for that child. The nurse should demonstrate sensitivity, objectivity, and confidentiality. The child will be more forthcoming if he or she feels that the nurse is listening carefully and is interested in what he or she has to say.

Child and Parent Observation

Because the child's primary environment is with the parent, child–parent interactions provide important data about the child–parent attachment and parenting practices. The nurse's observations focus on both the child *alone* and the child *within* the family. Nurses can actually make such observations while the family is in the waiting area. Nurses should observe the following:

- How the child and parent talk to each other, including how frequently each initiates conversation
- How the parent disciplines the child
- How attached the parent and child appear
- How the child and parent separate
- If the parent and child play together
- How the child gets the parent's attention, and how responsive the parent is to the child's attention-seeking initiatives
- How the parent and child show affection to each other

Interviewing Techniques

The nurse should interview the child and parent separately because each can provide unique meaningful information. Research has supported that when parent and child are interviewed separately in a structured interview about the child's psychopathology, they rarely agree on the presence of diagnostic criteria, regardless of the diagnostic type (Jensen et al., 1999). Generally, children provide better information about internalizing symptoms (eg, mood, sleep, suicide ideation), and parents provide better information about externalizing symptoms (eg, behavior disturbances, oppositionality, relationship with parents). Therefore, to get an accurate picture of the child, the nurse must interview both parent and child alone because each gives a unique perspective.

Discussion With the Child

After talking with the parent and child together, the nurse should ask to speak with the child alone for awhile.

Young children may fear separating from their parents. The nurse can reassure children by showing them where the waiting area is and telling them that, if they get scared, the nurse will accompany them to check on their parents. Introducing a toy or game or allowing the child to hold a transitional object may help. Remember that observing how the child separates from the parent is part of the data needed to complete the assessment.

Adolescents may act indifferent or even hostile when nurses ask to speak with them alone. Teens tend to be skeptical that adults can really understand their experience, suspicious that they will be blamed for their problems, and fearful that their thoughts and feelings are abnormal. Nurses should be patient with adolescents and say something like, "I can see you're pretty angry about being here. What are you particularly angry about? Perhaps there is some way I can help you" (Lewis, 1996). Another useful and reassuring question is, "During the last few minutes, you've been quiet. I'm wondering what you are feeling." Or the nurse may ask, "It can be uncomfortable to tell personal information to someone you don't know. Do you feel this way?" (Sattler, 1998).

To begin the initial assessment of a child, nurses introduce themselves and explain briefly what they will be doing. For children younger than 11 years of age, nurses should explain that they help worried or upset children by talking, playing, and giving advice to them and their parents. They should then ask about the child's understanding of why he or she is there. This question often helps to identify children's misperceptions (eg, believing nurses are going to give them an injection, thinking they have done something bad) that could create barriers to working with them.

Nurses must adapt communication to the child's age level (Text Box 11-1). The challenge is to avoid using overly complex vocabulary or talking down to children. Young children often express themselves more easily in the context of play than through adult-like conversation. For example, a child may reenact a conversation that he had with a sibling or parent using puppets. Children respond well to third-person conversation prompts, such as "Some kids don't like being compared to their brothers and sisters," or "I know a kid who was so sad when he lost his dog that he thought he would never be happy again."

Early in the interview, the goal is to explain the nurse's purpose, elicit any concerns the child may have about what is happening, and establish rapport with the child by engaging in unthreatening discussion. Many adults rarely ask children about things that truly interest them but expect children to respond readily to adult conversation. Nurses can establish a high degree of credibility simply by taking note of and asking about things that are obviously important to children (eg, a sport they participate in, a rock group displayed on a

TEXT BOX 11.1

Strategies for Interviewing Children

- Use a simple vocabulary and short sentences tailored to the child's developmental and cognitive levels.
- Be sure that the child understands the questions and that you do not lead the child to give a particular response. Phrase your questions so that the child does not receive any hint that one response is more acceptable than another.
- Select the questions for your interview on an individual basis, using judgment and discretion and considering the child's age and developmental level.
- Be sure that the manner and tone of your voice do not reveal any personal biases.
- Speak slowly and quietly, and try to allow the interview to unfold, using the child's verbalizations and behavior as guides.
- Use simple terms (eg, sad for depressed) in exploring affective reactions, and ask the child to give examples of how he or she behaves or how other people behave when emotionally aroused.
- Assume an accepting and neutral attitude toward the child's communications.
- Learn about children's current interests by looking at Saturday morning television programs, talking with parents, visiting toy stores, looking at children's books, and visiting day care centers and schools to observe children in their natural habitat (Sattler, 1998).

shirt, a toy they have brought with them). Children, however, have an uncanny natural "radar" for phony adult behavior. Attempts to establish rapport work only when the nurse is genuinely interested in the child's life.

Discussion With the Parents

After meeting alone with the child, nurses should spend some time alone with the parents and ask for a detailed description of their view of the problem. When alone, parents may feel comfortable discussing their children in depth and sharing frustrations with their behavior. Parents need this opportunity to speak freely without being constrained by concern for the child's feelings. In some cases, it would be detrimental for the child to hear the full force of the parents' complaints and feelings, such as helplessness, anger, or disappointment. Parents need nurses to allow them to express their feelings without passing judgment. This is the nurse's opportunity to enlist the help of parents as partners in the child's evaluation and treatment. Also, this time is good for filling in any gaps in the history and clarifying the data obtained from the interview with the child.

Parents need the chance to describe the presenting problem in their own words. Nurses can encourage

them by asking general questions, such as, "What brings you here today?" or "How have things been in your family?" Nurses should then reflect their understanding of the problem, showing empathy and respect for both parent and child. Asking any other family members about their view of the problem is always a good idea to clarify discrepant points of view, obtain additional data, and communicate awareness that different family members experience the same problem in different ways.

Building Rapport

To reduce anxiety about the evaluation, the nurse must develop rapport with the family members. Establishing rapport can be facilitated by maintaining appropriate eye contact; speaking slowly, clearly, and calmly with friendliness and acceptance; using a warm and expressive tone; reacting to communications from interviewees objectively; showing interest in what the interviewees are saying; and making the interview a joint undertaking (Sattler, 1998). Suggestions for building rapport with children and adolescents will continue to be addressed in each of the developmental sections. Text Box 11-2, Semi-Structured Interview for School-Aged Children and Adolescents, can serve as a guide to asking specific questions during a comprehensive assessment.

Preschool-Aged Children

When interviewing preschool-aged children, nurses should understand that these children may have difficulty putting feelings into words and that their thinking is very concrete. For example, a preschool-aged child might assume that a tall container holds more water than a wide container, even if both containers hold the same amount of fluid.

Nurses can achieve rapport with preschool-aged children by joining their world of play. Play is an activity by which the child transforms an experience from real life into a symbolic, nonliteral representation. Play encourages verbalizations, promotes manual strength, teaches rules and problem-solving, and helps children master control over their environment (Moore et al., 2000). With children younger than 5 years of age, nurses may conduct the assessment in a playroom. Useful materials are paper, pencils, crayons, paints, paint brushes, easels, clay, blocks, balls, dolls, doll houses, puppets, animals, dress-up clothes, and a water supply. Nurses must inform preschool-aged children about any rules for the play. For example, the nurse must tell the child that the nurse must ensure safety, so that there will be no hitting in the playroom.

When observing the child in a free play setting, the nurse should pay attention to initiation of play, energy level, manipulative actions, tempo, body movements,

Text Box 11.2

Semi-Structured Interview With School-Aged Children

Precede the questions below with a preliminary greeting, such as the following: "Hi, I am (your name and title). You must be Tom Brown. Come in."

For All School-Aged Children

1. Has anyone told you about why you are here today?
2. (If yes) Who?
3. (If yes) What did he (she) tell you?
4. Tell me why *you* think you are here. (If child mentions a problem, explore it in detail.)
5. How old are you?
6. When is your birthday?
7. Your address is. . .?
8. And your telephone number is. . .?

School

9. Let's talk about school. What grade are you in?
10. What is your teacher's name?
11. What grades are you getting?
12. What subjects do you like the best?
13. And what subjects do you like least?
14. What subjects give you the most trouble?
15. And what subjects give you the least trouble?
16. What activities are you in at school?
17. How do you get along with your classmates?
18. How do you get along with your teachers?
19. Tell me how you spend a usual day at school.

Home

20. Now, let's talk about your home. Who lives with you at home?
21. Tell me a little about each of them.
22. What does your father do for work?
23. What does your mother do for work?
24. Tell me what your home is like.
25. Tell me about your room at home.
26. What chores do you do at home?
27. How do you get along with your father?
28. What does he do that you like?
29. What does he do that you don't like?
30. How do you get along with your mother?
31. What does she do that you like?
32. What does she do that you don't like?
33. (Where relevant) How do you get along with your brothers and sisters?
34. What do (does) they (he/she) do that you like?
35. What do (does) they (he/she) do that you don't like?
36. Who handles the discipline at home?
37. Tell me about how they (he/she) handle (handles) it.

Interests

38. Now, let's talk about you. What hobbies and interests do you have?
39. What do you do in the afternoons afterschool?
40. Tell me what you usually do on Saturdays and Sundays.

Friends

41. Tell me about your friends.
42. What do you like to do with your friends?

Moods and Feelings

43. Everybody feels happy at times. What things make you feel happiest?
44. What are you most likely to get sad about?
45. What do you do when you are sad?
46. Everybody gets angry at times. What things make you angriest?
47. What do you do when you are angry?

Fears and Worries

48. All children get scared sometimes about some things. What things make you feel scared?
49. What do you do when you are scared?
50. Tell me what you worry about.
51. Any other things?

Self-Concerns

52. What do you like best about yourself?
53. Anything else?
54. What do you like least about yourself?
55. Anything else?
56. Tell me about the best thing that ever happened to you.
57. Tell me about the worst thing that ever happened to you.

Somatic Concerns

58. Do you ever get headaches?
59. (If yes) Tell me about them. (How often? What do you usually do?)
60. Do you get stomach aches?
61. (If yes) Tell me about them. (How often? What do you usually do?)
62. Do you get any other kinds of body pains?
63. (If yes) Tell me about them.

Thought Disorder

64. Do you ever hear things that seem funny or usual?
65. (If yes) Tell me about them. (How often? How do you feel about them? What do you usually do?)
66. Do you ever see things that seem funny or unreal?
67. (If yes) Tell me about them. (How often? How do you feel about them? What do you usually do?)

TEXT BOX 11.2 *(Continued)*

Memories and Fantasy

68. What is the first thing you can remember from the time you were a very little baby?

69. Tell me about your dreams.

70. Which dreams come back again?

71. Who are your favorite television characters?

72. Tell me about them.

73. What animals do you like best?

74. Tell me about these animals.

75. What animals do you like least?

76. Tell me about these animals.

77. What is your happiest memory?

78. What is your saddest memory?

79. If you could change places with anyone in the whole world, who would it be?

80. Tell me about that.

81. If you could go anywhere you wanted to right now, where would you go?

82. Tell me about that.

83. If you could have three wishes, what would they be?

84. What things do you think you might need to take with you if you were to go to the moon and stay there for 6 months?

Aspirations

85. What do you plan on doing when you become an adult?

86. Do you think you will have any problem doing that?

87. If you could do anything you wanted when you become an adult, what would it be?

Concluding Questions

88. Do you have anything else that you would like to tell me about yourself?

89. Do you have any questions that you would like to ask me?

For Adolescents

These questions can be inserted after number 67.

Heterosexual Relations

1. Do you have any special girlfriend (boyfriend)?

2. (If yes) Tell me about her (him).

3. What kind of sexual concerns do you have?

4. (If present) Tell me about them.

Drug and Alcohol Use

5. Do your parents drink alcohol?

6. (If yes) Tell me about their drinking. (How much, how frequently, and where?)

7. Do your friends drink alcohol?

8. (If yes) Tell me about their drinking.

9. Do you drink alcohol?

10. (If yes) Tell me about your drinking.

11. Do your parents use drugs?

12. (If yes) Tell me about the drugs they use. (How much, how frequently, and for what reasons?)

13. Do your friends use drugs?

14. (If yes) Tell me about the drugs they use.

15. Do you use drugs?

16. (If yes) Tell me about the drugs you use.

(Sattler, 1998)

---

tone, integration, creativity, products, age appropriateness, and attitudes toward adults. In addition, themes of play, expression of emotions, and temperament are important to observe. Nurses must allow children to direct and initiate these themes.

The nurse's roles are to be a good listener; to use appropriate vocabulary; to tolerate a child's anxious, angry, or sad behavior; and to use reflective comments about the child's play. Through play, the nurse can assess the child's sensorimotor skills, cognitive style, adaptability, language functioning, emotional and behavioral responsiveness, social level, moral development, coping styles, problem-solving techniques, and approaches to perceiving and interpreting the surrounding world. Analysis of fairy tales can provide the clinician with clues to culture, problems, solutions, and elements of mental functioning (Trad, 1989). The Devereux Early Childhood Assessment (DECA) instrument measures protective factors of attachment, self-control, and initiative in children aged 2 to 5 years. The DECA tool is used in the preschool classroom setting with the goal of promoting positive resilience in children.

School-Aged Children

Unlike preschool-aged children, school-aged (5 to 11 years) children can use more constructs, provide longer descriptions and make better inferences of others, and acquire more complete conceptions of various social roles. Children in middle school are more capable of verbal exchange and can tolerate limited periods of direct questioning (see Text Box 11-1). Nurses can establish rapport with school-aged children by using competitive board games such as checkers and playing cards. A therapeutic game helpful in assessing the child's perceptions, cognition, and emotions and in establishing rapport between clinician and child is the thinking–feeling–doing game. In this game, the clinician and child take turns drawing cards that pose hypothetical situations and ask what a person might think, feel, or do in such scenarios. For example, one card might say, "A boy has something on his mind that he is afraid to tell his father. What is he scared to talk about?" Another might read, "A girl heard her parents fighting. What were they fighting about? What was the girl thinking while she listened to her parents?"

Adolescents

Adolescents have an increased command of language concepts and have developed the capacity for abstract and formal operations thinking. Their social world is also more complex. Some early adolescents tend to assume that their subjective experiences are real and congruent with objective reality, which can lead to egocentrism (Shave & Shave, 1989). **Egocentrism** is a preoccupation with one's own appearance, behavior, thoughts, and feelings. For example, a preteen may think that he caused his parents to divorce because he fought with his father the day before the parents announced their decision to separate. Because teenagers have a heightened sense of self-consciousness, they may be preoccupied during the interview with applying makeup or other self-grooming tasks.

During early adolescence, cognitive changes include increased self-consciousness, fear of being shamed, and demands for privacy and secrecy. An adolescent's willingness to talk to a nurse will depend partly on his or her perception of the degree of rapport between them. The nurse's ability to communicate respect, cooperation, honesty, and genuineness is important. Rejection by the adolescent, even outright hostility, during the first few interactions is not uncommon, especially if the teen is having behavior problems at home, at school, or in the community. Nurses should be patient and avoid jumping to conclusions. Hostility or defiance may be a test of how much the teen can trust the nurse, a defense against anxiety, or a transference phenomenon (see Chap. 6).

Adolescents are likely to be defensive in front of their parents and concerned with issues of confidentiality. At the start of the interview, nurses should clearly convey to adolescents what information they will and will not share with parents (ie, nurses will need to alert parents to any information that concerns the teenager's safety, such as suicidal or homicidal intentions). Adolescents generally prefer a straightforward, candid approach to the interview because they often distrust those in authority. Mentioning to adolescents that they do not have to discuss anything that they are not ready to reveal is also a good idea, so that they will feel in control while they gradually build trust.

BIOPSYCHOSOCIAL PSYCHIATRIC NURSING ASSESSMENT OF CHILDREN AND ADOLESCENTS

As discussed, the comprehensive assessment of the child or adolescent includes interviews with the child and parents, child alone, and parents alone. After completing these components, the nurse should bring the child and parents back together to summarize his or her view of their concerns and to ask for feedback regarding whether the nurse's perceptions agree with theirs. The nurse must give the family a chance to share additional information and ask questions. Then, the nurse should thank them for their willingness to talk and give them some idea of the next steps. Use of an assessment tool such as that provided in Text Box 11-3 is helpful in organizing data for mental health planning and intervention.

When interviewing both child and parents, directly asking the child as many questions as possible is generally the best way to get accurate, first-hand information and to reinforce interest in the child's viewpoint. Asking the child questions about the history of the current problem, previous psychiatric experiences (both good and bad), family psychiatric history, medical problems, developmental history (to get an idea of what the child has been told), school adjustment, peer relationships, and family functioning is particularly important. If necessary, the nurse can ask some or all of these same questions of the parents to verify the accuracy of the data, attain supplemental information, or both. Keep in mind that trends in developmental research show moderate to low correlation between parent and child reports of family behavior.

Biologic Domain

Nurses should include a thorough history of psychiatric and medical problems in any comprehensive assessment. A physical assessment is necessary to rule out any medical problems that could be mistaken for psychiatric symptoms (eg, weight loss resulting from diabetes versus depression, drug-induced psychosis). Pharmacologic assessment should include prescription and over-the-counter (OTC) medications. Nurses should ask about any allergies to food, medications, or environmental triggers.

Genetic Vulnerability

The line between nature and nurture is not always clear. Characteristics that appear to be inborn may influence parents and teachers to respond differently toward different children, thus creating problems in the family environment. A phenomenon called **assortative mating**, the tendency for individuals to select mates who are similar in genetically linked traits such as intelligence and personality style, may contribute to the genetic transmission of psychiatric disorders. Research increasingly shows that major psychiatric disorders (eg, depression, anxiety disorder, schizophrenia, bipolar disorder, substance abuse) run in families. Thus, having a parent or sibling with a psychiatric disorder usually

TEXT BOX 11.3

Biopsychosocial Psychiatric Nursing Assessment of Children and Adolescents

1. **Identifying Information**
   Name

   Sex

   Date of birth

   Age

   Birth order

   Grade

   Ethnic background

   Religious preference

   List of others living in household

2. **Major Reason for Seeking Help**
   Description of presenting problems or symptoms

   When did the problems (symptoms) start?

   Describe both the child's and the parent's perspective.

3. **Psychiatric History**
   Previous mental health contacts (inpatient and outpatient)

   Other mental health problems or psychiatric diagnosis (besides those described currently)

   Previous medications

   Family history of depression, substance abuse, psychosis, etc., and treatment

4. **Current and Past Health Status**
   Medical problems

   Current medications

   Surgery and hospitalizations

   Allergies

   Diet and eating habits

   Height and weight

   Hearing and vision

   Menstrual history

   If sexually active, birth control method used

   Date of last physical examination

   Pediatrician or nurse practitioner's name and telephone number

5. **Medications**
   Prescription (dosage, side effects)

   Over-the-counter drugs

6. **Neurologic History**
   Right handed, left handed, or ambidextrous

   Headaches, dizziness, fainting

   Seizures

   Unusual movement (tics, tremors)

   Hyperactivity

   Episodes of weakness or paralysis

   Slurred speech, pronunciation problems

   Fine motor skills (eating with utensils, using crayon or pencil, fastening buttons and zippers, tying shoes)

   Gross motor skills and coordination (walking, running, hopping)

7. **Responses to Mental Health Problems**
   What makes problems (symptoms) worse or better?

   Feelings about those experiences (what helped and did not help)

   What interventions have been tried so far?

   Major loss or changes in past year

   Fears, including punishment

8. **Mental Status Examination**
   Appearance

   Interaction with nurse

   Psychosis, hallucinations, delusions

   Mood, affect, anxiety

   Speech (clarity, speed, volume), language

   Thought patterns (organization, thought content)

   Intellectual ability, judgment, insight

   Activity level, stereotypes, mannerisms, obsessions or compulsions

9. **Developmental Assessment**
   Physical maturation

   Psychosocial

   Language

10. **Attachment, Temperament/Significant Behavior Patterns**
    Attachment

    Concentration, distractability

    Eating and sleeping patterns

    Ability to adjust to new situations and changes in routine

    Usual mood and fluctuations

    Excitability

    Ability to wait, tendency to interrupt

    Responses to discipline

    Lying, stealing, fighting, cruelty to animals, fire-setting

11. **Self-Concept**
    Beliefs about self

    Body image

    Self-esteem

    Personal identity

12. **Risk Assessment**
    History of suicidal thoughts, attempts

    Suicide ideation

    History of violent, aggressive behavior

    Homicidal ideation

13. **Family Relationships**
    Relationship with parents

    Family conflicts (nature and content)

(continued)

TEXT BOX 11.3 (*Continued*)

Disciplinary methods

Quality of sibling relationship

Sleeping arrangements

Who does the child relate to or trust in the family?

14. School and Peer Adjustment
Learning difficulties

Behavior problems at school

School attendance

Relationship with teachers

Special classes

Best friend

Relationships with peers

Dating

Drug and alcohol use

Participation in sports, clubs, other activities

Afterschool routine

15. Community Resources
Professionals or agencies working with child or family

Day care resources

16. Functional Status
Global Assessment of Functioning Scale (GAF)

17. Stresses and Coping Behaviors
Psychosocial stresses

Coping behaviors (strengths)

18. Summary of Significant Data

indicates increased risk for the same or another closely related disorder in a child or adolescent. In addition, many childhood psychiatric disorders, such as autism, mental retardation, developmental learning disorders, some language disorders (eg, dyslexia), attention deficit hyperactivity disorder (ADHD), Tourette's syndrome, and enuresis (bed wetting), appear to be genetically transmitted (American Psychiatric Association, 2000; Rutter et al., 1999; State et al., 2000). Certain disorders (eg, ADHD, enuresis, stuttering) are more common in boys than in girls.

Neurologic Examination

A full neurologic evaluation is beyond the scope of practice for a baccalaureate-level or masters-level nurse without specific neuropsychiatric training. A screening of neurologic soft signs, however, can help establish a database that will clarify the need for further neurologic consultation. Nurses should ask the brief neurologic screening questions listed in Text Box 11-3 directly of the child. They also should note any soft signs of neurologic dysfunction, such as slurred speech, unusual movements (eg, tics, tremors), hyperactivity, and coordination problems. Nurses can ask young children to hop on one foot, skip, or walk from toe to heel to assess their gross motor coordination and to draw with a crayon or pencil or play pick-up-sticks or jacks to assess their fine motor coordination.

Psychological Domain

Children can usually identify and discuss what improves or worsens their problems. The assessment may be the first time that someone has asked the child to explain his or her view of the problem. It is also a perfect opportu-

nity to discuss any life changes or losses (eg, death of grandparents or pets, parental divorce) and fears, especially of punishment.

Mental Status Examination

The mental status examination of children combines observation and direct questioning. Nurses should note the child's general appearance, including size, cleanliness, dress, masculinity or femininity, and level of attractiveness. Although it perhaps should not be so, social-psychological research shows that appearance and attractiveness of both children and adults strongly influence their social relationships (Eagly et al., 1991). Also, nurses should note the child's nonverbal behavior, including posture, tone of voice, eye contact, and mannerisms. How active is the child? Does he or she seem to have difficulty focusing on the interview, sitting still, refraining from impulsive behavior, and listening without interrupting (possible signs of ADHD)? Does the child seem underactive, lethargic, distant, or hopeless (possible signs of depression)?

Nurses should observe the child's sentence structure and vocabulary for a general sense of his or her intellectual functioning. Does the child seem able to form a relationship with the examiner, or does the child seem distant, uninterested, or in his or her own world? Speech patterns, such as rate (overly fast or slow), clarity, and volume, and any speech dysfluencies (eg, stuttering, halting) are important in screening for mood disorders (eg, depression, mania), language disorders, psychotic processes, and anxiety disorders (see Chap. 29).

Asking children general questions about their everyday lives and observing the content and process of their play (eg, ability to focus on an activity, play themes, boundaries between themselves and others) helps to reveal the level of organization and content of their thinking. Nurses should also note the level of organization of speech. Young children normally shift subjects rather abruptly, but adolescents should continue with one train of thought before moving to another. Nurses should note any morbid or eccentric thoughts, violent fantasies, and self-deprecating statements that could reflect a poor self-concept. Assessment of preteens and adolescents should address substance use and sexual activity because responses may provide useful information about high-risk behavior or substance abuse. Also, nurses should inquire about any obsessions or compulsions (eg, worries about germs, severe hand washing).

Developmental Assessment

Children are not miniature adults. They respond to life's stresses in different ways, according to their developmental level. Knowing the difference between normal child development and psychopathology is crucial in helping parents view their children's behavior realistically and respond appropriately. The key areas for assessment include maturation, psychosocial development, and language.

Maturation. Healthy development of the brain and nervous system during childhood and adolescence provides the foundation for successful functioning throughout life. Such development, called **maturation**, unfolds through sequential and orderly growth processes. These processes are biologically and genetically based but depend on constant interactions with a stimulating and nurturing environment. If trauma or neglect impairs the process of normal biologic maturation, **developmental delays** and disorders that may not be fully reversible can result. For example, babies born with fetal alcohol syndrome suffer permanent brain damage, often resulting in mental retardation (Roebuck et al., 1999). A pregnant woman's use of crack cocaine deprives the fetus of nutrients and oxygen, leading to developmental delays, deformities, and behavior disorders (eg, impulsivity, withdrawal, hyperactivity).

The nurse can assess for developmental delays by asking questions from specific sections of the mental status examination:

Intellectual functioning: Evaluate the child's creativity, spontaneity, ability to count money and tell time, academic performance, memory, attention, frustration tolerance, and organization.

Gross motor functioning: Ask the child to hop on one foot, throw a ball, walk up and down the hall, and run.

Fine motor functioning: Ask the child to draw a picture or pick up sticks.

Cognition: Testing such as the Wechsler Intelligence Scale for Children (WISC-III) provides measures of Intelligence Quotient (IQ). A psychologist usually performs such tests. The nurse can request cognitive testing if he or she has concerns about developmental delays or learning disabilities.

Thinking and perception: Evaluate level of consciousness; orientation to date, time, and person; thought content; thought process; and judgment.

Social interactions and play: Assess the child's ability to follow rules, organization, creativity, and drawing capacity. Children experiencing developmental delays may remain engaged solely in parallel play instead of moving to reciprocal play. They may consistently play with toys designed for younger children. Nurses must understand that children with developmental delays may draw cruder body pictures. These children may also have receptive or expressive language problems.

Psychosocial Development. Assessment of psychosocial development is very important for children with mental health problems. Various theoretical models are available from which to choose; the most commonly used model is Erikson's stages of development. When considering this model, the nurse should examine the child's sex and cultural background for appropriateness. The nurse also may use the Baker Miller's model for girls (see Chap. 6).

Language. At birth, infants can emit sounds of all languages. Maturation of language skills begins with babbling, or the utterance of simple, spontaneous sounds. Babbling is not a mere imitation of adult speech. By the end of the first year, babies can make one-word statements, usually naming objects or people in the environment. By age 2 years, they should speak in short, telegraphic sentences consisting of a verb and noun (eg, "want cookie"). Between ages 2 and 4 years, vocabulary and sentence structure rapidly develop. In fact, the preschooler's ability to produce language often surpasses motor development, sometimes causing temporary stuttering when the child's mind literally works faster than the mouth.

Language development depends on the complex interaction of physical maturation of the nerves, development of head and neck musculature, hearing abilities, cognitive abilities, exposure to language, educational stimulation, and emotional well-being. Social needs create a natural inclination toward communication, but the child needs reinforcement to develop correct pronunciation, vocabulary, and grammar.

Before a diagnosis of a communication disorder (ie, impairment in language expression, comprehension, or both) can be made, the child must be tested to rule out hearing, visual, or other neurologic problems. Brain damage, especially to the left hemisphere (dominant for language in most individuals), can seriously impair the development of communication abilities in children.

Any child who has experienced brain damage from anoxia at birth, congenital trauma, head injury, infection, tumor, or drug exposure should be closely monitored for signs of a communication disorder. Before age 5 years, the brain has amazing plasticity, and sometimes other intact areas of the brain can take over functions of damaged areas, especially with immediate speech therapy. Genetically based disorders such as autism cause language delays that are sometimes permanent and severe. Children with language delays need particular encouragement to communicate properly because they tend to compensate by using nonverbal signals (Tanguay, 2000).

Nurses need to recognize normal variations in child development and assess lags in the development of vocabulary and sentence structure during the critical preschool years. Delays in this area can seriously affect other areas, such as cognitive, educational, and social development. Many children who receive psychiatric treatment have speech and language disorders that are sometimes undetected, either leading to or compounding their emotional problems. Cantwell and Baker (1991) studied 600 consecutive child referrals to an urban community clinic for speech and language disorders and found the psychiatric prevalence was 50% for any diagnosis, 26% for behavior disorders, and 20% for emotional disorders. The most common individual psychiatric diagnoses were ADHD (19%), oppositional defiant disorder (7%), and anxiety disorders (10%). Beitchman and colleagues (1996) found that children with receptive language disorders also had a high prevalence of ADHD (59%).

Attachment

Studies of **attachment** show that the quality of the emotional bond between the infant and parental figures provides the groundwork for future relationships. The need to touch and be close to a parental figure appears biologically driven and has been demonstrated in classic studies of monkeys who bonded with a terrycloth surrogate mother (Harlow & Harlow, 1971). A secure attachment is based on the caretaker's consistent, appropriate response to the infant's attachment behaviors (eg, crying, clinging, calling, following, protesting). Children who have developed a secure attachment protest when their parents leave them (beginning at about age 6 to 8 months), seek comfort from their parents in unfamiliar situations, and playfully explore the environment in the parent's presence. When parents are unresponsive to a child's attachment behaviors, the child may develop an insecure attachment, evidenced by clinging and lack of exploratory play when the parent is present, intense protest when the parent leaves, and indifference or even hostility when the parent returns (Ainsworth, 1989). Although the importance of the parent's responsiveness is unquestionable in determining the devel-

opment of a secure attachment, the process works both ways. Some babies seem to encourage attachment naturally with their parents by responding positively to holding, cuddling, and comforting behaviors. Others, such as those with developmental delays or autistic disorders, may respond less readily and even reject parental attempts at bonding.

Bowlby's early studies (1969) of maternal deprivation formed the initial framework for attachment theory, based on the notion that the infant tends to bond to one primary parental figure, usually the mother. Although this pattern is common, recent studies show that children make multiple attachments to parents and other caretakers, but high-quality, intense bonds remain essential for healthy development. Contemporary nursing theories, such as Barnard's parent–child interaction model, have stressed the importance of the interaction between the child's spontaneous behavior and biologic rhythms and the mother's ability to respond to cues that signal distress (Baker et al., 1994). Responses of fathers to the Adult Attachment Interview are less clearly related to attachment than are those of mothers, perhaps because fathers typically spend less time with infants (van Ijzendoorn & Bakermans-Krakenburg, 1996).

Disrupted attachments resulting from deficits in infant attachment behaviors, lack of responsiveness by caretakers to the child's cues, or both may lead to reactive attachment disorder, feeding disorder, failure to thrive, or anxiety disorder. A reactive attachment disorder is a state in which a child younger than 5 years of age fails to initiate or respond appropriately to social interaction and the caregiver subsequently disregards the child's physical and emotional needs. O'Connor and Rutter (2000) studied 163 adopted children with early severe deprivation at 4 years of age and again at 6 years of age. Longitudinal findings were that attachment disorder behaviors were correlated with attention and conduct problems. Solomon and George (1999) have reviewed the research on a new classification of attachment disorder titled attachment disorganization. **Attachment disorganization** is a consequence of extreme insecurity that results from feared or actual separation from the attached figure. Disorganized infants appear to be unable to maintain the strategic adjustments in attachment behavior represented by organized avoidant or ambivalent attachment strategies, with the result that both behavioral and physiological dysregulation occurs. Frightening and frightened caregivers can contribute to the disorganized attachment in infants. Preschoolers with disorganized attachment manifest behaviors of fear, contradictory behavior, and/or disorientation/disassociation in the caregivers' presence.

Temperament and Behavior

Temperament is a person's characteristic intensity, activity level, threshold of responsiveness, rhythmicity, adaptability, energy expenditure, and mood. According to research findings, temperamental differences can be observed early in life, suggesting that they are at least partly biologically determined, and patterns of temperament can be correlated with emotional and behavioral problems (Kagan et al., 1999). One basic aspect of temperament, the tendency to approach or avoid unfamiliar events, appears moderately stable over time and has been associated with distinct, apparently genetically based, physiologic profiles in 2-year-old children (Schwartz et al., 1999; Caspi & Silva, 1995; Snidman et al., 1995).

The classic New York Longitudinal Study (Thomas et al., 1968) identified three main patterns of temperament seen in infancy that often extend into childhood and later life:

- **Easy temperament,** characterized by a positive mood, regular patterns of eating and sleeping, positive approach to new situations, and low emotional intensity
- **Difficult temperament,** characterized by irregular sleep and eating patterns, negative response to new stimuli, slow adaptation, negative mood, and high emotional intensity
- **Slow-to-warm-up temperament,** characterized by a negative, mildly emotional response to new situations that is expressed with intensity and initially slow adaptation but evolves into a positive response

On the positive side, an easy temperament can serve as a protective factor against the development of psychopathology. Children with easy temperaments can adapt to change without intense emotional reactions. Difficult temperament places children at high risk for adjustment problems, such as with adjustment to school or bonding with parents.

Temperament has a major influence on the chances that a child may experience psychological problems; however, temperament is not unchangeable, and environmental influences can change or modify a child's emotional style. Kerr and coauthors (1994) found that temperament remained stable from childhood to adulthood only in those children who were extremely inhibited or uninhibited.

The concept of temperament provides an excellent example of the interaction between biologic-genetic and environmental factors in producing child psychopathology. Although a child may be born with a particular temperament, studies show that the temperament itself is less influential than the "goodness of fit" between the child's temperament and the reactions of parents and significant others. Difficult children in particular may evoke negative reactions in parents and teachers, thereby creating environments that exacerbate their biologically based behavior problems, initiating a vicious cycle. Vanden Boom and Hoeksma (1994) found that infants with difficult temperaments received less sensitive caring than other children, and parents of 2-year-old children with difficult temperaments often resorted to angry, punitive discipline.

Most research in temperament has focused on the child with a difficult temperament. Studies show that the difficult temperament is correlated with the development of child psychopathology, but only if such temperament persists beyond 3 years of age. Furthermore, the effects of a difficult temperament are more significant in psychiatric populations than in nonpsychiatric populations (Tubman et al., 1992). Extremely difficult temperament has been associated with the development of oppositional and conduct disorders as well as ADHD (Dulcan & Martini, 1999).

Nurses working with parents of young children need to understand temperament so that they can educate families about this concept, particularly because many parents of children with difficult temperaments blame themselves for their children's behavior. Parents may compare the child with a difficult temperament to children with easier temperaments and wonder what they have done wrong or attribute negative motives to the child. Nurses can help parents accept biologically based differences in their children and learn to adapt their behavior to each child's needs.

Self-Concept

For young children, eliciting their view of themselves and the world by using some projective techniques is helpful. For example, nurses should ask them what they would wish for if they had three wishes. Answers can be revealing. Inability to wish for anything beyond a nice meal or place to live may reflect hopelessness, whereas wishes to conquer the world or put one's teacher in jail may indicate feelings of grandiosity. Another technique is to tell a story and ask the child to make up an ending for it. For example, a baby bird fell out of a nest—what happened to it? Nurses may design stories to elicit particular fears or concerns that they suspect may be relevant for the individual child.

Drawings also provide an excellent window into the child's internal world. Asking the child to draw a picture of a person can provide data about the child's self-concept, sexual identity, body image, and developmental level. By age 3 years, children should be able to draw some facial features and limbs, but their drawings may have an "x-ray" quality, in which clothing is transparent and the body can be seen underneath. Older children should produce more sophisticated drawings unless they are resistant to the task. After the child has finished the drawing, the nurse can ask what the person in the drawing is thinking and feeling, using this device to assess the child's mental processes. For example, one adolescent with school phobia drew a person fully dressed, in great detail, but with no feet. When asked about the drawing, he said that the boy could not go anywhere because his mother was afraid to let him leave home.

Other ways to assess children's self-concepts include asking them what they want to do when they grow up, what their best subjects are in school, what things they are really good at, and how well-liked they are at school. Before concluding the individual interview with children, nurses should always ask if they have any other information to share and whether they have any questions.

Risk Assessment

Nurses must ask the child about any suicidal or violent thoughts. The best way to assess these areas is to ask straightforward questions, such as, "Have you ever thought about hurting yourself? Have you ever thought about hurting someone else? Have you ever acted on these thoughts? Have you thought about how you would do it? What did you think would happen if you hurt yourself? Have you ever done anything to hurt yourself before?" Contrary to popular belief, even young children attempt suicide, and they are capable of violent acts toward other children, adults, and animals. When a child shares the intent to commit a suicidal or violent act, nurses must remind him or her that they will need to discuss this concern with the parent to keep the child and others safe.

Social Domain

Family Relationship

Children depend on adults to create a safe, nurturing, and appropriate environment to support their development. The nurse should assess the quality of the home, including living space, sleeping arrangements, safety, cleanliness, and child care arrangements either through a home visit or by discussing these issues with the family. To understand fully the family's values, goals, and beliefs, nurses must consider the family's ethnic, cultural, and economic background throughout the assessment (Carter & McGoldrick, 1999). A comprehensive family assessment should be considered (see Chapter 16).

School and Peer Adjustment

The child's adjustment to school is also significant. Often, children are referred for a mental health assessment as a result of changes in behavior at school. Falling grades, loss of interest in normal activities, decreased concentration, or withdrawal from or aggression toward peers may indicate that the child is suffering from emotional problems. It is very important that the nurse obtain signed permission from the parents to talk to the child's teacher for his or her observations of the child. If feasible, the nurse may want to observe the child in school to see how the child functions there. The parent can request a treatment planning conference in which the teacher, parent, and nurse discuss the child's school performance and strategize ways to promote the child's emotional, cognitive, and social functioning in school. Suggestions may range from having the child tested for learning disabilities to designing behavior plans that include rewards for improvements and functioning, such as computer time at the end of the day.

Community

Blyth and Leffert (1995) undertook a cross-sectional, longitudinal study of 112 different communities of 300 youths in grades 9 through 12. The study showed that youth in healthy communities were more likely to attend religious services, to feel their schools were places of caring and encouragement, to be involved in structured activities, and to remain committed to their own learning.

Children and adolescents function better if they are linked to community supports, such as churches, recreational programs, park district programming, and after-school programming. The Big Brother/Big Sister program fosters mentoring relationships for children. A parent or child may call the local Big Brother/Big Sister organization to request a mentor for the child. The mentor may perform a wide range of services, from taking a child to community events, helping with homework, or talking about how the child can achieve his or her dreams and goals. Some towns offer community-based juvenile justice programs to rehabilitate children who have had an altercation with the legal system. Juvenile justice programs provide support, such as individual and family counseling and prosocial recreational activities; teach children how to make positive choices about spending free time; and closely monitor their behaviors.

Functional Status

Functional status is evaluated in children and adolescents using the Global Assessment of Functioning (GAF) scale. The GAF scale ranges from 0 to 100; the lower the score, the higher is the level of impairment indicated in psychiatric symptoms and level of general functioning. Functional status is evaluated in children by noting behaviors in the domains of school, peers, activity level, mood, speech, family relationships, behavioral problems, self-care skills, and self-concept. For example, a score of 30 may indicate that the child is severely homicidal or suicidal and has made previous attempts; that hallucinations or delusions influence the child's behavior; or that the child has serious impairment in communication or judgment. Moderate symptom impairment scores usually fall in the range of 51 to 69. Indications of moderate symptom impairment include difficulty in one area, such as school phobia, that impairs school attendance or performance, but that the child is functioning well within other areas, such as with family and peers. Children in this category are not homicidal or suicidal and usually respond well to outpatient interventions. A score of 70 to 100 usually indicates that the child is functioning well in the areas of school, peers, family, and community. The GAF is always measured at the initial assessment so that treatment can be evaluated in terms of symptom improvement.

Stresses and Coping Behaviors

Biologic, behavioral, and personality predispositions, family, and community environment may affect a child's ability to cope with stressful life events. Stressful experiences for children include the death of a loved person or pet, parental divorce, violence, physical illness (especially chronic illness), mental illness, social isolation, racial discrimination, neglect, and physical and sexual abuse. If a child discloses neglect or physical or sexual abuse during the assessment process, the nurse must let the parent or caregiver know that the nurse must call DCF and report the child's disclosure. DCF will then investigate. Federal law mandates reporting to DCF any disclosure of abuse (Research Box 11-1).

The number of stressful events a child experiences, supports that the child has in place, and the child's developmental stage may also influence his or her ability to cope with stressors. Werner (1989) performed a longitudinal study of 500 high-risk Hawaiian youths. Children identified at risk were those born into poverty, homelessness, or families whose parents had little education or were alcoholic, mentally ill, or headed by a single parent. Other risk factors included low birth weight, difficult temperament, mental retardation, childhood trauma, exposure to racism, poor schools, and community and domestic violence. One third of the children born at risk did not develop mental health problems by age 18 years. The protective factors identified in these children included the following:

- Individual attributes, such as resilience, problem-solving skills, sense of self-efficacy, accurate processing of interpersonal cues, positive social orientation, and activity level
- A supportive family environment, including bonding with adults in the family, low family conflict, and supportive relationships
- Environmental supports, including those that reinforce and support coping efforts and recognize and reward competence

RESEARCH BOX 11.1

Screening Tool for Abuse Potential

This work involves the development of a tool for assessing levels of risk for child abuse and neglect in families of children aged 3 years and younger. The nurses who developed the tool undertook a comprehensive review of the literature on risk factors for child maltreatment and combined these data with ideas from other screening and research tools. The result was a 19-question interview protocol that can be administered in 5 minutes or less. The researchers' goal was to provide a tool that could be used efficiently in primary care settings because other available tools are more cumbersome and impractical. The nurse researchers piloted the instrument in a primary care clinic, and the nurses who administered it reported that it was concise and easy to use. The tool includes an interview screening protocol with carefully worded questions designed to avoid accusatory attitudes and with a scoring guide that indicates the need for referral to community resources.

Utilization in Clinical Setting: The nurses who developed this tool assert that assessment of risk for abuse and neglect should be a standard of practice in child health care programs. Screening for possible risk for maltreatment allows nurses to identify families who are most in need of tracking and preventive intervention. This maximizes the efficient use of resources by both families and health care providers; however, assessment tools must be brief and designed with specific, helpful questions that both experienced and novice professionals can adapt. Because primary care providers may be a family's only formal source of support in the early years of childrearing, this is a key setting for assessment. The development of this tool is a useful contribution to nursing practice, and it provides the potential to intervene with families early enough to make a difference.

Murry, S. K., Baker, A. W., & Lewin, L. (2000). Screening families with young children for child maltreatment potential. *Pediatric Nursing, 26,* 47–54.

Summary of Key Points

➤ Mental health assessment of children and adolescents includes evaluating the child's biologic, psychological, and social factors.

➤ Assessment of children and adolescents differs from assessment of adults in that the nurse must consider the child's developmental level, specifically addressing the child's language, cognitive, social, and emotional skills. Establishing a treatment alliance and building rapport are essential to obtaining a good mental health history.

➤ The mental status examination includes observations and questions about the child's appearance, speech, language, vocabulary, orientation, knowledge base (including reading, writing, and math skills), attention level, activity level, social skills, peer relationships, relationship to interviewer, mood, affect, suicidal or homicidal tendencies, thinking (presence or absence of hallucinations or delusions), substance use, and behaviors.

➤ Assessment of the child and caretaker together provides important information regarding child–parent attachment and parenting practices.

➤ The three main types of temperament include the easy temperament, difficult temperament, and slow-to-warm-up temperament. Temperament can be evaluated by assessing the child's sleep and eating habits, mood, emotional intensity, and responses to new stimuli.

➤ A child's self-concept can be evaluated using tools such as play, stories, asking three wishes, and asking the child to draw a picture of himself or herself.

➤ If a child reveals suicidal ideation in the interview, the nurse must assess whether the child has a plan, let the parent know the child is suicidal, and make a plan to keep the child safe, such as an inpatient hospitalization.

➤ If a child reports to the nurse neglect or physical or sexual abuse, the nurse must by law report the child's disclosure to the state DCF.

➤ Protective factors that promote resiliency in children are ability to problem solve, sense of self-efficacy, accurate processing of social cues, supportive family environment, and environmental supports that promote coping efforts and recognize and reward competence.

Critical Thinking Challenges

1. An adolescent is hostile and refuses to talk in an interview. How would you respond?
2. What are some strategies for building rapport with children?
3. A child reports that he is suicidal. What would be your next question? What measures would you take next?
4. What are some techniques and mediums for obtaining information about a child's inner world, such as self-concept, sexual identity, body image, and developmental level?
5. Explain why it may be detrimental to interview a child in front of his parent. Why may it be detrimental to interview a parent in front of her child?
6. Why is obtaining the mental health histories of parents relevant to the child's mental health assessment?

WEB LINKS

www.nncc.org/Child.dev.page.html This site gives detailed accounts of expected developmental milestones from birth through adulthood and links to numerous articles on child development and parenting.
www.aacap.org/publications/factsfam/index.htm This website of the American Academy of Child & Adolescent Psychiatry provides an exhaustive list of links to short articles on many mental health issues and is geared toward families and consumers.

REFERENCES

Ainsworth, M. D. S. (1989). Attachments beyond infancy. *American Psychologist, 44,* 709–716.

American Nurses Association. (2000). *Statement on psychiatric-mental health clinical practice and standards of psychiatric-mental health clinical nursing practice.* Washington, DC: American Nurses Publishing.

American Psychiatric Association. (2000). *Diagnostic and statistical manual of mental health disorders* (4th ed., Text revision). Washington, DC: Author.

Baker J. K., Borchers, D. A., Cochran, D. T., et al. (1994). Parent-child interaction model (of Kathryn Barnard). In A. Marriner-Tomey (Ed.), *Nursing theorists and their work.* St. Louis: Mosby.

Beitchman, J. H., Cohen, N. J., Konstantareas, M. M., & Tannock, R. (Eds.). (1996). *Language, learning, and behavior disorders: Developmental, biological, and clinical perspectives.* New York: Cambridge University Press.

Blyth, D. A., & Leffert, N. (1995). Communities as contexts for adolescent development: An empirical analysis. *Journal of Adolescent Research, 10*(1), 64–87.

Bowlby, J. (1969). *Attachment* (Vol. 1 of *Attachment and loss*). New York: Basic Books.

Cantwell, D. P., & Baker, L. (1991). *Psychiatric and developmental disorders in children with communication disorders.* Washington, DC: American Psychiatric Press.

Carter, B., & McGoldrick, M. (1999). *The expanded family life cycle: Individual, family, and social perspectives* (3rd ed.). Needham Heights, MA: Allyn & Bacon.

Caspi, A., & Silva, P. A. (1995). Temperamental qualities at age 3 predict personality traits in young adulthood: Longitudinal evidence from a birth cohort. *Child Development, 66,* 486–498.

Dulcan, M., & Martini, D. R. (1999). *Child and adolescent psychiatry.* Washington, DC: American Psychiatric Press.

Eagly, A. H., Ashmore, R. D., Makhijani, M. G., & Kennedy, L. (1991). What is beautiful is good, but . . . : A meta-analytic review of research on physical attractiveness stereotype. *Psychological Bulletin, 110,* 109–128.

Harlow, H. F., Harlow, M. K., & Suomi, S. J. (1971). From thought to therapy: Lessons from a private laboratory. *American Scientist, 59* (5), 538–549.

Jensen, P., Rubio-Stipac, M., Carnio, G., et al. (1999). Parents and child contributions to diagnosis of mental disorder: Are both informants always necessary? *Journal of the American Academy of Child and Adolescent Psychiatry, 38*(12), 1569–1579.

Kagan J. (1999). The concept of behavioral inihibition. In L. Schmidt & J. Schulkin (Eds.), *Extreme fear, shyness, and social phobia: Origins, biological mechanisms, and clinical outcomes.* Series in affective science. New York, NY: Oxford University Press.

Le Buffe, P. A., & Naglievi, J. (1988). *Devereux early childhood assessment.* The Devereux Foundation. Lewisville, NC: Kaplan Press.

Lewis, M. (1996). Psychiatric assessment of infants, children and adolescents. In M. Lewis (Ed.), *Child and adolescent psychiatry: A comprehensive textbook* (2nd ed.). Baltimore: Williams & Wilkins.

Moore-Taylor, K. M., Menarchek-Fetkovich, M., & Day, C. (2000). In K. Gillin-Weiner, A. Sandgrund, & C. Scafer (Eds.), The play history, interview play diagnosis and assessment (2nd ed.) New York, NY: Wiley Publishers.

Murry, S. K., Baker, A. W., & Lewin, L. (2000). Screening families with young children for child maltreatment potential. *Pediatric Nursing, 26,* 47–54.

O'Connor, T., & Rutter, M. (2000). Attachment disorder behavior following early severe deprivation: Extension and longitudinal follow-up. *Journal of the American Academy of Child and Adolescent Psychiatry, 39*(6), 709–712.

Roebuck, T. M., Mattson, S. N., & Riley, E. P. (1999). Behavioral and psychosocial profiles of alcohol-exposed children. *Alcoholism: Clinical and Experimental Research, 23*(6), 1070–1076.

Rutter, M., Silberg, J., O'Connor, T., & Simonoff, E. (1999). Genetics and child psychiatry. I. Advances in qualitative and molecular genetics. *Journal of Psychological Psychiatry, 40,* 3–18.

Sattler, J. (1998). *Clinical and forensic interviewing of children and families.* San Diego: Jerome Sattler Publisher.

Schwartz, C., Snidman, N., & Kagan, J. (1999). Adolescent social anxiety as an outcome of inhibited temperament in childhood. *Journal of the American Academy of Child and Adolescent Psychiatry, 38*(8), 1008–1015.

Shave, D., & Shave, B. (1989). *Early adolescence and search for self: A developmental perspective.* New York, NY: Praeger Publishers.

Snidman, N., Kagan, J., Riordan, L., & Shannon, D. C. (1995). Cardiac function and behavioral reactivity. *Psychopathology, 32,* 199–207.

Solomon, J., & George, C. (1999). *Attachment Disorganization.* New York, NY: The Guilford Press.

State, M., Lombroso, P., Pauls, D., & Leckman, J. (2000). The genetics of childhood psychiatric disorders: A decade of progress. *Journal of the American Academy of Child and Adolescent Psychiatry, 39*(8), 946–962.

Tanguay, P. (2000). Pervasive developmental disorders: A 10-year review. *Journal of the American Academy of Child and Adolescent Psychiatry, 39,* 1079–1095.

Thomas, A., Chess, S., & Birch, H. G. (1968). *Temperament and behavior disorders in childhood.* New York: New York University Press.

Trad, P. (1989). *The preschool child assessment, diagnosis and treatment.* New York: Wiley Publishers.

Tubman, J. G., Lerner, R. M., Lerner. J. V., & Von Eye, A. (1992). Temperament and adjustment in young adulthood: A 15-year longitudinal analysis. *American Journal of Orthopsychiatry, 62,* 564–574.

Vanden Boom, D. C., & Hoeksma, J. B. (1994). The effect of infant irritability on mother-infant interaction: A growth curve analysis. *Developmental Psychology, 30,* 581–590.

van Ijzendoorn, M. H., & Bakermans-Krakenburg, M. J. (1996). Attachment representations in mothers, fathers, adolescents, and clinical groups: A meta-analytic search for normative data. *Journal of Consulting and Clinical Psychology, 64,* 8–21.

Werner, E. E. (1989). High-risk children in young adulthood: A longitudinal study form birth to 32 years. *American Journal of Orthopsychiatry, 59,* 72–81.

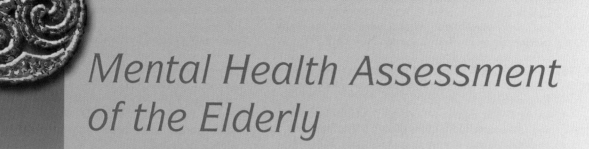

Mental Health Assessment of the Elderly

Mary Ann Boyd and Mickey Stanley

LEARNING OBJECTIVES

After studying this chapter, you will be able to:

➤ Compare changes in normal aging with those associated with mental health problems in elderly people.

➤ Select various techniques in assessing elderly people who have mental health problems.

➤ Delineate important areas of assessment for the biologic domain in completing the geropsychiatric nursing assessment.

➤ Delineate important areas of assessment for the psychological domain in completing the geropsychiatric nursing assessment.

➤ Delineate important areas of assessment for the social domain in completing the geropsychiatric nursing assessment.

KEY TERMS

dysphagia
functional activities
insomnia

instrumental activities
polypharmacy
xerostomia

KEY CONCEPTS

biopsychosocial geropsychiatric
  nursing assessment
normal aging

*T*he average life span in the United States has increased from 47 years in 1900 to more than 75 years in 2001. Health care providers will face new and increased challenges as the Baby Boomers move into the ranks of the elderly population. By the year 2010, projections are that more than 13% of the U.S. population will be older than age 65 years, with 1.9% older than age 85 years.

Normal aging is associated with some physical decline, such as decreased sensory abilities and decreased pulmonary and immune function, but many important functions do not change. Intellectual function, capacity for change, and productive engagement with life remain stable. Many myths exist about normal aging. Some people believe that "senility" is normal, or that depression or hopelessness is natural for elderly people. If family members believe these myths, they will be less likely to seek treatment for their elders with real problems. For example, although some cognitive changes contribute to a slower pace of learning, memory complaints are more likely related to depression than normal aging (U.S. Department of Health and Human Services, 1999).

Almost 20% of adults older than age 55 years experience specific mental disorders that are not part of "normal aging" (U.S. Department of Health and Human Services, 1999). Elders with mental health problems comprise different population groups. One group consists of those with long-term mental illnesses who have reached the ranks of the elderly population. These individuals are experienced usually understand their disorders and treatments. Unfortunately, the changes associated with aging can affect a patient's control of his or her chronic mental illness. Symp-

toms may reappear, and medications may need to be adjusted. Another group is comprised of those individuals who are relatively free of mental health problems until their elder years. These individuals, who may already have other health problems, develop late-onset mental disorders such as depression, schizophrenia, or dementia. For these individuals and their family members, the development of a mental disorder can be very traumatic.

Mental health problems in the elderly can be especially complex because of the effects of frequently coexisting medical problems and treatments. Many symptoms of somatic disorders mimic or mask psychiatric disorders. For example, fatigue may be related to anemia, but it also may be symptomatic of depression. Additionally, older individuals are more likely to report somatic symptoms rather than psychological ones, making identification of a mental disorder even more difficult.

The purpose of this chapter is to present a comprehensive geropsychiatric–mental health nursing assessment process that serves as the basis of care of elderly people (discussed in Chaps. 30 and 31.) A mental health assessment is necessary when psychiatric or mental health issues are identified or when patients with mental illnesses reach their later years (usually about age 65 years). The assessment generally follows the same format as described in Chapter 10. Because the overall health care issues for the elderly can be very complex, however, it follows that certain components of the geropsychiatric nursing assessment are unique. Thus, the geriatric assessment emphasizes some areas that are less critical to the standard adult assessment.

KEY CONCEPT   **Normal aging.** **Normal aging** is associated with some physical decline, such as decreased sensory abilities and decreased pulmonary and immune function, but many important functions do not change.

TECHNIQUES OF DATA COLLECTION

The nurse assesses the patient using an interview format that may take a few sessions to complete. He or she also may rely on self-report standardized tests, such as depression and cognitive functioning tools. A wide variety of physiologic disorders may cause changes in mental status for older adults; thus, results of laboratory tests are often significant. For example, urinalysis can detect a urinary tract infection that has affected a patient's cognitive status. Text Box 12-1 contains a representative listing of common physiologic causes of changes in mental status. Additionally, medical records from other health care providers are useful in developing a complete picture of the patient's health status.

An important source of patient data is family members, who often notice changes that the patient overlooks or fails to recognize. A patient with memory impairment may be unable to give an accurate history. By interviewing family members, the nurse expands the scope of the patient assessment. Moreover, the nurse has an opportunity to evaluate the caregivers themselves to determine whether they can care for the patient adequately and how they are coping with the situation. For example, a husband may be unable to care for his wife but is unwilling to admit it. If the nurse can establish rapport with the husband, the nurse may use the assessment interview as an opportunity to help the husband to examine his wife's care requirements realistically.

TEXT BOX 12.1

Common Causes of Changes in Mental Status

- Acid–base imbalance
- Dehydration
- Drugs (prescribed and over-the-counter)
- Electrolyte changes
- Hypothyroidism
- Hypothermia and hyperthermia
- Hypoxia
- Infection and sepsis

BIOPSYCHOSOCIAL GEROPSYCHIATRIC NURSING ASSESSMENT

KEY CONCEPT   **Biopsychosocial geropsychiatric nursing assessment.** A **biopsychosocial geropsychiatric nursing assessment** is the comprehensive, deliberate, and systematic collection and interpretation of biopsychosocial data that is based on the special needs and problems of elderly people to determine current and past health, functional status, and human responses to mental health problems, both actual and potential (Text Box 12-2).

At the beginning of the assessment, the nurse should determine the patient's ability to participate. For example, if a patient is using a wheelchair, he or she may have physical limitations that prevent full participation in the assessment. The patient must be able to hear the nurse. For a patient with compromised hearing, the nurse must attend to voice projection and volume. Shouting at the older patient is unnecessary. The nurse should remember to lower the pitch of his or her voice because higher-pitched sounds are often lost with presbycusis (loss of hearing sensitivity associated with aging). The nurse should eliminate distracting noises, such as from a television or radio, and ensure that the patient's hearing aid is in place and turned on. Facing the patient and using distinct enunciation will help lip-reading patients understand what is being said. Sometimes, deafness is mistaken for cognitive dysfunction. If a patient's hearing is questionable, the nurse should enlist the help of a speech and language specialist. Generally, the pace of the interview should mirror the patient's ability to move through the assessment. Usually, the pace will be slower than the nurse uses with younger populations.

Biologic Domain

Collecting and analyzing data for assessment of the biologic domain includes areas similar to those discussed in Chapter 10. The assessment components include present and past health status, physical examination results, physical functioning, and pharmacology review. When focusing on the biologic domain, the nurse pays special attention to the patient's general physical appearance as well as any observable manifestations of illness. The nurse should assess how all physical problems affect the patient's mental well-being. For example, pain and immobility are physical problems that can negatively affect mental health. Low energy level may be immediately apparent. Women with obvious osteoporosis are experiencing pain most of the time. Men undergoing radiation for prostate cancer worry about sexual functioning and urinary incontinence.

TEXT BOX 12.2

Biopsychosocial Geropsychiatric Nursing Assessment

I. Major reason for seeking help _____

II. Initial information

    Name _____

    Age _____ Current marital status _____

    Gender _____ Caregiver's name _____

    Living arrangements _____

III. Level of independence:

    High (needs no help) _____

    Moderate (lives independently, but needs some help with instrumental activities) _____

    Low (Relies on others for help in meeting functional and instrumental activities) _____

    Physical limitations _____

    Level of education completed _____

	Normal	Treated	Untreated
Physical functions: system review	☐	☐	☐
Activity/exercise	☐	☐	☐
Sleep patterns	☐	☐	☐
Appetite and nutrition	☐	☐	☐
Hydration	☐	☐	☐
Sexuality	☐	☐	☐
Existing physical illnesses	☐	☐	☐

List any chronic illnesses _____

Presence of pain (Use standardized instrument if pain is present.)   No _____   Yes _____

    Score _____ Treatment of pain _____

Medication (prescription and over-the-counter)	Dosage	Side Effects	Frequency

Significant Laboratory Tests	Values	Normal Range

(continued)

TEXT BOX 12.2 (*Continued*)

IV. Responses to mental health problems

    Major concerns regarding mental health problem _____

    Major loss/change in past year: No _____ Yes _____

    Fear of violence: No _____ Yes _____

    Strategies for managing problems/disorder _____

V. Mental status examination

    General observation (appearance, psychomotor activity, attitude) _____

    Orientation (time, place, person) _____

    Mood, affect, emotions (Geriatric Depression Scale should be used if evidence of depression)

    Speech (verbal ability, speed, use of words correctly) _____

    Thought processes (hallucinations, delusions, tangential, logic, repetition, rhyming of words, loose connections, disorganized) (*Describe content of hallucinations, delusions.*)

    Cognition and intellectual performance (*Use standardized test scores as well as observations.*)

    Attention and concentration _____

    Abstract reasoning and concentration _____

    Memory (recall, short-term, long-term) _____

    Judgment and insight _____

    (MMSE, CASI scores) _____

VI. Significant behaviors (psychomotor, agitation, aggression, withdrawn) (*Use standardized test if behaviors are problematic.*) _____

    When did problem behavior begin? Has it gotten worse? _____

VII. Self-concept (beliefs about self—body image, self-esteem, personal identity) _____

VIII. Risk assessment

    Suicide: High _____ Low _____ Assault/homicide: High _____ Low _____

    S*uicide* thoughts or ideation: No _____ Yes _____

      Current thoughts of harming self _____ Plan _____

      Means _____

      Means available

    Assault/homicide thoughts: No _____ Yes _____

      What do you do when angry with a stranger? _____

      What do you do when angry with family or partner? _____

      Have you ever hit or pushed anyone? No _____ Yes _____

      Have you ever been arrested for assault? No _____ Yes _____

      Current thoughts of harming others _____

IX. Functional status (*Use standardized test such as FAQ.*) _____

X. Cultural assessment

    Cultural group _____

    Cultural group's view of health and mental illness _____

    By what cultural rules do you try to live? _____

    Special, cultural foods that are important to you _____

XI. Stresses and coping behaviors _____

    Social support _____

    Family members _____

    Which members are important to you? _____

    On whom can you rely? _____

    Community resources _____

XII. Spiritual assessment _____

XIII. Economic status _____

TEXT BOX 12.2 (*Continued*)

XIV. Legal status_____

XV. Quality of life _____

Summary of significant data that can be used in formulating a nursing diagnosis:

SIGNATURE/TITLE_____ Date_____

Present and Past Health Status

A review of the patient's current health status includes examining health records as well as collecting information from the patient and family members. The nurse must identify chronic health problems that could affect mental health care. For example, the patient's management of diabetes mellitus could provide clues to the likelihood of complications such as retinopathy or neuropathy, which in turn will affect the patient's ability to follow a mental health treatment regimen. The must nurse must document a history of psychiatric treatment.

Physical Examination

The psychiatric nurse reviews the physical examination findings, paying special attention to recent laboratory values, such as urinalysis, white and red blood cell counts, and fasting blood glucose data (see Chap. 7). Results of neurologic tests could indicate compromise of the neuromuscular systems. Many psychiatric medications that may be prescribed lower the seizure threshold, making a history of seizures, which can cause behavior changes, an important assessment component. The nurse should note any evidence of movement disorders, such as tremors, abnormal movements, or shuffling. If a patient has been exposed to conventional antipsychotics, the nurse should consider assessment for symptoms of tardive dyskinesia, using one of the appropriate assessment tools (see Chap. 18 for further discussion of tardive dyskinesia).

The nurse should take routine vital signs during the assessment. He or she should note any abnormalities in blood pressure (ie, hypertension or hypotension) because many psychiatric medications affect blood pressure. Generally, these medications may cause orthostatic hypertension, which can lead to dizziness, unsteady gait, and falls. A baseline blood pressure is needed for future monitoring of medication side effects. Lying, sitting, and standing blood pressures are especially useful in assessing for orthostatic hypotension.

Physical Functions

The nurse must consider the patient's physical functioning within the context of the normal changes that accompany aging and the presence of any chronic disorders. The nurse should note the patient's use of any personal devices, such as canes, walkers, wheelchairs, or oxygen, or environmental devices, such as grab bars, shower benches, or hospital beds. Specific areas to consider are nutrition and eating, elimination, and sleep patterns.

Nutrition and Eating. Assessment of the type, amount, and frequency of food eaten is standard in any geriatric assessment. The nurse should note any weight loss of more than 10 pounds without trying. He or she must consider such nutrition changes in light of mental health problems. For example, is a patient's weight loss related to an underlying physical problem or to the patient's belief that she is being poisoned and is afraid to eat?

Eating is often difficult for elderly patients, who may suffer from lack of appetite. The nurse must assess eating and appetite patterns because many psychiatric medications can affect digestion and may further impair an already compromised gastrointestinal tract. A common problem of elderly people who live in nursing homes is **dysphagia**, or difficulty swallowing. Dysphagia can lead to dehydration, malnutrition, pneumonia, or asphyxiation. People who have been exposed to conventional antipsychotics (eg, haloperidol, chlorpromazine) are more likely to have symptoms of tardive dyskinesia. Swallowing can be difficult. Thus, the nurse should evaluate any patient who has been exposed to the older psychiatric medications for symptoms of tardive dyskinesia.

Xerostomia, or dry mouth, which is common in elderly people, also may impair eating. The nurse should pay particular attention to those who are currently receiving treatment for mental illnesses, particularly with medications that have anticholinergic properties. Dry mouth is also an anticholinergic side effect of many medications. Frequent rinsing with a nonalcohol-based mouthwash will help to correct the dry condition. Decreased taste or smell is common among elderly people and may reduce the pleasure of eating, so that the patient may eat less. Making meal times social and relaxing experiences can help the patient compensate for some of the loss of pleasure associated with decreased taste or smell. Preparing favorite foods will also enhance the quality of meals and meal times.

The nurse also must determine the patient's use of alcohol. Alcoholism is a growing problem in the elderly population. Estimates are that the prevalence of heavy drinking (12 to 21 drinks per week) in older adults is 3% to 9% (U.S. Department of Health and Human Services, 1999). The use of the CAGE questionnaire may be helpful in this area (see Chap. 25).

Elimination. The nurse must assess the patient's urinary and bowel functions. Elderly patients are more likely to experience constipation because the peristaltic movement of the bowels slows. Medications with anticholinergic properties can cause constipation, leading to fecal impaction. Abuse of laxatives is common among the elderly and requires evaluation. Adding fiber, although recommended for constipation, may cause bloating and excessive gas production. Elderly patients are also more likely to experience urinary frequency because the strength of the sphincter muscles decreases. Because many older adults reduce their fluid intake to manage urinary incontinence, fluid intake also becomes an important factor in assessing urinary functioning and constipation. The nurse should remember that urinary incontinence is a symptom of a disorder that requires follow-up and treatment.

Sleep. During the normal aging process, sleep patterns change, and patients often sleep less than they did when younger. The nurse must assess any recent changes in sleep patterns and evaluate whether they are related to normal aging or are symptomatic of an underlying disorder. **Insomnia**, the inability to fall or remain asleep throughout the night, can lead to increased risk for depression and regular use of sleep medications. Patients with insomnia report that they cannot sleep at night and do not feel rested in the morning. They often sleep during the day. In one study of 2,398 noninstitutionalized individuals aged 65 years and older, 36% of men and 54% of women had insomnia (Maggi et al., 1998). Sleep problems are also often linked to the use of alcohol. If a patient reports sleep problems, the nurse should ask about the patient's use of alcohol, over-the-

counter medications, and prescription drugs (Tabloski & Church, 1999) (Research Box 12-1).

Pain

Elders are more likely to experience pain than younger adults because they are at increased risk for chronic illness and may be suffering from the consequences of a lifetime of injuries. For many elders, pain is a constant companion. The experience of chronic pain often contributes to unexplained behavior and personality changes. To assess pain, the nurse can use many pain instruments. One of the most popular is the Wong-Baker faces pain rating scale initially developed for children but now used for all age groups (Fig. 12-1). This scale is especially useful in communicating with people from different cultures and languages than the nurse. See Chapter 34 for further discussion of pain.

Assessment of pain is especially critical for those elders who are cognitively impaired and living in long-term care institutions. One study determined the relationship between cognitive status of elderly people and

RESEARCH BOX 12.1

Insomnia, Alcohol, and Drug Use

Insomnia is a common complaint of older people, and they frequently use alcohol and over-the-counter or prescription medications as sedatives. The potential for adverse drug and alcohol interactions is a serious threat to health and functional status. This research study examined the use of alcohol and medications in a retrospective sample of community resident elderly people with sleep complaints. The sample consisted of 19 people ranging in age from 65 to 88 years who reported daily alcohol consumption. The most commonly voiced reason for seeking care was related to problems of the central nervous system, including depression, anxiety, and memory loss or forgetfulness. Other problems included urinary incontinence or retention, unexplained falls, bruises, trauma, and pain. Eighteen of the 19 people (95%) were using medications that adversely interact with alcohol. Sixteen of the 19 (84%) reported sleep problems, and sleep maintenance was the most common complaint.

Utilization in Clinical Setting: Nurses should ask patients aged 65 years and older who report insomnia about their use of alcohol, over-the-counter drugs, and prescription drugs. They should carefully assess patients for drug and alcohol interactions during the initial health history. Nurses should encourage patients to try nonpharmacologic sleep interventions first.

Tabloski, P. A., & Church, O. M. (1999). Insomnia, alcohol and drug use in community-residing elderly persons. *Journal of Substance Use, 4*(3), 147–154.

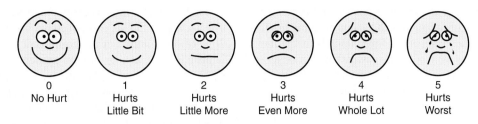

Wong-Baker Rating Scale

Each face represents a person who is happy or sad depending on how much or how little pain he/she has:

0   "a person who is very happy because he/she doesn't hurt at all"
1   "it hurts just a little bit"
2   "it hurts a little more"
3   "it hurts even more"
4   "it hurts a whole lot"
5   "it hurts as much as you can imagine, but you don't have to be crying to feel this bad"

Subject ID #:_____ Date: ___/___/___ Visit #_____

Pt. name:_____

RA:_____

FIGURE 12.1 Wong-Baker rating scale for pain assessment.

pain medication orders and administration through a retrospective medication review of residents' charts (Kaasalainen et al., 1998). The pain ratings of 25 registered nurses using a visual analogue scale were correlated with pain medications given to residents on the day of the ratings. Results indicated that the nurses' ratings of residents' pain and administration of pain medications were not significantly related. Residents with cognitive impairment were prescribed significantly fewer scheduled medications and received significantly fewer pain medications (either PRN or scheduled) than those without cognitive impairment. The study theorized that nurses based their medication administration on verbal reports of pain. Because residents with cognitive impairment could not verbalize their pain, they subsequently did not receive pain medication. These results indicate that pain is underrecognized and undertreated in elderly people with cognitive impairment.

Pharmacologic Assessment

One of the most important areas of the biologic domain is the pharmacologic assessment. **Polypharmacy**, the concurrent use of several different medications, is common in elderly people. The nurse must ask the patient and family to list all medications and times that the patient takes them. Asking family members to bring in all the medications the patient is taking, including over-the-counter medications, vitamins, and herbal supplements, is a good idea. Because elderly people are more sensitive to medications, the possibility of drug-to-drug interactions is greater. When considering potential drug interactions, the nurse should ask the patient about

the consumption of large amounts of grapefruit juice, which contains narginin, an inhibitor of the CYP3A4 enzyme involved in the metabolism of many medications (eg, antidepressants, antiarrhythmics, erythromycin, several statins).

Psychological Domain

Assessment of the psychological domain provides the nurse with the opportunity to identify limitations, behavior symptoms, and reactions to illness. The nurse assesses many of the same areas as in other adult assessments, but again, the emphasis may be different. The following discussion focuses on the responses of elderly patients to mental health problems, mental status examination, behavior changes, stress and coping patterns, and risk assessments.

Responses to Mental Health Problems

Many elderly patients are reluctant to admit that they have psychiatric symptoms, particularly if their culture stigmatizes mental illness. They may also fear that if they admit to any symptoms, they may be placed outside their home. If patients do not recognize or admit to having psychiatric symptoms, their vulnerability to being taken advantage of or injured increases.

Throughout the assessment, the nurse evaluates the patient's verbal reports, obvious symptoms, and family reports. It is not unusual for a patient to deny having any mental or emotional problems. If a patient flatly denies any psychiatric symptoms (eg, depression, mood swings, outbursts of anger, memory problems), the nurse should respectfully accept the patient's answer and avoid arguments or confrontation (see the accompanying Therapeutic Dialogue: Assessment Interview). If the patient's family members contradict the patient's report or symptoms are obvious during the interview, the nurse can approach the issue while planning care.

Mental Status Examination

The areas of special interest in the mental status examination are mood and affect, thought processes, and cognitive functioning. The nurse should interpret the results in light of any accompanying physical problems, such as chronic pain, or life changes, such as loss of a spouse.

Mood and Affect. Depression in elderly people is common and associated with the following risk factors: loss of spouse, physical illness, education below high school, impaired functional status, and heavy alcohol consumption. In older people, other disorders may mask depression. When symptoms are present, they may be attributed to normal aging or atherosclerosis or other age-related problems. Older patients are less likely to report feeling sad or worthless than are younger patients. As a result, family members and primary care providers often overlook depression in elderly patients.

Depressive symptoms are much more common than a full-fledged DSM-IV depressive disorder. Eight to 20% of older adults in the community and up to 37% in primary care settings suffer from depressive symptoms (U.S. Department of Health and Human Services, 1999). The term *late-onset depression* refers to the development of depression or depressive symptoms that impair functioning after 60 years of age. In late-onset depression, the risk for recurrence is relatively high. Once identified, treatment is effective in 60% to 80% of cases, but the response generally takes longer than that for other adults (U.S. Department of Health and Human Services, 1999).

The Geriatric Depression Scale (GDS) is a useful screening tool with demonstrated validity and reliability (Hyer & Blount, 1984). The GDS was designed as a self-administered test, although it has been used in observer-administered formats as well. One advantage of the test is its "yes/no" format, which may be easier for older adults than the Hamilton Rating Scale for Depression (HAM-D), which uses a scale from 0 to 4 (see Chap. 20). The original GDS developed by Brink and Yesavage in 1982 consisted of 30 items. In 1986, Sheikh and Yesavage developed the shorter 15-item GDS to improve efficiency with no important loss of accuracy. This tool is easy to ad-

---

THERAPEUTIC DIALOGUE | **Assessment Interview**

Tom, 79-years-old, is being seen for the first time in a geropsychiatric clinic because of recent changes in his behavior and his accusations that family members are trying to steal his house and car. He locked his wife out of the house, accusing her of being unfaithful. When Susan, the psychiatric nurse assigned to his case, is conducting the assessment interview, Tom cooperates and is very pleasant until the nurse begins to assess the psychological domain.

Ineffective Approach

Nurse: Have there been times when you have had problems with any members of your family?
Patient: No. (Silence)
Nurse: Have you noticed that lately you have been getting more upset than usual?
Patient: No. Who has been talking to you?
Nurse: Your wife seems to think that you may be getting a little more upset than usual.
Patient: You are just like her. She keeps telling me something is wrong with me. (Getting very agitated)
Nurse: Please, I'm trying to help you. I understand that you locked your wife out of the house last week.
Patient: Leave me alone. (Gets up and leaves)

Effective Approach:

Nurse: How have things been going at home?
Patient: All right.
Nurse: (Silence)
Patient: Well, my wife and I sometimes argue.

Nurse: Oh. Most husbands and wives argue. Any special arguments?
Patient: No, just the usual. I don't pick up after myself enough. I don't dress right to suit her. But, lately, she's gone a lot.
Nurse: She is gone a lot?
Patient: Yeah! A lot.
Nurse: The way you say that, it sounds like you have some feelings about her being gone.
Patient: You're damned right I do—and you would, too.
Nurse: I'm missing something.
Patient: Well, if you must know, I think she's having an affair with the man next door.
Nurse: Really? That must upset you to think your wife is having an affair.
Patient: I am devastated. I feel so bad.
Nurse: Would you say that you are depressed?
Patient: Well, wouldn't you be? Yes, I'm feeling pretty low.

Critical Thinking Challenge

- How do the very first questions differ in the two interviews?

- What therapeutic techniques did the nurse use in the second interview to avoid the pitfalls the nurse encountered in the first scenario?

- How did the nurse in the second scenario elicit the patient's delusion about his wife's affair?

- From the data that the second nurse gathered, how many patient problems can be identified?

minister and provides valuable information about the possibility of depression (Text Box 12-3). If results are positive, the nurse should refer the patient to a psychiatrist or advanced practice nurse for further evaluation.

Among nursing home residents, the usefulness of the GDS depends on the degree of cognitive impairment. Residents who are mildly impaired may be able to answer yes/no questions; however, moderately to severely impaired patients will be unable to do the same. The best validated scale for patients with dementia is the Cornell Scale for Depression in Dementia (CSDD) (Alexopoulos et al., 1998). The CSDD is an interview-administered scale that uses information both from the patient and an outside informant.

Anxiety is another important mood for nurses to assess in elderly people because it can interfere with normal functioning. In dementia, anxiety is common, with prevalence rates varying from 12% to 50% (Absher & Cummings, 1994). The Rating Anxiety in Dementia (RAID) scale was developed as a global scale to assess anxiety in patients with dementia (Shankar et al., 1999). The domains that the RAID scale assesses include worry, apprehension and vigilance, motor tension, autonomic hyperactivity, and phobias and panic attacks (see Appendix D for a copy of the RAID scale).

Thought Processes. Thought processes and content are critical in the assessment of elderly patients. Can the patient express ideas and thoughts logically? Can the patient understand questions and follow the conversation of others? If the patient shows any indication of hallucinations or delusions, the nurse should explore the content of the hallucination or delusion. If the patient has a history of mental illness such as schizophrenia, these symptoms may be familiar to family members, who can validate whether they are old or new problems. If this is the first time the patient has experienced these abnormal thought processes, the nurse should further evaluate the content. Suspicious and delusional thoughts that characterize dementia often include some of the following beliefs:

- People are stealing my things.
- The house is not my house.
- My relative is an impostor.

If a patient shares any such thoughts, the nurse can complete further assessment by using the Behavioral Pathology in Alzheimer's Disease rating scale (BEHAVE-AD). This 25-item scale is based on caregivers' reports within the previous 2 weeks (Reisberg & Ferris, 1985). The BEHAVE-AD measures thought and behavior disturbances in seven major categories, with each item scored on a four-point scale of severity (0 to 3), including delusions, hallucinations, activity disturbances, aggressiveness, diurnal rhythm disturbances, mood disturbances, and anxieties and phobias. The BEHAVE-AD also contains a four-point global assessment of the overall magnitude of the behavior symptoms in terms of disturbance to the caregiver, dangerousness to the patient, or both. The reliability of the BEHAVE-AD (.95 and .96; $p < .01$) is comparable to that of the Mini-Mental State Examination (Reisberg et al., 1996). A copy of the BEHAVE-AD is found in Appendix E.

TEXT BOX 12.3

Geriatric Depression Scale (Short Form)

1. Are you basically satisfied with your life?	Yes	No
2. Have you dropped many of your activities and interests?	Yes	No
3. Do you feel that your life is empty?	Yes	No
4. Do you often get bored?	Yes	No
5. Are you in good spirits most of the time?	Yes	No
6. Are you afraid that something bad is going to happen to you?	Yes	No
7. Do you feel happy most of the time?	Yes	No
8. Do you often feel helpless?	Yes	No
9. Do you prefer to stay at home rather than go out and do new things?	Yes	No
10. Do you feel you have more problems with memory than most?	Yes	No
11. Do you think it is wonderful to be alive now?	Yes	No
12. Do you feel pretty worthless the way you are now?	Yes	No
13. Do you feel full of energy?	Yes	No
14. Do you feel that your situation is hopeless?	Yes	No
15. Do you think that most people are better off than you are?	Yes	No

*Score:*___/15   One point for "No" to questions 1, 5, 7, 11, 13

One point for "Yes" to other questions

Normal	3 ± 2
Mildly depressed	7 ± 3
Very depressed	12 ± 2

Adapted from Sheikh, J. I., & Yesavage, J. A. Geriatric depression scale (GDS): Recent evidence and development of a shorter version. In T. L. Brink (Ed.), *Clinical gerontology: A guide to assessment and intervention* (pp. 165–173). Binghamton, NY: Haworth Press, 1986. © By The Haworth Press, Inc. All rights reserved. Reprinted with permission.

Cognition and Intellectual Performance. Cognitive functioning includes such parameters as orientation, attention, short- and long-term memory, consciousness, and executive functioning. Intellectual functioning, also considered a cognitive measure, is rarely formally assessed with a standardized intelligence test in elderly people. Considerable variability among individuals depends on lifestyle and psychosocial factors (Gottlieb, 1995).

Some changes in cognitive capacity accompany aging, but important functions are spared. Normal cognitive changes during aging include a slowing of information processing and memory retrieval. Abnormalities of consciousness, orientation, judgment, speech, or language are not related to age, but to underlying neuropathologic changes. Cognitive changes in elderly people are associated with delirium or dementia (see Chap. 31) or schizophrenia (see Chap. 18).

The assessment includes the number of years of education. An inverse relationship between Alzheimer's disease and the number of years of education exists. When assessing cognitive functioning, the nurse should use standardized instruments and not rely on observations or chart documentation (Research Box 12-2) (Souder & Sullivan, 2000). Of such instruments, the

RESEARCH BOX 12.2

Nursing Documentation Versus Standardized Assessment

Although the literature discusses the importance of assessing cognitive status, few studies have explored the concordance of nurses' documentation of cognitive status and standardized assessment. This study examined nurses' documentation of cognitive status in 42 medically hospitalized individuals (mean age, 51.9 years; SD, 10.1 years) using various standardized measures. Although the chart review revealed no documentation of impaired cognitive status, it identified impaired performance in 24% to 67% of the cognitive measures. This study suggests nurses are missing cognitive impairment in hospitalized patients by limiting assessment to orientation. Use of a combination of several brief screening measures, such as the clock-drawing test and the standardized Mini-Mental State Examination (MMSE), would provide timely, effective, and inexpensive assessment of cognitive status (abstract).

Utilization in Clinical Setting: This article supports the use of standardized instruments in assessing cognitive status.

Souder, E., & O'Sullivan, P. S. (2000). Nursing documentation versus standardized assessment of cognitive status in hospitalized medical patients. *Applying Nursing Research, 13*(1), 29–36.

Mini-Mental State Examination (MMSE) discussed in Chapter 10 is most widely used in screening for cognitive functioning related to dementia. Various studies suggest that an MMSE score below 24 of 30 has a reasonable sensitivity (80% to 90%) and specificity (80%) for discriminating between those with dementia and those without. Some data, however, suggest that the MMSE may have a built-in bias against those with fewer than 8 years of education or among those who belong to ethnic minority groups (Mulgrew et al., 1999).

Evidence suggests that severe cognitive deterioration may occur in elderly people with schizophrenia. In assessing the cognitive status of this population, the Cognitive Abilities Screening Instrument (CASI) demonstrates greater specificity than the MMSE (Sherrell et al., 1999). The CASI is a 25-item instrument test developed and piloted in Japan and the United States (Teng et al., 1994). The total score ranges from 0 to 100, with a suggested cutoff of 74 for classifying dementia. The CASI provides quantitative assessment of nine domains: attention, concentration, orientation, long-term memory, short-term memory, language, visual construction (copying pentagons), fluency (naming four-legged animals), and abstraction and judgment. Developed as a research instrument, it is now being recommended as a useful clinical assessment tool in determining level of cognitive impairment and could be used in establishing individualized care plans. A copy of the CASI is found in Appendix F.

Behavior Changes

Behavior changes in elderly people can indicate neuropathologic processes and thus require nursing assessment. If such changes occur, it is most likely that family members will notice them before the patient. Apraxis (inability to initiate motor movement) is not attributed to age, but indicates an underlying disease process such as Alzheimer's disease, Parkinson's disease, or other disorders. Various other behavior problems are associated with psychiatric disorders in elderly people, including irritability, agitation, apathy, and euphoria. Other behaviors in elderly people who are experiencing psychiatric problems include wandering, aggressive behaviors. The BEHAVE-AD identifies these behaviors.

The Neuropsychiatric Inventory (NPI) was developed in 1994 to assess behavior problems associated with dementia. The scale assesses 10n behavior problems: delusions, hallucinations, dysphoria, anxiety, agitation/aggression, euphoria, inhibition, irritability/lability, apathy, and aberrant motor behavior (Cummings et al., 1994). This very popular tool is used in many medication clinical trials. There are two versions. The standard version is used when the patient is still at home, whereas a different version is used when the patient is in a nursing home.

Stress and Coping Patterns

Identifying stresses and coping patterns is just as important for elderly patients as it is for younger adults. Unique stresses for elderly patients include living on a fixed income, handling declining health, losing partners and friends, and ultimately confronting death. Coping ability varies among patients depending on their unique circumstances. For example, some patients respond to stressful events with amazing adaptability, whereas others become depressed and suicidal.

Loss of a spouse is common in late life. Estimates are that 800,000 older Americans lose their spouses each year (U.S. Department of Health and Human Services, 1999). Bereavement, a natural response to the death of a loved one, includes crying and sorrow, anxiety and agitation, insomnia, and loss of appetite. These symptoms, while overlapping with major depression, do not constitute a mental disorder. Only when these symptoms persist for 2 months or longer can a diagnosis of either adjustment disorder or major depressive disorder be made (American Psychiatric Association, 2000). Although a normal response, the nurse must identify bereavement and develop interventions to help the individual successfully resolve the loss. Bereavement is an important and well-established risk factor for depression. At least 10% to 20% of widows and widowers develop symptoms of depression during the first year of bereavement. Without interventions, depression can persist, become chronic, and lead to further disability (U.S. Department of Health and Human Services, 1999). It also can lead to other serious health problems.

Risk Assessment

Suicide is a major mental health risk for the elderly. Suicide rates increase with age, with older white men having a rate of suicide six times that of the general population. The highest suicide rates are for white men older than 85 years of age (68.2 per 100,000). Most elderly people who commit suicide have visited their primary care physician in the month before their death (see Web Links for the Centers for Disease Control and Prevention website).

When caring for the elderly patient with mental health problems, the nurse always should consider the patient's potential to commit suicide. Depression is the greatest risk factor for suicide. In assessing an elderly patient, the nurse should consider the following characteristics as indications of high risk for committing suicide:

- Depression
- Attempted suicide in the past
- Family history of suicide
- Firearms in the home
- Abuse of alcohol or other substances
- Unusual stress

- Chronic medical condition (eg, cancer, neuromuscular disorders)
- Social isolation

Social Domain

Assessment of the social domain includes determining the patient's interactions with others in his or her family and community. The nurse targets social support because it is so important to the well-being of older adults, functional status because of the potential physical changes that can affect this area, and social systems, which encompasses all community resources.

Social Support

Remaining active throughout one's life is one of the best predictors of mental health and wellness in an elderly patient. People obtain their sense of self-worth through their interactions with others in their environment. A sense of "who one is" is closely tied to the roles that a person plays in life. When older adults relinquish such roles because of physical disabilities, become isolated from friends and family, or begin to sense that they are a burden to those around them rather than contributing members of society, a sense of hopelessness and helplessness often follows.

The role of social support is critical to assess in this age group. Social support is a reciprocal concept, meaning that simply receiving assistance increases the person's sense of being a burden. Those elders who also believe that they contribute to the welfare of others are most likely to remain mentally healthy. For this reason, pets are often "life savers" for older adults who live alone. Nothing can be more understanding and accepting of an older adult's behavior or disabilities than a beloved pet.

The nurse should assess the patient's number of formal and informal social contacts. The nurse should ask about the frequency of contacts with others (in person and through telephone, letters, and cards) that the patient has (see Chap. 6). Determining whether these contacts are actually satisfying and supporting to the patient is essential. If family members are important to the patient's well-being, the nurse should complete a more in-depth family assessment (see Chap. 16).

The nurse can use the following questions to focus on social support (Kane, 1995):

- In the past 2 weeks, how often would you say that others let you know that they care about you?
- In the past 2 weeks, how often has someone provided you with help, such as giving you a ride somewhere or helping around the house?
- Do you have any one special person you could call or contact if you needed help? Who?
- In general, other than your children, how many relatives do you feel close to and have contact with at least once a month?

For patients who are isolated with few social contacts, the nurse can develop interventions to improve social support.

Functional Status

As part of a complete assessment, the nurse will need to assess the older adult's functional status. **Functional activities** or activities of daily living (ADLs) are those activities necessary for self-care (ie, bathing, toileting, dressing, and transferring). **Instrumental activities** of daily living (IADLs) include those that facilitate or enhance the performance of ADLs (ie, shopping, using the telephone, using transportation). These aspects are critical to consider for any older adult living alone. The most common tools used to assess functional status are the Index of Independence in Activities of Daily Living and the Instrumental Activities of Daily Living scale (Katz, 1976). The Functional Activities Questionnaire (FAQ) measures the adult's functional abilities based on information from family members and caregivers. The older person is rated on 10 complex, higher-order activities, such as writing checks, assembling tax records, and driving (Costa et al., 1996).

Social Systems

Community resources are essential to an older adult's ability to maintain mental health and wellness as well as to his or her ability to remain at home throughout the later years. Senior centers are federally funded community resources that provide a wide array of services to the nation's elderly. They provide daily balanced meals at a nominal cost. In addition, they provide opportunities for socialization, which is key to combating loneliness and social isolation. Many senior centers provide annual influenza and pneumonia vaccination clinics and education opportunities on such topics as fall prevention and recognition and prevention of elder abuse. Additional community resources that are specific to elderly people include geriatric assessment clinics and adult day care centers.

During the assessment, the nurse must determine which community resources are available and if the elderly patient uses them. Lack of transportation to and from these community resources may be a barrier to their effective use. Most communities have buses available for elderly or handicapped individuals. The nurse may need to assist the elder in accessing this important resource.

Many elderly citizens rely on the Social Security Administration for their monthly income. For many elders, this financial support, although less than adequate in most instances, is their only source of income. In addition to Social Security, the federal government provides basic health care coverage in the form of the state-administered Medicare program. Together, these programs contribute to the patient's ability to live independently and receive health care. The nurse should assess a patient's sources of financial support. Sometimes, nurses are uncomfortable asking for financial information, fearing that they are invading the patient's privacy. Such data, however, are important for the nurse to determine whether a patient's resources adequately meet his or her needs. The source of financial support is also important. For example, a patient whose income is adequate and from personal resources is more likely to be independent than the patient who depends on family members for income.

The nurse should ask the patient about accessible clinics, support groups, and pharmaceutical services. Information about available health care resources can provide useful data regarding the patient's ability to access services and can also provide potential referral sources. In urban areas that are likely to have adequate health care resources, cultural and language barriers may prohibit access. People who live in rural areas where health care resources are limited are less likely to enjoy the full range of health care resources than those in urban areas. Even in rural areas with mental health services, the use of these services by elderly people with mental illnesses is low (Neese et al., 1999). If elders are married and have insurance, they are more likely to seek mental health services.

Spiritual Assessment

Spiritual needs are basic for all age groups and are requirements for establishing meaning and purpose, love and relatedness, and forgiveness. The 1971 White House Conference on Aging affirmed that all people are spiritual, even if they do not rely on religious institutions or practice no personal pieties (Fish & Shelly, 1978). Aging is a process that can bring one closer to understanding the finite nature of existence. With advanced age, many people begin to reflect on their successes and failures. During such reflection, many seek out God or a higher being to make sense of the past and establish hope for the future.

The process of spiritual assessment involves active listening, thoughtful observing, and sensitive questioning. The nurse may simply ask if the elder would find comfort from a visit from a spiritual leader. Many forms of religion use various rituals that are important to the elder's daily routine. The nurse should explore and honor these aspects to the extent possible.

Legal Status

A growing trend in the United States is to view the elderly as a special population whose rights deserve increased attention. Instances of elder abuse are far too common. Every nurse must consider himself or herself a patient advocate and be vigilant in recognizing the signs of neglect or abuse, such as unexplained injuries.

TEXT BOX 12.4

Rights of Older Adults

- Right to individualized care
- Right to be free from neglect and abuse
- Right to privacy
- Right to be free from discrimination
- Right to visit and freely associate
- Right to have access to community resources
- Right to vote
- Right to sue
- Right to enter into contracts
- Right to obtain a will
- Right to practice religion of choice
- Right to marry
- Right to control funds

Adapted from Aiken, T. D. (1999). Legal issues affecting older adults. In M. Stanley & P. Beare (Eds.), *Gerontological nursing: A health promotion/ protection approach* (p. 44). Philadelphia: F. A. Davis.

At times, abuse can take the form of another individual usurping the rights of the older person. Unless an individual is determined to be incompetent, he or she has the same rights to personal decision making as any other adult, including the right to refuse treatment. Text Box 12-4 lists many of the common rights of older adults (Aiken, 1999).

Quality of Life

Sense of quality of life is closely tied to values and beliefs. For many elders, quality of life is not reflected in material possessions or physical health. At this stage, quality of life is connected more with contentment over how the person has lived life and the extent to which his or her life has had meaning and purpose. Keeping close personal contacts with friends and family and having the opportunity to shares stories of lifetime experiences are essential to maintaining mental health and wellness for older adults. For elderly people, physical illnesses may affect the quality of life more than psychiatric disorders. The assessment of quality of life becomes especially important when assessing a patient living in a nursing home or isolated in his or her own home. The assessment of quality of life of the elderly is similar to that for younger adults (see Chap. 10).

Summary of Key Points

➤ Normal aging is associated with some physical decline, but most functions do not change. Intellectual functioning, capacity for change, and productive engagement with life remain stable.

➤ Mental health assessments are necessary when elderly patients face psychiatric or mental health issues. The biopsychosocial geropsychiatric nursing assessment examines many sources of data, including self-reports, laboratory test results, and reports from family members.

➤ The biopsychosocial geropsychiatric nursing assessment is based on the special needs and problems of the elderly. This assessment examines current and past health, functional status, and human responses to mental health problems.

➤ Assessment of the biologic domain involves collecting data about past and present health status, physical examination findings, physical functions (ie, nutrition and eating, elimination patterns, sleep), pain, and pharmacologic information.

➤ Assessment of the psychological domain includes the patient's responses to mental health problems, mental status examination, behavioral changes, stress and coping patterns, and risk assessment.

➤ When conducting an assessment, the nurse may find several tools useful. For patients with possible depression, the Geriatric Depression Scale (GDS) may be helpful. For patients with anxiety, nurses can use the Rating Anxiety in Dementia (RAID) scale. In addition to a careful interview, the nurse can use the Rating Anxiety in Dementia (BEHAVE-AD) scale to determine delusions, hallucinations, activity disturbances, aggressiveness, diurnal rhythm disturbances, mood disturbances, anxieties, or phobias.

➤ The nurse can conduct cognitive assessment using the Mini-Mental State Examination (MMSE) or the Cognitive Abilities Screening Instrument (CASI).

➤ Coping with the stresses of aging varies among patients. Determining stresses and coping skills for dealing with stresses is important.

➤ Social support is critical to patients in this age group and requires assessment.

➤ Determination of the patient's ability to perform functional and instrumental activities of daily living is critical in the assessment of the elderly. The Functional Activities Questionnaire (FAQ) measures the functional abilities based on information from others.

➤ Social systems, spiritual assessment, legal information, and quality of life are components within the social domain that the nurse should consider.

Critical Thinking Challenges

1. You are asked to provide a 1-hour presentation to your community senior citizens group on mental health and wellness. Describe the key points you would emphasize in your presentation.

2. An older adult brings 60, 70, or 80 years of history to the assessment. Describe the approach you would take to elicit the most important information needed to develop an individualized plan of care for your elderly patient.

3. An older adult is telling you that children are in her room at night. She does not mind that they are there, but they keep her up all night. How would you assess this perceptual experience? What other data should you gather from this patient?

4. A caregiver brings a sack of medications to the patient's assessment interview. What information should you obtain from the caregiver regarding the patient's use of these medications?

5. A woman brings her father, who has a long history of frequent psychiatric hospitalizations for depression, to the clinic. The patient's wife recently died, and the daughter fears that her father is becoming depressed again. What approach would you use in assessing for changes in mood?

6. Obtain a listing of the social services available in your community. Examine the list for areas of duplication and omission of services needed by an older adult living alone in his or her own home.

WEB LINKS

www.alzheimers.org   The Alzheimer's Association website contains assessment tools.

www.cdc.gov   The Centers for Disease Control and Prevention website contains up-to-date statistical demographic and health data.

www.aarp.org   The American Association of Retired Persons has a wealth of links on this website.

www.surgeongeneral.com   The Surgeon General's website contains all major documents related to health care published by the U.S. government.

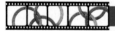

MOVIES

On Golden Pond: 1981. In this classic film, Henry Fonda portrays a crotchety, retired professor named Norman Thayer. Norman is angry that he is 80-years-old and scared that he may lose his cognitive abilities. His wife, played by Katherine Hepburn, provides support and encouragement in maintaining his independence. The story revolves around Norman's relationship with his estranged daughter (played by Jane Fonda) as they try finally to understand each other during Norman's later years.

Viewing Points: Identify the physical impairments that are obvious throughout the movie. Identify specific memory problems that Norman experiences. Are these problems part of normal aging? If you were Norman Thayer's nurse, what key assessment areas would you explore?

REFERENCES

Absher, J. R., & Cummings, J. L. (1994). Cognitive and non-cognitive aspects of dementia syndrome: An overview. In A. Burns & R. Levy (Eds.), *Dementia* (pp. 59–76). London: Chapman & Hall.

Aiken, T. D. (1999). Legal issues affecting older adults. In M. Stanley & P. Beare (Eds.), *Gerontological nursing: A health promotion/protection approach* (p. 44). Philadelphia: F. A. Davis.

Alexopoulos, G. S., Abrams, R. C., Young, R. C., et al. (1998). Cornell scale for depression in dementia. *Biological Psychiatry, 23,* 271–284.

American Psychiatric Association (APA). (2000). *Diagnostic and statistical manual of mental disorders* (4th ed., Text revision). Washington, DC: Author.

Costa, P. T., Williams, R. F., Somerfield, M., et al. (1996). Recognition and initial assessment of Alzheimer's disease and related dementias. No. 19, AHCPR Publication No. 97-0703. Rockville, MD: U.S. Department of Health and Human Services. Public Health Service, Agency for Health Care Policy and Research.

Cummings, J. L., Mega, M., Gray, K., et al. (1994). The Neuropsychiatric Inventory: Comprehensive assessment of psychopathology in dementia. *Neurology, 44*(12), 2308–2314.

Fish, S., & Shelley, J. A. (1978). *Spiritual care: The nurse's role.* Downers Grove, IL: InterVarsity.

Gottlieb, G. L. (1995). Geriatric psychiatry. In H. H. Goldman (Ed.), *Review of general psychiatry* (4th ed., pp 483–491). Norwalk, CT: Appleton & Lange.

Hyer, L., & Blount, J. (1984). Concurrent and discriminant validities of the geriatric depression scale with older psychiatric inpatients. *Psychological Reports, 54,* 611–616.

Kaasalainen, S., Middleton, J., Knezacek, S., et al. (1998). Pain and cognitive status in the institutionalized elderly: Perceptions and interventions. *Journal of Gerontological Nursing, 24*(8), 24–31, 50–51.

Kane, R. A. (1995). Assessment of social functioning: Recommendations for comprehensive geriatric assessment. In Z. Rubenstein, D. Wieland, & R. Bernabei (Eds.), *Geriatric assessment technology: The state of the art* (pp. 91–110). New York: Springer.

Katz, S., & Akpom, A. (1976). A measure of primary socio-biological functions. *International Journal of Health Science, 6,* 493.

Maggi, S., Langlois, J. A., Minicuci, N., et al. (1998). Sleep complaints in community-dwelling older persons: Prevalence, associated factors, and reported causes. *Journal of the American Geriatric Society, 46*(2), 161–168.

Mulgrew, C., Morgenstern, N., Shetterly, S., et al. (1999). Cognitive functioning and impairment among rural elderly Hispanics and Non-Hispanic whites as assessed by the Mini-Mental State Examination. *Journal of Gerontology, 54B*(4), 223–230.

Neese, J. B., Abraham, I. L., & Buckwalter, K. C. (1999). Utilization of mental health services among rural elderly. *Archives of Psychiatric Nursing, 13*(1), 30–40.

Reisberg, B., & Ferris, S. (1985). A clinical rating scale for symptoms of psychosis in Alzheimer's disease. *Psychopharmacology Bulletin, 21*, 101–104.

Reisberg, B., Auer, S., & Monteiro, I. (1996). Behavioral pathology in Alzheimer's disease (BEHAVE-AD) rating scale. *International Psychogeriatrics, 8*(3), 301–308.

Shankar, K. K., Walker, M., Frost, D., & Orrell, M. W. (1999). The development of a valid and reliable scale for rating anxiety in dementia (RAID). *Aging & Mental Health, 3*(1), 39–49.

Sheikh, J. I., & Yesavage, J. A. (1986). Geriatric depression scale (GDS): Recent evidence and development of a shorter version. In T. L. Brink (Ed.), *Clinical gerontology: A guide to assessment and interventions* (pp. 165–177). Binghamton, NY: Haworth Press.

Sherrell, K., Buckwalter, K., Bode, R., & Strozdas, L. (1999). Use of the cognitive abilities screen instrument to assess elderly persons with schizophrenia in long-term care settings. *Issues in Mental Health Nursing, 20*, 541–558.

Souder, E., & O'Sullivan, P. S. (2000). Nursing documentation versus standardized assessment of cognitive status in hospitalized medical patients. *Applying Nursing Research, 13*(1), 29–36.

Tabloski, P. A., & Church, O. M. (1999). Insomnia, alcohol and drug use in community-residing elderly persons. *Journal of Substance Use, 4*(3), 147–154.

Teng, E., Kazuo Hasegawa, K., Homma, A., et al. (1994). The cognitive abilities screen instrument (CASI): A practical test for cross-cultural epidemiological studies of dementia. *International Psychogeriatrics, 6*(1), 45–58.

U.S. Department of Health and Human Services. (1999). *Mental health: A report of the Surgeon General.* Rockville, MD: U.S. Department of Health and Human Services, Substance Abuse and Mental Health Services Administration, Center for Mental Health Services. National Institutes of Health, National Institute of Mental Health.

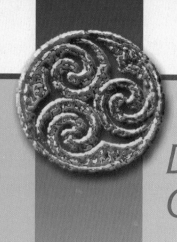

Diagnosis and Outcomes Development

Doris Bell

DERIVING NURSING DIAGNOSES

DEVELOPING PATIENT OUTCOMES
Evolution of Patient Outcomes

Purpose of Patient Outcomes and Indicators
Nursing Process and Patient Outcomes
Types of Patient Outcomes

EVALUATION

After studying this chapter, you will be able to:

- ➤ Discuss the use of nursing diagnosis.
- ➤ Define patient outcomes.
- ➤ Discuss the relationship between development of patient outcomes and quality care.
- ➤ Describe the steps in identification of outcomes.
- ➤ Identify the American Nurses Association psychiatric–mental health nurse standards for outcome identification.
- ➤ Define indicators and their use.
- ➤ Describe nurse-sensitive outcomes.
- ➤ Describe the relationship between patient outcomes and indicators.
- ➤ Discuss use of patient outcomes in psychiatric–mental health nursing.
- ➤ Describe measurement of patient outcomes.
- ➤ Write patient outcome statements for psychiatric–mental health nursing.

CHAPTER 13

KEY TERMS

clinical domain outcome
  statements
clinical paths
defining characteristics
diagnosis-specific
  outcomes
discharge outcomes
discipline-specific
  outcomes
humanitarian domain
  outcome statements

indicators
initial outcomes
provider domain
  outcome statements
public welfare domain
  outcome statements
rehabilitative domain
  outcome statements
related factors
revised outcomes

KEY CONCEPT

outcomes

After completing an assessment of the patient, the nurse chooses appropriate nursing diagnoses based on the assessment data. As the nurse gains experience, he or she begins to cluster the assessment data into areas that nursing interventions can affect positively. Basing them on the nursing diagnoses, the nurse develops outcomes and connects them with nursing interventions. Carrying out the appropriate interventions is only the beginning. It is the patient outcomes that tell the story—did the nursing interventions make a difference? Success outcomes, related to nursing interventions, give nursing the clout to share in health care dollars paid. What this means is that nursing can share in or receive some money for health care if the profession can prove that its contributions are making a positive difference. Patient outcomes tell the nurse, patient, family, and third-party payers if the nursing interventions were successful. Understanding the importance of patient outcomes is an important part of the professional nursing role. Nursing research to develop valid outcomes for specific nursing interventions can only increase the profession's contribution to health care.

DERIVING NURSING DIAGNOSES

When choosing nursing diagnoses for a particular patient, the nurse refers to objective signs and subjective symptoms found during the nursing assessment. The complete list of NANDA diagnoses can be found in Appendix G. These **defining characteristics**, the clues given by the signs and symptoms, join together in the nurse's mind to form a cluster. This cluster leads the nurse to choose certain diagnoses over others. For example, when assessing a patient, the nurse notices that the patient's responses are often self-negating (eg, "I always mess things up," "I never get it right"). The nurse also notices that the patient shows indecisiveness and lacks problem-solving abilities (eg, "I can never decide what is the right thing to do, and when I do finally choose, it is always wrong"). By noting and thinking about such defining characteristics, the nurse can determine that the nursing diagnosis Self-Esteem Disturbance is appropriate.

In addition to defining characteristics, the nurse also turns to related factors to further and help establish the

TABLE 13.1   Outcome Continuum

Outcome	Continuum				
Anxiety Control	Never Demonstrate	Rarely Demonstrate	Sometimes Demonstrate	Often Demonstrate	Consistently Demonstrate
	d 1	d 2	d 3	d 4	d 5

From Johnson, M., & Maas, M. (1997). *Nursing outcomes classification: Iowa Outcome Project.* St. Louis: Mosby.

nursing diagnosis. **Related factors** are those factors that have influenced the change in the patient's health status. The related factors may be grouped into four categories: biologic or psychological, which are called *pathophysiologic*; maturational; social, which are called *situational* or *contextualized*; and treatment-related. To continue with the assessment example, the nurse hears the patient discuss the loss of three jobs within the past year and related financial problems. These situational related factors further strengthen the nursing diagnosis of Self-Esteem Disturbance.

As the nurse moves from novice to expert, he or she clusters information gathered from the patient using all the senses (sight, smell, hearing, touch, and taste). Not only the answers the patient gives but also what the nurse perceives influence the selection of nursing diagnoses. For example, the nurse notices that the patient is sitting with her head down. The patient makes no eye contact and is dressed in dirty clothes. Such findings may lead the nurse to conclude that the patient's diagnosis should be Self-Esteem Disturbance.

DEVELOPING PATIENT OUTCOMES

Outcomes can be defined as a patient's response to the care he or she has received. Outcomes are the end result of a process, in this case the process of nursing. Merwin and Mauck (1995) state that these responses can be seen as changes in the patient's behavior or knowledge as well as his or her degree of satisfaction with the health care

provided. A second way to define outcomes is as "variable client or caregiver states, behavior or perceptions that are responsive to nursing intervention" (Maas et al., 1996, p. 296).

Outcomes were developed as variable concepts, not goals, so that nurses could document and monitor them over time and across clinical settings, providing more information than whether a goal was met. A third and more recent definition has evolved from work with nurse-sensitive outcomes. This definition indicates that "outcomes can be neutral (no change) and can be measured along a continuum (Johnson & Maas, 1997, p. 82) (Table 13-1). Measuring outcomes not only demonstrates clinical effectiveness but also helps to promote rational clinical decision making on the nurse's part (Tusaie-Mumford, 1996).

KEY CONCEPT   Outcomes. Outcomes are the patient's response to nursing care at a given point in time. An outcome is concise, stated in few words and in neutral terms. Outcomes do not describe a nurse's behavior or intervention. An outcome is not a nursing diagnosis. Outcomes describe a patient's state, behavior, or perception that is variable and can be measured (Table 13-2).

Outcome identification has moved away from the clinical symptoms and laboratory signs that medicine has traditionally used to describe patient knowledge, behaviors, and quality of life. These outcomes can be used to evaluate the effect of nursing interventions.

TABLE 13.2   Example of Outcomes

Diagnosis	Outcome	Intervention
Impaired Social Interaction (isolates self from others)	Social involvement	Using a contract format, explain role and responsibility of patients
	Indicators a. Interact with other patients. b. Attend group meetings.	

Evolution of Patient Outcomes

The concept of patient outcomes is not new to nursing. Florence Nightingale analyzed patient outcomes during the Crimean War. As early as 1962, Mildred Adelotte published one of the first nursing studies involving patient outcomes (Maas et al., 1996). In the 1980s, several researchers identified different categories of nursing outcomes (Johnson & Maas, 1997). Lang and Clinton (1984) proposed the following outcomes: physical health status, mental health status, social and physical functioning, health attitude, knowledge and behavior, use of professional health resources, and patient perception of the quality of nursing care. Marek (1989) identified 15 categories: physiologic measures; symptom control; frequency of service; home maintenance; psychosocial measures; well-being; functional status; goal attainment; patient behaviors; patient satisfaction; patient knowledge; rehospitalization; safety; cost; and resolution of nursing diagnoses. In the 1990s, McCormick, Brown, Naylor, Lalande, Daybert, and colleagues and the Omaha Visiting Nurse Association all developed outcomes that could be used to evaluate nursing effectiveness. The Omaha Visiting Nurse Association outcomes are for both individuals and families (Johnson & Maas, 1997).

Although the importance of identifying outcomes of nursing interventions has been the subject of several nursing research studies since the 1960s, managed care has forced the issue of determining the cost and quality of care that patients receive and measuring the results of nursing interventions using outcomes. According to Davies and coworkers (1994), the health care process has several goals: avoid adverse effects of care; improve a patient's physiologic status; reduce a patient's signs and symptoms; improve a patient's functional status and well-being; achieve patient satisfaction; minimize cost of care; and maximize revenues. Nursing interventions can affect all these goals. Patient outcomes can help to determine the importance of nursing interventions to the patient's care and to improve the quality of that care by identifying which interventions have worked and which have not been beneficial. Outcomes can be used to show the accountability and value of nursing service or practice and can be incorporated into the reimbursement formula for organizational services and the financial survival of the nursing profession. When the nursing profession uses and links nursing interventions, diagnoses, and outcomes, it will truly affect the nation's health care process in meeting goals.

As nursing continues to evolve, the nursing profession develops tools to help document nursing's contribution. Quality of patient care, cost-effectiveness, and resource use have contributed to the development of clinical paths, of which outcomes are an integral part. **Clinical paths** (critical pathways) are flow charts that usually contain assessment parameters, nursing diagnoses, nursing interventions, and outcomes for a specific diagnosis. Facilities continue to develop and refine clinical paths for the typical patient served (Table 13-3).

Purpose of Patient Outcomes and Indicators

The purpose of patient outcomes and indicators is to evaluate the effectiveness of nursing interventions or strategies. Outcomes answer the question, "What are the expected results of the nurse's actions or interventions?" (Table 13-4.)

Psychiatric–mental health nurses work as members of interdisciplinary teams. Therefore, patient outcomes in psychiatric nursing are important in assessing the quality of care provided by nursing and in determining the results that came from nursing interventions only. From an economic viewpoint, the results of psychiatric nursing interventions are important. Increasingly, cost reduction is a guiding principle for health care, and financing the care is based on outcomes. Identifying nursing interventions sensitive to patient outcomes can show the psychiatric nurse's contribution to multidisciplinary care. If the nursing contribution is not visible, it will not be counted and therefore may become dispensable.

TABLE 13.3 Clinical Path: Depression

Day	Assessment Parameters	Nursing Diagnosis	Nursing Interventions	Patient Outcomes
Day 1	Patient admits to having a suicide plan.	High Risk for Violence, Self-Directed	Institute suicide precautions.	Suicide: self-restraint
Day 2			Maintain suicide precautions.	Suicide: self-restraint
Day 3	Patient is apathetic, doesn't wash or dress self.	Impaired Health Maintenance	Help patient with personal hygiene, exhibit patience.	Self-care: dressing and bathing

TABLE 13.4 Results of Nursing Interventions

Diagnosis	Patient Outcome	Nursing Intervention
Grieving, Anticipatory	Grief resolution (adjusting to impending loss) **Indicators** a. Express feelings about loss. b. Express feelings about how life will change due to loss. c. Maintain relationships until death occurs. d. Maintain nutrition. e. Maintain social support. f. Practice skills and role function needed in the future.	Provide supportive feedback to verbal concerns and feelings.

Outcomes can be used as a tool of communication when working with other nurses, case managers, caregivers, insurance companies, and policy makers and to conduct program evaluations and develop research databases. Standardized labels (outcomes) provide effective and efficient ways to deliver the nurse's message that nursing is part of the health care system.

According to Johnson and Maas (1997, p. 7), there are several categories of patient outcomes:

1. Global, multidisciplinary patient outcomes tend to measure patient satisfaction and general health status. These were developed to evaluate the effectiveness of managed care systems and to provide information about health care providers. These outcomes are not specific enough to determine accountability that leads to improvement, (eg, behavioral control, use of restraints), or diagnosis- or condition-specific outcomes related to a specific diagnosis that are usually found in clinical pathways (Table 13-5).
2. System-specific outcomes are used to evaluate the efficiency and effectiveness of a particular organization or managed care system. They usually have a multidisciplinary focus and provide information about the effects of care but cannot help determine accountability for outcomes, for example, the number of patients who have movement disorders (occurrence) (Table 13-6).

3. **Discipline-specific outcomes** are based on the standards of the discipline and can be used to evaluate the individual practitioner's practice (Table 13-7). The outcome knowledge of medication effects can be based on the psychiatric nursing standards listed in Table 13-8.

Nurses are accountable for documentation of patient outcomes, nursing interventions, and any changes in diagnosis, care plan, or both. This documentation is important for further research, cost, and continuity and quality of care studies. The measurement of patient outcomes helps to meet the goal of continuous quality improvement (CQI). By identifying variations in patient outcomes and working to reduce or eliminate these variations, CQI occurs. Thus, outcomes drive the CQI process (Fig. 13-1).

Indicators answer the question, "How close is the recipient moving toward the outcome?" The indicator represents the dimensions of the outcome. Outcome indicators represent or describe patient status, behaviors, or perceptions evaluated during a patient's assessment.

TABLE 13.5 Example of Condition: Diagnosis-Specific Outcomes

Diagnosis	Outcome
Anxiety	a. Anxiety control b. Aggression control

TABLE 13.6 Example of System-Specific Outcome

Diagnosis	Outcome
Altered Sensory Perception (hallucination)	Movement disorder occurrence **Indicators** a. Initiation of antipsychotic drugs b. Demonstration of choreic movement c. Demonstration of pelvic gyrations d. Increase or decrease in dosage of antipsychotic drugs

TABLE 13.7	Example of Discipline-Specific Outcome
Diagnosis	**Outcome**
Deficient Knowledge	Knowledge: medication
	Indicator
	Description of side effects of medications

Indicators are a measurement of patient progress in relation to the patient outcomes and can serve as intermediate outcomes in a clinical pathway or standardized care plan. Indicators are sensitive to nursing interventions; therefore, if other disciplines use the outcome, the indicators that are sensitive to nursing can be monitored to provide nursing accountability for care (see Table 13-4). Indicators are responsive to nursing interventions, and in a multidisciplinary setting, they can be used to provide nursing accountability. When both disciplines use the same outcomes (Table 13-9), both of the indicators are related to the outcome; however, one is more sensitive to nursing intervention, and the other in more sensitive to interventions from another discipline. For example in Table 13-9, "descriptions of side effects of medication" is more sensitive to nursing intervention, whereas "description of potential adverse reactions when taking multiple drugs" is a pharmacy indicator.

In addition, outcomes motivate the patient by providing a sense of achievement when he or she reaches them. They provide guidelines for what is expected of the patient and direction for continuity of care that reflects current knowledge in the field of mental health nursing. Outcomes can be **initial outcomes** (those written after the initial patient interview and assessment), **revised outcomes** (those written after each evaluation), and **discharge outcomes** (those outcomes to be met before discharge). Because of the decreased length of stay or days of service, discharge outcomes may not be met, and they often are passed along to the community nurse, who will continue to help the patient meet them if they remain relevant. In fact, the outcomes that were discharge outcomes to the hospital, clinic, or program nurse may become initial outcomes to the community or home care nurse. Outcomes and indicators provide excellent nurse-to-nurse communication, which leads to good continuity of care.

Nursing Process and Patient Outcomes

Outcomes are the results of planning, which is the fourth step in the nursing process, and are derived from the nursing diagnoses that provide the basis for selecting nursing interventions. Nursing interventions are the activities that nurses do to produce patient outcomes. The term *patient* is a broad concept when used with outcomes. In this case, patient can refer to individuals, families, communities, and organizations.

The *Scope and Standards of Psychiatric–Mental Health Nursing Practice* (American Nurses Association et al., 2000) (see Chap. 5 for a review of the standards) set the stage for the focus on outcomes by stating the following:

Standards of care pertain to professional nursing activities that are demonstrated by the nurse through nursing process. These involve assessment, diagnosis, outcome identification, planning, implementation, and evaluation. The Nursing Process is the foundation of clinical decision making and encompasses all significant action taken by nurses in providing developmentally and culturally relevant psychiatric mental health care to all patients.

Patient outcomes and nursing diagnosis, which are part of the nursing process, can be combined. When they are combined or linked, they provide a way to monitor nursing practice and facilitate clinical decision making and knowledge development (Table 13-10).

Types of Patient Outcomes

Nursing has made great strides in defining its role in health care. Nurses have started to describe expected results of their interventions or care given to patients. The linking of nursing diagnosis with interventions

TABLE 13.8	Standards of Care for Psychiatric Nurses
Standards	**Outcome**
V_E: Health teaching V_D: Psychobiologic interventions V_I: Prescriptions of pharmacologic agents	Knowledge: medication

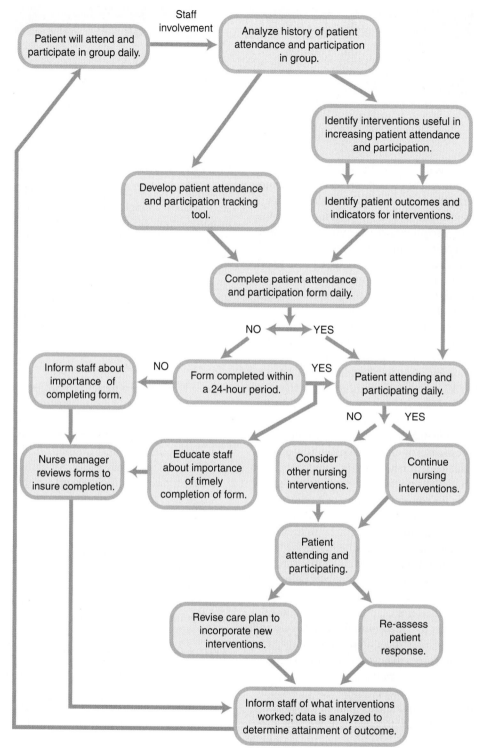

Outcomes and CQI

Figure 13.1 Outcomes and continuous quality improvement.

TABLE 13.9 Outcome With Multidisciplinary Indicators

Standards	Outcome	Continuum				
V_E: Health teaching V_D: Psychobiologic interventions V_I: Prescriptions of pharmacologic agents	Knowledge: medication	Never 1	Limited 2	Moderate 3	Substantial 4	Extensive 5

Indicators*
a. Description of side effects of medication
a. Know the name and dosage of medication
b. Know the therapeutic effect of medication
b. Description of potential of an adverse reaction when taking multiple drugs

* a, Nurse indicator; b, pharmacy indicator.

and outcomes of care will support the push by the nursing profession to gain respect and a stronger place in decision making in the health care arena.

Now, two different types of outcomes show nursing's potential. These are the National Institute of Mental Health outcomes and the specific nursing-sensitive outcomes developed by the Iowa Outcome Project in 1996 (Table 13-11).

In 1991, the National Institute of Mental Health defined four categories of outcome statements that are not necessarily nurse sensitive: humanitarian domain, public welfare domain, rehabilitative domain, and clinical domain. In their review of nursing outcome research, Merwin and Mauck (1995) felt it necessary to add a fifth category, that of provider domain. Definitions and examples of each of the five categories of outcome statements are as follows:

1. **Humanitarian domain outcome statements** spell out behaviors or responses that show a sense of well-being of patients and personal fulfillment of patients and family members (Table 13-12).
2. **Public welfare domain outcome statements** show responses or behaviors that provide exam-

ples for preventing harm to self, family, and community (Table 13-13).
3. **Rehabilitative domain outcome statements** provide examples of improvement or restoration of social and vocational functioning and lead to independent living (Table 13-14).
4. **Clinical domain outcome statements** indicate reduction in symptoms of illness or cure of a specific mental illness (Table 13-15).
5. **Provider domain outcome statements** describe behaviors and attitudes of nursing staff and responses to nurse–patient relationships (Table 13-16).

In the late 1990s, the Iowa Outcome Project was the first group to produce nurse-sensitive outcomes that described patient outcomes and their indications for measurement that are affected by nursing practice and linked to nursing diagnoses. These outcomes were written as neutral concepts, so that they could be measured on a continuum rather than as discrete met or unmet goals. The outcomes focus on the individual recipient of care (patient or family caregivers) and include patient states, behaviors, or perceptions that are sensitive to or influ-

TABLE 13.10 Example—Linkage of Nursing Diagnosis and Outcomes

Diagnosis	Outcome
1. Disturbed Body Image	Self-mutilation restraint
2. Confusion, Chronic	Improved thought control
3. Ineffective Denial	Anxiety control

From Johnson, M., & Maas, M. (1997). *Nursing outcome classification: Iowa Outcome Project.* St. Louis: Mosby.

TABLE 13.11   Expected Outcomes From Nursing Interventions

Nursing Intervention	Expected Outcome
Provide educational information about mental illness	Knowledge: disease process
Educational group in caregiving	Caregiver: patient relationship
Group therapy	Improved thought control
Weight control counseling	Knowledge: diet
Health teaching	Knowledge: medication
Teaching limit setting	Coping
Reality orientation	Identity: self
Life review	Hope
Teaching anger management	Impulse control

From Johnson, M., & Maas, M. (1997). *Nursing outcomes classification: Iowa Outcome Project.* St. Louis: Mosby.

TABLE 13.12   Example of Humanitarian Domain Outcome

Diagnosis	Outcome	Intervention
Family: Coping Potential for Growth	Parents and adolescents talk to each other at breakfast about feelings and concerns.	Encourage family to spend time listening to each other's concerns and feelings.

TABLE 13.13   Example of Public Welfare Domain Outcome

Diagnosis	Outcome	Intervention
Risk for Violence Directed at Others (Hitting)	Patient verbalizes feelings (not act out).	Encourage patient to talk about feelings.

TABLE 13.14   Example of Rehabilitative Domain Outcome

Diagnosis	Outcome	Intervention
Ineffective Coping (not attending school)	Patient demonstrates responsibility for behavior (graduation from high school).	Assist patient in identifying stressors that hinder attendance in school.

Adapted from Brooker, C. (1999). Evaluating clinical outcome and staff morale in a rehabilitating team for people with serious mental health problems. *Journal of Advance Nursing, 29*(1), 44–51.

TABLE 13.15   Example of Clinical Domain Outcome

Diagnosis	Outcome	Intervention
Disturbed Sensory Perception (auditory hallucinations)	Patient questions validity of voices.	Discuss possible explanations for the voices.

TABLE 13.16 Example of Provider Domain Outcome		
Diagnosis	**Outcome**	**Intervention**
Fear Related to Assault (patient violence)	Nurses discuss fear of recurrence of event.	Supportive counseling (crisis intervention)

enced by nursing interventions. The outcomes are organized into six domains: functional health, psychosocial, behavior, physiologic health, perceived health, and family health (Keenan & Aquilino, 1998). Whether nurses use the five categories of the National Institute of Mental Health, the Iowa Outcome Project Nursing Classification, or the biopsychosocial model to develop outcome statements (see Table 13-11), they can cover all aspects of the patient and how he or she relates to the family and community (Fig. 13-2).

EVALUATION

Evaluation of patient outcomes involves answering the following questions:

- What is the cost-effectiveness of the intervention?
- What benefits did the patient receive?
- What was the patient's level of satisfaction?
- Was the outcome diagnosis specific or nonspecific?

Diagnosis-specific outcomes show that the intervention resolved the problem or nursing diagnosis (Table 13-17). At other times, the outcome is not diagnosis-specific, meaning it does not show resolution of the diagnosis. In that case, the outcome is abstract or general (Table 13-18). When measuring outcomes, nurses must consider the time frame. Identifying the intermediate outcome indicators that may be achieved in one setting versus what outcome indicators can be achieved in a second setting provides for a measurement of progression and enhances continuity of care. For example, in Table 13-19, the patient may be able to satisfy the first set of indicators: resolution of depression, demonstration of confidence, demonstration of self-esteem, and decreased suicide attempts during his or her stay in an organized health care setting (hospital). Nevertheless, not until discharge or movement to a community setting can the patient satisfy the second set of indicators: demonstration of confidence when alone at home, demonstration of positive interpersonal relationship with opposite sex; demonstration of confidence in role skills (worker/mother), and demonstration of self-advocacy behavior. The first set of indicators, together with the second set, can provide measurement of the patient's progress.

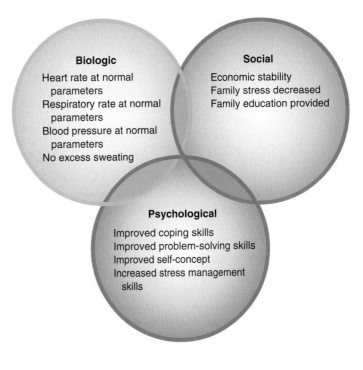

FIGURE 13.2 Biopsychosocial outcomes for a patient with anxiety.

TABLE 13.17   Example of Diagnosis-Specific Outcome

Diagnosis	Outcome	Intervention
Disturbed Sleeping Pattern (inability to sleep)	a. Sleep b. Resting **Indicator** Determine number of hours of sleep. Describe factors that prevent sleep. Describe factors that promote sleep.	Teach patient relaxation techniques to use at bedtime.

TABLE 13.18   Nonspecific Outcomes

Diagnosis	Outcome	Intervention
Chronic Low Self-Esteem	Open communication	Attend group with patient and provide support and feedback to verbal concerns.

TABLE 13.19   Progression in Care

Diagnosis	Outcome	None 1	Limited 2	Moderate 3	Substantial 4	Extensive 5
Family Violence: Individual	Abuse recovery: emotional **Indicators** a. Resolution of depression; demonstration of confidence; demonstration of self-esteem; decreased suicide attempts b. Demonstration of confidence when alone in home; demonstration of positive interpersonal relationship with opposite sex; demonstration of confidence in role skills (worker, mother); self-advocacy behavior					

Outcomes can be measured immediately after the nursing intervention or after time passes. Remember that outcomes based on health prevention and health promotion diagnoses can occur after considerable time has passed.

Accountability is an important concept in current health care. Nursing and other disciplines have been pressured to justify their practice, control health care costs, and demonstrate to consumers that they deliver quality care. Measurement of outcomes can be used to determine quality of care during a single episode of illness, across the continuum of care, and can assist in discharge planning. Also, outcomes can be used to determine quality of care in different systems and between systems (DePalma, 1999; Nowell-Kleinpell & Weiner, 1999; Smith, 1999).

Summary of Key Points

➤ With the advent of managed care, patient outcomes have become important in the evaluation of care.

➤ Statements in the American Nurses Association (2000) *Scope and Standards of Psychiatric–Mental Health Nursing Practice* support the importance of outcome identification.

➤ Outcomes must be measurable.

➤ More research is needed to identify patient outcomes as they relate to nursing interventions and nursing diagnosis.

➤ Nursing diagnoses, nursing interventions, and patient outcomes are initially derived from the assessment data.

➤ Outcome indicators provide measurement of patient progress.

➤ Initial, revised, and discharge outcomes can be included in a nursing care plan.

➤ Outcome statements can cover the biopsychosocial domains.

Critical Thinking Challenges

1. Create a nursing care plan with outcomes for a patient who has a substance abuse problem.
2. Create a teaching plan that shows linkage of diagnoses and outcomes.

REFERENCES

American Nurses Association, American Psychiatric Association, & International Society of Psychiatric–Mental Health Nurses. (2000). *Scope and standards of psychiatric–mental health nursing practice*. Washington, DC: American Nurses Publishing.

Brooker, C. (1999). Evaluating clinical outcome and staff morale in a rehabilitating team for people with serious mental health problems. *Journal of Advance Nursing, 29*(1), 44–51.

Davies, A. R., Doyle, M. A., Lansky, D., et al. (1994). Outcome assessment in clinical settings: A consensus statement on principles and best practice in project management. *Journal of Quality Improvement, 20*(1), 6–16.

Denehy, J. (1998). Integrating nursing outcomes classification in nursing education. *Journal of Nursing Care Quality, 12*(5), 73–84.

DePalma, J. (1999). Measuring outcomes related to nursing. *Home Health Care Manage Practice, 11*(4), 67–68.

Johnson, M., & Maas, M. (1997). *Nursing outcomes classification: Iowa outcome project.* St. Louis: Mosby.

Keenan, G., & Aquilino, M. (1998). Standardized nomenclatures: Keys to community of care, nursing accountability and nursing effectiveness. *Outcome Management for Nursing Practice, 2*(2), 81–86.

Lang, N. M., & Marek, K. D. (1990). The classification of patient outcomes. *Journal of Professional Nursing, 6*, 153–163.

Maas, M., Johnson, M., & Morehead, S. (1996). Classifying nursing-sensitive patient outcomes. *Image—The Journal of Nursing Scholarship, 28*(4), 295–301.

Marek, K. D. (1989). Outcome measurement in nursing. *Journal of Nursing Quality Assurance, 4*(1), 1–9.

Merwin, E., & Mauck, A. (1995). Psychiatric nursing outcome research: The state of the science. *Archives of Psychiatric Nursing, 9*(6), 311–331.

Nowell-Kleinpell, R., & Weiner, T. (1999). Measuring advance practice nursing outcomes. *American Association of Clinical Nursing: Clinical Issues, 10*(3), 356–368.

Smith, G. B. (1999). Practice guidelines and outcome evaluation. *Outcome Management for Nursing Practice, 2*(3), 24–29.

Tusaie-Mumford, K. (1996). Practice outcome evaluation: Patient behavioral health care demonstration project. *Issues in Mental Health Nursing, 17*, 59–71.

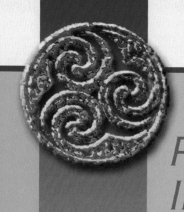

Psychiatric Nursing Interventions Overview

Mary Ann Boyd

NURSING INTERVENTIONS AND PSYCHIATRIC–MENTAL HEALTH NURSING

INTERVENTIONS FOR THE BIOLOGIC DOMAIN
Promotion of Self-Care Activities
Activity and Exercise Interventions
Sleep Interventions
Nutrition Interventions
Relaxation Interventions
Hydration Interventions
Thermoregulation Interventions
Pain Management
Medication Management

INTERVENTIONS FOR THE PSYCHOLOGICAL DOMAIN
Counseling Interventions
Conflict Resolution

Conflict Resolution Process
Cultural Brokering in
*   Patient–System Conflicts*
Bibliotherapy
Reminiscence
Behavior Therapy
    Behavior Modification
    Token Economy
Cognitive Interventions
Psychoeducation
Health Teaching
Spiritual Interventions

INTERVENTIONS FOR THE SOCIAL DOMAIN
Social Behavior and Privilege
    Systems in Inpatient Units
Milieu Therapy
    Containment
    Validation

Structured Interaction
Open Communication
Milieu Therapy in
    Different Settings
Promotion of Patient Safety on
    Psychiatric Units
    Observation
    De-escalation
    Seclusion
    Restraints
Home Visits
Community Action

LEARNING OBJECTIVES

After studying this chapter, you will be able to:

➤ Discuss the basis for selection of psychiatric–mental health nursing interventions.

➤ Discuss the application of nursing interventions for the biologic domain.

➤ Discuss the application of nursing interventions for the psychological domain.

➤ Discuss the application of nursing interventions for the social domain.

CHAPTER 14

KEY TERMS

automatic thinking
behavior modification
behavior therapy
bibliotherapy
chemical restraint
cognitive interventions
conflict resolution
containment
counseling
cultural brokering
de-escalation
distraction
guided imagery
home visits

illogical thinking
milieu therapy
observation
open communication
physical restraint
psychoeducation
reminiscence
seclusion
simple relaxation
  techniques
spiritual support
structured interaction
token economy
validation

KEY CONCEPT

nursing interventions

*N*ursing interventions are nursing activities that promote and foster health, assess dysfunction, assist patients to regain or improve their coping abilities, or prevent further disabilities (American Nurses Association [ANA] et al., 2000). Nursing interventions include any treatment that a nurse performs to enhance patient outcomes. Nurses base these interventions on clinical judgment and knowledge. These interventions are direct (performed through interaction with the patient) or indirect (performed away from, but on behalf of, the patient) (McCloskey & Bulechek, 1999). Interventions can be either nurse-initiated treatment, which is an autonomous action in response to a nursing diagnosis, or physician-initiated treatment, which is a response to a medical diagnosis as a result of a "physician's order." In psychiatric nursing, the Scope and Standards of Psychiatric–Mental Health Nursing Practice describes the scope of practice, differentiates levels of practice, delineates nursing roles, and guides the selection of interventions for implementation in the plan of care (ANA et al., 2000) (see Chap. 5).

KEY CONCEPT   **Nursing interventions.** **Nursing interventions** are nursing activities that promote and foster health, assess dysfunction, assist patients to regain or improve their coping abilities, or prevent further disabilities (ANA et al., 2000).

After considering many different factors, selection of nursing approaches involves integrating biologic, psychological, and social interventions into a comprehensive plan of care. This chapter presents an overview of the interventions that nurses can use in caring for patients with psychiatric disorders (Fig. 14-1). Psychiatric–mental health nurses deliver care in various roles. In some settings, such as an acute care hospital or the home, the nurse provides direct nursing care. In other settings, the nurse may assume the role of a case manager, who primarily coordinates care for all disciplines as well as nursing. In this instance, the nurse may be responsible for all or part of direct nursing care as well as for ensuring that agreed-on care is appropriate for the patient, even if other providers deliver it. The nurse may also be the

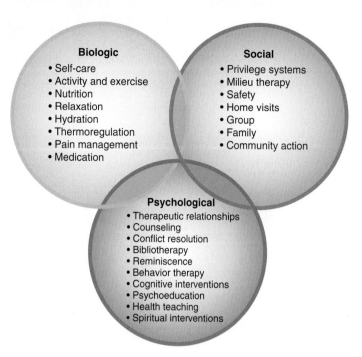

Biologic
- Self-care
- Activity and exercise
- Nutrition
- Relaxation
- Hydration
- Thermoregulation
- Pain management
- Medication

Social
- Privilege systems
- Milieu therapy
- Safety
- Home visits
- Group
- Family
- Community action

Psychological
- Therapeutic relationships
- Counseling
- Conflict resolution
- Bibliotherapy
- Reminiscence
- Behavior therapy
- Cognitive interventions
- Psychoeducation
- Health teaching
- Spiritual interventions

FIGURE 14.1 Psychiatric nursing interventions.

leader or manager of a nursing unit and thus responsible for delegating the care to paraprofessional and nonprofessional providers; however, he or she remains accountable for the patient's care. In all these instances, the nurse plans and initiates interventions that are safe and appropriate for the patient.

NURSING INTERVENTIONS AND PSYCHIATRIC–MENTAL HEALTH NURSING

The Nursing Interventions Classification (NIC) is an extensive system consisting of 433 specific interventions, with discrete activities for each (McCloskey & Bulechek, 1999). The NIC system is based on data collected from surveys of practicing nurses. These nurses identified the interventions that were ultimately classified. The NIC taxonomy includes classes or groups of interventions categorized according to six domains: physiologic basic, physiologic complex, behavioral, safety, family, and health system. The intention of the NIC taxonomy is to represent both basic and specialty advanced nursing practice. For example, both basic and specialist nurses use interventions such as reinforcing positive behavior; however, the advanced practice psychiatric nurse may actually develop the plan and also use it as part of psychotherapy with the patient. This text uses many NIC interventions and those identified

in the *Scope and Standards of Psychiatric–Mental Health Nursing* (ANA et al., 2000) as well as others reported in the psychiatric nursing literature (Text Box 14-1).

INTERVENTIONS FOR THE BIOLOGIC DOMAIN

Biologic interventions focus on physical functioning and are directed toward the patient's self-care, activities and exercise, sleep, nutrition, relaxation, hydration, and thermoregulation as well as pain management and medication management. In the NIC taxonomy, these interventions are found within the physiologic basic and complex domains.

Promotion of Self-Care Activities

Self-care is the ability to perform activities of daily living successfully. Many patients with psychiatric–mental health problems can manage self-care activities such as bathing, dressing appropriately, selecting adequate nutrition, and sleeping regularly. (Even though maintaining adequate nutrition and promoting normal sleep hygiene are considered self-care activities, they are discussed in separate sections because of their significance in mental health care.) Others cannot manage such self-care activities, either because of their symptoms or as a result of the side effects of medications. Because nursing is concerned with maintaining the patient's health and

TEXT BOX 14.1

Nursing Intervention Classification Taxonomy

I. PHYSIOLOGIC: BASIC—Care That Supports Physical Functioning

A. Activity and exercise management: Interventions to organize or assist with physical activity and energy conservation and expenditure

B. Elimination management: Interventions to establish and maintain regular bowel and urinary elimination patterns and manage complication due to altered patterns

C. Immobility management: Interventions to manage restricted body movement and the sequelae

D. Nutrition support: Interventions to modify or maintain nutritional status

E. Physical comfort promotion: Interventions to promote comfort using physical techniques

F. Self-care facilitation: Interventions to provide or assist with routine activities of daily living

II. PHYSIOLOGIC: COMPLEX—Care That Supports Homeostatic Regulation

G. Electrolyte and acid–base management: Interventions to regulate electrolyte/acid–base balance and prevent complications

H. Drug management: Interventions to facilitate desired effects of pharmacologic agents

I. Neurologic management: Interventions to optimize neurologic function

J. Perioperative care: Interventions to provide care before, during, and immediately after surgery (ECT)

K. Respiratory management: Interventions to promote airway patency and gas exchange

L. Skin/wound management: Interventions to maintain or restore tissue integrity

M. Thermoregulation: Interventions to maintain body temperature within a normal range

N. Tissue perfusion management: Interventions to optimize circulation of blood and fluids to the tissues

III. BEHAVIORAL—Care That Supports Psychosocial Functioning and Facilitates Lifestyle Changes

O. Behavioral therapy: Interventions to reinforce or promote desirable behaviors or alter undesirable behaviors

P. Cognitive therapy: Interventions to reinforce or promote desirable cognitive functioning or alter undesirable cognitive functioning

Q. Communication enhancement: Interventions to facilitate delivering and receiving verbal and nonverbal messages

R. Coping assistance: Interventions to assist another to build on own strengths, adapt to a change in function, or achieve a higher level of function

S. Patient education: Interventions to facilitate learning

T. Psychological comfort promotion: Interventions to promote comfort using psychological techniques

IV. SAFETY—Care That Supports Protection Against Harm

U. Crisis management: Interventions to provide immediate, short-term help in both psychological and physiologic crises

V. Risk management: Interventions to initiate risk reduction activities and continue monitoring risks over time

V. FAMILY—Care That Supports the Family Unit

W. Childbearing care: Interventions to assist in understanding and coping with the psychological and physiologic changes during the childbearing period

X. Life span care: Interventions to facilitate family unit functioning and promote the health and welfare of family members throughout the life span

VI. HEALTH SYSTEM—Care That Supports Effective Use of the Health Care Delivery System

Y. Health system mediation: Interventions to facilitate the interface between patient/family and the health care system

  a. Health system management: Interventions to provide and enhance support services for the delivery of care

  b. Information management: Interventions to facilitate communication among health care providers

From McCloskey, J., & Bulechek, G. (1996). *Nursing interventions classification (NIC)* (pp. 56–68). St. Louis: Mosby.

---

well-being, a focus on routine, basic activities of daily living can become a nursing priority.

Dorothea Orem's general nursing model is based on the concept of self-care deficit (see Chap. 6). This model promotes the ideas that self-care is learned and that these behaviors regulate human integrity, functioning, and development. This theory actually consists of three nursing theories: self-care deficit, self-care (the core theory), and nursing system. This model is often used in psychiatric nursing, particularly in the areas of rehabilitation, self-care, and patient education (Burks, 1999; Campbell & Soeken, 1999). The emphasis on helping

the individual develop independence is consistent with patient outcomes in psychiatric nursing.

In the inpatient setting, the psychiatric nurse structures the patient's activities so that basic self-care activities are completed. During acute phases of psychiatric disorders, the inability to attend to basic self-care tasks such as getting dressed is very common. Ability to complete personal hygiene activities (eg, dental care, grooming) is monitored, and patients are assisted in completing such activities. In a psychiatric facility, patients are encouraged and expected to develop independence in completing these basic self-care activities.

In the community, monitoring these basic self-care activities is always a part of the nursing visit or clinic appointment.

Activity and Exercise Interventions

In some psychiatric disorders (eg, schizophrenia), people become sedentary and appear to lack the motivation to complete daily activities, such as getting up in the morning, showering, dressing, and going to work. This lack of motivation is part of the disorder and requires nursing intervention. Additionally, side effects of medication include sedation and lethargy.

The nurse must attend to the patient's level of activity. Encouraging regular activity and exercise can improve overall general well-being and physical health. In some instances, exercise behavior becomes an abnormal focus of attention, such as in some patients with anorexia nervosa. Usually, however, exercise can keep patients active and engaged in life.

When assuming the responsibility of direct care provider, the nurse can help patients identify realistic activities and exercise goals. As leader or manager of a psychiatric unit, the nurse can influence ward routine. Alternately, the nurse can delegate activity and exercise interventions to nurses' aides. Some institutions have other professionals (eg, recreational therapists) available for the implementation of exercise programs. As a case manager, the nurse should consider the activity needs of individuals when coordinating care.

Sleep Interventions

Many psychiatric disorders and medications are associated with sleep disturbances. Some disorders are specifically related to sleep (see Chap. 26). Sleep is also disrupted in patients with dementia; such patients may have difficulty falling asleep or may frequently awaken during the night. In dementia of the Alzheimer's type, individuals may reverse their sleeping patterns by napping during the day and staying awake at night. Nonpharmacologic interventions are always used first because of the side-effect risks associated with the use of sedatives and hypnotics (see Chap. 8). Sleep interventions to use with patients include the following:

- Go to bed only when tired or sleepy.
- Establish a consistent bedtime routine.
- Avoid stimulating foods, beverages, or medications.
- Avoid naps in the late afternoon or evening.
- Eat lightly before retiring and limit fluid intake.
- Use bed only for sleep or intimacy.
- Avoid emotional stimulation before bedtime.
- Use behavioral and relaxation techniques.
- Limit distractions.

Nutrition Interventions

For people who are emotionally deprived, food, the universal symbol for nurturing, becomes of paramount importance, providing a means of self-nourishment and security. Psychiatric disorders and medication side effects can affect eating behaviors. Some patients eat too little, whereas others eat too much. Homeless patients with mental illness have difficulty maintaining adequate nutrition because of their deprived lifestyle. Substance abuse also interferes with maintaining adequate nutrition. Nutrition interventions should be specific and relevant to the individual's mental health. Recommended daily allowances are important in the promotion of physical and mental health, and nurses should consider them when planning care.

Some psychiatric symptoms involve changes in perceptions of food, appetite, and eating habits. If a patient believes that food is poisonous, he or she may eat sparingly or not at all. Interventions are then necessary to address the suspiciousness as well as to encourage adequate intake of recommended daily allowances. Allowing patients to examine foods, participate in preparations, and test the safety of the meal by eating slowly or after everyone else may be necessary.

Obesity is common is people with mental disorders. Antipsychotics, antidepressants, and mood stabilizers are associated with weight gain, which is thought to be related to changes in metabolism and appetite that some of these types of medications cause. Many patients stop taking medications because of the weight gain. Excessive weight gain can be especially stressful to the individual's emotional well-being as well as detrimental to physical health. Nurses should encourage patients, however, to avoid quick weight loss programs. The recidivism rate for people who have lost weight only to regain more approaches 95% to 99%. Most diets do not work. For example, no evidence supports very-low-calorie diets (500 to 800 calories daily). Instead, the dieter runs the risk of caloric deprivation that can lead to intermittent hypoglycemia, ketosis, and muscle loss. Hypoglycemia can exacerbate a depressed mood and lead to suicidal thoughts. If weight gain is a problem, careful monitoring of current intake and helping the patient develop realistic strategies for changing eating patterns is the best approach.

Relaxation Interventions

Relaxation promotes comfort, reduces anxiety, alleviates stress, eases pain, and prevents aggression. It can diminish the effects of hallucinations and delusions. The many different relaxation techniques used as mental health interventions range from simple deep breathing to biofeedback to hypnosis. Even though some techniques such as biofeedback require additional training and, in some instances, certification, nurses can easily apply simple relaxation, distraction, and imagery techniques.

Simple relaxation techniques encourage and elicit relaxation to decrease undesirable signs and symptoms. **Distraction** is the purposeful focusing of attention away from undesirable sensations, and **guided imagery** is the purposeful use of imagination to achieve relaxation or direct attention away from undesirable sensations (Table 14-1). These interventions are helpful for people experiencing anxiety; guided imagery is especially useful in stress management. As a direct care provider,

TABLE 14.1 Relaxation Techniques: Descriptions and Implementation

Simple Relaxation Techniques	Distraction	Guided Imagery
• Create a quiet, nondisrupting environment with dim lights and a comfortable temperature. • Instruct the patient to assume a relaxed position, wearing loose and comfortable clothing. • Instruct the patient to relax and to let the sensations happen. • Use a low tone of voice with a slow, rhythmic pace of words. • Instruct the patient to take an initial slow, deep breath (abdominal breathing) while thinking about pleasant events. • Use soothing music (without words) to enhance relaxation. • Reinforce the use of relaxation by praising efforts and helping the patient to schedule time regularly for it. • Evaluate and document the patient's response to relaxation.	• Distraction techniques include music, counting, television, reading, play, and exercise. Help the patient choose a technique that will work for him or her. • Advise the patient to practice the distraction technique before he or she will need to use it. • Have the patient develop a specific plan for how and when he or she will use distraction. • Evaluate and document the patient's response to distraction.	• Help the patient choose a particular guided imagery technique (alone or with others). • Discuss an image the patient has experienced as pleasurable and relaxing, such as lying on a beach, watching snow fall, floating on a raft, or watching the sun set. • Individualize the images chosen, considering religious or spiritual beliefs, artistic interests, or other individual preferences. • Make suggestions to induce relaxation (eg, peaceful images, pleasant sensations, or rhythmic breathing). • Use modulated voice when guiding the imagery experience. • Have the patient travel mentally to the scene, and assist in describing the setting in detail. • Use permissive directions and suggestions when leading the imagery, such as "perhaps," "if you wish," or "you might like." • Have the patient slowly experience the scene: How does it look? smell? sound? feel? taste? • Use words or phrases that convey pleasurable images, such as floating, melting, and releasing. • Develop cleansing or clearing portion of imagery (eg, all pain appears as red dust and washes downstream in a creek as you enter). • Assist the patient in developing a method of ending the imagery technique, such as counting slowly while breathing deeply. • Encourage expression of thoughts and feelings regarding the experience. • Prepare the patient for unexpected (but often therapeutic) experiences, such as crying. • Evaluate and document the patient's response.

the nurse may teach the patient relaxation exercises. As a case manager, nurses can include relaxation exercises in the plan of care; the unit leader can be responsible for ensuring that appropriately prepared staff implement relaxation exercises.

Relaxation techniques that involve physical touch (eg, back rubs) are usually not used for people with mental disorders. Touching and massaging usually are not appropriate for patients with mental disorders, especially those who have a history of physical or sexual abuse. Such patients may find touching too stimulating or misinterpret it as sexual or aggressive.

Hydration Interventions

Overhydration or underhydration can be a symptom of a disorder. Assessing fluid status and monitoring fluid intake and output are often important interventions. Some patients with psychotic disorders experience chronic fluid imbalance. For these individuals, a treatment protocol that includes a target weight procedure can help prevent both overhydration and water intoxication and promote self-control (see Chap. 18). The nurse functions as the direct care provider (teaching patient), unit leader (delegating weighing of the patient to staff), or coordinator of the protocol.

Many psychiatric medications affect fluid and electrolyte balance (see Chap. 8). For example, when taking lithium carbonate, patients must have adequate fluid intake, with special attention paid to serum sodium levels. When sodium levels drop through perspiration, lithium is used in place of sodium, which in turn leads to lithium toxicity. Many psychiatric medications cause dry mouth, which in turn causes individuals to drink fluids excessively. Interventions that help patients understand the relationship of medications to fluid and electrolyte balance are important in their overall care.

Thermoregulation Interventions

Many psychiatric disorders can disturb the body's normal temperature regulation. Patients, then, cannot sense temperature increases or decreases and, consequently, cannot protect themselves from extremes of hot or cold. This problem is especially difficult for people who are homeless or live outside the protected environments of institutions and boarding homes. Additionally, many psychiatric medications affect the ability to regulate body temperature.

Interventions include educating patients about the problem of thermoregulation, identifying potential extremes in temperatures, and developing strategies to protect the patient from the adverse effects of temperature changes. For example, reminding patients to wear coats and sweaters in the winter or to wear loose, light-weight garments in the summer may prevent frostbite or heat exhaustion, respectively.

Pain Management

Emotional reactions are often manifested as pain. In somatization disorder, chronic, unexplained pain is one of the main symptoms (see Chap. 23). Psychiatric nurses are more likely to provide care to patients experiencing chronic pain than acute pain. Chronic pain is particularly problematic because often no cause for it is found. The use of a single intervention is seldom successful for chronic pain. In some instances, pain is managed by medication; in other instances, nonpharmacologic techniques are used, such as simple relaxation techniques, distraction, or imagery.

Relaxation is one of the most widely used cognitive and behavior approaches to pain. Education, stress management techniques, hypnosis, and biofeedback are also used in pain management. Physical agents include heat and cold therapy, exercise, and transcutaneous nerve stimulation.

The key to managing pain is identifying how the pain is disrupting the patient's personal, social, professional, and family life. Education focusing on the pain, use of medications for treatment, and development of cognitive skills are important pain management components. In some cases, redefining treatment success as improvement in functioning rather than alleviation of pain may be necessary. The interaction between stress and pain is important. Increased stress leads to increased pain. Patients can better manage their pain when stress is reduced.

Medication Management

The psychiatric–mental health nurse uses many medication management interventions to help patients maintain therapeutic regimens. Medication management involves more than the actual administration of medications. Nurses must always assess a medication's effectiveness and side effects. They also need to consider drug–drug interactions. Treatment with psychopharmacologic agents can be lengthy because of the chronic nature of many disorders; many patients remain on medications for years, never becoming medication free. Thus, medication education is an ongoing intervention that requires careful documentation. Medication follow-up may include home visits as well as telephone calls.

INTERVENTIONS FOR THE PSYCHOLOGICAL DOMAIN

A major emphasis in psychiatric–mental health nursing is on the psychological domain: emotion, behavior, and cognition. The nurse–patient relationship serves as the basis of interventions directed toward the psychological domain. Because the therapeutic relationship was extensively discussed in Chapter 9, it is not covered in this chapter. This section does cover counseling, conflict resolution, bibliotherapy, reminiscence, behavior therapy, cognitive interventions, psychoeducation, health teaching, and spiritual interventions. Chapter 6 presents the theoretic basis for many of these interventions.

Counseling Interventions

Counseling interventions are specific, time-limited interactions between a nurse and a patient, family, or group experiencing immediate or ongoing difficulties related to their health or well-being. Counseling is usually short-term and focuses on improving coping abilities, reinforcing healthy behaviors, fostering positive interactions, or preventing illness and disability. Counseling strategies are discussed throughout the text. Psychotherapy, which differs from counseling, is generally a long-term approach aimed at improving or helping patients regain previous health status and functional abilities. Mental health specialists such as advanced practice nurses use psychotherapy.

Conflict Resolution

A conflict involves an individual's perception, emotions, and behavior. In a conflict, the person believes that his or her own needs, interests, wants, or values are incompatible with someone else's. The individual experiences fear, sadness, bitterness, anger, hopelessness, or some combination of these emotions in response to the perceived threat. Consequently, the individual takes action to meet his or her own needs, a course of action that can potentially interfere with the other person's ability to do the same (Mayer, 2000).

    Conflict resolution is a specific type of intervention by which the nurse helps patients resolve disagreements or disputes with family, friends, or other patients. Conflict can be positive if individuals see the problem as solvable and providing an opportunity for growth and interpersonal understanding. The nurse may be in the position of actually resolving a family conflict or teaching family members how to resolve their own conflicts positively. Additionally, because nurses are in positions of leadership, they often need conflict resolution skills to settle employee conflicts.

Conflict Resolution Process

Calmness and objectivity are important in resolving any patient or family conflict. The desired outcome of successful conflict resolution is a "win-win" situation—that is, each party feels good about the outcome. Conflict resolution includes the following steps: (1) helping those

involved identify the problem; (2) developing expectations for a win-win situation; (3) identifying interests; (4) fostering creative brainstorming; and (5) combining options into a win-win situation (Littlefield et al., 1993) (Fig. 14-2).

    The first step is identifying the problem. Because the conflict exists, with each party thinking he or she has the solution, each party must state his or her view of the problem and solution. During this phase, de-escalation of emotions may be necessary. The next step is developing expectations for a win-win situation by creating an atmosphere of mutual respect and trust. The nurse should avoid taking sides and reassure the involved parties that there may be a way to solve the problem by which everyone feels positive about the outcome. Next, an exploration of underlying issues is important to elicit interest and response. Questions such as, "What do you really want?" or "What are you worried about?" often identify the real issues and target what could become acceptable outcomes. The nurse also needs to determine whether he or she has any underlying issues by asking the same questions. The next step, brainstorming creative options, can then occur. The nurse directs participants to create potential solutions. The nurse writes them down without allowing any criticism; deferring any judgment of what has been said helps prevent premature rejection of good ideas. The final step is combining the generated ideas into a win-win situation. The group develops solutions that meet many of the participants' key interests and usually represent new approaches that are acceptable to all (Littlefield et al., 1993).

Cultural Brokering in Patient–System Conflicts

At times, patients who are politically and economically powerless find themselves in conflict with the health care system. Differences in cultural values and languages between patients and health care organizations contribute to feelings of powerlessness. For example, migrant farm workers, people who are homeless, and people who need to make informed decisions under stressful conditions may be unable to negotiate the health care system. The nurse can help to resolve such conflicts through **cultural brokering,** the act of bridging, linking, or mediating messages, instructions, and belief systems between groups or people of differing cultural systems to reduce conflict or produce change (Tripp-Reimer et al., 1999).

    For the "nurse-as-broker" to be effective, he or she attempts to establish and maintain a sense of connectedness or relationship with the patient. In turn, the nurse also establishes and cultivates networks with other health care facilities and resources. Cultural sensitivity enables the nurse to be aware of and sensitive to the needs of culturally diverse patients. Cultural competence is necessary for the brokering process to be effective.

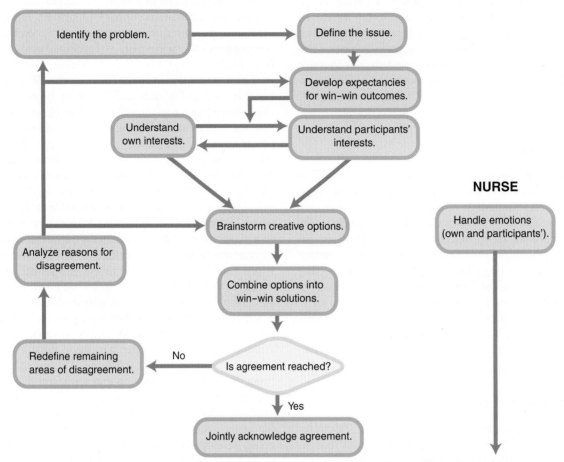

FIGURE 14.2 Conflict resolution model. (Adapted from Littlefield, L., Love, A., Peck, C., & Wertheim, E. [1993]. A model for resolving conflict: some theoretical, empirical, and practical applications. *Australian Psychologist, 28*(3), 80–85.)

Bibliotherapy

Bibliotherapy, sometimes referred to as *bibliocounseling*, is the reading of selected written materials to express feelings or gain insight under the guidance of a health care provider. The provider assigns and discusses with the patient a book, story, or article. The provider makes the assignment because he or she believes that the patient can receive therapeutic benefit from the reading. (It is assumed that the provider who assigned the reading has also read it.) The provider needs to consider the patient's reading level before making an assignment. If a patient has limited reading ability, the provider should not use bibliotherapy.

Literary works serve as a projective screen through which people see themselves in the story. Literature can help patients identify with characters and vicariously experience their reality. It can also expose patients to situations that they have not personally experienced, but the vicarious experience allows growth in self-knowledge and compassion. Through reading, patients can enrich their lives in the following ways:

Catharsis: expression of feelings stimulated by parallel experiences

Problem solving: development of solutions to problems in the literature from practical ideas about problem solving

Insight: increased self-awareness and understanding as the reader explores personal meaning from what is read (Lanza, 1996)

Reminiscence

Reminiscence, thinking about or relating past experiences, is used as a nursing intervention to enhance life review in older patients. The use of reminiscence encourages patients, either in individual or group settings, to discuss their past and review their lives. Through reminiscence, individuals can identify past coping strategies that can support them in current stressful situations. Patients can use reminiscence to maintain self-esteem, stimulate thinking, and support the natural healing process of life review. Activities that facilitate reminiscence include writing an account of past events, making a tape recording and playing it back, explaining pictures in old family albums, drawing a family tree, and writing to old friends.

Behavior Therapy

Behavior therapy interventions focus on reinforcing or promoting desirable behaviors or altering undesirable ones. The basic premise is that, because most behaviors are learned, new functional behaviors can also be learned. Behaviors—not internal psychic processes—are the targets of the interventions. The models of behavioral theorists serve as a basis for these interventions (see Chap. 6).

Behavior Modification

Behavior modification is a specific, systematized behavior therapy technique that can be applied to individuals, groups, or systems. The aim of behavior modification is to reinforce desired behavior responses and extinguish undesired ones. Desired behavior is rewarded to increase the likelihood that patients will repeat it, and over time, replace the problematic behavior with it. Behavior modification is used for various problematic behaviors, such as dysfunctional eating and addictions, and often with children and adolescents.

Token Economy

A **token economy** is the application of behavior modification to multiple behaviors and is used in inpatient settings. In a token economy, patients are rewarded with tokens for selected desired behaviors. They can use these tokens to purchase meals, leave the unit, watch television, or wear street clothes. In less restrictive environments, patients use tokens to purchase additional privileges such as attending social events. Token economy systems have been especially effective in reinforcing positive behaviors in people who are developmentally disabled or have severe and persistent mental illnesses. The strategy also works with aggressive psychiatric inpatients.

Cognitive Interventions

Cognitive interventions are verbally structured interventions that reinforce and promote desirable or alter undesirable cognitive functioning. The belief underlying this approach is that thoughts guide emotional reactions, motivations, and behaviors. Cognitive interventions do not solve problems for the patient but help the patient develop new ways of viewing situations so that they can solve their problems themselves. Nurses may use several models as the basis for cognitive interventions, but all models assume that, by changing the cognitive appraisal of a situation (view of the world) and by examining the meaning of events, patients can reinterpret situations. In turn, emotional changes will follow the cognitive changes, and ultimately, behaviors will change.

Because people develop their thinking patterns throughout their lifetime, many thoughts become so automatic that they are outside the individual's awareness. Thus, a person may be unaware of the automatic thoughts that influence his or her actions or other thoughts. **Automatic thinking** is often subject to errors, or tangible distortions of reality that contradict objective appraisals. For example, a patient with depression may be convinced that not one living soul cares about him. In fact, his large, extended family is deeply concerned. **Illogical thinking,** another thinking error, occurs when a person draws a faulty conclusion. For example, a college student is so devastated by failing an examination that she perceives that her college career is over.

To engage in cognitive treatment, the patient must be capable of introspection and reflection on thoughts and fantasies. Cognitive interventions are used in a wide range of clinical situations from short-term crises to persistent mental disorders. Cognitive interventions also include thought stopping, contracting, and cognitive restructuring. These specific interventions are discussed in Unit IV.

Psychoeducation

Psychoeducation uses educational strategies to teach patients the skills they lack because of a psychiatric disorder. The goal in psychoeducation is a change in knowledge and behavior. Nurses use psychoeducation to meet the educational needs of patients through adapting teaching strategies to their disorder-related deficits. As patients gain skills, functioning improves. Some patients may need to learn how to maintain their morning hygiene. Others may need to understand their illness and cope with hearing voices that others do not hear.

Specific psychoeducation techniques are based on adult learning principles, such as beginning at the point the learner is currently at and building on his or her current experiences. Thus, the nurse assesses the patient's readiness to learn and current skills. From there, the nurse individualizes a teaching plan for each patient. He or she can conduct such teaching in a one-to-one situation or group format.

Psychoeducation is a continuous process of assessing, setting goals, developing learning activities, and evaluating for changes in knowledge and behavior. Nurses use it with individuals, groups, families, and communities. Psychoeducation serves as a basis for psychosocial rehabilitation (PSR), a service-delivery approach for those with severe and persistent mental illness (see Chap. 17).

Health Teaching

One of the standards of care for the psychiatric nurse is health teaching (ANA et al., 2000). Psychoeducation (discussed in the previous section) is an approach that is consistent with the health teaching standard. According to this standard, "the psychiatric–mental health nurse, through health teaching, assists patients in achieving satisfying, productive, and healthy patterns of living" (ANA et al., 2000, p. 36). Health teaching is based on principles of learning and involves transmitting new information and providing constructive feedback and positive rewards, practice sessions, homework, and experimental learning. In health teaching, the psychiatric nurse is challenged to attend to potential health care problems other than mental disorders and emotional problems.

For example, if a person has diabetes mellitus and is taking insulin, the nurse needs to provide the health care teaching related to diabetes and the interaction of this problem with the mental disorder. According to the *Scope and Standards,* health teaching is the integration of principles of teaching and learning with the knowledge of health and illness (ANA et al., 2000) (Fig. 14-3).

Spiritual Interventions

Spiritual care is based on an assessment of the patient's spiritual needs. The development of a nonjudgmental relationship and just "being with" (not doing for) the patient are key to providing spiritual intervention. In some instances, patients ask to see a religious leader. Nurses should always respect and never deny these requests. To

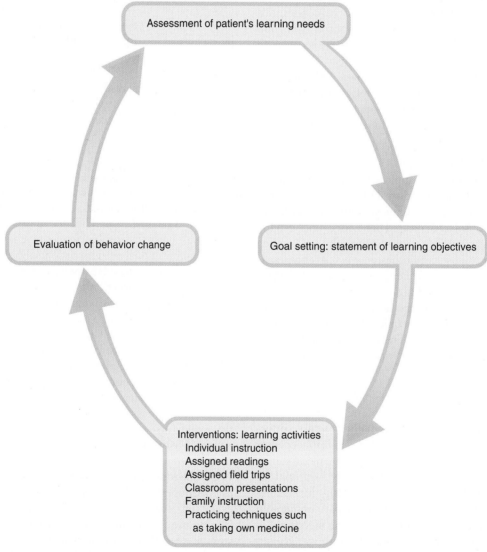

FIGURE 14.3 Teaching evaluation model. (Adapted from Rankin, S., & Stallings, K. [1990]. *Patient education* [p. 252]. Philadelphia: J. B. Lippincott.)

assist people in spiritual distress, the nurse should know and understand the beliefs and practices of various spiritual groups. **Spiritual support,** assisting patients to feel balance and connection within their relationships, involves listening to expressions of loneliness, using empathy, and providing patients with desired spiritual articles.

INTERVENTIONS FOR THE SOCIAL DOMAIN

The social domain can be understood as including the individual's environment and its affect on the patient's responses to mental disorders and distress. Interventions encompassing the social domain are geared toward couples, families, friends, and large and small social groups with special attention to ethnicity and community interactions. In some instances, nurses design interventions that affect a patient's environment, such as helping a family member make the decision to place a loved one in long-term care. In other instances, the nurse actually modifies the environment to promote positive behaviors. Group and family interventions are discussed in Chapters 15 and 16.

Social Behavior and Privilege Systems in Inpatient Units

In psychiatric units, unrelated strangers who have problems interacting are expected to live together in close quarters. For this reason, most psychiatric units develop a list of behavioral expectations, called *unit rules*, that staff members post and explain to patients upon admittance. The purpose is to facilitate a comfortable and safe living environment and has little to do with the patients' reasons for admission. Getting up at certain times, showering before breakfast, making the bed, and not visiting in others' rooms are typical expectations. Patients who follow the unit behavioral expectations usually gain more privileges.

Most psychiatric facilities use a privilege system to reinforce appropriate behavior. Privileges are either assigned by the admitting mental health provider or are inherent within the unit operations. Privileges are based on the assessment of a patient's risk to harm self or others and ability to follow treatment regimens. A privilege system is also effective in shaping appropriate social activity and can be used instead of a token economy. A patient with few privileges may be required to stay on the unit and eat only with other patients. A patient with full privileges may have complete freedom to leave the unit and go outside the hospital and into the community for short periods.

Milieu Therapy

Milieu therapy provides a stable and coherent social organization to facilitate an individual's treatment. The terms milieu therapy and *therapeutic environment* are often used interchangeably. In milieu therapy, the design of the physical surroundings, structure of patient activities, and promotion of a stable social structure and cultural setting enhance the setting's therapeutic potential. A therapeutic milieu facilitates patient interactions and promotes personal growth. Milieu therapy is the responsibility of the nurse in collaboration with the patient and other health care providers. The key concepts of milieu therapy include containment, validation, structured interaction, and open communication.

Containment

Containment is the process of providing safety and security and involves the patient's access to food and shelter. In a well-contained milieu, patients feel safe from their illnesses and protected against social stigma. The physical surroundings are important in this process and should be clean and comfortable, with special attention paid to promoting a noninstitutionalized environment. Pictures on walls, comfortable furniture, and soothing colors help patients relax. Most facilities encourage patients and nursing staff to wear street clothes, which helps decrease the formalized nature of hospital settings and promotes nurse–patient relationships. Therapeutic milieus emphasize patient involvement in treatment decisions and operation of the unit; nurses should encourage freedom of movement within the contained environment. Patients participate in maintaining the quality of the physical surroundings, assuming responsibility for making their own beds, attending to their own belongings, and keeping an acceptable living area. Families are viewed as a part of the patient's life, and ties are maintained. In most inpatient settings, specific times are set for family interaction, education, and treatment. Family involvement is many times a criterion for admission for treatment, and the involvement may include regular family attendance at therapy sessions.

Validation

In a therapeutic environment, **validation** is another process that affirms patient individuality. Staff–patient interactions should constantly reaffirm the patient's humanity and human rights. Any interaction a staff member initiates with a patient should reflect his or her underlying respect for that patient. Patients must believe that staff members truly like and respect them. The staff should encourage group and social interaction among patients.

Patients should be actively involved in and participate in the decisions made about the treatment process. When possible, the roles between patients and nurses are blurred, and nurses view patients as responsible human beings in charge of their own treatment decisions. Such expectations validate the humanity of patients.

Structured Interaction

One of the most interesting milieu concepts is **structured interaction,** purposeful interaction that allows patients to interact with others in a useful way. The daily community meeting provides the structure to explain unit rules and consequences of violations. Ideally, patients who are either elected or volunteer for the responsibility assume leadership for these meetings. In the meeting, the group discusses behavioral expectations, such as making beds daily, appropriate dress, and rules for leaving the unit. Usually, there are other rules, such as no fighting or name calling (Table 14-2).

In some instances, the treatment team assigns structured interactions to specific patients as a part of their treatment. Specific attitudes or approaches are directed toward individual patients who benefit from a particular type of interaction. Nurses consistently assume indulgence, flexibility, passive or active friendliness, matter-of-fact attitude, casualness, watchfulness, or kind firmness when interacting with specific patients. For ex-

ample, if a patient is known to overreact and dramatize events, the staff may provide a matter-of-fact attitude when the patient engages in dramatic behavior. Staff may approach another patient in a firm matter whenever he or she requests special privileges.

Open Communication

In **open communication,** staff and patient willingly share information. Staff members invite patient self-disclosure within the support of a nurse–patient relationship. Additionally, they provide a model of effective communication when interacting with one another as well as with patients. They arrange an environment to facilitate optimal interaction and resocialization. Support, attention, praise, and reassurance that staff gives to the patients improves self-esteem and increases confidence. Patient education is also a part of this support, as are directions to foster coping skills.

Milieu Therapy in Different Settings

In long-term care settings, the therapeutic milieu becomes essential because patients may reside in a facility for months or years. These patients typically have a diagnosis of schizophrenia or developmental disabilities. Structure in daily living is important to the successful functioning of the individuals and the overall group but must be applied within the context of individual needs.

TABLE 14.2   Patient–Staff Community Meeting

Goal	Implementation
Plan ahead.	• Designate leader and several deputy leaders. • Hold brief meeting with staff.
Operate the meeting.	• Establish rules and norms. • Announce the purpose, format, and rules (include patients who know the routine). • Keep meeting brief. • Refer treatment questions to outside of meeting.
Get everyone involved.	• Ask everyone to introduce themselves. • Address individuals by name. • Use structured exercises to engage all patients. • Delegate tasks of meeting to individuals.
Infuse energy.	• Use exercises to mobilize energy. • Use humor and empathy. • Maintain a lively and interesting approach.
Choose relevant topics.	• Focus on discussion of issues that affect all. • Deal with difficult issues calmly and frankly. • Affirm rules and norms.
Address unit process.	• Discuss needs of unit each meeting: containment, structure, support, involvement, validation. • Discuss strategies.

From Kahn, F., (1994). The patient–staff community meeting: Old tools, new rules. *Journal of Psychosocial Nursing, 32*(8). 23–26.

For example, if a patient cannot get up one morning in time to complete assigned tasks (eg, showering or making a bed) because of a personal crisis the night before, the nurse should consider the context compassionately and flexibly, not applying the "consequences" rule or taking away the patient's privileges. In turn, the nurse must weigh individual needs against the collective needs of all the patients. For the patient who is consistently late for treatment activities, the nurse should apply the rules of the unit even if it means taking away privileges.

Recently, concepts of milieu therapy have also been applied to short-term inpatient and community settings. In inpatient, acute care settings, nursing actions provide limits and controls on patient behavior and provide structure and safety for the patients. Milieu treatments on the unit are based on the individual needs of the patients and include relaxation groups, discussion groups, and medication groups. Spontaneous and planned activities are possible on a short-term unit as well as in a long-term setting. In the community, it is possible to apply milieu therapy approaches in day treatment centers, group homes, and single dwellings.

Promotion of Patient Safety on Psychiatric Units

Although the use of social rules of conduct and privilege systems can enhance smooth operation of a unit, some potentially serious problems can be associated with these practices. One of the most critical aspects of psychiatric–mental health nursing is the promotion of patient safety, especially on the inpatient units. This section discusses interventions that are designed for the protection of patients.

Observation

Observation is an ongoing assessment of the patient's mental status to identify and subvert any potential problem. An important process in all nursing practice, observation is particularly important in psychiatric nursing. In psychiatric settings, patients are ambulatory and thus more susceptible to environmental hazards. Judgment and cognition impairment are symptoms of many psychiatric disorders. Often, the patient has been admitted because of being a danger to self or others. In psychiatric nursing, observation is more than just seeing the patient. It means continually monitoring the patient for any indication of harm to self or others.

All patients who are hospitalized for psychiatric reasons are continually monitored. The intensity of the observation depends on their risk to themselves and others. Some patients are merely asked to "check in" at different times of the day, whereas others have a staff member assigned to only them, such as in instances of potential suicide. Mental health facilities and units all have policies that specify levels of observation for patients of varying degrees of risk.

De-escalation

De-escalation is an interactive process of calming and redirecting a patient who has an immediate potential for violence, directed toward either self or others. This intervention involves assessing the situation and preventing it from escalating to one in which injury occurs to the patient, staff, or other patients. Once the nurse has assessed the situation, he or she calmly calls to the patient and asks the individual to leave the situation. The nurse must avoid rushing toward the patient or giving orders (see Chap. 36). Nurses can use various interventions in this situation, including distraction, conflict resolution, and cognitive interventions. The goal of de-escalation is avoiding further confrontation and injury.

Seclusion

Seclusion is the involuntary confinement of a person in a room or an area where the person is physically prevented from leaving (Health Care Finance Administration [HCFA], 2000). A patient is placed in seclusion for purposes of safety or behavioral management. The seclusion room has no furniture except a mattress and a blanket. Walls are usually padded. The room is environmentally safe, with no hanging devices, electrical outlets, or windows from which the patient could jump. Once a patient is placed in seclusion, he or she is observed at all times. There are several types of seclusion arrangements. The use of seclusion must follow the same guidelines as the use of restraints (discussed in the next section). Some facilities have seclusion rooms next to the nurses' stations that have an observation window. Other facilities use a modified patient room and assign a staff member to view the patient at all times.

Seclusion is an extremely negative patient experience; consequently, its use is seriously questioned (Meehan et al., 2000), and many facilities have completely abandoned its practice (Research Box 14-1). Patient outcomes may actually be worse if seclusion is used. In one study, secluded subjects exhibited poorer attitudes toward the hospital and had longer lengths of stay than their nonsecluded cohorts (Legris et al., 1999). If units are adequately staffed and personnel are trained in dealing with assaultive patients, seclusion is rarely needed.

Restraints

The most restrictive safety interventions are restraints, which are used only in the most extreme circumstances.

RESEARCH BOX 14.1

Patients' Perceptions of Seclusion: A Qualitative Investigation

Twelve patients receiving acute inpatient psychiatric care participated in semistructured interviews to elicit their perceptions of seclusion. Assessed areas of interest included perceptions of the reasons for seclusion, feelings while in seclusion, perceptions of staff about the seclusion experience, and attitudes to the seclusion environment.

Results: Five themes recurred. Most patients felt that they were secluded inappropriately and experienced seclusion as punishment. The experience generated negative emotions. Patients reported feeling angry before, during, and after the seclusion episode and directed their anger primarily toward the staff involved. Anger usually gave way to a sense of powerlessness. The social isolation and physical characteristics of the seclusion room combined to distort reality, making some patients feel as if they were "going mad" or "losing control." Patients did develop several strategies to assist them in coping with their restricted environment, including talking to themselves, singing, and pacing. Finally, the level of interaction with staff during and following seclusion was a source of dissatisfaction. Patients believed that if communication had been more effective, they would not have ended up in seclusion.

Utilization in Clinical Setting: This study further supports avoiding the seclusion of patients. The experience is negative and does not foster positive mental health. Patients view seclusion as punishment, blocking effective nurse–patient communication.

Meehan, T., Vermeer, C., & Windsor, C. (2000). Patients' perceptions of seclusion: A qualitative investigation. *Journal of Advanced Nursing, 31*(2), 370–377.

TEXT BOX 14.2

Summary of Restraint and Seclusion Guidelines

- The patient has the right to be free from restraints of any form that are not medically necessary or that staff use as a means of coercion, discipline, convenience, or retaliation.
- A restraint can be used only if needed to improve the patient's well-being and if less restrictive interventions have been determined ineffective.
- The use of restraint must be (1) selected only when less restrictive measures have been found ineffective to protect the patient or others from harm, (2) in accordance with the order of a physician or other licensed independent practitioner (LIP) permitted by the state and hospital.
- The order must (1) never be written as a standing or on an as needed basis, and (2) must be followed by consultation with the patient's treating physician in accordance with the patient's plan of care.
- The LIP orders the use of restraint or seclusion. The LIP must see and evaluate the need for restraint or seclusion within 1 hour after the initiation of this intervention.
- Each written order for a physical restraint or seclusion is limited to 4 hours for adults, 2 hours for children and adolescents aged 9 to 17 years, or 1 hour for patients younger than 9 years.
- Written or verbal orders for initial and continuing use of restraint are time limited.
- Patients in restraint or seclusion continually must be assessed, monitored, and re-evaluated.
- Restraint and seclusion may not be used simultaneously unless the patient is monitored face to face by an assigned staff member.

Adapted from Health Care Finance Administration. (2000). *Quality of information, quality standards.* Hospital Interpretative Guidelines. Patients Rights. A 182–195. www.hcfa.gov.

Chemical restraint is the use of medication to control patients or manage their behavior. Chemical restraints are added to the patient's regular drug regimen. A **physical restraint** is any manual method or physical or mechanical device attached or adjacent to the patient's body that restricts freedom of movement or normal access to one's body, material, or equipment and cannot be easily removed. Holding a patient in a manner that restricts movement constitutes restraint for that patient (HCFA, 1999).

The use of seclusion and restraints must follow the Quality Standards regulation contained in the *Patients' Rights Condition of Participation* (CoP) (HCFA, 1999). Agencies that do not follow the regulations may lose their Medicare and Medicaid certification and, consequently, funding (Text Box 14-2).

The application of physical restraints should follow nursing standards and hospital policies. Nurses should document all the previously tried de-escalation interventions before the application of restraints. They should limit use of restraints to times when an individual is judged to be a danger to self or others; they should apply restraints only until the patient has gained control over behavior. When a patient is in physical restraints, the nurse should closely observe the patient and protect him or her from self-injury.

Different types of restraints are available. Wrist restraints restrict arm movement. Walking restraints, or ankle restraints, are often used if a patient cannot resist the impulse to run from a facility but is safe to go outside and to activities. Three-point and four-point restraints are applied to the wrist and ankles in bed. When five-point restraints are used, all extremities are secured, and another restraint is placed across the chest.

Home Visits

Psychiatric home health services become more available as reimbursement for them increases. Delivery of psychiatric nursing services has moved from the hospital into the community. Usually, these patients have been hospitalized or have received treatment for acute psychiatric symptoms before being referred to the psychiatric home service. The goal of home care is to maximize the patient's functional ability within the nurse–patient relationship and with the family or significant other as appropriate (Finkelman, 1997). The psychiatric nurse who makes home visits needs to be able to work independently, is skilled in teaching patients and families, can administer and monitor medications, and uses community resources for the patient's needs.

For many years, **home visits**, or delivery of nursing care in the patient's living environment, had fallen out of favor with most specialties in the United States, including psychiatric–mental health care. In the past, home visits were viewed as an inefficient use of professional time, and transporting supplies was seen as inconvenient. The costs of home visits today, however, are much lower than are the costs of hospitalization. With managed care and practice guidelines, home visits are now favorably viewed as an efficient and cost-effective way to deliver mental health care. Some states have set up their public mental health services to include home visits on a team basis. Managed care private payers also support home visits.

Home visits are especially useful in several different situations, including helping reluctant patients enter therapy, conducting a comprehensive assessment, strengthening a support network, and maintaining patients in the community when their condition has deteriorated. Home visits are useful in helping individuals become compliant in taking medication. One major advantage of home visits is the opportunity to provide family members information and education and to engage them in planning and interventions.

Home visits also help providers develop cultural sensitivity to families from diverse backgrounds. Home-based interventions allow the nurse to assess the family structure and interaction, including the roles members play, how the family functions in terms of responsibilities, and the family life cycle. A family's cultural background will influence all these factors; culture is important to consider when planning interventions.

The home visit process consists of three steps: (1) the previsit phase, (2) the home visit, and (3) the postvisit phase (Gerace et al., 1990). During previsit planning, the nurse sets goals for the home visit based on data received from other health care providers or the patient; the nurse and patient agree on the time of the visit. As the nurse travels to the home, he or she should assess the neighborhood for access to services, socioeconomic factors, and safety.

The actual visit can be divided into four parts (Wayman et al., 1990). The first is the greeting phase, in which the nurse establishes rapport with family members. Greetings, which are usually brief, establish the communication process and the atmosphere for the visit. Greetings should be friendly but professional. In cultures that consider greetings important, this phase may involve more formal interactions, such as taking food or tea with family members. The next phase is the establishment of the focus of the visit. In some instances, the purpose of the visit is administration of medication, health teaching, or counseling. These visits typically last 30 to 90 minutes, and the patient and family must be clear regarding the purpose. The implementation of the service is the next phase and should use most of the visit time. If the purpose of the visit is problem solving or decision making, the family's cultural values may determine the types of interaction and decision-making approaches.

Closure is the last phase, the end of the home visit. It is a time to summarize and clarify important points and bring closure to the visit. The nurse should schedule any additional visits and reiterate patient expectations between visits. Usually, the nurse is the only provider to see the patient regularly. The nurse should acknowledge family members on leaving if they were not a part of the visit.

The postvisit phase includes documentation, reporting, and follow-up planning. This time is also when the nurse meets with the supervisor and presents data from the home visit at the team meeting (Gerace et al., 1990).

Community Action

Nurses have a unique opportunity to be involved in the promotion of mental health awareness and to support humane treatment for people with mental disorders. Activities range from being an advisor to support groups to participating in the political process through lobbying efforts and serving on community mental health boards. These unpaid activities are usually outside the realm of a particular job. An important role of professionals, however, is to provide community service in addition to service through income-generating positions.

Summary of Key Points

➤ Nurses develop nursing interventions from assessment data and organize them around nursing diagnoses. The patient outcomes and the *Scope and Standards of Psychiatric–Mental Health Nursing Practice* guide their selection (ANA et al., 2000).

➤ The ability of patients with psychiatric disorders to manage self-care activities varies. The Orem self-care model is often used in conceptualizing patient needs and implementing interventions.

➤ Interventions focusing on the biologic areas include activity and exercise; sleep, nutrition, relaxation, hydration, and thermoregulation interventions; pain management; and medication management. Nutritional interventions are used with most patients with psychiatric disorders. Medication management is a priority because of the long-term nature of the disorders and the importance of medication compliance.

➤ Interventions focusing on the psychological dimensions include counseling, behavior therapy, cognitive interventions, psychoeducation, health teaching, and others. Implementation of these interventions requires a broad theoretic knowledge base.

➤ Interventions focusing on the social dimensions include group and family approaches, milieu therapy, safety interventions, home visits, and community action. On an inpatient psychiatric unit, the nurse uses milieu therapy to maximize the treatment effects of the patient's environment.

Critical Thinking Challenges

1. Review Standard V, Implementation, in the *Scope and Standards of Psychiatric–Mental Health Nursing Practice* in Chapter 5. Develop an argument as to whether or not the interventions in the psychiatric–mental health nursing standards are compatible with the Nursing Interventions Classification. Justify your argument.

2. Tom, a 25-year-old man with schizophrenia, lives with his parents, who want to retire to Florida. Tom goes to work each day but relies on his mother for meals, laundry, and reminders about taking his medication. Tom believes that he can manage the home, but his mother is concerned. She asks the nurse for advice about leaving her son to manage on his own. Identify a nursing diagnosis and interventions that would meet some of Tom's potential responses to his changing lifestyle.

3. Joan, a 35-year-old married woman, is admitted to an acute psychiatric unit for stabilization of her mood disorder. She is extremely depressed but refuses to consider a recommended medication change. She asks the nurse what to do. Using a conflict resolution intervention, explain how you would approach Joan's problem.

4. A nurse reports to work for the evening shift. The unit is chaotic. The television in the day room is loud; two patients are arguing over the program. Visitors are mingling in patients' rooms. The temperature of the unit is hot. One patient is running up and down the hall yelling, "Help me, help me." Using a milieu therapy approach, what would you do to calm the unit?

5. A patient is admitted to the unit and becomes extremely agitated, endangering himself and others. After trying to de-escalate the patient, the nurse decides that the best approach is to put the patient into restraints. Outline a procedure that the nurse must follow to meet the Health Care Finance Administration guidelines regarding restraints and seclusion contained in the *Patients' Rights Condition of Participation*.

 WEB LINKS

www.hcfa.gov   The Health Care Finance Administration website contains the regulations regarding the use of seclusion and restraint.

www.nic.com   This Nursing Interventions Classification (NIC) website explains the development of the NIC and answers questions related to its use.

www.apna.com   The American Psychiatric Nurses Association site contains conference information and literature related to nursing.

REFERENCES

American Nurses Association, American Psychiatric Nurses Association, & International Society of Psychiatric–Mental Health Nurses. (2000). *Scope and standards of psychiatric–mental health nursing practice*. Washington, DC: American Nurses Publishing.

Burks, K. J. (1999). A nursing model for chronic illness. *Rehabilitation Nursing, 24*(5), 197–200.

Campbell, J. C., & Soeken, K. L. (1999). Women's responses to battering: A test of the model. *Research in Nursing & Health, 22*(1), 49–58.

Finkelman, A. (1997). *Psychiatric home care*. Gaithersburg, MD: Aspen.

Gerace, L., Tiller, J., & Anderson, J. (1990). Development of a psychiatric home visit module for student training. *Hospital and Community Psychiatry, 41*(9), 1015–1017.

Health Care Finance Administration. (2000). *Interpretive guidelines for hospital CoP for patient rights*. Quality of Care Information, Quality Standards. **www.hcfa.gov.**

Health Care Finance Administration. (2000). *Hospital conditions of participation for patients' rights*. Quality of Care Information, Quality Standards. **www.hcfa.gov/quality/4b2.htm.**

Kahn, E. (1994). The patient–staff community meeting: Old tools, new rules. *Journal of Psychosocial Nursing, 32*(8), 23–26.

Lanza, M. (1996). Bibliotherapy and beyond. *Perspectives in Psychiatric Care, 32*(1), 12–14.

Legris, J., Walters, M., & Browne, G. (1999). The impact of seclusion on the treatment outcomes of psychotic in-patients. *Journal of Advanced Nursing*, *30*(2), 448–459.

Littlefield, L., Love, A., Peck, C., & Wertheim, E. (1993). A model for resolving conflict: Some theoretical, empirical and practical implications. Special issue: The psychology of peace and conflict. *Australian Psychologist*, *28*(2), 80–85.

Mayer, B. (2000). *The dynamics of conflict resolution.* San Francisco: Jossey-Bass.

McCloskey, J., & Bulechek, G. (1999). *Nursing interventions: Effective nursing treatments.* Philadelphia: W. B. Saunders.

Meehan, T., Vermeer, C., & Windsor, C. (2000). Patients' perceptions of seclusion: A qualitative investigation. *Journal of Advanced Nursing, 3*(2), 370–377.

Tripp-Reimer, T., Brink, P., & Pinkham, C. (1999). Cultural brokerage. In J. McCloskey, & G. Bulechek (Eds.), *Nursing interventions: Effective nursing treatments* (pp. 637–649). Philadelphia: W. B. Saunders.

Wayman, K., Lynch, E., & Hanson, M. (1990). Home-based early childhood services: Cultural sensitivity in a family systems approach. *Topics in Early Childhood Special Education, 10*(4), 56–75.

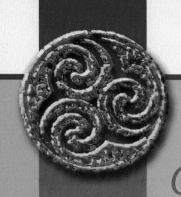

Group Interventions

Mary Ann Boyd

GROUP: DEFINITIONS AND CONCEPTS
Open Versus Closed Groups
Group Size
Group Development
  Beginning Stage
  Working Stage
  Termination Stage
Roles of Group Members
Group Communication
  Verbal Communication
  Nonverbal Communication
Group Norms and Standards
Group Cohesion
Groupthink and Decision Making

GROUP LEADERSHIP
Choosing Leadership Styles
Selecting the Members
Arranging Seating
Dealing With Challenging
  Group Behaviors
  Monopolizer
  "Yes, but"
  Disliked Member
  Group Conflict

TYPES OF GROUPS
Psychoeducation Groups
Supportive Therapy Groups
Psychotherapy Groups
Self-Help Groups

COMMON NURSING INTERVENTION GROUPS
Medication Groups
Symptom Management Groups
Anger Management Groups
Self-Care Groups

LEARNING OBJECTIVES

After studying the chapter, you will be able to:

➤ Discuss group concepts that are useful in leading groups.

➤ Compare the roles that group members can assume.

➤ Identify important aspects of leading a group, such as member selection, leadership skills, seating arrangements, and ways of dealing with challenging behaviors of group members.

➤ Identify four types of groups: psychoeducation, supportive therapy, psychotherapy, and self-help.

➤ Describe common nursing intervention groups.

Group interventions can have powerful treatment effects on patients who are trying to develop self-understanding, conquer unwanted thoughts and feelings, and change behaviors. They are efficient because several patients can receive treatment at once. For interventions to be effective, the nurse must possess leadership skills that can shape and monitor group interactions. The psychiatric–mental health nurse uses group interventions in all roles, including direct care provider, case manager, and unit leader. Additionally, all nurses can use group interventions, such as when conducting patient education or leading support groups. This chapter presents relevant group concepts that the psychiatric nurse will use. It explores group leadership, with special emphasis on the groups that nurses commonly lead.

GROUP: DEFINITIONS AND CONCEPTS

There are many different definitions of a group. In the psychoanalytic tradition, a group is a collection of individuals who identify with the leader and then with one another but who act, for the most part, independently. According to systems theory, a group consists of parts or components that exist to perform some activity or purpose. As members of a group interact, subsystems form, which challenges the leader to understand the effect of these components on the total system and to improve channels of communication. A global but rather simple definition of a group is two or more people who are in an interdependent relationship with one another. The simplicity of the definition is misleading because interactions within groups, or **group dynamics,** are anything but simple. Group dynamics influence the group's development and process. In fact, it takes an astute observer to determine the real dynamics of a group and their effects on individuals. No matter the type of group, its theoretic orientation, or its purpose, group dynamics influence the success or failure of a group intervention.

In this text, a group is defined as two or more people who develop interactive relationships and share at least one common goal or issue. Groups can be further defined according to the number of people or the relationship of members. A **dyad** is a group of only two people who are usually related, such as a married couple, siblings, or parent and child. A **triad** is a group of three people who may or may not be related. A family is a special type of group and will be discussed in Chapter 16.

KEY CONCEPT Group. A **group** is defined as two or more people who develop interactive relationships and share at least one common goal or issue.

277

Open Versus Closed Groups

A group can be viewed as either an open or a closed system. In an **open group**, new members may join, and old members may leave the group at different sessions. For example, a newly admitted patient may join an anger management group that is part of an ongoing program in an inpatient unit. As a new member, the individual is at a disadvantage because the other members already know one another and have established relationships. The advantage of an open group is that participants can join at any time and stay in the group as long as they need. Also, these groups can function on an ongoing basis and thus can be available to more people.

In a **closed group**, members begin the group at one time, and no new members are admitted. If a member of a closed group leaves, no replacement joins. Advantages of a closed group are that the participants get to know one another at the same time, the group is more cohesive, and members move through the group process concurrently. Most clinicians prefer closed groups because such groups facilitate the best treatment results. Implementing closed-group interventions is often difficult, however, because patients are not always available at the same time.

Group Size

Group size is an important consideration in forming group programs. Many mental health professionals favor small groups, but large groups can also be effective. Whether to form a large or small group depends on the purpose, abilities, and availability of the participants and the skills of the leader. Small groups (usually no more than 8 to 10 members) become more cohesive, are less likely to form subgroups, and can provide a richer interpersonal experience than large groups. Small groups function nicely with one group leader, although many small groups are led by two people. An ideal small group is about seven to eight people in addition to the leader or leaders. Five is the minimum number of members necessary for therapeutic group process to develop (Yalom, 1995).

Small groups often are used for patients who are trying to deal with complex emotional problems such as sexual abuse, eating disorders, or trauma. Small groups are ideal for individuals who have special learning needs or others who need much individual attention. These groups work best if they are closed to new members or if new members are gradually introduced. The disadvantage of small groups is that they cannot withstand the loss of members and can quickly dissolve if members leave. Additionally, if places are unfilled, the group's dynamics change, which may interfere with the therapeutic process. A large group (more than 10 members) can

also be therapeutic as well as cost-effective in clinical settings. Some research suggests that large treatment groups are as effective as small groups for certain patient populations, such as those with alcoholism (Klein, 1993). A large group can be ongoing and open ended. It can be effective without the development of intense transference and countertransference issues. A disadvantage is that participants of large groups are more likely to feel alienated from one another.

Leading a large group is more complex than leading a small group because of the number of potential interactions and relationships that can form. The leader needs both presentation and group leadership skills. In a large group, determining the feelings and thoughts of the participants can be difficult. The leader of a large group usually views the group as a system and identifies the various subgroups that form. If subgroups form, the leader changes the structure and function of communication within the subgroups by rearranging seating and encouraging the subgroup to interact with the rest of the group.

Group Development

The development of a group is a process, just as is the development of the therapeutic relationship (see Chap. 9). The term group process is used to describe the culmination of the session-to-session interactions of the members that move the group toward its goal. Some maintain that there is no normal sequence of group phases (Cissna, 1984; Gersick, 1988) or that growth continues as the group becomes more cohesive (Barker, 1991). Many researchers, however, view group development as a sequence of phases, particularly in small groups (Table 15-1). Although models of group development differ, most follow a pattern of a beginning, middle, and ending phase (Agazarian, 1999). These stages should be thought of not as a straight line with one preceding another, but as a dynamic process that is constantly revisiting and re-examining group interactions and behaviors, as well as progressing forward.

> **KEY CONCEPT**   **Group process.** **Group process** is the culmination of the session-to-session interactions of the members that move the group toward its goals.

Beginning Stage

The beginning of a group is a time when group members get to know one another and the group leader. The length of the beginning stage depends on, among other variables, the purpose of the group, number of members, and skill of the leader. The beginning stage may last for only a few sessions or several. "Honeymoon" behavior characterizes this stage in the beginning, but "conflict"

TABLE 15.1 Comparison of Models of Group Development

Robert Bales (1955)	Bruce Tuckman (1965)	William Schutz (1960)
• *Orientation:* What is the problem? • *Evaluation:* How do we feel about it? • *Control:* What should we do about it?	• *Forming:* Get to know one another and form a group. • *Storming:* Tension and conflict occur; subgroups form and clash with one another. • *Norming:* Develop norms of how to work together. • *Performing:* Reach consensus and develop cooperative relationships.	• *Inclusion:* Deal with issues of belonging and being in and out of the group. • *Control:* Deal with issues of authority (who is in charge?), dependence, and autonomy. • *Affection:* Deal with issues of intimacy, closeness, and caring, versus dislike and distancing.

dominates at the end. During the initial sessions, members usually display polite, congenial behavior typical of those in new social situations. They are "good patients" and often intellectualize their problems. That is, these patients deal with emotional conflict or stress by excessively using abstract thinking or generalizations to minimize disturbing feelings. Members are usually anxious and sometimes display behavior that does not truly represent their feelings. In the first few sessions, members test whether they can trust one another. Sometime after the initial sessions, group members usually experience a period of conflict, either among themselves or with the leader. This conflict is a normal part of group development, and many believe that conflict is necessary to move into any working phase. Sometimes, one or more group members become the scapegoat. Such situations challenge the leader to guide the group during this period by avoiding taking sides and treating all members respectfully.

Working Stage

The working stage of groups involves a real sharing of ideas and the development of closeness. A group personality may emerge that is distinct from the individual personalities of its members. The group develops its own rules and rituals and has its own behavioral norms. For example, groups develop regular patterns of seating and interaction. During this stage, the group realizes its purpose. If the purpose is education, the participants engage in learning new content or skills. If the aim of the group is to share feelings and experiences, these activities consume group meetings. During this phase, the group starts on time, and the leader often needs to remind members when it is time to stop.

Termination Stage

Termination can be difficult for a group, especially a successful one. During the final stages, members begin to grieve for the loss of the group's closeness and begin to reestablish themselves as individuals. Individuals terminate from groups as they do from any relationship. One person may not show up at the last session, another person may bring up issues that the group has already addressed, and others may demonstrate anger or hostility. Most members of successful groups are sad as the group terminates. During the last meetings, members may make arrangements for meeting after group. These plans rarely materialize or continue. Leaders should recognize these plans as part of the farewell process—saying good-bye to the group.

Roles of Group Members

There are two official or **formal group roles**, the leader and the members; however, individuals in small groups may have many informal roles. Members often assume **informal group roles**, or positions in the group with rights and duties that are directed toward one or more group members. These roles can either help or hinder the group's process. One of the oldest models is Benne and Sheats' (1948) list of task, maintenance, and individual roles. **Task functions** involve the business of the group or "keeping things focused." Individuals who provide this function keep the group focused on a main purpose. For any group to be successful, it must have members who assume some of these roles. Frequently assumed task roles include *information seeker* (asks for clarification), *coordinator* (spells out relationships between ideas), and *recorder* (keeper of the minutes). **Maintenance functions** help the group stay together by ensuring it starts on time, assisting individuals to compromise, and determining membership. These individuals are more interested in maintaining the group's cohesiveness than focusing on the group's tasks. The *harmonizer, compromiser,* and *standard setter* are examples of maintenance roles. In a successful group, members assume both group task and maintenance functions (Table 15-2).

TABLE 15.2 Roles and Functions of Group Members

Task Roles	Maintenance Roles	Individual Roles
Initiator-contributor suggests or proposes new ideas or a new view of the problem or goal.	*Encourager* praises, agrees with, and accepts contributions of others.	*Aggressor* deflates the status of others; expresses disapproval of the values, acts, or feelings of others; attacks the group or problem; jokes aggressively; tries to take credit for the work.
Information seeker asks for clarification of the values pertinent to the group activity.	*Harmonizer* mediates differences among members and relieves tension in conflict situations.	
Information giver offers "authoritative" facts or generalizations or gives own experiences.	*Compromiser* operates from within a conflict and may yield status or admit error to maintain group harmony.	*Blocker* tends to be negative and resistant, disagrees and opposes without or beyond "reason," and attempts to bring back an issue after group has rejected it.
Opinion giver states belief or opinions with emphasis on what should be the group's values.	*Gate-keeper* attempts to keep communication channels open by encouraging or facilitating the participation of others or proposes regulation of the flow of communication through limiting time.	*Recognition-seeker* calls attention to self through such activities as boasting, reporting on personal achievements, acting in unusual ways.
Elaborator spells out suggestions in terms of examples, develops meanings of ideas and rationales, tries to deduce how an idea would work.		
Coordinator shows or clarifies the relationships among various ideas and suggestions.	*Standard setter* expresses standards for the group to achieve.	*Self-confessor* uses group setting to express personal, non–group-oriented feelings or insights.
Orienter defines the position of the group with respect to its goals.	*Group observer* keeps records of various aspects of group processes and interprets data to group.	*Playboy* makes a display of lack of involvement in group's processes.
Evaluator-critic measures the outcome of the group against some standard.	*Follower* goes along with the movement of the group.	*Dominator* tries to assert authority or superiority in manipulating the group or certain members of the group through flattery, being directive, interrupting others.
Energizer attempts to stimulate the group to action or decision.		
Procedural technician expedites group movement by doing things for the group such as distributing copies, arranging seating.		*Help-seeker* attempts to call forth sympathy from other group members through expressing insecurity, personal confusion, or depreciation of self beyond reason.
Recorder writes suggestions, keeps minutes, serves as group memory.		*Special interest pleader* speaks for a special group, such as "grass roots," usually representing personal prejudices or biases.

From Benne, K., & Sheats, P. (1948). Functional roles of group members. *Journal of Social Issues, 4*(2), 41.

Individual roles are those member roles that either enhance or detract from the group's functioning. These roles have nothing to do with the group's purpose or cohesion. For example, someone who monopolizes the group inhibits the group's work. People who are participating in the group may be meeting personal needs, such as feeling important or being an expert on a subject. When individual roles predominate, however, the risk is that dominant individuals may contribute to neither the task nor the maintenance of the group.

In selecting members and analyzing the progress of the group, the leader must pay attention to the balance between the task and maintenance functions. If too many group members assume task functions and too few assume maintenance functions, the group may have difficulty developing cohesion. If too many members assume maintenance functions, the group may never finish its work. Although it is usually impossible to select individuals only because of their group role, tracking the group in terms of how well it functions and how much it actually gets done is important.

Group Communication

One of the responsibilities of the group leader is to facilitate both verbal and nonverbal communication to meet the treatment goals of the individual members and the entire group. Because of the number of people involved, developing trusting relationships within groups is more complicated than is developing a single relationship with a patient. The communication techniques used in establishing and maintaining individual relationships are the same for groups, but the leader also attends to the communication patterns among the members.

Verbal Communication

Communication Network. Group interaction can be viewed as a communication network that becomes patterned and predictable. In a group, verbal comments are linked in a chain formation. Asking a colleague to observe and record the content and interaction is a useful technique in determining the interaction pattern within a group; the leader may also use an audio or video recorder. In some groups, one person may always change the subject when another raises a sensitive topic. One person may always speak after another. People who sit next to each other tend to communicate among themselves. By analyzing the content and patterns, the leader can determine the existence of communications pathways—who is most liked in the group, who occupies a position of power, what subgroups have formed, and who is isolated from the group. Moreno's (1953) sociometric diagrams of interpersonal choice provide a way to identify stars, isolates, and overchosen and underchosen group members. Usually, those who are well liked or display leadership abilities tend to be chosen for interactions more often than those who are not (Fig. 15-1). In one study of communication networks, members who exhibited more dominant behaviors or who the group perceived as being dominant emerged as more central to the group's communication networks and both sent and received more messages. The study also found that the task at hand affects the communication network. Groups that worked on low-complexity tasks had more centralized communication than when they worked on high-complexity tasks (Brown & Miller, 2000).

Group Themes. Group themes are the collective conceptual underpinnings of a group and express the members' underlying concerns or feelings, regardless of the group's purpose. Themes that emerge in groups help members to understand group dynamics. Different groups have different themes. For example, in a support group for parents whose children were being treated for HIV infection, the predominant group themes were guilt, anger, and loss of control (Mayers & Spiegel, 1992). In another couples group in which one partner in each couple had cancer, the themes that emerged were anger, role changes, impairment in sexual relationships, and diminished communication (Knakal, 1988). Although some predictable themes occur in groups, the obvious or assumed themes at the beginning may actually wind up differing from reality as the process continues. In one hospice support group, the members seemed to be focusing on the memories of their loved ones. Upon examination of the content of their interactions, however, discussions were revolving around financial planning for the future (Text Box 15-1).

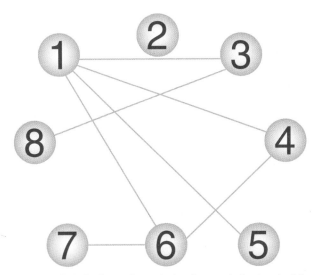

FIGURE 15.1 Sociometric analysis of group behavior. In this sociometric structure, response pattern was recorded during member interaction. Group members interacted with number 1 the most. Therefore, number 1 is the overchosen person. Numbers 5 and 7 are underchosen. Number 2 is never chosen and is determined to be the isolate.

TEXT BOX 15.1

Group Themes

A large symptom-management group is ongoing at a psychiatric facility. It is co-led by two nurses who are skilled in directing large groups and knowledgeable about the symptoms of mental disorders. Usually 12 people attend. The usual focus of the group is on identifying symptoms that indicate an impending reemergence of psychotic symptoms, medication side effects, and managing the numerous symptoms that medication is not controlling.

The nurses identified the appearance of the theme of powerlessness based on the following observations:

Session 1: TL expressed his frustration at being unable to keep a job because of his symptoms. The rest of the group offered their own experiences of being unable to work.

Session 2: CR is late to group and announces that she was late because the bus driver forgot to tell her when to get off and she missed her stop. She is irritated with the new driver.

Session 3: NT is out of medication and says that he cannot get more because he is out of money, again. He asks the nurses to lend him some money and make arrangements to get free medication.

Session 4: GM relies on his family for all transportation and refuses to use public transportation.

In all these sessions, participants expressed feelings that are consistent with loss of power.

Nonverbal Communication

Nonverbal communication is important to understanding group behavior. All members, not just the group leader, observe the eye contact, posture, and body gestures of the participants. What is expressed is the result of individual and group, as well as internal and external, processes. For example, if one member is explaining a painful experience and another member looks away and tries to engage still another, the self-disclosing member may feel devalued and rejected because he or she interprets the disruptive behavior as disinterest. If the leader interprets the disruptive behavior as anxiety over the topic, however, he or she may try to engage the other member in discussing the source of the anxiety.

The leaders should monitor the nonverbal behavior of group members during each session. Often, one or two people can set the overall mood of the group. Someone who comes to a session very sad or angry can set a tone of sadness or anger for the whole group. An astute group leader recognizes the effects of an individual's mood on the total group. If the purpose of the group is to deal with emotions, the group leader may choose to discuss the member's problem at the beginning of the session. The leader thus limits the mood to the one person experiencing it. If the group's purpose is inconsistent with self-disclosure of personal problems, the nurse should acknowledge the individual member's distress and offer a private session after the group. In this instance, the nurse would not encourage repeated episodes of self-disclosure from that member or others.

Group Norms and Standards

Groups develop norms or rules and standards that establish acceptable group behaviors. Some norms are formalized, such as beginning group on time, but others are never really formalized. These standards encourage conformity of behavior among group members. The group discourages deviations from these established norms. A member must quickly learn the norms or be ostracized.

Group Cohesion

One of the goals of most group leaders is to foster **group cohesion**, the forces that act on the members to stay in a group. Leaders can encourage cohesiveness by placing participants in situations that promote social interaction with minimal supervision, such as refreshment periods, and through team-building exercises. Cohesiveness is especially important in groups that focus on health maintenance behaviors such as exercise and weight control. These groups typically have high dropout rates, but members are more likely to attend when a group is cohesive (Annesi, 1999).

Without cohesiveness, the group's true existence is questionable. In cohesive groups, members are committed to the existence of the group. In large groups, cohesiveness tends to be decreased, with subsequent poorer performance among group members in completing tasks. When members are strongly committed to completing a task and the leader encourages equal participation, cohesiveness promotes quality decision making (Miranda, 1994; Mullen et al., 1994). Cohesiveness, however, can be a double-edged sword. In very cohesive groups, members are more likely to transgress personal boundaries. Dysfunctional relationships may develop that are destructive to the group process and ultimately not in the best interests of individual members.

Groupthink and Decision Making

Groupthink is the tendency of many groups to avoid conflict and adopt a normative pattern of thinking that is often consistent with the ideas of the group leader (Janis, 1972, 1982). In groupthink, striving for unanimity overrides the motivation of members to appraise realistically alternative courses of action. Many catastrophes, such as the *Challenger* explosion and Bay-of-Pigs Invasion, have been attributed to groupthink, but empiric evidence of groupthink's negative implications in organizations is small. Studies have shown that closed leadership style and external threat, particularly time pressure, appear to promote symptoms of groupthink and defective decision making (Neck & Moorhead, 1995). The relationship between cohesiveness and groupthink is still inconclusive. Current research suggests that groupthink can have positive effects on the group. In one study, groupthink was positively associated with group activities and team performance and negatively associated with concurrence (pressure for everyone to agree) and defective decision making (Choi & Kim, 1999). The question that remains unanswered is whether more cohesive groups are more likely to experience groupthink.

The psychiatric nurse often leads decision-making groups that decide activities, unit governance issues, and learning materials. The nurse who is leading a decision-making group should observe the process for any signs of groupthink. There may be instances in which groupthink can lead to a reasonable decision—for example, a group decides to arrange a going-away party for another patient. In other situations, groupthink may inhibit individual thinking and problem solving; for example, a team is displaying groupthink if it decides that a patient should lose privileges based on the assumption that the patient is deliberately exhibiting bizarre behaviors. In this case, the team is failing to consider or examine other evidence that suggests the bizarre behavior is really an indication of psychosis.

GROUP LEADERSHIP

In either a small or large group, the leader (1) obtains and receives information; (2) helps determine group goals, obstacles, and consequences of decisions; (3) facilitates communication; (4) helps integrate the various perspectives and alternative possibilities; and (5) tests and evaluates proposals and decisions (Sampson & Marthas, 1990). To carry out these functions, the leader must process the group interactions by staying objective and viewing what occurs as well as participating in the group. The leader reflects on, evaluates, and responds to just-completed interactions. Using various techniques enhances the leader's ability to lead the group effectively and to help the group meet its goals (Table 15-3).

One of the most important leadership skills is listening. A leader who practices active listening provides group members with someone who is responsive to what they say. A group leader who listens also models listening behavior for others, helping them improve their skills. Listening enables the leader to process events and track interactions. The leader should be able to listen to the group members and formulate responses based on an understanding of the discussion. Members may need to learn to listen to one another, track discussions without changing the subject, and not speak while others are talking (Belcher & Johnson, 1995).

The leader tracks the verbal and nonverbal interactions throughout the group. Depending on the group's purpose, the leader may keep this information to himself or herself to understand the group process or may share the observations with the group. For example, if the purpose of the group is psychoeducation, the leader may use the information to facilitate the best learning environment. If the purpose of the group is to improve the self-awareness and interaction skills of members, the leader may point out the observations. The leader needs to be clear about the purpose of the group and tailor leadership strategies accordingly.

The leader maintains a neutral, nonjudgmental style and avoids showing preference to one member over another. This may be difficult because some members may naturally seek out the leader's attention or ask for special favors. These behaviors are divisive to the group, and the leader should discourage them. Other important skills include providing everyone with an opportunity to contribute and respecting everyone's ideas. A leader who truly wants group participation and decision making does not reveal his or her beliefs.

There are generally accepted guidelines in leading groups that facilitate smooth functioning, including setting start and stop times, arranging for the introduction of new members, and listening while other people talk. Leaders should explain these rules at the first group meeting and reemphasize them at different points. A group should always begin at its scheduled time. Otherwise, members who tend to be late will not their change behavior, and those who are on time will resent waiting for the others. A group should also end on time. Members should understand from the beginning that either new people can attend without the group knowing about it or that the group will discuss the introduction of new members before their attendance. Whatever the group decides, the leader must also follow the rules.

Choosing Leadership Styles

A group is led within the context of the group leader's theoretic background and the group's purpose. For example, a leader with training in cognitive-behavioral therapy may focus on treating depression by asking members to think differently about situations, which in turn leads to feeling better. A leader with a psychodynamic orientation may focus on the feelings of depression by examining situations that generate the same feelings. Whatever the leader's theoretic background, his or her leadership behavior can be viewed on a continuum of direct to indirect. In **direct leadership behavior**, the leader controls the interaction by giving directions and information and allowing little discussion. The leader literally tells the members what to do. On the other end of the continuum is the **indirect leader**, who primarily reflects the group members' discussion and offers little guidance or information to the group. Sometimes, the group needs more direct leadership; other times, it needs a leader who is indirect. The challenge of providing leadership is to give sufficient direction that the group can meet its goals and develop its own group process but enough freedom that members can make mistakes and recover from their thinking errors in a supportive, caring, learning environment.

Selecting the Members

Individuals can refer themselves or be referred to groups by treatment teams or clinicians. The leader is responsible for assessing the individual's suitability to the group. In instances when a new group is forming, the leader selects and invites members so that the group can be well functioning and successful. The leader should consider the following criteria when selecting members:

- Does the purpose of the group match the needs of the potential member?
- Does the potential member have the social skills to function comfortably in the group?
- Will the other group members accept the new group member?
- Can the potential member make a commitment to attending group meetings?

TABLE 15.3 Techniques in Leading Groups

Technique	Purpose	Example
Support: giving feedback that provides a climate of emotional support	Helps a person or group continue with ongoing activities Informs group about what the leader thinks is important Creates a climate for expressing unpopular ideas Helps the more quiet and fearful members speak up	"We really appreciate your sharing that experience with us. It looked like it was quite painful."
Confrontation: challenging a participant (needs to be done in a supportive environment)	Helps individuals learn something about themselves Helps reduce some forms of disruptive behavior Helps members deal more openly and directly with one another	"Tom, this is the third time that you have changed the subject when we have talked about spouse abuse. Is something going on?"
Advice and suggestions: sharing expertise and knowledge that the members do not have	Provides information that members can use once they have examined and evaluated it Helps focus group's task and goals	"The medication that you are taking may be causing you to be sleepy."
Summarizing: statements at the end of sessions that highlight the session's discussion, any problem resolution, and unresolved problems	Provides continuity from one session to the next Brings to focus still-unresolved issues Organizes past in ways that clarify; brings into focus themes and patterns of interaction	"This session we discussed Sharon's medication problems, and she will be following up with her physicians."
Clarification: restatement of an interaction	Checks on the meanings of the interaction and communication Avoids faulty communication Facilitates focus on substantive issues rather than allowing members to be side tracked into misunderstandings	"What I heard you say was that you are feeling very sad right now. Is that correct?"
Probing and questioning: a technique for the experienced group leader that asks for more information	Helps members expand on what they were saying (when they are ready to) Gets at more extensive and wider range of information Invites members to explore their ideas in greater detail	"Could you tell us more about your relationship with your parents?"
Repeating, paraphrasing, highlighting: a simple act of repeating what was just said	Facilitates communication among group members Corrects inaccurate communication or emphasizes accurate communication	*Member:* "I forgot about my wife's birthday." *Leader:* "You forgot your wife's birthday."
Reflecting feelings: identifying feelings that are being expressed	Orients members to the feelings that may lie behind what is being said or done Helps members deal with issues they might otherwise avoid or miss	"You sound upset."
Reflecting behavior: identifying behaviors that are occurring	Gives members an opportunity to see how their behavior appears to others and to evaluate its consequences Helps members to understand others' perceptions and responses to them	"I notice that when the topic of sex is brought up, you look down and shift in your chair."

Adapted from Sampson, E., & Marthas, M. (1990). *Group process for the health professions* (pp. 222–224). Albany, NY: Delmar.

Arranging Seating

Spatial and seating arrangements contribute to group communication. Group members tend to sit in the same places. Those who sit close to the group leader are more likely to have more power in the group than those who sit far away. Communication flows better when no physical barriers, such as tables, are between members. Arranging a group in a circle with chairs comfortably close to one another without a table enhances group work. No one should sit outside the group. If a table is necessary, a round table is better than a rectangular one, which implicitly increases the power of those who sit at the ends.

The session should be held in a quiet, pleasant room with adequate space and privacy. Holding a session in too large or too small a room inhibits communication. Group sessions should not be held in rooms in which nonparticipants have access because of compromised confidentiality and potential distractions. Usually, group leaders do not permit eating during group sessions.

Dealing With Challenging Group Behaviors

Problematic behaviors occur in all groups. They can be challenging to the most experienced group leaders and frustrating to new leaders. In dealing with any problematic behavior or situation, the leader must remember to support the integrity of the individual members and the group as a whole.

Monopolizer

Some people tend to monopolize a group by constantly talking or interrupting others. This behavior is common in the beginning stages of group formation and usually represents anxiety that the member displaying such behavior is experiencing. Within a few sessions, this person usually relaxes and no longer attempts to monopolize the group. For some people, however, monopolizing discussions is part of their normal personality and will continue. Other group members usually find the behavior mildly irritating in the beginning and eventually extremely annoying. Members may drop out of the group to avoid that person. The leader needs to decide if, how, and when to intervene. The best case scenario is when savvy group members remind the monopolizer to let others speak. The leader can then support the group in establishing rules that allow everyone the opportunity to participate. Often, however, the group waits for the leader to manage the situation. There are a few ways to deal with the situation. The leader can interrupt the monopolizer by acknowledging the member's contribution but redirecting the discussion to others. The leader can also become more directive and limit the discussion time per member.

"Yes, but"

Some people have a patterned response to any suggestions from others. Initially, they agree with suggestions others offer them, but then they add "yes, but" and give several reasons why the suggestions will not work for them. Leaders and members can easily identify this patterned response. In such situations, it is best to avoid problem solving *for* the member and encourage the person to develop his or her own solutions. The leader can serve as a role model of the problem-solving behavior for the other members and encourage them to let the member develop a solution that would work specifically for him or her.

Disliked Member

In some groups, members clearly dislike one particular member. This situation can be challenging for the leader because it can result in considerable tension and conflict. This person could become the group's scapegoat. The group leader may have made a mistake by placing the person in this particular group, and another group may be a better match. One solution may be to move the person to a better-matched group. Whether the person stays or leaves, the group leader must stay neutral and avoid displaying negative verbal and nonverbal behaviors that indicate that he or she too dislikes the group member or that he or she is displeased with the other members for their behavior. Often, the group leader can manage the situation by showing respect for the disliked member and acknowledging his or her contribution. In some instances, getting supervision from a more experienced group leader is useful. Defusing the situation may be possible by using conflict resolution strategies and discussing the underlying issues.

Group Conflict

Most groups experience periods of conflict. The leader first needs to decide whether the conflict is a natural part of the group process or whether the group needs to address some issues. Member-to-member conflict can be handled through the previously discussed conflict resolution process (see Chap. 14). Leader-to-member conflict is more complicated because the leader has the formal position of power. In this instance, the leader can use conflict resolution strategies but should be sensitive to the power differential between the leader's role and the member's role.

TYPES OF GROUPS

Psychoeducation Groups

Psychoeducation groups include (1) task groups that focus on completion of specific activities, such as planning a week's menu, and (2) teaching groups used to enhance knowledge, improve skills, or solve problems. Learning how to give medication or control angry outbursts is often the aim of teaching groups. Psychoeducation groups are formally planned, and members are purposefully selected. Members are asked to join specific groups because of the focus of the group. In a time-management group, the members need help with time management. The group leader develops a lesson plan for each session that includes objectives, content outline, references, and evaluation tools. These groups are time-limited and last for only a few sessions.

Supportive Therapy Groups

Supportive therapy groups are usually less intense than psychotherapy groups and focus on helping individuals cope with their illnesses and problems. Implementing supportive therapy groups is one of the basic functions of the psychiatric nurse, but leading psychotherapy groups is reserved for nurses and other clinicians prepared at least at the master's degree level. In supportive therapy groups, nurses use counseling interventions.

Psychotherapy Groups

Psychotherapy groups actually treat individuals' emotional problems and can be implemented from various theoretic perspectives, including psychoanalytic, behavioral, and cognitive. These groups focus on examining emotions and helping individuals face their life situations. At times, these groups can be extremely intense. Psychotherapy groups provide an opportunity for patients to examine and resolve psychological and interpersonal issues within a safe environment. Mental health specialists who have a minimum of a master's degree and are trained in group psychotherapy lead such groups. Patients can be treated in psychotherapy and still be members of other nursing groups. Communication with the therapists is important for continuity of care.

Self-Help Groups

Self-help groups are led by people who are concerned about coping with a specific problem or life crisis. These groups do not explore psychodynamic issues in depth. Professionals usually do not attend these groups or serve as consultants. Alcoholics Anonymous, Overeaters Anonymous, and One Day at a Time (grief group) are examples of self-help groups.

COMMON NURSING INTERVENTION GROUPS

Common intervention groups that nurses lead include medication, symptom management, anger management, and self-care groups. Additionally, nurses lead many other groups, including stress management, relaxation groups, and women's groups. The key to being a good leader is to integrate group leadership, knowledge, and skills with nursing interventions that fit a selected group.

Medication Groups

Nurse-led medication groups are common in psychiatric nursing. Not all medication groups are alike; hence, the nurse must be clear regarding the purpose of each specific medication group (Text Box 15-2). A medication group can be used primarily to transmit information about medications, such as action, dosage, and side effects, or it can focus on issues related to medications, such as compliance, management of side effects, and lifestyle adjustments. Many nurses incorporate both perspectives.

Assessing a member's medication knowledge is important before he or she joins the group to determine what the individual would like to learn. People with mental illness may have difficulty remembering new information; therefore, assessment of cognitive abilities is important. Assessing attention span, memory, and problem-solving skills gives valuable information that nurses can use in designing the group. The nurse should determine the members' reading and writing skills to select effective patient education materials.

An ideal group is one in which all members use the same medication. In reality, this situation is rare. Usually, the group members are using various medications. The nurse should know which medications each member is taking, but to avoid violating patient confidentiality, the nurse needs to be careful not to divulge that information to other patients. If group members choose, they can share the names of their medications with one another. A small group format works best, and the more interaction, the better. Using a lecture method of teaching is less effective than involving the members in the learning process. The nurse should expose the members to various audio and visual educational materials, including workbooks, videotapes, and handouts. The nurse should ask members to write down information to help them remember and learn through various modes. Evaluation of the learning outcomes begins with the first class. Nurses can develop and give pretests and posttests. Using the pretest, they can measure learning outcomes.

Symptom Management Groups

Nurses often lead groups that focus on helping patients deal with a severe and persistent mental illness. Handling hallucinations, being socially appropriate, and staying motivated to complete activities of daily living are a few common topics. In symptom management groups, members also learn when a symptom indicates that relapse is imminent and what to do about it. Within the

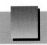

TEXT BOX 15.2

Medication Group Protocol

Purpose	Develop strategies that reinforce a self-medication routine.
Description	The medication group is an open, ongoing group that meets once a week to discuss topics germane to self-administration of medication. Members will not be asked to disclose the names of their medications.
Member selection	The group is open to any person taking medication for a mental illness or emotional problem who would like more information about medication, side effects, and staying on a regimen. Referrals from mental health providers are encouraged. Each person will meet with the group leader before attending the group to determine if the group will meet the individual's learning needs.
Structure	Format is a small group, with no more than eight members and one psychiatric nurse group leader facilitating a discussion about the issues. Topics are rotated.
Time and location	2:00–3:00 PM, every Wednesday at the Mental Health Center
Cost	No charge for attending
Topics	How Do I Know If My Medications Are Working? Side Effect Management: Is It Worth It? Hints for Taking Medications Without Missing Doses! Health Problems That Medications Affect (Other topics will be developed to meet the needs of group members.)
Evaluation	Short pretest and posttest for instructor's use only

context of a symptom management group, patients can learn how to avoid relapse.

Anger Management Groups

Anger management is another common topic for a nurse-led group, often in the inpatient setting. The purposes of an anger management group are to discuss the concept of anger, identify antecedents to aggressive behavior, and develop new strategies to deal with anger besides verbal and physical aggression (see Chap. 36). The treatment team refers individuals with histories of being verbally and physically abusive, usually to family members, to these groups for better understanding of their emotions and behavioral responses. Impulsiveness and emotional lability are problems for many of the group members. Anger management usually includes a discussion of associated stressful situations, events that trigger anger, feelings about the situation, and unmet personal needs.

Self-Care Groups

Another common nurse-led psychiatric group is a self-care group. People with psychiatric illnesses often have self-care deficits and benefit from the structure that a group provides. These groups are challenging because members usually know how to perform these daily tasks (eg, bathing, grooming, performing personal hygiene), but their illnesses cause them to lose the motivation to complete them. The leader not only reinforces the basic self-care skills but also, and more importantly, helps identify strategies that can motivate the patients and provide structure to their daily lives.

Summary of Key Points

➤ The definition of group can vary according to theoretic orientation. A general definition is that a group is two or more people who have at least one common goal or issue. Group dynamics are the interactions within groups that influence the group's development and process.

➤ Groups can be open, with new members joining at any time, or closed, with members admitted only once. Either small or large groups can be effective, but dynamics change in different sized groups.

➤ The process of group development occurs in phases: beginning, middle, and termination. These stages are not fixed, but dynamic. The process challenges the leader to guide the group. During the working stage, the group addresses its purpose.

➤ Although there are only two formal group roles, leader and member, there are many informal group roles. These roles are usually categorized according to purpose—task functions, maintenance functions, and individual roles. Members who assume task functions encourage the group members to stay focused on the group's task. Those who assume maintenance functions worry more about the group working together than the actual task itself. Individual roles can either enhance or detract from the work of the group.

➤ Verbal communication includes the communication network and group themes. Nonverbal communication is more complex and involves eye contact, body posture, and mood of the group. Decision-making groups can be victims of groupthink, which can have either positive or negative outcomes. Groupthink research is ongoing.

➤ Leading a group involves many different functions from obtaining and receiving information to testing and evaluating decisions. The leader should explain the rules of the group at the beginning of the group.

➤ Seating arrangements can affect group interaction. The fewer physical barriers there are, such as tables, the better the communication is. Everyone should be a part of the group, and no one should sit outside of it. In the most interactive groups, members face one another in a circle.

➤ Leadership skills involve listening, tracking verbal and nonverbal behaviors, and maintaining a neutral, nonjudgmental style.

➤ The leader should address behaviors that challenge the leadership, group process, or other members to determine whether to intervene. In some instances, the leader redirects a monopolizing member; at other times the leader lets the group deal with the behavior. Group conflict occurs in most groups.

➤ There are many different types of groups. Psychiatric nurses lead psychoeducation and supportive therapy groups. Mental health specialists who are trained to provide intensive therapy lead psychotherapy groups. Consumers lead self-help groups, and professionals assist only as requested.

➤ Medication, symptom management, anger management, and self-care groups are common nurse-led groups.

Critical Thinking Challenges

1. Group members are very polite to one another and are superficially discussing topics. You would assess the group as being in which phase? Explain your answer.

2. After three sessions of a supportive therapy group, two members begin to share their frustration with having a mental illness. The group is moving into which phase of group development? Explain your answer.

3. Define the roles of the task and maintenance functions in groups. Observe your clinical group, and identify classmates who are assuming task functions and maintenance functions.

4. Observe a patient group for at least five sessions. Discuss the seating pattern that emerges. Identify the communication network and the group themes. Then identify the group's norms and standards.

5. Discuss the conditions that lead to groupthink. When is groupthink positive? When is groupthink negative? Explain.

6. List at least six behaviors that are important for a group leader. Justify your answers.

7. During the first meeting, one member seems very anxious and tends to monopolize the conversation. Discuss how you would assess the situation and whether you would intervene.

8. At the end of the fourth meeting, one group member angrily accuses another of asking too many questions. The other members look on quietly. How would you assess the situation? Would you intervene? Explain.

 WEB LINKS

www.mentalhelp.net/selfhelp   This website serves as an online self-help resource containing information on many different self-help groups.

www.princeton.edu   This site includes an *Outdoor Action Guide to Group Dynamics and Leadership*, which reviews how to teach a skill, leadership concepts, and group dynamics.

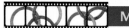 **MOVIES**

12 Angry Men: 1998. In this excellent film, a young man stands accused of fatally stabbing his father. A jury of his "peers" is deciding his fate. This jury is portrayed by an excellent cast, including Jack Lemmon, George C. Scott, Tony Danza, and Ossie Davis. At first, the case appears to be "open and shut." This film depicts an intense struggle to reach a verdict and is an excellent study of group process and group dynamics. *Viewing Points:* Identify the leaders in the group. How does leadership change throughout the film? Do you find any evidence of groupthink? How does the group handle conflict?

References

Agazarian, Y. (1999). Phases of development in the Systems-Centered Psychotherapy group. *Small Group Research,* *30*(1) 82–107.

Annesi, J. (1999). Effects of minimal group promotion on cohesion and exercise adherence. *Small Group Research,* *30*(5), 542–557.

Barker, D. (1991). The behavioral analysis of interpersonal intimacy in group development. *Small Group Research,* *2*(1), 76–91.

Belcher, C., & Johnson, S. (1995). Leadership and listening: A study of member perceptions. *Small Group Research,* *26*(1), 77–85.

Benne, K., & Sheats, P. (1948). Functional roles of group members. *Journal of Social Issues, 4*(2), 41–49.

Brown, T., & Miller, C. (2000). Communication networks in task-performing groups: Effects of task complexity, time, pressure, and interpersonal dominance. *Small Group Research, 31*(2), 131–157.

Choi, J., & Kim, M. (1999). The organizational application of groupthink and its limitations in organizations. *Journal of Applied Psychology, 84*(2), 297–306.

Cissna, K. (1984). Phases of group development. *Small Group Behavior, 15*(1), 3–32.

Gersick, C. (1988). Time and transition in work teams. *Academy of Management Journal, 1*, 9–41.

Janis, I. (1972). *Victims of groupthink*. Boston: Houghton-Mifflin.

Janis, I. (1982). *Groupthink* (2nd ed.). Boston: Houghton-Mifflin.

Klein, E. (1993). Large groups in treatment and training settings. Special issue: The large group. *Group, 17*(4), 198–209.

Knakal, J. (1988). A couples group in oncology social work practice: An innovative modality. *Dynamic Psychotherapy, 6*(2), 153–156.

Mayers, A., & Spiegel, L. (1992). A parental support group in a pediatric AIDS clinic: Its usefulness and limitations. *Health and Social Work, 17*(3), 183–191.

Miranda, S. (1994). Avoidance of groupthink: Meeting management using group support systems. *Small Group Research, 25*(1), 105–136.

Moreno, J. (1953). *Who shall survive?* Beacon, NY: Beacon House.

Mullen, B., Anthony, T., Salas, E., & Driskell, J. (1994). Group cohesiveness and quality of decision making: An integration of tests of the groupthink hypothesis. Special issue: Social cognition in small groups. *Small Group Research, 25*(2), 189–204.

Neck, C. P., & Moorhead, G. (1995). Groupthink remodeled: The importance of leadership, time pressure, and methodical decision-making procedures. *Human Relations, 48*(5), 537–557.

Sampson, E., & Marthas, M. (1990). *Group process for the health professions*. Albany, NY: Delmar.

Yalom, I. (1995). *The theory and practice of group psychotherapy*. New York: Basic Books.

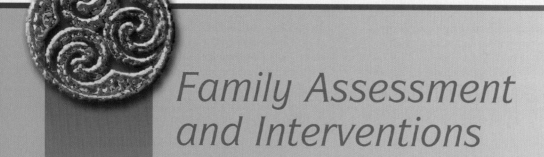

Family Assessment and Interventions

Mary Ann Boyd

**MENTAL HEALTH
OF FAMILIES AND
FAMILY DYSFUNCTION**
Effects of Mental Illness on
   Family Functioning
Influence of Cultural Beliefs
   and Values

**COMPREHENSIVE FAMILY
ASSESSMENT**
Relationship Building With Families
Genograms
   Analyzing Genograms
   Using Genograms as
      Intervention Tools

Family Biologic Domain
   Health Status
   Mental Disorders
Family Psychological Domain
   Family Development
   Family Life Cycles
   Communication Patterns
   Stress and Coping
   Problem-Solving Skills
Family Social Domain
   Family Systems
   Social and Financial Status
   Formal and Informal
      Support Networks

**IDENTIFYING FAMILY
NURSING DIAGNOSES**

FAMILY INTERVENTIONS
Counseling
Promoting Self-Care Activities
Supporting Family Functioning
   and Cohesiveness
Providing Education
   and Health Teaching
Using Family Therapy

**LEARNING
OBJECTIVES**

After studying this chapter, you will be able to:

➤ Discuss the balance of family mental health with family dysfunction.

➤ Develop a genogram that depicts the family history, relationships, and mental disorders
   across at least three generations.

➤ Develop a plan for a comprehensive family assessment.

➤ Apply family nursing diagnoses to families who need nursing care.

➤ Discuss nursing interventions that are useful in caring for families.

A family is a group of people connected emotionally, by blood, or in both ways that has developed patterns of interaction and relationships. Family members have a shared history and a shared future (Carter & McGoldrick, 1999b). A nuclear family is two or more people living together and related by blood, marriage, or adoption. An extended family is several nuclear families whose members may or may not live together and function as one group. Families are unique in that, unlike all other organizations, they incorporate new members only by birth, adoption, or marriage, and members can leave only by death.

> **KEY CONCEPT** **Family.** A **family** is a group of people connected emotionally, by blood, or in both ways that has developed patterns of interaction and relationships. Family members have a shared history and a shared future (Carter & McGoldrick, 1999b).

The psychiatric nurse interacts with families in various ways. Because of the interpersonal and chronic nature of many mental illnesses, psychiatric nurses often have frequent and long-term contact with families. Involvement may range from meeting family members only once or twice to treating the whole family as a patient. Unlike a therapeutic group (see Chap. 15), the family system has a history and continues to function when the nurse is not there. The family is reacting to past, present, and anticipated future relationships within at least a three-generation family system. The purpose of this chapter is to integrate important family concepts into the nursing process when providing psychiatric nursing care to families experiencing mental health problems.

MENTAL HEALTH OF FAMILIES AND FAMILY DYSFUNCTION

In a mentally healthy family, members live in harmony among themselves and within society. These families support and nurture their members throughout their lives. Dysfunction and mental illness, however, can affect a family's overall mental health.

A **dysfunctional family** is one whose interactions, decisions, or behaviors interfere with the positive development of the family and its individual members. Sometimes, a mentally healthy family becomes dysfunctional after a crisis or a stressful situation that the family lacks the coping skills to handle. A family can be mentally healthy and at the same time have a member who has a mental illness. Conversely, a family can be dysfunctional and have no member with a diagnosable mental illness.

Effects of Mental Illness on Family Functioning

Families of people with persistent mental disorders have special needs. Many of these adults continue to live with their parents well into their 30s and 40s. For adults with persistent mental illness, the family serves several functions that those without mental illness do not need. Such functions include the following:

Providing support. People with mental illness have difficulty maintaining outside or nonfamilial support networks and may rely exclusively on their families.

Providing information. Families often have complete and continuous information about care and treatment over the years.

Monitoring services. Families observe the progress of their relative and report concerns to those in charge of care.

Advocating for services. Family groups advocate for money for residential care services.

Conflicts can occur between parents and mental health workers who place a high value on independence. Members of the mental health care system may criticize families for being "overly protective." In reality, the patient with mental illness may face real barriers to independent living. Housing may be unavailable; when available, the quality may be lacking. The patient may fear leaving home, may be at risk for relapse if he or she does leave, or may be too comfortable at home to want to leave (Hatfield, 1992). On a long-term basis, when caregivers die, patients with mental illness experience housing disruptions and potentially traumatic transitions. Few families actually plan for this difficult eventuality (Smith et al., 2000).

Nurses must use an objective and rational approach about independence and dependence. Emotions often obscure the underlying issues. The nurse can diffuse the emotions that surround the issue of independence so that everyone can explore the alternatives comfortably. Although separation must eventually occur, the timing and process vary according to each family's particular situation. Parents may be highly anxious when their adult children first leave home and will need reassurance and support.

Influence of Cultural Beliefs and Values

Conceptualizations of normal family functioning vary among different cultural groups. For example, some Asian cultures expect for a mother-in-law to move in with her married child and his or her spouse to help care for the couple's children. In some families of European descent, a mother-in-law's presence is construed as unusual or an interference with the family's functioning. One of the challenges of psychiatric nursing is to avoid classifying certain family patterns as pathologic just because they deviate from either dominant cultural norms or the nurse's theoretically based or theoretically driven values. On the other hand, the nurse has to be careful not to overattribute symptoms and dysfunctional patterns to culture when such difficulties reflect actual problems. For example, the nurse might overlook a patient's withdrawal as a symptom of depression if he or she attributes such behavior as a "cultural" tendency.

Beliefs about seeking help for mental health problems are also culturally based and vary among groups. Generally, help-seeking patterns include the following:

- African American and Latino families tend to seek support from extended family and other community members rather than from health or mental health professionals in the initial stages of a family problem (Celano & Kaslow, 2000).
- Although most families experience some discomfort in sharing family problems with outsiders, the stigma of disclosure is particularly prominent in families from ethnic minority groups (Celano & Kaslow, 2000).
- African American families have higher rates of attrition and earlier termination of family therapy than do white families (McGoldrick & Giordano, 1996).

COMPREHENSIVE FAMILY ASSESSMENT

A comprehensive family assessment is the collection of all relevant data related to family health, psychological well-being, and social functioning to identify problems for which the nurse can generate nursing diagnoses. Nurses conduct a comprehensive family assessment when they care for patients and their families over an extended period. They also use them when the patient's mental health problems are so complex that family support is important for optimal care (Text Box 16-1). The assessment is a face-to-face interview with family members, and nurses can conduct it over several different sessions.

KEY CONCEPT Comprehensive family assessment. A **comprehensive family assessment** is the collection of all relevant data related to family health, psychological well-being, and social functioning to identify problems for which the nurse can generate nursing diagnoses.

Text Box 16.1

Family Mental Health Assessment

I. Family members present

Name	Age	Relationship
_____	_____	_____
_____	_____	_____
_____	_____	_____

II. Health Status

Member	Disorder and current treatment
_____	_____
_____	_____

III. Mental health status

Member	Disorder and current treatment
_____	_____
_____	_____

IV. Impact of mental illness on family function

Describe the changes that occur in the family as a result of the family member's disorder:

_____

_____

_____

V. Family life cycle

Describe the family life cycle stage and any transitions that are occurring.

_____

_____

_____

VI. Communication patterns

Describe the family communication patterns in terms of usual times of communication (morning, dinner, etc.), which family members talk to each other, who communicates the family rules, who carries out discipline. Identify triangulated messages. _____

_____

_____

_____

VII. Stress and coping

Identify current family stressful events and family coping mechanisms. _____

_____

_____

_____

VIII. Problem-solving skills

Determine who solves problems in the family. Are the problem-solving skills of the family able to manage most family problems? _____

_____

_____

_____

IX. Family system (from the genogram)

Family composition_____

_____

_____

(continued)

TEXT BOX 16.1 (*Continued*)

Health and illness patterns _____

_____

Relationship patterns _____

_____

Social functioning patterns _____

_____

Financial and legal status _____

_____

Formal and informal network _____

_____

X. Nursing diagnoses

_____

_____

_____

Relationship Building With Families

In preparing for a family assessment, nurses must give time and attention to developing a relationship with the family. Although necessary when working with any family, relationship development is particularly important for families from minority cultures. Developing a relationship takes time; hence, the nurse may need to complete the assessment over several meetings rather than just one.

In developing a positive relationship with families, nurses must attend to two important areas. The first is establishing credibility with the family. The family must see the nurse as knowledgeable and skillful. Possessing culturally competent nursing skills and projecting a professional image are crucial to establishing credibility. The second area is addressing the family's immediate intervention needs. For example, a family who needs shelter or food is not ready to discuss a member's medication regimen until the first needs are met. The nurse will make considerable progress in establishing a relationship with the family when he or she helps members meet their immediate needs.

Genograms

Families contain various structural configurations (eg, single-parent, multigenerational, same-gender relationships). The nurse can facilitate taking the family history by completing a **genogram,** which is a multigenerational schematic diagram that lists family members and their relationships. The genogram is a skeleton of the family that the nurse can use as a framework for exploring relationships and patterns of health and illness.

The genogram includes the ages, dates of marriage, deaths, and geographic locations of all members. Squares represent men, and circles represent women; ages are listed inside the squares and circles. Horizontal lines represent marriages with dates; vertical lines connect parents and children. Genograms can be particularly useful in understanding family history, composition, relationships, and illnesses (Fig. 16-1).

Genograms vary from simple to elaborate. Depending on the level of detail, nurses can collect various data. They can study important events such as marriages, divorces, deaths, and geographic movements. They can include cultural or religious affiliations, education and economic levels, and the nature of the work of each family member. They should include mental disorders and other significant health problems in the genogram. The patient and family's assessment needs guide the level of detail of the genogram. In a small family with limited problems, the genogram can be rather general. In a large family with multiple problems, the genogram should reflect these complexities.

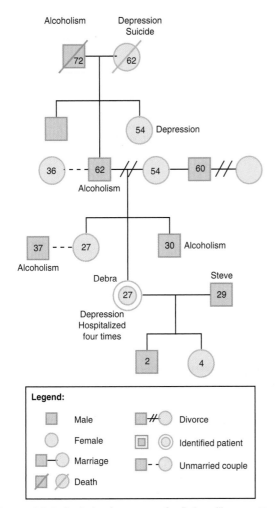

FIGURE 16.1 Analysis of genogram for Debra. Illness patterns are depression (maternal aunt, grandmother [suicide]) and alcoholism (brother, father, grandfather). Relationship patterns show that parents are divorced and neither sibling is married.

Analyzing Genograms

For a genogram to be useful, the nurse needs to analyze the data for family composition, relationship problems, and mental health patterns. A place to start in analyzing the data is with the composition. How large is the family? Where do family members live? A large family whose members live in the same city is more likely to have support than a family in which distance separates members. Of course, this is not always the case. Sometimes, even when family members live geographically close, they are still emotionally distant from one another.

The nurse should also study the genogram for relationship and illness patterns. For example, alcoholism, often transmitted across several generations, may be prevalent in men on one side of a family. The nurse can then hypothesize that alcoholism is one of the mental health risks for the family and design interventions to reduce the risk. The nurse may find in a genogram that

members of a family's previous generation were in "state hospitals" or had "nerve problems." They may also find a history of divorces or family members who have never been seen.

Using Genograms as Intervention Tools

Genograms not only are useful in assessment but also can be used as intervention strategies. Nurses can use genograms in helping family members understand current feelings and emotions as well as the family's evolution over several generations. The development of a genogram allows the family to examine relationships from a factual, objective perspective. Often, family members gain new insights. In many instances, they can begin to understand their problems within the context of their family system. For example, families may begin to view depression in an adolescent daughter with a new seriousness when they see it as part of a pattern of several generations of women who have had lifelong struggles with depression. A husband, raised as an only child in a small Midwestern town, may better understand his feelings of being overwhelmed after comparing his family structure with that of his wife, who comes from a large family of several generations living together in the urban Northeast (Text Box 16-2).

Family Biologic Domain

The family assessment includes a thorough picture of health status and mental disorders and their effects on family functioning. The health status of family members is an indication not only of their physical status but also of the stress currently being placed on the family and its resources. The family with multiple health problems will be trying to manage these problems as well as to obtain the many financial and health care resources it needs.

Health Status

The family health status includes physical illnesses and disabilities of any members. The nurse can record such information on the genogram and include physical illnesses and disabilities of other generations. The nurse should pay particular attention to any physical problems that affect family functioning. For example, if a member requires frequent visits to a provider or hospitalizations, the whole family will feel the effects of focusing excessive time and financial resources on that member. The nurse should explore how such situations affect other members.

Mental Disorders

Detecting mental disorders in families may be difficult because these disorders are often hidden or the "family secret." Very calmly, the nurse should ask family members to identify anyone who has had a mental illness. He or she should record the information on the genogram

TEXT BOX 16.2

John and Judy Jones

John and Judy Jones were married 3 years ago after their graduation from a small liberal arts college in the Midwest. Judy's career choice required that she live on the East Coast near her large family. John willingly moved with her and quickly found a satisfying position. After about 6 months of marriage, John became extremely irritable and depressed. He kept saying that his life was not his own. Judy was very concerned but could not understand his feelings of being overwhelmed. His job was going well, and they had a very busy social life, mostly revolving around her family, whom John loved. They decided to seek counseling and completed the following genogram:

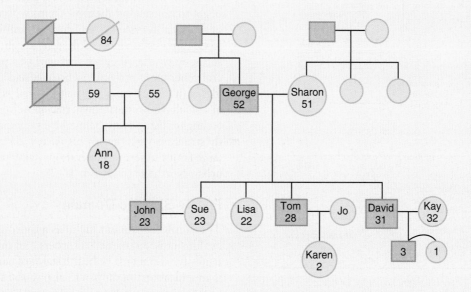

After looking at the genogram, both John and Judy began to realize that part of John's discomfort had to do with the number of family members who were involved in their lives. Judy and John began to re-define their social life, allowing more time with friends and each other.

as well as in the narrative. If family members do not know if mental illness is in the family, the nurse should ask if anyone in the family was treated for "nerves" or had a "nervous breakdown." Overall, a good family history of mental illness across multiple generations helps the nurse to understand the significance of mental illness in the current generation.

Family Psychological Domain

Assessment of the family's psychological domain focuses on the family life cycle, communication patterns, stress and coping, and problem-solving skills. One aim of the assessment is to grasp the relationships within the fam-ily. Even though family roles and structures are impor-tant, the true value of the family is in its relationships, which are irreplaceable. For example, if a parent leaves or dies, another person (eg, stepparent, grandparent) can assume some parental functions, but this person can never really replace the emotional relationship with the missing parent.

Family Development

Family development is a broad term that refers to all the processes connected with the growth of a family, including changes associated with work, geographic location, migration, acculturation, and serious illness.

In optimal family development, family members are relatively differentiated (capable of autonomous functioning) from one another, anxiety is low, and the parents have good emotional relationships with their own families of origin.

Family Life Cycles

Family development differs from the concept of the family life cycle. Family life cycle refers to family stages based on significant events related to the arrival and departure of family members, such as birth or adoption, childrearing, departure of children from home, occupational retirement, and death. These traditional models are being challenged, modified, and redesigned to address contemporary structural and role changes. These

models also may not fit many cultural groups. This section highlights selected life-cycle models and the issues that are important in assessing the family from a life-cycle perspective.

The **family life cycle** is a process of expansion, contraction, and realignment of relationship systems to support the entry, exit, and development of family members in a functional way (Carter & McGoldrick, 1999b) (Table 16-1). A family's life cycle is conceptualized in terms of stages throughout the years. To get from one stage to the next, the family system undergoes some changes. Problems within stages can usually be handled by rearranging the system (first-order changes), whereas transition from one stage of the family life cycle to the next requires changes in the system itself (second-order changes). In first-order changes, the family system is

TABLE 16.1 Stages of the Family Life Cycle

Family Life Cycle Stage	Emotional Transition	Required Family Changes
1. Leaving home: single young adults	Accepting emotional and financial responsibility for self	Differentiation of self in relation to family of origin Development of intimate peer relationships Establishment of self regarding work and financial independence
2. The joining of families through marriage: the new couple	Commitment to new system	Formation of marital system Realignment of relationships with extended families and friends to include spouse
3. Families with young children	Accepting new members into the system	Adjusting marital system to make space for children Joining in childrearing, financial, and household tasks Realignment of relationships with extended family to include parenting and grandparenting roles
4. Families with adolescents	Increasing flexibility of family boundaries to include children's independence and grandparents' frailties	Shifting of parent–child relationships to permit adolescent to move in and out of system Refocus on midlife marital and career issues Beginning shift toward joint caring for older generation
5. Launching children and moving on	Accepting a multitude of exits from and entries into the family system	Renegotiation of marital system as a dyad Development of adult–adult relationships between grown children and their parents Realignment of relationships to include in-laws and grandchildren Dealing with disabilities and death of parents (grandparents)
6. Families in later life	Accepting the shifting of generational roles	Maintaining own and couple functioning interests in face of physiologic decline; exploration of new familial and social role options Support for a more central role of middle generation Making room in the system for the wisdom and experience of the elderly, supporting the older generation without over functioning for them Dealing with loss of spouse, siblings, and other peers and preparation for own death

From Carter, B., & McGoldrick, M. (1999b). Overview: The changing family life cycle. In B. Carter & M. McGoldrick (Eds.), *The expanded family life cycle: Individual, family, and social perspectives* (p. 2). New York: Allyn & Bacon.

rearranged, such as when all the children are finally in school and the stay-at-home parent returns to work. The system is rearranged, but the structure remains the same. In second-order changes, the family structure does change. When a member moves away from the family home to live independently, the whole family structure changes.

The nurse should not view this model as the "normal" life cycle for every family and should limit its use to those families it clearly fits. Variations of the family life cycle are presented for the divorced family (Table 16-2) and the remarried family (Table 16-3) as well.

A new cycle begins at the young adult stage, when the individual is coming to terms with his or her family of origin; deciding when, how, and whether to marry; and determining how to carry out the family life cycle.

Transition times are any times of addition, subtraction, or change in status of family members. During transitions, family stresses are more likely to cause symptoms or dysfunction. Significant family events, such as the death of a member or the introduction of a new member, also affect the family's ability to function. During these times, families may seek help from the mental health system.

Cultural Variations. The social science research community is being challenged to rethink and redefine conceptual frameworks that speak to varied family life-cycle changes and developmental transitions across and within diverse groups. In caring for families from diverse cultures, the nurse should examine whether the underlying assumptions and frameworks of life-cycle models apply. Even the concept of "family" varies among cultures. For example, the dominant middle-class culture definition of family has focused on the intact nuclear family. For Italian Americans, the entire extended network of aunts, uncles, cousins, and grandparents may be involved in family decision

TABLE 16.2 The Divorcing Family

Family Life Cycle Stage	Prerequisite Attitude	Developmental Issues
Divorce		
1. Decision to divorce	Acceptance of inability to resolve marital tensions sufficiently to continue relationship	Acceptance of one's own part in the failure of the marriage
2. Planning the breakup of the system	Supporting viable arrangements for all parts of the system	Working cooperatively on problems of custody, visitation, and finances Dealing with extended family about the divorce
3. Separation	Willingness to continue cooperative co-parental relationship and joint financial support of children Work on resolution of attachment to spouse	Mourning loss of intact family Restructuring marital and parent–child relationships and finances; adaptation to living apart Realignment of relationships with extended family; staying connected with spouse's extended family
4. The divorce	More work on emotional divorce: Overcoming hurt, anger guilt, etc.	Mourning loss of intact family: giving up fantasies of reunion Retrieval of hopes, dreams, expectations from the marriage Staying connected with extended families
Postdivorce Family		
1. Single-parent (custodial household or primary residence)	Willingness to maintain financial responsibilities, continue parental contact with ex-spouse, and support contact of children with ex-spouse and his or her family.	Making flexible visitation arrangements with ex-spouse and his family Rebuilding own financial resources Rebuilding own social network
2. Single-parent (noncustodial)	Willingness to maintain parental contact with ex-spouse and support custodial parent's relationship with children	Finding ways to continue effective parenting relationship with children Maintaining financial responsibilities to ex-spouse and children Rebuilding own social network

From Carter, B., & McGoldrick, M. (1999a). The divorce cycle: A major variation in the American family life cycle. In B. Carter & M. McGoldrick (Eds.), *The expanded family life cycle* (p. 375). New York: Allyn & Bacon.

TABLE 16.3   Remarried Family Formulations

Family Life Cycle Stage	Prerequisite Attitude	Developmental Issues
1. Entering the new relationship	Recovery from loss of first marriage (adequate "emotional divorce")	Recommitment to marriage and to forming a family with readiness to deal with the complexity and ambiguity
2. Conceptualizing and planning new marriage and family	Accepting one's own fears and those of new spouse and children about remarriage and forming a stepfamily Accepting need for time and patience for adjustment to complexity and ambiguity of: Multiple new roles Boundaries: space, time, membership, and authority. Affective issues: guilt, loyalty conflicts, desire for mutuality, unresolvable past hurts	Work on openness in the new relationships to avoid pseudomutuality Plan for maintenance of cooperative financial and co-parental relationships with ex-spouses Plan to help children deal with fears, loyalty conflicts, and membership in two systems Realignment of relationships with extended family to include new spouse and children Plan maintenance of connections for children with extended family of ex-spouses
3. Remarriage and reconstitution of family	Final resolution of attachment to previous spouse and ideal of "intact" family Acceptance of a different model of family with permeable boundaries	Restructuring family boundaries to allow for inclusion of new spouse-stepparent Realignment of relationships and financial arrangement throughout subsystems to permit interweaving of several systems Making room for relationships of all children with biologic (noncustodial) parents, grandparents, and other extended family Sharing memories and histories to enhance stepfamily integration

From Carter, B., & McGoldrick, M. (1999b). The divorce cycle: A major variation in the American family life cycle. In B. Carter & M. McGoldrick (Eds.), *The expanded family life cycle* (p. 377). New York: Allyn & Bacon.

---

making and share holidays and life-cycle transitions. For African Americans, the family may include a broad network of kin and community that includes long-time friends who are considered family members (McGoldrick & Giordano, 1996).

Cultural groups also differ in the importance they give to different life-cycle transitions. For example, Irish Americans emphasize the wake, viewing death as an important life-cycle transition. African Americans emphasize funerals, going to considerable expense and delaying services until family members arrive. Italian American and Polish American families place great emphasis on weddings (McGoldrick & Giordano, 1996).

Families in Poverty. The family life cycle of those living in poverty may vary from those with adequate financial means. People living in poverty are always struggling to make ends meet, and members may face difficulties in meeting their own or other members' basic developmental needs. To be poor does not mean that a family is automatically dysfunctional. But poverty is an important factor that can force even the healthiest families to crumble. In studying African American families living in poverty, Hines observed four distinguishing characteristics (1999):

Condensed life cycle. Family members leave home, mate, have children, and become grandparents at much earlier ages than their working-class and middle-class counterparts. Consequently, many individuals in such families assume new roles and responsibilities before they are developmentally capable.

Female-headed households of the extended-family type. A woman, her children, and her daughter's children often live together without clear delineation of their respective roles. This scenario can create economic and emotional burdens for the older women and difficulty for the younger women in assuming parental responsibilities.

Chronic stress and untimely losses. Families living in poverty are subject to family disruption through abrupt loss of members from unemployment, illness, death, imprisonment, or alcohol or drug addiction. Ordinary problems, such as transportation or a sick child, can become major crises because of a lack of resources to solve them.

Reliance on institutional supports. Poor families are often forced to seek public assistance, which ultimately can result in additional stress in having to deal with a governmental agency.

The condensed life cycle can be loosely divided into three overlapping stages: (1) adolescence and unattached adulthood, (2) family with young children, and (3) family in later life. In the African American family living in poverty, members may either push male adolescents out of the home or cling to them desperately as a source of assistance. Education subsequently becomes a low priority, and these teens often drop out of school. Peer relationships are powerful and can conflict with expectations at home. Male adolescents cannot differentiate themselves from either family or peers. They often cannot find employment, except for menial work. They may assert their masculinity in transient heterosexual relationships. Both the family burdens and peer pressure leave them ill equipped to handle later stages. They quickly move into the next stage of family with young children but often cannot assume their parental roles.

Often, the role of women living in poverty is conscripted to childrearing as pregnancies interrupt their education, and they eventually become dependent on public support. Then, older family members (usually the baby's new grandmother) become the primary sources of assistance. Subsequent pregnancies may increase the burden of caregiving. The next stage, family in later life, does not signal a decrease in daily responsibilities or a shift into concerns about retirement. Instead, elderly family members continue to work to make ends meet and support their children and grandchildren despite poor health. Men may die relatively young compared with their middle-class counterparts (Hines, 1999).

Communication Patterns

Family communication patterns develop over a lifetime. Some family members communicate more openly and honestly than others. Family subsystems develop from communication patterns. The nurse should assess the communication patterns of members during the interview and then investigate the typical, day-to-day family communication patterns. Just as in any assessment interview, the nurse should observe the verbal and nonverbal communication of the family members. Who sits next to each other? Who talks to whom? Who answers most questions? Who volunteers information? Who changes the subject? Which subjects seem acceptable to discuss? Which topics are not discussed? Can spouses be intimate with each other? Are any family secrets revealed? Does the nonverbal communication match the verbal communication? Nurses can use all this information to identify family problems and communication issues.

Nurses should also assess the family for its daily communication patterns. Identifying which family members confide in one another is a place to start examining ongoing communication. Other areas include how often children talk with parents, who talks to the parents most, and who is most likely to discipline the children. Can family members express positive and negative feelings? In determining how open or closed the family system is, the nurse explores the type of information that the family shares with nonfamily members. For example, one family may tell others about a member's mental illness, whereas another family may not discuss any illnesses outside the family.

Stress and Coping

One of the most important assessment areas is determining how family members deal with major and minor stressful events and their available coping skills. Some families seem able to cope with overwhelming stresses such as the death of a member, major illness, or severe conflict, whereas other families seem to fall apart over relatively minor events. It is important for the nurse to listen to which situations a family appraises as stressful and help the family identify usual coping responses. The nurse can then evaluate the coping responses. If the family's responses are maladaptive (eg, substance abuse, physical abuse), the nurse will discuss the need to develop coping skills that lead to family well-being (see Chap. 35).

Problem-Solving Skills

Nurses assess family problem-solving skills by focusing on the more recent problems that the family has experienced and determining the process that members used to solve them. For example, a child is sick at school and has to go home. Does the mother, father, grandparent, or babysitter receive the call from the school? Who then cares for the child? Underlying the ability to solve problems is the decision-making process. Who makes and implements decisions? How does the family handle conflict? All these data provide information regarding the family's problem-solving abilities. Once identified, the nurse can build on these strengths in helping families deal with additional problems.

Family Social Domain

The assessment of the family's social domain provides important data regarding the operation of the family as a system and its interaction within its environment. Areas of concern include the system itself, social and financial status, and formal and informal support networks.

Family Systems

A family has many different roles including responsibility for individual growth, economic support, protection of members, promotion of health, and maintenance of the organization and system despite constant individual, family, and societal change. Just like any group can be viewed as a system, a family can also be understood as a system with interdependent members. Family system theories view the family as an open system whose members interact with their environment as well as among themselves. One family member's change in thoughts or behavior can cause a ripple effect and change everyone else. For example, a mother who decides not to pick up her children's clothing off their bedroom floors anymore forces the children to deal with cluttered rooms and dirty clothes in a different way than before.

One very common scenario in mental health is the effect of a patient's improvement on the family. With new medications and treatment, patients are more likely to be able to live independently, which subsequently changes the responsibilities and activities of family caregivers. Although on the surface, the members may seem relieved that their caregiving burden is lifted, in reality, they must adjust their time and energies to fill the remaining void. This transition may not be easy because it is often less stressful to maintain familiar activities than to venture into uncharted territory. Families may seem as though they want to keep an ill member dependent, but in reality, they are struggling with the change in their family system.

Two models, Bowen's family system and Minuchin's structural family system, are often used to explain how the family as a system works. Nurses can use both models in assessing families and developing interventions.

Family Systems Therapy Model. Murray Bowen recognized the power of a system and believed that there is a balance between the family system and the individual (see Chap. 6). He believed that, for an individual to develop into a mature adult, he or she had to stay connected to the family, yet separate from the emotional chaos that is inherent in many family systems. Bowen developed several concepts that professionals often use today when working with families (Bowen, 1975, 1976):

Differentiation of self. For Bowen, the individual must resolve attachment to his or her family's emotional chaos before he or she can differentiate into a mature, healthy personality. Differentiation of self involves two processes: intrapsychic and interpersonal. Intrapsychic differentiation means separating thinking from feeling. A differentiated individual can distinguish between thoughts and feelings and can consequently think through

behavior. For example, even though a family member is angry, he or she will think through the underlying issue before acting if he or she has experienced intrapsychic differentiation. An undifferentiated individual cannot separate thoughts from feelings; consequently, feelings, rather than rational thoughts, govern his or her behavior. The feeling of the moment will drive this family member's behavior. Interpersonal differentiation is the process of freeing oneself from the family's emotional chaos. That is, the individual can recognize the family turmoil but avoid reentering the arguments and issues.

Triangles. According to Bowen, the triangle is a three-person system and the smallest stable unit in human relations. Cycles of closeness and distance characterize a two-person relationship. When anxiety is high during periods of distance, one party "triangulates" a third person or thing into the relationship. For example, two partners may have a stable relationship when anxiety is low. When anxiety and tension rise, one partner may be so uncomfortable that he or she confides in a friend instead of the other partner. In these cases, triangulating reduces the tension but freezes the conflict in place. In families, triangulating occurs when a husband and wife diffuse tension by focusing on the children. The two parties avoid conflict as long as there is triangulation. To maintain the status quo and avoid the conflict, one of the parents develops an overly intense relationship with one of the children, which tends to produce symptoms in the child (eg, bed wetting, fear of school).

Family projection process. Through this process, the triangulated member becomes the center of the family conflicts. The family projects its conflicts onto the child or spouse. Projection is anxious, enmeshed concern. For example, a husband and wife are having difficulty deciding how to spend money. One of the children is having difficulty with interpersonal relationships in school. Instead of the parents resolving their differences over money, one parent focuses on the child's needs and becomes intensely involved in the child's issues. The other parent then relates coolly and distantly to the involved parent.

Nuclear family emotional process. Emotional forces in families recur over the years. This concept describes patterns of emotional functioning in a family in a single generation. For example, a spouse may stay emotionally distant from his partner, just like his father was with his mother. This emotional distance is a patterned reaction in daily interactions with the spouse.

Multigenerational transmission process. Bowen believed that one generation transferred its emotional processes to the next generation. Certain basic patterns between parents and children are replicas of those of past generations, and generations to follow will repeat them as well. The child who is the most involved with the family is least able to differentiate from his or her family of origin and passes on conflicts from one generation to another.

Sibling position. Children develop fixed personality characteristics based on their sibling position in their families. For example, a first-born child may have more confidence and be more outgoing than the second-born child, who has grown up in the older child's shadow. Conversely, the second-born child may be more inclined to identify with the oppressed and be more open to other experiences than the first-born child. These attitudinal and behavioral patterns become fixed parts of both children's personalities. Knowledge of these general personality characteristics is helpful in predicting the family emotional process and family patterns.

Emotional cutoff. If a member cannot differentiate from his or her family, that member may just flee from the family either by moving away or avoiding personal subjects of conversation. Yet, a brief visit from parents can render these individuals helpless.

In using this model, the nurse can observe family interactions to determine how differentiated family members are from one another. Are members autonomous in thinking and feeling? Do triangulated relationships develop during periods of stress and tension? Are the family members interacting in the same manner as their parents or grandparents? How do the personalities of older siblings compare with those of younger siblings? Who lives close to one another? Does any family member live in another city? The Bowen model can provide a way of assessing the system of family relationships.

Family Structure Model. Salvador Minuchin emphasizes the importance of family structure (see Chap. 6). In his structural family system model, the family consists of three essential components: structure, subsystems, and boundaries (Minuchin et al., 1996). **Family structure** is the organized pattern in which family members interact. As two adult partners come together to form a family, they develop the quantity of the interactions. For example, a newly married couple may establish their evening interaction pattern by talking to each other during dinner but not while watching television. The quality of the interactions also becomes patterned. Some topics are appropriate for dinner conversation (eg, reciting daily events), whereas controversial or emotionally provocative topics are relegated to other times and places.

Family rules are important influences on interaction patterns. For example, "family problems stay in the family" is a common rule. Both the number of people in the family and its development also influence the interaction pattern. The interaction between a single mother and her children changes when she remarries and introduces a stepfather. Over time, families repeat interactions, which develop into enduring patterns. For example, if a mother tells her son to pick up his room and the son refuses until his father yells at him, the family has initiated an interactional pattern. If this pattern continues, the child will come to see the father as the disciplinarian and the mother as incompetent. The mother, however, will be more affectionate to her son, and the father will remain as the disciplinarian on the "outside."

Subsystems develop when family members join together for various activities or functions. Minuchin views each member, as well as dyads and other larger groups that form, as a subsystem. Families develop different groupings. Obvious groups are parents and children. Sometimes, there are "boy" and "girl" systems. Such systems become obvious in an assessment when family members talk about "the boys going fishing with dad" and "the girls going shopping with mother." Family members belong to several different subgroups. A mother may also be a wife, sister, and daughter. Sometimes, these roles can conflict. It may be acceptable for a woman to be very firm as a disciplinarian in her role as mother. In her sister, wife, or daughter role, however, the similar behavior would provoke anger and resentment.

Boundaries are the invisible barriers with varying permeabilities that surround individuals and subsystems (see Chap. 9). They regulate the amount of contact a person has with others. In a family, boundaries protect the separateness and autonomy of the family and its subsystems. If family members do not take telephone calls at dinner, they are protecting themselves from outside intrusion. When parents do not allow children to interrupt them, they are establishing a boundary between themselves and their children. According to Minuchin, the spouse subsystem must have a boundary that separates it from parents, children, and the outside world. A clear boundary between parent and child enables children to interact with their parents but excludes them from the spouse subsystem.

Boundaries vary from being rigid to diffuse. If boundaries are too rigid and permit little contact from outside subsystems, disengagement results. Disengaged individuals are relatively isolated and autonomous. On the other hand, rigid boundaries permit independence, growth, and mastery within the subsystem, particularly if parents do not hover over their children, telling them what to do or fighting their battles for them. Enmeshed subsystems result when boundaries are diffuse. When boundaries are too relaxed, parents may become too involved with their children, and the children learn to rely on the parents to make decisions, resulting in decreased independence. If children see their parents as friends and treat them as they would peers, Minuchin would say that enmeshment exists.

In the family structural theory view, what distinguishes normal families is not the absence of problems but a functional family structure to handle them. Normal husbands and wives must learn to adjust to each other, rear their children, deal with their parents, cope with their jobs, and fit into their communities. The types of struggles change with developmental stages and situational crises. The psychiatric nurse assesses the family structure and the presence of subsystems or boundaries. He or she uses these data to determine how the subsystems and boundaries affect the family's functioning. Helping family members change a subsystem, such as including girls in the boys activities, may improve family functioning.

Social and Financial Status

Social status is often linked directly to financial status. The nurse should assess the occupations of the family members. Who works? Who is primarily responsible for the family's financial support? Families of low social status are more likely to have limited financial resources, which can place additional stresses on the family. Cultural expectations and beliefs about acceptable behaviors may cause additional stress. Nurses can use information regarding the family's financial status to determine whether to refer the family to social services.

Cultural expectations and beliefs about acceptable behaviors also may cause additional stress. For example, in one qualitative study of 12 black West Indian depressed women who emigrated to Canada or were first-born Canadians, the women rarely sought professional help because of the strong culturally defined stigma against mental disorders. Instead, they managed depression by "being strong," which meant that they tried not to dwell on their feelings, focused on diversions, tried to regain composure, or used other approaches. The researchers concluded that "being strong" may be a factor in inducing depression or slowing or preventing recovery for some women (Schreiber et al., 2000).

Formal and Informal Support Networks

According to balance theory, both formal and informal networks are important in providing support to individuals and families (see Chap. 6). The networks are the link among the individual, families, and the community. Assessing the extent of formal support (eg, hospitals, agencies) and informal support (eg, extended family, friends, neighbors) will give a clearer picture of the availability of support. In assessing formal support, the nurse should

ask about the family's involvement with government institutions and self-help groups such as Alcoholics Anonymous. Assessing the informal network is particularly important in cultural groups with extended family networks or close friends because these individuals can be major sources of support to patients. Without asking about the informal network, these important people may be missed. Do any family members volunteer at schools, local hospitals, or nursing homes? Does the family attend religious services or activities? Investigating the role of extended family members, friends, and neighbors in daily activities will provide useful information regarding the family network.

IDENTIFYING FAMILY NURSING DIAGNOSES

From the assessment data, nurses can choose several possible nursing diagnoses. Interrupted Family Processes, Ineffective Therapeutic Regimen Management, or Compromised, Disabling, or Ineffective Family Coping are all possibilities. Nurses choose Interrupted Family Processes if a usually supportive family is experiencing stressful events that challenge its previously effective functioning. They choose Ineffective Management of Therapeutic Regimen if the family is experiencing difficulty integrating into daily living a program for the treatment of illness and the sequela of illness that meets specific health goals. They select Ineffective Family Coping when the supportive primary person is providing insufficient, ineffective, or compromised support, comfort, or assistance to the patient in managing or mastering adaptive tasks related to the individual's health challenge (Carpenito, 2000).

The assessment data may also reveal other nursing diagnoses of individual family members, such as Caregiver Role Strain, Ineffective Denial, or Dysfunctional Grieving. If the nurse finds that any other nursing diagnosis is appropriate, the individual family member should have an opportunity to explore ways of managing these problems.

FAMILY INTERVENTIONS

Family interventions focus on supporting the biopsychosocial integrity and functioning of the family as defined by its members. Whereas family therapy is reserved for mental health specialists, the generalist psychiatric–mental health nurse can implement several biopsychosocial interventions. They include counseling, promotion of self-care activities, supportive therapy, and education and health teaching.

In implementing any family intervention, flexibility is essential, particularly when working with culturally diverse groups. To implement successful culturally competent family interventions, nurses need to modify the structure and format of the sessions. Longer sessions are often useful, especially when a translator or interpreter is used. Nurses also need to respect and work with the changing family composition of family and non-family participants (eg, extended family members, intimate partners, friends and neighbors, community helpers) in sessions. Because of the stigma that some cultural groups associate with seeking help, nurses may need to hold intervention sessions in community settings (eg, churches and schools) or at the family's home. Finally, termination may need to be gradual or delayed (Celano & Kaslow, 2000).

Counseling

The nurse will encounter families with various needs. Nurses often use counseling when working with families because it is a short-term problem-solving approach that addresses current issues. If the assessment reveals complex, long-standing relationship problems, the nurse needs to refer the family to a family therapist. If the family is struggling with psychiatric problems of one or more family members or the family system is in a life-cycle transition, the nurse should use short-term counseling. The counseling sessions should focus on specific issues or problems using sound group process theory. Usually, a problem-solving approach works well once an issue has been identified (see Chap. 14).

Promoting Self-Care Activities

Families often need support in changing behaviors that promote self-care activities. For example, families may inadvertently reinforce a family member's dependency out of fear of the patient being taken advantage of in work or social situations. A nurse can help the family explore how to meet the patient's need for work and social activity and at the same time help alleviate family fears.

Caregiver distress or role strain can also occur in families who are responsible for the care of people with long-term illness. Family interventions can help families deal with the burden of caring for members with psychiatric disorders. An analysis of 16 studies indicated that family interventions can affect relatives' burden, psychological distress, and relationship between patient and relative and family functioning. These interventions varied from education sessions to intensive family treatment. In most interventions, information on mental illness was presented, as well as discussion. Interventions with more than 12 sessions had larger effects than shorter interventions (Cuijpers, 1999). Identifying community resources, groups, and volunteers that can assist in caring for the caregiver will help alleviate this distress (Cuellar & Butts, 1999).

Supporting Family Functioning and Cohesiveness

Supporting family function involves various nursing approaches. In meeting with the family, the nurse should identify and acknowledge the family's values. In developing a trusting relationship with the family, the nurse should confirm the senses of self and worth as individuals among all members. Supporting family subsystems, such as encouraging the children to play while meeting with the spouses, reinforces family boundaries. Based on the analysis of the family system's operation and communication patterns, the nurse can reinforce open, honest communication.

In communicating with the family, the nurse needs to observe boundaries constantly and avoid becoming triangulated into family issues. An objective, empathic leadership style can set the tone for the family sessions.

Providing Education and Health Teaching

One of the most important family interventions is education and health teaching, particularly in families with mental illness. Families have a central role in the treatment of mental illnesses. Members need to learn about mental disorders, medications, actions, side effects, and overall treatment approaches and outcomes. Families are often reluctant to have members take psychiatric medications because they believe that the medications will "drug" the patient or become addictive. The family's beliefs about mental illnesses and treatment can affect whether patients will be able to manage their illness.

The nurse can also teach families about how a family system works. Using genograms to track the development of illnesses and relationship patterns across several generations can help family members gain insight into how their family system works.

Using Family Therapy

Family therapy is useful for families who are having difficulty in maintaining family integrity. Various theoretic perspectives are used in family therapy, but the Minuchin and Bowen models discussed in the assessment section serve as the basis for most approaches. Family therapy can be short-term or long-term and is conducted by mental health specialists, including advanced practice psychiatric–mental health nurses.

Summary and Key Points

➤ A family is a group of people who are connected emotionally, by blood, or in both ways that has developed patterns of interactions and relationships.

Families come in various compositions, including nuclear, extended, multigenerational, single-parent, and same-gender families. Cultural values and beliefs define family composition and roles.

➤ Nurses complete a comprehensive family assessment when they care for families over extended periods or if a patient has complex mental health problems.

➤ In building relationships with families, families must view the nurse as credible and competent. Unless the nurse addresses the family's immediate needs first, the family will have difficulty engaging in the challenges of caring for someone with a mental disorder.

➤ The genogram is an assessment and intervention tool that is useful in understanding health problems, relationship issues, and social functioning across several generations.

➤ In assessing the family biologic domain, the nurse determines health status and mental disorders and their effects on family functioning.

➤ Family members are often reluctant to discuss the mental disorders of family members because of the stigma associated with mental illness. In many instances, family members do not know whether mental illnesses were present in other generations.

➤ The family psychological assessment focuses on family development, the family life cycle, communication patterns, stress and coping, and problem-solving skills. An aim of the assessment is to begin to understand family interpersonal relationships.

➤ Family life cycle is a process of expansion, contraction, and realignment of the relationship system to support the entry, exit, and development of family members in a functional way. The nurse should determine whether a family fits any of the life-cycle models. Families living in poverty may have a condensed life cycle.

➤ In assessing the family social domain, the nurse includes data collection about the system itself, social and financial status, and formal and informal support networks.

➤ The family system model proposes that a balance should exist between the family system and the individual. A person needs family connection but also needs to be differentiated as an individual. Important concepts include triangles, family projection process, nuclear family emotional process, multigenerational transmission, sibling position, and emotional cutoff.

➤ The family structure model explains patterns of family interaction. Subsystems develop that also influence interaction patterns. Boundaries can vary from rigid to relaxed. The rigidity of the boundaries affects family functioning.

➤ Family interventions focus on supporting the family's biopsychosocial integrity and functioning as defined by its members. Family psychiatric nursing interventions include counseling, promotion of self-care activities, supportive therapy, and education and health teaching. Mental health specialists, including advanced practice nurses, conduct family therapy.

➤ Family counseling should focus on specific issues or problems using group process theory.

➤ Promotion of family self-care activities involves helping family members identify community resources, groups, or volunteers that can assist the self-care activities.

➤ Education of the family is one of the most useful interventions. Teaching the family about mental disorders, life cycles, family systems, and family interactions can help the family develop a new understanding of family functioning and the effects of mental disorders on the family.

Critical Thinking Challenges

1. Differentiate between a nuclear and extended family. How can a group of people who are unrelated by blood consider themselves a family?
2. Interview a family with a member who has a mental illness and identify who provides support to the individual and family during acute episodes of illness.
3. Interview someone from another culture regarding family beliefs about mental illness. Compare them to your own.
4. Develop a genogram for your family. Analyze the genogram in terms of its pattern of health problems, relationship issues, and social functioning.
5. Differentiate the terms *family development* and *family life cycle*.
6. Compare and contrast the family life cycle of a traditional nuclear family with that of a single-parent family.
7. A female patient, divorced with two small children, reports that she is considering getting married again to a man whom she met 6 months ago. She asks for help in considering the pros and cons of remarriage. Using the remarried family formulations life-cycle model, develop a plan for structuring the counseling session.
8. Define the following terms and give examples: differentiation of self, triangles, family projection process, nuclear family emotional process, multigenerational transmission process, sibling position, and emotional cutoff.
9. Define Minuchin's term *family structure* and use that definition in observing your own family and its interaction.
10. Discuss what happens to a family who has rigid boundaries.

11. A family is finding it difficult to provide transportation to a support group for an adult member with mental illness. The family is committed to his treatment but is also experiencing severe financial stress because of another family illness. Using a problem-solving approach, outline a plan for helping the family explore solutions to the transportation problem.

WEB LINKS

www.aamft.org   The American Association for Marriage and Family Therapy website offers help in finding a therapist and information on families and health. It provides resources for practitioners.

www.bcfamily.com   B-C Family Productions provides training products for use by advocates and providers to be successful in developing comprehensive systems of care for children and families.

www.fame.volnetmmp.net   The Family Association for Mental Health Everywhere (FAME) is an organization for family support when mental illness of any form is an issue. FAME is run for and by families to reduce the stress of coping with mental illness by strengthening and supporting family members in their role as caregivers.

www.mc-mlmhs.org   Family Dynamics Across Cultures: Mental Health Perspectives provides information about different cultural groups and their family dynamics.

http://mentalhelp.net   Mental Help Net is one of the oldest mental health Internet guides for education and resources.

MOVIES

American Beauty: 1999. This film depicts the life of a family undergoing structural change. Lester and Carolyn Burnham are a seemingly ordinary couple in an anonymous suburban neighborhood whose lives and marriage are slowly unraveling. Their lack of communication and anger toward each other sets the stage for a cascade of events that estranges their daughter and psychologically damages everyone. Lester's behavior shows how a family member can lose his or her good sense while undergoing the stresses of a dysfunctional marriage.

Viewing Points: Identify the life cycle phase of the Burnham family. Identify the triangulation that occurs within the family. How does Lester's attraction to his daughter's friend represent a violation of boundaries among family members? How would you describe the communication between Lester and Carolyn?

The Godfather: 1972. The film is the first of a trilogy (Godfather II, 1975 and Godfather III, 1990) depicting the violent lives and times of Mafia patriarch Vito Corleone and his son (and successor) Michael. Violence, corruption, and crime in America are examined within the context of family loyalties. In this film, the family dynamics and cultural practices are the basis for decisions in all aspects of life.

Viewing Points: Identify how beliefs about family affect its functioning. Who are the important family members? How are decisions made? Look for triangulation in interactions that occur throughout the film. If this film were made today, how do you think it would be different?

REFERENCES

Bowen, M. (1975). Family therapy after twenty years. In S. Arieti, D. Freedman, & J. Dyrud (Eds.), *American handbook of psychiatry* (2nd ed., Vol. 5, pp. 379–391). New York: Basic Books.

Bowen, M. (1976). Theory in the practice of psychotherapy. In P. Guerin (Ed.), *Family therapy: Theory and practice* (pp. 42–90). New York: Gardner Press.

Carpenito, L. (2000). *Nursing diagnosis: Application to clinical practice* (8th ed.). Philadelphia: Lippincott Williams & Wilkins.

Carter, B., & McGoldrick, M. (1999a). The divorce cycle: A major variation in the American family life cycle. In B. Carter & M. McGoldrick (Eds.), *The expanded family life cycle* (pp. 373–398). New York: Allyn & Bacon.

Carter, B., & McGoldrick, M. (1999b). Overview: The expanded family life cycle. Individual, family, and social perspectives. In B. Carter & M. McGoldrick (Eds.), *The expanded family life cycle* (pp. 1–26). New York: Allyn & Bacon.

Celano, M., & Kaslow, N. (2000). Culturally competent family interventions: Review and case illustrations. *American Journal of Family Therapy, 28,* 217–228.

Cuellar, N., & Butts, J. (1999). Caregiver distress: What nurses in rural settings can do to help. *Nursing Forum, 34*(3), 24–30.

Cuijpers, P. (1999). The effects of family interventions of relatives' burden: A meta-analysis. *Journal of Mental Health, 8*(3), 275–285.

Hatfield, A. (1992). Leaving home: Separation issues in psychiatric illness. *Psychosocial Rehabilitation Journal, 15*(4), 37–47.

Hines, P. M. (1999). The family life cycle of African American families living in poverty. In B. Carter &

M. McGoldrick (Eds.), *The expanded family life cycle* (pp. 327–345). New York: Allyn & Bacon.

McGoldrick, M., & Giordano, F. (1996). Overview: Ethnicity and family therapy. In M. McGoldrick, J. Giordano, & J. K. Pearce (Eds.), *Ethnicity and family therapy* (pp. 1–27). New York: The Guilford Press.

Minuchin, S., Lee, W., & Simon, G. (1996). *Mastering family therapy: Journey of growth and transformation.* New York: John Wiley & Sons.

Schreiber, R., Noerager Stern, P., & Wilson, C. (2000). Being strong: How Black West-Indian Canadian women manage depression and its stigma. *Journal of Nursing Scholarship, 32*(1), 39–45.

Smith, G. C., Hatfield, A. B., & Miller, D. C. (2000). Planning by older mothers for the future care of offspring with serious mental illness. *Psychiatric Services, 51*(9), 1162–1166.

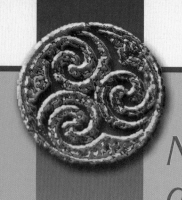

Nursing Practice Within a Continuum of Care

Denise M. Gibson, Robert B. Noud,
Kimberly H. Littrell, Carol D. Peabody

**DEFINING THE
CONTINUUM OF CARE**
Least Restrictive Environment
Coordination of Care
  and Nursing Process
Components of the
  Continuum of Care
  Inpatient Care
  Outpatient Care

MANAGED CARE
Public and Private Collaboration
Role of the Nurse

**PSYCHIATRIC
REHABILITATION**
Role of the Nurse
Assessment and Selection
  of Level of Care
Discharge Planning

**LEARNING
OBJECTIVES**

After studying the chapter, you will be able to:

➤ Identify the different treatment settings and associated programs along the continuum of care.

➤ Discuss the role of the nurse at different points along the continuum of care.

➤ Compare the stages of the nursing process with the phases of coordination of care in the continuum.

➤ Describe current health care trends in inpatient and outpatient psychiatric services.

➤ Explain how the concept of the least restrictive environment influences the assessment of patients for placement in different treatment settings.

➤ Discuss the factors that determine the level of care to be provided to a patient seeking voluntary or involuntary treatment.

➤ Discuss the influence of managed care on services and use of services in the continuum of care.

CHAPTER 17

KEY TERMS

assertive community
    treatment
board-and-care homes
case management
clubhouse model
continuum of care
coordination of care
crisis intervention
in-home mental
    health care
intensive outpatient
    program
least restrictive
    environment
managed care
    organizations

outpatient
    detoxification
partial hospitalization
psychiatric
    rehabilitation
    programs
referral
reintegration
relapse
residential treatment
    facility
stabilization
therapeutic foster care
transfer
23-hour beds

Behavioral health care continues to evolve into a system of care that is responding to the needs of a complex and dynamic population. A demand exists for a comprehensive, holistic approach to care that encompasses all levels of health care needs. Consumers, families, providers, advocacy groups, and third-party payers of mental health care no longer accept long-term hospitalization and institutionalization, once the hallmark of psychiatric care. Instead, they advocate for short-term treatment in an environment that promotes the patient's dignity and well-being while meeting his or her biologic, psychological, and social needs.

Beginning with the introduction of neuroleptic medications and the deinstitutionalization of patients with chronic mental illness in the 1950s, a myriad of treatment alternatives and options have enhanced mental health care. Reimbursement issues and regulatory bodies that govern hospital

lengths of stay, however, have influenced health care. Health maintenance organizations (HMOs), preferred provider organizations (PPOs), Medicaid, and Medicare regulate the type and quality of treatment that can be received. This results in fragmentation of services, limits available financial and treatment resources, and moves the patient through various treatment programs that do not adequately address individual needs or promote independent functioning. Today, psychiatric–mental health nurses face the challenge of providing mental health care within a complex system that is affected by financial constraints and narrowed treatment requirements. To provide mental health care and treatment, the psychiatric–mental health care nurse must understand the vast and diverse components of mental health care that will meet the individual needs of patients based on their level of illness and recovery.

DEFINING THE CONTINUUM OF CARE

The concept of the **continuum of care** began in 1956 when Congress passed the Health Amendments Act. This act led to better access to comprehensive community mental health center legislation through pilot projects, demonstrations, and applied research and evaluation studies. In 1963, President Kennedy submitted to Congress a "Special Message on Mental Illness and Mental Retardation" that called for a new approach to these two health problems. President Kennedy noted that these health problems "occur more frequently, affect more people, require more prolonged treatment, cause more suffering by families of the afflicted, waste more of our human resources, and constitute more financial drain upon the public treasury and the personal finances of the individual families than any other single condition" (Geller, 2000, p. 43). President Kennedy endorsed the Mental Retardation Facilities and Community Mental Health Centers Construction Act of 1963, which allocated funds for constructing community mental health centers.

During the 1980s, the focus of care shifted to other areas of concern, including needs assessment, after-care specialty services, case management, residential care, community mental health centers, autonomy, family care, crisis care, and continuity of care. This shift in focus gave rise to the concept of continuum of care. The Joint Commission on Accreditation of Healthcare Organizations (JCAHO) defined the continuum of care as matching an individual's ongoing needs with the appropriate level and type of medical, psychological, health, or social care or services within an organization or across multiple organizations. Continuing care is provided over an extended time, within an integrated system of settings, services, health care practitioners, and care levels, spanning the illness-to-wellness continuum that makes up a continuum of care. The continuum facilitates the stability, continuity, and comprehensiveness of service to an individual and maximizes the coordination of care or services.

Given the levels of treatment that can occur along the continuum of care, patient care and services must be integrated and coordinated to best meet the patient's needs. The patient care needs should be facilitated within clinically appropriate levels of treatment across an entire episode of illness (Kiser et al., 1999a, 1999b). This chapter discusses the different components of the continuum of care and its effects on the delivery of mental health care. It will explore and identify the nurse's role across different levels of treatment services (Fig. 17-1).

Least Restrictive Environment

Today's treatment options for the person with mental illness span many treatment settings with various levels of patient care. The continuum spans from court-

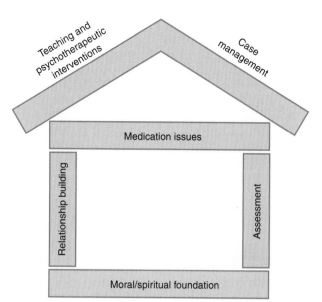

FIGURE 17.1 The Bay Area model for psychiatric home care. (Adapted from Carson, V. B. [1994]. *Bay Area psychiatric home care manual*. Baltimore, MD: Bay Area Health Care.)

ordered involuntary treatment to at-home mental health treatment with minimal community involvement. In 1964, the case of Dixon vs. Weinberger first introduced the concept of **least restrictive environment**. This case proposed that patients have a statutory right to treatment in a setting consistent with suitable treatment that does not disrupt their lifestyle or interfere with their support network. Choices and decisions made regarding treatment services and programs must consider the least restrictive environment that will promote care beyond stabilization toward continuous personal growth (Wilbur & Arns, 1998). The primary goal of the continuum of care is to provide treatment that allows the patient to achieve the highest level of functioning in the least restrictive environment that will meet his or her immediate safety needs.

Coordination of Care and Nursing Process

Coordination of care and services is defined as the process by which care is provided by a health care organization, including referral to appropriate community resources and liaisons with others (eg, physician, other health care organizations, community services) to meet a person's ongoing identified needs, to ensure implementation of the plan of care, and to avoid unnecessary duplication of services (JCAHO, 1999). The components of coordination of care are interchangeable with the nursing process. The components include assessment, nursing diagnosis and outcome development, planning and implementation of nursing interventions, and evaluation of outcomes. Coordination of care requires collaborative and cooperative relationships among many agencies, including public health, mental health, social services, housing, education, and criminal justice to name a few. Coordination of care has four phases:

- *Preadmission phase*: identification and use of available information sources about the patient's needs
- *Admission phase*: services available within the organization and through other settings or organizations, with referrals and transfer of patient services based on individual needs
- *Predischarge phase*: assessment of continuing patient needs and coordination of them among practitioners
- *Discharge phase*: reassessment of continuing patient care needs with referral to practitioners, settings, or organizations that can meet the patient's continuing needs

Components of the Continuum of Care

The continuum of care for mental health services falls into the inpatient and outpatient settings. Within these two domains, there are different levels of specialized services available. This section of the continuum of care will begin with inpatient treatment.

Inpatient Care

Inpatient hospitalization is considered the most restrictive setting in the continuum. Inpatient treatment is reserved for acutely ill patients who, because of a mental illness, meet one or more of three criteria: (1) are at high risk for harming themselves, (2) are at high risk for harming others, or (3) cannot care for their basic needs (Akhavain et al., 1999). Delivery of inpatient care can occur in a psychiatric hospital, psychiatric unit within a general hospital, or state-operated mental hospital. The state-operated mental hospital is typically viewed as the most restrictive of these options.

Inpatient care results from an involuntary admission or a voluntary admission. In the case of an involuntary admission, either a mental health professional or the judicial system has initiated the determination for commitment. A voluntary patient agrees to seek inpatient treatment. The average length of stay for an involuntary admission can range between 24 hours to several days, whereas length of stay for a voluntary admission depends on the acuity of symptoms and the patient's ability to pay the costs of treatment. Nevertheless, the interdisciplinary treatment team, led by the treating psychiatrist, must determine that the patient is no longer at risk to self or others before discharge can occur.

People with mental illness should be treated on an outpatient basis whenever possible to reduce reliance on hospital-based services (Foster, 1998; Wasylenki et al., 2000). Intensive and comprehensive local services include the use of 24-hour inpatient services should the patient require this setting. The setting for the delivery of mental health services is shifting from an inpatient to outpatient focus. Inpatient length of stay has continually decreased since the 1980s, a trend that has been primarily attributed to managed care and treatment advances, especially medications (Sturm & Bao, 2000). In response to pressure to reduce hospital length of stay, various cost-containment mechanisms have been developed, including strict admission criteria, utilization review, case management, and contracting arrangements with third-party payers that limit psychiatric services (Leslie & Rosenheck, 2000). The average length of stay for inpatient care has decreased from 38.74 days in 1985 to 6.51 days (Hughes, 1999).

Long-Term Care. Long-term inpatient care involves a minimum stay of 3 months and can extend beyond 6 months. This type of treatment is used only under circumstances in which a person continues to demonstrate high risk to injure himself or herself or is at risk for harming someone else. Care centers that have inpatient stays beyond 6 months are classified as **residential treatment facilities**. This form of treatment combines residential care and mental health services. It is designed to provide rehabilitation and therapy to people with serious and persistent mental illnesses, including chronic schizophrenia, bipolar illnesses, and unrelenting depression (Callahan, 1999). Other patients with organic pathologies, such as mental retardation or with traumatic brain injuries may require long-term inpatient hospitalization as well.

Nursing plays an important role in the care of people with chronic mental illnesses who require long-term stays at inpatient treatment facilities. Nurses are involved with psychoeducation groups, including basic social skills training, aggression management, activities of daily living (ADLs) training, and group living. Education on symptom management, understanding mental illnesses, and medication education are essential to recovery.

Short-Term Care. When inpatient care is necessary, the dominant type of treatment in the continuum of care is short-term treatment. This type of treatment has become the focus, as stringent admission criteria and diminished funding have changed mental health care. Short-term care is a continuum that extends from immediate crisis intervention to traditional inpatient care and is generally classified according to length of hospital stay. The classification of short-term care according to the length of stay is as follows:

- Average—10 to 12 days
- Short-term—7 to 10 days
- Brief or respite—fewer than 7 days

Crisis Stabilization. This type cares is usually very short-term, lasting fewer than 7 days, and has a symptom-based indication for hospital admission. The primary purpose of **stabilization** is control of precipitating symptoms through medications, behavioral interventions, and coordination with other agencies for appropriate aftercare. The major focus of nursing care in a short-term inpatient setting is symptom management (Buccheri & Underwood, 1993).

Medication stabilization and monitoring for efficacy and side effects are major components of nursing care during stabilization. Nurses may also provide focused group psychotherapy designed to develop and strengthen the personal management strategies of patients (Kanas, 1991). When treating aggressive or violent patients, the nurse monitors the appropriate use of seclusion and restraints.

23-Hour Beds. The use of **23-hour beds** is a type of short-term treatment that serves the patient in immediate but short-term crisis. This type of care admits individuals to an inpatient setting for crisis stabilization but then discharges them within 24 hours (Weissberg, 1991). The nurse's role in this treatment modality is generally limited to monitoring vital signs, administering medications, and transferring care to an inpatient unit or to a less restrictive outpatient setting. This type of treatment modality is used to treat acute trauma, such as rape, alcohol, and narcotic detoxification, and individuals with Axis II personality disorders presenting with self-injurious behaviors.

Crisis Intervention. An organized system is required to treat individuals in crisis, including a mechanism for rapid access to care (within 24 hours), a referral for hospitalization, or an access to outpatient services (Kiser et al., 1999a). **Crisis intervention** treatment is brief, usually less than 6 hours. A multidisciplinary approach attains the focus of consistent, therapeutic goal setting (Kelly & Stephens, 1999). This type of short-term care focuses on crisis stabilization, symptom reduction, and prevention of relapse requiring inpatient services.

Crisis intervention units can be found in the emergency department of a general or psychiatric hospital or in crisis centers within a community mental health center. Patients in crisis demonstrate severe symptoms of acute mental illness, including labile mood swings, suicidal ideation, or self-injurious behaviors. Therefore, this treatment option commands a high degree of nursing expertise. Patients in crisis usually require medications such as anxiolytics or benzodiazepines for symptom management. Nurses provide care in the form of assessment and medication administration as ordered. They also facilitate admission referral for hospitalization or outpatient services.

Intermediate Care. This type of treatment setting offers careful, comprehensive, psychiatric, and psychosocial diagnosis and treatment in a hospital environment for new patients as well as for those patients experiencing recurrence of illness who cannot be assessed or treated at a lesser level of care. The primary objective is to provide treatment in a short time, within 10 to 14 days (occasionally up to 30 days). The next step is to assist with appropriate follow-up care to facilitate adherence and successful treatment, rehabilitation in a less restrictive environment, or both.

The intermediate care setting offers 24-hour staff supervision and intensive intervention. Nurses assume the responsibility of monitoring patient safety because patients present with severe, disabling symptoms that they cannot adequately manage. Because of the symptoms of their mental illnesses, they are at imminent risk for harming themselves or others, cannot care for their basic physical needs, and may lack family or community resources to assist them.

If the patient is at risk for escalation toward aggressiveness, violence, or both, the nurse will be involved with the application of restraints or seclusion and subsequent monitoring of the patient. Nursing care will also include monitoring vital signs, monitoring medications for efficacy and side effects, behavioral management, and coordination of referrals to outpatient services upon discharge.

Rehabilitation. This type of inpatient care has been referred to as long-term care for those patients who were not receiving care in the expectation of an improved status or rehabilitation. It includes specialized treatment and rehabilitation programs generally found in larger psychiatric hospitals. Treatment is actively directed toward a return to former or improved levels of functioning, and health and is rehabilitative rather than custodial. Length of stay is usually less than 90 days.

An example of a rehabilitation treatment program is substance abuse rehabilitation. This program provides an inpatient rehabilitation setting for patients with serious chemical dependency who require more than detoxification or intermediate care because of significant risk for resumption of abuse on return to the community. Upon completion of treatment, discharge planning includes linkage with outpatient services and caregiver support.

Role of the Nurse. The nurse–patient relationship is central to the treatment process. The nurse is instrumental in developing and implementing the plan of care (treatment plan) and evaluating treatment outcomes (Yurkovich & Smyer, 1998). The Scope and Standards of Psychiatric–Mental Health Nursing Practice guide the nurse in the delivery of patient care (American Nurses Association, 2000). Nurses have the greatest level of contact with patients and are in the critical position of monitoring the patient's response to and the effectiveness of the treatment plan and interventions. The treatment plan is the clinical care pathway that the nurse uses to guide and monitor patient care. Jones and Norman (1998) discuss the assessment components of the treatment plan as follows:

- Functional physical assessment
- Mental health status assessment
- Response to nursing interventions and treatment plan of care
- Monitoring for the absence of, presence of, or change in symptoms of illness
- Response to medications for efficacy and potential side effects
- Response to implementation of other treatment modalities
- Monitoring patient's adherence to treatment plan of care and medication
- Clinical documentation of patient's progress and response to the treatment plan of care
- Statement of discharge goals and referral to appropriate outpatient services

Because individuals receiving inpatient care are in crisis, the nurse will face clinical decisions regarding the use of seclusion and the application of restraints to prevent harm to the patient who is acting out or others in his or her proximity. Nurses should use restraints and seclusion only in emergencies to prevent such harm. Using restraints or seclusion as a form of punishment for the acting-out person is unethical. Patients with mental illnesses may have comorbid physical illnesses, and the nurse should perform a physical assessment before the application of restraint devices to ensure that the use of restraints or seclusion does not pose undue risk to the patient.

Nurses must be conscious of the standards, policies, and procedures that govern the use of restrictive devices. Moreover, nurses promote a therapeutic environment that minimizes the potential for situations that can lead to the use of restraint and seclusion. The astute professional nurse uses nonviolent interventions such as verbal de-escalation, limit setting, and emergency medication proactively before the patient escalates and requires physically restrictive interventions.

Outpatient Care

Outpatient care is considered a level of care that occurs beyond the confines of a hospital or institution. Outpatient services are a less intensive level of care provided to those patients who do not require an inpatient environment or residential setting. Many patients are enrolled into outpatient services immediately upon discharge from an inpatient setting to assist with community reintegration, medication management and compliance, and symptom management. The concept of outpatient ser-

vices resulted from the advances in psychiatry that made it possible for clinicians to provide treatment and care without hospitalization. As a result of deinstitutionalization in the 1950s, treatment of patients with severe mental illness shifted from hospitals to community-based systems of care. Alternative community resources, however, were not in place when deinstitutionalization occurred, and individuals with mental illness were not integrated into the community (Pickens, 1998). Symptoms in many of these people immediately worsened without a social or community network in place to assist them.

During this period in mental health care, funding was allocated for the development of outpatient clinics, halfway houses, day hospitals, emergency services programs, family care, mental health house calls, and integration of services across different organizations. The concept of community treatment began to emerge in the 1960s when therapeutic and supportive programs were designed and developed to meet the ever-changing needs of patients at different levels of symptom intensity during the course of their illness (Geller, 2000).

In response to the challenges of providing treatment to patients with severe mental illness, outpatient care shifted toward a more humanistic and individualized approach. Patients were afforded the right to choose home as a placement option, became more involved in aftercare support services that were individualized to the level of care required, and became more socially integrated into society (Friedrich et al., 1999).

The continuum of outpatient care extends from prevention of inpatient treatment to long-term maintenance. Its focus is to create a three-tiered support network to provide primary, secondary, and tertiary prevention of mental illness symptoms. Primary prevention focuses on preventing the onset of mental health symptoms. Secondary prevention rehabilitates the individual to optimal functioning. Tertiary prevention seeks to minimize the chronic deterioration of mental functioning inherent in mental illnesses (Aday et al., 1999).

The Association for Ambulatory Behavioral Healthcare proposed a collaborative continuum of care that extends from 24-hour inpatient care to traditional outpatient modes of care. It recognized the clinical and economic value and benefits in support of partial hospitalization, intensive outpatient programs, and other emerging types of intermediate treatment. By establishing a set of six unifying principles, the continuum of Behavioral Health Services uses levels of care to address treatment of an illness episode.

1. The continuum of Behavioral Health Services defines various levels of care designed for people in need of treatment for psychiatric illness, chemical dependency, or both regardless of age.

2. An individualized treatment plan provides services based on patient needs and level placement in the continuum of care.

3. Effective clinical process and management of resources maximize access to care at all levels of intensity.

4. The patient and clinician collectively share decision making regarding the course of care.

5. Treatment requires the active involvement of the service team, patient with family, and community resources.

6. Targeting interventions based on patient needs within the most appropriate and least restrictive environment relies on the patient's strengths, family, and community support systems and promotes cost-efficient services (Kiser et al., 1999b).

This continuum of care model identifies discrete service and patient variables. Table 17-1 defines the six levels of service variables along the continuum; Table 17-2 outlines the patient variables. This chapter addresses discrete outpatient services that patients may receive separately or simultaneously and within a variety of settings.

Partial Hospitalization. **Partial hospitalization** was developed to complement the existing traditional inpatient mental health care and outpatient services. It provides services to patients who spend a minimum of 4 hours per day in programming and is scheduled 4 to 6 days a week. This level of care does not provide overnight hospital stay; however, the patient can achieve admission to inpatient stay within 24 hours.

The American Association for Partial Hospitals defines partial hospitalization as a time-limited, ambulatory, active treatment program that offers therapeutically intensive, coordinated, and structured clinical services within a stable milieu. All partial hospital programs pursue the goal of stabilization with the intention of averting inpatient hospitalization or reducing the length of a hospital stay. It should be used as an alternative to inpatient treatment only within a system of care that includes effective triage and crisis service that can evaluate patients' needs and resources (Akhavain et al., 1999). Partial hospitalization provides short-term intensive treatment for patients with acute psychiatric symptoms who are experiencing a decline in their social or occupational functioning, cannot function autonomously on a day-to-day basis, or do not pose imminent danger to themselves or others.

Referrals for partial hospitalization treatment primarily originate from the inpatient unit. A highly integrated, collaborative team of mental health disciplines provides treatment, including psychiatrists, nurses, social workers, therapeutic recreational specialists, substance abuse counselors, vocational and rehabilitation counselors, and mental health counselors. The interdisciplinary treatment team devises and executes a comprehensive plan of care that encompasses modalities such as behavioral therapy, social skills training, basic living skills training, education regarding illness and symptom identification and relapse prevention, community survival skills training, relaxation training, nutrition and exercise counseling, and other forms of expressive therapy. Partial hospitalization exemplifies the most intensive form of nursing care compared with other outpatient treatment programs.

Outpatient Detoxification. Except for situations involving severe or complicated withdrawal, alcohol and drug rehabilitation is now almost exclusively outpatient based. The development of community and domiciliary-based alcohol and substance detoxification services has proved effective in providing accessible and convenient treatment options, with only a small percentage of severely alcohol-dependent patients requiring hospitalized detoxification (Bennie, 1998).

Outpatient detoxification provides a specialized form of partial hospitalization for patients requiring medical supervision. During the initial phase of withdrawal, use of a 23-hour bed may be a treatment option depending on the stage of alcohol withdrawal and the type of addictive substance abused. If the 23-hour bed is not used, the patient may be required to attend a detoxification program 4 to 5 days per week until symptoms resolve. The length of participation depends on the severity of addiction.

Outpatient detoxification includes the 12-step recovery model, such as Alcoholics Anonymous (AA) and Narcotics Anonymous (NA), which provides outpatient involvement with professionals experienced in addiction counseling. It encourages abstinence and provides training in stress management and relapse prevention. Ala-Non and Ala-Teen provide 12-step support for families of substance abusers, who are usually included in the treatment program (Prater et al., 1999).

Intensive Outpatient Programs. The primary focuses of **intensive outpatient programs** are stabilization and relapse prevention for highly vulnerable individuals who function autonomously on a daily basis. People who meet these criteria have returned to their previous lifestyle, such as interacting with family, resuming work, or returning to school. Attendance in this type of program is appropriate for those individuals who still require frequent monitoring and support within a therapeutic milieu that extends beyond the treatment setting and enables the individual to maintain their community network. The duration of treatment and level of services rendered is based on the patient's immediate needs.

TABLE 17.1 The Continuum of Behavioral Health Care: Service Variables

	Service Variables					
	Primary Care	Outpatient	Multimodal Outpatient	Intermediate Ambulatory	Acute Ambulatory	Inpatient Residential
Service function	Provision of screening, early identification, and education; medication management	Decrease in symptoms related to mild to moderate disorders; maintenance of stable, severe disorders	Coordinated treatment for prevention of decline in functioning when outpatient service cannot meet patient need	Stabilization, symptom reduction, and prevention of relapse	Crisis stabilization and acute symptom reduction; serves as alternative to and prevention of hospitalization	Provision of 24-hour monitoring, supervision, and intensive intervention
Scheduled programming	Incorporated with visits for general medical care	Sessions scheduled as needed with maximum of 3 hours per week.	A minimum of 4 hours per week	Minimum of 3–4 hours per day, at least 2–3 days per week	Minimum of 4 hours per day scheduled 4–7 days	24 hours per day
Crisis backup availability	Decision-assistance programs; established liaison with behavioral health specialty care, warm lines	On-call coverage	A 24-hour crisis and consultation service	A 24-hour crisis and consultation service	An organized, integrated 24-hour crisis backup system with immediate access to current clinical and treatment information	24-hour-per-day staffing with personnel skilled in crisis intervention
Medical involvement	Not applicable	Medical consultation PRN	Medical consultation PRN	Medical consultation	Medical supervision	Medical management
Accessibility	Regular appointments scheduled within 3–5 days	Regular appointments scheduled within 3–5 days	Capable of admitting within 72 hours	Capable of admitting within 48 hours	Capable of admitting within 24 hours	Capable of admitting within 1 hour
Milieu	Relationship between provider and patient	Within the session and relationship between therapist and patient	Active therapeutic; primarily within home and community	Active therapeutic within both treatment setting and home and community	Preplanned, consistent, and therapeutic; primarily within treatment setting	Preplanned, consistent and therapeutic within treatment setting
Structure	Minimal structure afforded through scheduled appointments	Minimal structure afforded through scheduled appointments	Individualized and coordinated	Regularly scheduled, individualized	High degree of structure and scheduling	High degree of structure, security, and supervision

(continued)

TABLE 17.1 The Continuum of Behavioral Health Care: Service Variables (Continued)

	Service Variables					
	Primary Care	**Outpatient**	**Multimodal Outpatient**	**Intermediate Ambulatory**	**Acute Ambulatory**	**Inpatient Residential**
Responsibility and control	Patient functions independently with support from family and community	Patient functions independently with support from family and community	Monitoring and support placed primarily with patient, family, and support system	Monitoring and support shared with patient, family, and support system	Staff aggressively monitors and supports patient and family	Staff assumes responsibility for safety and security of patient
Service examples	Regular medical check-up	Outpatient office visit; specialty group; psychotherapy	After-care; clubhouse programs	Psychosocial rehabilitation; day-treatment programs; intensive outpatient; 23-hour respite beds	Partial hospital programs; intensive in-home crisis intervention; outpatient detoxification; 23-hour observation beds	Acute inpatient unit; crisis stabilization bed

From http://www.aabh.org/public/detailpgs/continuum.html.

Treatment duration is usually time limited, with sessions offered 3 to 4 hours per day and 2 to 3 days per week. The treatment activities of the intensive outpatient program are similar to those offered in the partial hospitalization program. Partial hospitalization emphasizes social skills training, whereas the intensive outpatient program promotes education in the areas of stress management, illness, medication, and relapse prevention.

In-Home Mental Health Care. As a result of deinstitutionalization, the treatment environment for patients with severe mental illness has shifted from hospital to community based. The shift is toward homes, not residential treatment settings; choices, not placement; physical and social integration, not segregated and congregate grouping by disability; and individualized flexible services and support, not standardized levels of service (Friedrich et al., 1999). Additionally, psychiatric home care services continue to grow as the result of efforts to contain increasing hospital costs. With this trend, the number of home care provider organizations has grown significantly to meet the demands of the growing number of patients receiving home care.

In-home mental health care uses case management skills to increase the functionality of the patient within the home and decreases hospital stays (Green & Lydon, 1998; Littrell, 1996). Therefore, individuals most appropriate for in-home mental health care services include those patients diagnosed with chronic, persistent mental illness or patients with mental illness who have comorbid medical conditions that require ongoing monitoring.

The provision of in-home mental health care services, as prescribed by a psychiatrist or physician, relies on the skills of the mental health nurse in providing ongoing assessment and implementing a comprehensive, individualized treatment plan of care. Development of the care plan and the ongoing assessment should include mental health status, the environment, medication compliance, family dynamics and home safety, supportive psychotherapy, psychoeducation, case management in the coordination of services delivered by other home care staff, and communication of clinical issues to the patient's psychiatrist. Additionally, the treatment plan of care should also address the provision of care as related to collection of laboratory specimens and crisis intervention to reduce rehospitalization.

The in-home mental health care service requires a comprehensive approach and is illustrated in the Bay Area model for psychiatric home care. Based on the

TABLE 17.2   The Continuum of Behavioral Health Care: Patient Variables

	Patient Variables					
	Primary Care	**Outpatient**	**Multimodal Outpatient**	**Intermediate Ambulatory**	**Acute Ambulatory**	**Inpatient Residential**
Level of functioning	At-risk, sub-clinical, or mild impairment	Mild to moderate impairment in at least one area of daily life	Moderate impairment in at least one area of daily life	Marked impairment in at least one area of daily life	Severe impairment in multiple areas of daily life	Significant impairment with inability to maintain activities of daily living without 24-hour assistance
Psychiatric signs and symptoms	At-risk, sub-clinical presentation, or mild symptoms related to behavioral health disorder	Mild to moderate symptoms related to acute condition or exacerbation of severe or persistent disorder	Moderate symptoms related to acute condition or exacerbation of severe or persistent disorder	Moderate to severe symptoms related to acute condition or exacerbation of severe or persistent disorder	Severe to disabling symptoms related to acute condition or exacerbation of severe or persistent disorder	Disabling symptoms related to acute condition or exacerbation of severe or persistent disorder
Risk, dangerousness	At-risk or limited with minimal need for confinement	Limited, transient dangerousness and minimal risk for confinement	Mild instability with limited dangerousness and low risk for confinement	Moderate instability and/or dangerousness with some risk for confinement	Marked instability and/or dangerousness with high risk for confinement	Significant danger to self or others
Commitment to treatment follow-through	Ability to form and maintain treatment contract	Ability to form and sustain treatment contract	Ability to sustain treatment contract with intermittent monitoring and support	Limited ability to form extended treatment contract; requires frequent monitoring and support	Inability to form more than initial treatment contract; requires close monitoring and support	Inability to form treatment contract; requires constant monitoring and supervision
Social support system	Ability to form and maintain relationships outside of treatment	Ability to form and maintain relationships outside of treatment	Ability to form and maintain relationships outside of treatment	Limited ability to form relationships or seek support	Impaired ability to access or use caretaker, family, or community support	Insufficient resources and/or inability to access or use caretaker, family, or community support

From http://www.aabh.org/public/detailpgs/continuum.html.

structure of a house, the model establishes six principles in providing in-home treatment: moral and spiritual qualities of the nurse; assessment; building relationships; medication issues; patient education and psychotherapeutic interventions; and case management (Carson, 1995). The moral and spiritual qualities of the nurse are the foundation of the house and enable the nurse to respect the patient regardless of the behaviors or problems the patient may exhibit. Forming the supporting walls of the house are assessment and relationship, essential structures in providing psychotherapeutic interventions to promote change and improvement, which is the goal of treatment. The key supporting structure of the house is medication issues. Medication issues are a major challenge for the nurse and patient because medications involve issues such as denial of illness, need for medication, management of medication side effects, and effects of coexisting physical health problems. The roof is configured with teaching and psychotherapeutic interventions and case management, the remaining components that influence the total house. According to the model, almost all therapy issues can be transformed to opportunities for patient education. Because mental illness can disrupt all areas of an individual's life, case management and coordination of care are critical factors in assisting a patient to gain other supportive care, such as vocational training or linkage with social services.

In-Home Detoxification. There is an increasing shift toward outpatient detoxification of patients with alcohol addiction. Although a reported 15 million Americans have alcohol problems and more than 100,000 deaths are attributed to alcoholism, fewer than 5% of people with alcohol problems receive formal treatment (Prater et al., 1999). Except for situations involving severe or complicated withdrawal, alcohol detoxification is now almost exclusively an outpatient process. It is not recommended for adolescents because of safety and compliance issues. The nurse will be required to visit the patient daily for medication monitoring during the patient's first week of sobriety. Daily visits are necessary until the patient has completed detoxification and is medically stable. Referrals may come from primary care physicians, court mandates, or employee assistance programs (a program provided by the employer for the provision of mental health services).

Case Management Services. **Case management** for patients with severe mental illness originated in the United States in the late 1970s (Test & Stein, 1980) as a method of coordinating agencies providing community care. Since then, it has become an integral part of mental health services. Case management can be viewed as a therapeutic tool in providing clinical services or as a brokerage system for coordinating the total package of care (Ward et al., 1999).

Case management can be delivered in several ways, and theoretic models include the pure brokerage model, the extended brokerage model, and the assertive community treatment (ACT) model (Chan et al., 2000). Although the models of case management may differ, the fundamental elements of case management are consistent. They include a comprehensive needs assessment, development of a plan of care to meet those needs, a method of ensuring the individual has access to care, and a method of monitoring the care provided.

The goal of case management is to act as a patient advocate by increasing access to care through coordinated efforts that reduce fragmentation of care and diminish health care costs (Sabin, 1998). Nurses employed in the role of case manager usually provide case management services by the ACT model or the Generalist Case Management model.

Assertive Community Treatment. The **assertive community treatment** model emphasizes a multidisciplinary team approach that provides a comprehensive range of treatment, rehabilitation, and supportive services to help patients meet the requirements of community living. One goal of ACT is to reduce recurrences of hospitalization. The rationale for ACT is that concentrating services for high-risk patients within a single multiservice team enhances continuity and coordination of care, improving both the quality of care and its cost-effectiveness (Lehman et al., 1999). Patients initially will receive direct assistance on a daily or frequent basis while reintegrating into the community. Emergency phone numbers, or crisis numbers, are shared with patients and their families in the event that a patient is in need of immediate assistance. The ACT program is staffed 24 hours a day for emergency referral (Soden & Wogan 1999).

Drs. Len Stein and Mary Ann Test introduced the concept of ACT into the literature in 1980. They developed the ACT program with core elements that promote the functional needs of the patient over time: (1) a core interdisciplinary team responsible for a small group of patients (staff-to-patient ratio of 1:10); (2) assertive outreach treatment to patients living in the community that assist the patient with ADLs (eg, buying groceries, doing laundry, making medical appointments); (3) a treatment plan of care that addresses the patient's individual needs; and (4) ongoing treatment and support.

Generalist Case Management Services. Generalist case management services, or broker case management, is a relatively common method in which services are provided to people with serious mental illness. The generalist case management services model does not necessarily provide needed services, but links the individual with community service providers (Bigelow & Young, 1991; Morse et al., 1997). Patients served in this model are typically outpatients with high levels of service use. The staff-to-patient ratio is about 1:30, with contact usually once every 1 to 2 weeks. Although little empiric evidence suggests that the generalist case management services method is effective, it remains popular because of its low operational costs and high patient-to-staff ratios (Morse et al., 1997). Figure 17-2 compares the ACT and generalist case management services models.

The Nurse as Case Manager. Psychiatric nurses serve in various pivotal functions across the continuum of care. The nurse as case manager is a role in which the nurse must have commanding knowledge and special training in individual and group psychotherapy, psychopharmacology, and psychosocial rehabilitation. Not only must the nurse have expertise in psychopathology and up-to-date treatment modalities, but he or she must also have expertise in treating the mentally ill family as a unit. Such modalities include the therapeutic use of self, networking and social systems, crisis intervention, pharmacology, physical assessment, psychosocial and functional assessment, and psychiatric rehabilitation. The repertoire of skills needed by the nurse for effective case management includes collaborative skills, teaching skills, management and leadership skills, group skills, and research skills. The nurse as case manager is probably the most diverse role within the psychiatric continuum.

Alternative Housing Arrangements. Patients with psychiatric disabilities who are homeless are a vulnerable population. One of the largest hurdles to overcome in the treatment of the chronically mentally ill patient is finding appropriate housing that will meet the patient's immediate social, financial, and safety needs. The course of chronic mental illness, as symptoms wax and wane, preys on the stamina of families and caregivers. The prevalence of mental illness among homeless people may range as high as 35% (Tsemberis & Eisenberg, 2000). Most individuals live in some form of supervised or supported community living situation, which ranges from highly supervised congregate settings to independent apartments. Those who lack the resources to find housing suffer higher rates of substance abuse, physical illness, incarceration, and victimization (Tsemberis & Eisenberg, 2000). The following discussion focuses on four models of alternative housing and the role of the nurse. These include personal care homes, board-and-care homes, supervised apartments, and therapeutic foster care.

Personal Care Homes. Personal care homes are programs operating within houses in the community with 6 to 10 people living in one house. A health care attendant provides 24-hour supervision to assist with medication monitoring or other minor activities, including transportation to appointments, meals, and self-care skills.

The clientele are generally heterogenous and include elderly, mildly mentally retarded, and mentally ill patients whose severity of illness is chronic and subacute. Most states require these homes to be licensed.

Board-and-Care Homes. **Board-and-care homes** provide 24-hour supervision and assistance with medication, meals, and some self-care skills. Individualized attention to self-care skills and other ADLs is generally not available. These homes are licensed to house 50 to 150 people in one location. Rooms are shared with two to four occupants per bedroom.

Therapeutic Foster Care. **Therapeutic foster care** is indicated for patients in need of a family-like environment and a high level of support. This level of care actually places patients in residences of families specially trained to handle individuals with mental illnesses. Therapeutic foster care is available for child, adolescent, and adult populations. The training usually consists of crisis management, medication education, and illness education. The family provides supervision, structure, and support for the individual living with them. The person who receives these services shares the responsibility of completing household chores and may also be required to attend an outpatient program during the day.

Supervised Apartments. In a supervised apartment setting, individuals live in their own apartments, usually alone or with one roommate, and are responsible for all household chores and self-care. A staff member or "supervisor" stops by each apartment routinely to evaluate how well the patients are doing, make sure they are taking their medications, and ensure household chores are being completed. The supervisor may also be required to mediate disagreements between roommates.

Role of the Nurse. The professional registered nurse is not typically employed in alternative housing settings. Nurses play a pivotal role, however, in the successful reintegration of patients from more restrictive inpatient settings into society. Nurses are employed in partial hospitalization programs, inpatient units, and as case managers. Therefore, nurses act as liaisons for the residential placement of patients. Nurses are employed directly as consultants or provide consultation to treatment teams during discharge planning in determining appropriate outpatient settings, evaluating medication follow-up needs, and making recommendations for necessary medical care for existing physical conditions. Feedback from the residential care providers and follow-up by the treatment team regarding the patient's response to treatment interventions are essential. Rehospitalization can be curtailed if the residential care operators identify and forward specific problems to the treatment teams. Patient interventions can be modified in an outpatient setting.

Program of Assertive Community Treatment   **Community Mental Health Center**

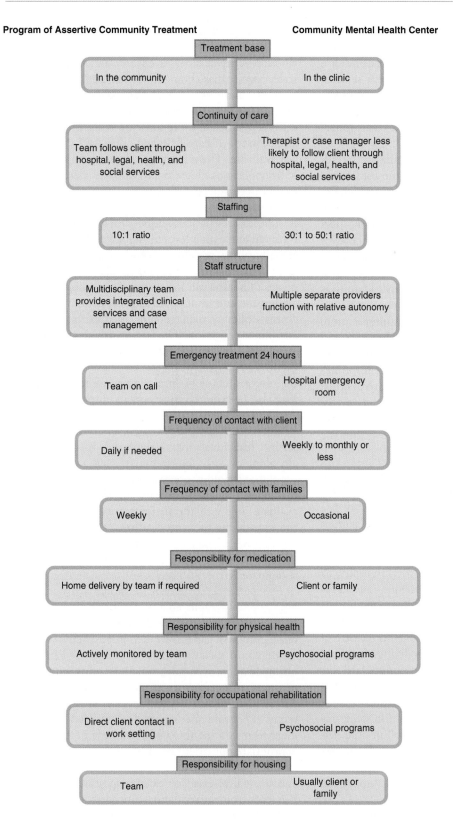

Treatment base

In the community   In the clinic

Continuity of care

Team follows client through hospital, legal, health, and social services   Therapist or case manager less likely to follow client through hospital, legal, health, and social services

Staffing

10:1 ratio   30:1 to 50:1 ratio

Staff structure

Multidisciplinary team provides integrated clinical services and case management   Multiple separate providers function with relative autonomy

Emergency treatment 24 hours

Team on call   Hospital emergency room

Frequency of contact with client

Daily if needed   Weekly to monthly or less

Frequency of contact with families

Weekly   Occasional

Responsibility for medication

Home delivery by team if required   Client or family

Responsibility for physical health

Actively monitored by team   Psychosocial programs

Responsibility for occupational rehabilitation

Direct client contact in work setting   Psychosocial programs

Responsibility for housing

Team   Usually client or family

FIGURE 17.2 Comparison between the Program of Assertive Community Treatment (PACT) model and traditional community mental health center services.

Clubhouse Model. The **clubhouse model** is a form of psychosocial rehabilitation that aims to reintegrate a person with mental illness into the community. Fountain House in New York City developed the clubhouse model in the 1940s. Its belief system is one of belonging to a membership—being wanted, needed, and expected (Farrell & Deeds, 1997). Additional fundamental beliefs include that (1) all members of society can be productive, (2) every human being aspires to achieve gainful employment, (3) humans require social contacts, and (4) programs are incomplete if they offer recreational, social, and vocational opportunities but neglect housing needs (Farrell & Deeds, 1997).

The Fountain House seeks to improve its members' quality of life by organizing daytime support, providing meaningful daytime activities, and offering opportunities for paid labor. Clubhouses are a unique form of treatment because they are entirely run by patients with psychiatric illnesses with minimal assistance from mental health professionals. Patients who join a clubhouse are voluntary "members," and they are expected to help in the operation of the house. Membership is not time limited. Generally, members do not live in the clubhouse; however, the clubhouse may have formed relationships with providers of low-cost housing. Open 365 days a year, services are available anytime an individual needs them. The Fountain House remains the model on which other clubhouses are built. Today, about 200 clubhouses are found across the United States (Torrey, 1995).

Clubhouses establish liaisons with various businesses and services within the community to provide services for its members. Clinical services, such as psychiatric visits, routine medical care, and low-rent, Section 8 (government-subsidized housing for disabled individuals who meet specific criteria) housing arrangements are made with private providers. Most social and vocational services, however, are provided through members' activities associated with the clubhouse.

Members of the clubhouse are expected to assist with household chores, follow instructions of others, volunteer for tasks, and above all, be punctual (Farrell & Deeds, 1997). Most new members begin vocational training by participating in work units at the clubhouse, such as janitorial services, meal preparation, clerical services, public relations, and maintenance services. As members improve, they may move on to transitional employment, which is part-time paid work outside the clubhouse setting. When vocational skills have been acquired, members move into competitive employment.

The role of the staff person in this unique setting is different than in other inpatient and outpatient settings. Because a clubhouse is operated by its members, staff roles are limited. The focus of the staff member is to accentuate the skills and performance of the members.

The employee works with rather than for the member. The clubhouse model requires the employee nurse to function as a member of the clubhouse and be active in all components of the program. Although the nurse has expertise in pathology of mental illness, the focus is strictly on the individual's recovery. Case management in the clubhouse setting requires staff to participate in work units or transitional employment settings with members. More commonly, a nurse plays a pivotal role in urging a patient's participation in a clubhouse program and may actually refer patients to the program.

Relapse Prevention After-Care Programs. Relapse of mental illness symptoms and substance abuse is the major reason for rehospitalization in this country. The term **relapse** refers to the recurrence or marked increase in severity of the symptoms of a disease, especially following a period of apparent improvement or stability. Many issues can affect the status of a person's well-being. First and foremost, patients must feel that their lives are meaningful and worthwhile. Homelessness and unemployment create tremendous threats to a person's identity and feelings of wellness. Donegan and Palmer-Erbs (1998) stated that 85% to 95% of the severe and persistent mentally ill population are unemployed. This frightening statistic affects the stability of people with mental illness.

Much effort has been directed at the creation of relapse prevention programs for the major mental illnesses and addiction disorders. Relapse prevention programs generally seek to (1) provide an understanding of the illness for patients and families, (2) enable patients and families to come to terms with the chronic nature of the illness, (3) teach patients and families to recognize early warning signs of relapse, (4) educate patients and families about prescribed medication and the importance of compliance, and (5) provide information about other disease management strategies (ie, stress management, exercise) in the prevention of relapse (Goldstein, 1994).

The Prelapse (Prevent Relapse) program is for relapse prevention for adults with schizophrenia. It has shown a high degree of success in preventing rehospitalization. Developed in Germany by Dr. Werner Kissling, the program is a highly structured 8-week after-care program for patients with schizophrenia and their families. Nurses conduct the programs, which are highly didactic in format, with audiovisual and written materials, and pretests and posttests (Kissling, 1994). Prelapse focuses on patient education about the illness, early warning signs of relapse, and medication information such as side effects, dosing, and need for medication adherence. Patients are referred to the program on readmission for a psychotic episode. They may begin the program while they are still inpatients or immediately after discharge.

Supported employment programs are new, highly individualized, and competitive. They provide on-site support and job-coaching services on a one-to-one basis. They occur in real work settings and are used for patients with severe mental illnesses. The primary focus is to maintain attachment between the mentally ill person and the workforce (Donegan & Palmer-Erbs, 1998). Transitional employment programs offer the same support as supported employment programs, but the employment is temporary. This type of work has a time frame and agreed on by the employer and the participant. The person works at the temporary position until he or she can find permanent, competitive employment (Donegan & Palmer-Erbs, 1998).

The nurse becomes involved in relapse prevention programs in several different ways. He or she can act as a referral source for the programs, trainer or leader of the programs, or an after-care source for patients when the program is completed. Additionally, mental health nurses can help the patient and family by promoting optimism, sticking to goals and aspirations, and focusing on the person's strengths. All mental health nurses must know the latest trends in effective treatment and available community resources. They must appreciate the stigmas that may hinder psychiatric rehabilitation. Above all, psychiatric nurses demonstrate patient advocacy by networking with community agencies and vocational specialists to ensure that the patient has available resources in the community to lessen the chances of symptom relapse.

MANAGED CARE

Managed care continues to tailor the delivery of health care in all settings. The concept of managed care emerged in efforts to coordinate patient care efficiently and cost-effectively. Federal expenditures are dramatically rising as a large proportion of the aging population needs either nursing home care or home health visits (Bartels et al., 1999). Managed care companies are large companies that contract with private employers, health care plans, and government agencies to manage mental health care on an "at-risk" basis (Mechanic, 1999). By 1997, a handful of behavioral health care companies had monopolized the behavioral health care market, serving 120 million people alone (Mechanic, 1999).

The goals of **managed care organizations** are to increase access to care and to provide the most appropriate level of services in the least restrictive setting. They focus efforts on providing more outpatient and alternative treatment programs and try to avoid costly inpatient hospitalizations. When properly conducted and administered, managed care allows patients better access to quality services, while using health care dollars wisely.

Today, managed behavioral health care has succeeded in standardizing admissions criteria, reducing length of patient stay, and directing patients to the proper level of care—inpatient and outpatient—all while attempting to control the costs. Across the continuum of care nurses will encounter managed care organizations in their work with patients, and they must be familiar with the policies, procedures, and clinical criteria established by managed care organizations.

Managed care organizations typically provide two or three services across the continuum of care, including the following:

Utilization management. This Review process establishes clinical criteria that help health care providers render appropriate, accessible, and affordable treatment across the continuum of care.
Care management. This fully integrated health care model offers clinical standards and guidelines and a management network of credentialed and specialty behavioral health providers who are members of the network.
Employee assistance program. This is designed to help employees of sponsoring companies with personal and workplace problems at no cost, including such services as confidential assessment, counseling, and referral problems (Green Spring Health Services, 1995).

Unfortunately, as managed care continues to regulate the delivery of mental health care, services become more limited (Mallik et al., 1998). For example, as the population ages, more people will require nursing home placement while the trend is to offer more outpatient or community resources. Additionally, many older adults with mental illness currently receive no other community services than medication monitoring (Bartels et al., 1999). Increasing home health care services for people with mental illness is an important alternative to institutionalization. Medicare, however, currently covers only acute symptom management and not long-term illness management (Bartels et al., 1999).

Public and Private Collaboration

Managed Medicaid behavioral health care is an emerging reform within the managed care arena. With Medicaid expenditures doubling since 1988, more than 24 states are actively involved in Medicaid reforms (Sternbach & Waters, 1995). These reform efforts have been characterized by many public–private sector collaborations. The impetus behind this movement is to preserve the strength of public mental health systems while bringing the technologies and strengths of the private sector to public mental health reform efforts. The need for public–private collaboration prompted the National

Association of State Mental Health Program Directors (NASMHPD), an organization representing the 55 state and territorial public mental health systems, and the American Managed Behavioral Healthcare Association (AMBHA), an organization representing 19 private managed behavioral health care firms, to set forth guidelines for this type of joint venture (NASMHPD-AMBHA, 1994). Nurses can expect to see more strategic alliances and joint ventures between the public and private sectors.

Role of the Nurse

Because of decreases in length of inpatient stays, the psychiatric–mental health nurse must maximize the short time he or she has to educate the mental health patient about his or her illness, available community resources, and medications to minimize the potential for relapse. The nurse should focus on teaching social skills and self-reliance and creating empowering environments that, in turn, build self-confidence (Clement, 1997).

The interface of psychiatric–mental health nurses with managed care organizations is primarily in the form of providing information regarding the progress of individual patients to the managed care organization utilization managers. In many instances, managed care organizations hire psychiatric nurses for crisis intervention and as case managers. Nurses may also advocate for funding to place patients in other portions of the continuum and be required to provide substantiating documentation and information regarding the medical necessity of the transfer.

PSYCHIATRIC REHABILITATION

Psychiatric rehabilitation programs, also termed psychosocial rehabilitation, are focused on the **reintegration** of people with psychiatric disabilities into the community through work, educational, and social avenues while addressing their medical and residential needs (Littrell, 1995). These programs are designed to increase functioning of patients with psychiatric disabilities so that they are successful and satisfied in their environments of choice with the least amount of ongoing professional intervention necessary (Palmer-Erbs & Anthony, 1995). Psychiatric rehabilitation programming provides a highly structured environment, similar to a partial hospitalization program, but is conducted in a variety of settings: professional office buildings, outpatient units of hospitals, free-standing buildings, and large, renovated houses. Its goal is to empower the patients to achieve the highest level of functioning possible (Adams & Jenkins-Partee, 1998). Programming emphasizes acquiring skills such as communication skills or vocational skills that can help patients function in the community.

Table 17-3 presents an example of a schedule from a rehabilitation program for adults with schizophrenia.

Role of the Nurse

The psychiatric–mental health nurse's role in the delivery of psychosocial rehabilitation continues to adapt to the changing needs of persons with mental illness. As behavioral health care delivery switches from the inpatient to more of an outpatient setting, the traditional inpatient nurse role will move into diverse outpatient, rehabilitative, and community-based settings (Furlong-Norman et al., 1997). Most rehabilitation programs have a full-time nurse who functions as part of the multidisciplinary team.

For psychiatric–mental health nurses, a psychiatric rehabilitation approach is concerned with matching the details of an accurate diagnosis and engaging in an appropriate trial of medication to target symptoms. Furthermore, nurses are concerned with the holistic evaluation of the person and must assess and educate the patient on compliance issues, necessary laboratory work, and environmental and lifestyle issues. This evaluation assesses the five dimensions of a person—physical, emotional, intellectual, social, spiritual—with the focus toward developing a psychiatric rehabilitation emphasis. Issues of psychotropic medication also fall to the nurse—evaluation of response, monitoring of side effects, and connection with pharmacy services.

Assessment and Selection of Level of Care

Psychiatric–mental health nurses will encounter mentally ill individuals at varying phases in recovery and will practice in many different treatment settings across the continuum of care. Regardless of the situation or setting, the nurse must perform an assessment at the point of first contact with an individual. The individual's needs are matched with the most appropriate setting, service, or program that will meet his or her needs.

The selection of the level of care required begins with an initial assessment of the patient. The nurse must assess the individual's biologic, psychological, and social functioning to determine the need for care, the type of care to be provided, and the need for further assessment. The nurse must discuss with the patient suicidal and homicidal thoughts. Nurses should consider financial issues because funding considerations may play a part in placement options. Other factors affecting the selection of care include the type of treatment the individual is seeking, the individual's current physical condition, the individual's ability to agree to or consent to treatment, and the organization's ability to provide directly or to deflect the care of the person to another service provider.

TABLE 17.3 Schedule From a Rehabilitation Program for Adults With Schizophrenia

Time	Monday	Tuesday	Wednesday	Thursday	Friday	Saturday	Sunday
0900–0920	Community meeting	Community meeting	Community meeting	Community meeting	Community meeting		
0930–1010	Group therapy	Group therapy	Group therapy	Group therapy	Group therapy		
1010–1030	Break	Break	Break	Break	Break		
1030–1130	Relapse prevention	Chemical dependency	Psycho-educational training	Psycho-educational training	Psycho-educational training		
1130–1215	Lunch	Lunch	Lunch	Lunch	Lunch	1200–1700 Therapeutic recreational outing to a community event	1400–1900 Therapeutic recreational outing to a community event
1215–1315	Therapeutic recreation	Therapeutic recreation	Therapeutic recreation	Therapeutic recreation	Therapeutic recreation		
1315–1330	Break	Break	Break	Break	Break		
1330–1430	Expressive arts therapy	Psychosocial training	Prevocational training	Psychosocial training	Expressive arts therapy		
1430–1445	Wrap up	Wrap up	Wrap up	Wrap up	Wrap up		
1500–1700	Staff time	Multidisciplinary treatment team meeting	Staff time	Staff time	Staff time		

Based on the results of the assessment performed at first contact, the nurse may admit the patient into services provided at that agency or initiate a referral or transfer to provide the intensity and scope of treatment required by the individual at that point in time (Fig. 17-3). **Referral** is sending an individual from one clinician to another or from one service setting to another for either care or consultation. **Transfer** is formally shifting responsibility for the care of an individual from one clinician to another or from one care unit to another. The processes of referral and transfer to other levels of care are integral for effective use of services along the continuum. These processes are based on the individual's assessed needs and the organization's capability to provide the care. Figure 17-3 graphically depicts the process of assessment, treatment, transfer, and referral when considering appropriate levels of care.

Discharge Planning

Discharge planning begins upon admission of the individual at any level of health care. Most facilities have a written procedure for the discharge planning process. This procedure often provides for a transfer of clinical care information when a person is referred, transferred, or discharged to another facility or level of care. All discharge planning activities should be recorded in the clinical record, including the patient's response to proposed after-care treatment, follow-up for psychiatric and physical health problems, and discharge instructions. Medication education, food–drug interactions, drug–drug interactions, and special diet instructions (if applicable) are extremely important in providing patient safety.

Discharge planning is an integral part of psychiatric nursing care and should be considered a part of the psychiatric rehabilitation process. In addressing an individual's biopsychosocial needs, one can coordinate after-care and discharge interventions that produce optimal outcomes. The overall goal of discharge planning is to provide the patient with all the resources he or she needs to function as independently as possible in the least restrictive environment and to avoid rehospitalization.

Recognizing that individuals may have psychiatric rehabilitation needs in more than one domain, Hochberger (1995) developed a discharge checklist. She stipulated that six domains are pertinent to the successful discharge of psychiatric patients: (1) medications, (2) ADLs, (3) mental health after-care, (4) residence, (5) follow-up in physical health care, and (6) special education, financial, or other needs. Hochberger's discharge checklist (Text Box 17-1) is not meant to substitute for a nursing assessment or any other professional assessment. Instead, its use is intended as a tool to facilitate interdisciplinary planning for after-care and discharge.

The nurse can optimize discharge plan compliance by involving the patient at various levels. This is espe-

Continuum flowchart

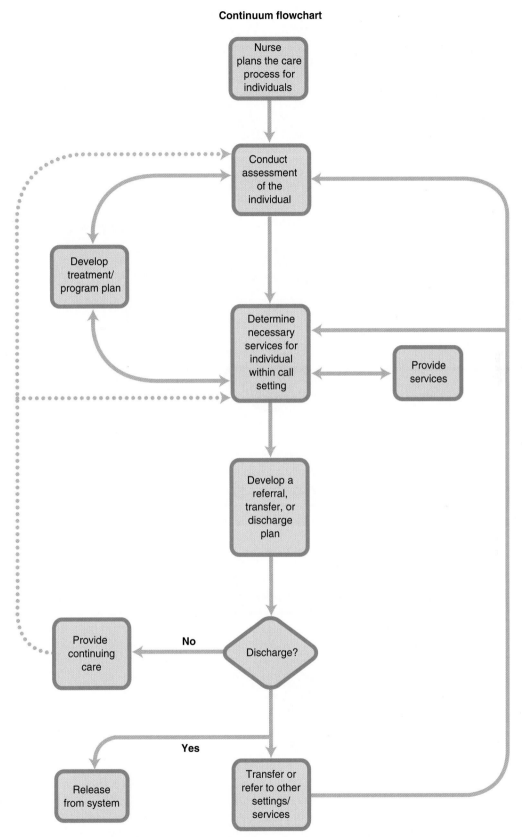

Figure 17.3 Continuum flowchart and selection of care flowchart.

Selection of care flowchart

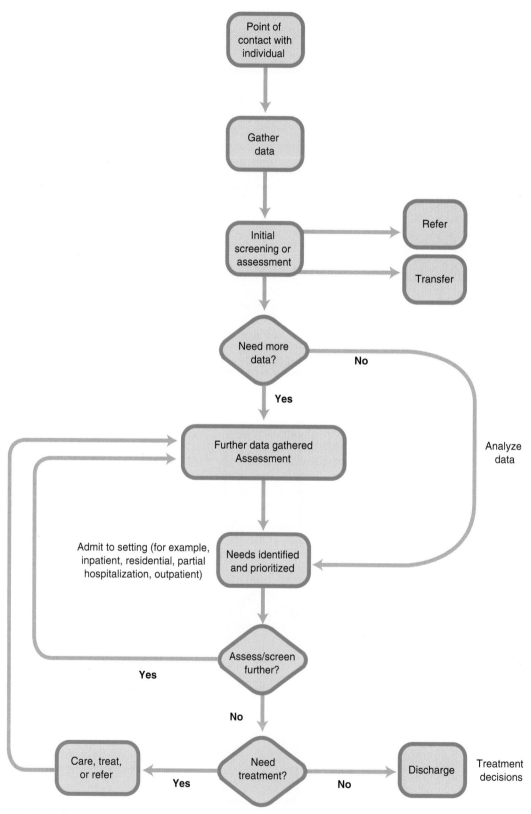

FIGURE 17.3 *(continued)*

TEXT BOX 17.1

Mental Health Discharge Checklist

Name:

Number:

Medication

   Medication supply or prescription

   Number of days medication supplied for

   Medication education—drug dosage, time, how to take

   Special instructions

Activities of daily living

   Hygiene instructions

   Activities requiring assistance

   Safety instructions

   Work, work training

   Activity, rest

   Special instructions

Mental health after-care

   Psychiatrist or therapist

   Community mental health center or agency

   Nurse specialist or visiting nurse

   Psychiatric social worker

   Community support group

   Day care program referral

Residence

   Boarding home

   Group home

   Hotel

   Nursing home

   Family residence

   Residential health care facility

   Own home or lives alone

   Other

Follow-up medical care

   Appointment with medical doctor

   Visiting nurse or nurse practitioner

   Medical clinic appointment

   Diet or fluid instructions

   Dental care

Special needs

   Sexually transmitted diseases and AIDS prevention
     education

   Symptom recognition education

   Transportation needs

   Financial assistance

Additional comments

From Hochberger, J. M. (1995). A discharge checklist for psychiatric patients. *Journal of Psychosocial Nursing, 33*(12), 36.

cially important in the psychiatric setting. Because patients with mental illnesses may have limited cognitive abilities and residual motivational and anxiety problems, nurses should explain all after-care plans and instructions to the patient in detail. It is helpful to make all after-care appointments before the patient leaves the facility. The nurse should then give the patient written instructions about where and when to go for the appointment and a contact person's name and telephone number at the after-care placement. Finally, the nurse should review emergency telephone numbers and contacts and medication instructions with the patient.

Summary of Key Points

➤ The continuum of care is a comprehensive system of services and programs designed to match the needs of the individual with the appropriate treatment in settings that vary according to levels of service, structure, and intensity of care.

➤ The psychiatric–mental health nurse's specific responsibilities vary according to the setting. In most settings, nurses function as members of a multidisciplinary team and assume responsibility for assessment and selection of level of care, education, evaluation of response to treatment, referral or transfer to a more appropriate level of care, and discharge planning. Discharge planning provides patients with all the resources they need to function effectively in the community and avoid rehospitalization.

➤ Managed care is influencing the continuum of care by standardizing admissions criteria and clinical guidelines for practitioners, encouraging alternative treatment programs that avoid costly inpatient hospitalizations, and providing consumers with an integrated network of credentialed specialty behavioral health providers to help meet their needs within the community.

Critical Thinking Challenges

1. Discuss the difference between long-term and short-term care as components of inpatient treatment.
2. Differentiate the role of the nurse in each of the following continuum settings:
   a. Short-term care-stabilization
   b. In-home mental health
   c. Psychosocial rehabilitation program
   d. Assertive community treatment
3. Compare nursing management with the coordination of care framework in the continuum of care.
4. How and when did the concept of the least restrictive environment emerge in mental health? Describe how it affects the current continuum of care.

5. Discuss how managed care has affected the types and availability of services provided in the continuum of care.

6. Discuss the various patient safety-related factors that determine which level of care is most appropriate for an individual within the continuum of care.

REFERENCES

Adams, S., & Jenkins-Partee, D. (1998). Integrating psychosocial rehabilitation in a community-based faculty nursing practice. *Journal of Psychosocial Nursing, 36*(4), 24–29.

Aday, L., Begley, C., Lairson, D., et al. (1999). A framework for assessing the effectiveness, efficiency, and equity of behavioral healthcare. *American Journal of Managed Care, 5*(Special Issue), 25–44.

Akhavain, P., Amaral, D., Murphy, M., & Uehlinger, K. (1999). Collaborative practice: Perspective of the psychiatric interdisciplinary treatment team. *Holistic Nurse Practice, 13*(2), 1–11.

American Nurses Association, American Psychiatric Nurses Association. (2000). International Society for Psychiatric-Mental Health Nursing Practice. Washington, D.C.: American Nurses Publishing.

Bartels, S., Levine, K., & Shea, D. (1999). Community-based long-term care for older persons with severe and persistent mental illness in an era of managed care. *Psychiatric Services, 50*(9), 1189–1197.

Bennie, C. (1998). A comparison of home detoxification and minimal intervention strategies for problem drinkers. *Alcohol & Alcoholism, 33*(2), 157–163.

Bigelow, D., & Young, D. (1991). Effectiveness of a case management program. *Community Mental Health Journal, 27*, 115–123.

Buccheri, R., & Underwood, P. (1993). Nursing management: Inpatient nursing care of persons with schizophrenia. *New Directions for Mental Health Services, 58*, 23–31.

Callahan, D. (1999). Balancing efficiency and need in allocating resources to the care of persons with serious mental illness. *Psychiatric Services, 50*(5), 664–666.

Carson, V. B. (1995). Bay Area health care model of psychiatric home care. *Home Healthcare Nurse, 13*(4), 26–32.

Chan, S., Mackenzie, A., Tin-Fu, N. G. D., & Ka-yi Leung, J. (2000). An evaluation of the implementation of case management in the community of psychiatric nursing service. *Journal of Advanced Nursing, 31*(1), 144–156.

Clement, J. (1997). Managed care and recovery: Opportunities and challenges for psychiatric nursing. *Archives of Psychiatric Nursing, 11*(5), 231–237.

Donegan, K., & Palmer-Erbs, V. (1998). Promoting the importance of work for persons with psychiatric disabilities: The role of the psychiatric nurse. *Journal of Psychosocial Nursing, 36*(4), 13–22.

Farrell, S., & Deeds, E. (1997). The clubhouse model as exemplar. *Journal of Psychosocial Nursing, 35*(1), 27–34.

Foster, M. (1998). Does continuum of care improve the timing of follow-up services? *Journal of the American Academy of Child and Adolescent Psychiatry, 37*(8), 805–814.

Friedrich, R., Hollingsworth, B., Hradek, E., et al. (1999). Family and client perspectives on alternative residential settings for persons with severe mental illness. *Psychiatric Services, 50*(4), 509–514.

Furlong-Norman, K., Palmer-Erbs, V., & Jonikas, J. (1997). Exploring the field: Strengthening psychiatric rehabilitation nursing practice with new information and ideas. *Psychiatric Rehabilitation Nursing, 35*(1), 35–37.

Geller, J. (2000). The last half-century of psychiatric services as reflected ion psychiatric services. *Psychiatric Services, 51*(1), 41–67.

Goldstein, M. J. (1994). Psychoeducational and family therapy in relapse prevention. *Acta Psychiatrica Scandinavica, 89*, 54–57.

Green, K., & Lydon, S. (1998). The continuum of patient care. *American Journal of Nursing, 98*(10), 16BBB–16DDD.

Green Spring Health Services, Inc. (1995). *Directory of services and providers*. Columbia, MD: Author.

Hochberger, J. (1995). A discharge checklist for psychiatric patients. *Journal of Psychosocial Nursing and Mental Health Services, 33*(12), 35–38.

Hughes, W. (1999). Managed care, meet community support: Ten reasons to include direct support services in every behavioral health plan. *Health and Social Work, 24*(2), 103–111.

Joint Commission on the Accreditation of Healthcare Organizations. (1999). *Accreditation manual for mental health, chemical dependency, and mental retardation/ developmental disabilities services, Vol. 1: Standards.* Oakbrook Terrace, IL: Author.

Jones, A., & Norman, I. (1998). Managed mental health care: Problems and possibilities. *Journal of Psychiatric Mental Health Nursing, 5*, 21–31.

Kanas, N. (1991). Group therapy with schizophrenic patients: A short-term homogenous approach. *International Journal of Group Psychotherapy, 41*(1), 33–48.

Kelly, J., & Stephens, I. (1999). Community case management for mentally illness. *Australian Nursing Journal, 6*(10), 24–26.

Kiser, L., King, R., & Lefkovitz, P. (1999a). A comparison of practice patterns and a model continuum of ambulatory behavioral health services. *Psychiatric Services, 50*(5), 605–606.

Kiser, L., Lefkovitz, P., Kennedy, L., et al. (1999b). *The continuum of behavioral healthcare services: A position paper from the Association for Ambulatory Behavioral Healthcare.* Alexandria, VA: American Association for Ambulatory Behavioral Healthcare.

Kissling, W. (1994). Compliance, quality assurance and standards for relapse prevention in schizophrenia. *Acta Psychiatrica Scandinavica, 89*, 16–24.

Lehman, A., Dixon, L., Hoch, J., et al. (1999). Cost-effectiveness of assertive community treatment for homeless persons with severe mental illness. *British Journal of Psychiatry, 174*, 346–352.

Leslie, D., & Rosenheck, R. (2000). Comparing quality of mental health care for public-sector and privately insured populations. *Psychiatric Services, 51*(5), 650–655.

Littrell, K. H. (1995). Maximizing schizophrenia treatment outcomes: A model for reintegration. *Psychiatric Rehabilitation Journal, 19*(7), 75–77.

Littrell, K. H. (1996, August). Emerging roles for case management in public mental health. In *Shared horizons: The Ohio public mental health forum.* Symposium conducted in Open Minds educational seminar, Columbus, OH.

Mallik, K., Reeves, R., & Dellario, D. (1998). Barriers to community integration for people with severe and persistent psychiatric disabilities. *Psychiatric Rehabilitation Journal, 22*(2), 175–180.

Mechanic, D. (1999). The state of behavioral health in managed care. *American Journal of Managed Care, 5,* sp17–sp20.

Morse, G., Calsyn, R., Klinkenberg, W., et al. (1997). An experimental comparison of three types of case management for homeless mentally ill persons. *Psychiatric Services, 48*(4), 497–503.

National Association of State Mental Health Program Directors and American Managed Behavioral Healthcare Association. (1994). *Draft white paper: Public mental health systems, Medicaid re-structuring and managed behavioral healthcare.* Arlington, VA: Author.

Palmer-Erbs, V. K., & Anthony, W. A. (1995). Incorporating psychiatric rehabilitation principles into psychiatric–mental health nursing practice: An opportunity to develop a full partnership among nurses, consumers, and families. *Journal of Psychosocial Nursing and Mental Health Services, 33*(3), 36–44.

Pickens, J. (1998). Formal and informal care of persons with psychiatric disorders: Historical perspectives and current trends. *Journal of Psychosocial Nursing, 36*(1), 37–43.

Prater, C., Miller, K., & Zylstra, R. (1999). Outpatient detoxification of the addicted or alcoholic patient. *American Family Physician, 60*(4), 1175–1182.

Sabin, J. (1998). Public-sector managed behavioral health care. I. Developing an effective case management program. *Psychiatric Services, 49*(1), 31–33.

Soden, J., & Wogan, E. (1999). The benefits of assertive community treatment. *Nursing Times, 95*(16), 50–52.

Sternbach, K. O., & Waters, R. (1995, July/August). Anatomy of Medicaid behavioral managed care program: Green Spring's AdvoCare of Tennessee. *Behavioral Health Management Magazine, 15*(4), 14–18.

Sturm, R., & Bao, Y. (2000). Psychiatric care expenditures and length of stay: Trends in industrialized countries. *Psychiatric Services, 51*(3), 7.

Test, M. A., & Stein, L. I. (1980). Alternative to mental hospital treatment: I. Conceptual model, treatment program, and clinical evaluation. *Archives of General Psychiatry, 37,* 392–397.

Torrey, E. F. (1995). *Surviving schizophrenia: A manual for families, consumers, and providers* (3rd ed.). New York: Harper Perennial.

Tsemberis, S., & Eisenberg, R. (2000). Pathways to housing: Supported housing for street-dwelling homeless individuals with psychiatric disabilities. *Psychiatric Services, 51*(4), 487–493.

Ward, M., Armstrong, C., Lelliott, P., & Davies, M. (1999). Training, skills and caseloads of community mental health support workers involved in case management: Evaluation from the initial UK demonstration sites. *Journal of Psychiatric and Mental Health Nursing, 6,* 187–197.

Wasylenki, D., Goering, P., Cochrane, J., Durbin, J., Rogus, J., & Prendergast, P. (2000). Tertiary mental health services. I. Key concepts. *Canadian Journal of Psychiatry, 45*(2), 179–184.

Weissberg, M. (1991). Chained in the emergency department: The new asylum for the poor. *Hospital and Community Psychiatry, 42*(3), 317–319.

Wilbur, S., & Arns, P. (1998). Psychosocial rehabilitation nurses: Taking our place on the multidisciplinary team. *Journal of Psychosocial Nursing, 36*(4), 33–41.

Yurkovich, E., & Smyer, T. (1998). Strategies for maintaining optimal wellness in the chronic mentally ill. *Perspectives in Psychiatric Care, 34*(3), 17–24.

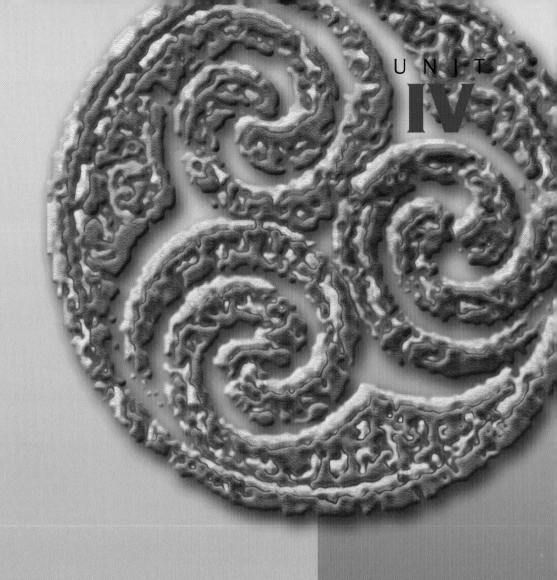

Care of Persons With Psychiatric Disorders

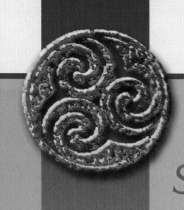

Schizophrenia

Andrea C. Bostrom and Mary Ann Boyd

**LEARNING
OBJECTIVES**

After studying this chapter, you will be able to:

➤ Distinguish key symptoms of schizophrenia.

➤ Analyze the prevailing biologic, psychological, and social theories that are the basis for understanding schizophrenia.

➤ Analyze human response to schizophrenia with emphasis on hallucinations, delusions, and social isolation.

➤ Formulate nursing diagnoses based on a biopsychosocial assessment of people with schizophrenia.

➤ Formulate nursing interventions that address specific diagnoses based on a continuum of care.

➤ Analyze special concerns within the nurse–patient relationship common to treating those with schizophrenia.

➤ Identify expected outcomes and their evaluation.

KEY TERMS

affective flattening
   or blunting
affective lability
aggression
agitation
agranulocytosis
akathisia
alogia
ambivalence
anhedonia
apathy
autistic thinking
avolition
catatonic excitement
circumstantiality
clang association
concrete thinking
confused speech and
   thinking
delusions
echolalia
echopraxia
expressed emotion
extrapyramidal side
   effects
flight of ideas

hallucinations
hypervigilance
hypofrontality
illusions
loose associations
metonymic speech
neologisms
neuroleptic malignant
   syndrome
oculogyric crises
paranoia
paranoid schizophrenia
polyuria
pressured speech
prodromal
referential thinking
regressed behavior
retrocollis
stereotypy
stilted language
tangentiality
tardive dyskinesia
torticollis
verbigeration
waxy flexibility
word salad

KEY CONCEPTS

disordered water balance
disorganized symptoms
negative symptoms
neurocognitive impairment
positive symptoms

*S*chizophrenia has fascinated and confounded healers, scientists, and philosophers for centuries. Its symptoms have been attributed to possession by demons, considered punishment by gods for evils done, or accepted as evidence of the inhumanity of its sufferers. These explanations resulted in enduring stigma for those who were diagnosed with the disorder. Even today, much of the stigma persists, although it has less to do with demonic possession than with society's unwillingness to shoulder the tremendous costs associated with housing, treating, and rehabilitating patients with schizophrenia.

Schizophrenia is one of the most severe mental illnesses. It occurs in about 1.3% of the population in the United States, or more than 3 million people (U.S. Department of Health and Human Services [USDHHS], 1999). Its economic costs are enormous. Direct costs, such as treatment expenses, were estimated at 2.5% of the total health care budget in 1990 (American Psychiatric Association [APA], 1997), the last year for which these data were available (USDHHS, 1999). In 1996, this would account for $23.6 billion of health care dollars spent. The indirect costs, such as lost wages, premature death, and incarceration, were estimated to be $46 billion in the first half of the 1990s (APA, 1997). Further, unemployment among people with schizophrenia may be as high as 80%, whereas permanent disability is 10% (APA, 1997). The costs of schizophrenia in terms of individual and family suffering are probably inestimable.

CLINICAL COURSE

In the late 1800s, Emil Kraeplin was the first to describe the course of the disorder he called "dementia praecox." In the early 1900s, Eugen Bleuler renamed the disorder "schizophrenia," meaning *split minds*, and began to determine that there was not just one type of schizophrenia, but rather a group of schizophrenias. More recently, Kurt Schneider began to differentiate behaviors associated with schizophrenia as "first rank" symptoms (psychotic delusions, hallucinations) and "second rank" symptoms (all other experiences and behaviors associated with the disorder). These pioneering physicians had a great influence on the present diagnostic conceptualizations of schizophrenia that emphasize the heterogeneity of the disorder in terms of symptoms, course of illness, and existence of positive and negative symptoms (Andreasen & Carpenter, 1993; Boyle, 1990).

Diagnostic Criteria

The current definition outlined in the APA's *Diagnostic and Statistical Manual of Mental Disorders*, 4th edition, Text revision (*DSM-IV-TR*) (APA, 2000) states that schizophrenia is a mixture of both positive and negative symptoms that present for a significant portion of a 1-month period, but with continuous signs of disturbance persisting for at least 6 months. Positive symptoms reflect an excess or distortion of normal functions, including delusions and hallucinations. Negative symptoms reflect a lessening or loss of normal functions, such as restriction or flattening in the range and intensity of emotion (**affective flattening or blunting**); reduced fluency and productivity of thought and speech (**alogia**); withdrawal and inability to initiate and persist in goal-directed activity (**avolition**); and inability to experience pleasure (**anhedonia**). Positive symptoms can be thought of as those symptoms that exist but should not, and negative symptoms as ones that should be there but are not.

Schizophrenia is a complex mixture of both positive and negative symptoms. Positive or excessive characteristics include delusions and hallucinations. Negative characteristics are ones that are lacking, such as lack of speech (alogia), lack of goal-directed behavior (avolition), lack of feelings (affective flattening or blunting), and lack of happiness or pleasure (anhedonia).

KEY CONCEPT Positive Symptoms. **Positive symptoms** reflect an excess or distortion of normal functions, including delusions and hallucinations.

KEY CONCEPT Negative Symptoms. **Negative symptoms** reflect a lessening or loss of normal functions, such as restriction or flattening in the range and intensity of emotion (affective flattening or blunting); reduced fluency and productivity of thought and speech (alogia); withdrawal and inability to initiate and persist in goal-directed activity (avolition); and inability to experience pleasure (anhedonia).

The criteria for the diagnosis of schizophrenia outlined in the *DSM-IV-TR* (APA, 2000) include necessary symptomatology, duration of symptoms, evaluation of functional impairment, and elimination of alternate hypotheses that might account for the symptoms. Several schizophrenia subtypes are currently recognized: paranoid, disorganized, catatonic, undifferentiated, and residual. There is a growing belief that this subtyping is not useful for predicting the course and response to treatment. The APA is exploring subtyping that is more consistent with the symptom clusters described earlier: positive (psychotic), disorganized, and negative (APA, 2000). The diagnostic criteria and current subtypes are listed in Table 18-1 and Text Box 18-1, respectively.

Positive Symptoms of Schizophrenia

Delusions are erroneous fixed beliefs that usually involve a misinterpretation of experience. For example, the patient believes someone is reading his or her thoughts, monitoring him or her, or plotting against him or her. There are many types of delusions, including the following:

TABLE 18.1 Key Diagnostic Characteristics of Schizophrenia	
Diagnostic Criteria and Target Symptoms	**Associated Findings**
Diagnostic Criteria • Two or more of the following characteristic symptoms present for a significant portion of time during a 1-month period: delusions; hallucinations; disorganized speech; grossly disorganized or catatonic behavior; negative symptoms • One or more major areas of social or occupational functioning (such as work, interpersonal relations, self-care) markedly below previously achieved level • Continuous signs persisting for at least 6 months • Absence or insignificant duration of major depressive, manic, or mixed episodes occurring concurrently with active symptoms • Not a direct physiologic effect of a substance or medical condition • Prominent delusions or hallucinations present when a prior history of autistic disorder or another pervasive developmental disorder exists *Target Symptoms and Associated Findings* • Inappropriate affect • Loss of interest or pleasure • Dysmorphic mood (anger, anxiety, or depression) • Disturbed sleep patterns • Lack of interest in eating or refusal of food • Difficulty concentrating • Some cognitive dysfunction, such as confusion, disorientation, memory impairment • Lack of insight • Depersonalization, derealization, and somatic concerns • Motor abnormalities	*Associated Physical Examination Findings* • Physically awkward • Poor coordination or mirroring • Motor abnormalities • Cigarette-related pathologies, such as emphysema and other pulmonary and cardiac problems *Associated Laboratory Findings* • Enlarged ventricular system and prominent sulci in the brain cortex • Decreased temporal and hippocampal size • Increased size of basal ganglia • Decreased cerebral size • Slowed reaction times • Abnormalities in eye tracking

Grandiose: the belief that one has exceptional powers, wealth, skill, influence, or destiny

Nihilistic: the belief that one is dead or a calamity is impending

Persecutory: the belief that one is being watched, ridiculed, harmed, or plotted against

Somatic: beliefs about abnormalities in bodily functions or structures

Hallucinations are perceptual experiences that occur in the absence of actual external sensory stimuli. They can involve any of the five senses, but they are usually auditory or visual in nature. Auditory hallucinations are more common than visual. For example, the patient hears voices carrying on a discussion about his or her own thoughts or behaviors.

Negative Symptoms of Schizophrenia

Negative symptoms are not as dramatic as positive symptoms, but they can interfere greatly with the patient's ability to function day to day. Because of the difficulty in expressing emotion, people with schizophre-

nia laugh, cry, and get angry less often. Their affect is flat, and they show little or no emotion when personal loss occurs. They also suffer from **ambivalence,** which is the concurrent experience of opposite feelings that are equally strong, so that it is impossible to make a decision. The avolition may be so profound that simple activities of daily living, such as dressing or combing hair, may not get done. Anhedonia prevents the person with schizophrenia from enjoying activities. People with schizophrenia have the limited speech of alogia; they have trouble saying anything new or carrying on a conversation. These negative symptoms cause the person with schizophrenia to withdraw and suffer feelings of severe isolation.

Neurocognitive Impairment

There is now evidence that neurocognitive impairment exists in schizophrenia and may be independent of the positive and negative symptoms. Neurocognition includes memory (short and long-term), vigilance or sustained attention, verbal fluency or the ability to generate new words, and executive functioning, which

TEXT BOX 18.1

*Key Diagnostic Characteristics
of Schizophrenia Subtypes*

Paranoid Type: *DSM-IV-TR* 295.30
- Preoccupation with delusions or auditory hallucinations
- Lacks disorganized speech, disorganized or catatonic behavior, or flat or inappropriate affect

Disorganized Type: *DSM-IV-TR* 295.10
- Disorganized speech, disorganized behavior, and flat or inappropriate affect

Catatonic Type: *DSM-IV-TR* 295.20
At least two of the following characteristics present:
- Motor immobility or stupor
- Excessive purposeless motor activity
- Extreme negativism
- Posturing, stereotyped movements, prominent mannerisms, or prominent grimacing
- Echolalia or echopraxia

Undifferentiated Type: *DSM-IV-TR* 295.90
- Only characteristic symptoms present, but does not meet criteria for other subtypes

Residual Type: *DSM-IV-TR* 295.60
- Absence of prominent delusions, hallucinations, disorganized speech, and grossly disorganized or catatonic behavior
- Negative symptoms persist or two or more positive symptoms are present in attenuated form such as odd beliefs or unusual perceptual experiences.

includes volition, planning, purposive action, and self-monitoring behavior. Working memory is a concept that includes short-term memory and the ability to store and process information. Neurocognitive impairment in memory, vigilance, and executive functioning is related to poor functional outcome in schizophrenia (Green et al., 2000).

KEY CONCEPT   **Neurocognitive Impairment. Neurocognitive impairment** in memory, vigilance, and executive functioning is related to poor functional outcome in schizophrenia (Green et al., 2000).

This impairment is independent of the positive symptoms. That is, cognitive dysfunction can exist even if the positive symptoms are in remission. Not all areas of cognitive functioning are impaired. Long-term memory and intellectual functioning are not necessarily affected. Many people with the disorder, however, appear to have low intellectual functioning, which may be related to lack of educational opportunities that are common for people with mental illnesses.

Neurocognitive dysfunction is often manifested in disorganized symptoms: those things that make it difficult for the person to understand and respond to the ordinary sights and sounds of daily living. Disorganized symptoms include **confused speech and thinking** and disorganized behavior.

KEY CONCEPT   Disorganized Symptoms. **Disorganized symptoms** of schizophrenia are those things that make it difficult for the person to understand and respond to the ordinary sights and sounds of daily living. These include confused speech and thinking and disorganized behavior.

Disorganized Thinking. The following are examples of confused speech and thinking patterns:

- **Echolalia**—repetition of another's words that is parrot-like and inappropriate
- **Circumstantiality**—extremely detailed and lengthy discourse about a topic
- **Loose associations**—absence of the normal connectedness of thoughts, ideas, and topics; sudden shifts without apparent relationship to preceding topics
- **Tangentiality**—the topic of conversation is changed to an entirely different topic that is a logical progression but causes a permanent detour from the original focus
- **Flight of ideas**—the topic of conversation changes repeatedly and rapidly, generally after just one sentence or phrase
- **Word salad**—string of words that are not connected in any way
- **Neologisms**—words that are made up that have no common meaning and are not recognized
- **Paranoia**—suspiciousness and guardedness that are unrealistic and often accompanied by grandiosity
- **Referential thinking**—belief that neutral stimuli have special meaning to the individual, such as the television commentator speaking directly to the individual
- **Autistic thinking**—restricts thinking to the literal and immediate so that the individual has private rules of logic and reasoning that make no sense to anyone else
- **Concrete thinking**—lack of abstraction in thinking; inability to understand punch lines, metaphors, and analogies
- **Verbigeration**—purposeless repetition of words or phrases
- **Metonymic speech**—use of words interchangeably with similar meanings
- **Clang association**—repetition of words or phrases that are similar in sound but in no other way, for example, right, light, sight, might

- **Stilted language**—overly and inappropriately artificial formal language
- **Pressured speech**—speaking as if the words are being forced out

Disorganized perceptions often create an oversensitivity to colors, shapes, and background activities. **Illusions** occur when the person misperceives or exaggerates stimuli that actually exist in the external environment. This is in contrast to hallucinations, which are perceptions in the absence of environmental stimuli. Ancillary symptoms that may accompany schizophrenia include anxiety, depression, and hostility.

Disorganized Behavior. Disorganized behavior (which may manifest as very slow, rhythmic, or ritualistic movement) coupled with disorganized speech makes it difficult for the person to partake in daily activities. Examples of disorganized behavior include the following:

- **Aggression**—behaviors or attitudes that reflect rage, hostility, and the potential for physical or verbal destructiveness (usually comes about if the person believes someone is going to do him or her harm)
- **Agitation**—inability to sit still or attend to others, accompanied by heightened emotions and tension
- **Catatonic excitement**—a hyperactivity characterized by purposeless activity and abnormal movements like grimacing and posturing
- **Echopraxia**—involuntary imitation of another person's movements and gestures
- **Regressed behavior**—behaving in a manner of a less mature life stage; childlike and immature
- **Stereotypy**—repetitive, purposeless movements that are idiosyncratic to the individual and to some degree outside of the individual's control
- **Hypervigilance**—sustained attention to external stimuli as if expecting something important or frightening to happen
- **Waxy flexibility**—posture held in odd or unusual fixed position for extended periods of time

Phases of Schizophrenia

The natural progression of schizophrenia is usually described as deteriorating over time, with an eventual plateau in the symptoms. Only for elderly patients with schizophrenia has it been suggested that improvement might occur. In reality, no one really knows what the course of schizophrenia would be if patients were able to adhere to a treatment regime throughout their lives. Only recently have the medications been relatively effective, with manageable side effects. At this point, it is understood that the symptoms of schizophrenia combine in various numbers and degrees. The clinical picture of schizophrenia is complex; individuals differ from each other, and the experience for a single individual may be different from episode to episode. The typical course of the illness appears to have phases. For this discussion, three phase categories are presented.

Phase I: Initial Diagnosis and Early Schizophrenia

During this initial phase of diagnosis and early symptoms, the behaviors may be both confusing and frightening to the patient and the family. Often, the changes are subtle. However, at some point, the changes in thought and behavior become so disruptive or bizarre that they can no longer be overlooked. These might include episodes of staying up all night for several nights, incoherent conversations, or aggressive acts against self or others. For example, one patient's parents reported their son walking around the apartment for several days holding his arms and hands as if they were a machine gun, pointing them at his parents and siblings, and saying "rat-a-tat-tat, you're dead."

Another father described his son's first delusional-hallucination episode as "so convincing that I was frightened" and described it as follows: He believed he had been visited by space aliens who wanted to unite their world with earth and assured him that he would become Speaker of the House and then President following the deaths of the President and Vice President. He began visiting cemeteries and making "mind contact" with the deceased. He also believed that he saw his deceased grandmother walking around in the home. He was certain that there were pipe bombs in objects in his parents' home and that a sniper was outside aiming at him (Willwerth, 1993, p. 40).

As symptoms progress, the patient is less and less able to care for basic needs, such as eating, sleeping, and bathing. Usually, the person cannot attend and function at school or a job, resulting in dependency on family and friends. Because delusions or hallucinations seem so real, the individual is generally unable to recognize the need for treatment. Usually, hospitalization or some type of intensive outpatient treatment must be initiated by family and friends.

Phase II: Adaptation

After the initial diagnosis of schizophrenia and the successful initiation of treatment, the patient enters a period in which symptoms may be less acute and require less drastic measures to control. This, however, is not a period of quiescence, and both positive and negative symptoms may actually be worse (Breier et al., 1991).

McGlashan (1994) describes this period as having two subphases: (1) the subacute and postpsychotic depression phase, and (2) the moratorium or adaptive plateau. The subacute phase has waning positive symptoms and leads to a period of depression in which patients withdraw to conserve resources and become "defensive, nonfunctional, and . . . [susceptible] to symptom exacerbation under stress" (p. 195). Functional deficits persist during this period, and the patient and family must learn to cope with these. Deficits in the patient's ability to function may be found in all areas. Emotional blunting diminishes the ability and desire to engage in hobbies, vocational activities, and relationships. Limited participation in social activities spirals into numerous skill deficits, such as difficulty engaging others interpersonally because of behaviors such as gaze avoidance, difficulty perceiving and recognizing emotional expressions of others, and difficulty with problem-solving behaviors like negotiation and compromise (Bellack, 1992). Cognitive deficits lead to problems recognizing patterns in situations and transferring learning and behaviors from one circumstance to another similar one. Sometimes treatments, especially medications, are discontinued without consultation with mental health professionals. This is extremely detrimental to the patient's outcome and puts the person at significant risk for relapse.

If patients are able to adhere to the treatment regimen, they begin to adjust to having a severe, chronic illness. The moratorium or adaptive plateau is a period "of relative stability [in] which [patients learn through treatment] to slowly reconstitute identity, accumulate supports, and strengthen skills" (McGlashan, 1994, p. 195) (Text Box 18-2).

Phase III: Relapse

Relapse is "a return of the illness symptoms, [which are] severe enough to disrupt daily activities . . . or require unscheduled inpatient or outpatient intervention" (Murphy & Moller, 1993, p. 227). Relapse is not inevitable; however, it occurs with sufficient regularity to be a major concern in the treatment of schizophrenia. Reported relapse rates vary from 25% to 90%, and relapse affects both those who were being treated and those who were not (Zubin et al., 1992). The lower relapse rates were, for the most part, among groups who were following a treatment regimen.

Many factors converge to effect relapse: the degree of impairment in cognition and coping that leaves patients vulnerable to stressors; the accessibility of community resources, such as public transportation, housing, entry-level and low-stress employment, and social services and income supports that buffer the day-to-day stressors of living; the degree of stigmatization that the community holds for mental illness that attacks the self-concept of patients; and the responsiveness of relationships with family, friends, and supportive others (like peers and professionals) when patients need help. It is clear that support and involvement of family are extremely impor-

TEXT BOX 18.2

Clinical Vignette: Parent Describes His Son With Schizophrenia

Dr. Willick (1994) described his reactions and observations of his son diagnosed with schizophrenia:

> . . . Struggling as he does with many of what we now call the "negative symptoms," he has lost that gleam in his eye, that joyous good humor, that zest for life which he once showed. Today, it is hard for him to feel things strongly, or to enjoy his music, sports, or being with the family. . . . There has also been a significant cognitive impairment. Things that he was easily able to grasp when he was 14-years-old are now much harder for him. He has lost considerable capacity for abstract thinking. His language is very concrete and has lost the richness and subtlety of expression it once had. He has a hard time following a moderately complicated plot of an article he reads or a movie he sees, and he can describe it only in a superficial and concrete way (pp. 8–9).

> I know that I should be most proud of Gary, and I can often feel that. The problem is that it is not easy to see that he is displaying great courage in coping with what has happened to him. The symptoms of the illness make him appear lacking in motivation, initiative, and will, and even he accuses himself of not trying hard enough. It is hard for an observer to see how difficult it must be for him to get up every day, hoping to feel different, only to awake with the same feeling of anhedonia. In some ways, those admirable qualities that he possessed before he became ill are no doubt serving him well as he tries to fight an illness that none of us, let alone Gary himself, can really comprehend (pp. 11–12).

tant at this time. From the initial period when the diagnosis is made, patients and families must be educated to anticipate and expect relapse and know how to cope with it. This is one of the important themes throughout the nursing process for people with schizophrenia.

Medication treatment of schizophrenia has generally contributed to an improvement in the lifestyle of people with this disease. However, no medication has proved curative for schizophrenia. The life-long course described previously applies to people whether they follow their medication management or not. Faithful medication management tends to make the impairments in functioning less severe when they occur and to diminish the extremes an individual might experience. This is particularly true of some of the more newly marketed antipsychotic medications. Stopping medications almost certainly leads to a relapse and may actually be an iatrogenic stressor that causes a severe and rapid relapse (Baldessarini, 1997). Combining medications and psychosocial treatment greatly diminishes the severity and frequency of recurrent relapse.

Schizophrenia in Special Populations

Children

The diagnosis of schizophrenia is rare in children before the onset of adolescence. When it does occur in children aged 5 or 6 years, the symptoms are essentially the same as in adults. In this age group, hallucinations tend to be visual and delusions less developed. Because disorganized speech and behavior may be explained better by other disorders that are more common in childhood, those disorders should be considered before applying the diagnosis of schizophrenia to a child (APA, 2000).

Elderly People

People with schizophrenia grow old. The 1-year prevalence for schizophrenia among those 65 years of age and older was estimated in the Surgeon General's report (USDHHS, 1999) to be 0.6% (about half the percentage for adults 18 to 54 years of age). For elderly patients who have had schizophrenia since young adulthood, this may be a time in which they experience some improvement in symptoms or relapse fluctuations. However, their lifestyle is probably dependent on the effectiveness of earlier treatment, the support systems that are in place (including relationships with family members and professionals), and the interaction between environmental stressors and the patient's functional impairments.

In late-onset schizophrenia, the diagnostic criteria are met after the age of 45 years. Women are affected in a higher proportion than men. The presentation of late-onset schizophrenia is most likely to include positive symptoms, particularly paranoid or persecutory delusions. Cognitive deterioration and affective blunting occur less frequently. Social functioning is more intact. Many individuals diagnosed with late-onset schizophrenia have alterations in sensory functions, primarily hearing and vision losses (APA, 2000; USDHHS, 1999). The cost of caring for elderly patients with schizophrenia remains high because of deinstitutionalization; community-based treatment has developed more slowly for this age group than for younger adults.

EPIDEMIOLOGY

Schizophrenia occurs in all cultures and countries. The incidence and prevalence rates are similar across studies, with variations explained by the definition of schizophrenia and the sampling method used. The estimated prevalence rate ranges from 0.5% to 1.5% (APA, 2000); the United States Surgeon General estimates a 1.3% 1-year prevalence rate among adults 18 to 54 years of age (USDHHS, 1999). The incidence has been estimated to range from 0.5 to 5.0 in 10,000 per year (APA, 2000). Birth cohort studies suggest that the incidence may be higher among individuals born in urban settings versus rural and may be somewhat lower in later-born birth cohorts (APA, 2000).

People with schizophrenia tend to cluster in the lowest social classes in industrialized countries and urban communities. This finding has been consistent in studies of schizophrenia. Two causes are hypothesized to explain this finding. The first is the downward drift of individuals so diagnosed. The second is genetic selection. In agrarian and rural societies, this is less the case. Explanations for this difference between urban and rural cultures include decreased demands for vulnerable individuals and closer support networks in agrarian societies (McGlashan, 1994).

Homelessness is a problem for the severely mentally ill (ie, people with schizophrenia or manic-depressive illness). In 1992, the severely mentally ill were estimated to be one third of the 4 million homeless (Leshner et al., 1992). Of the estimated 600,000 severely mentally ill, specific numbers of people with schizophrenia were not estimated (see Chap. 32).

Risk Factors

The study of risk factors has attempted to explain stressors that might contribute to the vulnerability-stress model of causation. The Surgeon General's report (USDHHS, 1999) summarizes these. Stressors, as risk factors, in the perinatal period include many circumstances that can be categorized as maternal stressors: maternal prenatal poverty, poor nutrition, depression, exposure to influenza outbreaks, war zone exposure, and Rh-factor incompatibility. Infants affected by these maternal stressors may demonstrate conditions that create their own risk: low birth weight, short gestation, and early developmental difficulties. In childhood, stressors may include central nervous system infections caused by crowded living conditions and influenza. As earlier, however, research support for these factors is inconsistent. In general, poverty and minority social status affect the life-time course of schizophrenia.

Age of Onset

Most people who develop schizophrenia are diagnosed in late adolescence and early adulthood. When schizophrenia begins earlier than the age of 25 years, several observations have been made (USDHHS, 1999). Symptoms seem to develop more gradually, and negative symptoms predominate over the course of the disease. People with early-onset schizophrenia suffer a greater number of neuropsychological problems. Finally, disruptions occur in milestone events of early adulthood, such as achieving in education, work, and long-term relationships.

Gender Differences

A gender difference for age of onset exists, with men diagnosed earlier than women. The median age of onset for men is in the middle 20s, whereas the median age of onset for women is in the late 20s (APA, 2000). These sex differences have received attention because of hypotheses about sex-linked genetic etiologies. For instance, estrogen may play a protective role against the development of schizophrenia that disappears as estrogen levels drop during menopause (USDHHS, 1999). This would account for the higher median age of onset and a more favorable treatment outcome in women. However, there seems to be a subgroup of women who develop schizophrenia at the same time as men. For this group, the outcome is not as favorable as for those women with later onset (Gureje & Bamidele, 1998).

Ethnic and Cultural Differences

Increasingly, efforts are being made to consider culture and ethnic origin when diagnosing and treating individuals who display symptoms of schizophrenia (USDHHS, 1999; APA, 2000). While symptoms of schizophrenia appear to be clearly defined, it is possible to find cultures in which what appears to be a hallucination may be considered a vision or a religious experience. Behaviors such as averting eyes during a conversation or minimizing emotional expression may be culturally bound yet easily misinterpreted by clinicians of a different cultural or ethnic background.

Some racial groups are diagnosed more often with schizophrenia. It is not clear, however, if these findings represent correct diagnosis or overdiagnosis of the disorder based on a cultural bias of the clinician. In the United States and the United Kingdom, studies have found that schizophrenia is more often diagnosed among African Americans and Asian Americans (APA, 2000).

Familial Differences

First-degree biologic relatives (children, siblings, parents) of an individual with schizophrenia have a 10 times greater risk for schizophrenia than the general population (APA, 2000). Other relatives may have an increased risk for disorders that are within the "schizophrenia spectrum" (a group of disorders with some similarities of behavior, like schizoaffective disorder and schizotypal personality disorder) (APA, 2000).

Comorbidity

Several somatic and psychological disorders coexist with schizophrenia. It is estimated that nearly 50% of patients with schizophrenia have a comorbid medication condition, but many of these illnesses are misdiagnosed or undiagnosed (Goldman, 1999). Recently, more attention has been paid to the causes of mortality among people with schizophrenia, and several physical disorders have been identified. These include vision and dental problems, hypertension, diabetes, and sexually transmitted diseases (USDHHS, 1999).

Substance Abuse and Depression

Among the behavioral comorbidities, substance abuse is common. Depression may also be observed in patients with schizophrenia. This is an important symptom for several reasons. First, depression may be evidence that the diagnosis of a mood disorder is more appropriate (see Chaps. 20 and 25). Second, depression is not an unusual occurrence in chronic stages of schizophrenia and deserves attention. Third, the suicide rate (10%) among individuals with schizophrenia is elevated over that of the general population. Risk factors for suicide are male gender, chronic illness with frequent relapses, frequent short hospitalizations, a negative attitude toward treatment, impulsive behavior, parasuicide, psychosis, and depression (De Hert et al., 2001).

Diabetes Mellitus

There is a renewed interest in the relationship of diabetes mellitus and schizophrenia. Years ago, an association was established between glucose regulation and psychiatric disorders (Schimmelbusch et al., 1971; Franzen, 1970). In fact, insulin shock therapy was used in the treatment of severe disorders. Recently, there has been an interest in the effect of glucose on cognitive function in schizophrenia. There is evidence that glucose availability improves cognitive performance (Newcomer et al., 1999).

Disordered Water Balance

Water intoxication, a severe form of disordered water balance, is a major cause of death in institutionalized psychiatric patients (Goldman et al., 1988). This potentially fatal medical emergency is characterized by abnormally high water intake followed by a rapid drop in serum sodium levels and the development of diverse neurologic signs ranging from ataxia to coma. Patients with schizophrenia, especially schizophrenia of early onset, are most often affected (Jos et al., 1986; Lawson et al., 1985), but the disorder is also common in patients with bipolar disorder, psychotic depression, alcohol abuse, and mental retardation (Riggs et al., 1991). Other risk factors include extended hospitalizations with a minimal response to neuroleptics, a high frequency of tardive dyskinesia, heavy tobacco use, and structural brain abnormalities (Kirch et al., 1985).

KEY CONCEPT Disordered Water Balance. **Disordered water balance** is a state of chronic water imbalance common in psychiatric patients with chronic illnesses.

Prevalence. Prevalence rates of disordered water balance are surprisingly high, varying from about 6% (Mercier-Guidez, et al., 2000; Jos et al., 1986;) to 17.5% (Blum et al., 1983). In a frequently cited study by Vieweg and others, more than 60% of the 100 patients in a chronic care unit of a state mental hospital had abnormal fluid weight gains associated with disordered water balance; in 7% of those patients, intermittent water intoxication occurred (Vieweg et al., 1989a; Vieweg et al., 1989b). In a separate study of mortality rates in institutionalized mentally ill patients who died before the age of 53 years, Vieweg and colleagues (1985) found that 18.5% of the 60 patients studied had died of complications of self-induced water intoxication. These data indicate that water intoxication is common among patients who are undergoing long-term psychiatric treatment.

Etiology of Disordered Water Balance. The specific cause of water intoxication is unknown. Recent studies suggest that it has multiple causes, including impaired renal excretion because of increased production of the antidiuretic hormone (ADH) arginine vasopressin, an abnormality in the hippocampal area resulting in the stereotypical repetitive behavior of drinking, faulty osmoregulation of fluid intake (Delva & Crammer, 1988; Goldman, 1991; Snider & Boyd, 1991), and a neurobiologic dysfunction that affects the ADH thirst and salt-appetite mechanisms (Boyd & Lapierre, 1996).

Clinical Characteristics. Water intoxication is generally preceded by a prolonged period or recurrent periods of disordered water balance. These patients display a characteristic daily pattern of excessive fluid intake or compulsive water drinking that begins in the morning, followed by diurnal weight gain (weight gained during the daytime) in the afternoon. The fluid that is retained produces generalized edema, cellular dysfunction, diminished serum osmolality, and dilution of serum sodium. As fluid volumes peak by midday and the concentration of serum sodium begins to drop, symptoms of chronic hyponatremia (decreased sodium concentration) appear (Table 18-2). These symptoms generally resolve overnight as excess fluid is excreted and sodium levels gradually rise (Baier et al., 1989; Boyd & Lapierre, 1996; Snider & Boyd, 1991).

Disordered water balance and resulting hyponatremia may vary from mild to severe, depending on the amount of fluid intake, the ability of the kidneys

TABLE 18.2 Signs and Symptoms of Hyponatremia

Condition	Signs and Symptoms
Chronic hyponatremia	Generalized weakness
	Giddiness
	Headache
	Irritability
	Loss of appetite
	Muscle cramps
	Nausea
	Restlessness
	Slight confusion
	Vomiting
Acute hyponatremia	Coma
	Confusion
	Decreased serum osmolality
	Decreased urine osmolality
	Increased urinary volume
	Lethargy
	Muscle twitching
	Seizures
	Specific urine gravity <1.010
	Weakness

From Riggs, A., Dyksen, M., Kim, S., & Opsahl, J. (1991). A review of disorders of water homeostasis in psychiatric patients. *Psychosomatics, 32*(2), 133–148.

to excrete urine, or both (Riggs et al., 1991). The severity of the symptoms depends on the degree of hyponatremia and how rapidly it develops. Usually a benign condition, disordered water balance often goes undetected, sometimes continuing for months or even years. Ingesting large amounts of water over a prolonged period of time may cause physical complications, including renal dysfunction, urinary incontinence, flaccid bladder, hydronephrosis, cardiac failure, malnutrition, hernia, dilation of the gastrointestinal tract, or permanent brain damage (Goldman, 1991; Boyd & Lapierre, 1996). Disordered water balance may also lead to the life-threatening complication of water intoxication, which occurs when unusually large volumes of fluid are ingested, overwhelming the capacity of the kidneys to excrete water (Wyngaarden et al., 1992). As a result, serum sodium levels rapidly fall from a normal range of 135 to 145 mEq/L to 120 mEq/L or below. This rapid decrease in sodium produces muscle twitching, irritability, and even the risk for seizures or coma.

The classic feature of disordered water balance is *polydipsia*, or excessive fluid intake. Patients are literally "driven to drink" and may consume more than 4 to 10 liters of water daily. They are often seen carrying soda cans or water cups around the ward or making frequent trips to the bathroom. They may also horde water cups or other containers for storing fluid, or take fluids from other unsuspecting patients. In addition, these patients may drink from water fountains, toilets, or showers and may become highly agitated and injure others if their pursuit of water is interrupted (Baier et al., 1989; Boyd & Lapierre, 1996; Riggs et al., 1991; Snider & Boyd, 1991).

Polyuria, the excessive excretion of urine, is a sign that the kidneys are overloaded with fluid. The amount of urine excreted corresponds with the amount ingested and can easily exceed 3 to 5 liters a day. Patients with polyuria may have such embarrassing problems as urgency and incontinence, especially at night. Their rooms may smell strongly of urine, and their clothing or bed linens may have to be changed frequently.

Lowered serum sodium levels are responsible for most of the emotional manifestations of disordered water balance. As the concentration of serum sodium begins to drop, patients display an increase in psychotic symptoms or become more irritable and labile. The emotional symptoms they exhibit vary with the degree of change in sodium values. As excess water builds up, the intracellular movement of water causes the brain cells to swell, resulting in neurologic dysfunction and behavioral changes.

Reduced concentrations of serum sodium are an important physiologic sign of disordered water balance. Changes in these levels relate directly to the progression of the disorder. When serum sodium levels fall below the normal range of 135 to 145 mEq/L, signs and symptoms of hyponatremia begin to appear. The severity of the symptoms is related more to the rate of change in the sodium value than to the actual value itself (Boyd & Lapierre, 1996). As a result, when serum sodium levels fall more gradually, clinical signs and symptoms of chronic hyponatremia appear; when serum sodium levels drop rapidly, however, symptoms of acute hyponatremia appear. It is important to remember that patients with chronic disordered water balance have a more prolonged, benign condition than patients with acute cases. In chronic cases, the patient's sodium level falls gradually to 120 mEq/L or below, allowing the patient to tolerate lower levels of sodium than would be possible if the drop were more rapid.

Urinary dilution is also an important physiologic marker of disordered water balance. Excessive fluid intake overloads the kidneys, producing changes in the degree of urine concentration, or urine specific gravity. An indication of urinary volume can also be obtained by testing the urine specific gravity. Hyposthenuria, a condition in which the urine specific gravity is below 1.008, is a sign of the early stages of disordered water balance (Boyd & Lapierre, 1996). Changes in the urine specific gravity that reflect the

progression of disordered water balance are presented in Text Box 18-3.

ETIOLOGY

Since the 1970s, hypotheses about the causes of schizophrenia have changed dramatically. Purely psychological theories have been replaced by a neurobiologic model that says that patients with schizophrenia have a biologic predisposition or vulnerability that is exacerbated by environmental stressors (see the diathesis-stress model discussed in Chapter 6). Those with schizophrenia are thought to have a genetically or biologically determined sensitivity that leaves them vulnerable to an overwhelming onslaught of stimuli from without and within (US-DHHS, 2000). These inherent vulnerabilities include cognitive, psychophysiologic, social competence, and coping deficits that alter the individual's ability, both cognitively and emotionally, to manage life events and interpersonal situations (Text Box 18-4 and Fig. 18-1).

O'Connor (1994) adapted this diathesis-stress model to a nursing model for intervention that acknowledges both the patient's inherent vulnerabilities and the inability to manage the environmental and interpersonal stressors (Research Box 18-1).

TEXT BOX 18.3

Physiologic Signs and Symptoms of Disordered Water Balance

Mild Disordered Water Balance
- Increased diurnal weight gain
- Urine specific gravity (1.011–1.025)
- Normal serum sodium (135–145 mEq/L)

Moderate Disordered Water Balance
- Increased diurnal weight gain
- Urine specific gravity (1.010–1.003)
- Possible facial puffiness
- Periodic nocturia

Severe Disordered Water Balance
- Possible evidence of stomach or bladder dilation
- Urine specific gravity (1.003–1.000)
- Frequent signs of nausea, vomiting
- Possible history of major motor seizure
- Possible change in blood pressure or pulse
- Polyuria
- Polydipsia
- Urinary incontinence during the night

From Snider, K., & Boyd, M. (1991). When they drink too much: Nursing interventions for patients with disordered balance. *Journal of Psychosocial Nursing, 29*(7), 13.

TEXT BOX 18.4

Deficits That Cause Vulnerability in Schizophrenia

Cognitive Deficits
- Deficits in processing complex information
- Deficits in maintaining a steady focus of attention
- Inability to distinguish between relevant and irrelevant stimuli
- Difficulty forming consistent abstractions
- Impaired memory

Psychophysiologic Deficits
- Deficits in sensory inhibition
- Poor control of autonomic responsiveness

Social Skills Deficits
- Impairments in processing interpersonal stimuli, such as eye contact or assertiveness
- Deficits in conversational capacity
- Deficits in initiating activities
- Deficits in experiencing pleasure

Coping Skills Deficits
- Overassessment of threat
- Underassessment of personal resources
- Overuse of denial

Adapted from McGlashan, T. H. (1994). Psychosocial treatments of schizophrenia: The potential relationships. In N. C. Andreasen (Ed.), *Schizophrenia: From mind to molecule* (pp. 189–215). Washington, DC: American Psychiatric Press.

Biologic Theories

The theories and research about the biologic vulnerability for schizophrenia have focused on incorporating multiple observations into a coherent explanation. These observations include the course of the illness already described, possible brain structure changes found through postmortem and neuroimaging techniques, familial patterns, and pharmacologic effects on behavior and neurotransmitter functions in the brain. One of the more recent theories about the cause of schizophrenic vulnerability focuses on neurodevelopment of the brain from the prenatal period through adolescence. This section describes the various observations and current theories about the cause of schizophrenia. The exact cause of schizophrenia, however, remains elusive.

Neuroanatomic Findings

Postmortem and neuroimaging brain studies of patients diagnosed with schizophrenia have shown four consistent changes in brain anatomy. These changes include (a) decreased blood flow to the left globus pallidus early in the disease; (b) absence of normal blood flow increase in frontal lobes during tests of frontal lobe functioning, such as working memory tasks; (c) a thinner cortex of the medial temporal lobe and a smaller anterior portion of the hippocampus; and (d) enlarged lateral and third ventricles and widened sulci (Stevens, 1997; Kandel et al., 2000). Although these are regular findings among patients with schizophrenia, they were not found among all patients with a diagnosis of schizophrenia who were studied. For instance, ventricle enlargement has been found in only 15% to 30% of patient subjects when compared with control subjects in various studies (Stevens, 1997).

Ventricular enlargement suggests that brain atrophy occurs in schizophrenic patients and that this tissue loss occurs after the cranium has fully developed (Stevens, 1997). This atrophy has not consistently been found to be progressive over the course of the illness and is not generalized throughout the brain (Stevens, 1997). Prefrontal cortical and limbic structures that articulate with the ventricles have been examined. These include the temporal lobe gray matter, hippocampus, entorhinal cortex, and cortex gray matter (Keltner et al., 1998). Associations between anatomic findings and premorbid functioning, stage, and duration of illness and the type of treatment have not been consistently found (Stevens, 1997).

Familial Patterns

Evidence supports a familial or genetic base for schizophrenia. First-degree relatives (including siblings and children) are 10 times more likely to develop schizophrenia than the general population (APA, 2000; USDHHS, 2000). Concordance for schizophrenia is higher among monozygotic twins than among dizygotic twins, although the rate is not perfectly concordant.

Genetic research has sought to identify specific genes responsible for schizophrenia, but no replicated results have emerged from this work (Moldin & Gottesman, 1997). The absence of reproducible results in this area of study is likely due to the heterogeneity of the disorder, which may not be consistent with a single gene theory. A model that includes several genes is more likely to explain the development of schizophrenia (USDHHS, 2000). Two possible locations are on the long arm of chromosome 22 and on chromosome 6 (Kandel et al., 2000).

Neurodevelopment

Current theory and research are attempting to explain how genes or events early in life (especially perinatal events such as infections or obstetric irregularities) would cause schizophrenia yet manifest symptoms only after years—in adolescence or young adulthood. The neurodevelopmental theory explains and reconciles the inconsistent neuroanatomic brain changes

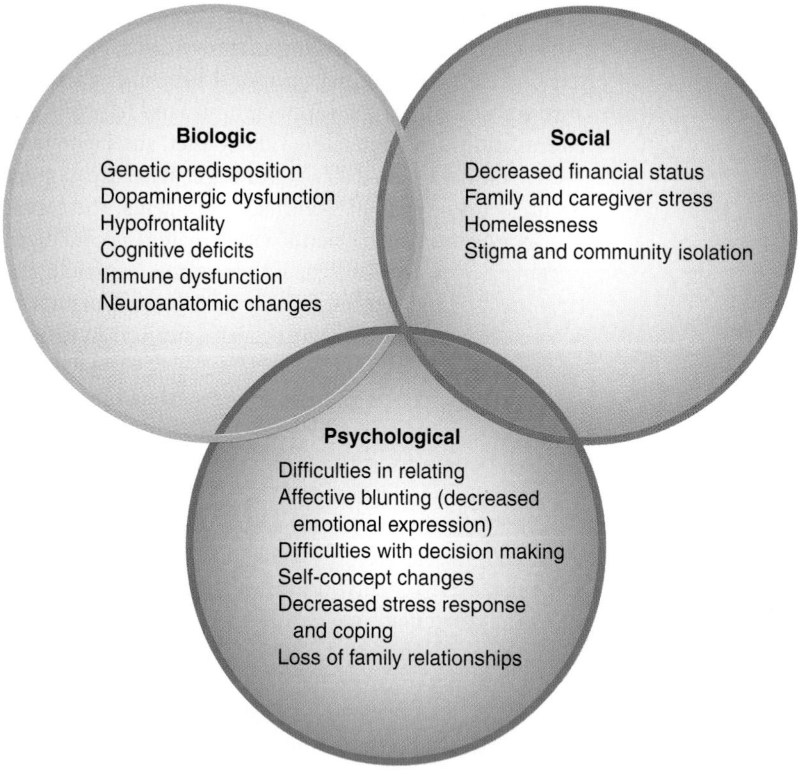

Biologic

Genetic predisposition
Dopaminergic dysfunction
Hypofrontality
Cognitive deficits
Immune dysfunction
Neuroanatomic changes

Social

Decreased financial status
Family and caregiver stress
Homelessness
Stigma and community isolation

Psychological

Difficulties in relating
Affective blunting (decreased
  emotional expression)
Difficulties with decision making
Self-concept changes
Decreased stress response
  and coping
Loss of family relationships

FIGURE 18.1 Biopsychosocial etiologies for patients with schizophrenia.

RESEARCH BOX 18.1

Stress of Schizophrenia

This author adapted a stress–vulnerability model of causation for schizophrenia, which suggests that exacerbated psychotic symptoms are a result of unmanaged stress. She proposed that this stress–vulnerability model be used as a basis for developing appropriate clinical interventions to help patients manage stress.

The author categorized the factors that determine a patient's stress as *stressors* or *moderators*. *Stressors* include such factors as neurologic dysfunction (modified mesocortical and mesolimbic dopamine activity), psychobiologic stressors (amount and frequency of drug and alcohol abuse, number of symptoms, and negative appraisal of symptoms and life events), and environmental or interpersonal stressors (stressful life events or hassles, environmental stimulation, and critical attitudes of family or staff). *Moderator* dimensions include ability to measure symptom levels and use coping strategies (symptom-regulation skill competencies); instrumental and expressive support of family, peers, and clinicians (perception of social support); and effectiveness of antipsychotic medication. The author proposed that these stressors and moderators interact continuously, and when moderators are insufficient to manage stressors, stress and psychotic symptoms result.

From this stress–vulnerability framework, the author concluded that to reduce symptoms and prevent relapse, clinical interventions should be directed at both: (1) reducing risk factors such as the environmental and interpersonal stressors and (2) enhancing moderators such as symptom-regulation skills. Interventions come from several sources and include family and residential staff support, peer support, and clinician intervention, consultation, and support.

Utilization in the Clinical Setting: For the nurse working with patients in a clinical setting, interventions can be directed both at reducing stressors and enhancing moderators. Two stressor areas that can be targeted for intervention include environmental stimulation and interpersonal conflict, with interventions such as helping patients learn problem-solving and teaching techniques to manage interpersonal conflicts. Interventions that help enhance moderators of stress include educating patient groups in symptom management, reinforcing the taking of medications, teaching families strategies for managing the patient, and promoting peer support and social support.

O'Connor, F. W. (1994). A vulnerability–stress framework for evaluating clinical interventions in schizophrenia. *Image—The Journal of Nursing Scholarship 26,* 231–237.

that have been found and links them to early development. Brain development from prenatal periods through adolescence requires several coordinated molecular activities, including cell proliferation, cell migration, axonal outgrowth, pruning of neuronal connections, programmed cell death, and myelination. All of these activities require coordinated development, usually through activation and inactivation of proteins by genes. Any of these processes could be disrupted by (a) inherited genes that place the individual at risk for schizophrenia, (b) a wild-type allele of this gene that is activated in adolescence or early adulthood; or (c) genetic sensitizing that leaves the individual susceptible to environmental causes or lesioning during some adverse perinatal event. Further, several maturational events normally occur during puberty that may affect brain development: (a) changes in dopaminergic, serotonergic, adrenergic, glutamatergic, γ-aminobutyric acid (GABA)–ergic, and cholinergic neurotransmitter systems and substrates; (b) a complex combination of synaptic pruning along with substantial brain growth in some areas of the cortex, and (c) changes in the steroid-hormonal environment (Weickert & Weinberger, 1998).

Neurotransmitters, Pathways, and Receptors

Theories about the cause and pathophysiology of schizophrenia have been generated from decades of pharmacologic research and management of the disorder. For years, the leading hypothesis about the neurobiology of schizophrenia has been based on observations of drug actions. The *dopamine hypothesis* of schizophrenia arose from observations that antipsychotic drugs, which so successfully ameliorate or reduce the positive symptoms of schizophrenia, act primarily by blocking postsynaptic dopamine receptors in the brain (Table 18-3). In addition, other drugs that enhance dopamine function, such as amphetamines or cocaine, cause behavioral symptoms similar to **paranoid schizophrenia** in humans and bizarre stereotyped behavior in monkeys. Antipsychotic drugs stop these drug-induced behaviors. Based on these observations, researchers concluded that schizophrenia was a syndrome of hyperdopaminergic action in the brain.

This old, straightforward hypothesis of dopamine hyperactivity is clearly complicated by recent findings. Positron emission tomography (PET) scan findings suggest that in schizophrenia, there is a general reduction in

TABLE 18.3   Types of Antipsychotic Drugs

Generic Name	Trade Name	Dosage Range for Adults (mg/d)
Selected Conventional Antipsychotic Drugs Used to Treat Psychosis in the United States		
Chlorpromazine	Thorazine	30–800
Chlorprothixene	Taractan	12–64
Fluphenazine	Prolixin; Permitil	0.5–20
Haloperidol	Haldol	1–15
Loxapine	Loxitane	20–250
Mesoridazine	Serentil	100–300
Molindone	Moban	15–225
Perphenazine	Trilafon	4–32
Pimozide	Orap*	1–10
Prochlorperazine	Compazine[†]	15–25
Thioridazine	Mellaril	150–800
Thiothixene	Navane	5–25
Trifluoperazine	Stelazine	5–25
Triflupromazine	Vesprin	60–150
Second-Generation		
Clozapine	Clozaril	200–600
Risperidone	Risperdal	4–16
Olanzapine	Zyprexa	10–20
Quetiapine	Seroquel	300–400
Ziprasidone	Geodon	40–160

*Approved in the United States for Tourette's syndrome.
[†]Adapted from Stahl, S. (2000). *Essential psychopharmacology: Neuroscientific basis and practical application* (2nd ed., p. 404). Cambridge, UK: Cambridge University Press.

brain metabolism with a relative hypermetabolism in the left side of the brain and in the left temporal lobe. Abnormalities exist in specific areas of the brain, such as in the left globus pallidus (Sedvall, 1994). These findings support further exploration of differential brain hemisphere function in schizophrenia (Fig. 18-2). Other PET studies show **hypofrontality,** or a reduced cerebral blood flow and glucose metabolism in the prefrontal cortex of people with schizophrenia and hyperactivity in the limbic area (Buchsbaum, 1990) (Figs. 18-3 and 18-4). Also, we now understand that there are several types dopamine receptors (labeled D_1, D_2, D_3, D_4, and D_5) and that dopamine is found in four pathways (mesolimbic, mesocortical, nigrostriatal, and tuberoinfundibular) that enervate different parts of the brain (Kandel et al., 2000) (see Chap. 8). Based on the current understanding of schizophrenia, the following discussion relates the neurobiologic changes to the clinical symptoms.

Positive Symptoms: Hyperactivity of Mesolimbic Tract. Positive symptoms of schizophrenia (hallucinations and delusions) are thought to be caused by dopamine *hyperactivity* in the mesolimbic tract, which regulates memory and emotion. It is hypothesized that this hyperactivity could be a result of overactive modulation of neurotransmission from the nucleus accumbens (Kandel et al., 2000). Another possible explanation for dopaminergic hyperactivity in the mesolimbic tract is hypoactivity of the mesocortical tract, which normally inhibits dopamine activity in the mesolimbic tract by some type of feedback mechanism. In schizophrenia, the primary defect may be in the mesocortical tract, where dopaminergic function is diminished, thereby decreasing the inhibitory effects on the mesolimbic tract. This disinhibition may be responsible for the overactivity of dopamine in the mesolimbic tract, resulting in the positive symptom cluster (Kandel et al., 2000). Support for this interconnection between mesocortical and mesolimbic tracts has been found in laboratory animals. Destruction of the mesocortical tract of animals resulted in increased activity in the mesolimbic tract, especially in the nucleus accumbens. A compensatory increase in mesolimbic neurons is a suggested mechanism by which this overactivity occurs.

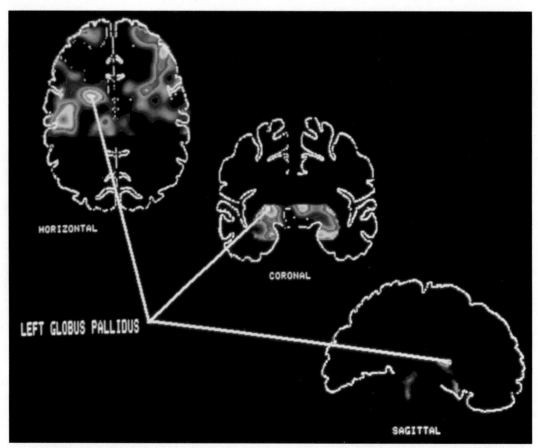

FIGURE 18.2 Area of abnormal functioning in a person with schizophrenia. These three views show the excessive neuronal activity in the left globus pallidus (portion of the basal ganglia next to the putamen). (Courtesy of John W. Haller, PhD, Departments of Psychiatry and Radiology, Washington University, St. Louis, MO.)

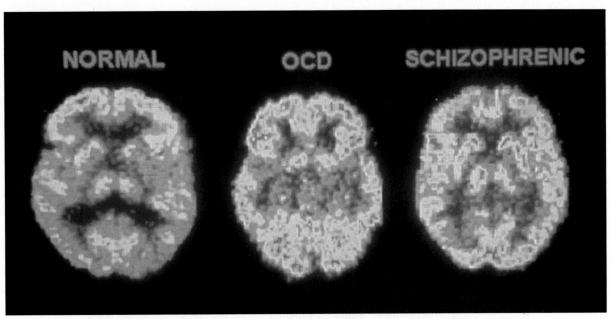

FIGURE 18.3 Metabolic activity in a control subject (*left*), a subject with obsessive-compulsive disorder (center), and a subject with schizophrenia (*right*). (Courtesy of Monte S. Buchsbaum, MD, The Mount Sinai Medical Center and School of Medicine, New York, NY.)

Negative Symptoms and Cognitive Impairment: Hypoactivity of the Mesocortical Tract. Negative symptoms and cognitive impairment are thought to be related to *hypoactivity* of the mesocortical dopaminergic tract, which by its association with the prefrontal and neocortex, contributes to motivation, planning, sequencing of behaviors in time, attention, and social behavior (Kandel et al., 2000; Jibson & Tandon, 2000). Negative symptoms, such as poor motivation and planning, and flat affect are remarkably similar to symptoms of patients who underwent lobotomy procedures in the late 1940s and early 1950s to disconnect the frontal cortex from the rest of the brain. Monkeys who have had dopamine in the prefrontal cortex depleted have difficulty with cognitive tasks. Finally, PET scans of energy metabolism suggest a reduced metabolism in frontal and prefrontal areas (Sedvall, 1994).

Role of Other Dopamine Pathways. The tuberoinfundibular dopaminergic tract is active in prolactin regulation and may be the source of neuroendocrine changes observed in schizophrenia. The nigrostriatal dopaminergic tract functions include modulation of motor activity. This is believed to be the site of the **extrapyramidal side effects** of antipsychotic drugs, such as pseudoparkinsonism and tardive dyskinesia. This may also be the site of some motor symptoms of schizophrenia, such as stereotypical behavior.

Role of Other Receptors. Other receptors are also involved in dopamine neurotransmission, especially serotonergic receptors. It is becoming clear that schizophrenia does not result from dysregulation of a single neurotransmitter or biogenic amine (eg, norepinephrine, dopamine, or serotonin). Investigators are also hypothesizing a role for glutamate and GABA (Gray, 1998) because of the complex interconnections of neuronal transmission and the complexity and heterogeneity of schizophrenia symptoms. The *N*-methyl-D-aspartate (NMDA) class of glutamate receptor is being explored because of the actions of phencyclidine (PCP) at these sites and the similarity of the psychotic behaviors that are produced when someone takes PCP (Kandel et al., 2000; Keltner & Folks, 2001). See Figures 18-2 to 18-4.

Psychological Theories

Several psychological frameworks have been used to explain the etiology of schizophrenia. Before new biologic and neurochemical discoveries, these psychological theories, held by the mental health community, viewed the primary cause of schizophrenia to be dysfunctional parenting in early childhood development. Families often were blamed and alienated by mental health professionals. Although these theories are no longer thought valid and have given way to the neurochemical-biologic theories, they are presented here so that the nurse might understand the prejudices, biases, and misunderstandings that once plagued families regarding the origins of schizophrenia.

Psychoanalytic theories hypothesize that schizophrenia originates from frustration or oversatisfaction

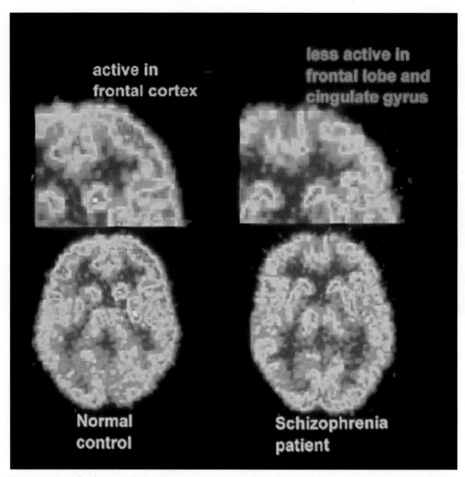

FIGURE 18.4 Position emission tomography scan with 18F-deoxyglucose shows metabolic activity in a horizontal section of the brain in a control subject (*left*) and in an unmedicated patient with schizophrenia (*right*). Red and yellow indicate areas of high metabolic activity in the cortex; green and blue indicate lower activity in the white-matter areas of the brain. The frontal lobe is magnified to show reduced frontal activity in the prefrontal cortex of the patient with schizophrenia (Courtesy of Monte S. Buchsbaum, MD, The Mount Sinai Medical Center and School of Medicine, New York, NY.)

of the infant during the oral stage of development. Anxiety generated by the inability to control basic urges of the id for sexual and aggressive drive satisfaction result in use of some of the most primitive defense mechanisms (eg, regression, projection, and denial). Homosexual panic was considered operational in many patients with schizophrenia who had difficulty controlling sexual drives except with severe psychotic symptoms.

Harry Stack Sullivan, an early pioneer of interpersonal theories of schizophrenia, focused his work on the personality's attempts to organize interpersonal experiences and language development. He accounted for the bizarre language in schizophrenia:

[T]he schizophrenic does not have our pleasant illusions that speech will help him to satisfactions, because he is quite sure there are none. He uses speech exclusively for counteracting his

feeling of insecurity among other people. The schizophrenic's speech shows characteristic peculiarities because of recurrent severe disturbances in his relationships with other people and the result of a confusion of the critical faculties concerning the structure of spoken and written language (Sullivan, 1964, p. 15).

This emphasis on the interpersonal characteristics of disturbances increased the attention by researchers on communication patterns in the family as the origin of mental illness. Bateson and colleagues (1956) proposed a theory of schizophrenia based on communication analysis of families. They believed that many of the speech and thought disturbances resulted from a particular type of family interaction called the "double bind communication" in which the "victim" is the child who repeatedly receives sets of contradictory messages from an adult who is vitally important to the child, to behave in a particular fashion. But the "victim" is confused by the contradictory messages and is unable to escape the situation or comment on the contradictory messages being sent. Hence, the person with schizophrenia tries to cope with these messages by attempting to concoct meaning from them, ignoring them or withdrawing from the world, or responding only to the literal meaning of the messages.

Social Theories

There are no social theories believed to be the cause of schizophrenia, but some theories focus on patterns of family interaction that seem to affect the eventual outcome and social adjustment of individuals with schizophrenia. The theory of **expressed emotion** (EE) correlates certain family communication patterns with an increase in symptoms and relapse in patients with schizophrenia. Families are classified as high-EE families when one or more of the following are exhibited within a 2-hour interview session: (1) six or more critical comments about family members or aspects of speech that connote criticism, (2) hostile and negative remarks about who the patient is, and (3) emotional overinvolvement with the patient, such as overprotectiveness or self-sacrifice. Low-EE families make fewer negative comments and show less overinvolvement with the patient (Mintz et al., 1987, p. 228). Families that rate high in the areas of criticism, hostility, and battles for control are associated with increases in the patient's positive symptoms and relapse. The emotional overinvolvement factor in high-EE families does not seem to correlate as clearly (King & Dixon, 1996; McCarrick, 1996). Because much of the research is correlational, some question whether mental health professionals can conclude that these negative family interactions are truly the cause of increased symptoms and relapse in the patient, or whether the interactions develop in response to coping with a family member who is schizophrenic (Kanter et al., 1987). Although this research might help to understand the impact of negative family interaction on the patient, there are drawbacks to categorizing families in this manner. It might cause professionals to assign blame to families for causing the schizophrenia or to limit the patient's contact with family and thus further alienate families who are so vital to the care and support of the patient.

INTERDISCIPLINARY TREATMENT

The most effective treatment approach for individuals with schizophrenia involves a variety of disciplines, including nursing (both generalist and advanced practice psychiatric nurses), psychiatry, psychology, social work, occupational and recreational therapy, and pastoral counselors. Often, individuals with general education in psychology, sociology, and social work serve as case managers, nursing aids or technicians, and various other supportive roles within both hospital and community treatment agencies. These varied types of professionals and paraprofessionals are necessary because of the complex nature of the symptoms and chronic course of schizophrenia.

Among these professionals, there is considerable overlap of the types of therapeutic interventions they may deliver. Advanced practice nurses may monitor or prescribe psychoactive medications, along with psychiatrists, depending on state nurse practice acts. Individual, group, and family counseling may be performed by advanced practice nurses, psychiatrists, psychologists, certified social workers, and pastoral counselors. Nurses, along with occupational and recreational therapists, can help patients with schizophrenia cope with the disruptions in their day-to-day functioning caused by cognitive and social deficits associated with negative symptoms. Teams of professionals working from all of these perspectives create the best environment for stabilizing and enhancing the lives of people who have schizophrenia.

Unfortunately, the current health care environment creates many barriers to this type of treatment. Community mental health agencies often have inadequate funding to hire all the members of the interdisciplinary team and have huge caseloads to manage. The managed care environment encourages competition for limited reimbursement rather than cooperation among professionals who can provide medication management or supportive and insight therapies to patients and their families. Psychiatric hospitals have shorter lengths of stay and less emphasis on creating a team of staff because of decreasing insurance reimbursement or decreasing state funding (as the insurers of last resort for the chronically and persistently mentally ill).

Despite of these barriers, nurses can play a central role on these multidisciplinary teams because of nursing's emphasis on (a) patients' responses to their illnesses, (b) patients' functional adaptation, and (c) patients' holistic needs, including their physical and psychosocial requirements. Unfortunately, this role is not often realized. As nursing curricula have integrated psychiatric nursing content and minimized contact with patients who have severe mental illness, fewer nurses have selected mental health nursing as a career path, and many avoid caring for severely mentally ill patients. The rewards of contributing to and participating on a multidisciplinary team to care for some of our most profoundly needful patients should not be avoided because of stigmatization within nursing education.

PRIORITY CARE ISSUES

Several special concerns exist when working with people with schizophrenia. About 20% to 50% of people diagnosed with schizophrenia attempt suicide, and 10% commit suicide either as a result of psychosis in acute stages or in response to depression in the chronic phase (De Hert et al., 2001). Suicide assessment always should be done with a person who is experiencing his or her first psychotic episode. In an inpatient unit, patient safety concerns extend to potential aggressive actions toward staff and other patients during episodes of psychoses. A priority in care is antipsychotic therapy.

➡ FAMILY RESPONSE TO DISORDER

Few families have had experience with mental illness to help them deal with the manifestations of schizophrenia. The initial episodes are often accompanied by mixed emotions of disbelief, shock, fear, and care and concern for the family member. Hope that this is an isolated or transient episode may also be present. They may initially try to seek reasons, such as the episode being a reaction to taking illicit drugs or a result of some extraordinary stress or fatigue. They do not know how to comfort their disturbed family member and may even find themselves becoming fearful of his or her behaviors. If the patient is hostile and aggressive toward family members, the family may respond with anger and hostility along with fear. During these episodes, families often find it necessary to call law enforcement to help control the situation.

The initial period of illness for a patient and family who receive a diagnosis of schizophrenia is an extraordinarily difficult one. Families may attempt to deny the severity and chronicity of the illness, try to engage in the activities of their previous lifestyle, and only partially engage in treatment within the mental health system. Often, in the initial phase of treatment, there may be minimal explanation to the patient and family; they may experience extreme confusion, fear, and anxiety. As they gradually learn of the severity of this diagnosis and the long-term care and extensive rehabilitation required, they may feel overwhelmed, angry, and depressed.

The following is one parent's feelings regarding early reactions to the diagnosis of schizophrenia in a child:

> A feeling that was present in the early years of his illness was a profound disbelief that this was really happening to him and to us. As young parents with four children we occasionally worried, like all parents do, about catastrophes that might befall the children: accidents, leukemia, brain tumor. We never thought of schizophrenia. For a long time this sense of disbelief continued, as-

sociated with bewilderment. We did not know what hit us; this could not be happening to him and to us (Willick, 1994, p. 10).

People with schizophrenia marry and have children, just like everyone else.

NURSING MANAGEMENT: HUMAN RESPONSE TO DISORDER

The nursing management of the patient with schizophrenia lasts many years. Different phases of the illness require various nursing interventions. During exacerbation of symptoms, the patient will most likely be hospitalized for stabilization. During periods of relative stability, the nurse helps the patient maintain a therapeutic regimen, develop positive mental health strategies, and cope with the stress of having a severe, chronic illness.

Because of the complexity of this major psychiatric disorder, the nursing management for each domain is discussed separately. In reality, the nursing process steps overlap in all domains. For example, medication management is a direct biologic intervention; however, the effects of medications are seen in psychological functioning as well. In the clinical area, effective nursing management requires an integration of the assessment data from all domains into meaningful interventions. Nursing interventions should cover all aspects of functioning, including biologic, psychological, social, and family functioning. See Nursing Care Plan 18-1 and the Interdisciplinary Treatment Plan that follows.

There are many nursing diagnoses that apply to a person who has developed schizophrenia. This is particularly true given that schizophrenia affects so many aspects of an individual's functioning and that symptoms can be observed in cognitive, emotional, family, social, and physical functioning. The applicable diagnoses can be categorized into the phases in which they are most likely to appear. It is important to note, however, that just because they have been sorted into these categories, they may still represent problems in other phases. It is also important to note that the quieter periods between exacerbations of symptoms are actually very active and important phases for intervention.

Biologic Domain

Biologic Assessment

The following discussion highlights the important assessment areas for people with schizophrenia. Assessment guidelines can be found in Chapters 10 to 12.

Present and Past Health Status and Physical Examination. It is important to conduct a thorough history and physical examination to rule out medical illness or substance abuse that could cause the psychiatric
(text continues on page 355)

NURSING CARE PLAN 18.1
Patient With Schizophrenia

JT is a 19-year-old African American man who was brought to the hospital following his return from college, where he had locked himself in his room for 3 days. He was talking to nonexistent people in a strange language.

His room was covered with small pieces of taped paper with single words on them. His parents immediately made arrangements for him to be hospitalized.

SETTING: PSYCHIATRIC INTENSIVE CARE UNIT

Baseline Assessment: JT is a 6'1", 145-lb young man whose appearance is disheveled. He has not slept for 4 days and appears frightened. He is hypervigilant, pacing, and mumbling to himself. He is vague about past drug use, but his parents do not believe that he has used drugs. He appears to be hallucinating, conversing as if someone is in the room. He is confused and unable to write, speak, or think coherently. He is disoriented to time and place. Lab values are within normal limits except Hgb, 10.2 and Hct, 32. He has not eaten for several days.

Associated Psychiatric Diagnosis	*Medications*

Axis I: Schizophrenia, paranoid
Axis II: None
Axis III: None
Axis IV: Educational problems (failing)
    Social problems (withdrawn from peers)
GAF = Current 25
    Potential?
	Risperidone (Risperdal), 2 mg bid, then titrate
	    to 3 mg if needed.
	Lorazepam (Ativan) 2mg PO or IM for
	    agitation PRN

NURSING DIAGNOSIS 1: DISTURBED THOUGHT PROCESSES

Defining Characteristics	*Related Factors*

Inaccurate interpretation of stimuli
    (people thinking his thoughts)
Cognitive impairment—attention, memory,
    and executive function impairment
Suspiciousness
Hallucinations
	Uncompensated alterations in brain activity

OUTCOMES

Initial	*Long-Term*

Decrease or eliminate hallucinations
Accurate interpretation of environment
    (stop thinking people are thinking his thoughts)
Improvement in cognitive functioning
    (improved attention, memory, executive functioning)
	Use coping strategies to deal with
	    hallucinations or delusions if reappear
	Communicate clearly with others
	Maintain cognitive functioning

INTERVENTIONS

Interventions	*Rationale*	*Ongoing Assessment*
Initiate a nurse–patient relationship by using an accepting, nonjudgmental approach. Be patient.	A therapeutic relationship will provide patient support as he begins to deal with a devastating disorder. Be patient because his brain is not processing information normally.	Determine the extent to which JT is willing to trust and engage in a relationship.
Administer risperidone as prescribed. Observe for effect, side effects, and adverse effects. Begin teaching about the medication and its importance, once symptoms subside.	Risperidone is a D_2 and $5\text{-}HT_{2A}$ antagonist and is indicated for the management of psychotic disorders.	Make sure JT swallows pills. Monitor for relief of positive symptoms and assess side effects, especially extrapyramidal. Monitor BP for orthostatic hypotension and body temperature increase (NMS).

NURSING CARE PLAN 18.1 (Continued)

INTERVENTIONS

Interventions	Rationale	Ongoing Assessment
During hallucinations and delusional thinking, assess significance (is it frightening, voices telling him to hurt himself or others?). Reassure JT that you will keep him safe. (Do not try to convince JT that his hallucinations are not real.) Redirect to the here-and-now.	It is important to understand the context of the hallucinations and delusions to be able to provide the appropriate interventions. By avoiding arguments about the content, the nurse will enhance communication.	Assess the meaning of the hallucination or delusion to the patient. Determine whether he is a danger to himself or others. Determine whether patient can be redirected.
Assess ability for self-care activities.	Disturbed thinking may interfere with JT's ability to carry out ADLs.	Continue to assess. Determine whether patient can manage own self-care.

EVALUATION

Outcomes	Revised Outcomes	Interventions
Hallucinations and delusions began to decrease within 3 days. Is oriented to time, place, and person. Attention and memory improving.	Participate in unit activities according to ITP. Agree to continue to take antipsychotic medication as prescribed.	Encourage attendance at treatment activities. Teach JT about medications. Teach JT about schizophrenia.

NURSING DIAGNOSIS 2: RISK FOR VIOLENCE

Defining Characteristics	Related Factors
Assaultive toward others, self, and environment Presence of pathophysiologic risk factors: delusional thinking	Frightened, secondary to auditory hallucinations and delusional thinking Poor impulse control Dysfunctional communication patterns

OUTCOMES

Initial	Long-Term
Avoid hurting self or assaulting other patients or staff. Decrease agitation and aggression.	Control behavior with assistance from staff and parents.

INTERVENTIONS

Interventions	Rationale	Ongoing Assessment
Acknowledge patient's fear, hallucinations, and delusions. Be genuine and empathetic.	Hallucinations and delusions change an individual's perception of environmental stimuli. Patient who is frightened will respond out of his need to stay safe.	Determine whether patient is able to hear you. Assess his response to your comments and his ability to concentrate on what is being said.
Offer patient choices of maintaining safety: keeping distance from others, medication for relaxation.	By having choices, he will begin to develop a sense of control over his behavior.	Observe patient's nonverbal communication for evidence of increase agitation.
Administer Lorazepam 2 mg for agitation. Oral route is preferable over injection.	Exact mechanisms of action are not understood, but medication is believed to potentiate the inhibitory neurotransmitter γ-aminobutyric acid, relieving anxiety and producing sedation.	Observe for decrease in agitated behavior.

(continued)

NURSING CARE PLAN 18.1 (Continued)

EVALUATION

Outcomes	Revised Outcomes	Interventions
JT gradually decreased agitated behavior. Lorazepam was given regularly for first 2 days.	Demonstrate control of behavior by resisting hallucinations and delusions.	Teach JT about the effects of hallucinations and delusions. Problem solve ways of controlling hallucinations if they occur. Emphasize the importance of taking medications.

INTERDISCIPLINARY TREATMENT PLAN 18.1
Patient With Schizophrenia

Admission Date:	Date of This Plan:	Type of Plan: Check Appropriate Box					
		☐ Initial	☐ Master	☐ 30	☐ 60	☐ 90	☐ Other

Treatment Team Present:
A. Barton, MD; J. Jones, RNC; C. Anderson, CNS; B. Thomas, PhD; T. Toon, Mental Health Technician (MHT); J. Barker, MHT.

DIAGNOSIS (*DSM-IV-TR*):

AXIS I: Schizophrenia, paranoid
AXIS II: None
AXIS III: None
AXIS IV: Educational problems (failing)
           Social problems (withdrawn from peers)
AXIS V: Current GAF:
           Highest-Level GAF This Past Year: 90

ASSETS (MEDICAL, PSYCHOLOGICAL, SOCIAL, EDUCATIONAL, VOCATIONAL, RECREATIONAL):

1. First episode of psychosis. No evidence of drug use.
2. Premorbid functional level appears to be normal.
3. Maintained good grades in high school.
4. Has supportive family members.

Prob. No.	Date	Problem	Code	Change Code	Date
1	3/5/01	Is hallucinating and had delusional thoughts. Unable to communicate with parents or staff.		T	
2	3/5/01	Is aggressive and is hitting out at staff and unfamiliar people.		T	
3	3/5/01	Dropped out of college because of thoughts and behaviors.		X	
4	3/5/01	Family members are very upset about their son's psychiatric symptoms.		T	

CODE T = Problem must be addressed in treatment.
        N = Problem noted and will be monitored.
        X = Problem noted, but deferred/inactive/no action necessary.
        O = Problem to be addressed in aftercare/continuing care.
        I = Problem incorporated into another problem.
        R = Resolved.

INDIVIDUAL TREATMENT PLAN PROBLEM SHEET

#1 Problem/Need:	Date Identified	Problem Resolved/Discontinuation Date
	3/5/01	

Is hallucinating and has delusional thoughts. Unable to communicate with parents or staff.

Objective(s)/Short-Term Goals:	Target Date	Achievement Date
1. Reduce report and observations of hallucinations and delusions.	3/15/01	

Treatment Interventions:	Frequency	Person Responsible
1. Antipsychotic therapy for hallucinations and delusions. Administer and monitor for adherence, effect, and side effects.	As prescribed	MD/RN
2. Monitor frequency of hallucinations and delusions.	Close observation for 24–48 hours, then according to RN judgment	RN/MHT
3. Attend Symptom Management group as symptoms subside.	Daily	PhD, RN

#2 Problem/Need:	Date Identified	Problem Resolved/Discontinuation Date
	3/5/01	

Is aggressive and is hitting out at staff and unfamiliar people.

Objective(s)/Short-Term Goals:	Target Date	Achievement Date
1. De-escalate aggressive behavior.	3/15/01	

Treatment Interventions:	Frequency	Person Responsible
1. Keep patient in a quiet, nonstimulating environment. Assign private room.	Ongoing	RN
2. Administer antianxiety medication as needed.	PRN	MD/RN
3. Use de-escalation techniques when approaching patient.	Ongoing	Everyone
4. Assign to anger management group if needed when psychotic symptoms decrease.	In 1 week	CNS

#3 Problem/Need:	Date Identified	Problem Resolved/Discontinuation Date
	3/5/01	

Family members are very upset about their son's psychiatric symptoms.

Objective(s)/Short-Term Goals:	Target Date	Achievement Date
Increase family's comfort levels with mental illness.	3/15/01	

Treatment Interventions:	Frequency	Person Responsible
1. Meet with family each time they visit. Provide counseling and education to family.	Ongoing	CNS/RN/MD/PhD
2. Encourage to attend family support group.	Weekly	PhD
3. Provide community resources for the treatment of mental illness.	When visiting	CNS

Responsible QMHP   **Client or Guardian**   **Staff Physician**

Signature   Date   Signature   Date   Signature   Date

symptoms. It is also important to screen for comorbid medical illnesses that need to be treated. The presence or family history of diabetes mellitus, hypertension, and cardiac disease should be identified. People with schizophrenia have a higher mortality rate from physical illness and often have smoking-related illnesses, such as emphysema, and other pulmonary and cardiac problems. The nurse should determine whether the patient smokes or chews tobacco, which not only affects the patient's health but also can affect the clearance of medications.

Physical Functioning. The negative symptoms of schizophrenia are often manifested in terms of impairment in physical functioning. Self-care often deteriorates, and sleep may be nonexistent during acute phases. Information regarding physical functioning may best be collected from family members.

Nutritional Assessment. A nutritional history should be completed to determine baseline eating habits and preferences. Medications can alter normal nutrition, and the patient may need to limit calories or fat consumption.

Fluid Imbalance Assessment. The nurse should remain alert for signs of polydipsia and polyuria in order to identify patients with disordered water balance. Patients with these symptoms make frequent trips to the water fountain or display other excessive water-drinking behaviors; their excessive water intake may cause them to become disoriented, confused, or agitated. Polydipsia is difficult to detect in patients who do not drink fluid more often than normal but simply consume large volumes (Boyd & Lapierre, 1996).

Patients who are thought to have disordered water balance should be assessed for signs and symptoms of hyponatremia, water intoxication, excessive urination, incontinence, or periodically elevated blood pressure. Signs and symptoms of hypervolemia that may be evident include puffiness of the face or eyes, abdominal distention, and hypothermia (Snider & Boyd, 1991). Also, patients who are suspected of having disordered water balance should be weighed daily, and their urine specific gravity and serum sodium levels should be monitored.

Pharmacologic Assessment. Baseline information about initial psychological and physical functioning should be obtained before initiation of medication (or as early as possible). Side effects of medications should be assessed. Patients are often physically awkward and have poor coordination, motor abnormalities, and abnormalities in eye tracking. Before medications are begun, standardized assessment of abnormal motor movements should be conducted using one of several assessment tools designed for that purpose, such as the Abnormal Involuntary Movement Scale (AIMS) (see Appendix I) (Guy, 1976), the Dyskinesia Identification System (DISCUS) (Sprague & Kalachnik, 1991) (Table 18-4), or the Simpson-Angus Rating Scale (Appendix H) (Simpson & Angus, 1970), which is designed for Parkinson's symptoms.

Nursing Diagnoses Related to Biologic Domain

Typical nursing diagnoses focusing on the biologic domain for the person with phases of schizophrenia include Self-Care Deficit and Disturbed Sleep Pat-

TABLE 18.4 The Dyskinesia Identification System (DISCUS)

NAME		I.D.

_____
(facility)

Dyskinesia Identification System:
Condensed User Scale (DISCUS)

CURRENT PSYCHOTROPICS/ANTI-
CHOLINERGIC AND TOTAL MG/DAY

_____ _____ mg

_____ _____ mg

_____ _____ mg

_____ _____ mg

See Instructions on Other Side

EXAM TYPE (check one)
☐ 1. Baseline
☐ 2. Annual
☐ 3. Semi annual
☐ 4. D/C—1 mo
☐ 5. D/C—2 mo
☐ 6. D/C—3 mo
☐ 7. Admission
☐ 8. Other

COOPERATION (check one)
☐ 1. None
☐ 2. Partial
☐ 3. Full

SCORING
0—**Not Present** (movements not observed or some movements observed but not considered abnormal)
1—**Minimal** (abnormal movements are difficult to detect or movements are easy to detect but occur only once or twice in a short non-repetitive manner)
2—**Mild** (abnormal movements occur infrequently and are easy to detect)
3—**Moderate** (abnormal movements occur frequently and are easy to detect)
4—**Severe** (abnormal movements occur almost continuously **and** are easy to detect)
NA—**Not assessed** (an assessment for an item is not able to be made)

ASSESSMENT
DISCUS Item and Score (circle one score for each item)

FACE
1. Tics . . . . 0 1 2 3 4 NA
2. Grimaces . . . . 0 1 2 3 4 NA

EYES
3. Blinking . . . . 0 1 2 3 4 NA

ORAL
4. Chewing/Lip Smacking . . . . 0 1 2 3 4 NA
5. Puckering/Sucking/Thrusting Lower Lip . . . . . . 0 1 2 3 4 NA

LINGUAL
6. Tongue Thrusting/Tongue in Cheek . . . . 0 1 2 3 4 NA
7. Tonic Tongue . . . . 0 1 2 3 4 NA
8. Tongue Tremor . . . . 0 1 2 3 4 NA
9. Athetoid/Myokymic/Lateral Tongue . . . . 0 1 2 3 4 NA

HEAD/NECK/TRUNK
10. Retrocollis/Torticollis . . . . . 0 1 2 3 4 NA
11. Shoulder/Hip Torsion . . . . . 0 1 2 3 4 NA

UPPER LIMB
12. Athetoid/Myokymic Finger–Wrist–Arm . . . . 0 1 2 3 4 NA
13. Pill Rolling . . . . 0 1 2 3 4 NA

LOWER LIMB
14. Ankle Flexion/Foot Tapping . . . . 0 1 2 3 4 NA
15. Toe Movement . . . . 0 1 2 3 4 NA

COMMENTS/OTHER

TOTAL SCORE (items 1–15 only)

EXAM DATE

EVALUATION (see other side)

1. Greater than 90 days neuroleptic exposure? : YES NO
2. Scoring/intensity level met? : YES NO
3. Other diagnostic conditions? : YES NO (if yes, specify)

4. Last exam date: _____
   Last total score: _____
   Last conclusion: _____

Preparer signature and title for items 1–4 (if different from physician):

5. Conclusion (circle one):
A. No TD (if scoring prerequisite met, list other diagnostic condition or explain in comments)
B. Probable TD
C. Masked TD
D. Withdrawal TD
E. Persistent TD
F. Remitted TD
G. Other (specify in comments)

6. Comments:

RATER SIGNATURE AND TITLE	NET EXAM DATE	CLINICIAN SIGNATURE	DATE

From Sprague, R. L., & Kalachnik, J. E. (1991). Reliability, validity, and a total score cutoff for the Dyskinesia Identification System, Condensed User Scale (DISCUS) with mentally ill and mentally retarded populations. *Psychopharmacology Bulletin, 27*(1), 51–58.

tern. During the relapse phase, Ineffective Therapeutic Regimen Management, Imbalanced Nutrition, Excess Fluid Volume, and Sexual Dysfunction are possible diagnoses. Constipation may occur if taking anticholinergic medications.

Biologic Interventions

Nursing interventions during the initial acute phase of schizophrenia include prompt, safe, and informed administration of antipsychotic medications. During any stage, attention to self-care needs and the patient's ability to maintain hygiene and adequate nutrition are important.

Promotion of Self-Care Activities. For many with schizophrenia, the plan of care will include specific interventions to enhance self-care, nutrition, and overall health knowledge. Because of the negative symptoms, patients are often unable to initiate these seemingly simple activities. Developing a daily schedule of routine activities (showering, shaving, and so forth) can help the patient structure the day. Most patients actually know how to perform self-care activities (eg, hygiene, grooming) but are not motivated (avolition) to carry them out consistently. Interventions include developing a schedule with the patient regarding times for various hygiene activities and emphasizing the importance of maintaining appropriate self-care activities. Given the problems related to attention and memory in people with schizophrenia, education about these areas requires careful planning.

Activity, Exercise, and Nutritional Interventions. Encouraging activity and exercise is necessary, not only to maintain a healthy lifestyle, but also to counteract the side effects of those psychiatric medications that cause weight gain. Because the diagnosis is usually made in late adolescence or early adulthood, it is possible to establish a solid exercise patterns early on.

During episodes of acute psychosis, patients are unable to focus on eating. When patients begin antipsychotic medication, these normal satiety and hunger responses are often changed, and overeating or weight gain can become a problem. Promoting healthy nutrition is a key intervention. Maintaining healthy nutrition and monitoring calorie intake also becomes important because of the effect many medications have on changing eating habits. Patients report that appetite increases and cravings for food develop when some medications are initiated.

Thermoregulation Interventions. Patients with schizophrenia may have disturbed body regulation. In winter, they may seem to be oblivious to cold weather. In the heat of summer, they may dress for winter. Observing patients' responses to temperatures helps in identifying problems in this area. In patients who are taking psychiatric medications, body temperature needs to be monitored, and the patient need to be protected from extremes in temperature.

Promotion of Normal Fluid Balance and Prevention of Water Intoxication. It is possible to help patients who are at risk for fluid imbalance to regulate fluid intake by teaching about disordered water balance and assisting in developing self-monitoring skills (fluid intake and weight gain) as a way of controlling fluid intake (Boyd, 1995). When both measures are instituted, the potential for the development of water intoxication is greatly reduced.

The signs and symptoms of disordered water balance can be classified as mild, moderate, or severe (Snider & Boyd, 1991) (see Text Box 18-3). Patients with mild disordered water balance benefit from teaching interventions aimed at helping them monitor and control their fluid intake. These patients may be successfully managed in outpatient settings or general inpatient psychiatric units. They benefit from educational programs about their disorder and can be successfully taught to monitor their own urine specific gravity and daily weight gains.

Although patients with moderate disordered water balance are less able to control their fluid intake than those with a milder disorder, they respond positively to teaching. The use of a targeted weight procedure is helpful with these patients (Boyd et al., 1992; Boyd & Lapierre, 1996; Delva & Cramer, 1988). This procedure entails establishing a baseline weight for the patient, calculating the patient's target weight, and weighing the patient throughout the day (see Text Box 18-5). Patients are taught that gaining 5 to 7 lb in 2 to 3 hours indicates that they have taken in too much fluid. Patients who reach their designated target weight should be observed closely and have their fluids restricted. Patients who exceed their targeted weight could develop water intoxication (Boyd & Lapierre, 1996).

Patients with severe disordered water balance who continually try to "sneak fluids" are at high risk for water intoxication. These patients are unable to control their drive to drink fluids and may even become combative if their access to water is denied. The goal of nursing care of these patients is to restrict their fluid intake (Boyd & Lapierre, 1996; Snider & Boyd, 1991). Their continual water-seeking behavior create considerable disruption in inpatient treatment settings and is challenging for nursing staff members. By placing these patients under continuous one-on-one observation, nursing staff may be able to redirect their fluid seeking behavior. For more information, see Research Box 18-2.

TEXT BOX 18.5

Water Intoxication Protocol

I. Observation: evidence of polydipsia and polyuria

II. Assessment of fluid balance

   A. History of polydipsia and polyuria

   B. Presence of hyponatremia:
      serum Na$^+$ >135 mEq/L

   C. Hyposthenuria: urine specific gravity <1.005

III. Interventions:

   A. If the above symptoms are present, the following
      interventions should be instituted.

     1. Target weight procedure

     2. Daily assessment of behavioral changes

     3. Monitor urine specific gravity daily

     4. Identify specific interventions for helping
        patient develop control over fluid intake and
        learn self-monitoring skills

       a. Cognitive therapy approaches

       b. Individual or group therapy approaches

       c. Arrange access to sugarless candies, gum,
          and fruit to reduce feelings of thirst

       d. Limit access to fluids during the day

   B. If weight equal to or greater than patient's target
      weight, the following should be initiated:

     1. Prohibit fluid intake

     2. Restrict to program and residential area

     3. Assess vital signs q1h × 2

     4. Provide low-fluid diet after symptoms subside

   C. If more severe symptoms develop, notify physician
      and transfer to a medical unit.

IV. Evaluation

   A. Patient gains control over fluid balance as evi-
      denced by developing strategies to stay under
      target weight.

   B. If there is no evidence of water intoxication and
      there is evidence that patient is gaining control
      over fluid balance, the target weight procedure
      and daily assessments of behavior and urine
      specific gravity can be discontinued.

Pharmacologic Interventions. Early in the 20th century, somatic treatment of schizophrenia included treatments such as hydrotherapy (baths), wet-pack sheets, insulin shock therapy, electroconvulsive therapy, psychosurgery, and even occupational and physical therapy. But in the early 1950s, treatment of schizophrenia drastically changed with the accidental discovery that a drug, chlorpromazine, used for anesthesia induction also caused calming in patients with schizophrenia. Optimism persists as older medications continue to be used effectively while offering clues into the workings of the brain and as new discoveries about the brain have led to more precise medications for treating schizophrenia.

Antipsychotic drugs have the general effect of blocking dopamine transmission in the brain by blocking D$_2$ receptors to some degree (see Chap. 8). Some also block other dopamine receptors and receptors of other neurotransmitters to varying degrees. For the most part, the antidopamine effects are not specific to the mesolimbic and mesocortical tracts associated with schizophrenia, but instead travel to all the dopamine receptor sites

RESEARCH BOX 18.2

Disordered Water Balance

The St. Louis Target Weight Procedure (STWP) was developed to help patients with disordered water balance control their fluid intake. It required the establishment of baseline and target weights and monitoring weight throughout the day. The baseline weight was determined as an early morning weight before dressing, after voiding, and before any oral intake. The target weight was calculated to be 105% of the baseline weight. The purpose of this study was to determine whether the STWP was useful in controlling hyponatremia. Patients with disordered water balance were weighed throughout the day; when their target weight was elevated, fluids were restricted.

Thirty subjects hospitalized in a long-term care facility who met the criteria for disordered water balance volunteered for the 6-week study. The subjects were randomly assigned to one of two groups. Urine specific gravities served as the dependent variable and were collected daily at 4:00 PM. It was reasoned that urine specific gravities would approach normal if fluid balance was normalized. Baseline data on both groups were collected for the first 3 weeks. During weeks 4 through 6, the STWP was used for the treatment group. This group was weighed throughout the day and was restricted from drinking when their target weight was reached. The other group served as a control. The results of the study showed that the STWP group significantly increased its urine specific gravities, thus improving fluid balance. These findings demonstrated the clinical utility of the STWP.

Utilization in the Clinical Setting: A nurse working in a long-term psychiatric setting used the results of this study to introduce a target weight procedure as a new nursing intervention for patients with water intoxication or fluid imbalance. The procedure was modified for use in this particular institution and was piloted on one unit before being introduced to the whole hospital.

Boyd, M., Williams, L., Evenson, R., et al. (1992). Target weight procedure for disordered water balance in long term care facilities. *Journal of Psychosocial Nursing, 30*(12), 22–27.

throughout the brain. This results in desirable antipsychotic effects but also creates some unpleasant and undesirable side effects. Additional side effects are accounted for by the effects of these drugs on other neurotransmitter systems.

The newer antipsychotic drugs risperidone (Risperdal) (see Drug Profile: Risperidone), olanzapine (Zyprexa), quetiapine (Seroquel), and ziprasidone (Geodon) appear to be more efficacious and safer than conventional antipsychotics. They are effective in treating negative symptoms as well as positive. These newer drugs also affect several other neurotransmitter systems, including serotonin. This is believed to contribute to their antipsychotic effectiveness (see Chap. 8).

Monitoring and Administering Medications. Antipsychotic medications are the treatment of choice for patients with psychosis. The use of conventional antipsychotics (eg, haloperidol, thioridazine) has dramatically decreased with the introduction of the second-generation of antipsychotics. Generally, it takes about 1 to 2 weeks to begin to effect change in symptoms. During the stabilization period, the type of drug selected should be given an adequate trial, generally 6 to 12 weeks, before considering a change in the drug prescription. If treatment effects are not seen, another antipsychotic may be tried. Clozaril may be initiated in instances in which no other atypical antipsychotic is effective (see Drug Profile: Clozapine).

Adherence to a prescribed medication regime is the best approach to prevention of relapse. When conventional antipsychotics were the only treatment options, patients would often stop taking their medication because of the side effects. With the atypical antipsychotics, discontinuation of medication is not as likely. In those instances in which patients cannot take or refuse to take daily oral medications. For these individuals long-acting antipsychotic decanoates, such as haloperidol decanoate, may be more suitable. To date, no atypical antipsychotic is manufactured in decanoate form.

In the past, patients were stabilized on medications before discharge from the hospital. In these days of managed care, even state and veterans' facilities are discharging patients before a judgment can be made about the efficacy of a given drug treatment. It is incumbent on nurses and other mental health professionals to ensure continuation of these stabilization protocols and to ensure that outpatient caregivers assume responsibility for maintaining this stabilization phase of treatment and continue to monitor and manage the patient's symptoms. Outpatient systems should avoid the immediate manipulation of dosages and drugs during the stabilization phase unless a medical emergency ensues.

Generally, patients with schizophrenia face a lifetime of taking antipsychotic medications. Rarely is discontinuation of medications prescribed; however, many

---

DRUG PROFILE: Risperidone
(Atypical Antipsychotic Agent)
Trade Name: Risperdal

Receptor affinity: Antagonist with high affinity for D_2 and $5-HT_2$, also histamine (H_1), and α_1-, α_2-adrenergic receptors, weak affinity for D_1 and other serotonin receptor subtypes; no affinity for acetylcholine or β-adrenergic receptors.

Indications: Psychotic disorders, such as schizophrenia, schizoaffective illness, bipolar affective disorder, and major depression with psychotic features.

Routes and dosage: 1-, 2-, 3-, and 4-mg tablets and liquid concentrate (1 mg/mL).

Adult: Initial dose: typically 1 mg bid. Maximal effect at 6 mg/d. Safety not established above 16 mg/d. Use lowest possible dose to alleviate symptoms.

Geriatric: Initial dose, 0.5 mg/d, increase slowly as tolerated.

Children: Safety and efficacy with this age group have not been established.

Half-life (peak effect): mean, 20 h (1 h, peak active metabolite = 3–17 h).

Select adverse reactions: Insomnia, agitation, anxiety, extrapyramidal symptoms, headache, rhinitis, somnolence, dizziness, headache, constipation, nausea, dyspepsia, vomiting, abdominal pain, hypersalivation, tachycardia, orthostatic hypotension, fever, chest pain, coughing, photosensitivity, weight gain.

Warning: Rare development of neuroleptic malignant syndrome. Observe frequently for early signs of tardive dyskinesia. Use caution with individuals who have cardiovascular disease; risperidone can cause ECG changes. Avoid use during pregnancy or while nursing. Hepatic or renal impairments increase plasma concentration.

Specific patient/family education:

- Notify prescriber if tremor, motor restlessness, abnormal movements, chest pain, or other unusual symptoms develop.
- Avoid alcohol and other CNS depressant drugs.
- Notify prescriber if pregnancy is possible or planning to become pregnant. Do not breast-feed while taking this medication.
- Notify prescriber before taking any other prescription or OTC medication.
- May impair judgment, thinking, or motor skills; avoid driving or other hazardous tasks.
- During titration, the individual may experience orthostatic hypotension and should change positions slowly.
- Do not abruptly discontinue.

DRUG PROFILE: Clozapine
(Atypical Antipsychotic Agent)
Trade Name: Clozaril

Receptor affinity: D_1 and D_2 blockade, antagonist for 5-HT$_2$, histamine (H$_1$), α-adrenergic, and acetylcholine. These additional antagonist effects may contribute to some of its therapeutic effects. Produces fewer extrapyramidal effects than standard antipsychotics with lower risk for tardive dyskinesia.
Indications: Severely Ill individuals who have schizophrenia and have not responded to standard antipsychotic treatment. Unlabeled use for other psychotic disorders, such as schizoaffective disorder and bipolar affective disorder.
Routes and dosage: Available only in tablet form, 25- and 100-mg doses.
Adult Dosage: Initial dose 25 mg PO bid or qid, may gradually increase in 25–50 mg/d increments, if tolerated, to a dose of 300–450 mg/d by the end of the second week. Additional increases should occur no more than once or twice weekly. Do not exceed 900 mg/d. For maintenance, reduce dosage to lowest effective level.
Children: Safety and efficacy with children under 16 years have not been established.
Half-life (peak effect): 12 h (1–6 h).
Select adverse reactions: Drowsiness, dizziness, headache, hypersalivation, tachycardia, hypo/hypertension, constipation, dry mouth, heartburn, nausea/vomiting, blurred vision, diaphoresis, fever, weight gain, hematologic changes, seizures, tremor, akathisia.
Warning: Agranulocytosis, defined as a granulocyte count of <500 mm^3 occurs at about a cumulative 1-year incidence of 1.3%, most often with 4–10 weeks of exposure, but may occur at any time. Required registration with the clozapine *Patient Management System,* a WBC count before initiation, and weekly WBC counts while taking the drug and for 4 weeks after discontinuation. Rare development of neuroleptic malignant syndrome. No confirmed cases of tardive dyskinesia, but remains a possibility increased seizure risk at higher doses. Use caution with individuals who have cardiovascular disease; clozapine can cause ECG changes. Cases of sudden, unexplained death have been reported. Avoid use during pregnancy or while nursing.
Specific patient/family education:
- Need informed consent regarding risk for agranulocytosis. Weekly blood draws are required. Notify prescriber immediately if lethargy, weakness, sore throat, malaise, or other flu-like symptoms develop.
- Notify prescriber if pregnancy is possible or planning to become pregnant. Do not breast-feed while taking this medication.
- Notify prescriber before taking any other prescription or OTC medication. Avoid alcohol or other CNS depressant drugs.
- May cause drowsiness and seizures; avoid driving or other hazardous tasks.
- During titration, the individual may experience orthostatic hypotension and should change positions slowly.
- Do not abruptly discontinue.

patients stop taking medications on their own. Some situations require stopping medications, such as after neuroleptic malignant syndrome (see later) when medications must be stopped either permanently or for a circumscribed period or when agranulocytosis develops. Discontinuation is an option when tardive dyskinesia develops. Discontinuation of medications, other than in circumstances of a medical emergency, should be achieved by gradually lowering the dose over time. This diminishes the likelihood of withdrawal symptoms, which include withdrawal dyskinesias and withdrawal psychosis.

Monitoring Side Effects

Extrapyramidal Side Effects. Parkinsonism that is caused by antipsychotic drugs is identical in appearance to Parkinson's disease and tends to occur in older patients. The symptoms are believed to be caused by the blockade of D_2 receptors in the basal ganglia, which throws off the normal balance between acetylcholine and dopamine in this area of the brain and effectively increases acetylcholine. These symptoms are managed by reestablishing the balance between acetylcholine and dopamine by reducing the dosage of the antipsychotic (increasing dopamine activity) or adding an anticholinergic drug (decrease acetylcholine activity), such as benztropine (Cogentin) or trihexyphenidyl (Artane). Discontinuation of anticholinergic drugs should never be

abrupt, which can cause a cholinergic rebound and result in a variety of withdrawal symptoms including vomiting, excessive sweating, and altered dreams and nightmares. Hence, anticholinergic drugs should be tapered over several days. If a patient develops akathisia, the use of an anticholinergic medication will only worsen the akathisia. Table 18-5 lists anticholinergic side effects and interventions to manage them.

Dystonic reactions are also believed to result from the imbalance of dopamine and acetylcholine, with the latter dominant. Young men seem to be more vulnerable to this particular extrapyramidal side effect. Generally, this side effect develops rapidly and dramatically. It can be very frightening for patients as their muscles tense and their body becomes contorted. Often, the experience starts with **oculogyric crisis,** in which the muscles that control eye movements tense and pull the eyeball so that the patient is looking toward the ceiling. This may be followed rapidly by **torticollis,** in which the neck muscles pull the head to the side, or **retrocollis,** in which the head is pulled back, or orolaryngeal-pharyngeal hypertonus, in which the patient has extreme difficulty swallowing (Casey, 1994). The patient may also experience contorted extremities. These symptoms occur early in antipsychotic drug treatment when the patient may still be experiencing psychotic symptoms. This com-

TABLE 18.5	Nursing Interventions for Anticholinergic Side Effects of Antipsychotic Drugs
Effect	**Intervention**
Dry mouth	Sips of water; hard candies and chewing gum (preferably sugar free)
Blurred vision	Avoid dangerous tasks; teach patient that this side effect will diminish in a few weeks
Decreased lacrimation	Artificial tears if necessary
Mydriasis	May aggravate glaucoma; teach patient to report eye pain
Photophobia	Sunglasses
Constipation	High-fiber diet; increased fluid intake; laxatives as prescribed
Urinary hesitancy	Privacy; run water in sink; warm water over perineum
Urinary retention	Regular voiding (at least every 2–3 h) and whenever urge is present; catheterize for residual; record intake and output; evaluate benign prostatic hypertrophy
Tachycardia	Evaluate for pre-existing cardiovascular disease; sudden death has occurred with thioridazine (Mellaril)

pounds the patient's fear and anxiety and requires a quick response. The immediate treatment is to administer benztropine, 1 to 2 mg, or diphenhydramine (Benadryl), 25 to 50 mg, intramuscularly or intravenously. This is followed by daily anticholinergic drugs and, possibly, by a decrease in antipsychotic medication (see Drug Profile: Benztropine Mesylate).

Akathisia is motor restlessness that appears to be caused by the same biologic mechanism as other extrapyramidal side effects. Patients display restlessness and complain of an internal sense of feeling almost driven to keep moving. They are very uncomfortable. Frequently, this response is misinterpreted as anxiety or increased psychotic symptoms, and the patient may be inappropriately given increased dosages of antipsychotic drug, which only perpetuates this side effect. If possible, the dose of antipsychotic drug should be reduced. A β-adrenergic blocker such as propranolol (Inderal), 20 to 120 mg, may be required.

Tardive dyskinesia (impairment of voluntary movement, resulting in fragmented or incomplete movements), tardive dystonia, or tardive akathisia are less likely to appear in individuals taking atypical than conventional antipsychotics. Table 18-6 describes theses as well as associated motor abnormalities. Tardive dyskinesia is late-appearing abnormal involuntary movements (dyskinesia). It can be viewed as the opposite of parkinsonism both in observable movements and in etiology. Whereas in parkinsonism there is muscle rigidity and absence of movement, in tardive dyskinesia, there is almost constant movement. The characteristic movements are in the mouth, tongue, and jaw and include lip smacking, sucking, puckering, tongue protrusion, the bon-bon sign (where the tongue rolls around in the mouth and protrudes into the cheek as if the patient were sucking on a piece of hard candy), athetoid (worm-like) movements in the tongue, and chewing. Other facial movements, such as grimacing and eye blinking, may be present. Movements in the trunk and limb are frequently observable. These include rocking from the hips, athetoid movements of the fingers and toes, jerking movements of the fingers and toes, guitar strumming movements of the fingers, and foot tapping. The long-term health problems for people with tardive dyskinesia are choking because of loss of control of muscles responsible for swallowing and compromised respiratory functioning leading to infections and possibly respiratory alkalosis.

In etiology, because the movements resemble the dyskinetic movements of some patients with idiopathic Parkinson's disease who have received long-term treatment with L-dopa (a direct-acting dopamine agonist that crosses the blood–brain barrier), the suggested hypothesis for tardive dyskinesia includes the overactivity of dopamine in the basal ganglia. Although this hypothetical cause is not entirely satisfactory, the suggestion is that after long-term (months to years) treatment with antipsychotic drugs, the receptor side of the synapse up-regulates and creates more receptor sites to compensate for the antipsychotic drug's blockade of dopamine. When patients become tolerant to the dose of drug, have a smaller dose prescribed, or discontinue the drug (either by prescription or by nonadherence), the supersensitive dopamine neurons display a relative overactivity of dopaminergic transmission in comparison to cholinergic transmission in the basal ganglia. Thus, the characteristic movements become evident only after some time has passed, at least 3 to 6 months

DRUG PROFILE: Benztropine Mesylate
(Antiparkinson Agent [anticholinergic])
Trade Name: Cogentin and various generic formulations

Receptor affinity: Blocks cholinergic (acetylcholine) activity, which is believed to restore acetylcholine/dopamine imbalance in the basal ganglia.

Indications: Used in psychiatry to reduce extrapyramidal symptoms (acute medication-related movement disorders), including pseudoparkinsonism, dystonia, and akathisia (not tardive syndromes) due to neuroleptic drugs such as haloperidol. Most effective with acute dystonia.

Routes and dosage: Available in tablet form, 0.5-, 1-, and 2-mg doses, also injectable 1 mg/mL.

Adult Dosage: For acute dystonia, 1–2 mg IM or IV usually provides rapid relief. No significant difference in onset of action after IM or IV injection. Treatment emergent symptoms may be relieved in 1 or 2 days, with 1–2 mg orally 2–3 times/d. Maximum daily dose is 6 mg/d. After 1–2 weeks withdraw drug to see if continued treatment is needed. Medication-related movement disorders that develop slowly may not respond to this treatment.

Geriatric: Older adults and very thin patients cannot tolerate large doses.

Children: Do not use in children under 3. Use with caution in older children.

Half-life: 12–24 h, very little pharmacokinetic information is available.

Select adverse reactions: Dry mouth, blurred vision, tachycardia, nausea, constipation, flushing or elevated temperature, decreased sweating, muscular weakness or cramping, urinary retention, urinary hesitancy, dizziness, headache, disorientation, confusion, memory loss, hallucinations, psychoses, and agitation in toxic reactions, which are more pronounced in the elderly and occur at smaller doses.

Warning: Avoid use during pregnancy or while breast-feeding. Give with caution in hot weather due to possible heatstroke. Contraindicated with angle-closure glaucoma, pyloric or duodenal obstruction, stenosing peptic ulcers, prostatic hypertrophy or bladder neck obstructions myasthenia gravis, megacolon, or megaesophagus. May aggravate the symptoms of tardive dyskinesia or other chronic forms of medication-related movement disorder. Concomitant use of other anticholinergic drugs may increase side effects and risk for toxicity. Coadministration of haloperidol or phenothiazines may reduce serum levels of these drugs.

Specific patient/family education:
- Take with meals to reduce dry mouth and gastric irritation.
- Dry mouth may be alleviated by sucking sugarless candies, adequate fluid intake, or good oral hygiene, increase fiber and fluids in diet to avoid constipation, stool softeners may be required. Notify prescriber if urinary hesitancy or constipation persists.
- Notify prescriber if rapid or pounding heartbeat, confusion, eye pain, rash, or other adverse symptoms develop.
- May cause drowsiness, dizziness, or blurred vision; use caution driving or performing other hazardous tasks requiring alertness. Avoid alcohol and other CNS depressants.
- Do not abruptly stop this medication because a flu-like syndrome may develop.
- Use caution in hot weather. Ensure adequate hydration. May increase susceptibility to heat stroke.

TABLE 18.6   Extrapyramidal Side Effects of Antipsychotic Drugs

Side Effect	Period of Onset	Symptoms
Acute Motor Abnormalities		
Parkinsonism or pseudoparkinsonism	5–30 d	Resting tremor, rigidity, bradykinesia/akinesia, mask-like face, shuffling gait, decreased arm swing
Acute dystonia	1–5 d	Intermittent or fixed abnormal postures of the eyes, face, tongue, neck, trunk, and extremities
Akathisia	1–30 d	Obvious motor restlessness evidenced by pacing, rocking, shifting from foot to foot; subjective sense of not being able to sit or be still; these symptoms may occur together or separately
Late-Appearing Motor Abnormalities		
Tardive dyskinesia	Months to years	Abnormal dyskinetic movements of the face, mouth, and jaw; choreothetoid movements of the legs, arms, and trunk
Tardive dystonia	Months to years	Persistent sustained abnormal postures in the face, eyes, tongue, neck, trunk, and limbs
Tardive akathisia	Months to years	Persisting, unabating sense of subjective and objective restlessness

Adapted from Casey, D. E. (1994). Schizophrenia: Psychopharmacology. In J. W. Jefferson & J. H. Greist (Eds.), *The Psychiatric Clinics of North America Annual of Drug Therapy* (Vol. 1, pp. 81–100). Philadelphia: W. B. Saunders.

and often years. The only patient factors that have been associated with tardive dyskinesia are increased age, female gender, and amount of antipsychotic drug received over time.

There is no consistently effective treatment; however, antipsychotic drugs mask the movements of tardive dyskinesia and have periodically been suggested as a treatment. This is counterintuitive because these are the drugs that cause the disorder. Newer antipsychotic drugs, such as clozapine, may be less likely to cause the disorder. The best management, however, remains prevention through prescription of the lowest possible dose of antipsychotic drug over time that minimizes the symptoms of schizophrenia, prescription of these drugs for psychotic symptoms only, and early case finding by regular systematic screening of everyone receiving these drugs.

Orthostatic hypotension is another side effect of antipsychotic drugs. The primary antiadrenergic effect is decreased blood pressure, which may be general or orthostatic. Patients must be protected from falls by teaching them to rise slowly and by monitoring blood pressure before doses of drug. The nurse should monitor and document lying, sitting, and standing blood pressure at the initiation of any antipsychotic.

Prolactinemia can also occur. When dopamine is blocked in the tuberoinfundibular tract, it can no longer repress prolactin, the neurohormone that regulates lactation and mammary function. The prolactin level increases and, in some individuals, side effects appear. Gynecomastia (enlarged breasts) can occur among both sexes and is understandably distressing to individuals who may be experiencing delusional or hallucinatory body image disturbances. Galactorrhea (lactation) may occur as well. Menstrual irregularities and sexual dysfunction are also possible. If these symptoms appear, the medication should be reduced or changed to another antipsychotic. Evidence for long-term consequences of hyperprolactinemia is lacking. Hyperprolactinemia is associated with haloperidol and risperidone.

Weight gain is related to antipsychotics, especially olanzapine and clozapine, that have major antihistiminic properties. Patients may gain up to 20 or 30 pounds within 1 year. Increased appetite and weight gain are often distressing to patients. Diet teaching and monitoring may have some effect on this side effect. Another solution is to increase the accessibility of healthy, easy-to-prepare food. Although nausea and vomiting can occur with these drugs, most often, these drugs mask nausea.

Sedation is another possible side effect of antipsychotic medication. Patients should be monitored for the sedating effects of antipsychotics that are antihistaminic. In elderly patients, sedation can be associated with falls.

New-onset diabetes should be looked for in patients taking antipsychotics. Recently, an association was made between new-onset diabetes mellitus and the administration of atypical antipsychotics, especially olanzapine and clozapine. Patients should be assessed and monitored for the appearance of clinical symptoms of diabetes. Fasting blood glucose is commonly ordered for these individuals.

Cardiac arrhythmias may also occur. Prolongation of the QTc interval is associated with torsades de pointes (polymorphic ventricular tachycardia) or ventricular fibrillation. The potential for drug-induced prolonged QT interval is associated with many drugs. The newly approved antipsychotic ziprasidone may be more likely than other drugs to prolong the QT interval and change the heart rhythm. For these patients, baseline electrocardiograms may be ordered. Nurses should observe these patients for cardiac arrhythmias.

Agranulocytosis is a reduction in the number of circulating granulocytes and decreased production of granulocytes in the bone marrow that limits one's ability to fight infection. Agranulocytosis can develop with all antipsychotic drugs, but it is most likely to develop with clozapine use. Although laboratory values below 500 cells/mm^3 are indicative of agranulocytosis, often granulocyte counts drop to below 200 cells/mm^3 with this syndrome (Gerson, 1990).

Patients taking clozapine should have regular blood monitoring of their white blood. White blood cells and granulocytes should be measured before initiating treatment and at least weekly or twice weekly after treatment has begun. Initial white blood cell counts should be above 3,500 cells/mm^3 to initiate treatment; in patients with counts 3,500 and 5,000 cells/mm^3, cell counts should be monitored three times a week if clozapine is prescribed. At any point that the white blood cell counts drop below 3,500 cells/mm^3 or granulocytes drop below 1,500 cells/mm^3, clozapine should be stopped, and the patient should be monitored for infection.

A faithfully implemented program of blood monitoring should not, however, replace careful observation of the patient. It is not unusual for blood cell counts to drop precipitously in a period of 2 to 3 days. This may not be discovered when the patient is on a strict weekly blood monitoring schedule. Any reported symptoms that are reminiscent of a bacterial infection (fever, pharyngitis, and weakness) should be cause for concern, and immediate evaluation of blood count status should be undertaken. Because patients are frequently discharged before the critical period of risk for agranulocytosis, patient education about these symptoms is also essential so that they will report these symptoms and obtain blood monitoring. In general, granulocytes return to normal in 2 to 4 weeks after discontinuing the medication.

Drug–Drug Interactions. Several potential drug–drug interactions are possible when administering antipsychotic medications. One of the cytochrome P450 enzymes responsible for the metabolism of olanzapine and clozapine is 1A2. If either olanzapine or clozapine is given with another medication that inhibits this enzyme, such as fluvoxamine (Luvox), the antipsychotic blood level would increase and possibly become toxic. On the other hand, cigarette smoking can also induce 1A2 and lower concentration of drugs metabolized by this enzyme, such as olanzapine and clozapine. Smokers may require a higher dose of these medications than nonsmokers (Stahl, 2000).

Several atypical antipsychotics, including clozapine, quetiapine, and ziprasidone, are metabolized by the 3A4 enzyme. Weak inhibitors of this enzyme include the antidepressants fluvoxamine, nefazodone, and norfluoxetine (an active metabolite of fluoxetine). Potent inhibitors of 3A4 enzyme include ketoconazole (antifungal), protease inhibitors, and erythromycin. If these drugs are given with clozapine, quetiapine, or ziprasidone, the antipsychotic level will rise. Additionally, the mood stabilizer carbamazepine (Tegretol) is a 3A4 inducer. When this drug is given with clozapine, quetiapine, or ziprasidone, the antipsychotic dose should be increased to compensate for the 3A4 induction. If carbamazepine is discontinued, the antipsychotic needs to be adjusted (Stahl, 2000).

Risperidone, clozapine, and olanzapine are substrates for the enzyme 2D6. Theoretically, antidepressants (fluoxetine and paroxetine) that inhibit this enzyme could increase these antipsychotics levels. However, this is not usually clinically significant (Stahl, 2000).

Teaching Points. Nonadherance to the medication regimen is an important factor in relapse; the family must be made aware of the importance of consistently taking medications. Medication education should cover the association between medications and the amelioration of symptoms (in general as well as individualized for the patient); side effects and their management; and interpersonal skills that help the patient and family report medication effects.

Medication Emergencies

Neuroleptic Malignant Syndrome. **Neuroleptic malignant syndrome** (NMS) is the development of severe muscle rigidity and elevated temperature accompanied by rapidly accelerating cascade of symptoms (occurring over the next 48 to 72 hours), which can include two or more of the following: hypertension, tachycardia, tachypnea, prominent diaphoresis, incontinence, mutism, leukocytosis, changes in level of consciousness ranging from confusion to coma, and laboratory evidence of muscle injury (eg, elevated creatinine phosphokinase) (Blair & Dauner, 1993; Sewell & Jeste, 1989). These symptoms suggest that all dopamine receptor tracts in the brain are reacting.

It is estimated that NMS occurs in about 1% of those who receive antipsychotic drugs (and other drugs that block dopamine, like metoclopramide), although some have suggested rates up to 2.4% (Adityanjee et al., 1999). Up to one third of these patients may die as a result of the syndrome. NMS is probably underreported and may well account for unexplained emergency room deaths of patients taking these drugs who are not diagnosed because their symptoms do not seem serious. The presenting symptom is usually an elevated temperature of greater than 99.58°F (usually between 101° and 103°F) with no apparent cause. The most important aspect of treating NMS is early recognition. Antidopaminergic drugs should be discontinued immediately. Care should be supportive for the symptoms displayed (eg, cooling blankets, antipyretic drugs, and intravenous fluids). Dopamine agonist drugs, such as bromocriptine, have been given with modest success. Muscle relaxants, such as dantrolene or benzodiazepine, have been used. Antiparkinsonism drugs are not particularly useful despite the similarity to extrapyramidal movement side effects. Some patients have improved with electroconvulsive therapy. NMS should be treated as a medical emergency that may require patients to be managed in a critical care unit.

The most important aspects of nursing care for patients with NMS relate to recognizing symptoms early, stopping the administration of any neuroleptic medications, and initiating supportive nursing care. Any patient with fever, fluctuating vital signs, abrupt changes in levels of consciousness, or any of the symptoms presented in Text Box 18-6 should be considered possibly to have NMS. The nurse should be especially alert for early signs and symptoms of NMS in high-risk patients, such as those who are agitated, physically exhausted, or dehydrated or who have an existing medical or neurologic illness. Patients who are receiving parenteral or higher doses of neuroleptic drugs or who are receiving lithium concurrently must also be carefully assessed. The nurse should carefully monitor fluid intake in these patients and also note their fluid and electrolyte status.

To prevent NMS from developing in a patient who shows signs or symptoms of the disorder, the nurse should immediately discontinue any neuroleptic drugs and notify the physician. Also, the nurse should "hold" any anticholinergic drugs that the patient may be taking. A common error made by nurses who fail to analyze the patient's total clinical picture (including vital signs, mental status changes, and laboratory values) is to

TEXT BOX 18.6

Diagnostic Criteria for Neuroleptic Malignant Syndrome*

1. Treatment with neuroleptics within 7 days of onset (2–4 weeks for depot neuroleptic medications).

2. Hyperthermia

3. Muscle rigidity

4. Five of the following:
   - Change in mental status
   - Tachycardia
   - Hypertension or hypotension
   - Tachypnea or hypoxia
   - Diaphoresis or sialorrhea
   - Tremor
   - Incontinence
   - Creatinine phosphokinase elevation or myoglobinuria
   - Leukocytosis
   - Metabolic acidosis

5. Exclusion of other drug-induced, systemic, or neuropsychiatric illnesses

---

* All five items are required concurrently.
From Caroff, S., & Mann, S. (1993). Neuroleptic malignant syndrome. *Medical Clinics of North America, 77*, 185–202 (with permission).

---

continue the use of neuroleptic drugs. Figure 18-5 is an algorithm that will help in deciding whether to withhold an antipsychotic medication.

The vital signs of the patient with symptoms of NMS must be monitored frequently. Also, it is important to check the results of the patient's laboratory tests for increased creatine phosphokinase, elevated white blood cell count, elevated liver enzymes, or myoglobinuria. The nurse must be prepared to initiate supportive measures or anticipate emergency transfer of the patient to a medical-surgical setting or an intensive care unit.

Treating high temperature (which frequently exceeds 103°F) is an important priority for these patients. High body temperature is reduced through the use of a cooling blanket and acetaminophen. Because many of these patients experience diaphoresis, temperature elevation, or dysphasia, it is important to monitor fluid hydration. Another important aspect of care for patients with NMS is patient safety. Also, joints and extremities that are rigid or spastic must be protected from injury (Waggoner, 1992). The treatment of these patients depends on the facility and availability of medical support services. Generally, patients in psychiatric inpatient units that

are separated from general hospitals are transferred to medical-surgical settings for treatment.

Anticholinergic Crisis. There is also potential for abuse of anticholinergic drugs. Some patients may find the anticholinergic effects of these drugs on mood, memory, and perception pleasurable. Although at toxic dosages, patients may experience disorientation and hallucinations, lesser doses may cause patients to experience greater sociability and euphoria. Anticholinergic crisis is a potentially life-threatening medical emergency caused by an overdose of or sensitivity to drugs with anticholinergic properties. This syndrome (also called *anticholinergic delirium*) may result from an accidental or intentional overdose of antimuscarinic drugs, including atropine, scopolamine, or belladonna alkaloids, which are present in numerous prescription drugs and over-the-counter medicines. The syndrome may also occur, however, in psychiatric patients who are receiving therapeutic doses of anticholinergic drugs, especially when they are combined with other psychotropic drugs that produce anticholinergic side effects. Numerous drugs commonly prescribed in psychiatric settings produce anticholinergic side effects, including tricyclic antidepressants and some antipsychotics. As a result of either drug overdose or sensitivity, these anticholinergic substances may produce an acute delirium or a psychotic reaction that resembles schizophrenia. More severe anticholinergic effects may occur in older patients, even at therapeutic levels (Stahl, 2000).

The signs and symptoms of anticholinergic crisis given in Text Box 18-7 are often dramatic and physically uncomfortable. This disorder is characterized by elevated temperature; parched mouth; burning thirst; hot, dry skin; decreased salivation; decreased bronchial and nasal secretions; widely dilated eyes (bright light is painful); decreased ability to accommodate visually; increased heart rate; constipation; difficulty urinating; and hypertension or hypotension. The face, neck, and upper arms may become flushed because of a reflex blood vessel dilation. In addition to peripheral symptoms, patients with anticholinergic psychosis may experience neuropsychiatric symptoms of anxiety, agitation, delirium, hyperactivity, confusion, hallucinations (especially visual), speech difficulties, psychotic symptoms, or seizures. The acute psychotic reaction that is produced resembles schizophrenia. The classic description of anticholinergic crisis is summarized in the following mnemonic: "Hot as a hare, blind as a stone, mad as a hatter, dry as a bone."

In general, episodes of anticholinergic crisis are self-limiting, usually subsiding in 3 days. If the condition is left untreated, however, the associated fever and delirium may progress to coma or cardiac and res-

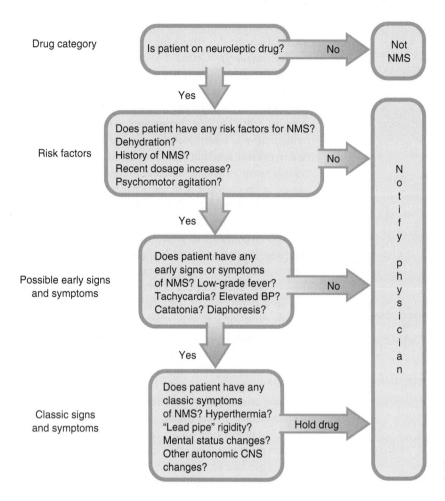

FIGURE 18.5 Action tree for whether the nurse "hold" a neuroleptic drug.

piratory depression. Although rare, death from this disorder has been reported. Death is generally due to hyperpyrexia and brain-stem depression.

This syndrome improves rapidly once the offending drug is discontinued; generally, improvement occurs within 24 to 36 hours. A specific and effective antidote,

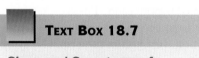

TEXT BOX 18.7

Signs and Symptoms of Anticholinergic Psychosis

Neuropsychiatric signs: confusion; recent memory loss; agitation; dysarthria; incoherent speech; pressured speech; delusions; ataxia; periods of hyperactivity alternating with somnolence, paranoia, anxiety, or coma

Hallucinations accompanied by "picking," plucking, or grasping motions; delusions; or disorientation

Physical signs: unreactive dilated pupils; blurred vision; hot, dry, flushed skin; facial flushing; dry mucous membranes; difficulty swallowing; fever; tachycardia; hypertension; decreased bowel sounds; urinary retention; nausea; vomiting; seizures; or coma

---

physostigmine, an inhibitor of anticholinesterase, is frequently used in the treatment and diagnosis of anticholinergic crisis. Administration of this drug rapidly reduces both the behavioral and physiologic symptoms of this syndrome. The usual adult dose of physostigmine is 1 to 2 mg intravenously given slowly over 5 minutes if no response is noted. Physostigmine is relatively short acting, so it may need to be given several times during the course of treatment. This drug provides relief from symptoms for a limited period of 2 to 3 hours. In addition to receiving physostigmine, patients who intentionally overdose on large amounts of anticholinergic drugs are treated by gastric lavage, administration of charcoal, and catharsis. Rapid injection of physostigmine may cause seizures, profound bradycardia, or heart block. The dose may be repeated after 20 or 30 minutes. It is important for the nurse to be alert for signs and symptoms of anticholinergic crisis, especially in elderly and pediatric patients, who are much more sensitive to the anticholinergic effects of drugs, and in patients who are receiving multiple medications with anticholinergic effects. If signs and symptoms of the syndrome occur, the nurse should discontinue the offending drug and notify the physician immediately.

Other Somatic Interventions. Electroconvulsive therapy is suggested as a possible alternative when the patient's schizophrenia is resistant to medications or when the patient cannot tolerate medications due to severe side effects (Zarate et al., 1995). For the most part, this is not indicated unless the patient is catatonic or has developed a depression that is not treatable by other means (Andreasen & Black, 1991).

Psychological Domain

Even though schizophrenia is a brain disorder, the psychological manifestations are the most difficult to assess and treat. Many of these psychological manifestations are improved with medications, but they are not necessarily eliminated.

Psychological Assessment

Several assessment scales have been developed and received considerable reliability and validity testing to help evaluate positive and negative symptom clusters in schizophrenia. Text Box 18-8 includes a listing of standardized instruments used in assessing symptoms of patients with schizophrenia. These include the Scale for the Assessment of Positive Symptoms (SAPS) (Text Box 18-9), the Scale for the Assessment of Negative Symptoms (SANS) (Text Box 18-10), and the Positive and Negative Syndrome Scale (PANSS) (Kay et al., 1987), which assesses both symptom clusters in the same instrument. Other tools that list symptoms, like the Brief Psychiatric Rating Scale (see Appendix C), SANS, or SAPS can also be used to help patients self-monitor their own symptoms.

Usually, information about prediagnosis experiences requires retrospective reporting by the patient or the family. This reporting is reliable for the frankly psychotic symptoms of delusions and hallucinations; however, negative symptoms are more difficult to date. In fact, negative symptoms vary from an imperceptible deviation from normal to a clear impairment. Negative symptoms probably occur earlier than positive symptoms and are less easily noted by the patient and patient's significant others.

Responses to Mental Health Problems. Schizophrenia robs people of their mental health and is socially stigmatizing. People with schizophrenia struggle to maintain control of their symptoms, which affect every aspect of their life. The person with schizophrenia displays a variety of interrelated symptoms and experiences deficits in several areas. Text Box 18-10 outlines these deficits. More than half of patients report the following **prodromal** symptoms (in order of frequency): tension and nervousness, lack of interest in eating, difficulty concentrating, disturbed sleep, decreased en-

TEXT BOX 18.8

Rating Scales for Use With Schizophrenia

Scale for the Assessment of Negative Symptoms (SANS)
Available from Nancy C. Andreasen, MD, PhD, Department of Psychiatry, College of Medicine, The University of Iowa, Iowa City, IA 52242. Copyright 1984. *See Text Box 18-10.*

Scale for the Assessment of Positive Symptoms (SAPS)
Available from Nancy C. Andreasen (see above). *See Text Box 18-9.*

Abnormal Involuntary Movement Scale (AIMS)
Guy, W. (1976). *ECDEU: Assessment manual for psychopharmacology* (DHEW Publication No. 76-338). Washington, DC: Department of Health Education and Welfare, Psychopharmacology Branch. *See Appendix I.*

Brief Psychiatric Rating Scale (BPRS)
Overall, J. E., & Gorham, D. R. (1988). The Brief Psychiatric Rating Scale (BPRS): Recent developments in ascertainment and scaling. *Psychopharmacology Bulletin, 24,* 97–99. *Included in Appendix C.*

Dyskinesia Identification System: Condensed User Scale (DISCUS)
Sprague, R. L., & Kalachnik, J. E. (1991). Reliability, validity, and a total score cutoff for the Dyskinesia Identification Scale System: Condensed User Scale (DISCUS) with mentally ill and mentally retarded populations. *Psychopharmacology Bulletin, 27(1),* 51–58. *See Table 18-4.*

Simpson-Angus Rating Scale
Simpson, G. M., Angus, J. W. S. L. (1970). A rating scale for extrapyramidal side effects. *Acta Psychiatrica Scandinavica (Suppl.) 212,* 11–19. Copyright 1970 Munksgaard International Publishers, Ltd. *Included in Appendix H.*

joyment and loss of interest, restlessness, forgetfulness, depression, social withdrawal from friends, feeling laughed at, more religious thinking, feeling bad for no reason, feeling too excited, and hearing voices or seeing things. Most of these are negative symptoms and are often the most subtle to describe (Keith & Matthews, 1991).

Because schizophrenia is a disorder of thoughts, perceptions, and behavior, it is sometimes not recognized as an illness by the person experiencing the symptoms. Many people with thought disorders do not believe that they have a mental illness. Their denial of a mental illness is very problematic for the family and clinicians because they are less likely to believe they need treatment. Ideally, in lucid moments, patients recognize that their thoughts are really delusions, that their perceptions are hallucinations, and that their behavior is disorganized. In reality, many patients do not believe

Text Box 18.9

Scale for the Assessment of Positive Symptoms (SAPS)

0 = None   1 = Questionable   2 = Mild   3 = Moderate
4 = Marked   5 = Severe

Hallucinations

1 *Auditory Hallucinations*   0 1 2 3 4 5
The patient reports voices, noises, or other sources that no one else hears.

2 *Voices Commenting*   0 1 2 3 4 5
The patient reports a voice that makes a running commentary on his behavior or thoughts.

3 *Voices Conversing*   0 1 2 3 4 5
The patient reports hearing two or more voices conversing.

4 *Somatic or Tactile Hallucinations*   0 1 2 3 4 5
The patient reports experiencing peculiar physical sensations in the body.

5 *Olfactory Hallucinations*   0 1 2 3 4 5
The patient reports experiencing unusual smells that no one else notices.

6 *Visual Hallucinations*   0 1 2 3 4 5
The patient sees shapes or people that are not actually present.

7 *Global Rating of Hallucinations*   0 1 2 3 4 5
This rating should be based on the duration and severity of the hallucinations and their effect on the patient's life.

Delusions

8 *Persecutory Delusions*   0 1 2 3 4 5
The patient believes he is being conspired against or persecuted in some way.

9 *Delusions of Jealousy*   0 1 2 3 4 5
The patient believes his spouse is having an affair with someone.

10 *Delusions of Guilt or Sin*   0 1 2 3 4 5
The patient believes that he has committed some terrible sin or done something unforgivable.

11 *Grandiose Delusions*   0 1 2 3 4 5
The patient believes he has special powers or abilities.

12 *Religious Delusions*   0 1 2 3 4 5
The patient is preoccupied with false beliefs of a religious nature.

13 *Somatic Delusions*   0 1 2 3 4 5
The patient believes that somehow his body is diseased, abnormal, or changed.

14 *Delusions of Reference*   0 1 2 3 4 5
The patient believes that insignificant remarks or events refer to him or have some special meaning.

15 *Delusions of Being Controlled*   0 1 2 3 4 5
The patient feels that his feelings or actions are controlled by some outside force.

16 *Delusions of Mind Reading*   0 1 2 3 4 5
The patient feels that people can read his mind or know his thoughts.

17 *Thought Broadcasting*   0 1 2 3 4 5
The patient believes that his thoughts are broadcast so that he himself or others can hear them.

18 *Thought Insertion*   0 1 2 3 4 5
The patient believes that thoughts that are not his own have been inserted into his mind.

19 *Thought Withdrawal*   0 1 2 3 4 5
The patient believes that thoughts have been taken away from his mind.

20 *Global Rating of Delusions*   0 1 2 3 4 5
This rating should be based on the duration and persistence of the delusions and their effects on the patient's life.

Bizarre Behavior

21 *Clothing and Appearance*   0 1 2 3 4 5
The patient dresses in an unusual manner or does other strange things to alter his appearance.

22 *Social and Sexual Behavior*   0 1 2 3 4 5
The patient may do things considered inappropriate according to usual social norms (eg, masturbating in public).

23 *Aggressive and Agitated Behavior*   0 1 2 3 4 5
The patient may behave in an aggressive, agitated manner, often unpredictably.

24 *Repetitive or Stereotyped Behavior*   0 1 2 3 4 5
The patient develops a set of repetitive actions or rituals that he must perform over and over.

25 *Global Rating of Bizarre Behavior*   0 1 2 3 4 5
This rating should reflect the type of behavior and the extent to which it deviates from social norms.

Positive Formal Thought Disorder

26 *Derailment*   0 1 2 3 4 5
A pattern of speech in which ideas slip off track onto ideas obliquely related or unrelated.

27 *Tangentiality*   0 1 2 3 4 5
Replying to a question in an oblique or irrelevant manner.

28 *Incoherence*   0 1 2 3 4 5
A pattern of speech that is essentially incomprehensible at times.

29 *Illogicality*   0 1 2 3 4 5
A pattern of speech in which conclusions are reached that do not follow logically.

30 *Circumstantiality*   0 1 2 3 4 5
A pattern of speech that is very indirect and delayed in reaching its goal idea.

31 *Pressure of Speech*   0 1 2 3 4 5
The patient's speech is rapid and difficult to interrupt; the amount of speech produced is greater than that considered normal.

32 *Distractible Speech*   0 1 2 3 4 5
The patient is distracted by nearby stimuli that interrupt his flow of speech.

(continued)

TEXT BOX 18.9 (*Continued*)

33 *Clanging*   0 1 2 3 4 5
    A pattern of speech in which sounds rather than
    meaningful relationships govern word choice.

34 *Global Rating of Positive Formal
    Thought Disorder*   0 1 2 3 4 5
    This rating should reflect the frequency of abnormality
    and degree to which it affects the patient's ability to
    communicate.

Inappropriate Affect

35 *Inappropriate Affect*   0 1 2 3 4 5
    The patient's affect is inappropriate or incongruous,
    not simply flat or blunted.

From Nancy C. Andreasen, MD, PhD, Department of Psychiatry, College of Medicine, The University of Iowa,
Iowa City, IA 52242. Copyright 1984 Nancy C. Andreasen. Reprinted with permission.

TEXT BOX 18.10

Scale for the Assessment of Negative Symptoms (SANS)

0 = None   1 = Questionable   2 = Mild   3 = Moderate
            4 = Marked   5 = Severe

Affective Flattening or Blunting

1 *Unchanging Facial Expression*   0 1 2 3 4 5
   The patient's face appears wooden, changes less than
   expected as emotional content of discourse changes.

2 *Decreased Spontaneous
   Movements*   0 1 2 3 4 5
   The patient shows few or no spontaneous movements,
   does not shift position, move extremities, etc.

3 *Paucity of Expressive Gestures*   0 1 2 3 4 5
   The patient does not use hand gestures, body position,
   etc., as an aid to expressing ideas.

4 *Poor Eye Contact*   0 1 2 3 4 5
   The patient avoids eye contact or "stares through"
   interviewer even when speaking.

5 *Affective Nonresponsivity*   0 1 2 3 4 5
   The patient fails to smile or laugh when prompted.

6 *Lack of Vocal Inflections*   0 1 2 3 4 5
   The patient fails to show normal vocal emphasis
   patterns, is often monotonic.

7 *Global Rating of
   Affective Flattening*   0 1 2 3 4 5
   This rating should focus on overall severity of symptoms, especially unresponsiveness, eye contact, facial
   expression, and vocal inflections.

Alogia

8 *Poverty of Speech*   0 1 2 3 4 5
   The patient's replies to questions are restricted in
   amount; tend to be brief, concrete, and unelaborated.

9 *Poverty of Content of Speech*   0 1 2 3 4 5
   The patient's replies are adequate in amount but tend
   to be vague, overconcrete, or overgeneralized, and
   convey little information.

10 *Blocking*   0 1 2 3 4 5
    The patient indicates, either spontaneously or with
    prompting, that his train of thought was interrupted.

11 *Increased Latency of Response*   0 1 2 3 4 5
    The patient takes a long time to reply to questions;
    prompting indicates that the patient is aware of the
    question.

12 *Global Rating of Alogia*   0 1 2 3 4 5
    The core features of alogia are poverty of speech and
    poverty of content.

Avolition–Apathy

13 *Grooming and Hygiene*   0 1 2 3 4 5
    The patient's clothes may be sloppy or soiled, and
    patient may have greasy hair, body odor, etc.

14 *Impersistence at Work or School*   0 1 2 3 4 5
    The patient has difficulty seeking or maintaining em-
    ployment, completing school work, keeping house,
    etc. If an inpatient, cannot persist at ward activities,
    such as OT, playing cards, etc.

15 *Physical Anergia*   0 1 2 3 4 5
    The patient tends to be physically inert. May sit for
    hours and does not initiate spontaneous activity.

16 *Global Rating of Avolition–Apathy* 0 1 2 3 4 5
    Strong weight may be given to one or two prominent
    symptoms if particularly striking.

Anhedonia–Asociality

17 *Recreational Interests
    and Activities*   0 1 2 3 4 5
    The patient may have few or no interests. Both the
    quality and quantity of interests should be taken into
    account.

18 *Sexual Activity*   0 1 2 3 4 5
    The patient may show a decrease in sexual interest
    and activity, or enjoyment when active.

(continued)

TEXT BOX 18.10 *(Continued)*

19 *Ability to Feel Intimacy
    and Closeness*   0 1 2 3 4 5
    The patient may display an inability to form close or
    intimate relationships, especially with the opposite
    sex and family.

20 *Relationships With
    Friends and Peers*   0 1 2 3 4 5
    The patient may have few or no friends and may pre-
    fer to spend all of time isolated.

21 *Global Rating of
    Anhedonia–Asociality*   0 1 2 3 4 5
    This rating should reflect overall severity, taking into
    account the patient's age, family status, etc.

Attention

22 *Social Inattentiveness*   0 1 2 3 4 5
    The patient appears uninvolved or unengaged. May
    seem "spacey."

23 *Inattentiveness During Mental
    Status Testing*   0 1 2 3 4 5
    Tests of "serial 7s" (at least five subtractions) and
    spelling "world" backward: Score: 2 = 1 error; 3 = 2
    errors; 4 = 3 errors.

24 *Global Rating of Attention*   0 1 2 3 4 5
    This rating should assess the patient's overall concen-
    tration, clinically and on tests.

From Nancy C. Andreasen, MD, PhD, Department of Psychiatry, College of Medicine, The University of Iowa,
Iowa City, IA 52242. Copyright 1984 Nancy C. Andreasen. Reprinted with permission.

that they have a mental illness but agree to treatment in order to please family and clinicians.

Mental Status

Appearance. The patient may look eccentric or disheveled or have poor hygiene and bizarre dress. The patient's posture may be one of lethargy or stupor.

Mood and Affect. Patients with schizophrenia often display altered mood states. In some cases, they may show heightened emotional activity; others may display severely limited emotional responses. Affect, the outward expression of mood, is categorized on a continuum: flat (emotional expression entirely absent), blunted (expression of emotions present but greatly diminished), and full range. Inappropriate affect is marked by incongruence between the emotional expression and the thoughts expressed.

Other common emotional symptoms include the following:

- **Affective lability**—abrupt, dramatic, unprovoked changes in type of emotions expressed
- **Ambivalence**—the presence and expression of two opposing forces, leading to inaction
- **Apathy**—reactions to stimuli are decreased, diminished interest and desire

Speech. Speech patterns may reflect obsessions, delusions, pressured thinking, loose associations, or flight of ideas and neologism. Speech is an indicator of thought content and other mental processes and is usually altered. An assessment of speech should note any difficulty articulating words (dysarthria) and difficulty swallowing (dysphagia) as indicators of medication side effects. In many instances, what an individual says is as important as how it is said. Both content and speech patterns should be noted.

Thought Processes

Delusions. Delusions can be distinguished from strongly held ideas by "the degree of conviction with which the belief is held despite clear contradictory evidence" (APA, 2000, p. 299). Culture must be considered when evaluating delusions. Delusional beliefs are those not sanctioned or held by a cultural or religious subgroup (Butler & Braff, 1991).

Bizarre delusions alone are sufficient to diagnose schizophrenia. It can often be difficult to distinguish between bizarre and nonbizarre delusions. Nonbizarre delusions generally have themes of jealousy and persecution and are derived from ordinary life experiences. For example, a woman believes that her husband, from whom she has recently separated, is trying to poison her, or a man believes that members of the Mafia are trying to kill him because, when he was in high school, he reported to the principal that several of his classmates were selling drugs at school (APA, 2000).

Bizarre delusions are those that are implausible, not understandable, and not derived from ordinary life experiences. Bizarre delusions often include delusions of control (that some outside force controls thoughts and actions), thought broadcasting (that others can read or hear one's thoughts), thought insertion (that someone has placed thoughts into one's mind), and thought withdrawal (that someone is removing thoughts from one's mind) (APA, 2000). For example, a patient who has been with a hypnotist for 2 months reports that the hypnotist continued to read his mind and was "picking his brain away piece by piece." Another patient was convinced that a computer chip was placed in her uterus during a gynecologic examination and that this somehow directly influenced her physical movements and her thoughts (Flaum et al., 1991, p. 63). Other behaviors may be present, such as aggression, agitation, regressed behavior, and psychomotor retardation. In some cases, behaviors that are observed need to be evaluated carefully to distinguish them from movements that are associated with medication side effects, such as grimacing, stereotypical behavior, or agitation.

Deciding which delusions, alone, are indicative of schizophrenia may be difficult even for the most experienced practitioner. In addition to assessing and judging the content of the delusion, exploration of other aspects of the delusional experience is helpful. These dimensions include looking at the conviction with which the delusion is held; examining how extensively other aspects of the individual's life are incorporated or affected by the delusion; determining the degree of internal consistency, organization, and logic evidenced in the delusion; and evaluating the amount of pressure (in terms of preoccupation and concern) individuals feel in their lives as a result of the delusion (Kendler et al., 1983) (see Therapeutic Dialogue: The Patient With Delusions).

Hallucinations. Hallucinations are the most common example of disturbances of sensory perception observed in patients with schizophrenia. Hallucinations can be experienced in all sensory modalities; however, auditory hallucinations are the most frequent in schizophrenia. Some specific hallucinations may be sufficient to diagnose schizophrenia, such as hearing voices conversing with each other or carrying on a discussion with someone who is not there. Because most individuals will not spontaneously share their hallucinatory experiences with an interviewer, the nurse may need to rely on indirect evidence in the patient's behavior, such as (1) pauses during conversations in which the individual seems preoccupied or appears to be listening to someone other than the interviewer, (2) looking toward the perceived source of a voice, or (3) responding to the voices in some manner (Trzepacz & Baker, 1993). Although patients may not spontaneously share their hallucinations, many validate observations of the examiner or admit to a his-

---

THERAPEUTIC DIALOGUE   The Patient With Delusions

John joined the nurse in a game of pool. The following conversation occurred as they played.

Ineffective Approach

John: The CIA put a transmitter in my molar, here. (Points to his right cheek.)
Nurse: No one would put a transmitter in your tooth; come on, the CIA isn't looking for you.
John: You get the striped ones. Yeah, they want to monitor me while I'm here. I know that they have the real Amy Carter here in the hospital. They are trying to get Jimmy Carter to intervene with the Michigan Militia. Mark from Michigan told me that.
Nurse: Amy Carter can't possibly be here, I saw her on television this morning.
John: Maybe—she does have darker hair and has different colored contacts to disguise her eyes. But they're just trying to keep people from knowing what they're doing.
Nurse: John, Amy Carter isn't in the hospital; if she were, I would know it because I work here.
John: (With anger.) You don't know anything! You are probably from the CIA also; I have nothing else to say to you.

Effective Approach

John: The CIA put a transmitter in my molar, here. (Points to his right cheek.)
Nurse: Oh. Which balls are mine?
John: You get the striped ones. Yeah, they want to monitor me while I'm here. I know that they have the real Amy Carter here in the hospital. They are trying to get Jimmy Carter to intervene with the Michigan Militia. Mark from Michigan told me that.
Nurse: I suppose it could be Amy Carter, but do you suppose that it could just be someone who looks like her?
John: Maybe—she does have darker hair and has different colored contacts to disguise her eyes. But they're

just trying to keep people from knowing what they're doing.
Nurse: You sound a little overwhelmed with all the information you have.
John: No, no. I can handle it. The CIA can't do anything to me. I'll never talk.
Nurse: I thought they could hear you when you talk to me.
John: Huh? Oh, that transmitter is so that they can send me misinformation. They send a tower of babble to my brain. They are trying to confuse me so that I stay away from Amy Carter. They all think they can keep me from my mission.
Nurse: Who's they?
John: Everyone in the government. The CIA, FBI, ATF, IRS— all those alphabets.
Nurse: So everyone in the government is trying to get to you.
John: Well, maybe not everybody. Just the ones that care about money and the militia. I don't think they care about me much in commerce or health and human services. Although they'd care too if they knew.
Nurse: I would think that's pretty frightening to have all these people out looking for you. You must be scared a lot.
John: It's scary but I can handle it. I've handled it all my life.
Nurse: You've been in scary situations all your life?
John: Yeah. I don't know. Maybe not scary, just hard. I never seemed to be able to do as well as my parents wanted—or as I wanted.

Critical Thinking Challenge

• How did the nurse's argumentative responses cause the patient to react in the first scenario?

• What effective communication techniques did the nurse use in the second scenario?

tory of hallucinations when asked (see Therapeutic Dialogue: The Patient With Hallucinations).

Disorganized Communication. The other aspect of thought content and processes that may be altered in schizophrenia is the organization of expressed thoughts. Impaired verbal fluency (ability to produce spontaneous speech) is often present. Abrupt shifts in the focus of conversation are a typical symptom of disorganized

thinking. The most severe shifts in focus may occur after only one or two words (word salad), after one or two phrases or sentences (flight of ideas or loose associations), or somewhat less severely as a shift that occurs when a new topic is repeatedly suggested and pursued from the current topic (tangentiality).

Cognitive Impairments. Although cognitive impairments in schizophrenia vary widely from patient to

---

THERAPEUTIC DIALOGUE | **The Patient With Hallucinations**

The following conversation took place in a dayroom with several staff in the room. The patient was potentially very violent. Although it is a good example of dealing with someone who is hallucinating, it is not a situation that should be taken lightly. Always make certain that you have a means to leave a situation (ie, that you are not in the corner of a room), that the patient does not have a potential weapon, and that you have sufficient staff close by so that you are safe.

Jason approached the nurse and asked to play pool. The nurse debated about playing but choose to play because the patient appeared very distracted, and the game might give him something to focus on.

Ineffective Approach

Nurse: Shall I break?

Jason: (Had been looking off to his right, but turns and looks directly at the nurse.) Yeah, go ahead. (Looks at the table briefly and then turns to look out the door and down the hallway.)

Nurse: (Breaking the pool balls without putting any in a pocket.) I guess it's your turn. You can hit any that you'd like.

Jason: (Turning back to the table.) Huh? (Shaking his head as he stared at the table.) What?

Nurse: You know, Jason, you really should pay attention.

Jason: (Hits a ball in and moves to the other side of the table. Stops in line with the next shot but doesn't bend down to take aim. Stands very still, then shakes his head slightly and quickly. Leans down to take aim and then stands up again.)

Nurse: Jason. (Looks at nurse.) Jason! Are you going to play or not, I don't have all day.

Jason: Oh yeah. (Leans down, takes aim, and misses.)

Nurse: (Moves to where the next shot is. Position is very close to where Jason is standing. Nurse watches him carefully, moving closer to him.) Please move over, Jason.

Jason: No. (Doesn't move. In peripheral vision, nurse sees Jason's lips move and he again looks to his right and shakes his head in a staccato motion, as if trying to shake something out of his head.)

Effective Approach

Nurse: Shall I break?

Jason: (Had been looking off to his right, but turns and looks directly at the nurse.) Yeah, go ahead. (Looks at the table briefly and then turns to look out the door and down the hallway.)

Nurse: (Breaking the pool balls without putting any in a pocket.) I guess it's your turn. You can hit any that you'd like.

Jason: (Turning back to the table.) Huh? (Shakes his head as he stares at the table.) What?

Nurse: You can hit any ball you like. I didn't get any.

Jason: (Hits a ball in and moves to the other side of the table. Stops in line with the next shot but doesn't bend down to take aim. Stands very still, then shakes his head slightly and quickly. Leans down to take aim and then stands up again.)

Nurse: Jason. (He looks at nurse.) Are you aiming at the 10 ball?

Jason: Oh yeah. (Leans down, takes aim, and misses.)

Nurse: (Moving to where her next shot is. The position is very close to where Jason is standing. Nurse watches him carefully while moving closer to him.) Here, let me take this shot.

Jason: Oh. (Moves back. In peripheral vision nurse sees Jason's lips move and again he looks to his right and shakes his head in a staccato motion, as if trying to shake something out of his head.)

Nurse: I missed again. (Moves away from table and turns to Jason, who moves up to the table. He leans down and then stands up again. His lips move again as he turns his head to the right and then looks over his back toward the doorway.) Jason. Jason. (He looks at the nurse.) You have the striped ones.

Jason: (Nods and leans down to take a shot, which he makes. He then misses the next shot. He stands up and moves back from the table, again looking back toward the doorway. He shakes his head and clearly says:) No!

Nurse: (Watches him closely and moves to the opposite side of the table, making the next shot. Lining up the next shot, Jason leans the pool cue against the table, looks past the nurse, and turns and walks away toward the door. Looks down the hallway, takes a few steps, stops for a minute or so, turns back into the room, and again looks past the nurse. Sits down and shakes his head again. Holds his head in his hands, with his hands covering his ears. The nurse picks up his pool cue and places both against the wall, out of the way. The nurse sits next to another staff member at a vantage point from which Jason can still be watched.)

Critical Thinking Challenge

- How did the nurse's impatience translate into Jason's behavior in the first scenario?

- What effective communicating techniques did the nurse use in the second scenario?

patient, several primary problems have been identified: (1) attention may be increased and sustained on external stimuli over a period of time (hypervigilance), (2) the ability to distinguish and focus on relevant stimuli may be diminished, (3) familiar cues may go unrecognized or be improperly encoded, and (4) information processing may be diminished, leading to inappropriate or illogical conclusions from available observations and information (Brenner et al., 1992; Liberman & Green, 1992).

Cognitive impairments are not easy to recognize. By relying only on clinical assessment, the nurse can miss the extent of the impairment. Using a standardized instrument such as the Mini-Mental Status Examination (MMSE), the Cognitive Assessment Screening Instrument (CASI), or the 7-minute screen can provide a screening measurement of cognitive function (see Chap. 10). If impairment exists, neuropsychological testing by a qualified psychologist may be necessary.

Memory and Orientation. Impairments in orientation, memory, and abstract thinking and orientation have been observed. Orientation to time, place, and person may remain relatively intact unless the patient is particularly preoccupied with delusions and hallucinations. Although all aspects of memory may be affected in schizophrenia, registration or the recall within seconds of newly learned information, may be particularly diminished. This affects the individual's short-term and long-term memory. The ability to engage in abstract thinking may be impaired.

Insight and Judgment. Individuals display insight when they display evidence of knowing their own thoughts, the reality of external objects, and their relationship to these. Judgment is the ability to formulate a decision or action about a situation. Insight and judgment are closely related to each other and depend on cognitive functions that are frequently impaired in people with schizophrenia (see Chap. 10).

Behavioral Responses. During periods of psychosis, unusual or bizarre behavior often occurs. These behaviors can usually be understood within the context of the patient's disturbed thinking. It is important for the patient to understand the significance of the behavior to the individual. One patient moved all of his family's furniture into the yard because he thought that the evil spirits were hiding in the furniture. His bizarre behavior was really an attempt to protect his family. Another patient painted a sequence of numbers on his bedroom walls. When asked about it, he said that the numbers were the languages of the angels. His bizarre thoughts were at the basis of his behavior.

Because of the negative symptoms, specifically, avolition, patients may not seem interested or organized to complete normal daily activities. They may stay in bed most of the day or refuse to take a shower. Many times, they will agree to get up in the morning and go to work, but they just never get around to it. Several specific behaviors are associated with schizophrenia, including stereotypy (idiosyncratic repetitive, purposeless movements), echopraxia (involuntary imitation of others' movements), and waxy flexibility (posture held in odd or unusual fixed position for extended periods).

Self-Concept. In schizophrenia, self-concept is usually poor. Patients often are aware that they are hearing voices others do not hear. They recognize that they are different than others and are often scared of "going crazy." The pervasive stigma associated with having a mental illness contributes to the poor self-concept. Body image can be disturbed, especially during periods of hallucinations or delusions. One patient believed that her body was infected with germs and she could feel them eating away her insides.

Stress and Coping Patterns. Stressful events are often linked to the appearance of psychiatric symptoms (See Chap. 6 for discussion of the stress-diathesis model). It is important to determine patient's stresses from their perspective. A stressful event for one person may not be stressful for another (see Chap. 35). It is also important to determine typical coping patterns, especially being aware of negative coping strategies such as the use of substances or aggressive behavior.

Risk Assessment. Because there is such a high rate of suicide and attempted suicides among patients with schizophrenia, it is important to assess for the risk for self-harm. The following question will help the nurse assess risk for self-injury: Does the patient speak of suicide, have delusional thinking that could lead to dangerous behavior, have command hallucinations telling him or her to harm self or others, or have homicidal ideations? Substance-related disorders are also common among patients with schizophrenia, and nurses should assess for substance abuse as well.

Nursing Diagnoses Related to Psychological Domain

There are many nursing diagnoses that can be generated from data collected assessing the psychological domain. Disturbed thought processes can be used for delusions, confusion, and disorganized thinking. Disturbed sensory perception is appropriate for hallucinations or illusions. Other examples of diagnoses include disturbed body image, low self-esteem, disturbed personal identity, risk for violence, ineffective coping, and knowledge deficit.

Psychological Interventions

All of the psychological interventions, such as counseling, conflict resolution, behavior therapy, and cognitive interventions, are appropriate for patients with schizophrenia. The following discussion focuses on the application of these interventions.

Special Issues in the Development of the Nurse–Patient Relationship. The development of the nurse–patient relationship with patients with schizophrenia centers on the development of trust and the acceptance of the person as a worthy human being. People with schizophrenia are often reluctant to engage in any relationship because of previous rejection by friends and society and, in some instances, an underlying suspiciousness that is a part of the illness. If they are having hallucinations, their images of other people may be distorted and frightening. They are struggling to trust their own thoughts and perceptions, and engaging in an interaction with another human being may prove too overwhelming. The nurse should approach the patient in a calm and caring manner. Engaging the patient in a relationship may take time. Short, time-limited interactions are best for a patient who is experiencing psychosis. Being consistent in interactions and following through on promises will help establish trust within the relationship.

The establishment of a therapeutic relationship is critical, especially in patients who deny that they have a mental illness. Patients are more likely to agree to treatment if these recommendations are made within the context of a safe, trusting relationship. Even if a patient denies having mental illness, the person may take the medication and attend treatment activities because he or she trusts the nurse.

Management of Disturbed Thoughts and Sensory Perceptions. Even though antipsychotic medications improves the positive symptoms, they do not always eliminate the hallucinations and delusions. The nurse will continue to help the patient develop creative strategies for dealing with these sensory and thought disturbances. Information about the content of the hallucinations and delusions is needed, not only to determine whether the medications are effective, but also to assess safety and the meaning of these thoughts and perceptions to the patient. In caring for a patient who is experiencing hallucinations or delusions, nursing actions should be guided by three general patient outcomes:

- Decrease the frequency and intensity of hallucinations and delusions.
- Recognize that hallucinations and delusions are symptoms of a brain disorder.
- Develop strategies to manage the recurrence of hallucinations or delusions.

When interacting with a patient who is experiencing hallucinations or delusions, it is important to remember that these experiences are real to the patient. The nurse should never tell a patient that his or her experiences are not real. By discounting the patient's experiences, the nurse blocks communication. On the other hand, it is dishonest to tell the patient that you also are having the same hallucinatory experience. It is best to validate that the patient is having these experiences and identify the meaning of these thoughts and feelings to the patient. For example, if a patient believes that he or she is under surveillance by the FBI, the person probably feels frightened and is very suspicious of everyone. By acknowledging how frightening it must be to always feel like you are being watched, the nurse focuses on the feelings that are generated by the delusion, not the delusion itself. The nurse can then offer to help the patient feel safe within his or her environment. The patient, in turn, begins to feel that someone understands him or her.

Teaching patients that hallucinations and delusions are part of the disorder becomes easier after the medication begins working. Once patients believe and acknowledge that they have a mental illness and that some of the some of their thoughts are delusions and some of their perceptions are hallucinations, they are then able to develop strategies to manage their symptoms.

Self-Monitoring and Relapse Prevention. Patients can greatly benefit by learning techniques of self-regulation, symptom monitoring, and relapse prevention. By monitoring the events, time, place, stimuli, and so forth surrounding the appearance of symptoms, the patient can begin to predict high-risk times for symptom recurrence. One group of researchers interviewed 51 patients with schizophrenia to determine what indicators they used to predict the onset of symptoms and what strategies they used to manage their symptoms. All patients felt some predicting feelings, such as anxiety (41%) or depression (28%); 49 of the 51 engaged in more than three activities to help manage their symptoms, such as getting busy, self-talk or withdrawal, medications, and substance use or acting out (in order of frequency) (Hamera et al., 1991).

The Moller-Murphy Symptom Management Assessment Tool (MM-SMAT) can be used as a systematic assessment of symptoms that could indicate relapse (Murphy & Moller, 1993). Using a list of behaviors typical of schizophrenia (other disorders are also included), the patients select the behaviors that typically occur before their relapse. These behaviors can be rated on frequency, duration, and intensity at regular intervals or follow-up appointments.

Discussions of how the patient manages or copes with these behaviors gives the nurse an opportunity to reinforce symptom-specific interventions that can promote greater health. Additionally, each patient will discover activities that help manage their symptoms. For example, using headsets with music works for some people, avoiding crowded places works for others, and yelling at the voices to go away may also work.

Another important nursing intervention is to help the patient identify who and where to talk about delusional or hallucinatory material. Because self-disclosure of these symptoms immediately labels someone as having a mental illness, patients should be encourage to evaluate the environment for negative consequences of disclosing these symptoms. For example, it may be fine to talk about it at home, but not at the grocery store.

Enhancement of Cognitive Functioning.
After deficits in cognitive functioning are identified, the next step is to develop interventions with the patient that target specific deficits. To be effective, the whole treatment team should be involved. If the ability to focus or attend is an issue, patients can be encouraged to select activities that improve attention, such as computer games. For memory problems, patients can be encouraged to make lists and to write down important information.

Executive functioning problems are the most challenging for these patients. Patients who are unable to manage daily problems may have impairment in the areas of planning and problem solving. For these patients, interventions should be developed that closely simulate real-world problems. Through coaching, the nurse can teach and support the development of problem-solving skills. For example, during hospitalizations, patients are given medications and reminded to take them on time. They are often instructed in a classroom setting but rarely have an opportunity to practice self-medication and figure out what to do if their prescription expires, the medications are lost, or they forget their medications. Yet, when discharged, patients are expected to take medication at the prescribed dose at the prescribed time. Interventions designed to have patients actively engage in problem-solving behavior with real problems are needed.

Another approach to helping patients solve problems and learn new strategies for dealing with problems is solution-focused therapy, which focuses on the strengths and positive attributes that exist within each person. This is a therapy that involves years of training to master, but there are techniques that can be used. For example, patients can be asked to identify the most important problem from their perspective. This focuses the patient on an important issue for that patient (Research Box 18-3).

Behavioral Interventions.
Behavioral interventions can be very effective in helping the patients improve motivation and organize routine, daily activities, such as maintaining a regular schedule and completing activities. Reinforcement of positive behaviors (getting up on time, completing hygiene, going to treatment activities) can easily be included in a treatment plan. In

RESEARCH BOX 18.3

Might Within the Madness: Solution-Focused Therapy and Thought-Disordered Patients

This article presents the use of solution-focused therapy (SFT) to help thought-disordered patients better cope with some of their negative experiences and symptomatology. The authors provided an overview of SFT, with a focus on how these techniques might be used on an inpatient psychiatry setting with patients experiencing thoughts. Three cases are presented: a 26-year-old man admitted to an inpatient hospital psychiatric unit with intrusive auditory and visual hallucinations, a 67-year-old woman who lived most of her life on a farm and managed her symptoms well until a recent move to the city, and a 49-year-old woman who was suffering from paranoid delusions about bombers and planes. Through the use of SFT, the nurses were able to see the individual as a person with hopes, dreams, and strengths. They also concluded that the process of SFT was an important as the outcome.

Utilization in the Clinical Setting: This article is interesting to read and can have direct clinical application for those interested in developing solution-focused techniques. Using some of the SFT techniques can help the nurse see past the disorder and view the patient as a human being with strengths.

Hagen, B. F., & Mitchell, D. (2001). Might within the madness: Solution-focused therapy and thought-disordered clients. *Archives of Psychiatric Nursing, 15*(2), 86–93.

the hospital, patients gain ward privileges by following an agreed-on treatment plan.

Stress and Coping Skills.
Developing skills to cope with personal, social, and environmental stresses is important to everyone, but particularly to those with a severe mental illness. Stresses can easily trigger symptoms that patients are trying to avoid. Establishing regular counseling sessions to support the development of positive coping skills is helpful for both the hospitalized patient and those in the community.

Patient Education.
Cognitive deficits (difficulty in processing complex information, maintaining steady focus of attention, distinguishing between relevant and irrelevant stimuli, and forming abstractions), can be a challenge to the nurse planning educational activities. There is evidence that people with schizophrenia learn best in an errorless learning environment (O'Carroll et al., 1999). These individuals learn best when the correct information is given directly to them, and they are encouraged to write it down. Asking

questions that encourage guessing is not as effective in helping them retain information.

Teaching and explaining should be done in an environment where distractions are minimized. Terminology should be clear and unambiguous. Visual aids can supplement verbal information, but these materials should have simple information stated in simple language. Care should be taken not to overcrowd the visual material or incorporate images that draw attention away from important content. Teaching should be done in small segments with frequent reinforcement. Most important of all, teaching should occur when the patient is ready. Regular assessments of cognitive abilities with standardized instruments can help determine this readiness. These suggestions can be adapted for teaching during any phase of the illness.

Skill-training interventions should be designed to compensate for these cognitive deficits. To help these patients to learn to process complex activities, like catching a bus, preparing a meal, or shopping for food or clothes, nurses should break the activity into a series of small component parts or steps and list them for the patient's reference, for example the following:

- Leave apartment with keys in hand.
- Make sure you have correct bus fare in pocket.
- Close the door.
- Walk to the corner.
- Turn right and walk 3 blocks to bus stop.

Family Education. Because a diagnosis of schizophrenia is a life-changing event not only for patients but also for the family and friends who must care for and support them, educating patients and their families is crucial. It is a primary concern for the psychiatric–mental health nurse. Family support is crucial to help patients maintain treatment and education and should include information about the disease course, treatment regimens, support systems, and life management skills (see Psychoeducation Checklist: Schizophrenia).

It is crucial that the patient and family understand that schizophrenia is a lifetime disorder involving many phases with regularly occurring relapses and periodic hospitalizations and that the disorder requires continual treatment and continual family help and support. Family members should be educated regarding the three phases of schizophrenia, the expected behaviors and emotional reactions in each, and the importance of maintenance of treatment even during the phases when symptoms seem to be reasonably controlled.

The most important factor to stress during patient and family education is the consistent taking of medication. Moller and Wer (1989) have adapted the traditional psychoeducational approach and termed it *health education* because they believe the term *psychoeducation* may be stigmatizing to patients and their families. A

PSYCHOEDUCATION CHECKLIST
Schizophrenia

When caring for the patient with schizophrenia, be sure to include the caregiver as appropriate and address the following topic areas in the teaching plan:

- Psychopharmacologic agents, including drug action, dosage, frequency, and possible adverse effects. Stress importance of adherence to the prescribed regimen.
- Management of hallucinations
- Coping strategies, such as self-talk, getting busy
- Management of the environment
- Use of contracts that detail expected behaviors, with goals and consequences
- Community resources

---

group of patients and their families meet together for 3-hour sessions twice a week for a period of 3 weeks. In contrast to traditional approaches in which patients were excluded from these sessions for fear that they might be disruptive or too anxious to participate, Moller and Wer found that although patients exhibit some symptoms during the sessions, they make valuable contributions by commenting on their experiences and validating the content included in the course. Each session has a particular focus (listed in order of sessions): introductions and information to facilitate the discussion of the overall experience of schizophrenia; biologic theories of cause and explanations of the *DSM-IV-TR* categorizations; levels of anxiety and their manifestations; hallucinations and how to manage them; psychotropic medications and their effects on the brain; and coping, environmental management, and relapse. These educational classes effectively bring families into the treatment continuum, decrease isolation, and teach about the illness.

Social Domain

Social Assessment

Several difficulties with social functioning occur in schizophrenia. As the disorder progresses, individuals can become increasingly socially isolated. On a one-to-one basis, this occurs as the individual seems unable to connect with people in his or her environment. Several aspects of the symptoms already discussed can contribute to this, for example, emotional blunting and anhedonia (the inability to form emotional attachment and experience pleasure). Cognitive deficits that contribute to difficult social functioning include problems with face and affect recognition, deficiencies in recall of past interactions, problems with decision making and judgment in conflictual interactions, and poverty of speech and language. Poor functioning and the inability to complete activities of daily living are manifested in poor hygiene, malnutrition, and social isolation.

Functional Status. Functional status of patients with schizophrenia should be assessed initially and at regular periods. The usual assessment instrument is the Global Assessment of Functioning (GAF). If the GAF score is below 60, interventions should be designed to enhance social or occupational functioning.

Social Systems. In schizophrenia, support systems become very important in maintaining the patient in the community. The individual may become socially isolated if the treatment and management occur in long-term care facilities and group homes away from family and friends. One challenge in the treatment of schizophrenia is to identify and maintain the patient's links with family and significant others. Assessment of the formal support (eg, family, providers) and informal support (eg, neighbors, friends) should be conducted (see Chap. 6 for discussion of the balance theory).

Quality of Life. People with schizophrenia often have a poor quality of life, especially older people, who may have spent many years in a long-term hospital. The nurse should assess the patient's quality of life and how it could be improved. Simple changes, such as arranging for a different roommate or improving access to social activities by meeting transportation needs, can greatly improve a patient's quality of life.

Family Assessment. The assessment of the family could take many forms, and the family assessment guide presented in Chapter 16 can be used. In some instances, the patient will be young and living with his or her parents. Often, the nurse's first contact with the patient and family is in the initial phases of the disorder. The family is dealing with the shock and disbelief of seeing a child develop a mental illness that has lifelong consequences. In this instance, the assessment process may be extended over several sessions to provide the family with support and education about the disorder.

Because women with schizophrenia generally have better treatment outcomes than men, many will marry and have children. These women experience the same life stresses as other women and may find themselves single parents, raising children in poverty-stricken conditions. Managing a psychiatric illness and trying to be an effective parent in a socially stigmatizing society is almost an impossibility because of the lack of financial resources and social support. This family will need an extensive assessment of financial need and social support. The family life cycle model presented in Chapter 12 can also be used as a framework for the assessment.

Nursing Diagnoses Related to Social Domain

The nursing diagnoses generated from the assessment of the social domain are typically Social Problems, Ineffective Role Performance, Disabled Family Coping, or Interrupted Family Processes. Outcomes will depend on the specific problem area.

Social Interventions

Promotion of Patient Safety on Psychiatric Units. Although violence is not a consistent behavior of people with schizophrenia, it is always a concern during the initial phase when hallucinations or delusions may put patients at risk for harming themselves or others. Nonviolent patients who are experiencing hallucinations and delusions can also be at risk for victimization by more aggressive patients. The patient who is hallucinating needs to be protected. This protection may include increased staff monitoring and, if necessary, a safer environment in a secluded area.

The nurse's best approach to avoiding violence or aggression is to administer medications as ordered, to assess and monitor for signs of fear and agitation, to demonstrate respect for the patient and the patient's personal space, and to use preventive interventions before the patient loses control. Because medications take 1 to 2 weeks to begin to moderate behavior, the nurse must be vigilant during this interim period.

Reducing environmental stimulation is particularly important for individuals who are experiencing hallucinations but can be helpful for all patients when signs of fear and agitation are observed. Allowing patients to use private rooms or seclusion for brief periods can be an important preventive method.

Other techniques of managing the environment (milieu management) have been found to be helpful in inpatient settings. One researcher who examined aggression and violence in psychiatric hospitals found violent behavior to be associated with the following predictors: history of violence, a coercive interaction style of using violence to obtain what is desired, and an environment in which violence is inadvertently rewarded. The latter situation may be an environment in which violent or aggressive acts gain the attention of staff, or an environment in which the patient lacks privacy and may act out or use violence to avoid treatment activities or obtain the privacy of seclusion (Morrison, 1992, 1993). Morrison proposed the following as interventions that help avoid acts of violence or aggression:

- Taking a thorough history that includes information about the patient's past use of violence

- Helping the patient to talk directly and constructively with those with whom they are angry, rather than venting anger to staff about a third person
- Setting limits with consistent and justly applied consequences
- Involving the patient in formulating a contract that outlines patient and staff behaviors, goals, and consequences
- Scheduling brief but regular time-outs to allow the patient some privacy without the attention of staff either before or after the time-out (these time-outs may be patient activated)

If the patient loses control and is a danger to self or others, restraints and seclusion may be used as a last resort. Health Care Financing Administration guidelines and hospital policy must be followed (see Chap. 4). Staff should be trained in the proper use of seclusion and restraints. Further, staff need to have planned sessions following all incidents of violence or physical management in which the event is analyzed. These sessions allow staff to learn how better to manage these situations and evaluate patients' cues. With sensitive leadership, these sessions can help staff to learn more about the interaction of patient and staff characteristics that can contribute to these incidents.

Support Groups. People with mental illness benefit from support groups that focus on daily problems and the stress of dealing with a mental illness. These groups are useful throughout the continuum of care. In the hospital setting, the focus of the group can be simply sharing the experience of living with a mental illness. In the community, a regular support group can provide interaction with people with similar problems and issues. Friendships often develop from these groups.

Milieu Therapy. Individuals with schizophrenia can be hospitalized or live in group homes for a long period of time. Expecting people who have an illness that interferes with their ability to live with family members to live with complete strangers in peace and harmony is unrealistic. Arranging the treatment environment to maximize therapy is crucial to the rehabilitation of the patient.

Psychiatric Rehabilitation. Rehabilitation strategies are used to support the individual's recovery and integration into the community (see Chap. 17). Community-based psychosocial rehabilitation programs usually offer long-term intensive case management services to adults with schizophrenia. Programs provide a continuum of services to meet the changing needs of people with psychiatric disabilities. Patients set rehabilitation goals, and services are then provided to help "clients" (most programs do not use the term

patients) reach their goals. Services range from daily home visits, providing transportation, occupational training, and group support. Social skills training has shown much promise for schizophrenia patients, both individually and in groups. This is a method for teaching patients specific behaviors needed for social interactions. The skills are taught with didactic lecture, demonstration, role playing, and homework assignments (see Chaps. 14 and 15). Nurses have become involved in principles of psychiatric rehabilitation, which promotes and supports normalized living. They may be team members and involved in case management or providing services. These and other psychological treatment approaches, combined with breakthroughs in biologic treatment, continue to help improve the functioning and quality of life for patients with schizophrenia.

Family Interventions. When schizophrenia first becomes apparent, the patient and family must negotiate the mental health system for the first time (in most cases), a challenge that almost equals that of confronting the family member's illness. In most states, the mental health system is huge and is usually ignored unless an adult foster care home moves into the neighborhood or a family member becomes seriously mentally ill. The system includes private inpatient and outpatient clinics supported by insurance, and public community mental health clinics and hospitals supported by public funds. Because mental health coverage in most insurance packages is woefully insufficient for someone with schizophrenia, most families eventually deal with the public mental health system. If the patient is aggressive, many private facilities encourage hospitalization in a public sector facility even for the first admission.

Family members should be encouraged to participate in support groups that help family members deal with the realities of living with a loved one with a mental illness (see Chap. 16). Family members should be given information about local community and state resources and organizations such as mental health associations and those that can help families negotiate the complex provider systems.

Evaluation and Treatment Outcomes

Outcome research related to schizophrenia has redefined previous ways of thinking about the course of the disorder. Where we once considered schizophrenia to have a progressively long-term and downward course, we now know that schizophrenia can be successfully treated and managed. In one older, but significant study, the researchers interviewed patients 20 to 25 years after diagnosis and found that 50% to 66% experienced significant improvement or recovery (Harding et al., 1987).

This study is important because it occurred before the development of atypical antipsychotics. Today, we can be hopeful that even more people can improve or recover from schizophrenia.

Continuum of Care

Continuity of care has been identified as a major goal of community mental health systems for patients with schizophrenia because they are at risk for becoming "lost" to services if left alone after discharge. Discharge planning encourages follow-up care in the community. In fact, many state mental health systems require an outpatient appointment before discharge. Treatment of schizophrenia occurs across a variety of settings (see Appendices M and N for clinical pathways). Not only inpatient hospitalization but also partial hospitalization, day treatment, and crisis stabilization can be used effectively.

Inpatient-Focused Care

Much of the previous discussion concerns the care in the inpatient setting. Today, inpatient hospitalizations are very short and focus on patient stabilization. Many times, these patients are involuntarily admitted for a short period of time (see Chap. 4). During the period of stabilization, the status is changed to one of a voluntary admission where the patient agrees to treatment.

Emergency Care

Emergency care ideally takes place in a hospital emergency room, but often the crisis occurs in the home. Patients are usually relapsing and do not recognize their bizarre or aggressive behaviors as symptoms. A specially trained crisis team is sent to assess the emergency and recommend further treatment. In the emergency room, patients are brought not only because of relapse but also because of medication side effects or water intoxication. Nurses should refer to the previous discussion for nursing management.

Community Care

Most of the care of patients with schizophrenia will be in the community through publicly supported mental health delivery systems. Community services include assertive community treatment, outpatient therapy, case management, and psychosocial rehabilitation, including clubhouse programs. While in the community, the mental health care should be integrated with the total health care of the individual. Nurses should be especially vigilant that patients with mental illnesses receive proper primary and medical health care.

Mental Health Promotion

It is often not the disorder itself that threatens the mental health of the person with schizophrenia but the stresses of trying to receive care and services. Health

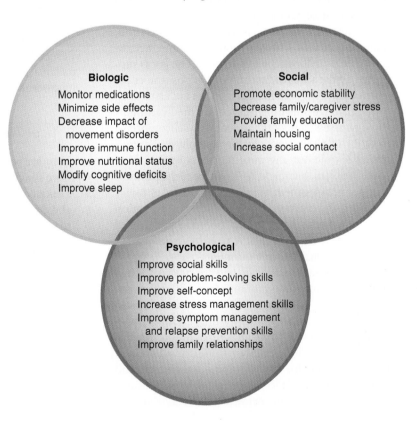

Biologic
Monitor medications
Minimize side effects
Decrease impact of
    movement disorders
Improve immune function
Improve nutritional status
Modify cognitive deficits
Improve sleep

Social
Promote economic stability
Decrease family/caregiver stress
Provide family education
Maintain housing
Increase social contact

Psychological
Improve social skills
Improve problem-solving skills
Improve self-concept
Increase stress management skills
Improve symptom management
    and relapse prevention skills
Improve family relationships

FIGURE 18.6 Biopsychosocial interventions for patients with schizophrenia.

care systems are complex and are often at the mercy of a system rule that is outdated. Development of assertiveness and conflict resolution skills can help the person in negotiating access to those systems that will provide services. Developing a positive support system for stressful periods will help promote a positive outcome (Fig. 18-6).

Summary of Key Points

➤ The patient with schizophrenia displays a complex myriad of symptoms typically categorized as positive symptoms (those that exist but should not exist), such as delusions or hallucinations and disorganized thinking and behavior, and negative symptoms (those characteristics that should be there but are lacking), such as alogia, avolition, anhedonia, and affective blunting.

➤ In the past, the diagnosis and treatment of schizophrenia have focused on more observable and dramatic positive symptoms (ie, delusions and hallucinations), but recently scientists have shifted their focus to the disorganizing symptoms of cognition.

➤ The clinical presentation of schizophrenia occurs over three phases: phase I entails initial diagnosis and first treatment; phase II includes periods of relative calm between episodes of overt signs and symptoms but during which the patient needs sustained treatment; and phase III includes periods of exacerbation or relapse that require hospitalization or more frequent contacts with mental health professionals and increased use of resources.

➤ There are several biologic theories of causation, including genetic, infectious-autoimmune, neuroanatomic, and dopamine hypotheses. The last is supported by the advanced technology of positron emission tomography scan findings and the understanding of the mechanisms of antipsychotic medications.

➤ Biologic assessment of the patient with schizophrenia must include a thorough history and physical examination to rule out any medical illness or substance abuse problem that might be the cause of the patient's symptoms, assessment of risk for self-injury or injury to others, and creation of baseline health information before medications are begun. Several standardized assessment tools are available to help assess characteristic abnormal motor movements.

➤ There are several nursing interventions that address the biologic domain—promotion of self-care activities, activity, exercise, nutritional, thermoregulation, and fluid balance interventions. The antipsychotic drugs used to treat schizophrenia have a general effect of blocking dopamine transmission in the brain but also cause some troublesome and sometimes serious side effects, primarily anticholinergic side effects and extrapyramidal side effects (motor abnormalities). Newer antipsychotics block serotonin as well as dopamine. The nurse should be familiar with these drugs, their possible side effects, and the interventions required to manage or control side effects.

➤ The extrapyramidal side effects of antipsychotic drugs can appear early in drug treatment and include acute parkinsonism or pseudoparkinsonism, acute dystonia, and akathisia; or they can appear late in treatment after months or years. The primary example of late-appearing extrapyramidal side effects is tardive dyskinesia, which is a severe syndrome of abnormal motor movements of the mouth, tongue, and jaw.

➤ Psychological assessment must include equal attention to manifestations of both positive and negative symptoms and a concentrated focus on the cognitive impairments that make it so difficult for these patients to manage their disorder. Several standardized assessment tools assess for positive and negative symptoms. Development of the nurse–patient relationship becomes key in helping patients manage the disturbed thoughts and sensory perceptions. Interventions should be designed to enhance cognitive functioning. Patient and family education are critical interventions for the person with schizophrenia.

➤ Because schizophrenia is a lifetime disorder and patients require the continued support and care of mental health professionals and family or friends, one of the primary nursing interventions is ensuring that patients and families are properly educated regarding the course of the disorder, importance of drug maintenance, and need for consistent care and support. Research is demonstrating that interaction between patients and their families is key to the success of long-term treatments and outcomes.

Critical Thinking Challenges

1. Why are positive symptoms easier to track than negative symptoms?
2. Describe ways in which medical illness or substance abuse could cause a patient to show symptoms similar to schizophrenia.
3. Suggest reasons that a higher rate of schizophrenia is found in lower classes of people from urban, industrialized communities.
4. The physical environment is important to the patient with schizophrenia. Think of the typical hospital unit. What environmental factors could be stress producing or misleading to the person with schizophrenia?
5. Compare therapeutic and nontherapeutic communication skills when dealing with a person with schizophrenia who is actively hallucinating.

WEB LINKS

www.nami.org   This is the website of the National Alliance for the Mentally Ill.

www.nimh.nih.gov/publicat/schioph.htm   The National Institute of Mental Health website presents all aspects of the diagnosis and treatment of schizophrenia.

www.narsad.org   This is the site of the National Alliance for Research on Schizophrenia and Depression, which is a national organization that raises and distributes money for research.

www.schizophrenia.ca   This is the site of the Schizophrenia Society of Canada, an organization committed to alleviating suffering caused by schizophrenia.

www.schizophrenia.com   This is a not-for-profit information, support, and education center.

www.mentalhealth.com   This site of the Mental Health Network provides extensive information on schizophrenia.

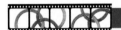

MOVIES

Benny and Joon: 1993. Joon is a young woman with schizophrenia who lives with her overprotective brother. In an attempt to keep her safe, Joon's brother unsuccessfully hires one housekeeper after another. After winning a bet in a poker game, Joon's brother acquires Benny, played by Johnny Depp, who entertains and cares for Joon. A romance develops that results in Benny and Joon attempting to run away. Joon's symptoms reappear. After treatment, Joon struggles with becoming independent from both her brother and boyfriend.

Viewing Points: How does Joon's brother's behavior interfere with her normal growth and development? When Joon's symptoms appeared, how would you classify them according to the *DSM-IV-TR?* What advise would you like to give to Joon and her brother?

References

Adityanjee, A. U. A., & Mathews, T. (1999). Epidemiology of neuroleptic malignant syndrome. *Clinical Neuropharmacology, 22*(3), 151–158.

American Psychiatric Association. (1997). Practice guidelines for the treatment of patients with schizophrenia. *American Journal of Psychiatry, 154*(4 Suppl.), 1–63.

American Psychiatric Association. (2000). *Diagnostic and statistical manual of mental disorders* (4th ed., Text revision). Washington, DC: Author.

Andreasen, N. C., & Black, D. W. (1991). *Introductory textbook of psychiatry.* Washington, DC: American Psychiatric Press.

Andreasen, N. C., & Carpenter, W. T. (1993). Diagnosis and classification of schizophrenia. *Schizophrenia Bulletin, 19,* 199–214.

Baier, M., Robinson, M., DeShay, E., & Snider, K. (1989). Issues in the nursing management of patients with water intoxication. *Archives of Psychiatric Nursing, 3*(6), 338–343.

Baldessarini, R. J., & Centorrino, F. (1996). *Results and limits of antipsychotic pharmacotherapy.* Unpublished manuscript.

Bateson, G., Jackson, D. D., Haley, J., & Weakland, J. H. (1956). Toward a theory of schizophrenia. *Behavioral Science, 1,* 251–264.

Bellack, A. S. (1992). Cognitive rehabilitation for schizophrenia: Is it possible? Is it necessary? *Schizophrenia Bulletin, 18,* 43–50.

Blair, D. T., & Dauner, A. (1993). Neuroleptic malignant syndrome: Liability in nursing practice. *Journal of Psychosocial Nursing, 31*(2), 5–12.

Blum, A., Tempey, F., & Lynch, W., (1983). Somatic findings in patients with psychogenic polydipsia. *Journal of Clinical Psychiatry, 44,* 55–56.

Boyd, M., & Lapierre, E. (1996). Fluid imbalance and water intoxication: The elusive syndrome. In A. McBride & J. Austin (Eds.), *Psychiatric mental health nursing: Integration of the biological into behavioral* (pp. 396–424). Philadelphia: W. B. Saunders.

Boyd, M., Williams, L., Evenson, R., et al. (1992). Target weight procedure for disordered water balance. *Journal of Psychosocial Nursing, 30*(12), 22–27.

Boyle, M. (1990). *Schizophrenia: A scientific delusion?* New York: Routledge.

Breier, A., Schreiber, J. L., Dyer, J., & Pickar, D. (1991). National Institute of Mental Health longitudinal study of chronic schizophrenia: Prognosis and predictors of outcome. *Archives of General Psychiatry, 48,* 239–246.

Brenner, H. D., Hodel, B., Roder, V., & Corrigan, P. (1992). Treatment of cognitive dysfunctions and behavioral deficits in schizophrenia. *Schizophrenia Bulletin, 18,* 21–26.

Buchsbaum, M. (1990). The frontal lobes, basal ganglia, and temporal lobes as a site for schizophrenia. *Schizophrenia Bulletin, 16,* 377–387.

Butler, R. W., & Braff, D. L. (1991). Delusions: A review and integration. *Schizophrenia Bulletin, 17,* 633–647.

Casey, D. E. (1994). Schizophrenia. Psychopharmacology. In J. W. Jefferson & J. H. Greist (Eds.), *The Psychiatric Clinics of North America annual of drug therapy* (Vol. 1, pp. 81–100). Philadelphia: W. B. Saunders.

De Hert, M., McKenzie, K., Peuskens, J. (2001). Risk factors for suicide in young people suffering from schizophrenia: a long-term follow-up study. *Schizophrenia Research, 47*(2–3), 127–134.

Delva, N., & Crammer, T., (1988). Polydipsia in chronic psychosis. Body weight and plasma sodium. *British Journal of Psychiatry, 152,* 242–245.

Flaum, M., Arndt, S., & Andreasen, N. C. (1991). The reliability of "bizarre" delusions. *Comprehensive Psychiatry, 32,* 59–65.

Franzen, G. (1970). Plasma free fatty acids before and after an intravenous insulin injection in acute schizophrenic men. *British Journal of Psychiatry, 116*(531), 173–177.

Gerson, S. L. (1990, April). *Clozapine and agranulocytosis.* Paper presented at the International Symposium of Schizophrenia and Clozapine, Cleveland, OH.

Goldman, L. S. (1999). Medical illness in patients with schizophrenia. *Journal of Clinical Psychiatry, 60*(Suppl. 21), 1015.

Goldman, M. (1991). A rational approach to disorders of water balance in psychiatric patients. *Hospital and Community Psychiatry, 42*(5), 488–493.

Goldman, M., Luchins, D., & Robertson, G. (1988). Mechanisms of altered water metabolism in psychotic patients with polydipsia and hyponatremia. *New England Journal of Medicine, 318*(7), 397–403.

Gray, J. A. (1998). Integrating schizophrenia. *Schizophrenia Bulletin, 24,* 249–266.

Green, M. F., Kern, R. S., Braff, D. L., & Mintz, J. (2000). Neurocognitive deficits and functional outcome in schizophrenia: Are we measuring the "right stuff"? *Schizophrenia Bulletin, 26*(1), 119–137.

Gureje, O., & Bamidele, R. W. (1998). Gender and schizophrenia: Association of age at onset with antecedent, clinical and outcome features. *Australia New Zealand Journal of Psychiatry, 32*(3), 415–423.

Guy, W. (1976). *ECDEU: Assessment manual for psychopharmacology* (DHEW Publication No. 76-338). Washington, DC: Department of Health, Education, and Welfare.

Hagen, B. R., & Mitchell, D. (2001). Might within the madness: Solution-focused therapy and thought-disordered clients. *Archives of Psychiatric Nursing, 15*(2), 86–93.

Hamera, E. K., Peterson, K. A., Handley, S. M., et al. (1991). Patient self-regulation and functioning in schizophrenia. *Hospital and Community Psychiatry, 42,* 630–631.

Harding, C., Zubin, J., & Strauss, J. (1987). Chronicity in schizophrenia: Fact, partial fact or artifact? *Hospital and Community Psychiatry, 38*(5), 477–486.

Jibson, M. D., & Tandon, R. (2000). Treatment of schizophrenia. In D. L. Dunner & J. E. Rosenbaum (Eds.), *The Psychiatric Clinics of North America annual of drug therapy* (Vol. 7, pp. 83–113). Philadelphia: W. B. Saunders.

Jos, C., Evenson, R., & Mallya, A. (1986). Self-induced water intoxication: A comparison of 34 cases with matched controls. *Journal of Clinical Psychiatry, 47*(7), 368–370.

Kandel, E. R., Schwartz, J. H., & Jessell, T. M. (2000). *Principles of neural science* (4th ed.). New York, NY: McGraw-Hill.

Kanter, J., Lamb, H. R., & Loeper, C. (1987). Expressed emotion in families: A critical review. *Hospital and Community Psychiatry, 38,* 374–380.

Keith, S. J., & Matthews, S. M. (1991). The diagnosis of schizophrenia: A review of onset and duration issues. *Schizophrenia Bulletin, 17,* 51–67.

Keltner, N., & Folks, D. G. (2001). *Psychotropic drugs* (3rd ed.). St. Louis: Mosby.

Keltner, N. L., Folks, D. G., Palmer, C. A., & Powers, R. E. (1998). *Psychobiological foundations of psychiatric care.* St. Louis: Mosby.

Kendler, K. S., Glazer, W. M., & Morgenstern, H. (1983). Dimensions of delusional experience. *American Journal of Psychiatry, 140,* 466–469.

King, S., & Dixon, M. (1996). The influence of expressed emotion, family dynamics and symptom type on the social adjustment of schizophrenic young adults. *Archives of General Psychiatry, 53,* 1098–1104.

Kirch, D., Bigelow, L., Weinberger, D., et al. (1985). Polydipsia and chronic hyponatremia in schizophrenic inpatients. *Journal of Clinical Psychiatry, 46*(5), 179–181.

Lawson, W., Kaison, C., & Bigelow, L. (1985). Increased urine volume in chronic schizophrenia patients. *Psychiatric Research, 14*(4), 323–331.

Leshner, A. I., Archer, L., Britten, G., et al. (1992). *Outcasts on Main Street* (DHHS Publication No. ADM 92-1904). Washington, DC: U.S. Government Printing Office.

McCarrick, A. (1996). Communication patterns and expressed emotion in families of persons with mental disorders. *Schizophrenia Bulletin, 22*(4), 671–690.

McGlashan, T. H. (1994). Psychosocial treatments of schizophrenia: The potential relationships. In N. C. Andreasen (Ed.), *Schizophrenia: From mind to molecule* (pp. 189–215). Washington, DC: American Psychiatric Press.

Mercier-Guidez, E., & Loas, G. (2000). Polydipsia and water intoxication in 353 psychiatric inpatients: An epidemiological and psychopathological study. *European Psychiatry, 15*(5), 306–311.

Mintz, L. I., Liberman, R. P., Miklowitz, D. J., & Mintz, J. (1987). Expressed emotion: A call for partnership among relatives, patients, and professionals. *Schizophrenia Bulletin, 13,* 227–235.

Moldin, S. O., & Gottesman, I. I. (1997). At issue: Genes, experience, and chance in schizophrenia—positioning for the 21st century. *Schizophrenia Bulletin, 23,* 547–561.

Moller, M. D., & Wer, J. E. (1989). Simultaneous patient/family education regarding schizophrenia: The Nebraska model. *Archives of Psychiatric Nursing, 3,* 332–337.

Morrison, E. F. (1992). A coercive interactional style as an antecedent to aggression in psychiatric patients. *Research in Nursing and Health, 15,* 421–431.

Morrison, E. F. (1993). Toward a better understanding of violence in psychiatric settings: Debunking the myths. *Archives of Psychiatric Nursing, 7,* 328–335.

Murphy, M. F., & Moller, M. D. (1993). Relapse management in neurobiological disorders: The Moller-Murphy symptoms management assessment tool. *Archives of Psychiatric Nursing, 7,* 226–235.

Newcomer, J., Craft, S., Fucetola, R., et al. (1999). Glucose-induced increase in memory performance in patients with schizophrenia. *Schizophrenia Bulletin, 25*(2), 321–335.

O'Carroll, R., Russell, H., Lawrie, S., & Johnstone, E. (1999). Errorless learning and the cognitive rehabilitation of memory-impaired schizophrenic patients. *Psychological Medicine, 29,* 105–112.

O'Connor, F. W. (1994). A vulnerability-stress framework for evaluating clinical interventions in schizophrenia. *Image—The Journal of Nursing Scholarship, 26,* 231–237.

Overall, J. E., & Gorham, D. R. (1962). The brief psychiatric rating scale. *Psychological Reports, 10,* 799–812.

Riggs, A., Dyksen, M., Kim, S., & Opsahl, J. (1991). A review of disorders of water homeostasis in psychiatric patients. *Psychosomatics, 32*(2), 133–148.

Schimmelbusch, W. H., Mueller, P. S., & Sheps, J. (1971). The positive correlation between insulin resistance and duration of hospitalization in untreated schizophrenia. *British Journal of Psychiatry, 118*(545), 42–36.

Sedvall, G. (1994). Positron-emission tomography as a metabolic and neurochemical probe. In N. C. Andreasen (Ed.), *Schizophrenia: From mind to molecule* (pp. 147–155). Washington, DC: American Psychiatric Press.

Sewell, D. D., & Jeste, D. V. (1989). Neuroleptic malignant syndrome: A review. *Japanese Journal of Psychopharmacology, 9*, 319–333.

Simpson, G. M., & Angus, J. W. S. (1970). A rating scale for extrapyramidal side effects. *Acta Psychiatrica Scandinavica, 212*(Suppl.), 11–19.

Snider, K., & Boyd, M. (1991). When they drink too much: Nursing interventions for patients with disordered water balance. *Journal of Psychosocial Nursing, 29*(7), 10–16.

Sprague, R. L., & Kalachnik, J. E. (1991). Reliability, validity, and a total score cut-off for the Dyskinesia Identification System: Condensed User Scale (DISCUS) with mentally ill and mentally retarded populations. *Psychopharmacology Bulletin, 27*, 51–58.

Stahl, S. (2000). *Essential psychopharmacology: Neuroscientific basis and practical application* (2nd ed.). Cambridge, UK: Cambridge University Press.

Stevens, J. R. (1997). Anatomy of schizophrenia revisited. *Schizophrenia Bulletin, 23*, 373–383.

Sullivan, H. S. (1964). The language of schizophrenia. In J. S. Kasanin (Ed.), *Language and thought in schizophrenia* (pp. 4–15). New York: Norton.

U.S. Department of Health and Human Services. (1999). *Mental health: A report of the Surgeon General.* Rockville, MD: Author.

Vieweg, W., Godleski, L., Graham, P., et al. (1989a). Diurnal weight gain in chronic psychosis. *Schizophrenia Bulletin, 15*(3), 501–505.

Vieweg, W., Godleski, L, & Graham, P. (1989b). Abnormal diurnal weight gain among long-term patients with schizophrenic disorders. *Schizophrenia Research, 1*, 67–71.

Vieweg, W., Rowe, W., & David, J. (1985). Patterns of urinary excretion among patients with self-induced water intoxication and psychosis. *Psychiatric Research, 15*, 71–79.

Weickert, C. S., & Weinberger, D. R. (1998). A candidate molecule approach to defining developmental pathology in schizophrenia. *Schizophrenia Bulletin, 24*(2), 303–316.

Willick, M. S. (1994). Schizophrenia: A parent's perspective-mourning without end. In N. C. Andreasen (Ed.), *Schizophrenia: From mind to molecule* (pp. 5–19). Washington, DC: American Psychiatric Press.

Willwerth, J. (1993, August 30). Tinkering with madness. *Time, 142*(9), 40–42.

Wyngarden, J., Smith, L., & Bennet, J. (Eds.), (1992). *Cecil textbook of medicine* (19th ed). Philadelphia: Saunders.

Zarate, C. A., Daniel, D. G., Kinon, B. J., et al. (1995). Algorithms for the treatment of schizophrenia. *Psychopharmacology Bulletin, 31*, 461–467.

Zubin, J., Steinhauer, S. R., & Condray, R. (1992). Vulnerability to relapse in schizophrenia. *British Journal of Psychiatry, 161*(Suppl. 18), 13–18.

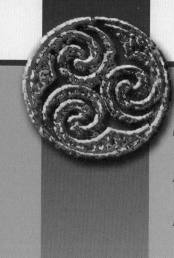

Schizoaffective, Delusional, and Other Psychotic Disorders

Nan Roberts

LEARNING OBJECTIVES

After studying this chapter, you will be able to:

➤ Define schizoaffective disorder and distinguish the major differences among schizophrenia, schizoaffective, and mood disorders.

➤ Discuss the important epidemiologic findings related to schizoaffective disorder.

➤ Explain the primary etiologic factors regarding schizoaffective disorder.

➤ Explain the primary elements involved in assessment, nursing diagnoses, nursing interventions, and evaluation of patients with schizoaffective disorder.

➤ Define delusional disorder and explain the importance of nonbizarre delusions in diagnosis and treatment.

384

CHAPTER 19

➤ Explain the important epidemiologic findings regarding delusional disorder.
➤ Discuss the primary etiologic factors of delusional disorder.
➤ Explain the various subtypes of delusional disorder.
➤ Explain the nursing care of patients with delusional disorder.

KEY TERMS

delusional disorder
delusions
erotomania
misidentification
nonbizarre delusions

persecutory delusions
psychosis
schizoaffective disorder
thymoleptic

*P*sychiatric–mental health nurses care for patients who
have psychiatric disorders involving underlying psychoses
other than schizophrenia and mood disorders. This chapter
introduces other psychotic disorders and describes the associated nursing care. Central to understanding the problems of
these patients is the concept of **psychosis**, a term used to describe a state in which an individual experiences positive
symptoms, also known as psychotic symptoms (hallucinations, delusions, or disorganized thoughts, speech, or behavior) (see Chap. 18). Other psychotic disorders defined by the
presence of psychosis include schizophreniform, schizoaffective, delusional, brief psychotic, and shared psychotic disorders. Still other psychotic disorders may be induced by drugs
or alcohol.

Schizoaffective disorder is one of the more complex psychotic disorders, but one of the more common diagnoses that
the generalist psychiatric nurse is likely to encounter. The
person with delusional disorder is more likely to be treated
in a medical-surgical setting and is rarely seen by a psychiatrist. This disorder often remains undiagnosed; therefore,
for nurses practicing in nonpsychiatric settings, recognizing
and understanding it are crucial to providing meaningful
care.

SCHIZOAFFECTIVE DISORDER

Definition and Clinical Course

Schizoaffective disorder is a complex and persistent
psychiatric diagnosis. This disorder was recognized
by Kasanin in 1933, who described varying degrees of
symptoms of both schizophrenia and mood disorders,
beginning in youth. All his patients were well adjusted
before the sudden onset of symptoms that erupted after
the occurrence of a specific environmental stressor.
Since Kasanin's time, there have been extensive debate
and controversy about the status of this disorder, resulting in many different definitions and classifications
that remain under consideration (Evans et al., 1999;
Maj et al., 2000).

Schizoaffective disorder is characterized by intervals of intense symptoms along with quiescent periods
during which psychosocial functioning is adequate.
The episodic nature of this disorder is characteristic of
this illness. There is general agreement that this disorder is at times marked by symptoms of schizophrenia; at other times, it appears to be a mood disorder.
In still other cases, both psychosis and pervasive
mood changes occur concurrently.

Patients with schizoaffective disorder are more likely to exhibit persistent psychosis with or without mood symptoms than those with a mood disorder (Strakowski et al., 1999). Patients with this disorder feel that they are on a "chronic roller coaster ride" of symptoms that are often more difficult to cope with than the individual problem of either schizophrenia or mood disorder (O'Connell, 1995). The diagnosis of this disorder is made only after these course-related characteristics are considered.

The long-term outcome of schizoaffective disorder is generally better than that of schizophrenia but worse than that of mood disorder (Evans et al., 2000). This group of patients is more like the mood disorder group in work function and the schizophrenia group in social function. When patients with this disorder were compared with those with a bipolar mood disorder, the schizoaffective patients were less likely to achieve recovery and more likely to have persistent psychosis, with or without mood symptoms (Strakowski et al., 1999).

Diagnostic Criteria

Mental health providers find schizoaffective disorder difficult to conceptualize, diagnose, and treat because of the varying clinical picture. Patients are often misdiagnosed as having schizophrenia. Others are diagnosed correctly with this disorder only because they do not easily fit the category of either schizophrenia or bipolar disorder. The difficulty in conceptualizing schizoaffective disorder is reflected in the controversy regarding the diagnostic criteria. For example, it has been argued that this disorder should be named either schizophrenia with mood symptoms or mood disorder with schizophrenic symptoms. More than 50 years after it was first described, the diagnosis of schizoaffective disorder was finally officially confirmed by the psychiatric community and included in the American Psychiatric Association's (APA's) *Diagnostic and Statistical Manual of Mental Disorders*, 3rd edition, Revision (*DSM-III-R*) (Table 19-1).

To be diagnosed with schizoaffective disorder, there is an uninterrupted period of illness when there is a major depressive, manic, or mixed episode along with two of the following symptoms of schizophrenia: delusions, hallucinations, disorganized speech, disorganized or catatonic behavior, or negative symptoms (eg, affective flattening, alogia, or avolition). Additionally, although the person experiences problems with mood most of the time, to be diagnosed with this disorder, the positive symptoms (delusions or hallucinations) have to be present *without* the mood symptoms at some time during this period (for at least 2 weeks) (Table 19-2). To clarify this disorder further, two related subtypes of schizoaffective disorder have been identified. In the bipolar type, the patient exhibits manic symptoms alone or a mix of manic and depressive symptoms. Patients di-

agnosed with the depressive type display only symptoms of a major depressive episode within the illness (APA, 2000; O'Connell, 1995). The most common disorders from which a differential diagnosis is required include mood disorders of manic, depressive, or mixed types and schizophrenia.

Epidemiology and Risk Factors

The lifetime prevalence of schizoaffective disorder is reported to be 0.5% to 13.6% (Kendler et al., 1995; Siris & Lavin, 1995). Occurrence of this disorder is less common than that of schizophrenia. The incidence of schizoaffective disorder is relatively constant across populations in wide geographic, climatic, industrial, and social environments. If environmental contributions exist, they are minimal.

Patients with schizoaffective disorder are at high risk for suicide. The lifetime frequency of suicide attempts has been reported to be 23% to 42% (Radomsky et al., 1999). The risk for dying by suicide in patients with psychosis is increased by the presence of depression. Risk for suicide is lower nearer the onset of the disorder and increases during the early years of the illness. Those at the greatest risk for suicide are young and socially isolated (Radomsky et al., 1999).

Lack of regular social contact may be a factor that has a long-term risk for suicidal behavior. Treatments designed to enhance social networks and contact may decrease the risk for suicidal behavior (Radomsky et al., 1999) and help patients to protect themselves against environmental stressors (Huxley et al., 2000). Cognition is more impaired with schizoaffective disorder than with nonpsychotic mood disorder (Evans et al., 1999).

Age of Onset

Schizoaffective disorder can be present in children and the elderly. In children, the disorder is rare and is often indistinguishable from schizophrenia. In the elderly,

TABLE 19.1	**History of the Diagnosis: Schizoaffective**
1933	Kasanin first coined the phrase *schizoaffective psychosis*.
1980	*DSM-III* did not include diagnostic criteria for Schizoaffective Disorder.
1987	Schizoaffective Disorder was first recognized as a separate diagnosis in the *DSM-III-R* that included length of time in relationship to symptoms.
1994	Schizoaffective Disorder was maintained as a separate disorder in the *DSM-IV*.
2000	Schizoaffective Disorder was maintained as a separate disorder in *DSM-IV-TR*.

TABLE 19.2 Key Diagnostic Characteristics of Schizoaffective Disorder 295.70

Diagnostic Criteria and Target Symptoms	Associated Findings
<ul><li>Uninterrupted period of illness with concurrent major depressive episode, manic episode, or mixed episode</li><li>Bipolar type: manic or mixed episode or manic or mixed episode and major depressive episode</li><li>Depressive type: only major depressive episode</li><li>Characteristic symptoms of schizophrenia (two or more) during a 1-month period<ul><li>Delusions</li><li>Hallucinations</li><li>Disorganized speech</li><li>Grossly disorganized or catatonic behavior or negative symptoms</li></ul></li><li>Delusions or hallucinations for at least 2 weeks without prominent mood symptoms</li><li>Symptoms of mood episode present for major portion of the active and residual periods of illness</li><li>Not a direct physiologic effect of a substance or medical condition</li></ul>	***Associated Behavioral Findings***<ul><li>Poor occupational functioning</li><li>Restricted range of social contact</li><li>Difficulties with self-care</li><li>Increased risk for suicide</li></ul>

this disorder becomes complicated because of frequent comorbid medical conditions. There is disagreement about the age of onset, although the difference may be related to the type of schizoaffective disorder exhibited. Age of onset can occur from late adolescence to late life. The typical age of onset for this disorder is early adulthood, and the most common type presented is bipolar. Other studies have reported a relatively late onset of schizoaffective disorder of mainly the depressive type (APA, 2000). With earlier age of onset, there is a longer duration of this disorder, and the illness is more severe with worse outcomes (APA, 2000; Berteisen & Gottesman, 1995; Henry & Coster, 1995).

Gender Differences

Gender differences may be helpful in understanding the nature of schizoaffective disorder. This disorder is more likely to occur in women than in men, which may be accounted for by an increased incidence of the depressive type in women (APA, 2000).

Ethnic and Cultural Differences

Most patients diagnosed with schizoaffective disorder are white. It has been reported that patients are usually of an elevated social class; however, others support no specific association with race, geographic area, or social class (Siris & Lavin, 1995).

Familial Differences

Some authorities support a familial association in schizoaffective disorder, but a clear familial pattern has not been established (Erlenmeyer et al., 1995). Relatives of patients diagnosed with schizoaffective disorder appear to be at increased risk for this disorder, schizophrenia, or both. Relatives are at a similar risk for mood disorder and are at some risk for schizophrenia

or other psychotic disorders. They are at increased risk for psychiatric disorders. Female relatives are at increased risk for mood disorders, whereas male relatives are at an increased risk for schizophrenia spectrum disorders (Kendler et al., 1995).

Comorbidity

Schizoaffective disorder may be associated with substance abuse. An increase in antisocial behavior in men has been reported. Panic disorder is also associated with this disorder. Twenty-five percent of patients diagnosed with schizoaffective disorder have a postpsychotic depression and experience panic attacks (APA, 2000).

Etiology

Biologic Theories

Although a large amount of research has investigated the etiology of schizophrenia and mood disorder, the etiology of schizoaffective disorder remains unresolved. Research to locate a biologic marker has been limited. Variables may be structural as well as neurochemical.

Neuropathologic. Magnetic resonance imaging (MRI) and computed tomography scans have shown midline brain abnormality, especially in women (Scott et al., 1993). Brain size is smaller in these patients, and there is asymmetry (Crow & Harrington, 1994). Men appear to have more volume loss or ventricular anomaly than white matter lesions, suggestive of differential neurologic mechanisms (Levine et al., 1995). Some degree of ventricular enlargement has been reported (Crow & Harrington, 1994). It is unclear whether the association of a midline structural abnormality is directly causal, indirectly contributory, or an intriguing phenomenon in schizoaffective disorder (Scott et al., 1993).

Genetic. The etiology is believed to be primarily genetic. Results from family, twin, and adoption studies are divergent but support a separate classification of broadly defined schizoaffective psychoses as possibly being phenotypic variations or expressions of a genetic interform between schizophrenia and affective psychoses (Berteisen & Gottesman, 1995; Evans et al., 1999). Concordance found in twin studies suggests a strong genetic factor (Berteisen & Gottesman, 1995).

Biochemical. Before 1999, overactivity of dopamine pathways was the prevailing neurochemical hypothesis. Whether patients undergo a primary disturbance of dopaminergic transmission remains unclear (Rietschel et al., 2000; Serretti et al., 2000; Serretti et al., 1999a; Serretti et al., 1999b). Different patterns of glucose metabolism have been found while studying deficit symptoms in schizoaffective disorder, causing increased neurobiologic and neurophysiologic impairments (Gerbaldo & Phillips, 1995). The season of birth has been studied in relation to schizoaffective disorder.

Psychological and Social Theories

Psychological, psychodynamic, environmental, and interpersonal factors may have a precipitating role when they coincide with a biomedical diathesis that creates vulnerability to this disorder (see Chap. 6 for explanation of the diathesis-stress theory). No psychodynamic behavioral, cognitive, or development theories of causation were found relating to schizoaffective disorder. Family dynamics do not appear to affect the development of this disorder, except for a strong genetic predisposition that is virtually unexplained.

Interdisciplinary Treatment

Patients with schizoaffective disorder benefit from a comprehensive treatment approach. Because of the persistent nature of this disorder, these individuals are constantly trying to manage the interaction of complex symptoms. Ideally, most of the treatment occurs within the patient's natural environment, and hospitalizations are limited to times of symptom exacerbation. There are times when symptoms are so severe or persistent that extended care in a protected environment, such as a hospital or residential facility, is necessary.

Pharmacologic intervention is always needed to stabilize the symptoms and presents specific challenges. Atypical antipsychotics on an ongoing basis are now the mainstay of pharmacologic treatment and are as effective as the traditional combination of a standard antipsychotic and antidepressant. Mood stabilizers, such as lithium or valproic acid (see Chap. 8), may also be ordered. In the clinical area, use of a combination of antipsychotics and antidepressants may be seen, but research support for this type of intervention is meager (Levinson et al., 1999).

After the patient has stabilized (ie, exhibits a decrease in positive and negative symptoms that were originally present) on a medication regimen, it is best to continue the treatment that led to remission of the acute symptoms. The downward titration of antipsychotics to the lowest dose that provides suitable protection may allow for optimal psychosocial functioning while slowing progression of new episodes even if the medication does not abort the episode entirely. It is unlikely that patients diagnosed with schizoaffective disorder will be medication free. Electroconvulsive therapy is considered when the patient appears to be refractory to other interventions or when the patient's life is at risk and a rapid response is required (Siris & Lavin, 1995).

The treatment plan is revised regularly as symptoms are monitored. Psychiatric nursing interventions are guided by the nursing diagnoses. Monitoring of psychiatric symptoms and medication management are always ongoing. After hospitalization, home visits may be needed. Psychotherapy by one of the mental health specialists (psychologist, advanced practice psychiatric nurse, social worker) may be beneficial in managing interpersonal relationships and changes in mood. Social services are often needed to assist the individual and family in obtaining disability benefits or other state or federal services.

Priority Care Issues

Patients with schizoaffective disorder may be especially susceptible to suicide. The rate of death by suicide is comparable to that associated with mood disorder (Tsuang & Coryell, 1993). Living with a persistent psychotic disorder that has a mood component makes suicide risk a real possibility.

NURSING MANAGEMENT: HUMAN RESPONSE TO DISORDER

Biologic Domain

Assessment

A careful history from the patient and family is crucial in obtaining an adequate assessment. The history contains a description of the full range of symptoms the patient has experienced and those observed by the family along with an accurate accounting of the length of time that the symptoms have been present; this information is important for predicting outcomes. It may be that a psychosis has a deteriorating affect on function (Henry & Coster, 1995). A patient who has had symptoms for a longer period of time has greater difficulty in overcoming effects of the psychosis. Assessment of patients with schizoaffective disorder would incorporate and be similar to that for those with schizophrenia and affective disorder.

A thorough systems assessment is important to discover any physiologic problems the patient is experiencing. Sleep pattern disturbances, difficulties with self-care, and poor nutritional habits may be present.

Nursing Diagnoses

Common nursing diagnoses for the biologic domain are Disturbed Thought Process, Disturbed Sensory Perception, and Disturbed Sleep Patterns. Because of the variety of problems in patients with schizoaffective disorder, almost any nursing diagnosis could be generated. The persistent nature of this disorder lends itself to numerous and varied problems that have been or will need to be addressed at one time or another (see Nursing Care Plan for a Patient With Schizoaffective Disorder.)

Interventions

Patient Education. Interventions are based on the needs identified in the biopsychosocial assessment (Fig. 19-1). Establishment of a regular sleep pattern by setting a routine can help to promote or reestablish normal patterns of rest. Educating the patient on the six food groups in the Food Guide Pyramid and what constitutes good nutrition is helpful in establishing improved nutritional status. Helping the patient to gain insight into the deficits related to self-care activities is valuable, especially if they are caused by lack of motivation. If the deficits are created by severe mood symptoms, helping the patient to establish a routine and set goals can be useful.

Pharmacologic Interventions. An in-depth history of the patient's medication is important in evaluating past medications and response to them along with the present medication regimen. Compliance with past treatment modalities is investigated to determine the probability of successful intervention. Based on past problems or issues related to medication adherence, a plan to increase compliance should be developed. Methods to increase adherence include use of medication boxes and calendars along with gaining help from others in managing the medication regimen. Early recognition of medication side effects and interventions to alleviate them will help maintain patient compliance. Helping patients gain insight into the need for medications and outlining the purpose of the medications for promoting wellness are essential.

The pharmacologic treatment of schizoaffective disorder is one of the least studied areas in psychiatry. Mood and psychotic symptoms should be considered equally important and evaluated throughout the course of treatment. In practice, atypical antipsychotics are

generally prescribed because of their efficacy in the treatment of schizophrenia and their safe side-effect profile. Clozapine efficacy in treating schizoaffective disorder has been reported by several authors. Use of clozapine can reduce hospitalizations and risk for suicide (Evans et al., 1999). Clozapine offers superior efficacy for patients who have been treatment resistant. A significant portion of patients with prior resistance to other neuroleptic agents improve on clozapine (Simpson et al., 1999). Atypical antipsychotics may have **thymoleptic** (providing mood stabilizing effects) as well as antipsychotic effects (Azorin, 1995; Zarate et al., 1995). Dosage is the same, but lower dosage ranges may also be effective.

In many cases, symptoms of depression disappear when psychotic symptoms decrease. If depressive symptoms persist, adjunctive use of an antidepressant may be helpful. Mood stabilizers, such as valproic acid, may be an alternative adjunctive medication for mood states associated with the bipolar type. This may be effective when added to the antipsychotics, lithium, or both. Valproic acid has a mood-stabilizing effect that may decrease the frequency and intensity of episodes. It may be effective in schizoaffective patients with concomitant panic attacks and as a first-line mood stabilizer because of its favorable side-effect profile and easy administration.

Monitoring and Administration of Medications. One of the greatest challenges in pharmacologic interventions is monitoring the target symptoms and identifying changes in symptom pattern. Patients can switch from being relatively calm to being very emotional. Determining whether the patient is overreacting to an environmental event or whether there is a change in mood symptoms requiring a medication change can be assessed only through careful observation and documentation.

Adherence to the medication regimen once discharged is critical to a successful outcome. Patients need an opportunity to discuss medications and compliance barriers.

Side-Effect Management. Monitoring medication side effects in patients with schizoaffective disorder is similar to that in patients with schizophrenia. Extrapyramidal side effects, weight gain, and sedation should be assessed and documented.

Drug–Drug Interactions. Agents observed to have potentially important interactions with valproic acid include aspirin, felbamate, rifampin, carbamazepine, clonazepam, diazepam, primidone, and phenytoin. Use of lithium along with an antipsychotic medication is cautioned against. There have been a few patients who developed an encephalopathic syndrome followed by irreversible brain damage with the combined use of haloperidol and lithium. The possibility of similar

(text continues on page 392)

NURSING CARE PLAN 19.1
Nursing Care Plan for a Patient With Schizoaffective Disorder

Mr. W is a 48-year-old white man who has lived in a residential care facility for the past several years. He was admitted to the hospital because of aggressive behavior (eg, fighting with another resident). The residential care facility has refused to take the patient back into the facility after hospitalization.

This is Mr. W's seventh hospital admission. He is agitated and verbalizing delusions related to OPEC. He thinks that he owns all the countries in OPEC, that he is a multibillionaire, and that OPEC has stolen all of his money. His delusions are ingrained, and attempts at reality feedback only agitate him more.

The patient's present medication regimen and the events leading up to the admission were reported by the residential care facility. Mr. W has recently become more agitated, with an increase in verbalization of delusions. He is unable to be calmed with reality feedback, which has only potentiated his agitation. Today, another resident told him that he was "full of it," which precipitated a fist fight between the two residents.

Mr. W has had numerous psychiatric admissions in the past 30 years. He has carried diagnoses of bipolar affective disorder, schizophrenia, and depression and is presently diagnosed with schizoaffective disorder. Medications have included antidepressants, neuroleptics (traditional and nontraditional), benzodiazepines, and mood stabilizers (eg, lithium, valproic acid). For the past several years, the patient has been compliant with medications, but on occasion, his agitation gets out of control, and he requires hospitalization to adjust medications.

Mr. W is single but has maintained a relationship with the same girlfriend for the past 5 years. His girlfriend is also mentally ill, but is able to function independently. They see each other frequently at the local day social club. Their families are also supportive of their relationship and allow Mr. W to visit on weekends and holidays. The patient's girlfriend has little influence over his behavior.

SETTING: INTENSIVE CARE PSYCHIATRIC UNIT IN A GENERAL HOSPITAL

Baseline Assessment: Mr. W is a 48-year-old white man admitted directly to the unit as a voluntary patient. He has been compliant with medications. The patient is well nourished and appropriately dressed. The patient is verbalizing delusions related to OPEC and becomes agitated when reality feedback is employed. Mr. W is oriented in all three spheres. He denies any problems.

Associated Psychiatric Diagnosis	*Medications*
Axis I: Schizoaffective disorder	Divalproex, 250 mg bid; 500 mg hs
Axis II: None	Olanzapine, 8 mg AM; 10 mg hs
Axis III: Hypertension, hyperlipidemia	Zestril, 20 mg bid
Axis IV: Social problem (social isolation)	Klonopin, 1 mg tid
Economic problem (low income)	
Occupation problem (unemployed)	
Axis V: Current, 36	
Potential, 54	

NURSING DIAGNOSIS 1: INEFFECTIVE INDIVIDUAL COPING

Defining Characteristics	*Related Factors*
Inability to meet role expectations	Chronicity of the condition
Agitation	Inadequate psychological resources secondary to delusions
Acting-out behavior	Inadequate psychological resources to adapt
Inability to problem solve	to residential setting

OUTCOMES

Initial	*Discharge*
1. Identify coping patterns	5. Manage own behavior
2. Identify acting out behavior	6. Identify inappropriate behavior
3. Identify personal strengths	
4. Accept support through the nursing relationship	

NURSING CARE PLAN 19.1 (Continued)

INTERVENTIONS

Interventions	Rationale	Ongoing Assessment
Initiate a nurse–patient relationship to develop trust.	Through the use of the nurse–patient relationship, the patient will be able to maintain compliance with the treatment plan.	Determine whether patient is able to relate to the nurse.
Facilitate the identification of stressors in patient's environment.	To be able to cope with stressors, they need to be identified by the patient.	Assess whether patient is able to identify and verbalize stressors.
Develop coping strategies to manage environmental stressors.	Patient needs to develop strategies that are realistic for him to handle environmental stressors.	Determine whether patient-identified strategies are realistic.
Help patient to identify personal strengths.	By identifying personal strengths, patient will increase confidence in using coping strategies.	Assess patient's ability to incorporate coping strategies into his daily routine.
Assist patient to understand the disorder and its management.	By understanding the disorder, patient can develop some insight into the chronicity of this disorder.	Assess the patient's level of understanding of the disease.
Facilitate emotional support from residential facility staff.	For the socially isolated patient, developing skills in seeking out emotional support can be learned within a helping relationship.	Assess patient's ability to seek emotional support from the residential care facility staff.
Teach stress management techniques.	By developing positive stress management skills, anxiety and agitation will decrease.	Assess patient's ability to learn the skills to manage stressors.

EVALUATION

Outcomes	Revised Outcomes	Interventions
Within the nursing relationship, Mr. W was able to understand acting-out behavior is controlled, there are fewer social difficulties.	Support the patient's ability to control behavior.	Refer to residential care facility staff.
Increased insight into what behavior is appropriate has helped the patient to decrease verbalization of delusions along with acting-out behavior.	Provide ongoing support to maintain present level of functioning.	Refer to residential care facility staff.

NURSING DIAGNOSIS 2: DISTURBED THOUGHT PROCESSES

Defining Characteristics	Related Factors
Delusions Impulsivity Inappropriate social behavior	Ingrained delusions Decreased ability to process secondary to delusions

OUTCOMES

Initial	Discharge
1. Maintain reality orientation 2. Communicate clearly with others. 3. Expresses delusional material less frequently.	4. Identify situations that occur before delusions. 5. Demonstrates knowledge of how verbalization of delusions affects others. 6. Use of coping strategies to deal with delusions. 7. Recognize changes in behavior.

(continued)

NURSING CARE PLAN 19.1 (Continued)

INTERVENTIONS

Interventions	Rationale	Ongoing Assessment
Administer olanzepine as ordered.	Antipsychotic medications decrease psychotic symptoms.	Assess for side effects: heat intolerance, neuroleptic malignant syndrome, renal failure, constipation, dry mouth, increased appetite, salivation, nausea, vomiting, tardive dyskinesia, seizures, somnolence, agitation, insomnia, dizziness.
Teach Mr. W about the action, effects, and side effects of olanzapine. Emphasize the importance of continuing medications.	The more knowledgeable patients are about medication, the more likely they will comply.	Assess ability to understand information.
Support reality testing through helping patient to differentiate thoughts and feelings in relationship to the outside world.	When comparing thoughts with the outside world, patients can develop skills to evaluate objectively and judge the world outside of self.	Assess the patient's ability to differentiate thoughts and the outside world.
Monitor verbalization of delusional material.	Olanzapine will decrease delusional thoughts. Verbalization of delusional thoughts should decrease.	Assess verbalization of delusional material.
Identify situations that occur before delusions.	If patient is able to identify stressors that result in the resurgence of disorganized thought processes, he can manage the stressors to effectively decrease altered thought processes.	Assess patient's ability to recognize stressors when they occur.
Assist patient in developing skills to deal with delusions (recognizing delusional themes can help the patient in distinguishing between reality- and nonreality-based patterns).	Even though medication can reduce the occurrence of delusions, they may continue in some people with decreased intensity. Cognitive-behavioral skills are important in dealing with these altered thoughts.	Monitor patient's ability to handle delusions.

EVALUATION

Outcomes	Revised Outcomes	Interventions
During hospitalization, Mr. W began to express delusions on a less frequent basis.	Continue to practice skills in reality orientation and communication.	Refer to residential care facility staff.
Patient verbalized action, effect, dosage, and side effects of olanzapine. Is accepting of taking medication.	Take medication prescribed regularly.	Refer to residential care facility staff.

Summary of Hospitalization: Mr. W was hospitalized for 10 days. A new residential care facility was located for him. He has been medication compliant. His behavior has been appropriate, with only minimal agitation and no acting-out behavior. The patient's level of agitation increases only when his delusions are directly challenged. His family will transport him to the new residential care facility.

interactions exists with other antipsychotics. The effects of neuromuscular blocking agents may be prolonged. Use of nonsteroidal, anti-inflammatory agents may increase plasma lithium levels. Caution should be used in prescribing diuretics and angiotensin-converting enzyme inhibitors with lithium.

Teaching Points. Patients should be instructed to take medication as prescribed. The nurse should de-

termine whether the patient has sufficient resources to purchase and obtain medications once discharged. The patient should write down the prescribed medication and time of administration. The nurse should explain the target symptom for each medication (eg, psychosis and mood for atypical antipsychotics, mood for antidepressants and mood stabilizers). Patients should be cautioned about orthostatic hypotension

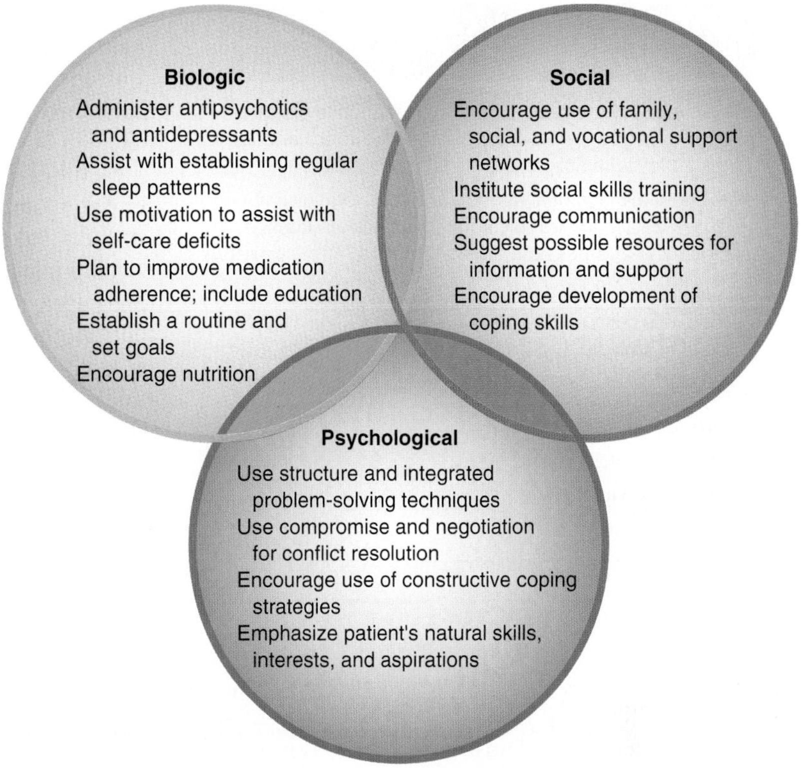

Biologic
Administer antipsychotics
  and antidepressants
Assist with establishing regular
  sleep patterns
Use motivation to assist with
  self-care deficits
Plan to improve medication
  adherence; include education
Establish a routine and
  set goals
Encourage nutrition

Social
Encourage use of family,
  social, and vocational support
  networks
Institute social skills training
Encourage communication
Suggest possible resources for
  information and support
Encourage development of
  coping skills

Psychological
Use structure and integrated
  problem-solving techniques
Use compromise and negotiation
  for conflict resolution
Encourage use of constructive coping
  strategies
Emphasize patient's natural skills,
  interests, and aspirations

FIGURE 19.1 Biopsychosocial interventions for patients with schizoaffective disorders.

and instructed to get up slowly from a lying or sitting position and to maintain an adequate fluid intake. Patients should be instructed to contact their case manager or health care provider if there are changes in body temperature (neuroleptic malignant syndrome [NMS]), ability to control motor movement (dystonia), or dizziness. Over-the-counter medications should be not be taken without consulting a prescriber. For olanzapine and clozapine, body weight should be monitored, and rapid weight gains should be reported.

Psychological Domain

Assessment

Determining the patient's level of insight into his or her illness may play a role in the course and treatment of schizoaffective disorder. Present stressors should be evaluated because they may trigger or precipitate symptoms. The nurse should also assess self-esteem because it is often low and self-worth is compromised. Patients with this disorder generally experience a wide range of problems. Uncovering or exploratory techniques are generally to be avoided, especially during the acute phase of the illness. Mental status and reality contact may be compromised. Assessment of anxiety level or reactions to stressful situations is important because the combination of these symptoms and psychosis place the patient at increased risk for suicide.

Nursing Diagnoses

In schizoaffective disorder, individuals vacillate between mood dysregulation and disturbed thinking. Typical nursing diagnoses for this domain include hopelessness, powerlessness, ineffective coping, and low self-esteem.

Interventions

Use of appropriate interpersonal modalities to help the patient, family, and social and vocational support networks cope with the onslaught of acute episodes and recuperative periods is important in these patients. Those with schizoaffective disorder have fewer awareness deficits than the group with schizophrenia. Structured, integrated, and problem-solving psychotherapeutic interventions are useful and should be used to develop or increase the patient's insight. Psychoeducational interventions can help to decrease symptoms, develop recognition of early regression, and develop psychosocial skills (see Psychoeducation Checklist: Schizoaffective Disorder).

Social Domain

Assessment

Social dysfunction is not uncommon in patients diagnosed with schizoaffective disorder. Premorbid adjustment, such as adolescent social adjustment and marital

When caring for the patient with schizoaffective disorder, be sure to include the caregiver as appropriate and address the following topic areas in the teaching plan:

- Psychopharmacologic agents (antipsychotic or antidepressants), if used, including drug action, dosage, frequency, and possible adverse effects
- Methods to enhance adherence
- Sleep measures
- Consistent routines
- Goal setting
- Nutrition
- Support networks
- Problem solving
- Positive coping strategies
- Social and vocational skills training

status, may influence the patient's prognosis. The nurse should assess for social skill deficits and problems with interpersonal conflicts. Antisocial behavior is reported to occur in men. Assessment of the patient's childhood, even though the person is an adult, may give a clue to the patient's present level of social functioning. The nurse assesses the patient's use of fantasy and fighting as a means of coping. Patients who report the most severe peer rejection present with the angriest dispositions and display antisocial behaviors. Patients with this disorder generally do not report family problems. Level of functioning at the time of diagnosis is related to premorbid social adjustment.

Nursing Diagnoses

Because of the mood and thought disturbances, these individuals will have significant problems in the social domain, yet they will usually function at a higher level than someone with schizophrenia. Typical nursing diagnoses include compromised family coping, impaired home maintenance, and social isolation.

Interventions

Social skills training is useful for remediating social deficits and may result in positive social adjustment. Positive results include improved interpersonal competence with a decrease in symptom severity. Help in identifying feelings and in developing realistic goals along with supportive therapy can integrate insight into the disease process (Higgins, 1995). Education focusing on skills to resolve conflict, which promotes expression of negative feelings along with compromise and negotiation, can help to achieve positive social adjustment. Improved

social skills can be attained through use of role play and assertiveness training. Supportive, nurturing, and nonconfrontational interventions help to minimize anxiety and improve understanding (see Therapeutic Dialogue: Mr. W's "Delusions").

Helping the patient to develop coping skills is essential. Communication skills are taught to decrease conflicts and environmental negativity. A link between development of social skills and memory has been identified. Psychotic symptoms may interfere with skill retention, resulting in slowed learning processes. These patients require long-term and more intense social training intervention.

Family members face many of the same issues as families of patients with schizophrenia. In addition, these families are often puzzled by the emotional overreaction to normal daily stresses. Frequent arguments may occur, leading to verbal and physical abuse. Families are at risk for ineffective coping.

Evaluation and Treatment Outcomes

It often takes longer to teach skills to patients with schizoaffective disorder. In evaluating progress related to interventions, one must be patient if outcomes are not completely met. Psychoeducation results in increased knowledge of the illness and treatment, increased medication compliance, a decrease in relapses and hospitalization, decreased inpatient stays, increased social function, a decrease in family tension, and the easing of family burden (Andres et al., 2000; Herz et al., 2000). Maintain realistic outcomes and praise small successes to promote positive outcomes (Fig. 19-2).

Continuum of Care

Inpatient-Focused Care

Hospitalization may be required at times of acute psychotic episodes or when suicidal ideations are present. This environment provides a structure that protects the patient from self-harm (ie, suicidal, assaultive, financial, legal, vocational, or social). During periods of acute psychosis, offering reassurance in a soft, nonthreatening voice and avoiding confrontational stances will help the patient begin to trust the staff and nursing care (see Chap. 9). Seclusion and restraint should be avoided. Environmental stimulation should be kept to a minimum. The nurse uses the patient's coping capabilities to reinforce constructive aspects to allow for a return to autonomy.

Emergency Care

Emergency care is needed during periods of symptom exacerbation. Psychosis, mood disturbance, and

THERAPEUTIC DIALOGUE | Mr. W's "Delusions"

Ineffective Approach

Nurse: Hello, Mr. W.
Patient: Is that doctor with you today?
Nurse: Yes, he is.
Patient: He lost his license and is thrown out of the hospital.
Nurse: No, he did not!
Patient: Yes, he did!
Nurse: He is not even on staff at the hospital you are talking about.
Patient: I'm not going to see him because he is in trouble.
Nurse: He is not in trouble and you will see him.

Effective Approach

Nurse: Hello, Mr. W.
Patient: Is that doctor with you?
Nurse: Yes, he will be here in a minute.
Patient: I am not going to see him today!
Nurse: Is there a problem?
Patient: He lost his license and has been thrown out of the hospital.
Nurse: I did not hear that.
Patient: I know it is true because I had to pay the fine. It cost me billions to get him out of trouble.

Nurse: I will see you today instead of the doctor if you wish.
Patient: That would be okay. If you ever get into trouble, all you have to do is call me, and I will bail you out.
Doctor: Hello, Mr. W. How are you today?
Patient: I have been doing okay.
Doctor: Are you ready to be seen?
Patient: Yes, that would be fine. I thought you had lost your license and were thrown off the hospital staff.
Doctor: No, I do not think that happened. (The doctor completed his evaluation.)
Patient: I knew all the money I spent on him was worth it.
Nurse: Is everything alright now?
Patient: Yes, we worked it out.

Critical Thinking Challenge

- How could the nurse's approach in the first scenario have prevented the patient from being seen by the doctor?

- How was the communication approach used in the second scenario beneficial in the patient being evaluated?

- Discuss the differences between the two approaches.

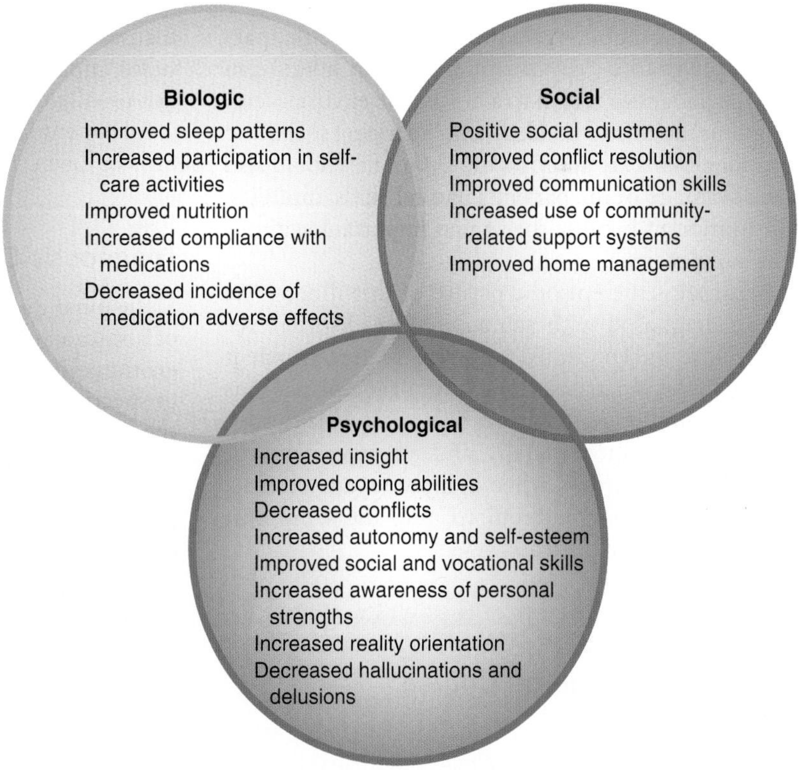

Biologic
Improved sleep patterns
Increased participation in self-care activities
Improved nutrition
Increased compliance with medications
Decreased incidence of medication adverse effects

Social
Positive social adjustment
Improved conflict resolution
Improved communication skills
Increased use of community-related support systems
Improved home management

Psychological
Increased insight
Improved coping abilities
Decreased conflicts
Increased autonomy and self-esteem
Improved social and vocational skills
Increased awareness of personal strengths
Increased reality orientation
Decreased hallucinations and delusions

Figure 19.2 Biopsychosocial outcomes for patients with schizoaffective disorder.

medication-related adverse effects account for most of the emergency situations. During an exacerbation of psychosis, patients may become agitated or aggressive. Assaultive behavior can be managed by using therapeutic techniques (see Chap. 36) and pharmacologic management. If medications are used to calm the patient during periods of acute agitation or aggression, benzodiazepines, such as lorazepam, are usually given. Patients are then evaluated for antipsychotic therapy. Possible medication-related adverse effects include NMS as a reaction to dopamine antagonists or serotonin intoxication, especially if the patient is taking an atypical antipsychotic and a selective serotonin reuptake inhibitor (see Chap. 18).

Family Intervention

Helping families support the patient in the home or a community placement is an integral part of nursing care. With patient permission, key family members can be included in home visits to learn about the symptoms, medications, and side effects. By collaborating with family members, the nurse can strengthen the patient's willingness to follow treatment regimen, monitor symptoms, and continue with rehabilitation and recovery efforts.

Community Treatment

After hospitalization, stepdown levels of care (ie, partial hospitalization, day treatment, group home) can help the patient to return to a normative environment. Programs that foster building and practicing social and vocational skills are appropriate. Programs should also take advantage of the patient's natural skills, interests, and aspirations because they are as important as problems and deficits.

Because of the episodic nature of this illness, the person diagnosed with schizoaffective disorder requires close and continued follow-up in the outpatient setting by psychiatrists, nurses, and therapists. This group requires ongoing medication management, supportive and cognitive therapy, and symptom management. During periods when symptoms are intense, hospitalization may be required until the symptoms are brought under control.

DELUSIONAL DISORDER

Definition and Clinical Course

Delusional disorder is a psychotic disorder characterized by nonbizarre, logical, stable, and well-systemized delusions that occur in the absence of other psychiatric disorders (Harmon et al., 1995). **Delusions** are false, fixed, and unbreakable beliefs that fall outside the person's social, cultural, or religious background. Although delusions are a symptom of many psychotic disorders, in delusional disorder, the delusions are **nonbizarre delusions**; that is, they are characterized by adherence to possible situations that could occur in real life and are plausible in the context of the person's ethnic and cultural background (Baker et al., 1995).

Examples of real-life situations include being followed, poisoned, infected, loved at a distance, or deceived by a spouse or lover. A diagnosis of delusional disorder is based on the presence of one or more nonbizarre delusion for at least 1 month (APA, 2000). Delusions are the primary symptom of this disorder.

The course of delusional disorder is variable. Onset can be acute or can occur gradually and become chronic. Patients with this disorder usually live with their delusions for years, rarely receiving psychiatric treatment. They are seldom brought to the attention of health care providers unless their delusion relates to their health (somatic delusion), or they act on the basis of their delusion and violate legal or social rules. Full remissions can be followed by relapses.

Apart from the direct impact of the delusion, psychosocial functioning is not markedly impaired. The person's clarity of thinking and behavior and emotional responses are usually consistent with the delusional focus. In general, behavior is not odd or bizarre. In fact, behavior is remarkably normal, except when the patient focuses on the delusion. At that time, thinking, attitudes, and mood may change abruptly. Personality does not usually change, but there is a gradual, progressive involvement with the delusional concern (APA, 2000; Siris & Lavin, 1995).

Diagnostic Criteria

Delusional disorder is characterized by the presence of nonbizarre delusions and includes several subtypes: erotomanic, grandiose, jealous, somatic, mixed, and unspecified (Table 19-3). These subtypes represents the prominent theme of the delusion. A patient who has met criteria A for schizophrenia is not diagnosed with this disorder (see Chapter 18 for criteria A). Although hallucinations may be present, they are not prominent (APA, 2000).

If mood episodes occur with this disorder, the total duration of the mood episode is relatively brief when compared with the total duration of the delusional period. The delusion is not caused by the direct physiologic effects of substances (ie, cocaine, amphetamines, marijuana) or a general medical condition (ie, Alzheimer's disease, systemic lupus erythematosus). Because delusional disorder is uncommon and possesses features that are characteristic of other illnesses, the differential diagnosis has clearcut logic. It is a diagnosis of exclusion requiring careful evaluation. Distinguishing this disorder

TABLE 19.3 Key Diagnostic Characteristics of Delusional Disorder 297.1	
Diagnostic Criteria and Target Symptoms	**Associated Findings**

• Nonbizarre delusions of at least 1 month's duration
• No presence of characteristic symptoms of schizophrenia
• Functioning not markedly impaired; behavior not odd or bizarre
• If concurrent with delusions, mood disorders relatively brief in comparison with delusional periods
• Not a direct physiologic effect of a substance or medical condition
   Erotomanic type: delusions that another person of usually higher status is in love with the person
   Grandiose type: delusions of inflated worth, power, knowledge, identity, or special relationship to a deity or famous person
   Jealous type: delusions that the individual's sexual partner is unfaithful
   Persecutory type: delusions that person or someone close to person is being malevolently treated in some way
   Somatic type: delusion that person has some physical defect or general medical condition
   Mixed type: delusions characteristic of more than one of the above types; no one theme predominates
   Unspecified type: delusion cannot be clearly identified or described
	• Social, marital, or work problems
	• Ideas of reference
	• Irritable mood
	• Marked anger and violent behavior (especially with jealous type)

from schizophrenia and mood disorders with psychotic features is difficult (APA, 2000; Siris & Lavin, 1995).

Subtypes

Erotomanic Delusions

The Concept of **erotomania** dates back to the 17th century. This disorder has also been referred to as *de Clérambault's syndrome.* Erotomanic delusions, in the pure or primary form, have also been known as *psychose passionelle* (Siris & Lavin, 1995). The pure or primary form, however, rarely appears. Secondary erotomania is more common and occurs in conjunction with other psychiatric conditions. Differential diagnosis is important in excluding other significant psychiatric disorders or histologic conditions.

The erotomanic subtype is characterized by the delusional belief that the patient is loved intensely by the "loved object," who is usually married, of a higher socioeconomic status, or otherwise unattainable. The patient believes that the loved object's position in life would be in jeopardy if his or her true feelings were known. Also, the patient is convinced that he or she is in amorous communication with the loved object. The loved object is often a public figure (eg, movie star, politician) but may also be a common stranger. The patient believes that the loved object was the first to make advances and fall in love. There may be some delusional beliefs about a sexual relationship with the loved object, but despite these, the patient remains chaste (Harmon et al., 1995). The delusion often idealizes romantic love and spiritual union rather that sexual at-

traction (APA, 2000). The delusion becomes the central focus of the patient's existence.

There may be minimal or no contact between the loved object and the patient. Often, the patient keeps the delusion secret and has no or minimal contact with the loved object, but efforts to contact the loved object through letters, telephone calls, gifts, visits, surveillance, and stalking are also common. The patient may in many cases transfer his or her delusion to another loved object (Harmon et al., 1995).

Patients with the erotomanic delusional disorder are generally unattractive in appearance; are often lower-level employees; lead withdrawn, lonely lives; are single with poor interpersonal relationships; and have limited sexual contacts or sexual repression. Clinical patients are mostly women, who do not usually act out their delusions. Forensic patients with erotomanic subtype delusional disorder are mostly men, who tend to be more aggressive and can become violent in pursuit of the loved object, although the loved object may not be the object of the aggression. Men in particular come into contact with the law in their pursuit of the loved object or in a misguided effort to rescue the loved object from some imagined danger. Orders of protection are generally ineffective, and criminal charges of stalking or harassment that lead to incarceration are ineffective as a long-term solution to the problem (Harmon et al., 1995). The result is repeated arrests and psychiatric examinations resulting in ineffective treatment. Patients are rarely motivated for psychiatric treatment. This disorder is difficult to control, contain, or treat. The patient seldom gives up the belief that he or she is loved by the loved object. Separation from the loved object is the only satisfactory means of intervention (APA, 2000; Siris & Lavin, 1995).

The prevalence rate of delusion disorder is about 3 per 10,000 general population. It is a rare disease even in psychiatric samples (Meloy, 1999) Research data are limited because of the small number of recorded case studies, which also have only a small number of participants. Studies lack a systematic description, assessment, and diagnosis of the participants (Munro et al., 1985).

Delusional disorder may be associated with dysfunction in the frontal-subcortical systems and with temporal dysfunction, particularly on the left side (Fujii et al., 1999). Cognitive rigidity may contribute to the maintenance of erotic delusions arising from frontal-subcortical dysfunction, which may result in an inability to alter a belief system (Fujii et al., 1999).

Grandiose Delusions

Patients presenting with grandiose delusions are convinced they have a great unrecognized talent or have made an important discovery. A less common presentation is the delusion of a special relationship with a prominent person (ie, an adviser to the President) or of actually being a prominent person (ie, the President). In the latter case, the person with the delusion may regard the actual prominent person as an impostor. Other grandiose delusions may be religious in nature, such as a delusional belief that he or she has a special message from a deity (APA, 2000; Siris & Lavin, 1995).

Jealous Delusions

The central theme of the jealous subtype is the unfaithfulness or infidelity of a spouse or lover. The belief is arrived at without cause and is based on incorrect inferences justified by "evidence" (ie, rumpled clothing, spots on sheets) the patient has collected. The patient usually confronts the spouse or lover with a host of such evidence. An associated feature is paranoia. The patient may attempt to intervene in the imagined infidelity by secretly following the spouse or lover or by investigating the imagined lover (APA, 2000; Siris & Lavin, 1995).

Delusions of jealousy are difficult to treat and may diminish only with separation, divorce, or the death of the spouse or lover. Except in the elderly, patients are generally male. Jealousy is a powerful, potentially dangerous emotion. Aggression, even violent behavior, may result. Litigious behavior is common, and symptoms with forensic aspects are seen repeatedly. Care in determining how to deal with this patient is essential.

A trend emerging with delusional jealousy is development in older patients. A Chinese study found jealousy delusions common in the elderly, with a prevalence rate of 1.4% (Chiu, 1995). In the elderly population this subtype is predominantly women (Chiu, 1995). In the

elderly, jealousy is characterized by a well-developed paranoid delusional system with or without hallucinations. The course may be variable with remissions and relapses, or it may be chronic with residual symptoms.

Somatic Delusions

Somatic delusions, a mix of psychotic and somatic symptoms, have been described for more than 100 years. The central theme of somatic delusions involves bodily functions or sensations. These patients believe they have a physical ailment. Delusions of this nature are fixed, inarguable, and intense, with the patient totally convinced of the physical nature of the somatic complaint (Siris & Lavin, 1995). The delusion occurs in the absence of other medical or psychiatric conditions. Medication or drug effects can cause tactile hallucinations that are the direct result of the physiologic effects of the medication or drug; when the medication or drug is removed, the symptoms disappear (Baker et al., 1995).

Somatic delusions are manifested in the following beliefs (APA, 2000):

- A foul odor is coming from the skin, mouth (delusions of halitosis), rectum, or vagina
- Insects have infested the skin
- Internal parasites have infested the digestive system
- A certain body part is misshapen or ugly (contrary to evidence)
- Parts of the body are not functioning (eg, large intestine, bowels)

Infestation of insects cannot occur in the absence of sensory perceptions, which constitute tactile hallucinations. The patient vividly describes crawling, itching, burning, swarming, and jumping on the skin surface or below the skin. The patient maintains the conviction that he or she is infested with parasites in the absence of objective evidence to the contrary.

Patients with somatic delusions present a dilemma for health care systems because of their excessive use of health care resources. They seek repeated medical consultations with dermatologists, entomologists, infectious disease specialists, and general practitioners. They seek treatment from primary care physicians and refuse psychiatric referral (Slaughter et al., 1998). Even if they seek psychiatric help, these patients typically do not comply with long-term psychiatric intervention. Patients often go through elaborate rituals to cleanse themselves or their surroundings of the perceived pests, collecting hair, scabs, and skin flakes as evidence of an infection. They insist on being given unnecessary medical tests and procedures and are consequently at risk for increased morbidity because of invasive evaluation. Anger and hostility are common among this group, and behavioral characteristics include shame, depression, and avoidance. Because of the anguish the person feels, suicide is not uncommon (Baker et al., 1995).

The occurrence of the somatic subtype is low, but this disorder may be underdiagnosed. Both genders are affected equally, and a positive family history is uncommon. When the onset occurs in late middle age, female patients tend to predominate (Baker et al., 1995; Siris & Lavin, 1995). Studies of somatic delusions have been marred by methodologic uncertainties, and factors limiting investigation include rarity of the disease, lack of contact with psychiatrists, and noncompliance with the medication regimen. A variant of the somatic subtype is body dysmorphic disorder, which is classified under somatoform disorders in the *Diagnostic and Statistical Manual of Mental Disorders*, 4th ed., Text revision (*DSM-IV-TR*) (see Chap. 23).

Unspecified Delusions

In the mixed subtype, there is no one predominant delusional theme, and the patient presents with two or more types of delusions. The delusional themes presented are not from a single subtype, and one theme is not predominant over the others. In the unspecified subtype, the delusional beliefs cannot be clearly determined, or the predominant delusion is not described in the other specific types. Patients are usually women who experience feelings of depersonalization and derealization and have negative associated paranoid features. The delusions can be short-lived, recurrent, or persistent. This subtype also includes delusions of **misidentification** (ie, illusions of doubles), wherein a familiar person is replaced by an impostor. For example, close family members may assume the persona of strangers, or people who are familiar to the patient can change into other people at their will. This type of delusion occurs rarely and is generally associated with schizophrenia, Alzheimer's disease, or other organic conditions (APA, 2000; Siris & Lavin, 1995).

Persecutory delusions are not listed as a separate subtype in the *DSM-IV-TR*, but they are addressed as a subtype of delusional disorder in the text. These delusions are the most common type seen (APA, 2000; Harmon et al., 1995; Siris & Lavin, 1995). The central theme of persecutory delusions is the patient's belief that he or she is being conspired against, cheated, spied on, followed, poisoned, drugged, maliciously maligned, harassed, or obstructed in pursuit of long-term goals. The patient exaggerates small slights, which become the focus of the delusion.

The focus of persecutory delusions is often on some injustice that must be remedied by legal action (querulous paranoia). Patients often seek satisfaction by repeatedly appealing to courts and other government agencies (Harmon et al., 1995). This litigious behavior sometimes leads to hundreds of letters of protest to government or judicial officials and to many court appearances. These patients are often angry and resentful and may even behave violently toward those people the patient believes are persecuting him or her. The course may be chronic, although waxing and waning of the patient's preoccupation with the delusional belief often occurs. The clarity, logic, and systematic elaboration of this delusional theme leaves a remarkable stamp on this condition (APA, 2000; Siris & Lavin, 1995).

Epidemiology and Risk Factors

Delusional disorder is relatively uncommon in clinical settings (APA, 2000), accounting for only 1% to 2% of psychiatric admission (Siris & Lavin, 1995). The best estimate of its prevalence in the population is about 0.03%, but precise information is lacking (APA, 2000). Lifetime morbidity is between 0.05% and 0.1% because of the late age of onset. Compared with patients with mood disorder, these people are more disadvantaged socially and educationally (Siris & Lavin, 1995). Several studies suggest that patients with delusional disorder come from poorer socioeconomic backgrounds.

There are few risk factors associated with delusional disorder. Patients can live with their delusions without psychiatric intervention because of the normalcy of behavior. When somatic delusions are present, there is a risk for unnecessary medical interventions. Acting on delusions carries a risk for intervention by law enforcement agencies or the legal system.

Age of Onset

Delusional disorder can begin in adolescence (Siris & Lavin, 1995). Generally, this disorder occurs in middle to later adulthood (APA, 2000). Most studies have found that delusional disorder has a later age of onset. An onset of age 40 years or later has been reported. Age of onset occurs later among this group than among schizophrenic patients (Siris & Lavin, 1995). A prevalence rate of 2% to 4% has been reported in the elderly (APA, 2000; Siris & Lavin, 1995).

Gender Differences

There do not appear to be major gender differences in the overall frequency of delusional disorder (APA, 2000). In erotomanic delusions, patients are generally women who do not act on their delusions. In forensic settings, those with this disorder are generally men, who tend to be more aggressive and tend to become violent in their pursuit of the loved object. Men tend to experience more jealous delusions, except in the elderly population, in which women outnumber men in this category. With somatic delusions, both genders are represented equally. Men usually come into conflict with the law and are found in forensic settings (Menzies et al., 1995).

Ethnic and Cultural Differences

A person's ethnic, cultural, and religious background must be considered in evaluating the presence of delusional disorder (APA, 2000). Some cultures have widely held and culturally sanctioned beliefs that other cultures consider delusional. The content of what is delusional varies between cultures and subcultures (APA, 2000). Evidence suggests that immigration may be associated with delusional disorder (Siris & Lavin, 1995).

Familial Differences

An increased familial risk and familial genetic factors may be present. Some evidence suggests family consistency in this disorder.

Comorbidity

Mood disorders are frequently found in patients with delusional disorder. Typically, the symptoms of depression are mild. Many people develop irritable or dysphoric mood as a reaction to the delusional belief. Delusional disorder may be associated with obsessive-compulsive disorder and paranoid, schizoid, or avoidant personality disorder (APA, 2000). Modest evidence indicates an increased risk for alcoholism (Kendler et al., 1995).

Etiology

The cause of delusional disorder is unknown. The only major feature of this condition is the formation and persistence of the delusions. There has been little investigation into the neurophysiologic and neuropsychological causes of delusional disorder. Causes are contradictory. No psychological or social theories of causation are addressed in the literature.

Biologic Theories

Neuropathologic. In patients with delusional disorder, there is a degree of temporal lobe asymmetry on MRI (Harrow et al., 1995). Because of only subtle differences found on MRI, however, it is suggested that delusional disorder involves a neurodegenerative component. The wide variety of dermatologic conditions seen in which tactile hallucinations occur may be caused by sensory alterations in the nervous system (Baker et al., 1995). Because of the late age of onset, sensory input may be misinterpreted because of the subtle cortical changes often associated with aging. There is no evidence of local brain pathology.

Genetic and Biochemical. Delusional disorder is probably biologically distinct from other psychotic disorders, yet little or no attention has been paid to these factors, resulting in a lack of studies addressing genetic factors. It is suggested that delusions involve faulty processing of essentially intact perceptions. The perception becomes linked with an interpretation that has deep emotional significance but no verifiable basis. It has been suggested that a complex dopaminergic system may lead to delusions. This could lead to the argument that a particular delusion depends on the "circuit" that is malfunctioning. Denial of reality has been linked to right posterior cortical dysfunction.

Interdisciplinary Treatment

Generally, few if any interdisciplinary treatments are associated with delusional disorder because patients rarely receive attention from health care providers. Pharmacologic intervention is often based on symptoms. For example, patients with somatic delusions are treated for the specific complaints with which they present on assessment. Use of benzodiazepines with this disorder may be prevalent because of the vagueness of complaints.

Priority Care Issues

By the time a patient diagnosed with delusional disorder is seen in a psychiatric setting, he or she has generally had the delusion for a long period of time. Keep in mind that the delusion with which the patient presents is deeply ingrained and many times unshakable, even with psychopharmacologic intervention. These patients rarely comply with continued use of psychotropic medications.

Male patients who have the erotomanic subtype are likely to require special care because they are more likely to act on their delusions (such as by continued attempts to contact the loved object, or stalking). This group is generally seen in forensic settings.

NURSING MANAGEMENT: HUMAN RESPONSE TO DISORDER

Biologic Domain

Assessment

A physical assessment of body systems is completed to evaluate any problems within various systems. In people with delusional disorder somatic subtype, assessment may be a tedious process because of the number and variety of symptoms with which these patients present. Complaints are explored to develop a complete history of the person's symptoms. Keeping in mind the importance of differential diagnosis in this disorder, it is easy to see the need to explore each complaint thoroughly to determine the origin (ie, Is there a true physical basis, or is the basis delusional?). Past history of each complaint should be explored because this information may affect the outcome of treatment. The more acute the onset, the more favorable the prognosis.

Most patients who are diagnosed with delusional disorder do not experience functional difficulties or impairments. There may be some interruption in normal self-care patterns in those with a diagnosis of the somatic subtype because of the elaborate processes used to treat their perceived disorder (eg, bathing rituals, creams). Sleep patterns may be disrupted because of the overpowering nature of the delusions, which can become the central focus of the person's existence.

A complete history of the person's past and present medication regimen is investigated. It is important to determine what the person's response has been to different medications and what agents the individual perceives as effective. The present medication regimen is obtained along with the patient's perception of present control of symptoms. Obtaining and assessing the patient's past medical records for tests and procedures may be helpful in substantiating the individual's complaints and symptoms.

Interventions

Interventions are based on problems that have been identified by assessment (Fig. 19-3). Problem areas are addressed individually. The nurse helps the patient to establish routines that can resolve problem areas and promote healthy functioning. A mechanism for managing the patient's medication regimen is developed.

Somatic Interventions. Delusional disorder has a reputation of being chronic and treatment resistant. Use of somatic treatment is difficult because of the patient's insistence that the problem is not psychiatrically related. Many patients with delusional disorder are never seen in psychiatric settings; they are seen by other specialists, who use expensive and ineffective treatments. Patients with this disorder may adhere poorly to the recommended psychiatric pharmacotherapy (Rockwell et al., 1995). Realistic and modest goals are the most sensible. The establishment of a therapeutic relationship between the provider and the patient is fundamental, although far from simple (Siris & Lavin, 1995).

Pharmacologic Interventions. Sparse literature is available related to the use of psychiatric medications in delusional disorder, and the available reports are conflicting. Antipsychotics may be effective, but little

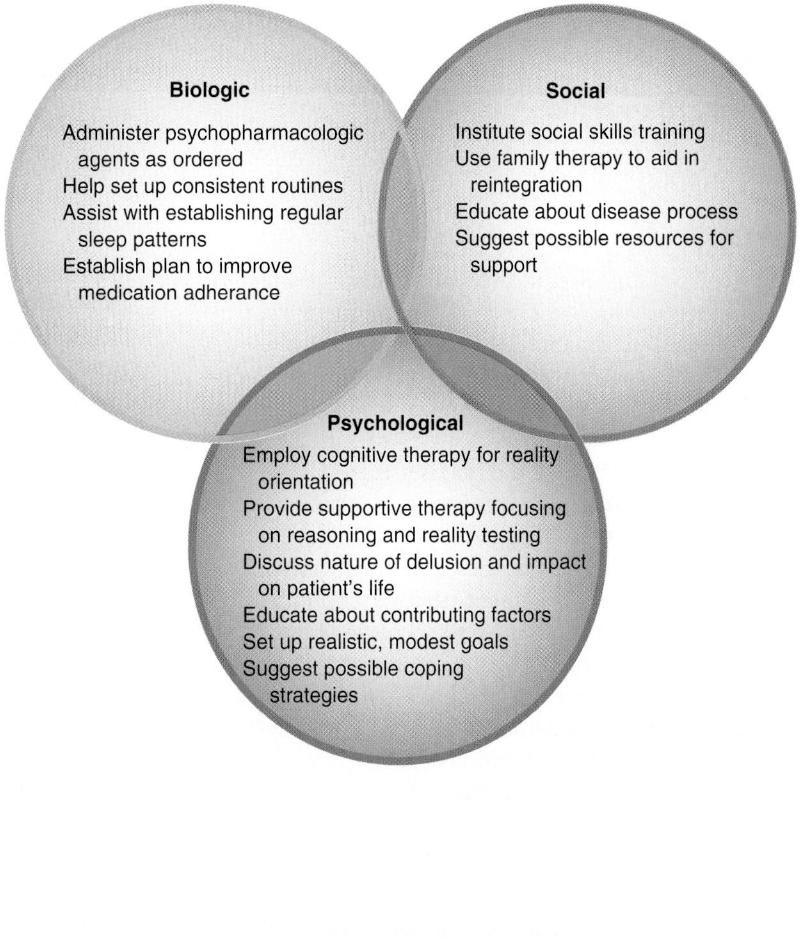

Biologic

Administer psychopharmacologic agents as ordered
Help set up consistent routines
Assist with establishing regular sleep patterns
Establish plan to improve medication adherance

Social

Institute social skills training
Use family therapy to aid in reintegration
Educate about disease process
Suggest possible resources for support

Psychological

Employ cognitive therapy for reality orientation
Provide supportive therapy focusing on reasoning and reality testing
Discuss nature of delusion and impact on patient's life
Educate about contributing factors
Set up realistic, modest goals
Suggest possible coping strategies

FIGURE 19.3 Biopsychosocial interventions for patients with delusional disorder.

if any formal information exists to support this theory. Antipsychotics are useful in improving acute symptoms by decreasing agitation and the intensity of the delusion.

Monitoring and Administration of Medications. Compliance is an issue with this population. Patients are noncompliant with medications and require monitoring of target symptoms. Patients need an opportunity to discuss medications and compliance barriers.

Side-Effect Management. Management of side effects is similar to that in other disorders that have a delusional component. The nurse assesses for NMS, extrapyramidal side effects, weight gain, and sedation.

Drug–Drug Interactions. Interactions would be similar to other disorders that have been discussed previously in other chapters. A detailed list of prior and current medications must be elicited from these patients because they may be receiving medications from many different practitioners.

Teaching Points. Patients should be instructed to take medication as prescribed. The nurse should determine whether the patient has sufficient resources to purchase and obtain medications and explain target symptoms for each medication. Over-the-counter medications should not be taken without consulting a prescriber.

Psychological Domain

Assessment

Patients with delusional disorder show few if any psychological deficits, and those that do occur are generally related directly to the delusion. In these patients, average or marginally low intelligence is characteristic. Use of the Minnesota Multiphasic Personality Inventory, which is a clinical scale that identifies paranoid symptom deviation, may be useful in substantiating the diagnosis (Siris & Lavin, 1995).

Mental status alteration is not generally affected. Thinking, orientation, affect, attention, memory, perception, and personality are generally intact. Presenting evidence that is reality based in an attempt to dissuade the person's delusion can be helpful in determining whether the belief can be altered with sufficient evidence. If mental status alteration is present, it is generally brought to the health professional's attention by a third party, such as police, family member, neighbor, physician, or attorney. In these cases, the person has usually acted in some manner to draw attention to himself or herself. It is important to spend time in discussion with the person to grasp the nature of the delusional thinking in terms of its theme, impact on life, complexity, systematization, and related features (Siris & Lavin, 1995). If the delusions are reactive, chances for positive outcomes are enhanced.

Interventions

Patients with delusional disorder are treated most effectively in outpatient settings. Supportive therapy that allays the person's anxiety may be most effective. Initiating discussion of the troubling experiences and consequences of the delusion and suggesting a means for coping may be successful. Assisting the person toward a more satisfying general adjustment is desirable (see Psychoeducation Checklist: Delusional Disorder).

Insight-oriented therapy is not generally used because there is no benefit in trying to prove the delusion is not present, arguing the person out of the delusion, or telling the individual that the delusion is imaginary. Cognitive therapy with supportive therapy that focuses on reasoning or reality testing of the person to decrease the delusional thinking or modifying the delusion itself may be helpful. Educational interventions can aid the patient in understanding how factors such as sensory impairment, social and physical isolation, and stress contribute to the intensity of this disorder.

In certain instances, hospitalization is needed in response to dangerous behavior that could include aggressiveness, poor impulse control, excessive psychological tension, unremitting anger, and threats. Suicide can be a concern, but most patients live a normal life span. People with the erotomanic, jealous, or persecutory subtypes are at the highest risk for difficulties (Siris & Lavin, 1995). If hospitalization is required, the person needs to be approached tactfully, and legal assistance may be necessary.

Social Domain

Assessment

A common characteristic of individuals with delusional disorder is the normalcy of their behavior and appear-

---

PSYCHOEDUCATION CHECKLIST
Delusional Disorder

When caring for the patient with delusional disorder, be sure to include the caregiver, as appropriate, and address the following topic areas in the teaching plan:

- Psychopharmacologic agents (antipsychotic or antidepressants), if used, including drug action, dosage, frequency, and possible adverse effects
- Identification of troubling experiences
- Consequences of delusions
- Realistic goal setting
- Positive coping strategies
- Safety measures
- Social training skills
- Family participation in therapy

ance unless their delusional ideas are being discussed or acted on (Siris & Lavin, 1995). The cultural background of the person with delusional disorder has to be evaluated in the context of the delusion itself. Ethnic and cultural systems have different beliefs that are accepted within their individual context but not outside their group. If the person's family or life partner is supportive, compliance is enhanced, with an overall improvement of outcomes.

Social function is generally impaired, and social isolation is common among this group. Most are employed, but they generally hold low-level jobs. Many are married. Problems can result in social, occupational, or interpersonal areas. In general, the person's social and marital functioning is more likely to be impaired than the intellectual or occupational functioning. Married women, rather than unmarried women, have a greater chance for a positive outcome.

When poor social or occupational functioning is present, it is related to the delusion itself. It is important to assess the person's capacity to act in response to the delusion. What is the person's level of impulsiveness (ie, related to behaviors of suicide, homicide, aggression, or violence)? Establishing as complete a picture of the person as possible, including the person's subjective private experiences and concrete psychopathologic symptoms, helps to reduce uncertainty in the assessment process (Siris & Lavin, 1995).

Interventions

People diagnosed with delusional disorder often experience a decrease in social functions, leading to social isolation. The secretiveness of their delusions and the focus the delusion has in their life are central to this phenomenon. Social skills training tailored to the specific deficits of the person can be helpful in improving social adaptation. Trying to help the person reintegrate into the family through family therapy is useful. Family education in conjunction with patient education is helpful to both the person and the family in their understanding of the person and the disease process. Group therapy would not be of benefit because of the lack of insight the person has related to the true origin of the delusion.

Families face many of the same issues as those in other disorders involving delusions. The stress of dealing with this disorder is not as high as in other disorders. Families are at risk for ineffective coping.

Evaluation and Treatment Outcomes

For patients with delusional disorders, the greater the lack of insight and the poorer the compliance, the more difficult it is to teach the individual. Resistance is typical, and the person is not amenable to interventions. It is important to remember that the person rarely, if ever, develops full insight, and the symptoms related to the original diagnosis are not likely to disappear completely. Maintaining realistic outcomes for the person helps in achieving successes and in promoting improved identification of positive outcomes (Fig. 19-4). In evaluating progress related to interventions, the nurse must remember that outcomes are often not met completely. The nurse should maintain realistic outcomes and praise small successes to promote positive outcomes.

Continuum of Care

Inpatient-Focused Care

Hospitalization rarely occurs and is usually initiated by the legal or social violations. The hospital environment protects the patient from further legal intervention. Insight-oriented interventions help the patient to understand his or her situation. Confrontational situations should be avoided. The nurse uses the patient's coping abilities to reinforce constructive aspects to allow for a return to autonomy.

Emergency Care

Emergency care is seldom required. Patients seen in emergency settings have usually had an altercation with the law or legal system. The patient may be agitated or aggressive because of the interruption of the delusion and their perception of the reality of the delusion.

Family Intervention

Helping families to understand the illness process and develop a supportive relationship with the patient is an important part of nursing care. By helping the family to develop mechanisms to cope with the patient's delusions, nurses help the family to be more supportive and understanding of the patient. Family therapy may be helpful.

Community Treatment

Patients diagnosed with delusional disorder are treated most effectively in an outpatient setting. They should be encouraged to seek psychiatric treatment. Insight-oriented therapy to develop an understanding of the patient's delusion may be helpful. Medications are not often used with delusional disorder, but use of antipsychotics or benzodiazepines is helpful during periods of exacerbation. Other treatments include supportive therapy, development of coping skills, cognitive therapy, and social skills training. Family therapy may be helpful.

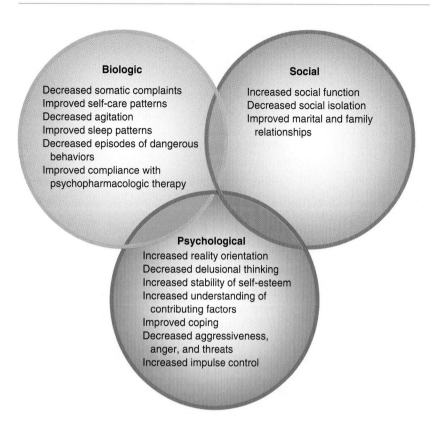

Biologic

Decreased somatic complaints
Improved self-care patterns
Decreased agitation
Improved sleep patterns
Decreased episodes of dangerous
   behaviors
Improved compliance with
   psychopharmacologic therapy

Social

Increased social function
Decreased social isolation
Improved marital and family
   relationships

Psychological

Increased reality orientation
Decreased delusional thinking
Increased stability of self-esteem
Increased understanding of
   contributing factors
Improved coping
Decreased aggressiveness,
   anger, and threats
Increased impulse control

FIGURE 19.4 Biopsychosocial outcomes for patients with delusional disorder.

OTHER PSYCHOTIC DISORDERS

Other disorders have psychoses as their defining features. Nursing care of patients with these disorders is not specifically discussed, but the generalist psychiatric nurse has the ability to apply care used with other disorders to the disorders presented here (Table 19-4).

Schizophreniform Disorder

The essential features of schizophreniform disorder are identical to those of criteria A for schizophrenia with the exception of the duration of the illness, which can be less than 6 months (APA, 2000). However, symptoms must be present for at least 1 month to be classified as a schizophreniform disorder (Table 19-5). This diagnosis is also used as provisional if symptoms have lasted more than 1 month but it is uncertain whether the person will recover before the end of the 6-month period.

Altered social or occupational functioning may occur but is not necessary (APA, 2000). An interruption in one or more areas of daily functioning is experienced by most patients. Of those receiving the diagnosis of schizophreniform disorder (provisional), one third recover, and two thirds progress to a diagnosis of schizoaffective disorder (APA, 1994).

Brief Psychotic Disorder

In brief psychotic disorder, the length of the episode is at least 1 day but less than 1 month. The onset is sudden and includes at least one of the positive symptoms of criteria A for schizophrenia found in Chapter 18 (see Table 19-5). Differential diagnosis is important in making this diagnosis.

The person generally experiences emotional turmoil or overwhelming confusion and rapid intense shifts of affect (APA, 2000). Even though episodes are brief, impairment can be severe, and supervision may be required to protect the person. Suicide is an increased risk, especially in younger patients. A predisposition to development of a brief psychotic disorder may include preexisting personality disorders (APA, 2000).

The person's ethnic and cultural background should also be considered in relation to the social or religious context of the symptoms presented. This disorder is uncommon but usually appears in early adulthood (APA, 2000).

Shared Psychotic Disorder

In shared psychotic disorder (*folie à deux*), a person develops a close relationship with another individual ("inducer" or "primary case") who has a psychotic disorder with prominent delusions (APA, 2000; Trabert, 1999)

TABLE 19.4 Other Psychotic Disorders

Disorder	Definition
Schizophreniform disorder	This disorder is identical to schizophrenia except the total duration of the illness can be less than 6 months (must be at least 1 month) and there may not be impaired social or occupational functioning.
Schizoaffective disorder	This disorder is characterized by an uninterrupted period of illness during which at some time there is a major depressive, manic, or mixed episode along with two of the following symptoms of schizophrenia: delusions, hallucinations, disorganized speech, disorganized or catatonic behavior, or negative symptoms (affective flattening, alogia, or avolition).
Delusional disorder	This disorder is characterized by the presence of nonbizarre delusion and includes several subtypes: erotomanic, grandiose, jealous, somatic, mixed, and unspecified.
Brief psychotic disorder	In this disorder, there is a sudden onset of at least one positive psychotic symptom that lasts at least 1 day but less than 1 month. Eventually, the individual has a full return to normal.
Shared psychotic disorders (folie à deux)	In this disorder, one person who is in a close relationship with another person who already has a psychotic disorder with prominent delusions also develops the delusion.
Other psychotic disorders due to substances such as drugs and alcohol	The prominent hallucinations or delusions are judged to be due to the physiologic effects of substances (drugs, alcohol).

American Psychiatric Association. (2000). *Diagnostic and statistical manual of mental disorders*, 4th ed., Text revision. Washington, DC: Author.

TABLE 19.5 Key Diagnostic Characteristics for Other Psychotic Disorders

Disorder	Diagnostic Characteristics and Target Symptoms

Schizophreniform disorder	Symptoms of schizophrenia present
	  Delusions, hallucinations, disorganized speech, grossly disorganized or catatonic behavior, and negative symptoms
	  Not due to schizoaffective or mood disorders
	  Not due to effects of substance or general medical condition
	Episode lasting at least 1 month but less than 6 months

Brief psychotic disorder	Presence of delusions, hallucinations, disorganized speech, and grossly disorganized or catatonic behavior (at least one) Duration of at least 1 day but less than 1 month; returns to preillness level of functioning Not the direct physiologic effect of a substance or general medical condition; not better accounted for by other mental disorders
Shared psychotic disorder (folie à deux)	Delusion developing in a person who is in a close relationship with another person who already has an established delusion Delusion similar in content to that of the other person Not the direct physiologic effect of a substance or general medical condition; not better accounted for by other mental disorders
Psychotic disorder due to a general medical condition	Prominent hallucinations or delusions Evidence from history, physical examination, or laboratory studies that disturbance is a result of the physiologic consequences of a general medical disorder Not occurring exclusively during delirium
Substance-induced psychotic disorders	Prominent hallucinations or delusions Symptoms developed during or within 1 month of substance intoxication or withdrawal or medication use related to the disturbance Not better accounted for by other mental disorders Not occurring exclusively during delirium

(see Table 19-5). With this disorder, the person believes and shares part or all of the inducer's delusional beliefs. The content of the delusions depends on the inducer, who is the dominant person in the relationship and imposes the delusions on the passive person (APA, 2000). Delusional beliefs are usually shared by people who have lived together for a long time in relative social isolation. When the relationship between the person and the inducer is interrupted, the person's delusional beliefs decrease or disappear (APA, 2000). However, family members rarely share the same delusional belief.

Treatment is infrequently sought (Trabert, 1999). When care is sought, the inducer usually brings the situation to clinical treatment (APA, 2000). This disorder is somewhat more common in women, and the age of onset is variable. If the passive person is removed from the setting, 93% have a favorable course even with no treatment (Trabert, 1999). If the inducer receives no intervention, the course is usually chronic.

Psychotic Disorders Due to Substance

Patients with a psychotic disorder due to a substance present with prominent hallucinations or delusions that are the direct physiologic effects of a substance (eg, drug abuse, toxin exposure) (APA, 2000) (see Table 19-5). During intoxication symptoms continue as long as the use of the substance continues. Withdrawal symptoms can occur for up to 4 weeks. Differential diagnosis is recommended.

Summary of Key Points

➤ Schizoaffective disorder is a separate disorder with a mix of symptoms typical of both schizophrenia and mood disorders. Although these patients suffer mood problems most of the time, to make the diagnosis of schizoaffective disorder, the patient must suffer positive symptoms (ie, delusions or hallucinations) *without* mood symptoms at some time during the uninterrupted period of illness.

➤ There has been much controversy and ongoing discussion about whether schizoaffective disorder is truly a separate disorder, but the *DSM-IV* now identifies schizoaffective disorder as a separate category.

➤ Patients with schizoaffective disorder have less awareness deficits and appear to have more insight than patients with true schizophrenia, a fact that can be used in teaching patients to control symptoms, recognize early regression, and develop some psychosocial skills.

➤ It is unlikely that patients with schizoaffective disorder will ever be medication free. Intermittent antipsychotic dosing is best for patients who can detect

recurrence of symptoms and institute their own drug therapy.

➤ Nursing care for patients with schizoaffective disorder is focused on minimizing psychiatric symptoms through promoting medication maintenance and helping patients maintain optimal levels of functioning. Interventions should be focused on developing social and coping skills through supportive, nurturing, and nonconfrontational approaches. The nurse must be constantly attuned to the mood state of the patient and help the patient learn to solve problems, resolve conflict, and cope with social situations that trigger anxiety.

➤ Delusional disorder is characterized by stable, well-systematized, and logical nonbizarre delusions that could occur in real life and are plausible in the context of the patient's ethnic and cultural background. These delusions may or may not interfere with an individual's ability to function socially. Patients typically deny any psychiatric basis for their problem and refuse to seek psychiatric care. These patients are often seen on medical-surgical units of hospitals when their delusions relate to various somatic complaints. Diagnosis is often made only when the delusions relate to their health or when they act on the basis of their delusions and violate the law or social rules.

➤ Delusional disorder is further classified as a particular subtype depending on the nature and content of the patient's delusions, including erotomanic, grandiose, jealous, somatic, mixed, and unspecified.

➤ Patients with delusional disorder usually do not experience functional difficulties or mental status impairments. Their thinking, orientation, effect, attention, memory, perception, and personality generally remain intact.

➤ The therapeutic relationship established with the patient with delusional disorder is crucial to successful treatment. Nurses must be aware of the patient's fragile self-esteem and unusual sensitivities and anxieties and try to establish a trusting relationship through a flexible, nonjudgmental approach that promotes empathy, trust, and support while keeping a physical and emotional detachment.

Critical Thinking Challenges

1. What differentiates schizoaffective disorder from true schizophrenia? What differentiates schizoaffective disorder from a true mood disorder? Why is it so important to have a separate disorder category of schizoaffective disorder?

2. Are there any significant differences in the epidemiologic factors (distribution, risk factors, age of onset, gender differences, ethnicity, comorbidity) between

schizoaffective disorder and delusional disorder? In what ways are these two disorders similar?

3. Discuss the etiologic theories of schizoaffective and delusional disorders.

4. Explain why ethnic and cultural differences are important in the assessment of a patient with delusional disorder.

5. Marion makes her first office visit to a mental health nurse after numerous trips to other providers in varying specialties. She describes an "uncomfortable, sometimes painful feeling of bugs crawling" on her. Discuss how you would conduct a comprehensive assessment of this patient.

6. Compare and contrast somatic subtype of delusional disorder with body dysmorphic disorder.

7. Explain what factors make the differential diagnosis of schizoaffective disorder and delusional disorder so difficult?

8. Give several factors that make the clinical management of the patient with schizoaffective disorder complex, and explain how this would affect psychiatric nursing care.

9. Give several factors that make the clinical management of the patient with delusional disorder difficult. What is one positive and hopeful advantage that the patient with delusional disorder has in regard to psychosocial skills?

 WEB LINKS

www.surgeongeneral.com Website for *Healthy People 2010* and *Report of the Surgeon General*

www.nami.com National Alliance for the Mentally Ill advocacy information

www.mentalhealth.com Internet mental health website that provides the American and European description of schizoaffective disorder and its treatment.

www.psycom.net Further defines the DSM-IV criteria for schizoaffective disorder and the ICD-10 criteria for schizoaffective disorder

www.geocities.com/CollegePark/Classroom/6237 Learn about what psychiatric nurses do and schizoaffective disorder

www.mhinfosource.com Questions about schizoaffective and other psychiatric disorders answered

MOVIES

Misery: 1990. Misery is a movie starring James Cahn as Paul Sheldon and Kathy Bates as Annie Wildes, and is about a writer with a popular mystery series who finishes his last novel in a secluded cabin in Col-

orado. After being rescued in a blizzard by Annie Wilkes, he becomes her prisoner when she prevents him from leaving his cabin. Annie is in love with him, but is demanding and possessive. She identifies with the heroine in the novel, and is outraged at the conclusion of his latest novel.

Significance: Annie demonstrates the thinking patterns associated with delusional disorder.

Viewing Points: Identify the disturbed thinking that Annie demonstrates. Part of Annie's behavior seems normal and other behaviors are illogical—how are they linked?

REFERENCES

American Psychiatric Association. (1980). *Diagnostics and statistical manual of mental disorders* (3rd ed.). Washington, DC: Author.

American Psychiatric Association. (2000). *Diagnostic and statistical manual of mental disorders* (4th ed., Text revision). Washington, DC: Author.

Andres, K., Plammatter, M., Garst, F. C., et al. (2000). Effects of a coping-oriented group therapy for schizophrenia and schizoaffective patients: A pilot study. *Acta Psychiatrica Scandinavica, 101*(4), 318–322.

Azorin, J. M. (1995). Long-term treatment of mood disorder in schizophrenia. *Acta Psychiatrica Scandinavica Supplementum, 388,* 20–23.

Baker, P. B., Cook, B. L., & Winokur, G. (1995). Delusional infestation: The interference of delusions and hallucinations. *Psychiatric Clinics of North America, 18*(2), 345–361.

Berteisen, A., & Gottesman, I. I. (1995). Schizoaffective psychosis: Genetical clues to classification. *American Journal of Medical Genetics, 60*(1), 7–11.

Chiu, H. R. (1995). Delusional jealousy in Chinese elderly psychiatric patients. *Journal of Geriatrics, Psychiatry and Neurology, 8*(1), 49–51.

Crow, T. J., & Harrington, C. A. (1994). Etiopathogenesis and treatment of psychosis. *Annual Review of Medicine, 45,* 219–234.

Erlenmeyer, K. L., Squires-Wheeler, E., Adama, U. H., et al. (1995). The New York High Risk Project: Psychoses and cluster A personality disorders in offspring of schizophrenic parents at 23 year follow-up. *Archives of General Psychiatry, 52*(10), 857–865.

Evans, J. D., Heaton, R. K., Paulsen, J. S., et al. (1999). Schizoaffective disorder: A form of schizophrenia or affective disorder? *Journal of Clinical Psychiatry, 60*(12), 874–884.

Fujii, D. E., Ahmed, I., & Takeshita, J. (1999). Neuropsychologic implications in erotomania: Two case studies. *Neuropsychiatry, Neuropsychology and Behavioral Management, 12*(2), 110–116.

Gerbaldo, H., & Phillips, M. (1995). The deficit syndrome in schizophrenic and nonschizophrenic patients: Preliminary studies. *Psychopathology, 28*(1), 55–63.

Harmon, R. B., Rosner, R., & Owens, H. (1995). Obsessional harassment and erotomania in a criminal court population. *Journal of Forensic Science, 41*(2), 188–196.

Harrow, M., MacDonald, A. W., Sands, J. R., & Silverstein, M. L. (1995). Vulnerability to delusions over time in schizophrenia and affective disorder. *Schizophrenic Bulletin, 21*(1), 95–105.

Henry, A., & Coster, W. (1995). Predictors of functional outcome among adolescents and young adults with psychotic disorder. *American Journal of Occupational Therapy, 50*(3), 171–181.

Herz, M. J., Lamberti, J. S., Mintz, J., et al. (2000). A program for relapse prevention in schizophrenia. *Archives of General Psychiatry, 57*(3), 277–283.

Higgins, P. (1995). Clozapine and the treatment of schizophrenia. *Health and Social Work, 20*(2), 124–132.

Huxley, N. A., Rendall, M., & Sederer, L. (2000). Psychosocial treatments in schizophrenia: A review of the past 20 years. *Journal of Nervous and Mental Disease, 188*(4), 187–201.

Kasanin, J. (1933). The acute schizo-affective psychoses. *American Journal of Psychiatry, 13*, 97–126.

Kendler, K. S., McGuire, M., Gruenberg, A. M., & Walsh, D. (1995). Examining validity of *DSM-III-R* schizoaffective disorder and its putative subtypes in the Roscommon Family Study. *American Journal of Psychiatry, 152*(5), 755–764.

Levine, R. R., Hudgins, P., Brown, R., et al. (1995). Differences in qualitative brain morphology findings in schizophrenia, major depression, bipolar disorder and normal volunteers. *Schizophrenia Research, 15*(3), 253–259.

Levison, D. F., Umapathy, C., & Mesthaq, M. (1999). Treatment of schizoaffective disorder and schizophrenia with mood symptoms. *American Journal of Psychiatry, 156*(8), 1138–1148.

Maj, M., Pirozzi, R., Formicola, A. M., et al. (2000). Reliability and validity of the *DSM-IV* diagnostic category of schizoaffective disorder: Preliminary data. *Journal of Affective Disorders, 57*(1–3), 95–98.

Meloy, J. R. (1999). Erotomania, triangulation and homicide. *Journal of Forensic Science, 44*(2), 421–424.

Menzies, R. P., Fedoroff, J. P., Green, C. M., & Isaacson, K. (1995). Prediction of dangerous behavior in male erotomania. *British Journal of Psychiatry, 166*(4), 529–536.

Munro, A., O'Brien, J. V., & Ross, D. (1985). Two cases of 'pure' or 'primary' erotomania successfully treated with pinozide. *Canadian Journal of Psychiatry, 30*(8), 619–622.

O'Connell, K. (1995). Schizoaffective disorder: A case study. *Journal of Psychosocial Nursing, 33*(10), 35–43.

Radomsky, E. D., Hass, G., Mann, J. J., & Sweeney, J. A. (1999). Suicidal behavior in patients with schizophrenia and other psychotic disorders. *American Journal of Psychiatry, 156*(10), 1590–1595.

Rietschel, M., Krauss, H., Muller, D. J., et al. (2000). Dopamine d3 receptor variant and tardive dyskinesia. *European Archives of Psychiatry and Clinical Neuroscience, 250*(1), 31–35.

Rockwell, E., Krull, A. J., Dimsdale, J., & Jeste, D. V. (1994). Late onset psychosis with somatic delusions. *Psychosomatics, 35*(1), 66–72.

Scott, T. F., Price, T. R., George, M. S., et al. (1993). Midline cerebral malformation and schizophrenia. *Journal of Neuropsychiatry and Clinical Neuroscience, 5*(3), 287–293.

Serretti, A., Cusin, C., Lattuada, E., et al. (1999a). No interaction between serotonin transporter gene and dopamine receptor d4 gene in symptomatology of major psychoses. *American Journal of Medical Genetics, 88*(5), 481–485.

Serretti, A., Lilli, R., DiBella, D., et al. (1999b). Dopamine receptor d4 gene is not associated with major psychoses. *American Journal of Medical Genetics, 88*(5), 486–491.

Serretti, A., Macciardi, F., Cusin, C., et al. (2000). Linkage of mood disorders with d2, d3 and th genes: A multicenter study. *Journal of Affective Disorders, 58*(1), 51–61.

Simpson, G. M., Josiassen, R. C., Stanilla, J. K., et al. (1999). Double-blind study of clozapine dose response in chronic schizophrenia. *American Journal of Psychiatry, 156*(11), 1744–1750.

Slaughter, J. R, Zanoi, K., Rezvani, J., & Flax, J. (1998). Psychogenic parasitosis: A case series and literature review. *Psychometrics, 39*(6), 491–500.

Siris, S. G., & Lavin, M. R. (1995). Other psychotic disorders. In H. Kaplan & B. Sadock (Eds.), *Comprehensive textbook of psychiatry* (6th ed.). Baltimore: Williams & Wilkins.

Strakowski, S. M., Keck, P. E., Jr., Sax, K. W., et al. (1999). Twelve-month outcome of patients with *DSM-III-R* schizoaffective disorder comparisons to matched patients with bipolar disorder. *Schizophrenia Research, 35*(2), 167–174.

Trabert, W. (1999). Shared psychotic disorder in delusional parasitosis. *Psychopathology, 32*(1), 30–34.

Tsuang, D., & Coryell, W. (1993). An eight-year follow-up of patients with *DSM-III-R* psychotic depression, schizoaffective disorder, and schizophrenia. *American Journal of Psychiatry, 150*(8), 1182–1188.

Zarate, G. A., Tohen, M., Banov, M. P., et al. (1995). Is clozapine a mood stabilizer? *Journal of Clinical Psychiatry, 56*(3), 108–112.

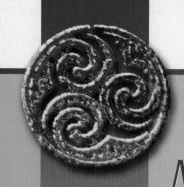

Mood Disorders

Katharine P. Bailey, Carol D. Sauer, and
Constance Herrell

After studying the chapter, you will be able to:

➤ Describe the global impact of underdiagnosed and untreated mood disorders as a major public health problem.

➤ Distinguish the clinical characteristics and course of depressive disorders and bipolar disorder.

➤ Analyze the prevailing biologic, psychological, and social theories that serve as a basis for caring for patients with mood disorders.

➤ Analyze the human responses to mood disorders with emphasis on concepts of mood, affect, depressed mood, and manic episode.

➤ Formulate nursing diagnoses based on a biopsychosocial assessment of patients with mood disorders.

➤ Formulate nursing interventions that address specific diagnoses based on a continuum of care.

➤ Identify expected outcomes and their evaluation.

➤ Analyze special concerns within the nurse–patient relationship common to treating people with mood disorders.

KEY TERMS

affect
bipolar
cyclothymic disorder
depressive episode
dysthymic disorder
euphoria
expansive mood

hypomanic episode
lability of mood
manic episode
mixed episode
rapid cycling
unipolar

KEY CONCEPTS

mania
mood
mood disorders

---

*The World Health Organization predicts that mood disorders will be the number-one public health problem in the 21st century. Major depression is currently the number one leading cause of disability worldwide (Murray & Lopez, 1996). Mood disorders are associated with high levels of impairment in occupation, social, and physical functioning and cause as much disability and distress to patients as chronic med-*ical disorders (USDHHS, 1999). Mood disorders often go undetected and untreated. Less than 50% of patients with major depressive disorder receive treatment for their condition, and of those treated, 57% receive all care from nonpsychiatric clinicians (Rosenbaum & Fava, 1998). Studies suggest that only about one third of people with bipolar disorder have been diagnosed, and at any given point in time, only 27% of these are *receiving treatment (Sachs, 1998). While health care resources are expended on working up these somatic complaints, the opportunity to make use of effective pharmaceutical and psychological treatments is often missed. The cost of mood disorders in the United States in 1990 was about $44 billion, about the same as the cost resulting from heart disease and about 30% of the total cost for all mental illness in that year (World Health Organization, 1997). In addition, because suicide is a significant risk in mood disorders, these disorders have a greater impact on premature mortality. Nurses practicing in any health care setting need to develop competence in assessing patients for the presence of a mood disorder and, if suspected, provide appropriate educational and clinical interventions or referral.*

KEY CONCEPT   **Mood. Mood** is a pervasive and sustained emotion that colors one's perception of the world and how one functions in it. Normal variations in mood occur as responses to specific life experiences. Normal mood variations, such as sadness, euphoria, and anxiety, are time limited and are not associated with significant functional impairment.

KEY CONCEPT   **Mood Disorder. Mood disorders,** as defined in the *Diagnostic and Statistical Manual of Mental Disorders, 4th edition, Text revision* ([DSM-IV-TR]; American Psychiatric Association [APA], 2000a), are recurrent disturbances or alterations in mood that cause psychological distress and behavioral impairment.

The primary alteration is in mood, rather than in thought or perception. There are several terms used to describe observable expressions of mood (called **affect**) (APA, 2000b). These include the following:

- *Blunted:* significantly reduced intensity of emotional expression
- *Flat:* absent or nearly absent affective expression
- *Inappropriate:* discordant affective expression accompanying the content of speech or ideation
- *Labile:* varied, rapid, and abrupt shifts in affective expression
- *Restricted or constricted:* mildly reduced in the range and intensity of emotional expression

What is considered the normal range of mood or affect varies considerably both within and between different cultures. (This issue is addressed later under Ethnic and Cultural Differences.)

Primary mood disorders include both depressive disorders (**unipolar**) and manic-depressive (**bipolar**) disorders. The *DSM-IV-TR* has established specific criteria for diagnostic classification of these disorders, including criteria for severity (a change from previous functioning), duration (at least 2 weeks), and clinically significant distress or impairment. Mood episodes are

the "building blocks" for the mood disorder diagnoses. The *DSM-IV-TR* describes four categories of mood episodes: major depressive episode, manic episode, mixed episode, and hypomanic episode. This chapter focuses on the depressive disorders and bipolar disorder. Even though depressive disorders are more common than bipolar disorder, the highlighted disorder is bipolar disorder because it has the characteristics of both mood disturbances—depression and mania.

The *DSM-IV-TR* categorizes mood disorders as follows:

- *Depressive disorders:* major depressive disorder, single or recurrent; dysthymic disorder; and depressive disorder not otherwise specified (NOS)
- *Bipolar disorders:* bipolar I disorder, bipolar II disorder, cyclothymic disorder, and bipolar disorder NOS
- *Mood disorder* due to a general medical condition
- *Substance-induced mood disorder*
- *Mood disorder NOS*

DEPRESSIVE DISORDERS

Clinical Course

The primary *DSM-IV-TR* criterion for major depression, or, more accurately, major depressive disorder, is the presence of one or more major depressive episodes. In a major **depressive episode,** either a depressed mood or a loss of interest or pleasure in nearly all activities must be present for at least 2 weeks. Four of seven additional symptoms must be present: disruption in sleep, appetite (or weight), concentration, energy; psychomotor agitation or retardation; excessive guilt or feelings of worthlessness; and suicidal ideation (see Table 20-1).

Individuals often describe themselves as depressed, sad, hopeless, discouraged, or "down in the dumps." If individuals complain of feeling "blah," having no feelings, or feeling anxious, the presence of a depressed mood can sometimes be inferred from their facial expression and demeanor (APA, 2000b).

Dysthymic disorder is considered to be a milder but more chronic form of major depressive disorder. The *DSM-IV-TR* criteria for dysthymic disorder are depressed mood for most days for at least 2 years and the presence of two or more of the following symptoms: poor appetite or overeating; insomnia or oversleeping; low energy or fatigue; low self-esteem; poor concentration or difficulty making decisions; and feelings of hopelessness. The NOS category includes disorders with depressive features that do not meet strict criteria for major depressive disorder.

Major depressive disorder is commonly a progressive, recurrent illness. Over time, episodes tend to be

TABLE 20.1 Key Diagnostic Characteristics for Major Depressive Disorder 296.xx
Major depressive disorder, single episode 296.2x
Major depressive disorder, recurrent 296.3x

Diagnostic Criteria and Target Symptoms	Associated Findings

• Change from previous level of functioning during a 2-week period
    Depressed mood
    Markedly diminished interest or pleasure in all or almost all activities
    Significant weight loss when not dieting, or weight gain or change in appetite
    Insomnia or hypersomnia
    Psychomotor agitation or retardation
    Fatigue or loss of energy
    Feelings of worthlessness or excessive or inappropriate guilt
    Diminished ability to think or concentrate, or indecisiveness
    Recurrent thoughts of death, recurrent suicidal ideation without a specific plan, or a suicide attempt or specific plan for committing suicide
• At least one symptom is depressed mood, or loss of interest or pleasure
• Significant distress or impairment of social, occupational, or other important areas of functioning
• Not a direct physiologic effect of substance or medical condition
• Not better accounted for by bereavement, schizoaffective disorder; not superimposed on schizophrenia, schizophreniform disorder, delusional disorder, or psychotic disorder not otherwise specified
	Associated Behavioral Findings
	• Tearfulness, irritability, brooding, obsessive rumination, anxiety, phobias, excessive worry over physical health, and complaints of pain
	• Possible panic attacks
	• Difficulty with intimate relationships
	• Difficulties with sexual functioning
	• Marital problems
	• Occupational problems
	• Substance abuse, such as alcohol
	• High mortality rate; death by suicide
	• Increased pain and physical illness
	• Decreased physical, social, and role functioning
	• May be preceded by dysthymic disorder
	
	Associated Physical Examination Findings
	• Chronic general medical conditions
	
	Associated Laboratory Findings
	• Sleep electroencephalographic abnormalities
	• Altered levels of neurotransmitters (norepinephrine, serotonin, acetylcholine, dopamine, and GABA)

more frequent, more severe, and of longer duration. About 25% of patients experience a recurrence in the first 6 months after a first episode, and about 50% to 75% have a recurrence within 5 years. The mean age of onset for major depressive disorder is about 40 years; 50% of all patients have an onset between the ages of 20 and 50 years. Over a 20-year period, the mean number of episodes is five or six. Symptoms usually develop over days to months. About 50% of patients have significant depressive symptoms before the first identified episode. An untreated episode typically lasts 6 to 13 months, regardless of age of onset. Ten to 15% of patients may not fully remit and will meet criteria for dysthymic disorder (Blazer et al., 1994). Suicide is the most serious complication and occurs in 10% to 15% of those formerly hospitalized for depression (Angst et al., 1999).

Depressive Disorders in Special Populations

Children and Adolescents

Depressive disorders in children have similar manifestations as in adults with a few exceptions. In major depres-

sive disorder, children are less likely to experience psychosis, but when they do, auditory hallucinations are more common than delusions. They are more likely to manifest anxiety symptoms, such as fear of separation, and somatic symptoms, such as stomach aches and headaches. Their mood may be irritable rather than sad. Suicide is a real risk in children and adolescents and peaks during the mid-adolescent years. Mortality from suicide, which increases steadily through the teens, is the third leading cause of death for that age group (USDHHS, 1999).

Elderly People

Most older patients with symptoms of depression do not meet the full criteria for major depression. However, it is estimated that 8% to 20% of older adults in the community and up to 37% in primary care settings suffer from depressive symptoms. Treatment is successful in 60% to 80%, but the response is slower than in younger adults. Depression in elderly people is often associated with chronic illnesses, such as heart disease, stroke, and cancer. Suicide is a very serious risk for the older adult.

People older than 65 years of age have the highest suicide rates of any age group. In those 85 years of age and older, the suicide rate is the highest, at 21 suicides per 100,000 (Report of the Surgeon General, 1999).

Epidemiology

The lifetime risk for major depressive disorder ranges from 7% to 12% in men and from 20% to 25% in women (Kessler et al., 1994). This percentage translates into an estimated 11 million people every year. It also appears that the chances of suffering from major depressive disorder are increasing in progressively younger age groups (Rosenbaum & Fava, 1998). Major depressive disorder is twice as common in adolescent and adult women as in adolescent and adult men. Prepubertal boys and girls are equally affected. Major depressive disorders often co-occur with other psychiatric and substance-related disorders. Depression is often associated with a variety of medical conditions, particularly endocrine disorders, cardiovascular disease, neurologic disorders, autoimmune conditions, viral or other infectious diseases, certain cancers, and nutritional deficiencies, or as a direct physiologic effect of a substance (eg, a drug of abuse, a medication, other somatic treatment for depression, or toxin exposure) (APA, 2000b).

Ethnic and Cultural Differences

Prevalence rates are unrelated to race (Agency for Health Care Policy and Research [AHCPR], 1993). Culture can influence the experience and communication of symptoms of depression. In some cultures, somatic symptoms may predominate rather than sadness or guilt. Complaints of "nerves" and headaches (in Hispanic and Mediterranean cultures); weakness, tiredness, or "imbalance" (in Chinese and Asian cultures); problems of the "heart" (in Middle Eastern cultures); or of being "heartbroken" (among Hopi Indians) may be the way of expressing the depressive experience. Although culturally distinctive experiences must be distinguished from symptoms, it is also imperative not to dismiss a symptom routinely because it is viewed as the norm for a culture (APA, 2000b).

Risk Factors

Depression is so common that it is sometimes difficult to identify risk factors. The generally agreed-on risk factors include the following (AHCPR, 1993):

- Prior episode of depression
- Family history of depressive disorder
- Lack of social support
- Stressful life event
- Current substance use
- Medical comorbidity

Etiology

Neurobiologic Theories

Genetics. Family, twin, and adoption studies demonstrate that genetic influences undoubtedly play a substantial role in the etiology of mood disorders. Major depressive disorder is 1.5 to 3 times more common among first-degree biologic relatives of people with this disorder than among the general population. Alcoholism in a biologic parent has been implicated as a probable marker for genetic vulnerability to depression (Cadoret et al., 1996). Currently, a major research effort is focusing on developing a more accurate paradigm regarding the contribution of genetic factors to the development of mood disorders (Nathan et al., 1995).

Biologic Hypotheses. Biologic theories of the etiology of depression emerged in the 1950s. These theories posit that major depression is caused by a deficiency or dysregulation in central nervous system (CNS) concentrations of the neurotransmitters norepinephrine, dopamine, and serotonin or in their receptor functions. These hypotheses arose in part from observations that some pharmacologic agents elevated mood, and subsequent studies identified their mechanisms of action. All antidepressants currently available have their therapeutic effects on these neurotransmitters or receptors. Current research that may eventually elucidate the etiology of depression is focused on the synthesis, storage, release, and uptake of these neurotransmitters as well as on postsynaptic events (eg, second-messenger systems) (Nathan et al., 1995).

Neuroendocrine and Neuropeptide Hypotheses. Major depressive disorder is associated with multiple endocrine alterations, specifically of the hypothalamic–pituitary–adrenal axis, the hypothalamic–pituitary–thyroid axis, the hypothalamic–growth hormone axis, and the hypothalamic–pituitary–gonadal axis. In addition, there is mounting evidence that components of neuroendocrine axes (eg, neuromodulatory peptides like corticotropin-releasing factor) may themselves contribute to depressive symptomatology. There is also evidence that the secretion of these hypothalamic and growth hormones is controlled by many of the neurotransmitters implicated in the pathophysiology of depression (Nathan et al., 1995).

Psychoneuroimmunology. Psychoneuroimmunology is a recently emerging major area of research involving the study of a diverse group of proteins that are known as *chemical messengers* between immune cells. These messengers, called *cytokines*, signal the brain and serve as mediators between immune and nerve cells. The brain is capable of influencing immune processes, and, conversely, immunologic response can result in changes in brain activity (Kronfol & Remick, 2000).

The specific role of these mechanisms in psychiatric disease pathogenesis is still unknown.

Psychological Theories

Psychodynamic Factors. Most psychodynamic theorists acknowledge some debt to Freud's original conceptualization of the psychodynamics of depression, which ascribes etiology to an early lack of love, care, warmth, and protection and resultant anger, guilt, helplessness, and fear regarding the loss of love. The ensuing conflict between wanting to be loved and fear of rejection engenders pathologic self-punitiveness (also conceptualized as aggression turned inward), self-rejection, low self-esteem, and depressive symptoms (see Chap. 6).

Behavioral Factors. The behavioral position holds that depression occurs primarily as the result of a severe reduction in rewarding activities or an increase in unpleasant events in one's life. The resultant depression then leads to further restriction of activity, thereby decreasing the likelihood of experiencing pleasurable activities, which, in turn, intensifies the mood disturbance (Thompson, 1996).

Cognitive Factors. The cognitive approach maintains that irrational beliefs and negative distortions of thought about the self, the environment, and the future engender and perpetuate depressive affects (Beck et al., 1979).

Developmental Factors. Developmental theorists posit that depression may be the result of loss of a parent through death or separation or lack of emotionally adequate parenting. These factors may delay or prohibit the realization of appropriate developmental milestones.

Social Theories

Family Factors. Family theorists ascribe maladaptive patterns in family interactions as a contributing factor to the onset of depression, particularly "ambivalent, abusive, rejecting, or highly dependent family relationships" (APA, 1993).

Social Factors. Major depression may follow adverse or traumatic life events, especially those which involve the loss of an important human relationship or role in life. Social isolation, deprivation, and financial deprivation are risk factors (APA, 2000b).

Interdisciplinary Treatment of Disorder

Even though depressive disorders are the most commonly occurring mental disorders, they are usually treated within the primary care setting, not the psychiatric setting. Individuals with depression enter mental health settings when their symptoms become so severe that hospitalization is needed, usually for suicide at-tempts, or if they self-refer because of being incapacitated. Interdisciplinary treatment of these disorders, which are often lifelong, needs to include a wide array of health professionals in all areas. The specific goals of treatment of major depressive disorder are as follows:

- Reduce and ultimately remove all signs and symptoms of the depressive syndrome.
- Restore occupational and psychosocial function to that of the asymptomatic state.
- Reduce the likelihood of relapse and recurrence.

Priority Care Issues

The overriding concern for people with mood disorders is safety. In depressive disorders, suicide risk should always be considered. Suicide assessments should be routine for these individuals (see Chap. 38).

 Family Response to Disorder

Depression in one member affects the whole family. Spouses, children, parents, siblings, and friends experience frustration, guilt, and anger when their family member is immobilized and unable to function. It is often hard for others to understand the depth of the mood and how disabling it can be. Financial hardship can occur when the family member cannot go to work and spends days in bed. The lack of understanding and difficulty of living with a depressed person can often lead to abuse. Women between the ages of 18 and 45 years constitute the majority of those suffering with depression (Report of the Surgeon General, 1999).

NURSING MANAGEMENT: HUMAN RESPONSE TO DISORDER

The diagnosis of major depressive disorder is made when *DSM-IV-TR* criteria are met. An awareness of the risk factors for depression, a comprehensive biopsychosocial assessment, and history of illness and past treatment are key to formulating a treatment plan and to evaluating outcomes. Interviewing a family member or close friend about the patient's day-to-day functioning and specific symptoms may be helpful in determining the course of the illness, current symptoms, and level of functioning.

Biologic Domain

Assessment

Because some symptoms of depression are similar to those of some medical problems or side effects of medications for treatment of medical problems, biologic assessment must include a physical systems review and thorough history of medical problems with special attention to CNS function, endocrine function, anemia, chronic pain, autoimmune illness, diabetes, or menopause. Additional medical information needed includes surgeries; medical hospitalizations; head injuries; episodes of loss of consciousness; pregnancies, childbirths, miscarriages, and abortions. A complete list of prescribed and over-the-counter medications should be compiled, including the reason a medication was prescribed or discontinued. A physical examination is recommended with baseline vital signs and baseline laboratory tests, including comprehensive blood chemistry panel, complete blood counts, liver function tests, thyroid function tests, urinalysis, and electrocardiograms (see Table 10-1 in Chap. 10). Biologic assessment also includes evaluating the patient for the characteristic neurovegetative symptoms of depression and associated behaviors (see Table 20-1). It is important to assess the following:

Appetite and weight changes. In major depression, changes from baseline include decrease or increase in appetite with or without significant weight loss or gain (ie, a change of more than 5% of body weight in 1 month). Weight loss occurs when not dieting and, in the presence of normal appetite, suggests medical illness. Older adults with moderate to severe depression need to be assessed for dehydration.

Sleep disturbance. The most common sleep disturbance associated with major depression is insomnia. *DSM-IV-TR* definitions of insomnia are divided into three categories: initial insomnia (difficulty falling asleep); middle insomnia (waking up during the night and having difficulty returning to sleep); or terminal insomnia (waking too early and being unable to return to sleep). Less frequently, the sleep disturbance is hypersomnia (prolonged sleep episodes at night or increased daytime sleep). The individual with either insomnia or hypersomnia usually complains of not feeling rested upon awakening.

Decreased energy, tiredness, and fatigue. Fatigue associated with depression is a subjective experience of feeling tired or enervated regardless of how much sleep or physical activity a person has had. Even the smallest tasks seem to require substantial effort.

An assessment of current medications should also be completed. As with any pharmacologic assessment, the frequency and dosage of prescribed and over-the-counter medications should be explored. In depression, the nurse must always assess the lethality of the medication the patient is taking. For example, if a patient has sleeping medications at home, the individual should be further queried about the number of pills in the bottle. Additionally, these patients need to be assessed for their use of alcohol, marijuana, and other mood-altering medications. The use of any herbal substances needs to be included because of the potential for drug–drug interactions. Patients would most likely be taking St. John's wort (hypericum perforatum).

Nursing Diagnoses for Biologic Domain

The nursing diagnoses associated with the biologic domain that are common in people with depression usually include Disturbed Sleep Pattern, Imbalanced Nutrition (more or less), and Fatigue. However, there may nursing diagnoses such as Failure to Thrive, Bathing/Hygiene Deficit, or Pain.

Interventions for Biologic Domain

Physical Care Nursing Interventions. Weeks or months of disturbed sleep patterns and nutrition imbalance only make the depression worse. It is important to provide counseling and education about re-establishing normal sleep patterns and nutrition. Encouraging patients to practice positive sleep hygiene and eat well-balanced meals regularly helps the patient move toward remission or recovery. Activity and exercise are also important for improving depressed mood state. Most people find that regular exercise is hard to maintain. People who are depressed may find it impossible. When providing education about exercise, it is important to start with the current level of patient activity and work up slowly. For example, if the patient is spending most of the time in bed, encouraging the patient to get dressed every day and walk for 5 or 10 minutes may be all that patient can tolerate. Gradually, patients should be encouraged to have a regular exercise program.

Pharmacologic Interventions. An antidepressant is primarily selected based on an individual patient's target symptoms and an individual agent's side-effect profile. Other factors that may influence choice are as follows:

- Prior medication response
- Drug interactions and contraindications
- Medication responses in family members
- Concurrent medical and psychiatric disorders
- Patient preference
- Patient age
- Cost of medication

Unlike many psychiatric disorders, in depressive disorders, medications are usually time limited. The treatment and clinical management of psychiatric disorders are divided into acute phase, continuation phase, maintenance phase, and, when indicated, discontinuation of medication.

Acute phase. The primary goal of the acute phase is symptom reduction or remission. The focus of this phase is choosing the right match of medication and dosage for the patient. Careful monitoring and follow-up are essential during this phase to assess patient response to medications, adjust dosage if necessary, identify and address side effects, and provide patient support and education.

Continuation phase. The goal of the continuation phase of treatment is to decrease the risk for relapse (a return of the current episode of depression). If a patient responds to an adequate trial of medication, it is generally continued at the same dosage for at least 4 to 9 months after return to a clinically well state (AHCPR, 1993).

Maintenance phase. As mentioned earlier, depression is typically a recurrent disorder with a worsening course. For patients who are at high risk for recurrence (see Risk Factors), the optimal duration of maintenance treatment is unknown but is measured in years, and full-dose therapy is required for effective prophylaxis (Arana & Rosenbaum, 2000).

Discontinuation of medication. The decision to discontinue active treatment should be based on the same factors considered in the decision to initiate maintenance treatment. These factors include the frequency and severity of past episodes, the persistence of dysthymic symptoms after recovery, the presence of comorbid disorders, and patient preference.

Antidepressant Medication. Antidepressant medications have been shown to be effective in all forms of major depression. To date, no single antidepressant drug has been shown in controlled trials to have greater efficacy in the treatment of major depressive disorder. Although relatively few controlled studies of antidepressant efficacy have been conducted in depressed patients older than 60 years of age, most antidepressants are believed to be equally efficacious for geriatric depression (Salzman, 1998). Antidepressant medications can be grouped as follows: (1) cyclic antidepressants, which include the tricyclic antidepressants (TCAs), and maprotiline (a tetracyclic); (2) selective serotonin reuptake inhibitors (SSRIs), which currently include fluoxetine, sertraline, fluvoxamine, paroxetine, and citalopram; (3) monoamine oxidase inhibitors (MAOIs), which include phenelzine and tranylcypromine; and (4) the "atypical" antidepressants, which include trazodone, bupropion, nefazodone, venlafaxine, and mirtazapine. Table 8-11 in Chap. 8 lists antidepressant medications, usual dosage range, half-life, and therapeutic blood levels. For examples, see Drug Profile: Nefazodone and Drug Profile: Mirtazapine in this chapter. Also see Figure 20-1.

The first-generation drugs, the TCAs and MAOIs, are being used less and less. The second-generation medications, the SSRIs and atypical antidepressants, selectively target neurotransmitters and receptors thought to be associated with depression and to minimize side effects. There are significant differences in the side-effect profiles of the two generations of drugs. The relative tolerability of the newer agents potentially enhances patient adherence. Table 20-2 compares the different side effects of various drugs.

The efficacy of the MAOIs has been well established, and evidence suggests that they show a distinct advantage in treatment of one specific subtype of depression, so-called atypical depression (characterized by increased appetite, reverse diurnal mood variation, and hypersomnia) or depression with panic symptoms (Arana & Rosenbaum, 2000). Side effects of the MAOIs, adverse interactions with certain foods and other drugs, and dietary restrictions are described in Chapter 8. Given the complexity of their use, MAOIs are usually reserved for patients who have failed trials of other antidepressants or have not been able to tolerate them.

Monitoring and Administration of Medication. Patients should be carefully observed when taking medications. In the depths of depression, saving medication for a later suicide attempt is quite common. During antidepressant treatment, there is ongoing monitoring of vital signs, plasma drug levels as appropriate, liver and thyroid function tests, complete blood counts, and blood chemistry. Responsibilities include ensuring that patients are receiving a therapeutic dosage, helping in the evaluation of compliance, monitoring side effects, and helping to prevent toxicity. (Therapeutic blood levels for antidepressant medications are listed in Table 8-11 in Chap. 8.) Table 20-3 indicates various pharmacologic and nonpharmacologic interventions for the various side effects of antidepressant medications. Table 8-13 in Chap. 8 lists diet restrictions for those taking MAOIs.

Baseline orthostatic vital signs should be obtained before initiation of any medication, and in the case of medications known to have an impact on vital signs, such as TCAs, MAOIs, or venlafaxine (Effexor), they should be monitored on a regular basis. If these medications are administered to children or elderly patients, the dosage should be lowered to accommodate the physiologic state of the individual.

Tools for monitoring medication effects are objective observations, monitoring of vital signs, the patient's subjective reports, and the administration of rating scales over the course of treatment. Responsibilities include ensuring that patients are receiving a therapeutic dosage (therapeutic blood levels for antidepressant medications are listed in Table 8-11 in Chap. 8), assessment of adherence to the medication regimen, and evaluation of compliance.

Individualizing dosages is essential for achieving optimal efficacy. When the newer antidepressants are used,

DRUG PROFILE: Nefazodone
(Antidepressant Agent)
Trade Name: Serzone

Receptor affinity: Inhibits uptake of serotonin and norepinephrine. Antagonist action at 5-HT$_2$ and α_1-adrenergic receptors. No significant affinity in vitro for acetylcholine, α_2- or β-adrenergic receptors, 5-HT$_{1a}$, dopamine, or benzodiazepine receptors.

Indications: Treatment of depression

Routes and dosage: 100-, 150-, 200-, and 250-mg scored tablets.

Adult: Initial dose: typically 100 mg bid. Increase as tolerated in 100–200-mg/d increments at no less than 1-week intervals. Effective dose in clinical trials was 300–600 mg/d. Several weeks may be required for full antidepressant response.

Geriatric: Initial dose = 50 mg bid, increase more slowly as tolerated.

Children: Safety and efficacy in children under 18 y has not been established.

Half-life (peak effect): 2–4 h (peak plasma concentration = 1 h); at least three active metabolites, mean half-life = 11–24 h. Steady-state plasma concentrations reached in 4–5 d. Food delays absorption and decreases bioavailability by 20%.

Select adverse reactions: Headache, drowsiness, dry mouth and throat, insomnia, nausea, agitation, dizziness, constipation, asthenia, blurred vision, weight loss, and postural hypotension. Although priapism was not reported during clinical trials, it is structurally similar to trazodone, which has been associated with priapism.

Warning: Allow 1 week before starting an MAOI after discontinuation or 14 days after MAOI discontinuation. Avoid use during pregnancy or while nursing because safety has not been established. Use cautiously in patients with a known cardiovascular or cerebrovascular disease that could be exacerbated by hypotension.

Specific patient/family education:

• Notify prescriber if headache, dizziness, agitation, or other unusual symptoms develop.

• Ensure hydration and see prescriber to monitor blood pressure during titration. Report any symptoms of light-headedness or dizziness when changing positions.

• Notify prescriber if pregnancy is possible or planning to become pregnant. Do not breastfeed while taking this medication.

• Notify prescriber before taking any other prescription or OTC medication.

• Use caution driving or performing other hazardous tasks until sure that nefazodone does not alter physical or mental alertness. Avoid alcohol or other CNS-depressant drugs.

• Monitor weight loss and report any significant change.

• Do not abruptly discontinue.

DRUG PROFILE: Mirtazapine
(Antidepressant)
Trade Name: Remeron

Receptor affinity: Believed to enhance central noradrenergic and serotonergic activity antagonizing central presynaptic α_2-adrenergic receptors. Exact mechanism of action unknown.

Indications: Treatment of depression.

Routes and dosage: Available as 15- and 30-mg tablets

Adults: Initially, 15 mg/d as a single dose preferably in the evening before sleeping. Dosage may be increased up to a maximum of 45 mg/d.

Geriatric: Use with caution; reduced dosage may be needed.

Children: Safety and efficacy not established.

Half-life (peak effect): 20–40 h (2 h)

Selected adverse reactions: Somnolence, dizziness, weight gain, elevated cholesterol/triglyceride and transaminase levels, malaise, abdominal pain, hypertension, vasodilation, vomiting, anorexia, thirst, myasthenia, arthralgia, hypoesthesia, apathy, depression, vertigo, twitching, agitation, anxiety, amnesia, increased cough, sinusitis, pruritus, rash, urinary tract infection, mania (rare), agranulocytosis (rare).

Warning: Contraindicated in patients with known hypersensitivity. Use with caution in the elderly, patients who are breastfeeding, and those with impaired hepatic function. Avoid concomitant use with alcohol or diazepam, which can cause additive impairment of cognitive and monitor skills.

Specific patient/family education:

• Take the dose once a day in the evening before sleep.

• Avoid driving or performing hazardous tasks requiring alertness.

• Notify prescriber before taking any OTC or other prescription drugs.

• Avoid alcohol or other CNS depressants.

• Notify prescriber if pregnancy is possible or planning a pregnancy.

• Monitor temperature and report any fever, lethargy, weakness, sore throat, malaise, or other "flu-like" symptoms.

• Maintain medical follow-up including any appointments for blood counts and liver studies.

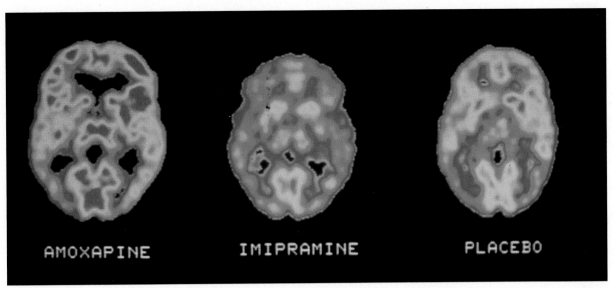

FIGURE 20.1 Acute effects of antidepressant medications in patients with affective disorder show widespread effects on the cortex that vary dramatically with the medication used. Position-emission tomography scanning is useful in revealing specific patterns of metabolic change in the brain and in providing clues to the mechanisms of antidepressant response. (Courtesy of Monte S. Buchsbaum, MD, The Mount Sinai Medical Center and School of Medicine, New York, NY)

this is usually done by fine-tuning medication dosage based on patient feedback. The TCAs (imipramine, desipramine, amitriptyline, and nortriptyline) have standardized valid plasma levels that can be useful in determining therapeutic dosages. Therapeutic plasma levels may vary from individual to individual. Blood samples should be drawn as close to 12 hours away from the last dose. The newer antidepressants do not have established standardized ranges, and optimal dosing is based on efficacy and tolerability.

Side-Effect Monitoring and Management

First-Generation Antidepressants. The most common side effects associated with TCAs are the antihistaminic (sedation and weight gain) and anticholinergic side effects: potentiation of CNS drugs, blurred vision, dry mouth, constipation, urinary retention, sinus tachycardia, and decreased memory. The TCA clomipramine, although used as an antidepressant in Europe, is indicated only for obsessive-compulsive disorder in the United States.

If possible, TCAs should not be prescribed for patients at risk for suicide. Lethal doses of TCAs are only three to five times the therapeutic dose, and more than 1 g of a TCAs is often toxic and may be fatal. Death may result from cardiac arrhythmia, hypotension, or uncontrollable seizures. Serum levels should be obtained when overdose is suspected. In acute overdose, almost all symptoms develop within 12 hours. Anticholinergic effects are prominent: dry mucous membranes, warm and dry skin, blurred vision, decreased bowel motility, and urinary retention. CNS suppression (ranging from drowsiness to coma) or an agitated delirium may occur. Basic management of overdose includes induction of emesis, gastric lavage, and cardiorespiratory supportive care.

Monoamine Oxidase Inhibitors. MAOIs have the potential to trigger a hypertensive crisis that may be fatal (see Chap 8). Symptoms of hypertensive crisis include sudden, severe pounding or explosive headache in the back of the head or temples, racing pulse, flushing, stiff neck, chest pain, nausea and vomiting, and increased sweating. An MAOI is generally given in divided doses to minimize side effects. These drugs are used cautiously in patients who are suicidal because of their relative lethality compared with the newer-generation antidepressants.

Select adverse reactions of MAOIs include headache, drowsiness, dry mouth and throat, insomnia, nausea, agitation, dizziness, constipation, asthenia, blurred vision, weight loss, and postural hypotension. Although priapism was not reported during clinical trials, the MAOIs are structurally similar to trazodone, which has been associated with priapism.

Serotonin Syndrome. Serotonin syndrome is a potentially serious side effect that is caused by drug-induced excess of intrasynaptic serotonin (5-hydroxytryptamine [5-HT]). First reported in the 1950s, it was relatively rare until the introduction of the SSRIs. Serotonin syndrome is most often reported in patients taking two or more medications that increase CNS serotonin levels by different mechanisms (Nolan et al., 2001). The most common drug combinations associated with serotonin syndrome involve the MAOIs, the SSRIs, and the TCAs.

TABLE 20.2   Comparison of Side Effects for Antidepressant Medications

Generic (Trade) Drug Name	Side Effects				
	Anticholinergic	Sedation	Orthostatic Hypotension	Gastrointestinal Distress	Weight Gain
Tricyclics: Tertiary Amines					
Amitriptyline (Elavil)	+4	+4	+2	0	+4
Clomipramine (Anafranil)	+3	+3	+2	+1	+4
Doxepin (Sinequan)	+2	+3	+2	0	+3
Imipramine (Tofranil)	+2	+2	+3	+1	+3
Trimipramine (Surmontil)	+2	+3	+2	0	+3
Tricyclics: Secondary Amines					
Amoxapine (Asendin)	+3	+2	+1	0	+1
Desipramine (Norpramin)	+1	+1	+1	0	+1
Nortriptyline (Aventyl, Pamelor)	+2	+2	+1	0	+1
Protriptyline (Vivactil)	+3	+1	+1	0	0
SSRIs					
Fluoxetine (Prozac)	0/+1	0/+1	0/+1	+3	0
Sertraline (Zoloft)	0	0/+1	0	+3	0
Paroxetine (Paxil)	0	0/+1	0	+3	0
Fluvoxamine (Luvox)	0/+1	0/+1	0/+1	+3	0
Citalopram (Celexa)	0/+1	0/+1	0/+1	+3	0
Others					
PHENETHYLAMINE					
venlafaxine (Effexor)	0	0	0	+3	0
TETRACYCLIC					
maprotiline (Ludiomil)	+1	+2	+1	0	+2
TRIAZOLOPYRIDINE					
trazodone (Desyrel)	0	+1	+3	+1	+1
PHENYLPIPERAZINE					
nefazodone (Serzone)	0/+1	+1	+2	+2	0/+1
AMINOKETONE					
bupropion (Wellbutrin)	+2	+2	+1	0	0/+1
PIPERAZINOAZEPINE					
mirtazapine (Remeron)	+3	+4	+3	+3	+2

0 = absent or rare
0/+1 = lowest likelihood
+4 = highest likelihood

It has also been reported in other drug interactions, including those between low-dose trazodone and paroxetine (Reeves & Bullen, 1995), clomipramine and lithium (Kojima et al., 1993), and fluoxetine and lithium (Muly et al., 1993).

Although serotonin syndrome can cause death, it is mild in most patients, who usually tend to recover with supportive care alone. Unlike neuroleptic malignant syndrome, which generally develops within 3 to 9 days after the introduction of neuroleptic medications (see Chap. 18), serotonin syndrome has a more rapid onset and tends to develop within hours or days after initiating or increasing the dose of serotoninergic medication

or adding a drug with serotomimetic properties. The symptoms include altered mental status, autonomic dysfunction, and neuromuscular abnormalities. At least three of the following must be present for a diagnosis: mental status changes, agitation, myoclonus, hyperreflexia, fever, shivering, diaphoresis, ataxia, and diarrhea. The presence of peripheral vascular disease and atherosclerosis may lead to severe vasospasm and hypertension in the presence of elevated serotonin levels. Additionally, a slow metabolizer of SSRIs may produce higher-than-normal levels of these antidepressants in the blood. Medications that are not usually considered serotoninergic, such as dextromethorphan and meperi-

TABLE 20.3 Interventions to Help Treat Side Effects of Antidepressant Medications

Side Effect	Pharmacologic Intervention	Nonpharmacologic Intervention
Dry mouth, caries, inflammation of the mouth	Bethanechol 10–30 mg tid Pilocarpine drops	Sugarless gum Sugarless lozenges 6–8 cups water per day Toothpaste for dry mouth
Nausea, vomiting	Cisapride 0.5 mg bid	Take medication with food Soda crackers, toast, tea
Weight gain	Change medication	Nutritionally balanced diet Daily exercise
Urinary hesitation	Bethanechol 10–30 mg tid	6–8 cups water per day
Constipation	Stool softener	Bulk laxative Daily exercise 6–8 cups water per day Diet rich in fresh fruits and vegetables, and grains
Diarrhea	OTC antidiarrheal	Maintain fluid intake
Orthostatic hypotension		Increase hydration Sit or stand up slowly
Drowsiness	Shift dosing time Lower medication dose Change medication	One caffeinated beverage at strategic time Do not drive when drowsy No alcohol or other recreational drugs Plan for rest time
Fatigue	Lower medication dose Change medication	Daily exercise
Blurred vision	Bethanechol 10–30 mg tid Pilocarpine eyedrops	Temporary use of magnifying lenses until body adjusts to medication
Flushing, sweating	Terazosin 1 mg qd Lower medication dose Change medication	Frequent bathing Lightweight clothing
Tremor	β-blockers	

dine, have been associated with the syndrome (Sporer, 1995). The most important emergency interventions are stopping the offending drug, notifying the physician, and providing necessary supportive care (eg, intravenous fluids, antipyretics, cooling blanket). Methysergide maleate, a nonspecific serotonin antagonist, has been used with some success; however, little research documents the effectiveness of this drug (Ames, 1993). The most common treatment involves the use of benzodiazepine, which has been shown to be effective in treating the myoclonus.

Drug–Drug Interactions. There are several potential drug interactions when administering antidepressants because these agents are metabolized by the cytochrome P450 systems. These potential interactions should be considered when children or elderly patients are treated (see Chap. 8). Five of the most important enzymes systems are 1A2, 2D6, 2C9, 2C19, 3A4. The 1A2 system is inhibited by the selective serotonin reuptake inhibitor fluvoxamine (Luvox). Thus, other drugs that use the 1A2 system will no longer be metabolized as efficiently. For

example, if fluvoxamine is given with theophylline, the theophylline dosage must be lowered, or else blood levels of theophylline will rise and cause possible side effects or toxic reactions, such as seizures. Fluvoxamine also effects the metabolism of atypical antipsychotics. On the other hand, smoking and caffeine can induce activity of the 1A2 system. This means that smokers may need to be given a higher dose of medications that are metabolized by this system (Stahl, 2000).

Fluoxetine (Prozac) and paroxetine (Paxil) have a potent inhibition of 2D6. One of the most significant drug interactions is caused by SSRI inhibition of 2D6 that in turn causes an increase in plasma levels of TCAs. If there is concomitant administration of an SSRI and a TCA, plasma drug level of the TCA should be monitored and probably reduced. In the 3A4 system, some SSRIs (fluoxetine [Prozac], fluvoxamine [Luvox], and nefazodone [Serzone]) will raise the levels of alprazolam [Xanax] or triazolam [Halcion] through enzyme inhibition, requiring reduction of dosage of the benzodiazepine. The use of fluoxetine, fluvoxamine, and nefazodone with any drugs that are substrates of 3A4 can result in increased levels of those drugs. Fluvoxamine and fluoxetine are potent inhibitors of both 2C9 and 2C19 (Stahl, 2000).

Teaching Points. Studies indicate that if depression goes untreated or is inadequately treated, episodes become more frequent, more severe, and of longer duration (Goodwin & Jamison, 1990). Patient education involves emphasizing this progressive, recurrent pattern and the importance of continuing medication after the acute phase of treatment to decrease the risk for relapse or future episodes. Patient concerns regarding long-term antidepressant therapy need to be assessed and addressed. Even after the first episode of major depression, medication should be continued for at least 6 months to 1 year after the patient achieves complete remission of symptoms. If the patient experiences a recurrence after tapering off the first course of treatment, the regimen should be reinstituted for at least another year, and if the illness reoccurs, medication should be continued indefinitely (Arana & Rosenbaum, 2000).

Patients should not take St. John's wort if also taking prescribed antidepressants. If St. John's wort is being used, the patient should be reminded that it should not be combined with nasal decongestants, hay fever and asthma medications, containing monoamines, amino acid supplements containing phenylalanine, and tyrosine, which may cause hypertension (Miller, 1998).

Other Somatic Therapies

Electroconvulsive Therapy. The efficacy of electroconvulsive therapy (ECT) has been established, although its therapeutic mechanism of action is unknown. ECT is an effective treatment for severe depression but is generally reserved for patients whose disorder is refractory or intolerant to initial drug treatments and who are so severely ill that rapid treatment is required (eg, patients with malnutrition, catatonia, or suicidality). ECT is contraindicated in the presence of increased intracranial pressure. Other high-risk patients include those with recent myocardial infarction, recent cerebrovascular accident, retinal detachment, or pheochromocytoma (tumor on the adrenal cortex) and those at risk for anesthesia complications. Although older age has been associated with a favorable response to ECT, many of these patients may have coexisting medical problems that place them at high risk for complications (APA, 1990).

Nursing Interventions for the Patient Undergoing Electroconvulsive Therapy. The American Nurses Association (2000) defined the role of the nurse in the care of the patient undergoing ECT to include providing educational and emotional support for the patient and family, assessing baseline or pretreatment level of function, preparing the patient for ECT process, and monitoring

and evaluating the patient's response to ECT, sharing it with the ECT team, and modifying treatment as needed. (Text Box 8-3 in Chap. 8 outlines specific interventions for patients receiving ECT.) The actual procedure, possible therapeutic mechanisms of action, potential adverse effects, contraindications, and nursing interventions are described in detail in Chapter 8.

Light Therapy (Phototherapy). Light therapy is described in Chapter 8. Given current modest research, light therapy is a treatment consideration for well-documented mild to moderate seasonal, nonpsychotic, winter depressive episodes in patients with recurrent major depressive or bipolar II disorders.

Psychological Domain

Assessment

The mental status examination is an effective clinical tool to evaluate the psychological aspects of major depression because the focus is on disturbances of mood and affect, thought processes and content, cognition, memory, and attention. The comprehensive mental status examination is described in detail in Chapter 10.

Mood and Affect. The person with depression will have a sustained period of feeling depressed, sad, or hopeless and may experience anhedonia (loss of interest or pleasure). The patient may report "not caring anymore" or not feeling any enjoyment in activities that were previously considered pleasurable. In some individuals, this may include decrease in or loss of libido (sexual interest or desire) and sexual function. Depressed mood may be severe enough to provoke thoughts of suicide.

Numerous scales are available for assessment of depression. Easily administered self-report questionnaires can be valuable detection tools. These questionnaires cannot be the sole basis for making a diagnosis of major depressive episode, but they are sensitive to depressive symptoms. The following are five commonly used self-report scales:

- General Health Questionnaire (GHQ)
- Center for Epidemiological Studies Depression Scale (CES-D)
- Beck Depression Inventory (BDI)
- Zung Self-Rating Depression Scale (ZSRDS)
- PRIME-MD (Pfizer)

Clinician-completed rating scales may be more sensitive to improvement in the course of treatment and may have a slightly greater specificity than do self-report questionnaires in detecting depression. These include the following:

- Hamilton Rating Scale for Depression (HRS-D) (see Appendix K)

- Montgomery-Asberg Depression Rating Scale (MADRS)
- National Institute of Mental Health Diagnostic Interview Schedule (DIS)

Thought Content. Depressed individuals often have an unrealistic negative evaluation of their worth or have guilty preoccupations or ruminations about minor past failings. Such individuals often misinterpret neutral or trivial day-to-day events as evidence of personal defects and have an exaggerated sense of responsibility for untoward events. The possibility of disorganized thought processes (eg, tangential or circumstantial thinking) and disturbances of perception (eg, hallucinations, delusions) should also be included in the assessment.

Suicidal Behavior. Patients with major depression are at increased risk for suicide. Suicide risk should be assessed initially and throughout the course of treatment. Suicidal ideation includes thoughts that range from a belief that others would be better off if the person were dead or thoughts of death (passive suicidal ideation) to actual specific plans for committing suicide (active suicidal ideation). The frequency, intensity, and lethality of these thoughts can vary and can help to determine seriousness of intent. The more specific the plan and the more accessible the means, the more serious the intent. Risk factors that must be carefully considered are the availability and adequacy of social supports, past history of suicidal ideation or behavior, presence of psychosis or substance abuse, and decreased ability to control suicidal impulses.

Cognition and Memory. Many individuals with depression report impaired ability to think, concentrate, or make decisions. They may appear easily distracted or complain of memory difficulties. In older adults with major depression, memory difficulties may be the chief complaint and may be mistaken for early signs of a dementia (pseudodementia) (APA, 2000). When the depression is fully treated, the memory problem often improves or fully resolves.

Nursing Diagnoses for Psychological Domain

Nursing diagnoses focusing on the psychological domain for the patient with a depressive disorder are numerous. If patient data lead to the diagnosis of Risk for Suicide, the patient should be further assessed for plan, intent, and accessibility of means. Other nursing diagnoses include Hopelessness, Low Self-Esteem, Ineffective Individual Coping, Decisional Conflict, Spiritual Distress, and Dysfunctional Grieving.

Interventions for Psychological Domain

Although pharmacotherapy is usually the primary modality of treatment of major depression, patients can bene-

fit from psychosocial and psychoeducational treatments as well. The most commonly used therapies are described. For patients with severe or recurrent major depressive disorder, the combination of psychotherapy (including interpersonal therapy, cognitive behavioral therapy, behavior therapy, or brief dynamic therapy) and pharmacotherapy has been found to be superior to treatment with a single modality. Adding a course of cognitive behavioral therapy may be an effective strategy for preventing relapse in patients who have had only a partial response to pharmacotherapy alone (APA, 2000b). The AHCPR guidelines suggest that the combination of medication and psychotherapy may be particularly useful in more complex situations (ie, depression in the context of concurrent, chronic general-medical, or other psychiatric disorders, or in patients who fail to respond fully to either treatment alone). Recent studies suggest that short-term cognitive and interpersonal therapies may be as effective as pharmacotherapy in milder depressions (Arana & Rosenbaum, 2000). Psychotherapy in combination with medication may also be used to address collateral issues, such as medication adherence or secondary psychosocial problems (Arana & Rosenbaum, 2000).

Therapeutic Nurse–Patient Relationship. One of the most effective therapeutic tools for treating any psychiatric disorder is the therapeutic alliance, a helpful and trusting relationship between clinician and patient. The alliance is built from a number of complex activities, including the following (Merriam & Karasu, 1996, p. 302):

- Establishment and maintenance of a supportive relationship
- Availability in times of crisis
- Vigilance regarding dangerousness to self and others
- Provision of education about the illness and the goals of treatment
- Provision of encouragement and feedback concerning the patient's progress
- Provision of guidance regarding the patient's interactions with his personal and work environment
- Realistic goal setting and monitoring

Interacting with individuals who are depressed is challenging because they tend to be withdrawn and have difficulty expressing feelings and engaging in interpersonal interactions. The development of the therapeutic alliance partly depends on winning the patient's trust through a warm and empathic stance within the context of firm professional boundaries (see Therapeutic Dialogue: Approaching the Patient With Depression).

Cognitive Therapy. Cognitive therapy directed at dispelling the patient's irrational beliefs and distorted attitudes has been successful in reducing depressive

THERAPEUTIC DIALOGUE — Approaching the Patient With Depression

Mr. Jones is a 35-year-old recently unemployed college professor who was admitted to an acute psychiatric unit in a general hospital following an attempted suicide. He is slumped in a chair across the dayroom, staring out the window with a very sad look on his face.

Ineffective Approach

Nurse: Hi, Mr. Jones, how are you today?
Mr. Jones: I don't know.
Nurse: Well, it's a beautiful day.
Mr. Jones: (Silence.)
Nurse: Have you had breakfast?
Mr. Jones: I'm not hungry.
Nurse: Oh. Mind if we talk for awhile?
Mr. Jones: I'd rather be left alone.
Nurse: OK, but you would feel better if you talked to other people.
Mr. Jones: (Silence. Continues to stare out the window.)
Nurse: I will talk to you later.

Effective Approach

Nurse: Hi. (Quietly.)
Mr. Jones: Hello.

Nurse: Mind if I sit down?
Mr. Jones: Suit yourself.
Nurse: (Nurse quietly pulls up chair and sits.)
Mr. Jones: What time is it? They took my watch.
Nurse: It's about 9:00 AM.
Mr. Jones: It's going to be a long day.
Nurse: Oh, how so?
Mr. Jones: I just feel so miserable.
Nurse: Can I help you?
Mr. Jones: Probably not. It's hard to get through the day.
Nurse: What are your days like?
Mr. Jones: Endless—especially now with no job, no future.
Nurse: No job?
Mr. Jones: I lost it, along with my wife who died in a car accident . . .

Critical Thinking Challenge

- How did the nurse's approach in the first scenario block communication?
- How was the communication approach utilized by the nurse in the second scenario beneficial to initiating a therapeutic relationship with Mr. Jones? Discuss the differences between the two approaches.

---

symptoms during the acute phase of less severe, non-melancholic forms of major depression (APA, 2000b) (see Chap. 12). In one study conducted by Persons and colleagues (1996), remission rates after cognitive therapy were comparable to those after pharmacotherapy. The use of cognitive therapy in the continuation and maintenance phase of depression has not been studied.

Behavior Therapy. Behavior therapy has been effective in the acute treatment of patients with mild to moderately severe depression, especially when combined with pharmacotherapy. Techniques include activity scheduling, self-control therapy, social skills training, and problem solving. The efficacy of behavior therapy in the continuation and maintenance phase of depression has not be subjected to controlled studies (APA, 2000b). Behavior therapy techniques are described in Chapter 12.

Interpersonal Therapy. Interpersonal therapy seeks to recognize, explore, and resolve the interpersonal losses, role confusion and transitions, social isolation, and deficits in social skills that may precipitate depressive states (Klerman et al., 1984). It maintains that losses must be mourned and related affects appreciated, that role confusion and transitions must be recognized and resolved, and that deficits in social skills must be overcome to permit the acquisition of social supports. Some evidence in controlled studies suggests that interpersonal therapy as a single agent is effective in reducing de-

pressive symptoms in the acute phase of nonmelancholic major depressive episodes and in the maintenance phase for psychosocial conflicts and work difficulties (Kupfer et al., 1992) (see Chap. 12).

Marital and Family Therapy. Parkerson and co-workers (1995) reported that patients who perceived high family stress were at risk for greater future severity of illness, higher utilization of health services, and higher health care expense. Marital and family problems are common among patients with mood disorders; comprehensive treatment requires that these problems be assessed and addressed. They may be a consequence of major depression but may also increase vulnerability to depression and in some instances retard recovery (Beach et al., 1990). Research suggests that marital and family therapy may reduce depressive symptoms and the risk for relapse in patients with marital and family problems. Marital and family approaches for the treatment of depression include behavioral approaches (Beach et al., 1990) and a "strategic marital therapy" approach (Coyne, 1988) as well as a psychoeducational approach. There are many family nursing interventions that the generalist psychiatric nurse can use when providing targeted family-centered care. These are discussed in detail in Chapter 12 and include some of the following activities:

- Monitor patient and family for indicators of stress.
- Teach stress management techniques.

- Counsel family members on coping skills for their own use.
- Provide necessary knowledge of options and support services.
- Facilitate family routines and rituals.
- Assist family to resolve feelings of guilt.
- Assist family with conflict resolution.
- Identify family strengths and resources with family members.
- Facilitate communication among family members.

Group Therapy. The role of group therapy in the treatment of depression is based on clinical experience rather than on systematic controlled studies. It may be particularly useful for depression associated with bereavement or chronic medical illness. Individuals may benefit from the example of others who have successfully dealt with the similar losses or challenges. Survivors can gain self-esteem as successful role models for new group members. Medication support groups can provide information to the patient and to family members regarding prognosis and medication issues, thereby providing a psychoeducational forum.

Patient and Family Education. Patients with depression and their significant others often incorrectly believe that their illness is their own fault and that they should be able to "pull themselves up by their boot straps and snap out of it." It is vital to educate patients and their families about the nature, prognosis, and treatment of depression to dispel these false beliefs and the unnecessary guilt that ensues. Patients need to know the full range of suitable treatment options before consenting to participate in treatment. The nurse can provide opportunities for them to question, discuss, and explore their feelings about past, current, and planned use of medications and other treatments (ANA, 2000). Developing strategies to enhance adherence and to raise awareness of early signs of relapse can be important aids to increasing treatment efficacy (see Psychoeducation Checklist: Major Depressive Disorder).

Social Domain

Assessment

Social assessment focuses on the individual's developmental history, family psychiatric history, patterns of relationships, quality of support system, education, work history, and impact of physical or sexual abuse on interpersonal function (see Chap. 10). Including a family member or close friend in the assessment process can be helpful. Changes in patterns of relating (especially social withdrawal) and changes in level of occupational functioning are commonly reported and may represent

---

PSYCHOEDUCATION CHECKLIST
Major Depressive Disorder

When caring for the patient with a major depressive disorder, be sure to include the following topic areas in the teaching plan:

- Psychopharmacologic agents, including drug action, dosing frequency, and possible adverse effects
- Risk factors for recurrence
- Adherence to therapy and treatment program
- Nutrition
- Sleep measures
- Self-care management
- Goal setting and problem solving
- Social interaction skills
- Follow-up appointments
- Community support services

---

a significant deterioration from baseline behavior. Increased use of "sick days" may occur. The family's level of support and understanding of the disorder also need to be assessed.

Nursing Diagnoses for Social Domain

Data collected from the biopsychosocial assessment often lead to the following nursing diagnoses: Ineffective Family Coping, Ineffective Role Performance, and Interrupted Family Processes. If the depressed patient is also a caregiver of a family member, Caregiver Role Strain can also be seen.

Interventions for Social Domain

Individuals experiencing depression have often withdrawn from the daily social activities such as engaging in family activities, attending work, and participating in community activities. During hospitalization, patients often withdraw to their rooms and refuse to participate in ward activity. Nurses are challenged to help the patient balance the need for privacy with the need to return to normal social functioning. Depressed patients should never be approached in an overenthusiastic manner—that approach will irritate them and block communication. On the other hand, patients should be encouraged to set realistic goals to reconnect with their families and communities. Explaining to the patients that attending the social activities, even though they do not feel like it, will facilitate the recovery process helps patients achieve those goals.

Milieu Therapy. On a psychiatric unit, depressed patients should be encouraged to attend groups and participate in all assigned treatment activities. These individuals have a decreased energy level and thus may be moving slower than others; however, their efforts should be praised.

Safety.   Patients are often admitted to the psychiatric hospital because of suicide attempt. Suicidality should continually be evaluated, and the patient should be protected from self-harm (see Chap. 10). During the depths of depression, patients may not have the energy to complete a suicide. As patients begin to feel better and have increased energy, they may even be at a greater for suicide. If a previously depressed patient appears to become energized overnight, he or she may have made a decision to commit suicide and thus may be relieved that the decision is finally made. The nurse may misinterpret the mood improvement as a positive move toward recovery; however, this patient may be very intent on completing a suicide. These individuals should be carefully monitored to maintain their safety (see Chap. 14).

Other Interventions.   Nurses are exceptionally well positioned to engage patients and their families in the active process of improving daily functioning, increasing knowledge and skill acquisition, and increasing independent living. Consumer-oriented support groups can help to enhance the self-esteem and the support network of participating patients and their families. Advice, encouragement, and the sense of group camaraderie may make an important contribution to recovery (APA, 2000b). Organizations providing support and information include the National Depressive and Manic Depressive Association (NDMDA), Depression Awareness, Recognition and Treatment (D/ART Program), National Alliance for the Mentally Ill (NAMI), and Recovery, Inc. (a self-help group).

Family Interventions

The family needs education and support during and after the treatment of family members. Because major depressive disorder is a recurring disorder, the family needs information about specific antecedents to a family member's depression and what steps to take. For example, one patient may routinely become depressed during the fall of each year, with one of the first symptoms being excessive sleepiness. For another patient, a major loss, such as a child going to college or a death of a pet, may precipitate a depressive episode. Families of elderly patients need to be aware of the possibility of depression and their related symptoms. Families of children who are depressed often misinterpret depression as behavior problems.

Evaluation and Treatment Outcomes

The major goals of treatment are to help the patient to be as independent as possible and to achieve stabilization, remission, and recovery from major depression. It is often a lifelong struggle for the individual. Ongoing evaluation of the patient's symptoms, functioning, and quality of life should be carefully documented in the patient's record in order to monitor outcomes of treatment.

Continuum of Care

Individuals with depressive disorders may initially present in inpatient and outpatient medical and primary care settings, emergency rooms, and inpatient and outpatient mental health settings. Nurses should be able to recognize depression in these patients and make appropriate interventions or referrals. The continuum of care beyond these settings may include partial hospitalization or day treatment programs; individual, family, or group psychotherapy; home visits, and, the mainstay of treatment, psychopharmacotherapy. Although most patients with major depression are treated in outpatient settings, brief hospitalization may be required if the patient is suicidal or psychotic. Nurses working on inpatient units provide a wide range of direct services, including dispensing and monitoring medications and target symptoms, conducting psychoeducational groups, and, more generally, structuring and maintaining a therapeutic environment. Nurses providing home care have an excellent opportunity to detect undiagnosed depressive disorders and make appropriate referrals.

Nursing practice requires a coordinated, ongoing interaction between patients, families, and providers to deliver comprehensive services. This includes using the complementary skills of both psychiatric and medical care colleagues for the formulation of overall goals, plans, and decisions and for the provision of continuity of care as needed (ANA, 2000). See Appendices M and N for patient clinical pathways for the treatment of depression. Collaborative care between the primary care provider and mental health specialist is also important to achieve remission of symptoms and physical well-being, restore baseline occupational and psychosocial functioning, and reduce the likelihood of relapse or recurrence (Fig. 20-2).

BIPOLAR DISORDERS (MANIC-DEPRESSIVE DISORDERS)
Diagnostic Criteria

Bipolar disorder is distinguished from depressive disorders by the occurrence of manic or hypomanic (ie, mildly

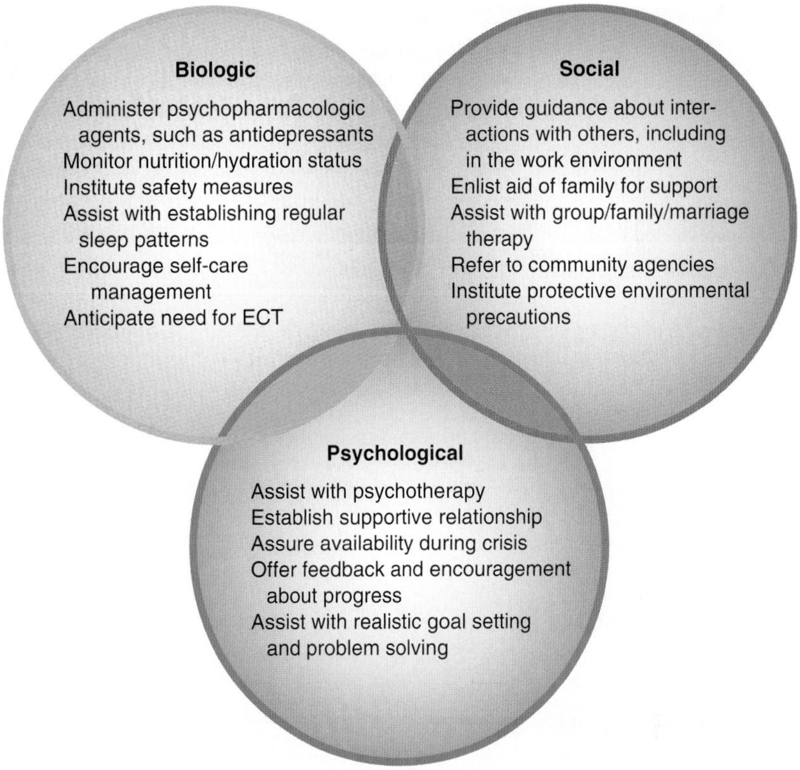

FIGURE 20.2 Biopsychosocial interventions for patients with major depressive disorder. ECT, electroconvulsive therapy.

manic) episodes in addition to depressive episodes. The *DSM-IV-TR* divides bipolar disorders into three major groups: bipolar I (periods of major depressive, manic, and/or mixed episodes); bipolar II (periods of major depression and hypomania); and **cyclothymic disorder** (periods of hypomanic episodes and depressive episodes that do not meet full criteria for a major depressive episode) (Table 20-4). These are described later. The specifiers describe either the most recent mood episode or the course of recurrent episodes, for example, "bipolar disorder I, most recent episode manic, severe with psychotic features."

KEY CONCEPT   **Mania. Mania** is primarily characterized by an abnormally and persistently elevated, expansive, or irritable mood for a duration of at least 1 week (or less, if hospitalized).

A **manic episode** is a distinct period (of at least 1 week, or less, if hospitalized) during which there is an abnormally and persistently elevated, expansive, or irritable mood (APA, 2000a). Elevated mood is characterized as **euphoria** (exaggerated feelings of well-being) or elation during which the person may describe feeling "high," "ecstatic," "on top of the world," or "up in the clouds." **Expansive mood** is characterized by inappropriate lack of restraint in expressing one's feelings and frequently overvaluing one's own impor-

tance. Expansive qualities include an unceasing and indiscriminate enthusiasm for interpersonal, sexual, or occupational interactions (Text Box 20-1). Manic episodes can also consist of irritable mood, in which the person is easily annoyed and provoked to anger, particularly when the person's wishes are challenged or thwarted. Additionally, manic episodes can consist of alterations between euphoria and irritability (**lability of mood**). To meet full *DSM-IV-TR* criteria, three (or four if the mood is irritable) of seven additional symptoms must be present: inflated self-esteem or grandiosity; decreased need for sleep; being more talkative or having pressured speech; flight of ideas or racing thoughts; distractibility; increase in goal-directed activity or psychomotor agitation; and excessive involvement in pleasurable activities that have a high potential for painful consequences. The disturbance must be severe enough to cause marked impairment in social activities, occupational functioning, and interpersonal relationships or to require hospitalization to prevent self-harm.

During a manic episode, decreased need to sleep is accompanied by increased energy and hyperactivity. The individual often remains awake during long periods of the night or wakes up several times full of energy. Increased motor activity and agitation, which may be purposeful at first (eg, cleaning the house), may deteriorate into inappropriate or disorganized actions.

TABLE 20.4 Key Diagnostic Characteristics of Bipolar I Disorder 296.xx
296.0x—Bipolar I, single manic episode
296.40—Bipolar I, most recent episode hypomanic
296.4x—Bipolar I, most recent episode manic
296.6x—Bipolar I, most recent episode mixed
296.5x—Bipolar I, most recent episode depressed
296.7—Bipolar I, most recent episode unspecified

Diagnostic Criteria and Target Symptoms	Associated Findings

Diagnostic Criteria and Target Symptoms

- Presence of one or more manic episodes or mixed episodes, including one or more major depressive episodes
  Manic episode
  - Abnormally and persistently elevated, expansive or irritable mood for at least 1 week
  - Persistence of inflated self-esteem and grandiosity
  - Decreased need for sleep
  - More talkative than usual or pressure to keep talking
  - Flight of ideas or racing thoughts
  - Distractibility
  - Increased goal-directed activity or psychomotor agitation
  - Excessive involvement in pleasurable activities with high potential for painful results (such as unrestrained buying sprees, foolish business investments)
  - Marked impairment in occupational functioning or in usual social activities or relationships; possible hospitalization to prevent harm; psychotic features
  Major depressive episode (symptoms appear nearly every day)
  - Depressed mood most of the day
  - Markedly diminished interest or pleasure in all or most all activities for most of the day
  - Significant weight loss when not dieting; weight gain or increase or decrease in appetite
  - Insomnia or hypersomnia
  - Psychomotor agitation or retardation
  - Fatigue or loss of energy
  - Feelings of worthlessness or excessive or inappropriate guilt
  - Diminished ability to concentrate or indecisiveness
  - Recurrent thoughts of death, suicidal ideation without a specific plan, suicide attempt or specific plan for committing suicide
  - Not bereavement
  - Clinically significant distress or impairment in social, occupational, or other important areas of functioning
  Mixed episode
  - Criteria for both manic and major depressive episodes nearly every day for at least 1 week
  - Hospitalization to prevent harm; psychotic features
  Hypomanic episode
  - Distinct period of persistently elevated, expansive, or irritable mood through at least 4 days
  - Clearly different from usual nondepressed mood
  - Same symptoms as that for manic episode but does not cause impairment in social or occupational functioning or necessitate hospitalization
  - Unequivocal change in function, uncharacteristic of person when asymptomatic
  - Change observable by others

Associated Findings

Associated Behavioral Findings

Manic episode
- Resistive to efforts for treatment
- Disorganized or bizarre behavior
- Change in dress or appearance
- Possible gambling and antisocial behavior

Major depressive episode
- Tearfulness, irritability
- Obsessive rumination
- Anxiety
- Phobia
- Excessive worry over physical symptoms
- Complaints of pain
- Possible panic attacks
- Difficulty with intimate relationships
- Marital, occupational, or academic problems
- Substance abuse
- Increased use of medical services
- Attempted or complete suicide attempts
Mixed episode
- Similar to those for manic and depressive episodes
Hypomanic episodes
- Sudden onset with rapid escalation within 1–2 d
- Possibly precede or are followed by major depressive episode

Associated Physical Examination Findings
Manic episode
- Mean age of onset for first manic episode after age 21–30 yrs
- Possible child abuse, spouse abuse, or other violent behavior during severe manic episodes
- Associated problems involving school truancy, school failure, occupational failure, divorce, or episodic antisocial behavior

Associated Laboratory Findings
Manic episodes
- Polysomnographic abnormalities
- Increased cortisol secretion

(*continued*)

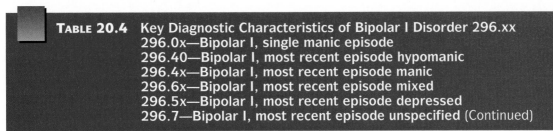

TABLE 20.4 **Key Diagnostic Characteristics of Bipolar I Disorder 296.xx**
296.0x—Bipolar I, single manic episode
296.40—Bipolar I, most recent episode hypomanic
296.4x—Bipolar I, most recent episode manic
296.6x—Bipolar I, most recent episode mixed
296.5x—Bipolar I, most recent episode depressed
296.7—Bipolar I, most recent episode unspecified (Continued)

Diagnostic Criteria and Target Symptoms	Associated Findings
• Not severe enough to cause marked impairment in social or occupational functioning or to require hospitalization; no psychotic features • Episode not better accounted for by other disorders such as schizoaffective disorder and not superimposed on schizophrenia, schizophreniform, delusional, or psychotic disorders • Not a direct physiologic effect of substance or other medical condition	• Absence of dexamethasone nonsuppression • Possible abnormalities with norepinephrine, serotonin, acetylcholine, dopamine, or GABA neurotransmitter *Major depressive episode* • Sleep electroencephalogram abnormalities • Possible abnormalities with norepinephrine, serotonin, acetylcholine, dopamine, or GABA neurotransmitter systems

The individual may get involved unrealistically in several new projects that may entail overspending, may overindulge in pleasurable activities including sexual encounters or drug or alcohol use, or may undertake high-risk activities such as driving too fast or taking up dangerous sports. The individual becomes overly talkative, feels pressured to continue talking, and at times is difficult to interrupt. Thoughts become disorganized and skip rapidly among topics that often have little relationship to each other. This decreased logical connection between thoughts is termed *flight of ideas*. Patients with mania have inflated self-esteem, which may range from unusual self-confidence to grandiose delusions. Other psychiatric disorders can have symptoms that mimic a manic episode. Schizophrenia, schizoaffective disorder, anxiety disorders, some personality disorders (borderline personality disorder and histrionic personality disorder), and adolescent conduct disorders should be considered (McDaniel et al., 1996).

The *DSM-IV-TR* criteria for a **mixed episode** are met when the criteria for both a manic episode and a major depressive episode are met and are present for at least 1 week. Individuals who are having a mixed episode usually exhibit high anxiety, agitation, and irritability. The criteria for a **hypomanic episode** are the same as for a manic episode except that the time criterion is at least 4 days rather than 1 week, and no marked impairment in social or occupational functioning is present.

Secondary Mania

Mania can be caused by medical disorders or their treatments or by certain substances of abuse (eg, certain metabolic abnormalities, neurologic disorders, CNS tumors, and medications) (McDaniel et al., 1996).

Rapid Cycling Specifier

Rapid cycling can occur in both bipolar I and bipolar II disorders. The essential feature of rapid cycling is the occurrence of four or more mood episodes that meet criteria for manic, mixed, hypomanic, or depressive episode during the previous 12 months.

The *DSM-IV-TR* criteria for **cyclothymic disorder** are the presence for at least 2 years of numerous periods

TEXT BOX 20.1

Clinical Vignette: Mr. Rizzo

Mr. Rizzo is a successful jewelry salesman who is well liked by his customers and coworkers. Normally a happy person, Mr. Rizzo has had bouts of depression that have lasted for a couple of months. Recently, he was feeling especially generous and bought his wife a new car. Even though the purchase stretched the family finances, Mrs. Rizzo was pleased. The following week, however, he bought a diamond ring for a woman with whom he had initiated a sexual liaison (the day after he bought his wife the car). The next weekend, he and a friend bought airline tickets to Las Vegas for a weekend of fun and games. He gambled and lost several thousand dollars. When Mr. Rizzo returned home, he had not slept for several days and was deeply in debt. He was confused and disoriented. His family admitted him to a local psychiatric facility.

with hypomanic symptoms and numerous periods with depressive symptoms that do not meet full criteria for a major depressive episode.

Clinical Course

Bipolar disorder is a chronic, cyclic disorder. There is general agreement that later episodes of illness occur more frequently than earlier episodes, and increased frequency of episodes or more continuous symptoms have been reported in patients who have had earlier age of illness onset and significant family history of illness. Some patients may have a predictable pattern moving from mania to depression or from depression to mania, but some patients may have an unpredictable and variable expression of the illness (Faedda et al., 1991). An additional feature of bipolar illness is rapid cycling, which in its most severe form, can include continuous cycling between subthreshold mania and depression or hypomania and depression (Post et al., 1990). It remains controversial whether mixed episodes result in poorer outcomes than pure mania, but mixed states have been associated with increased likelihood of comorbid substance abuse (Tohen et al., 1998) and with increased suicidal ideation compared with pure mania (Perugi et al., 1997). Bipolar disorder can lead to severe functional impairment as manifested by alienation from family, friends, and coworkers; indebtedness; job loss; divorce; and other problems of living (Rothbaum & Astin, 2000).

Bipolar Disorder in Special Populations

Children and Adolescents

Bipolar disorder in children has only recently been recognized. Although it is not well studied, depression usually appears first. Somewhat different than in adults, the hallmark of childhood bipolar disorder is intense rage. Children may display seemingly unprovoked rage episodes for up to 2 to 3 hours. The symptoms of bipolar disorder reflect the developmental level of the child. Children younger than 9 years of age exhibit more irritability and emotional lability; older children exhibit more classic symptoms, such as euphoria and grandiosity. The first contact with the mental health system often occurs when the behavior becomes disruptive, possibly 5 to 10 years after on its onset. These children often have other psychiatric disorders, such as attention deficit hyperactivity disorder and conduct disorder (Mohr, 2001) (see Chap. 29).

Elderly People

Geriatric mania patients demonstrate more neurologic abnormalities and cognitive disturbances (confusion and disorientation) than younger patients. It was generally believed that the incidence of mania decreases with age because this population was thought to consist of only those individuals who were diagnosed in younger years and managed to survive into old age. Recently, late-onset bipolar disorder was identified when researchers found evidence of an increased incidence of mania with age, especially in women after the age of 50 years and in men in the eighth and ninth decades. Late-onset bipolar disorder is more likely related to secondary mania and consequently has a poorer prognosis because of comorbid medical conditions (McDonald, 2000).

Epidemiology

Distribution and Age of Onset

Bipolar disorder has a lifetime prevalence of 0.4% to 1.6% in the general adult population (APA, 2000b). Most patients with bipolar disorder experience significant symptoms before the age of 25 years (Faedda et al., 1991). The estimated mean age of onset is between 21 and 30 years of age (Goodwin & Jamison, 1990). About 10% to 15% of adolescents with recurrent major depressive episodes go on to develop bipolar I disorder (APA, 2000b). Onset of symptoms after the age of 60 years is likely due to secondary medical causes, including major medical or neurologic illnesses (Hayes et al., 1998). However, some estimates of the prevalence of mania in elderly psychiatric patients are as high as 19%, with prevalence in nursing home patients estimated at about 10% (McDonald, 2000).

Gender and Ethnic and Cultural Differences

Although no significant gender differences have been found in the incidence of bipolar I and II diagnoses, gender differences have been reported in phenomenology, course, and treatment response (Liebenluft, 1996). Also, some data show that female bipolar patients are at greater risk for depression and rapid cycling than male patients, whereas male patients are at greater risk for manic episodes (Goodwin & Jamison, 1990). No significant differences have been found based on race or ethnicity (APA, 2000).

Comorbidity

The two most common comorbid conditions are anxiety disorders (most prevalent: panic disorder and social phobia) and substance use (most common: alcohol and marijuana). Individuals with a comorbid anxiety disorder are more likely to experience a more severe course. A history of substance abuse further complicates the course of illness and results in lower rates of remission and poor treatment compliance (Goldberg et al., 1999).

Etiology

Neurobiologic Theories

Neurotransmitter Hypotheses. Early biochemical theories of mood dysregulation focused on the neurotransmitters serotonin and norepinephrine. It was hypothesized that decreased levels of these two neurotransmitters in the brain caused depression and that excess amounts caused mania. Efforts to prove this theory have yielded inconsistent results. Current theories of the etiology of mood disorders are associated with chronic abnormalities of neurotransmission, which are thought to result in compensatory but maladaptive changes in brain regulation. Additionally, use of controlled structural and functional imaging studies of patients with mood disorders have generated hypotheses that dysfunction of the CNS is associated with specific structural brain abnormalities and functional CNS alterations (Nathan et al. 1995).

Chronobiologic Theories. Sleep disturbance is an important aspect of depression and mania. Sleep patterns appear to be regulated by an internal biologic clock center in the hypothalamus. Artificially induced sleep deprivation is known to alleviate depression or precipitate mania in some bipolar patients (Goodwin & Jamison, 1990). Because a number of neurotransmitter and hormone levels follow circadian patterns, sleep disruption may lead to biochemical abnormalities that affect mood. Seasonal changes in light exposure also trigger affective episodes in some patients, typically depression in winter and hypomania in the summer in the Northern Hemisphere (Cutler & Marcus, 1999).

Sensitization and Kindling Theory. Sensitization and the related phenomenon of kindling refer to animal models. Repeated chemical or electrical stimulation of certain regions of the brain produces stereotypical behavioral responses or seizures. The amount of the chemical or electricity required to evoke the response or seizure decreases with each experience. These phenomena have been used as models to explain why, over time, affective episodes, particularly those seen in patients with bipolar disorder, recur in shorter and shorter cycles and with less relation to environmental precipitants. It is hypothesized that repeated affective episodes might be accompanied by progressive alteration of brain synapses that lower the threshold for future episodes and increase the likelihood of illness.

Genetic Factors. First-degree biologic relatives of individuals with bipolar I disorder have elevated rates of bipolar I disorder (4% to 24%), bipolar II disorder (1% to 5%), and major depressive disorder (4% to 24%) (APA, 2000b). Results from family, adoption, and twin studies indicate that bipolar disorder is genetically transmitted (Goodwin & Jamison, 1990). Nevertheless, the mode of transmission and its genetic relationship to other affective disorders have not been identified (Tohen & Goodwin, 1995).

Psychological and Social Theories

Most psychological and social theories of mood disorders focus on loss as the cause of depression in genetically vulnerable individuals. Mania is considered to be a biologically rooted condition, but when viewed from a psychological perspective, mania is usually regarded as a condition that arises from an attempt to overcompensate for depressed feelings rather than a disorder in its own right. It is now generally accepted that environmental conditions contribute more to the timing of an episode of illness rather than cause the illness (Goodwin & Jamison, 1990).

Interdisciplinary Treatment of Disorders

Patients with bipolar disorder have a very complex set of issues and will likely be treated by an interdisciplinary treatment team. Nurses, physicians, social workers, psychologists, and activity therapists all have expertise that will be valuable to the person who has this disorder. If a child is diagnosed with bipolar disorder, school teachers and counselors will be included in the interdisciplinary team. In elderly patients, primary care physicians who have been treating existing chronic medical illnesses will also be a part of the team. An important goal of treatment is to minimize and prevent the occurrence of either a manic or depressive episode, which frequency tend to accelerate over time. The fewer the episodes, the more likely the person can live a normal, productive life. Another important goal is to help the patient and family to learn about the disorder and manage it throughout a lifetime.

Priority Care Issues

During a manic episode, protection of the patient is a priority. It is during a manic episode that poor judgment and impulsivity result in risk-taking behaviors that can have dire consequences for the patient and family. For example, one patient withdrew all the family money from the bank and gambled it away. Risk for suicide is always a possibility. During a depressive episode, the patient may feel that life is not worth living. During a manic episode, the patient may believe that he or she has supernatural powers, such as being able to fly. As patients recover from a manic episode, they may be so devastated by the consequences of impulsive behavior and poor judgment during the episode that suicide seems like a reasonable option.

Family Response to Disorder

Bipolar disorder can be devastating to families, whose members often feel that they are on an emotional merry-go-round. Unless familiar with the disorder, family members may have difficulty understanding the mood shifts. One of the major problems for family members is dealing with the consequences of the impulsive behavior during manic episodes, such as excessive debt, assault charges, and sexual infidelities.

NURSING MANAGEMENT: HUMAN RESPONSE TO DISORDER

The nursing management of patients with bipolar disorder is one of the most interesting yet greatest challenges in psychiatric nursing. These individuals generally have normal behavior between the mood episodes. The ideal nursing care occurs over a period of time when the nurse can see the patient in the acute illness phase and in remission. Nursing care of bipolar depression should be approached similarly as that of major depressive disorder described previously.

See Nursing Care Plan 20-1 and the Interdisciplinary Treatment Plan that follows.

Biologic Domain

Assessment

When focusing on the assessment of the biologic domain, the emphasis is on evaluation of symptoms of mania and, most particularly, changes in sleep patterns. The assessment should follow the guidelines in Chapter 10. In the manic phase of bipolar disorder, sleep may be practically nonexistent, resulting in irritability and physical exhaustion. Eating habits usually change during a manic or depressive episode; thus, the nurse should assess any changes in diet and body weight. Patients with mania can suffer from malnutrition and fluid imbalance. Laboratory studies should be completed, especially thyroid functioning. Abnormal thyroid functioning can be responsible for the mood and behavioral disturbances. During a manic phase, patients often become hypersexual and engage in risky sexual practices. Changes in sexual practices should be explored.

Pharmacologic Assessment. If a patient is in a manic state, the previous use of antidepressants should be assessed. It is not unusual for a manic episode to be triggered by antidepressant use. These antidepressants should be discontinued. Often, manic or depressive episodes occur after patients stop taking their mood stabilizer. The reason for stopping the medication should

be explored. Patients may stop their medications because of side effects or may stop because they no longer believe that they have a mental disorder. Special attention should also focus on the use of alcohol and other substances. Usually, a drug screen is done to determine current use of substances.

Nursing Diagnoses for Biologic Domain

The typical nursing diagnoses that will be generated include Disturbed Sleep Pattern, Sleep Deprivation, Imbalanced Nutrition, Hypothermia, and Deficit Fluid Volume. For patients who have stopped taking their medications, Noncompliance is a reasonable diagnosis. If patients are in the depressive phase of their illness, the previously discussed diagnoses for depression should be considered.

Interventions for Biologic Domain

Physical Care Nursing Interventions. In a state of mania, the physical needs of the patients are rest, adequate nutrition, and reestablishment of physical well-being. Self-care has usually deteriorated. For a patient who is unable to sit long enough to eat, snacks and high-energy foods should be provided that can be eaten while moving. Alcohol should be avoided. Sleep hygiene is a priority but may not be realistic until after medications take effect.

Once mood is stabilized, the nurse should focus on monitoring changes in physical functioning in sleep or eating behavior. Patients need to be taught to identify antecedents to mood episodes. A regular sleep routine should be maintained if at all possible. High-risk times for precipitating a manic episode, such as changes in work schedule (day to night), should be avoided if possible.

Pharmacologic Interventions. Pharmacotherapy is essential in bipolar disorder to achieve two goals: rapid control of symptoms in acute episodes of mania and depression, and prevention of future episodes or, at least, reduction in their severity and frequency.

Acute phase. The goal of the acute phase of treatment is symptom reduction and stabilization. Therefore, for the first few weeks of treatment, mood stabilizers may need to be combined with antipsychotics or benzodiazepines, particularly if the patient has psychotic symptoms, agitation, or insomnia. If the clinical situation is not an emergency, it is desirable to start patients on a low dose and gradually increase the dose until maximum therapeutic benefits are achieved. Once stabilization is achieved, the frequency of serum level

(*text continues on page 440*)

NURSING CARE PLAN 20.1
A Patient with Bipolar Disorder

JR, a 43-year-old, single female, lives in a metropolitan city and worked for a large travel agency booking corporate business trips. She has a history of alcohol abuse that began when she was in high school. Initially, she relied on alcohol for stress reduction, but gradually began abusing it. Her mother, grandfather, and sister all committed suicide within the past several years. JR's father has remarried and moved out of the area. JR does have one brother living in the same city, whom she occasionally sees.

Three years ago, JR left her husband after 15 years of an unhappy marriage and moved into a small condominium in a less affluent neighborhood. She began having symptoms of bipolar mixed disorder at that time, when she sold all her clothes, dyed her hair blonde, and began cruising the bars. She would consume excessive amounts of alcohol and often end up spending the night with a stranger. At first her behavior was attributed to her recent divorce. When she began missing work and charging excessively on her credit cards, her friends and two

children became concerned and convinced her to seek help for her behavior.

JR was diagnosed with a manic episode, and treatment with lithium carbonate was initiated. Her mood stabilized for a short period of time, but she had two more manic episodes within the next 18 months. Shortly after her last manic episode, she became severely depressed and attempted suicide. TCAs and MAOIs were tried, but she discontinued taking them after a significant weight gain. While she was being evaluated for ECT, she began to feel better. Once her depression lifted, her mood was stable for several months.

About 2 months ago, JR began missing work again because of depression. She refused to take any antidepressants and just wanted to "wait it out." She often boasted that her one success in life was helping people travel and have a good time. Last week she was told that her position was being eliminated because of a company issue. Now she believes that she is a failure as a wife, as an employee, and as a woman. She became despondent and finally took an overdose to "end it all."

SETTING: INTENSIVE CARE PSYCHIATRIC UNIT IN A GENERAL HOSPITAL

Baseline Assessment: Ms. R is a 43-year-old single woman transferred from ICU after a 3-day hospitalization following a suicide attempt with an overdose of multiple prescriptions and alcohol. She had her first manic episode 3 years before, and subsequently has had symptoms of a mixed bipolar mood disorder most of the time. Medication with lithium carbonate has not protected her from mood swings, and prior trials of TCAs and MAOIs have been unsuccessful. She is currently depressed, with pressured speech, agitation, irritability, sensory overload, inability to sleep, and anorexia.

Associated Psychiatric Diagnosis	*Medications*
Axis I: Bipolar I disorder, most recent episode mixed, severe, without psychotic features	Lithium carbonate 300 mg tid × 2 years
Axis II: Deferred (none apparent in her history and she is currently too ill for personality disorder to be assessed)	L-thyroxine 0.1 mg q AM × 1 d
	Clonazepam 0.5 mg bid for sleep and agitation
	Carbamazepine added on transfer to be titrated up to 400 mg tid
Axis III: Hypothyroidism	
Axis IV: Social problems (very poor marriage of 15 years, death by suicide of mother, grandfather, one sister)	
Axis V: GAF = Current 50	
Potential 85	

NURSING DIAGNOSIS 1: RISK SUICIDE

Defining Characteristics	*Related Factors*
Attempts to inflict life threatening injury to self	Feelings of helplessness and hopelessness secondary to bipolar disorder
Expresses desire to die	Depression
Poor impulse control	Loss secondary to finances/job, divorce
Lack of support system	

(continued)

NURSING CARE PLAN 20.1 (Continued)

OUTCOMES

Initial	Discharge
1. Develop a no self-harm contract. 2. Remain free from self-harm. 3. Identify factors that led to suicidal intent and methods for managing suicidal impulses if they return. 4. Accept treatment of depression by trying the SSRI antidepressants.	5. Discuss the complexity of bipolar disorder. 6. Identify the antecedents to depression.

INTERVENTIONS

Interventions	Rationale	Ongoing Assessment
Initiate a nurse–patient relationship by demonstrating an acceptance of Ms. Rothman as a worthwhile human being through the use of nonjudgmental statements and behavior.	A sense of worthlessness often underlies suicide ideation. The positive therapeutic relationship can maintain the patient's dignity.	Assess the stages of the relationship and determine whether a therapeutic relationship is actually being formed. Identify indicators of trust.
Initiate suicide precautions per hospital policy.	Safety of the individual is a priority with people who have suicide ideation. (See Chap. 34.)	Determine intent to harm self—plan and means.
Obtain a no self-harm contract.	A contract can help the patient resist suicide by providing a way of resisting impulses.	Determine patient's ability to commit to a contract.

EVALUATION

Outcomes	Revised Outcomes	Interventions
Has not harmed self, denies suicidal thought/intent after realizing that she is still alive.	Absence of suicidal intent will continue.	Discontinue suicide precautions; maintain ongoing assessment for suicidality.
Made a no self-harm contract with nurse, agrees to keep it after discharge.	Maintain a no self-harm contract with outpatient mental health provider.	Support and reinforce this contract.
JR agreed to try to treat her depression by initiating treatment with Prozac.		

NURSING DIAGNOSIS 2: CHRONIC LOW SELF-ESTEEM

Defining Characteristics	Related Factors
Long-standing self-negating verbalizations Expressions of shame and guilt Evaluates self as unable to deal with events Frequent lack of success in work and relationships Poor body presentation (eye contact, posture, movements) Nonassertive/passive	Failure to stabilize mood Unmet dependency needs Feelings of abandonment secondary to separation from significant other Feelings of failure secondary to loss of job, relationship problems Unrealistic expectations of self

OUTCOMES

Initial	Discharge
1. Identify positive aspects of self. 2. Modify excessive and unrealistic expectations of self.	3. Verbalize acceptance of limitations. 4. Report freedom from symptoms of depression. 5. Begin to take verbal and behavioral risks.

(continued)

NURSING CARE PLAN 20.1 (Continued)

INTERVENTIONS

Interventions	Rationale	Ongoing Assessment
Enhance JR's sense of self by being attentive, validating your interpretation of what is being said or experienced, and helping her verbalize what she is expressing nonverbally.	By showing respect for the patient as a human being who is worth listening to, the nurse can support the patient's sense of self.	Determine whether patient confirms interpretation of situation and if she can verbalize what she is expressing nonverbally.
Assist to reframe and redefine negative statements ("not a failure, but a setback").	Reframing an event positively rather than negatively can help the patient view the situation in an alternative way.	Assess whether the patient can actually view the world in a different way.
Problem solve with patient about how to approach finding another job.	Work is very important to adults. Losing a job can decrease self-esteem. Focusing on the possibility of a future job will provide hope for the patient.	Assess the patient's ability to problem solve. Determine whether she is realistic in her expectations.
Encourage positive physical habits (healthy food and eating patterns, exercise, proper sleep).	A healthy lifestyle promotes well-being, increasing self-esteem.	Determine JR's willingness to consider making lifestyle changes.
Teach patient to validate consensually with others.	Low self-esteem is generated by negative interpretations of the world. Through consensual validation, the patient can determine whether others view situations in the same way.	Assess JR's ability to participate in this process.
Teach esteem-building exercises (self-affirmations, imagery, use of humor, meditation/prayer, relaxation).	There are many different approaches that can be practiced to increase self-esteem.	Assess JR's energy level and ability to focus on learning new skills.
Assist in establishing appropriate personal boundaries.	In an attempt to meet their own needs, people with low self-esteem often violate other people's boundaries and allow others to take advantage of them. Helping patients establish their own boundaries will improve the likelihood of needs being met in an appropriate manner.	Assess patient's ability to understand the concept of boundary violation and its significance.
Provide an opportunity within the therapeutic relationship to express thoughts and feelings. Use open-ended statements and questions. Encourage expression of both positive and negative statements. Use movement, art, and music as means of expression.	The individual with low self-esteem may have difficulty expressing thoughts and feelings. Providing them with several different outlets for expression helps to develop skills for expressing thoughts and feelings.	Monitor thoughts and feelings that are expressed in order to help the patient examine them.
Explore opportunities for positive socialization.	Individuals with low self-esteem may be in social situations that reinforce negative valuation of self. Helping patient identify new positive situations will give other options.	Assess whether the new situations are potentially positive or are a re-creation of other negative situations.

(continued)

NURSING CARE PLAN 20.1 (Continued)

EVALUATION

Outcomes	Revised Outcomes	Interventions
JR began to identify positive aspects of self as she began to modify excessive and unrealistic expectations of self.	Strengthen ability to affirm positive aspects and examine expectations related to work and relationships.	Refer to mental health clinic for cognitive behavioral psychotherapy with a feminist perspective.
She verbalized that she would probably never work for the company again and that it would never be the same. She verbalized that she would need more assertiveness skills in her relationships.	Identify important aspects of job so that she can begin looking for a job that had those characteristics.	Attend a women's group that focuses on assertiveness skills.
As JR's mood improved, she was able to sleep through the night, and she began eating again—began feeling better about herself.	Maintain a stable mood to promote positive self-concept.	Monitor mood and identify antecedents to depression.

NURSING DIAGNOSIS 3: INEFFECTIVE INDIVIDUAL COPING

Defining Characteristics	Related Factors
Verbalization in inability to cope or ask for help Reported difficulty with life stressors Inability to problem solve Alteration in social participation Destructive behavior toward self Frequent illnesses Substance abuse	Altered mood (depression) caused by changes secondary to body chemistry (bipolar disorder) Altered mood caused by changes secondary to intake of mood-altering substance (alcohol) Unsatisfactory support system Sensory overload secondary to excessive activity Inadequate psychological resources to adapt to changes in job status

OUTCOMES

Initial	Discharge
1. Accept support through the nurse–patient relationship. 2. Identify areas of ineffective coping. 3. Examine the current efforts at coping. 4. Identify areas of strength. 5. Learn new coping skills.	6. Practice new coping skills. 7. Focus on strengths.

INTERVENTIONS

Interventions	Rationale	Ongoing Assessment
Identify current stresses in JR's life, including her suicide attempt and the bipolar disorder.	When areas of concern are verbalized by the patient, she will be able to focus on one issue at a time. If she identifies the mental disorder as a stressor, she will more likely be able to develop strategies to deal with it.	Determine whether JR is able to identify problem areas realistically. Continue to assess for suicidality.
Identify JR's strengths in dealing with past stressors.	By focusing on past successes, she can identify strengths and build on them in the future.	Assess if JR can identify any previous successes in her life.
Assess current level of depression using Beck's Depression Inventory or a similar one and intervene according to assessed level.	Severely depressed or suicidal individuals need assistance with decision making, grooming and hygiene, and nutrition.	Continue to assess for mood and suicidality.

(continued)

NURSING CARE PLAN 20.1 (Continued)

INTERVENTIONS

Interventions	Rationale	Ongoing Assessment
Involve JR in treatment and socialization activities. Stress importance of activity in helping recovery from depression and that she will have to make a conscious effort to fight it.	By keeping individuals who are depressed active, social withdrawal is prevented. Social activity helps the patient deal with the depression.	Assess for environmental withdrawal (time spent in room versus time spent with others).
Assist JR in discussing, selecting, and practicing positive coping skills (jogging, yoga, thought stopping).	New coping skills take a conscious effort to learn and will at first seem strange and unnatural. Practicing these skills will help the patient incorporate them into her coping strategy repertoire.	Assess whether JR follows through on learning new skills.
Educate regarding the use of alcohol and its relationship to depression.	Alcohol is an ineffective coping strategy because it actually exacerbates the depression.	Assess for the patient's willingness to address her drinking problem.
Assist patient in coping with bipolar disorder, beginning with education about it.	A mood disorder is a major stressor in a patient's life. To manage the stress, the patient needs a knowledge base.	Determine JR's knowledge about bipolar disorder.
Administer lithium as ordered (give with food or milk). Reinforce the action, dosage, and side effects. Review laboratory results to determine whether lithium is within therapeutic limits. Assess for toxicity. Recommend a normal diet with normal salt intake; maintenance of adequate fluid intake.	Lithium carbonate is effective in the treatment of bipolar disorder but must be managed. Patient should have a thorough knowledge of the medication and side effects.	Assess for target action, side effects, and toxicity.
Administer carbamazepine as ordered, to be titrated up to 400 mg tid. Observe for presence of hypersensitivity to the drug. Teach about action, dosage, and side effects. Emphasize the possibility of drug interaction with alcohol, some antibiotics, TCAs, and MAOIs.	Carbamazepine can be effective in bipolar disorder. However, it can increase CNS toxicity when given with lithium carbonate.	Assess for target action, side effects, and toxicity.
Administer thyroid supplement as ordered. Review laboratory results of thyroid functioning. Discuss the symptoms of hypothyroidism and how they are similar to depression. Emphasize the importance of taking lithium and L-thyroxine. Explain about the long-term effects of lithium on thyroid functioning.	Hypothyroidism can be a side effect of lithium carbonate and also mimics symptoms of depression.	Determine whether patient understands the relationship between thyroid dysfunction and lithium carbonate.
Clonazepam 0.5 mg bid for sleep and agitation.		

(continued)

NURSING CARE PLAN 20.1 (Continued)

EVALUATION

Outcomes	Revised Outcomes	Interventions
JR easily engaged in a therapeutic relationship. She examined the areas in her life where she coped ineffectively.	Establish a therapeutic relationship with a therapist at the mental health clinic.	Refer to mental health clinic.
She identified her strengths and how she coped with stressors and especially her illness in the past. She is willing to try antidepressants again, in hopes of not having the weight gain.	Continue to view illness as a potential stressor that can disrupt life.	Seek advice immediately if there are any problems with medications.
She learned new problem-solving skills and reported that she learned a lot about her medication. She is committed to complying with her medication regimen. She identified new coping skills that she could realistically do. She will focus on strengths.	Continue to practice new coping skills as stressful situations arise.	Discuss with therapist the outcomes of using new coping skills. Attend Alcoholics Anonymous if alcohol is used as a stress reliever.

INTERDISCIPLINARY TREATMENT PLAN 20.1
Patient With Bipolar Disorder

COMMUNITY MENTAL HEALTH CENTER TREATMENT PROGRAM FOR JR, A 43-YEAR-OLD FEMALE

Admission Date:	Date of This Plan:	Type of Plan: Check Appropriate Box					
		☐ Initial	☐ Master	☐ 30	☐ 60	☐ 90	☐ Other

Treatment Team Present:
M. Jones, MD; S. Smith, RNC; T. Thompson, PhD (psychologist); G. Bond, LCSW (social worker); V. Stevens, BA (rehabilitation counselor)

DIAGNOSIS (*DSM-IV-TR*):

AXIS I: Bipolar I
AXIS II: Deferred
AXIS III: Hypo
AXIS IV: Social Problems
AXIS V:
Current GAF: 50
Highest Level GAF This Past Year: 85

ASSETS (MEDICAL, PSYCHOLOGICAL, SOCIAL, EDUCATIONAL, VOCATIONAL, RECREATIONAL):

1. Controls illness through medication and monthly visits for brief counseling and stress management.
2. Lives independently in apartment.
3. Works at a library and has good relationships with boss and coworkers.
4. Easily makes friends.

INTERDISCIPLINARY TREATMENT PLAN 20.1 (Continued)
Patient With Bipolar Disorder

MASTER PROBLEM LIST

Prob. No.	Date	Problem	Code	Change Code	Change Date
1	1/12/98	Ineffective coping: Does not want to go to work because of intense grief for mother's death.		R	2/12/98
2	1/12/98	Mood disturbance. Patient is very depressed, not eating or sleeping.		R	4/14/98
3	6/12/98	Mood changes with the seasons. Needs monitoring of mood.		T	
4	6/12/98	Interpersonal issues interfering with ability to work at library.		T	

CODE T = Problem must be addressed in treatment.
        N = Problem noted and will be monitored.
        X = Problem noted, but deferred/inactive/no action necessary.
        O = Problem to be addressed in aftercare/continuing care.
        I = Problem incorporated into another problem.
        R = Resolved.

INDIVIDUAL TREATMENT PLAN PROBLEM SHEET

#1 Problem/Need:	Date Identified	Problem Resolved/Discontinuation Date
	3/12/98	Ongoing

Cyclic mood changes, usually according to the season.
Medication needs to be re-evaluated and adjusted
according to mood changes. Stress is often the precipitant
to mood changes. Needs updating on information about
bipolar disorder.

Objective(s)/Short-Term Goals:	Target Date	Achievement Date
1. Monitor mood changes.	Every 3 months	
2. Adjust medications as needed.		

Treatment Interventions:	Frequency	Person Responsible
1. Evaluate mood changes.	Every 3 months or as needed.	RN
2. Adjust medications.	Every 3 months or as needed.	MD
3. Medication education.	Weekly class.	RN
4. Stress management techniques.	Weekly class for 6 weeks.	Psychologist

Responsible QMHP   **Patient or Guardian**   **Staff Physician**

_____ _____   _____ _____   _____ _____
Signature   Date   Signature   Date   Signature   Date

monitoring should be every 1 to 2 weeks during the first 2 months and every 3 to 6 months during long-term maintenance. The medications most commonly used for mood stabilization in bipolar disorder are discussed here and in Chapter 8.

Continuation phase. The goal of this phase of treatment is to prevent relapse of the current episode or cycling into the opposite pole. It lasts about 2 to 9 months after acute symptoms have resolved. The usual pharmacologic procedure in this phase is to continue the mood stabilizer while closely monitoring the patient for signs or symptoms of relapse.

Maintenance phase. The goal of this phase of treatment is to sustain remission and to prevent new episodes. The great weight of evidence favors long-term prophylaxis against recurrence after effective treatment of acute episodes. It is recommended that long-term or lifetime prophylaxis with a mood stabilizer be instituted after two manic episodes or after one manic episode if it is severe or if there is a family history of bipolar disorder.

Discontinuation. Like major depressive disorder, the course of bipolar disorder is typically recurrent and progressive. Therefore, the same issues and principles regarding the decision to continue or discontinue pharmacotherapy apply.

Mood Stabilizers. The mainstays of somatic therapy are the mood-stabilizing drugs. The three agents that have shown significant evidence of efficacy in controlled trials are lithium carbonate (Lithium), divalproex sodium (Depakote), and carbamazepine (Tegretol) (Table 20-5). Both lithium and divalproex sodium have U.S. Food and Drug Administration indications for the treatment of acute mania, as does the atypical antipsychotic olanzopine (Zyprexa).

Lithium Carbonate. Lithium has been on the market in this country since 1970 and is the most widely used mood stabilizer (see Drug Profile: Lithium). Fifty-nine to 91% of patients with pure mania characterized by euthymic mood have been reported to have moderate or marked improvement during treatment with lithium (Prien et al., 1988). However, for most patients, lithium is not a fully adequate treatment for all phases of the illness, and, particularly during the acute phase, supplemental use of antipsychotics and benzodiazepines is often beneficial. During acute depressive episodes, supplemental use of antidepressants is most often indicated. Because of its significant side-effect burden (Table 20-6), lithium is poorly tolerated in at least one third of treated patients and has the narrowest gap between therapeutic and toxic concentrations of any routinely prescribed psychotropic agent (Bowden et al., 1994). Predictors of poor response to lithium in acute mania include a prior history of poor response, rapid cycling, dysphoric symptoms, mixed symptoms of depression and mania, psychiatric comorbidity, and medical comorbidity (Bowden, 1995b).

Lithium is a salt, and the interaction between lithium levels and sodium levels in the body and the relationship between lithium levels and fluid volume in the body remain crucial issues in its safe, effective use. The higher the sodium levels are in the body, the lower the lithium level will be, and vice versa. Thus, changes in dietary sodium intake can affect lithium blood levels that, in turn, may affect therapeutic results or increase the incidence of side effects. The same applies to fluid volume. If body fluid decreases significantly because of a hot climate, strenuous exercise, vomiting, diarrhea, or drastic reduction in fluid intake, then lithium levels can rise sharply, causing an increase in side effects, progressing to lethal lithium toxicity (see Table 20-6). See Table 20-7 for lithium interactions with other drugs. See Chapter 8 for further discussion of lithium's possible mechanisms of action, pharmacokinetics, side effects, and toxicity.

Divalproex sodium. Divalproex sodium, an anticonvulsant, has a broader spectrum of efficacy and has about equal benefit for patients with pure mania as for those with other forms of bipolar disorder (ie, mixed mania, rapid cycling, comorbid substance abuse, and secondary mania). Moreover, in contrast to lithium, the antimanic

TABLE 20.5 Mood Stabilizing Medications		
Generic (Trade) Drug Name	Usual Dosage Range (daily)	Half-life (h)
Lithium (Eskalith, Lithane)	600–1,800 mg	17–36
Divalproex sodium (Depakote)	15–60 mg/kg	6–16
Carbamazepine (Tegretol)	200–1,200 mg	25–65
Olanzapine (Zyprexa)	5–20 mg	21–54

DRUG PROFILE: Lithium
(Mood Stabilizer)
Trade Name: Eskalith, Lithane, Lithotabs, Lithonate, Lithium Carbonate, and various other generic preparations. Lithobid and Eskalith CR in slow-release preparations.

Receptor affinity: Alters sodium transport in nerve and muscle cells, increases norepinephrine uptake and serotonin receptor sensitivity, slightly increases intraneuronal stores of catecholamines, delays some second messenger systems. Mechanism of action is unknown.

Indications: Treatment and prevention of manic episodes in bipolar affective disorder. Used successfully in a number of unlabeled uses such as prophylaxis of cluster headaches, premenstrual tension, bulimia, etc.

Routes and dosage: 150-, 300-, and 600-mg capsules. Lithobid, 300-mg slow-release tablets; Eskalith CR, 450-mg controlled-release tablets. Lithium citrate, 300-mg/5 mL liquid form.

Adult: In acute mania, optimal response is usually 600 mg tid or 900 mg bid. Obtain serum levels twice weekly in acute phase. Maintenance: Use lowest possible dose to alleviate symptoms and maintain serum level of 0.6–1.2 mEq/L. In uncomplicated maintenance obtain serum levels every 2–3 months. Do not rely on serum levels alone.

Geriatric: Increased risk for toxic effects, use lower doses, monitor frequently.

Children: Safety and efficacy in children under 12 y has not been established.

Half-life (peak effect): mean, 24 h (peak serum levels in 1–4 h). Steady state reached in 5–7 d.

Select adverse reactions: Weight gain

Warning: Avoid use during pregnancy or while nursing. Hepatic or renal impairments increase plasma concentration.

Specific patient/family education:

- Avoid alcohol or other CNS depressant drugs.

- Notify prescriber if pregnancy is possible or planning to become pregnant. Do not breastfeed while taking this medication.

- Notify prescriber before taking any other prescription or OTC medication.

- May impair judgment, thinking, or motor skills; avoid driving or other hazardous tasks.

- Do not abruptly discontinue.

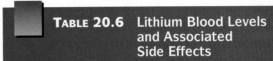

TABLE 20.6 Lithium Blood Levels and Associated Side Effects

Plasma Level	Side Effects or Symptoms of Toxicity
<1.5 mEq/L	Metallic taste in mouth Fine hand tremor (resting) Nausea Polyuria Polydipsia Diarrhea or loose stools Muscular weakness or fatigue Weight gain Edema Memory impairments
1.5–2.5 mEq/L	Severe diarrhea Dry mouth Nausea and vomiting Mild to moderate ataxia Incoordination Dizziness, sluggishness, giddiness, vertigo Slurred speech Tinnitus Blurred vision Increasing tremor Muscle irritability or twitching Asymmetric deep tendon reflexes Increased muscle tone
>2.5 mEq/L	Cardiac arrhythmias Blackouts Nystagmus Coarse tremor Fasciculations Visual or tactile hallucinations Oliguria, renal failure Peripheral vascular collapse Confusion Seizures Coma and death

effect of divalproex sodium may not be diminished by a history of repeated prior episodes (Bowden, 1995b). Whereas divalproex is usually initiated at 250 mg twice a day or lower, in the inpatient setting, it can be initiated in an oral loading dose using 20 to 30 mg/kg body weight. This may speed the reduction of manic symptoms and diminish the need for antipsychotics early in the course of therapy (McElroy et al., 1996) (see Drug Profile: Divalproex Sodium). Baseline liver function tests and a complete blood count with platelets should be obtained before starting therapy,

and patients with known liver disease should not be administered divalproex sodium. Optimal blood levels for mania are debated but appear to be in the range of 50 to 150 ng/mL. Levels may be obtained weekly until the patient is stable, and then every 6 months. Divalproex sodium is associated with increased risk for birth defects.

Carbamazepine. Carbamazepine, also an anticonvulsant, was found to have mood-stabilizing effects as early as the 1970s. Although few studies of carbamazepine for the treatment of bipolar disorder have been well designed, the data suggest that it may be effective in patients who fail to respond to lithium. Also, patients with secondary mania appear to be more responsive to carbamazepine than to lithium (Bowden, 1995).

TABLE 20.7 Lithium Interactions With Medications and Other Substances

Substance	Effect of Interaction
Angiotensin-converting enzyme inhibitors, such as: • captopril • lisinopril • quinapril	Increases serum lithium; may cause toxicity and impaired kidney function
Acetazolamide	Increases renal excretion of lithium, decreases lithium levels
Alcohol	May increase serum lithium level
Caffeine	Increases lithium excretion, increases lithium tremor
Carbamazepine	Increases neurotoxicity, despite normal serum levels and dosage
Fluoxetine	Increases serum lithium levels
Haloperidol	Increases neurotoxicity, despite normal serum levels and dosage
Loop diuretics, such as furosemide	Increases lithium serum levels, but may be safer than thiazide diuretics; potassium-sparing diuretics (amiloride, spirolactone) are safest
Methyldopa	Increases neurotoxicity without increasing serum lithium levels
Nonsteroidal antiinflammatory drugs, such as: • diclofenac • ibuprofen • indomethacin • piroxicam	Decreases renal clearance of lithium Increases serum lithium levels by 30%–60% in 3–10 d Aspirin and sulindac do not appear to have the same effect
Osmotic diuretics, such as: • urea • mannitol • isosorbide	Increases renal excretion of lithium and decreases lithium levels
Sodium chloride	High sodium intake decreases lithium levels; low sodium diets may increase lithium levels and lead to toxicity
Thiazide diuretics, such as: • chlorothiazide • hydrochlorothiazide	Promotes sodium and potassium excretion; increases lithium serum levels; may produce cardiotoxicity and neurotoxicity
Tricyclic antidepressants	Increases tremor; potentiates pharmacologic effects of tricyclic antidepressants

DRUG PROFILE: Divalproex Sodium
(Antimania Agent)
Trade Name: Depakote

Receptor affinity: Thought to increase level of inhibitory neurotransmitter, GABA to brain neurons. Mechanism of action is unknown.
Indications: Treatment of bipolar disorders.
Routes and dosage: Available in 125-mg delayed-release capsules, and 125-, 250-, and 500-mg enteric-coated tablets.
Adult dosage: Dosage depends on symptoms and clinical picture presented; initially, the dosage is low and gradually increased depending on the clinical presentation.
Half-life (peak effect): 6–16 h (1–4 h)
Select adverse reactions: Sedation, tremor (may be dose related), nausea, vomiting, indigestion, abdominal cramps, anorexia with weight loss, slight elevations in liver enzymes, hepatic failure, thrombocytopenia, transient increases in hair loss.
Warning: Use cautiously during pregnancy and lactation. Contraindicated in patients with hepatic disease or significant

hepatic dysfunction. Administer cautiously with salicylates; may increase serum levels and result in toxicity.
Specific patient/family education:
• Take with food if gastrointestinal upset occurs.
• Swallow tablets or capsules whole to prevent local irritation of mouth and throat.
• Notify prescriber before taking any other prescription or OTC medications.
• Avoid alcohol, sleep-inducing, or OTC products.
• Avoid driving or performing activities that require alertness.
• Do not abruptly discontinue.
• Keep appointments for follow-up, including blood tests to monitor response.

The most common side effects of carbamazepine are dizziness, drowsiness, nausea, and vomiting, which may be avoided with slow incremental dosing. Carbamazepine has both benign and severe hematologic toxicities. Frequent clinically unimportant decreases in white blood cell counts occur. Estimates of the rate of severe blood dyscrasias suggest an incidence of about 1 in 20,000 patients treated (Arana & Rosenbaum, 2000). Mild, nonprogressive elevations of liver function tests (LFTs) are relatively common. Carbamazepine is associated with increased risk for birth defects.

In patients older than 12 years of age, carbamazepine is begun at 200 mg once or twice a day. The dosage is increased by no more than 200 mg every 2 to 4 days, up to 800 to 1,000 mg a day, or until therapeutic levels or effects are achieved. It is important to monitor for blood dyscrasias and liver damage. Liver function tests and complete blood counts with differential are minimal pretreatment laboratory tests and should be repeated about 1 month after initiating treatment, and at 3 months, 6 months, and yearly. Other yearly tests should include electrolytes, blood urea nitrogen, thyroid function tests, urinalysis, and eye examinations. Carbamazepine levels are measured monthly until the patient is on a stable dose. Studies have suggested that blood levels in the range of 8 to 12 ng/mL correspond to therapeutic efficacy. See Table 20-8 for carbamazepine interactions with other drugs. See Chapter 8 for further discussion of carbamazepine's possible mechanisms of action, pharmacokinetics, side effects, and toxicity.

Both valproate and carbamazepine may be lethal if high doses are ingested. Toxic symptoms appear in 1 to 3 hours and include neuromuscular disturbances, dizziness, stupor, agitation, disorientation, nystagmus, urinary retention, nausea and vomiting, tachycardia, hypotension or hypertension, cardiovascular shock, coma, and respiratory depression.

Newer Anticonvulsants. Newer anticonvulsants have also shown promise as mood stabilizers in small clinical trials, case reports, and anecdotal evidence. Lamotrigine (Lamictal) has been shown to have efficacy in the treatment of mania, both as a single agent and in combination with lithium or valproate. Observations suggest that it may be particularly effective for rapid cycling and in the depressed phase of bipolar illness. Anecdotal evidence suggests that gabapentin (Neurontin) may be efficacious for acute mania and mood stabilization, including rapid cycling. Topiramate (Topamax) has been used mostly as add-on therapy in mixed patient samples with refractory mood disorders. A unique characteristic of topiramate is that it is more associated with weight loss than weight gain. Controlled trials are needed to evaluate further

TABLE 20.8	Selected Medication Interactions With Carbamazepine
Interaction	**Drug Interacting With Carbamazepine**
Increased carbamazemapine levels	Erythromycin
	Cimetidine
	Propoxyphene
	Isoniazid
	Calcium-channel blockers (Verapamil)
	Fluoxetine
	Danazol
	Diltiazem
	Nicotinamide
Decreased carbamazemapine levels	Phenobarbital
	Primidone
	Phenytoin
Drugs whose levels are decreased by carbamazepine	Oral contraceptives
	Warfarin, oral anticoagulants
	Doxycycline
	Theophylline
	Haloperidol
	Divalproex sodium
	Tricyclic antidepressants
	Acetaminophen—increased metabolism, but also increased risk for hepatotoxicity

the efficacy of these and other anticonvulsants in the treatment of bipolar disorder (Arana & Rosenbaum, 2000).

Antidepressants. Acute bipolar depression has received little scientific study in comparison with unipolar depression. Antidepressant drugs may cause either a switch to mania or a mixed state or may induce rapid cycling. Unfortunately, lithium or anticonvulsants are not as effective against depression as they are against mania. However, in a few patients, lithium or anticonvulsants can be used alone with good antidepressant effects. The most common treatment of bipolar depression is an antidepressant combined with a mood stabilizer to "protect" the patient against a manic switch. The antidepressant agents are the same as those used in unipolar illness, although they are sometimes given in lower dosages and for shorter periods of time as a precaution. Bupropion or an SSRI is the first-line choice. The TCAs may be more likely to cause mania than other antidepressants (Arana & Rosenbaum, 2000).

Antipsychotics. For patients who experience psychosis as a part of their bipolar disorder, antipsychotics are prescribed. If patients cannot tolerate mood stabilizers, antipsychotics may be given in place of antidepressants to stabilize the moods. Generally, the antipsychotic dosage is lower than what is prescribed for patients with schizophrenia.

Monitoring and Administration of Medication. During acute mania episodes, patients often do not believe that they have a psychiatric disorder and refuse to take medication. Because their energy is still high, they can be very creative in avoiding medication. Once patients begin to take medications, symptom improvement should be evident. If a patient is very agitated, a benzodiazepine may be given for a short period of time.

Side-Effect Monitoring and Management. It is unlikely that patients will be taking only one medication, and they may be taking several. In some instances, one agent will be used to augment the effects of another, such as supplemental thyroid hormone use to boost antidepressant response in depression. Possible side effects for each medication should be listed and cross-referenced. When a side effect appears, the nurse should document the side effect and notify the prescriber so that further evaluation can be made. In some instances, medication changes can be made. For example, one patient was having serious gastrointestinal symptoms (diarrhea, bloating) with lithium and was able to switch to valproic acid.

Drug–Drug Interactions. It is a well-established practice to combine mood stabilizers with antidepressants or antipsychotics. The previously discussed drug interactions should be considered when caring for a person with bipolar disorder. The biggest challenge is monitoring alcohol, drugs, over-the-counter medications, and herbal supplements. A complete list of all medications should be maintained and evaluated for any potential interaction.

Teaching Points. For patients who are taking lithium, it is important to explain that a change in salt intake can affect the therapeutic blood level. If there is a reduction in salt intake, the body will naturally retain lithium in order to maintain homeostasis. This increase in lithium retention can lead to toxicity. Once stabilized on a lithium dose, salt intake should remain constant. This is fairly easy to do, except during the summer, when excessive perspiration can occur. Patients should increase salt intake during periods of perspiration and dehydration.

Most of mood stabilizers and antidepressants can cause weight gain. Patients should be alerted to this potential side effect and should be instructed to monitor any changes in eating, appetite, or weight. Weight reduction techniques may need to be instituted.

Patients should be clearly instructed to check with the nurse or physician before taking any over-the-counter medication or herbal supplements.

Other Somatic Interventions: Electroconvulsive Therapy. ECT may be a valuable treatment alternative for severely manic patients who exhibit unremitting, frenzied physical activity. Other indications are acutely manic patients who are unresponsive to antimanic agents or who are at high risk for suicide. ECT is safe and effective in patients receiving antipsychotic drugs. Use of valproate or carbamazepine will elevate the seizure threshold, requiring some adjustments in treatment. If feasible, lithium should be stopped 48 hours before treatment to prevent the risk for neurotoxicity (Arana & Rosenbaum, 2000).

Psychological Domain

Assessment

The assessment of the psychological domain should follow the process explained in Chapter 10. Individuals with bipolar disorder can usually fully participate in this part of the assessment.

Mood. By definition, bipolar disorder is a disturbance of mood. If the patient is depressed, using one of the tools for depression may be useful in determining the severity of depression. If mania is the predominant symptom, evaluating the quality of the mood (elated, grandiose, irritated, or agitated) becomes important in understanding the patient. Usually, mania is determined by clinical observation.

Cognitive. In the depressive episode, the individual may not be able to concentrate in order to complete cognitive tools, such as the Mini Mental State Exam (MMSE). During the acute phase of a manic or depressive episode, the mental status may be abnormal. In a manic phase, the thinking may be so rapid, disjointed, and distorted that judgment is impaired. Feelings such as grandiosity can interfere with normal executive functioning.

Thought Disturbances. Psychosis commonly occurs in patients with bipolar disorder, especially during acute episodes of mania. Auditory hallucinations and delusional thinking are often apart of the clinical picture. In children and adolescents, the presence of psychosis will not easily be disclosed. In elderly people, the presence of psychosis will be easier to detect because they are more likely to verbalize their delusional or hallucinatory thinking.

Stress and Coping Factors. Stress and coping are critical assessment areas for a person with bipolar disorder. The antecedent to a manic or depressive episode is often a stressful event. In some instances, there are no particular stresses that preceded the episode, but it is important to discuss the possibility. Determining the patient's usual coping skills for stresses lays the groundwork for developing intervention strategies. Negative coping skills, such as the use of substances or aggression, should be identified because those are the one that need to be replaced with positive coping skills.

Risk Assessment. Patients with bipolar disorder are at high risk for injury to self and others, with 10% to 15% of patients completing suicide. Child abuse, spouse abuse, or other violent behaviors may occur during severe manic episodes; hence, patients should be assessed for suicidal or homicidal risk (APA, 2000b).

Nursing Diagnoses for Psychological Domain

The nursing diagnoses associated with the psychological domain of bipolar disorder include Disturbed Sensory Perception, Disturbed Thought Processes, Defensive Coping, Risk for Suicide, Risk for Violence, and Ineffective Coping.

Interventions for Psychological Domain

There is no question that pharmacotherapy is the treatment of choice for bipolar disorder. However, an integration of psychotherapeutic techniques with pharmacotherapy is strongly recommended (Hirschfield et al., 1994). The most common psychotherapeutic approaches include psychoeducation, individual cognitive-behavioral therapy, individual interpersonal therapy, and adjunctive therapies, such as those for substance abuse (Rothbaum & Astin, 2000).

A number of risk factors associated with bipolar disorders make patients more vulnerable to relapses and resistant to recovery. Among these are high rates of non-adherence to medications, marital conflict, separation, divorce, unemployment, and underemployment. The goals of psychosocial interventions are to address risk factors and associated features that are difficult to address with pharmacotherapy alone. Particularly important are improving medication adherence, decreasing the number and length of hospitalizations and relapses, enhancing social and occupational functioning, improving the patient's quality of life, increasing the patient's and family's acceptance of the disorder, and reducing the patient's suicide risk (Rothbaum & Astin, 2000).

Psychoeducation. Psychoeducation is designed to provide information on bipolar disorder and successful treatment and recovery and usually focuses on medication adherence. The nurse can provide education about the nature and course of the individual's illness and obstacles to recovery. Helping the patient to be able to identify warning signs and symptoms of relapse and to cope with residual symptoms and functional impairment are important interventions. Resistance to accepting the illness and to taking medication, the symbolic meaning of medication taking, and worries about the future can be discussed openly. In the interest of improved medication adherence, asking about and listening carefully to the patient's concerns about the medication, dosing schedules, and dose changes and addressing any side effects are helpful (see Psychoeducation Checklist: Bipolar I Disorder).

Psychotherapy. Psychotherapy is usually very helpful, particularly during high-risk stress periods. In a case study reported by Sauer and Ford (1995), the cost of care for a patient with bipolar disorder decreased from more than $40,000 (average hospital cost only) to less than $4,000 per year with the addition of psychotherapy provided by a psychiatric–mental health clinical nurse specialist. During the study period, the patient did not require a psychiatric hospitalization, demonstrated stabilization of mood with sustained absence of psychotic thinking or suicidal ideation, maintained abstinence from alcohol, and demonstrated improved family and social functioning.

Social Domain

Assessment

One of the real tragedies of bipolar disorder is its effect on social and occupational functioning. Cultural views of mental illness influence the patient's acceptance of the disorder. During illness episodes, patients often behave in ways that jeopardize their social relationships. Losing a job and going through a divorce are very common events. During the social domain assessment, social changes that have resulted from the a manic or depressive episode should be identified.

Nursing Diagnoses for Social Domain

Possible social domain nursing diagnoses include Ineffective Role Performance, Interrupted Family Processes, Impaired Social Interaction, Impaired Parenting, and Compromised Family Coping. In children and

---

PSYCHOEDUCATION CHECKLIST
Bipolar I Disorder

When caring for the patient with a bipolar I disorder, be sure to include the following topic areas in the teaching plan:

- Psychopharmacologic agents, including drug action, dosage, frequency, and possible adverse effects
- Adherence to medication regimens
- Measure strategies to decrease agitation and restlessness
- Safety measures
- Self-care management
- Follow-up laboratory testing
- Support services

adolescents, the diagnosis of Delayed Growth and Development should be considered. Caregiver Role Strain may be present in family members who are coping with a member with a bipolar disorder.

Interventions for Social Domain

Interventions focusing on the social domain are integral to nursing care for all ages. During mania, patients usually violate others' boundaries. While hospitalized, roommate selection for these patients needs to be carefully considered. They tend to irritate others, who quickly tire of the intrusiveness. These patients may miss the cues indicating anger and aggression from others. Patients in a mixed episode or depressive episode will need protection from self-harm.

Support groups are very helpful for people with this disorder. Participating in the groups allows the person to meet others with the same disorder and learn strategies to manage the disorder and prevent recurrence of the manic or depressive episodes. Support groups are very helpful in dealing with the stigma associated with mental illnesses.

Family Interventions

Marital and family interventions are often needed at different periods in the life of a person with bipolar disorder. For the family with a child with this disorder, additional parenting skills will be needed to manage the behaviors. The goal of family interventions is to help the family understand and cope with the disorder. These interventions may range from occasional counseling sessions to intensive family therapy.

Evaluation and Treatment Outcomes

Desired treatment outcomes are stabilization of mood and enhanced quality of life. Primary tools for evaluation of outcomes are nursing observation and patient self-report (see Nursing Care Plan 20-1 and the Interdisciplinary Treatment Plan that follows).

Continuum of Care

Inpatient Management

Inpatient admission is the treatment setting of choice for patients who are an immediate danger to themselves or others or who are severely psychotic. Medication management, including control of side effects (Fig. 20-3) and promotion of patient self-care, are major nursing responsibilities during inpatient hospitalization. Nurses should be familiar with several drug–drug interactions and with interventions to help control side effects (Table 20-9).

Intensive Outpatient Programs

Intensive outpatient programs for several weeks of acute-phase care during a manic or depressive episode

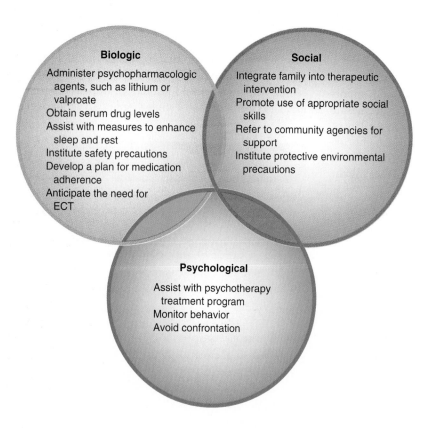

FIGURE 20.3 Biopsychosocial interventions for patients with bipolar I disorder. ECT, electroconvulsive therapy.

TABLE 20.9 Interventions for Lithium Side Effects

Side Effect	Intervention
Edema of feet or hands	Monitor intake and output, check for possible decreased urinary output. Monitor sodium intake. Patient should elevate legs when sitting or lying. Monitor weight.
Fine hand tremor	Provide support and reassurance, if it does not interfere with daily activities. Tremor worsens with anxiety and intentional movements; minimize stressors. Notify prescriber if it interferes with patient's work and compliance will be an issue. More frequent smaller doses of lithium may also help.
Mild diarrhea	Take lithium with meals. Provide for fluid replacement. Notify prescriber if becomes severe; may need a change in medication preparation or may be early sign of toxicity.
Muscle weakness, fatigue, or memory and concentration difficulties	Provide support and reassurance; this side effect will usually pass after a few weeks of treatment. Short-term memory aids such as lists or reminder calls may be helpful. Notify prescriber if becomes severe or interferes with the patient's desire to continue treatment.
Metallic taste	Suggest sugarless candies or throat lozenges. Encourage frequent oral hygiene.
Nausea or abdominal discomfort	Consider dividing the medication into smaller doses, or give it at more frequent intervals. Give medication with meals.
Polydipsia	Reassure patient that this is a normal mechanism to cope with polyuria.
Polyuria	Monitor intake and output. Provide reassurance and explain nature of side effect. Also explain that this causes no physical damage to kidneys.
Toxicity	Withhold medication. Notify prescriber. Use symptomatic treatments.

are used when hospitalization is not necessary or to prevent or shorten hospitalization. These programs are usually called *partial hospitalization* or *day hospitalization*. Close medication monitoring and milieu therapies that foster the restoration of an individual patient's previous adaptive abilities are the major nursing responsibilities in these settings.

Setting up frequent office visits and crisis telephone calls are additional nursing interventions that can help to shorten or prevent hospitalization during the acute phase of a manic episode. Family sessions or psychoeducation that includes the patient are second-line alternatives (Expert Consensus Panel, 1996). Severely and persistently ill patients may need ongoing intensive treatment, but the frequency of visits can be decreased in patients who stabilize and enter the continuation or the maintenance phase of treatment.

Spectrum of Care

In today's health care climate, with efforts to reduce hospitalization, most patients with bipolar disorder are treated as outpatients, except for those who are at

high risk for suicide or who are experiencing psychosis. Hospitalizations are usually brief, and treatment focuses on restabilization. Patients with mood disorders are likely to need long-term medication regimens and supportive psychotherapy to function in the community. Therefore, medication regimens and additional treatment planning need to be tailored to individual patients' needs. Patients need extended and continued follow-up to monitor medication trials and side effects, reinforce self-care management, and provide continued psychosocial support. See Appendices M and N for clinical pathways.

MENTAL HEALTH PROMOTION

Mental health promotion activities should be the focus during remissions. During this period, patients have an opportunity to learn new coping skills that promote positive mental health. Stress management and relaxation techniques can be practiced in order to use them when needed. A plan for managing emerging symptoms can also be developed during this period.

Summary of Key Points

➤ Mood disorders are characterized by persistent or recurring disturbances or alterations in mood that cause significant psychological distress and functional impairment. Moods can be broadly categorized as manic or dysphoric (typified by exaggerated feelings of elation or irritability) or depressive or dysthymic (typified by feelings of sadness, hopelessness, loss of interest, and fatigue).

➤ Primary mood disorders include both depressive disorders (unipolar depression) and manic-depressive disorders (bipolar disorders).

➤ Research demonstrates that genetic influences undoubtedly play a substantial role in the etiology of mood disorders. Risk factors include family history of mood disorders, prior mood episodes, lack of social support, stressful life events, substance use, and medical problems, particularly chronic or terminal illnesses.

➤ The recommended guidelines for treatment of depression include antidepressant medication, alone or with psychotherapeutic management or psychotherapy; electroconvulsive therapy for severe depression; or light therapy (phototherapy) for patients with seasonal depressive symptoms.

➤ Nurses must be knowledgeable regarding antidepressant medications, in particular, therapeutic effects and associated side effects, toxicity, dosage ranges, and contraindications. Nurses must also be familiar with electroconvulsive therapy protocols and associated interventions. Patient education and the provision of emotional support during the course of treatment are also nursing responsibilities.

➤ Many symptoms of depression, such as changes in weight and appetite, sleep disturbance, decreased energy, and fatigue, are similar to those of medical illnesses. Assessment includes a thorough medical history and physical examination to detect or rule out medical comorbidity.

➤ Biopsychosocial assessment includes assessing mood, speech patterns, thought processes and thought content, suicidal or homicidal thoughts, cognition and memory, and social factors, such as patterns of relationships, quality of support systems, and changes in occupational functioning. Several self-report scales are helpful in evaluating depressive symptoms.

➤ Establishing and maintaining a therapeutic nurse–patient relationship is key to successful outcomes. Nursing interventions that foster the therapeutic relationship include being available in times of crisis; providing understanding and education to patients and their families regarding goals of treatment; providing encouragement and feedback concerning the patient's progress; providing guidance in patient's interpersonal interactions with others and work environment; and helping to set and monitor realistic goals.

➤ Psychosocial interventions for mood disorders include self-care management, cognitive therapy, behavior therapy, interpersonal therapy, patient and family education regarding the nature of the disorder and treatment goals, marital and family therapy, and group therapy that includes medication maintenance support groups and other consumer-oriented support groups.

➤ Bipolar disorders are characterized by one or more manic episodes or mixed mania (co-occurrence of manic and depressive states) that cause marked impairment in social activities, occupational functioning, and interpersonal relationships and may require hospitalization to prevent self-harm.

➤ Manic episodes are periods in which the individual experiences abnormally and persistently elevated, expansive, or irritable mood characterized by inflated self-esteem, decreased need to sleep, excessive energy or hyperactivity, racing thoughts, easy distractibility, and inability to stay focused. Other symptoms can include hypersexuality and impulsivity.

➤ Similar to treatment of major depressive disorder, pharmacotherapy is the cornerstone of treatment of bipolar illness, but adjunctive psychosocial interventions are needed as well. Pharmacologic therapy includes treatment with mood stabilizers alone or in combination with antipsychotics or benzodiazepines if psychosis, agitation, or insomnia are present and antidepressants for unremitted depression. Electroconvulsive therapy is a valuable alternative for patients with severe mania.

➤ Recent major advances in bipolar disorder treatment research validate the efficacy of integrated psychosocial and pharmacologic treatment involving family or couples therapies, psychoeducational programs, and individual cognitive-behavioral or interpersonal therapies.

Critical Thinking Challenges

1. Discuss the prevalence of depression in the United States. Debate whether or not depression is truly a public health problem. Determine whether there is a greater prevalence of major depression or bipolar disorder.

2. Describe a typical clinical course of depression.

3. Compare the symptoms of major depression with those of bipolar disorder. How are they different and how are they similar?

4. Compare the biologic and psychological theories of depression. Using the biopsychosocial model, integrate the factors that are important in the experience of depression. Draw your model.

5. Compare the actions, therapeutic effects, and side effects of the tricyclic antidepressants, selective serotonin reuptake inhibitors, and monoamine oxidase inhibitors.

6. The development of a therapeutic relationship with a patient who is depressed requires different skills than with a patient with bipolar disorder. Based on your reading, develop two different approaches—one for a patient who is manic and one for a patient who is depressed.

7. A patient asks for information regarding the side effects of lithium carbonate. What are the critical points that should be included when developing a teaching plan?

8. Compare the action, therapeutic effects, and side effects of lithium carbonate and divalproex sodium.

 WEB LINKS

www.psycom.net *Go to Depression Central.* This site is the Internet's central clearinghouse for information on all types of depressive disorders and on the most effective treatments for individuals suffering from major depression, manic-depressive disorder (bipolar disorder), cyclothymia, dysthymia, and other mood disorders.

www.mhsource.com/bipolar This site provides an overview of bipolar disorder and comorbid illnesses.

www.nimh.nih.gov/publicat/bipolar.cfm This is a National Institutes of Health publication providing an overview of bipolar disorder.

www.home.att.net/~mercurial-mind This site provides an overview of bipolar disorder from a consumer perspective.

www.ndmda.org This website of the National Depressive and Manic-Depressive Association is provided by the organization to educate patients, families, professionals, and the public concerning the nature of depression and bipolar disorder.

www.depression-net.com *Depression Net.* This website, operated by Organon, provides an overview of depression and treatment.

www.narsad.org The National Alliance for Research on Schizophrenia and Depression is a national organization that raises and distributes funds to find the causes, cures, and better treatments of schizophrenia.

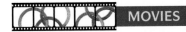 **MOVIES**

Scent of a Woman: 1992. A timid prep school student earns much-needed money on a long weekend taking a job as a companion to a crusty, blind, hard-drinking ex-Army Lt. Colonel Frank Slade played by Al Pacino. He has both a depressed mood and a loss of interest and pleasure in everyday activities. He is constantly angry. He spends his days in a drunken state or tormenting his 4-year-old niece. This film details the weekend in which the Lt. Colonel carries out his plans for his last few days before his suicide attempt.
Significance: Frank Slade demonstrates all of the symptoms of depression, but they are masked by his intense anger at the world and his heavy drinking.
Viewing Points: Identify your feelings about Frank Slade throughout the movie. Do they change? Identify his symptoms of depression. Focus on the interaction between the student and Frank Slade as the student attempts to prevent the suicide.

Mr. Jones: 1993. This film is about a musician, Mr. Jones, played by Richard Gere, and his psychiatrist. In his manic state, Mr. Jones is a charismatic, charming individual who persuades a contractor to hire him, proceeds to the roof of the building, and prepares to fly off the roof. He withdraws large sums of money from the bank. He knows that he has bipolar disorder but refuses to take his medication because of the side effects. He has episodes of depression during which he becomes suicidal. Once hospitalized, he struggles with trying to find a life on medication.
Significance: Viewers can gain insight into the impact of mental illness on the promising career of a classical musician. This film illustrates the ways in which interpersonal relationships are affected by a psychiatric disorder. Unfortunately, the unethical romantic relationship between Mr. Jones and his psychiatrist detracts from the quality of the movie content.
Viewing Points: Why does the diagnosis of paranoid schizophrenia not fit Mr. Jones' clinical picture in the admitting room? Identify the antecedents to the manic and depressive episodes. At what point is the doctor–patient relationship first compromised? Are there early warning signs that should have alerted the psychiatrist that she was violating professional boundaries?

REFERENCES

Agency for Health Care Policy and Research Depression Guideline Panel. (1993). *Clinical practice guidelines: Depression in primary care* (AHCPR Publications No. 93-0550 and 93-0551). Rockville, MD: U.S. Department of Health and Human Services.

American Nurses Association. (2000). *Scope and standards of psychiatric–mental health clinical nursing practice.* Washington, DC: Author.

American Psychiatric Association. (1993). Practice guideline for major depressive disorder in adults. *American Journal of Psychiatry, 150*(Suppl. 4), 1–26.

American Psychiatric Association. (2000a). *Diagnostic and statistical manual of mental disorders* (4th ed., Text revision). Washington, DC: Author.

American Psychiatric Association. (2000b). Practice guideline for the treatment of patients with major depressive disorder (revision). *American Journal of Psychiatry, 157*(Suppl. 4).

American Psychiatric Association Task Force on Electroconvulsive Therapy. (1990). *The practice of electroconvulsive therapy.* Washington, DC: Author.

Ames, D. (1993). Ecstasy, the serotonin syndrome, and neuroleptic malignant syndrome—a possible link? (Letter). *Journal of the American Medical Association, 269*(7), 869.

Angst, J., Angst, F., & Stassen, H. H. (1999). Suicide risk in patients with major depressive disorder. *Journal of Clinical Psychiatry, 60*(Suppl. 2), 57–62.

Arana, G. W., & Rosenbaum, J. F. (2000). *Handbook of psychiatric drug therapy* (4th ed.). Philadelphia: Lippincott Williams & Wilkins.

Beach, S. R. H., Sundeen, E. E., & O'Leary, K. D. (1990). *Depression in marriage.* New York: Guilford.

Beck, A. T., Rush, A. J., Shaw, B. F., & Emery G. (1979). *Cognitive therapy of depression.* New York: Guilford.

Blazer, D. G., Kessler, R. C., McGonagle, K. A., et al. (1994). The prevalence and distribution of major depression in a national community sample: The National Comorbidity Survey. *American Journal of Psychiatry, 151*, 979–986.

Bowden, C. L. (1995a). Treatment of bipolar disorder. In A. F. Schatzberg & C. B. Nemeroff (Eds.), *The American Psychiatric Press textbook of psychopharmacology* (pp. 603–614). Washington, DC: American Psychiatric Press.

Bowden, C. L. (1995b). Predictors of response to divalproex and lithium. *Journal of Clinical Psychiatry, 56*(Suppl 3):25–30.

Bowden, C. L., Brugger, A. M., Swann, A. C., et al. (1994). Efficacy of divalproex vx. Lithium and placebo in the treatment of mania. *Journal of the American Medical Association, 271*(12), 918–924.

Cadoret, R. J., Winokur, G., Langbehn, D., et al. (1996). Depression spectrum disease. I. The role of gene-environment interaction. *American Journal of Psychiatry, 153*, 892–899.

Coyne, J. C. (1988). Strategic therapy. In J. F. Clarkin, G. L. Haas, & I. D. Glick (Eds.), *Affective disorders and the family: Assessment and treatment* (pp. 89–113). New York: Guilford.

Cutler, J. L., & Marcus, E. R. (1999). Mood disorders. In *Psychiatry.* Philadelphia: W. B. Saunders.

Expert Consensus Panel for Bipolar Disorder. (1996). Treatment of bipolar disorder. *Journal of Clinical Psychiatry, 57*(Suppl. 12A), 1–84.

Faedda, G. L., Baldessarini, R. J., Suppes, T., et al. (1995). Pediatric onset bipolar disorder: A neglected clinical and public health problem. *Harvard Review of Psychiatry, 3*, 171–195.

Faedda, G. L., Baldessarini, R. J., Tohen, M., et al. (1991). Episode sequence in bipolar disorder and response to lithium treatment. *American Journal of Psychiatry, 148*, 1237–1239.

Goldberg, J. F., Garno, J. L., Leon, A. C., et al. (1999). A history of substance abuse complicates remission from acute mania in bipolar disorder. *Journal of Clinical Psychiatry, 60*, 733–740.

Goodwin, F. K., & Jamison, K. R. (1990). *Manic-depressive illness.* New York: Oxford University Press.

Hays, J. C., Krishnan, K. R., George, L. K., et al. (1998). Age of first onset of bipolar disorder: Demographic, family history, and psychosocial correlates. *Depression and Anxiety, 7*, 76–82.

Hirschfield, R. M. A., Clayton, P. J., Cohen, I., et al. (1994). Practice guideline for the treatment of patients with bipolar disorder. *American Journal of Psychiatry, 151*(Suppl. 12), 1–36.

Kessler, R. C., McGonagle, K. A., Zhao, S., et al. (1994). Lifetime and 12-month prevalence of *DSM-III-R* psychiatric disorders in the United States: Results from the National Comorbidity Survey. *Archives of General Psychiatry, 51*, 8–19.

Klerman, C. B., Weissman, M. M., Rounsaville, B. J., & Chevron, E. S. (1984). *Interpersonal psychotherapy of depression.* New York: Basic Books.

Kojima, H., Terao, T., & Yoshimura, R. (1993). Serotonin syndrome during clomipramine and lithium treatment. *American Journal of Psychiatry, 150*, 1877.

Kronfol, Z., & Remick, D. G. (2000). Cytokines and the brain: Implications for clinical psychiatry. *American Journal of Psychiatry, 157*(5), 683–694.

Kupfer, D. J., Frank, E., Perel, J. M., et al. (1992). Five-year outcome for maintenance therapies in recurrent depression. *Archives of General Psychiatry, 49*, 769–773.

Liberman, R. P., & Greene, M. F. (1992). Whither cognitive-behavioral therapy for schizophrenia? *Schizophrenia Bulletin, 18*(1), 27–35.

Liebenluft, E. (1996). Women with bipolar illness: Clinical and research issues. *American Journal of Psychiatry, 153*, 163–173.

McDaniel, J. S., Johnson, K. M., & Rundell J. R. (1996). Mania. In J. R. Rundell & M. G. Wise (Eds.), *Textbook of consultation-liaison psychiatry* (pp. 346–376). Washington, DC: American Psychiatric Press.

McDonald, W. M. (2000). Epidemiology, etiology, and treatment of geriatric mania. *Journal of Clinical Psychiatry, 2000*(61 Suppl. 13), 3–11.

McElroy, S., Keck, P., Stanton, S., et al. (1996). A randomized comparison of divalproex oral loading versus haloperidol in the initial treatment of acute psychotic mania. *Journal of Clinical Psychiatry, 57*(4), 142–146.

Merriam, A. E., & Karasu, T. B. (1996). Commentary. The role of psychiatry in the treatment of depression: Review of two practice guidelines. *Archives of General Psychiatry, 53*, 301–302.

Miller, L. G. (1998). Herbal medicinals: Selected clinical considerations focusing on known or potential drug–herb interactions. *Archives of Internal Medicine, 158*(20), 2200–2211.

Mohr, W. (2001). Bipolar disorder in children. *Journal of Psychosocial Nursing, 39*(3), 12–23.

Muly, E., McDonald, W., & Steffens, O. (1993). Serotonin syndrome produced by a combination of fluoxetine and lithium. *American Journal of Psychiatry, 150,* 1565.

Murray, J. L., & Lopez, A. D. (1996). *Global burden of disease and injury series.* Geneva: World Health organization.

Nathan, K. I., Mussellman, D. L., Schatzberg, A. F., & Nemeroff, C. B. (1995). Biology of mood disorders. In A. F. Schatzberg & C. B. Nemeroff (Eds.), *The American Psychiatric Press textbook of psychopharmacology* (pp. 439–478). Washington, DC: American Psychiatric Press.

Nolan, S. & Scoggin, J. A. (2001). Serotonin syndrome: Recognition and management. *US Pharmacist, 23*(2), **www.uspharmacist.com.**

Parkerson, G. R., Broadhead, W. E., & Tse, C. K. J. (1995). Perceived family stress as a predictor of health-related outcomes. *Archives of Family Medicine, 4,* 253–260.

Persons, J. B., Thase, M. E., & Crits-Cristoph, P. (1996). The role of psychotherapy in the treatment of depression: Review of two practice guidelines. *Archives of General Psychiatry, 53,* 283–290.

Perugi, G., Akiskal, H. S., Micheli, C., et al. (1997). Clinical subtypes of bipolar mixed states: Validating a broader European definition in 143 cases. *Journal of Affective Disorders, 43,* 169–180.

Post, R. M., Kramlinger, K. G., Altshuler, L. I., et al. (1990). Treatment of rapid cycling bipolar illness. *Psychopharmacology Bulletin, 26,* 37–47.

Prien, R. F., Himmelhoch, J. M., & Kupfer, D. J. (1988). Treatment of mixed mania. *Journal of Affective Disorders, 15,* 9–15.

Prien, R. F., & Rush, A. J. (1996). Commentary: National Institute of Mental Health Workshop report on the treatment of bipolar disorder. *Biological Psychiatry, 40*(3), 215–219.

Reeves, R., & Bullen, J. (1995). Serotonin syndrome produced by paroxetine and low dose trazodone. *Psychosomatics, 36*(2), 159–160.

Rosenbaum, J. F., & Fava, M. (1998). Approach to the patient with depression. In T. A. Stern, J. B. Herman, & P. L. Slavin (Eds.), *The MGH guide to psychiatry in primary care.* New York: McGraw-Hill.

Rothbaum, B. O., & Astin, M. C. (2000). Integration of pharmacotherapy and psychotherapy for bipolar disorder. *Journal of Clinical Psychiatry, 61*(Suppl. 9), 68–75.

Sachs, G. (1998). Approach to the patient with elevated, expansive, or irritable mood. In T. A. Stern, J. B. Herman, & C. Salzman (Eds.), *Clinical geriatric psychopharmacology.* Baltimore: Williams & Wilkins.

Sauer, C. D., & Ford, S. M. (1995). Quality, cost-effective psychiatric treatment: A CNS-MD collaborative practice model. *Archives of Psychiatric Nursing, 9*(6), 332–337.

Sporer, K. A. (1995). The serotonin syndrome: Implicated drugs, pathophysiology and management. *Drug Safety, 13*(2), 94–104.

Stall, S. (2000). *Essential psychopharmacology: Neuroscientific basis and practical applications.* Cambridge: Cambridge University Press.

Suppes, T., Dennehy, E. B., & Gibbons, E. W. (2000). The longitudinal course of bipolar disorder. *Journal of Clinical Psychiatry, 61*(Suppl. 9), 23–30.

Thompson, L. W. (1996). Cognitive-behavioral therapy and treatment for late-life depression. *Journal of Clinical Psychiatry, 57*(Suppl. 5), 29–37.

Tohen, M., & Goodwin, F. (1995). Epidemiology of bipolar disorder. In M. T. Tsuang, M. Tohen, & G. E. P. Zahner (Eds.), *Textbook in psychiatric epidemiology* (pp. 301–305). New York: Wiley-Liss.

Tohen, M., Greenfield, S. F., Weiss, R. D., et al. (1998). The effect of comorbid substance use disorders on the course of bipolar disorder: A review. *Harvard Review of Psychiatry, 6,* 133–141.

U.S. Department of Health and Human Services (USDHHS). (1999). *Mental Health: A report of the Surgeon General.* Rockville, MD: U.S. Department of Health and Human Services, Substance Abuse and Mental Health Services Administration, Center for Mental Health Services, National Institutes of Health, National Institute of Mental Health.

Waggoner, P. (1992). Case study: Neuroleptic malignant syndrome. *Critical Care Nurse, 10,* 32–34.

World Health Organization. (1997). *World health report 1997: Conquering suffering, enriching humanity.* Geneva: World Health Organization.

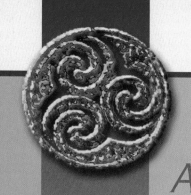

Anxiety Disorders

Robert B. Noud and Kathy Lee

*A*nxiety is a condition that all humans experience. Anxiety is an uncomfortable feeling of apprehension or dread that occurs in response to internal or external stimuli and can result in physical, emotional, cognitive, and behavioral symptoms. In fact, all of the symptoms of anxiety disorders can be found in healthy individuals given particular circumstances. It is when the symptoms of anxiety become so severe that they interfere with the individual's ability to function in work or interpersonal relationships that they considered to be symptomatic of an anxiety disorder. The anxiety disorders discussed in this chapter include panic disorder, generalized anxiety disorder, phobias, acute stress disorder, posttraumatic stress disorder (PTSD), and obsessive-compulsive disorder (OCD). Dissociative disorders are not *classified as anxiety disorders. However, they are included as part of this chapter because overwhelming anxiety is a cardinal symptom of these disorders.*

> **KEY CONCEPT** Anxiety. **Anxiety** is an uncomfortable feeling of apprehension or dread that occurs in response to internal or external stimuli and can result in physical, emotional, cognitive, and behavioral symptoms.

Panic disorder receives particular attention in this chapter, in part because of the frequency with which people suffering panic disorder or panic attacks are seen in medical facilities. There is also significant overlap of symptoms and interventions applicable to other anxiety disorders. OCD is highlighted because patients with this disorder often do not seek medical attention and because of the inherent difficulties in diagnosing and treating this condition.

NORMAL VERSUS ABNORMAL ANXIETY RESPONSE

Anxiety is an unavoidable, human condition that takes many forms and serves different purposes. The effects of the anxiety can be positive and serve as a motivator for an individual to take a needed action, or they can bring about fear in an individual and paralyze the person from taking any action. Normal anxiety is described as being of realistic intensity and duration for the situation and is followed by relief behaviors intended to reduce or prevent more anxiety (Peplau, 1989). Normal anxiety is appropriate to the situation, can be dealt with without repression by the patient, and can be used to help the patient identify what underlying problem has caused the anxiety.

During a perceived threat, rising anxiety levels cause physical and emotional changes in all individuals. A normal emotional response to anxiety consists of three parts: physiologic arousal, cognitive processes, and coping strategies. Physiologic arousal is composed of autonomic arousal, increased skeletal muscle tension, and increased ventilation of the lungs (commonly associated with the fight-or-flight response). Arousal is the signal that an individual is facing a threatening or challenging situation. Coping, or relief strategies, are triggered to resolve the threat. Cognitive processes decipher the situation and decide whether the perceived threat should be approached or avoided. Numerous physical, affective, cognitive, and behavioral symptoms may be associated with anxiety. Table 21-1 summarizes many of these symptoms.

The factors that determine whether anxiety is a symptom of a mental disorder are the intensity of anxiety to the situation, what causes the anxiety, and the particular symptom clusters that manifest the anxiety.

Table 21-2 describes the four degrees of anxiety and associated perceptual changes and patterns of behavior.

OVERVIEW OF ANXIETY DISORDERS

Anxiety disorders are the most common of the psychiatric illnesses that are treated by health care providers. It is estimated that 7.3% of people experience anxiety disorders at any given time and that 14.6% of people are affected by anxiety disorders during their lifetime. Anxiety disorders involve a variety of symptoms and behaviors. Women are twice as likely as men to experience anxiety disorders (Dickstein, 2000). Additionally, individuals younger than 45 years of age, those who are separated or divorced, those who have experienced childhood physical or sexual abuse, and those in low socioeconomic groups are at highest risk.

Anxiety disorders affect individuals across the life span. Of depressed elderly patients, 35% will have at least one anxiety disorder diagnosis (Lenze et al., 2000). In children and adolescents, anxiety disorders are prevalent and are often misdiagnosed, leading to a gradual worsening of symptoms. Untreated anxiety disorders have been implicated as increased risk factors for further maladaptive behaviors, including suicide.

It is not unusual for more than one anxiety disorder to be present in a single patient. Comorbid anxiety disorders include panic disorder (9.3%), phobias (15.4%), and generalized anxiety disorder (27.5%) (Lenze et al., 2000). Other mental disorders can also be present. In one study, 26.1% of people with anxiety disorders also met criteria for major depressive disorder (Beekman et al., 2000). On the other hand, people with a primary diagnosis of depression often have anxiety disorders. Anxiety disorder symptoms are reported to be as high as 35% in people with depression (Lenze et al., 2000).

PANIC DISORDER

Panic is an extreme, overwhelming form of anxiety often experienced when an individual is placed in a real or perceived life-threatening situation. Panic is normal during periods of threat, but when panic is experienced routinely and continuously in situations that pose no real physical or psychological threat, it is not normal. Panic can be so intense that the person experiences extreme anxiety about and fear of another panic attack. This type of panic can interfere with the individual's ability to function in everyday life and is characteristic of panic disorder.

> **KEY CONCEPT** Panic. **Panic** is a normal but extreme, overwhelming form of anxiety often experienced when an individual is placed in a real or perceived life-threatening situation.

TABLE 21.1 Symptoms of Anxiety

Physical

Cardiovascular

Sympathetic
Palpitations
Heart racing
Increased blood pressure

Parasympathetic
Actual fainting
Decreased blood pressure
Decreased pulse rate

Respiratory
Rapid breathing
Difficulty getting air
Shortness of breath
Pressure of chest
Shallow breathing
Lump in throat
Choking sensations
Gasping

Parasympathetic
Spasm of bronchi

Neuromuscular
Increased reflexes
Startle reaction
Eyelid twitching
Insomnia
Tremors
Rigidity
Spasm
Fidgeting
Pacing
Strained face
Unsteadiness
Generalized weakness
Wobbly legs
Clumsy motions

Skin
Face flushed
Face pale
Localized sweating (palm region)
Generalized sweating
Hot and cold spells
Itching

Gastrointestinal
Loss of appetite
Revulsion toward food
Abdominal discomfort
Diarrhea

Parasympathetic
Abdominal pain
Nausea
Heartburn
Vomiting

Eyes
Dilated pupils

Urinary Tract

Parasympathetic
Pressure to urinate
Increased frequency of urination

Affective

Edgy
Impatient
Uneasy
Nervous
Tense
Wound-up
Anxious
Fearful
Apprehensive
Scared
Frightened
Alarmed
Terrified
Jittery
Jumpy

Cognitive

Sensory-Perceptual
Mind is hazy, cloudy, foggy, dazed
Objects seem blurred/distant
Environment seems different/unreal
Feelings of unreality
Self-consciousness
Hypervigilance

Thinking Difficulties
Cannot recall important things
Confused
Unable to control thinking
Difficulty concentrating
Difficulty focusing attention
Distractibility
Blocking
Difficulty reasoning
Loss of objectivity and perspective
Tunnel vision

Conceptual
Cognitive distortion
Fear of losing control
Fear of not being able to cope
Fear of physical injury or death
Fear of mental disorder
Fear of negative evaluations
Frightening visual images
Repetitive fearful ideation

Behavioral

Inhibited
Tonic immobility
Flight
Avoidance
Speech dysfluency
Impaired coordination
Restlessness
Postural collapse
Hyperventilation

Adapted from Beck, A. T., & Emery, C. (1985). *Anxiety disorders and phobias: A cognitive perspective* (pp. 23–27). New York: Basic Books.

TABLE 21.2 Degrees of Anxiety

Degree of Anxiety	Effects on Perceptual Field and on Ability to Focus Attention	Observable Behavior
Mild	Perceptual field widens slightly. Able to observe more than before and to see relations (make connection among data).	Is aware, alerted, sees, hears, and grasps more than before. Usually able to recognize and name anxiety easily.
Moderate	Perceptual field narrows slightly. Selective inattention: does not notice what goes on peripheral to the immediate focus but can do so if attention is directed there by another observer.	Sees, hears, and grasps less than previously. Can attend to more if directed to do so. Able to sustain attention on a particular focus; selectively inattentive to contents outside the focal area. Usually able to state "I am anxious now."
Severe	Perceptual field is greatly reduced. Tendency toward dissociation: to not notice what is going on outside the current reduced focus of attention; largely unable to do so when another observer suggests it.	Sees, hears, and grasps far less than previously. Attention is focused on a small area of a given event. Inferences drawn may be distorted because of inadequacy of observed data. May be unaware of and unable to name anxiety. Relief behaviors generally used.
Panic (terror, horror, dread, uncanniness, awe)	Perceptual field is reduced to a detail, which is usually "blown up," ie, elaborated by distortion (exaggeration), or the focus is on scattered details; the speed of the scattering tends to increase. Massive dissociation especially of contents of self-system. Felt as enormous threat to survival.	Says, "I'm in a million pieces," "I'm gone." "What is happening to me?" Perplexity, self-absorption. Feelings of unreality. Flights of ideas, or confusion. Fear. Repeats a detail. Many relief behaviors used automatically (without thought). The enormous energy produced by panic must be used and may be mobilized as rage. May pace, run, or fight violently. With dissociation of contents of self-system, there may be very rapid reorganization of the self usually going along pathologic lines; eg, a "psychotic break" is usually preceded by panic.

From Peplau, H. (1989). Theoretical constructs: Anxiety, self, and hallucinations. In A. O'Toole, & S. Welt (Eds.), *Interpersonal theory in nursing practice: Selected works of Hildegard E. Peplau.* New York: Springer.

Clinical Course of Panic Disorder

Panic disorder is a lifelong disorder that typically peaks in the teenage years and then again in the 30s. The disorder can surface in childhood or after the fourth decade of life. However, it is unusual for the disorder to manifest after the third decade of life (American Psychiatric Association [APA], 2000). Even after treatment, many patients with panic disorder report that they continue to have panic symptoms or even have a worsening of symptoms. Studies have shown that even after years of treatment, many cases remain symptomatic (APA, 2000; Gardos, 2000).

Panic disorder is a chronic condition that has several exacerbations and remissions during the course of the disease. It is characterized by the appearance of disabling attacks of panic that often lead to other symptoms, such as phobias.

Panic Attacks

Panic attacks are sudden, discrete periods of intense fear or discomfort that are accompanied by significant physical and cognitive symptoms. The physical symptoms include palpitations, chest discomfort, rapid pulse, nausea, dizziness, sweating, paresthesias, trembling or shaking, and a feeling of suffocation or shortness of breath. Cognitive symptoms include disorganized thinking, irrational fears, depersonalization, and decreased ability to communicate. Feelings of impending doom or death, fear of going crazy or losing control, and desperation are common.

A panic attack usually peaks at 10 minutes but can last up to 30 minutes. There is a gradual return to normal functioning. Individuals with panic disorder experience recurrent, unexpected panic attacks, followed by persistent concern about experiencing subsequent panic attacks; they fear implications of the attacks; and they experience behavioral change related to attacks (APA, 2000).

Early panic attacks are often accompanied by a fear of having a heart attack because of similar physical symptoms, such as palpitations, heart racing, rapid breathing or shortness of breath, pressure in the chest, sweating, and feeling faint. Often, these individuals rush to the emergency rooms fearing a heart attack. It is estimated that up to 25% of emergency room visits for chest pain are by people with panic disorders (Fleet et al., 1998). It is estimated that up to 60% of patients who complain of cardiac symptoms and who have a negative workup for chest pain with cardiac origin have panic disorder (Rosenfeld, 1998). Additionally, people with panic attacks may believe that the attacks stem from an underlying major medical illness (APA, 2000). Even with sound medical testing and assurance of no underlying disease, these people often remain unconvinced. Panic attacks can occur in individuals first experiencing certain anxiety-provoking medical conditions, such as asthma, or in initial trials of substance use. However, individuals with panic disorder continue to experience panic attacks without predisposing conditions (Text Box 21-1).

Panic attacks are categorized into three types: unexpected cued, situational cued, and situationally predisposed. With unexpected cued panic attacks, the patient cannot connect the attack with a situational trigger. Situational cued attacks occur upon exposure to a trigger, and situationally predisposed attacks are not necessarily associated with the trigger and do not necessarily occur immediately when faced with the trigger.

All panic attacks are either internally or externally driven. Externally driven panic attacks may result, for example, from actually seeing a feared object. Internally driven panic attacks, however, result from an uncomfortable, internal feeling. Sensations of being too hot or cramped into a small room might provoke panic attacks. APA (2000) defines these categories.

AGORAPHOBIA AND OTHER PHOBIAS

Panic attacks can lead to the development of **phobias,** or persistent, unrealistic fears of situations, objects, or activities. People with phobias will go great lengths to avoid the feared objects or situations in order to deter panic attacks. Table 21-3 presents examples of common phobias. Common phobias include fear of heights (acrophobia) or fear of snakes (ophidiophobia).

Agoraphobia literally means fear of open spaces and commonly co-occurs with panic disorder and significantly affect the life of the person experiencing it. Agoraphobia may occur after experiencing panic attacks and leads to avoidance behaviors toward a cluster of situations. It begins with an intense, irrational fear of being in open spaces or of being alone or in public places where escape might be difficult or embarrassing. The person is afraid that if a panic attack occurred, there would be no help available. Then, the individual avoids similar situations. Such avoidance interferes with routine life functioning and eventually renders the person afraid to leave the safety of home. Some affected individuals continue to face feared situations, but with significant trepidation

---

TEXT BOX 21.1

Clinical Vignette: Leslie (Panic Disorder)

Leslie, a 24-year-old white woman, suddenly experienced chest pressure, pounding heart, shortness of breath, and sweating while attending a staff meeting at her new place of employment. Initially, Leslie tried to control these symptoms with deep breathing, but she became afraid she was experiencing a heart attack. She informed her supervisor that she felt ill and allowed a coworker to rush her to an emergency room. Within 20 minutes, Leslie's symptoms subsided. The doctor informed her that her heart was healthy and normal, but suggested that she see her regular physician. Leslie felt embarrassed and decided to tell her supervisor that she had "just a touch of food poisoning." Over the next few weeks, Leslie experienced several more episodes, at work, at home, in her car, and two while shopping with friends. During each of these episodes, she isolated herself and became extremely fearful that others would notice she was "losing her mind." She felt dread at going out in public or being trapped in a car.

TABLE 21.3 Common Phobias

Phobia
Acrophobia (fear of heights)
Agoraphobia (fear of open spaces)
Ailurophobia (fear of cats)
Algophobia (fear of pain)
Arachnophobia (fear of spiders)
Brontophobia (fear of thunder)
Claustrophobia (fear of closed spaces)
Cynophobia (fear of dogs)
Entomophobia (fear of insects)
Hematophobia (fear of blood)
Microphobia (fear of germs)
Nyctophobia (fear of night or dark places)
Ophidiophobia (fear of snakes)
Phonophobia (fear of loud noises)
Photophobia (fear of light)
Pyrophobia (fear of fire)
Topophobia (stage fright)
Xenophobia (fear of strangers)
Zoophobia (fear of animal or animals)

(ie, going in public only to pay bills, or to take children to school).

In many cases, agoraphobia quickly develops after a few episodes of panic attacks, but the resulting avoidance behaviors do not lead to a decrease in panic attacks (APA, 2000). Other patients can reduce panic attacks by dodging certain instances that precipitate attacks. Many of these individuals may be able to confront a situation if in the company of a companion, for example, going out in public with a friend close by.

Diagnostic Criteria

Panic disorder is characterized by the onset of panic attacks. Although panic attack is not a disorder with a specific *DSM* code, it does affect the person significantly. A person who is diagnosed with panic disorder has periods of intense fear, at which time at least four physical or psychological symptoms are manifested. These symptoms include palpitations, sweating, shaking, shortness of breath or smothering, sensations of choking, chest pain, nausea or abdominal distress, dizziness, derealization or depersonalization, fear of going crazy, fear of dying, paresthesias, and chills or hot flashes (APA, 2000).

There are two types of panic disorder: with and without agoraphobia. Both types include recurrent and unexpected panic attacks followed by 1 month or more of consistent concern about having another attack, worrying about the consequences of having another attack, or changing behavior because of fear of the attacks. See Table 21-4.

TABLE 21.4 Key Diagnostic Characteristics of Panic Disorder With or Without Agoraphobia	
Diagnostic Criteria	**Target Symptoms**
Panic Disorder Without Agoraphobia Recurrent unexpected panic attacks and 1 month or more (after an attack) of one of the following: • Persistent concern about additional attacks • Worry about the implications of the attack or its consequences • Significant change in behavior related to the attacks Absence of agoraphobia Not a direct physiologic effect of a substance or medical condition *Panic Disorder With Agoraphobia* Meets criteria for panic disorder, including panic attacks Experiences agoraphobia Not better accounted for by another mental disorder, such as a specific phobia or social phobia (eg, avoidance limited to social situations because of fear of embarrassment) *Agoraphobia:* Anxiety about being in places or situations from which escape might be difficult (or embarrassing) or in which help may not be available in the event of having an unexpected or situationally predisposed panic attack or panic-like symptoms Fears typically involve characteristic clusters of situations that include being outside the home alone; being in a crowd or standing in a line; being on a bridge; and traveling in a bus, train, or automobile Situations are avoided (eg, travel is restricted) or endured, with marked distress or anxiety about having a panic attack or panic-like symptoms; or the presence of a companion is required	*Panic Attacks* Discrete period of intense fear or discomfort with four (or more) of the following symptoms that develop abruptly and reach a peak within 10 minutes: • Palpitations, pounding heart, or accelerated heart rate • Sweating • Trembling or shaking • Sensations of shortness of breath or smothering • Feelings of choking • Chest pain or discomfort • Nausea or vomiting • Feeling dizzy, unsteady, lightheaded, or faint • Derealization (feeling of unreality) or depersonalization (being detached from oneself) • Fear of losing control or going crazy • Fear of dying • Paresthesias (numbness or tingling sensations) • Chills or hot flushes Great apprehension about the outcome of routine activities and experiences Loss or disruption of important interpersonal relationships Demoralization Possible major depressive episode *Associated Physical Examination Findings* • Transient tachycardia • Moderate elevation of systolic blood pressure *Associated Laboratory Findings* • Compensated respiratory alkalosis (decreased carbon dioxide, decreased bicarbonate levels, almost normal pH) *Other Targets for Treatment* • Loss or disruption of important interpersonal or occupational activities • Demoralization • Possible major depressive episode

Disorders in Special Populations

Prompt identification, diagnosis, and treatment of anxiety disorders may be difficult for special populations such as children and elderly patients. Often, the symptoms suggestive of anxiety disorders may go unnoticed by caretakers or are misdiagnosed because they mimic cardiac or pulmonary pathology rather than a psychological disturbance.

Children

Anxiety disorders are the most frequent of the psychiatric disorders that are treated in children, with the percentage of children affected comparable to that of asthma (Castellanos & Hunter, 1999). Young patients with anxiety disorders often suffer from separation anxiety disorder and OCD, and the symptoms can be insidious. During these stages in a young person's life, fear of strangers and other signs of anxiety are developmentally appropriate. If left undiagnosed and untreated, the condition typically worsens to the point that the child is unable to carry out his or her responsibilities.

Elderly People

Many people prescribe to the myth that elderly people do not suffer from depression or anxiety disorders because they have little to worry about. Many elderly people with depression also have comorbid anxiety disorders. This combination of depressive and anxiety symptoms has been shown to decrease social functioning, increase somatic (physical) symptoms, and increase depressive symptoms (Lenze et al., 2000). Because the elderly population is at risk for suicide, special assessment of anxiety symptoms is essential.

Epidemiology

Panic disorder is prevalent in as much as 1.6% of the general population (2.9 million) at any given time according to the Epidemiological Catchment Area survey. Authors have cited the prevalence of panic disorder to be as high as 6.8% in study populations (Wang et al., 2000). It is highly associated with depression, medical conditions including hypertension, and cigarette smoking. Patients experiencing panic disorder with agoraphobia tend to have more coexisting anxiety disorders, anxiety attacks, and anticipatory anxiety than patients with panic disorder without agoraphobia.

Studies of panic disorder in men and women have revealed gender-related differences. In one study, there were no significant differences between men and women in the number of or intensity of panic episodes (Yonkers et al., 1998). Women were more likely than men to experience panic disorder with agoraphobia. The same study revealed that women were more likely than men to experience panic symptoms after complete remission was attained. In the National Comorbidity Survey (8,098 participants), 3.5% of women experienced panic disorder in their lifetime, and 2.3% experienced panic disorder in the year preceding the survey. No difference in prevalence of panic disorders was found between African Americans and whites. However, the Epidemiological Catchment Area study did find lower lifetime rates of panic disorder among Hispanics (Kessler et al., 1994).

Etiology

Genetic Theories

There appears to be a substantial familial predisposition to panic disorder. The lifetime risk for panic disorder among the first-degree relatives of patients with panic disorder has been estimated to be as high as 25%, and the risk for women is twice that for men. Immediate family members of patients with panic disorder have eight times the risk for developing panic disorder than control groups. If the family member manifests panic disorder before 20 years of age, the risk in family members jumps to 20 times that of the general population (APA, 2000). Twin studies have found the occurrence of panic attacks to be as much as five times more frequent in monozygotic than dizygotic twins. Linkage studies have been promising but have not established the involvement of a particular gene. Higher familial prevalence of panic disorders that manifests in the teenage years may actually be a result of conditioning from early childhood. More research is needed to analyze this phenomenon.

Neuroanatomic Theories

Certain neurologic abnormalities have also been detected by magnetic resonance imaging tests of patients with panic disorder. The most common abnormalities are focal areas of abnormal activity in the fear network of the brain, which is believed to contribute to the development of panic disorder. These areas include the central nucleus of the amygdala, the hippocampus, and the periaqueductal gray area in the brain (Gorman et al., 2000). This may either indicate a genetic predisposition to panic disorder or may be the result of the disorder. Only further research can provide the answers to these and related questions.

Biochemical Theories

Identification of neurotransmitter involvement in panic disorder has evolved from neurochemical studies of the actions of substances known to produce panic attacks, such as yohimbine, fenfluramine, norepinephrine, epinephrine, sodium lactate, and carbon dioxide (CO_2). Substances that produce panic attacks are referred to as **panicogenic.** Also, by knowing the pharmacodynamics of medications that reduce panic episodes, investigators have been able to hypothesize which neurotransmitters are involved in panic disorder.

Norepinephrine. Norepinephrine is implicated in panic disorders because of its effects on the systems most affected during a panic attack—the cardiovascular, respiratory, and gastrointestinal systems. About half the norepinephrine neurons in the brain are located in the locus ceruleus, which is one of the internal regulators of numerous biologic rhythms. It has extensions to the cerebral cortex, cerebellum, limbic system, and spinal cord. Further support for the norepinephrine system involvement in producing anxiety is found in studies of monkeys. Electrical stimulation of the locus ceruleus in monkeys increases fear and anxiety. Norepinephrine effects are mediated by two types of receptors, α and β, which contribute to the complexities of understanding the role of norepinephrine in panic disorder. Some drugs, such as propranolol, act primarily on the β-adrenergic receptors, reducing the peripheral symptoms of anxiety, but with limited effectiveness against panic.

Accumulated evidence indicates that a dysregulation of the norepinephrine system may exist in panic disorder, but much research is needed to clarify the mechanisms. Drugs that increase activity of the locus ceruleus are often panicogenic in individuals who have panic disorder but not in healthy subjects. Yohimbine, an α_2-receptor antagonist of norepinephrine, increases norepinephrine release in the hippocampus area by increasing the rate of firing at the locus ceruleus, which increases anxiety symptoms (Sallee et al., 2000).

Drugs that inhibit the locus ceruleus are thought to be **anxiolytic,** meaning they reverse or diminish anxiety. Medications such as propranolol, morphine, endorphin, and tricyclic antidepressants (TCAs) decrease firing of the locus ceruleus. However, except for the TCAs, which affect the norepinephrine system in many ways, these drugs as a group appear to have limited effectiveness in reducing panic attacks. The benzodiazepines alprazolam and clonazepam have effectively controlled panic symptoms, but their effect on the locus ceruleus has not yet been determined.

Serotonin. Serotonin (5-HT) was implicated in the etiology of panic disorder when it was discovered that drugs that facilitate serotonergic neurotransmission are effective in relieving symptoms of panic disorder. Selective serotonin reuptake inhibitors (SSRIs) may impede the panic response by decreasing activity in the amygdala and interfering with transmission to extension sites in the hypothalamus (Gorman et al., 2000). Drugs that inhibit serotonin reuptake initially produce an increase in anxiety symptoms but begin to produce symptom relief after 2 to 6 weeks of pharmacotherapy. By blocking the reuptake of serotonin at the presynaptic cleft, more serotonin is available for presynaptic and postsynaptic binding, causing the medications' therapeutic effects. The initial response may be a result of hypersensitivity of postsynaptic 5-HT receptors caused by an increase in levels of synaptic 5-HT, and the therapeutic response occurs after compensatory down-regulation of postsynaptic receptors. At least 13 subtypes of 5-HT receptors exist, and each produces different therapeutic effects when acted on by different medications (Hoyer & Martin, 1997). The effects of serotonergic medications depend on the balance of these many pharmacologic actions and may differ during acute and chronic drug administration.

It seems evident that serotonin is involved in panic disorder. However, the data do not indicate which of the serotonin receptor subtypes is responsible in the pathogenesis of the disorder. Serotonin function is influenced by a number of different factors, such as gender, age, and season, which may contribute to inconsistencies in research findings (Johnson & Lydiard, 1995). Recent research is also beginning to provide an understanding of the interaction between norepinephrine and serotonin, indicating that serotonin connections from the raphe may have a regulatory function on norepinephrine in the locus ceruleus. Nonetheless, these possibilities provide some insight into the mechanisms by which SSRIs are also an effective treatment for panic disorder.

γ-Aminobutyric Acid. γ-Aminobutyric acid (GABA) is the primary inhibitory neurotransmitter in the brain. GABA receptor stimulation causes several effects, including neurocognitive effects, reduction of anxiety, and sedation. GABA stimulation also results in increased seizure threshold. These effects can be modulated by drugs that bind at receptor sites. Highly concentrated in cortical gray-matter areas, the benzodiazepine receptor exists in the same molecular complex as the GABA receptors. Benzodiazepines bind to these receptors and potentiate GABA effects by further facilitating the opening of the chloride ion channel.

Abnormalities in the benzodiazepine–GABA–chloride ion channel complex have been implicated in panic disorder (Taylor & Gorman, 1992). However, difficulties in directly measuring activity at these receptors in the brain have hindered research. Benzodiazepine receptor sites in the brain are pharmacologically different from those found in peripheral tissues, but the peripheral receptors are more accessible for study. Positron emission tomography and single-photon emission computed tomography may hold promise for providing more direct information about these receptors. However, magnetic resonance imaging has been used to provide superior resolution of anatomic brain structures and may be the only tool with which the physiology of a real-time panic attack can be captured (Gorman et al., 2000).

Corticotropin-Releasing Factor. Corticotropin-releasing factor (CRF) is a neuropeptide that acts as a neurotransmitter. It is essential to the function of the hypothalamic–pituitary–adrenal (HPA) axis. CRF and its receptors are found widely distributed in the forebrain, including in the frontal cortex, amygdala, hippocampus, and the locus ceruleus. Moreover, CRF is heavily involved in the production of cortisol, which is known found to be significantly elevated in individuals during panic attack episodes (Bandelow et al., 2000). Of note is that elevated cortisol levels alter the function of the HPA axis.

CRF is synthesized in the paraventricular nucleus of the hypothalamus and is transported down the axon to nerve terminals of the median eminence. From there, it is released into the hypothalamopituitary system and causes release of adrenocorticotropic hormone (ACTH), which then causes synthesis and release of adrenocortical glucocorticoids. CRF directly increases firing in the locus ceruleus, which increases fear and anxiety symptoms through the modulation of norepinephrine. In patients with panic disorder, the CRF stimulation test results in a blunted ACTH response, suggesting hyperactivity in the HPA axis. Other studies offer conflicting results of CRF stimulation tests. Pituitary ACTH responses most likely reflect hypothalamic CRF neuronal activity, whereas CRF neurons in limbic and cerebral cortical areas are probably involved in psychiatric disorders (Owens & Nemeroff, 1993). Long-term use of SSRI antidepressants may in fact inhibit the release of CRF in the hypothalamus.

Cholecystokinin. Cholecystokinin (CCK) is a neuropeptide that also functions as a neurotransmitter. CCK may be implicated in the etiology of panic disorders. High concentrations of CCK are found in the cerebral cortex, the amygdala, and the hippocampus. Two subtypes of CCK receptors have been identified: CCK-A and CCK-B. CCK-A receptors are predominant in the peripheral systems; CCK-B receptors are widely distributed throughout the brain, particularly in the limbic system and cortex. When administered in challenge tests, CCK tetrapeptide (CCK-4), a selective agonist for CCK-B receptors, induces panic attacks in patients with panic disorder and to a much lesser degree in people without panic disorder (Bradwejn et al., 1992). CCK has important interactions with other neurotransmitters, such as norepinephrine, implicated in panic disorder. CCK-B antagonists are under development as antipanic medications (Kunovac & Stahl, 1995).

Other Neuropeptides. Evidence of altered growth hormone (GH) activity in patients with panic disorder provides additional support for the role of the hypothalamus in panic disorder. GH secretion is regulated by two counterbalancing hypothalamic peptides: growth hormone-releasing factor and somatostatin. These peptides stimulate and inhibit the release of GH. Somatomedin C, which is stimulated by GH, is secreted from the liver and has feedback inhibitory effects on GH at the pituitary and hypothalamic levels.

In healthy subjects, α-adrenergic receptor simulation results in elevated GH. This process is blunted in individuals with panic disorders. This appears to be because of a sensitivity in α-adrenergic postsynaptic receptors resulting from chronic hyperactivity in the locus ceruleus. This leads to down-regulation of α-adrenergic receptors in the hypothalamus, which are responsible for GH mediation (Sallee et al., 2000).

Other Panicogenic Substances. In challenge tests, sodium bicarbonate, sodium lactate, and CO_2 induced panic attacks in people with panic disorders and in healthy people to some extent. CO_2 is the byproduct of both sodium bicarbonate and lactate. It readily crosses the blood–brain barrier, producing transient cerebral hypercapnia. This in turn stimulates CO_2 receptors, causing hyperventilation and panic. Individuals with panic disorder may have hypersensitivity to CO_2 and subsequently experience a sensation of suffocation immediately before panic attacks. This may be directly related to the action of CO_2 on the noradrenergic pathways in the brain (Ben-Zion et al., 1999).

Studies have been conducted to detect cerebral blood flow abnormalities during panic attacks in patients with panic disorder. Patients with panic disorder who panic during intravenous challenges with sodium lactate have exhibited asymmetry of blood flow to various regions of the brain. However, hyperventilation is inherent in the panic process, which causes hypocapnia-induced vasoconstriction of blood vessels. Therefore, measuring accurate rates of blood flow may be distorted. More research is necessary to measure the effects of elevated CO_2 levels on panic incidence (Gorman et al., 2000).

Psychoanalytic and Psychodynamic Theories

Freud originally believed that anxiety developed from a sexual energy that was externally constrained. Later, he said it resulted from unconscious repression of instinctual sexual drives. He thought that anxiety acted as a signal for the individual's ego to mobilize defense mechanisms such as repression to avoid a "dangerous" situation and to relieve the feelings of anxiety. Although psychoanalytic theories are not generally accepted as explaining the etiology of psychiatric disorders, the intrapsychic conflict model is the basis for many current psycho-analytic treatment approaches.

Psychodynamic theories contribute to the understanding of panic disorders by explaining the importance of the development of anxiety after separation and loss. Those with panic disorder report greater numbers and severity of recent personal losses at the time of onset of symptoms when compared with healthy control subjects. Many people with anxiety disorders, especially panic disorder, have experienced recent losses of family members, suffer more physical disability, and use emergency room services more often than healthy subjects (Roy-Byrne et al., 1999).

In a study of the background and personality traits of individuals with panic disorder, several commonalities were found, including (1) being fearful or shy as a child; (2) remembering their parents as angry, critical, or frightening; (3) having feelings of discomfort with aggression; (4) having long-term feelings of low self-esteem; and (5) experiencing a stressful life event associated with frustration and resentment that preceded the initial onset of symptoms (Shear et al., 1993). These researchers proposed the following theory of causation. The child may begin with a neurophysiologic vulnerability that predisposes one to fearfulness. This fearfulness is enhanced by parental behavior in some way, which results in disturbed parent–child relationships, causing the child to feel conflict about dependence and independence (separating from parent), self-doubt and confusion regarding self-identity, and personal control. These negative feelings of low self-esteem and powerlessness appear to make the individual feel extremely vulnerable to the stress of normal life events, such as going to school, getting married, or becoming a parent. As the person attempts to ignore these negative feelings and seems powerless to control them, he or she continues to experience distress in repeated stressful events. The chronic, intense fear and dread culminates in the first panic attack.

Cognitive-Behavioral Theories

Learning theory provides the basic underpinnings of most cognitive-behavioral theories of panic disorder. Classic conditioning theory suggests that one learns a fear response by linking an adverse or fear-provoking event, such as a car accident, with a previously neutral event, such as crossing a bridge. The person becomes conditioned into associating fear with crossing a bridge. There are limitations of applying this theory to those with panic disorder. Phobic avoidance is not always developed secondary to an adverse event.

Further development of this theory led to an understanding of **interoceptive conditioning**, which pairs a somatic discomfort, such as dizziness or palpitations, with an impending panic attack. For example, during a car accident, the individual may experience rapid heartbeat, dizziness, shortness of breath, and panic. Subsequent experiences of dizziness or palpitations, unrelated to an anxiety-provoking situation, incite anxiety and panic. Many cognitive theorists further expound that people with panic disorder may misinterpret mild physical sensations (sweating, dizziness) causing panic as a result of learned fear (catastrophic interpretation). For example, palpitations may be misinterpreted as an imminent heart attack.

Some researchers hypothesize that individuals with a low sense of control over their environment or with a particular sensitivity to anxiety are vulnerable to misinterpreting normal stress. It is accepted that controlled exposure to anxiety-provoking situations and cognitive countering techniques have been successful in reducing the symptoms of panic.

Risk Factors

Several risk factors have been implicated in the development of panic disorder, including family history, substance and stimulant use or abuse, and undertaking severe stressors. In addition to the potential genetic predisposition that was discussed earlier in the chapter, female gender has been implicated as a risk factor for this disorder because females have more panic symptoms than do males. People who have several anxiety symptoms and those who experience separation anxiety during childhood often present with panic disorder later in life (Hayward et al., 2000). Smoking tobacco products has been implicated in the risk for developing panic attacks as well.

Because panic disorder manifests predominantly in the teenage years, it would be prudent to determine which risk factors are highly associated with events occurring early in life. Early life traumas, history of physical or sexual abuse during childhood, and behavioral inhibition of children by adults have been associated with an increased risk for anxiety disorders in children (Castellas & Hunter, 2000; Marshall et al., 2000).

Comorbidity

Although people with panic disorder are thought to have more somatic complaints than the general population, there is a high correlation between panic disorder and certain medical conditions, including vertigo, cardiac disease, gastrointestinal disorders, and asthma (Rosenfeld, 1998). Patients with mitral valve prolapse, migraine headaches, and hypertension may also have an increased incidence of panic disorder. Research has not determined whether some of these medical conditions result from panic disorder or are discovered more often as a result of increased sensitivity to some of the physical symptoms. Whichever the case, people with panic disorder have reported to their health care providers that they feel as if they are in poor physical or psychological health (Mendlowicz & Stein, 2000).

Interdisciplinary Treatment of Panic Disorder

People with panic disorder require interdisciplinary treatment. Upon identifying an underlying anxiety disorder, several different disciplines take part in treating the individual. Nurses are the pivotal position of stabilizing the patient in the inpatient setting by providing a safe and therapeutic environment. The nurse also administers ordered medication and monitors its effects, and develops an individual care plan to meet the patient's needs. Advanced practice nurses, licensed clinical social workers, or licensed counselors provide individual psychotherapy sessions as appropriate. Often, a clinical psychologist administers psychological testing and interprets the test results to assist with appropriate diagnosis to tailor treatment approaches.

Priority Care Issues

Panic disorder and depression are highly associated with each other. Lenze and associates (2000) stated that 9.3% of patients with major depression have comorbid panic disorder. Additionally, Pilowsky and coworkers (1999) discovered that adolescents with panic disorder were three times as likely to express suicidal thoughts and were twice as likely to make suicide attempts than adolescents without panic disorder. As many as 15% of deaths of patients with panic disorder are by suicide, and women who have a dual diagnosis of panic disorder and depression or panic disorder and substance abuse are at higher risk.

Individuals with anxiety disorders require special attention because of issues surrounding comorbidity with other mental and physical illnesses. Patients with panic disorders have a high degree of comorbidity with other anxiety disorders, substance abuse and dependence, and depression. In one study of individuals with panic disorder, 70% had at least one comorbid anxiety disorder (Roy-Byrne et al., 1999). Common coexisting anxiety disorders in people with panic disorder include depression, schizophrenia, OCD, specific phobias, PTSD, and social phobias (Fleet et al., 1998; Lenze et al., 2000).

Because panic disorder manifests during the childbearing years, care should be taken to assess the pregnant patient for an underlying panic disorder. Although it is disputed that pregnancy may actually protect the mother from developing panic symptoms, postpartum onset of panic disorder requires particular attention. During a time that tremendous effort is spent on family, postpartum onset of panic disorder has been found to have a negative impact on lifestyle and to decrease self-esteem in affected women, leading to feelings of overwhelming personal disappointment (Beck, 1998).

NURSING MANAGEMENT: HUMAN RESPONSE TO DISORDER

Because panic disorder encompasses the physical, psychological, and social fields of the patient, assessment within a biopsychosocial framework is important. Physiologic symptoms tend to be the impetus for patients to seek medical assistance because the symptoms overlap with other medical and psychiatric illnesses. Often, patients are seen in emergency rooms as they seek treatment for their symptoms. Biologic, psychological, and social assessments unveil potential underlying pathology and guide the nurse to accurate diagnosis.

Biologic Domain

Assessment of Biologic Domain

Patients with panic disorder are often seen in a number of health care settings and present with an array of symptoms, and skillful assessment is required to rule out life-threatening causes, including cardiac or neurologic involvement. Physical examination, laboratory tests, and electrocardiography are performed to eliminate the possibility of an underlying physical cause of these symptoms.

After it is determined that the patient is not experiencing a life-threatening physical event, the nurse should assess for the characteristic symptoms of panic attack (Table 21-5). If the panic attack occurs in the presence of the nurse, direct assessment of the symptoms should be made and documented. Questions to ask the patient might include the following:

- What did you experience preceding and during a panic episode, including physical symptoms, feelings, and thoughts?
- When did you begin to feel that way?
- What is it that caused you to feel and think that way?
- Have you experienced these symptoms in the past? If so, under what circumstances?
- Has anyone in your family ever had similar experiences?
- What do you do when you have these experiences that helps you to feel safe? Have the feelings and sensations ever gone away on their own?

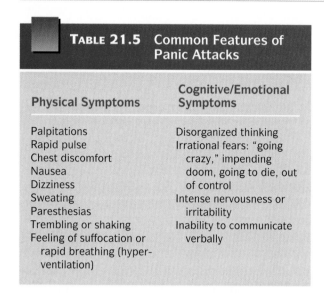

TABLE 21.5   Common Features of Panic Attacks

Physical Symptoms	Cognitive/Emotional Symptoms
Palpitations	Disorganized thinking
Rapid pulse	Irrational fears: "going
Chest discomfort	crazy," impending
Nausea	doom, going to die, out
Dizziness	of control
Sweating	Intense nervousness or
Paresthesias	irritability
Trembling or shaking	Inability to communicate
Feeling of suffocation or	verbally
rapid breathing (hyper-	
ventilation)	

Substance Use. Assessment for panicogenic substance use, such as sources of caffeine, pseudoephedrine, amphetamines, cocaine, or other stimulants, may rule out contributory issues either related or unrelated to panic disorder. Tobacco use is also considered to contribute to the risk for panic symptoms. Many individuals with panic disorder use alcohol or central nervous system (CNS) depressants in an effort to self-medicate anxiety symptoms, and withdrawal from CNS depressants may produce symptoms of panic. Binge drinking is associated with exacerbation of panic symptoms.

Sleep Patterns. Sleep is often disturbed in patients with panic disorder. In fact, panic attacks can occur during sleep. Individuals who experience spontaneous panic attacks during sleep may develop fear of going to sleep. Nurses should closely assess the impact of sleep disturbance because fatigue may increase anxiety and susceptibility to panic attacks.

Physical Activity. Active participation in a routine exercise program is an area that requires assessment. If the patient does not exercise routinely, define the barriers. If exercise is avoided because of chronic muscle tension, poor muscle tone, muscle cramps, general fatigue, exhaustion, or shortness of breath, the symptoms may be indicative of poor physical health.

Nursing Diagnoses Related to Biologic Domain

Appropriate nursing diagnoses for the individual with panic disorder include Anxiety, Risk for Self-Harm, Social Isolation, Powerlessness, and Ineffective Family Coping. Other diagnoses may apply after the nurse has completed a thorough psychiatric nursing assessment and an individual services plan (care plan) is developed.

Biologic Interventions

The course of panic disorder culminates in phobic avoidance as the inflicted person attempts to avoid situations that increase panic. Because identification and avoidance of anxiety-provoking situations is important in the therapy process, drastically changing one's lifestyle to avoid situations is not tremendously helpful in the recovery process. Interventions that focus of the physical aspects of anxiety and panic are particularly helpful in reducing the number and severity of the attacks, giving patients a rapid sense of accomplishment and control.

Breathing Control. Hyperventilation is a common symptom in many individuals who experience panic. Often, people are unaware that they begin to take rapid, shallow breaths when they become anxious. Assisting patients in learning breathing control can be a helpful tool. Focus on their breathing and help them to identify the rate, pattern, and depth. If their breathing is rapid and shallow, reassure the patient that exercise and breathing practice can help change their breathing pattern. Next, assist the patient in practicing abdominal breathing by performing the following exercises:

- Instruct the individual to focus on breathing deeply by having him or her place a hand on the abdomen just beneath the rib cage. Inhale slowly through the nose, attempting to fill the "bottom" of the lungs.
- Instruct the patient to observe that when one is breathing deeply, the hand on the abdomen will actually rise.
- After the patient seems to understand this process, ask him or her to inhale slowly through the nose counting to five, pause, and then exhale slowly through pursed lips.
- While exhaling, direct the attention to feeling the muscles relax, focusing on "letting go."
- Repeat the deep abdominal breathing for 10 breaths, pausing between each inhalation and exhalation. Count slowly. If the patient complains of lightheadedness, reassure him or her that this is a normal feeling while deep breathing. Instruct the individual to stop for 30 seconds, breathe normally, and then start again.
- The patients should stop between each cycle of 10 breaths and monitor normal breathing for 30 seconds.
- This series of 10 slow abdominal breaths followed by 30 seconds of normal breathing should be repeated for 3 to 5 minutes.
- Assist the patient in establishing a time for daily practice of abdominal breathing.

Abdominal breathing may also be used to interrupt an episode of panic as it begins. Once patients have learned to identify their own early signs of panic, they can learn the four-square method of breathing, which helps divert or decrease the severity of the attack. Patients should be instructed as follows:

- Practice at times when you are not overanxious.
- Begin by breathing in slowly through the nose, count to four, then hold the breath for a count of four.
- Exhale slowly through pursed lips to a count of four, and then rest for a count of four (no breath).
- Take two normal breaths and repeat the sequence.

After the skill is practiced, the nurse should assist patients in identifying the physical cues that will alert them to use this calming technique. The nurse may initially need to prompt those who are experiencing a panic attack in the nurse's presence.

Nutritional Planning. Maintaining regular and balanced eating habits reduces the likelihood of hypoglycemic episodes, light-headedness, and fatigue. The following are nursing interventions that can help educate the person in proper nutrition:

- Reduce or eliminate a number of substances in the diet that may promote anxiety and panic, such as caffeine, food coloring, or monosodium glutamate. Symptoms of caffeine withdrawal may stimulate panic. Patients need a plan to reduce consumption and then eliminate caffeine from their diet.

- Each substance should be assessed for the individual, noting symptoms of anxiety after consumption and monitoring for these same symptoms after the substances have been eliminated from the individual's diet.

Relaxation Techniques. Learning relaxation techniques is another important skill that can help many individuals with panic and anxiety disorders. Some individuals are unaware of the tension in their body and first need to learn to monitor their own tension. Isometric exercises and progressive muscle relaxation are helpful methods to learn to differentiate muscle tension from muscle relaxation (see Chap. 14). This method of relaxation is also helpful when patients have difficulty clearing the mind, focusing, or visualizing a scene, which are often required in other forms of relaxation, such as meditation. Text Box 21-2 provides one method of progressive muscle relaxation.

Increased Physical Activity. Physical exercise can diminish the occurrence of panic attacks by reducing muscle tension, increasing metabolism, and relieving stress. In a study comparing exercise, pharmacotherapy, and placebo in the reduction of panic symptoms, exercise proved much more effective than placebo in the reduction of symptoms (Broocks et al., 1998). Exercise programs reduce many of the precipitants of anxiety by improving circulation, digestion, endorphin stimulation,

---

TEXT BOX 21.2

Implementing Progressive Muscle Relaxation

Choose a quiet, comfortable location where you will not be disturbed for 20 to 30 minutes. Your position may be lying or sitting, but all parts of your body should be supported, including your head. Wear loose clothing, taking off restrictive items, such as glasses and shoes.

Begin by closing your eyes and clearing your mind. Moving from head to toe, focus on each part of your body and assess the level of tension. Visualize each group of muscles as heavy and relaxed.

Take two or three slow abdominal breaths, pausing briefly in between each breath. Imagine the tension flowing from your body.

Each muscle group listed below should be tightened (or tensed isometrically) for 5 to 10 seconds and then abruptly released, visualizing this group of muscles as heavy, limp, and relaxed for 15 to 20 seconds before tightening the next group of muscles. There are several methods to tighten each muscle group, and suggestions are provided below. Each muscle group may be tightened two to three times until relaxed. Do not overtighten or strain. You should not experience pain.

- Hands (tighten by making fists)
- Biceps (tighten by drawing forearms up and "making a muscle")

- Triceps (extend forearms straight, locking elbows)
- Face (grimace, tightly shutting mouth and eyes)
- Face (open mouth wide and raise eyebrows)
- Neck (pull head forward to chest and tighten neck muscles)
- Shoulders (raise shoulders toward ears)
- Shoulders (push shoulders back as if touching them together)
- Chest (take a deep breath and hold for 10 seconds)
- Stomach (suck in your abdominal muscles)
- Buttocks (pull buttocks together)
- Thighs (straighten legs and squeeze muscles in thighs and hips)
- Leg calves (pull toes carefully toward you, avoid cramps)
- Feet (curl toes downward and point toes away from your body)

Finally, repeat several deep abdominal breaths and mentally check your body for tension. Rest comfortably for several minutes, breathing normally, and visualize your body as warm and relaxed. Get up slowly when you are finished.

and tissue oxygenation. Additionally, exercise lowers cholesterol levels, blood pressure, and weight. After assessing for contraindications to physical exercise (ie, physical health issues), assist the patient in establishing a routine exercise program. Engaging in 10- to 20-minute sessions on treadmills or stationary bicycles two to three times weekly is ideal during winter months. Casual walking or bike riding during seasonal weather promotes health. Help the patient to identify community resources that promote exercise activity.

Psychopharmacologic Treatment. Several classes of pharmacologic agents are effective in treating panic disorder, including the SSRIs, TCAs, benzodiazepines, and monoamine oxidase inhibitors (MAOIs). Because the SSRIs are generally considered first-line treatment of panic disorder, other treatments are available for refractory or treatment-resistant symptoms.

Selective Serotonin Reuptake Inhibitors. The SSRIs are useful in treatment of panic attacks. Sertraline (Zoloft), paroxetine (Paxil), fluoxetine (Prozac), and fluvoxamine (Luvox) have all proved effective in the treatment of panic disorder in drug trials (Ballenger et al., 1998; Pohl et al., 1998; Saeed & Bruce, 1998). The SSRIs produce anxiolytic effects by increasing the transmission of serotonin by blocking serotonin reuptake at the presynaptic cleft. Although this initial increase in intrasynaptic 5-HT can lead to initial increases in panic symptoms, the chronic 5-HT stimulation at the postsynaptic receptor sites compensate by down-regulating 5-HT transmission (Grove et al., 1997). It is also postulated that as serotonin activity increases in the brain, there is a secondary decrease in biogenic amine activity—specifically, norepinephrine. The decreased norepinephrine activity diminishes cardiovascular symptoms of tachycardia and increased blood pressure that are associated with panic attacks (Gorman et al., 2000).

Monitoring and Administration of Medications. Overall, SSRI medications have more pleasant side-effect profiles, are safer to use, and are less lethal in the event of overdose. They produce fewer side effects but may cause an uncomfortable feeling of overstimulation when treatment is initiated.

Fluoxetine (Prozac) and sertraline (Zoloft) are known to cause feelings of overstimulation, but slow titration can help to alleviate this feeling. Morning dosing decreases interference with sleep, but at higher doses, some patients find the medication sedating. At this time, bedtime dosing is indicated. Paroxetine (Paxil) was the first of the SSRIs to be indicated for anxiety disorders. Dosing begins at 10 mg daily, usually in the morning, and then is increased 10 mg per week at weekly intervals, not to exceed 60 mg daily. Maximum daily doses of sertraline and fluoxetine are 200 mg and 100 mg, respectively.

Side-Effect Monitoring. The side effects of the SSRIs include anticholinergic effects (dry mouth, blurred vision, urinary hesitancy, constipation), dizziness, anxiety, nervousness, and sexual dysfunction. Although many of these side effects mimic those of the TCAs and MAOIs, they tend to be less pronounced. Sexual dysfunction is a common complaint in patients taking fluoxetine, sertraline, and paroxetine and must be weighed into the decision of which medication approach to treating panic disorder would be most advantageous.

Drug–Drug Interactions. Although each SSRI has certain drug–drug interactions, all carry similar concerns. All SSRIs interact violently with MAOIs by causing hypertensive crises and with tryptophan by causing serotonin syndrome. Fluoxetine interacts with flecainide, warfarin, phenytoin (Dilantin), carbamazepine (Tegretol), and vinblastine by increasing the serum levels of both drugs being taken. It also alters the action of insulin and antidiabetic agents. Fluoxetine further interacts with lithium and TCAs, causing adverse CNS affects by increasing the serum levels of one or both drugs being taken.

Paroxetine interacts with cimetidine (Tagamet), which decreases paroxetine's metabolism and might potentiate toxicity. It may also decrease digoxin levels and alter the actions of phenobarbitol and phenytoin. Paroxetine may also increase serum procyclidine levels; thus, monitoring for anticholinergic activity is indicated. People who use paroxetine and warfarin are at increased risk for bleeding because of their interaction.

Sertraline interacts specifically with diazepam and tolbutamide by decreasing their clearance. Warfarin may increase sertraline's serum plasma level when these two drugs are taken together.

Teaching Points. Warn patients of the use of over-the-counter medications, including St. John's wort, because of the risks of serotonin syndrome. The sedative effects of the medications may impede judgment while operating machinery. Avoid these circumstances until the medication effects are known. Foods containing high amounts of tryptophan should be avoided while taking fluoxetine. Assist the patient in recognizing these foods so that they can be avoided. These foods include: meats, poultry, organ meats, eggs, nuts, broad beans, and wheat germ.

Tricyclic Antidepressants. The TCAs imipramine (Tofranil) and clomipramine (Anafranil) reduce panic symptoms in patients (Broocks, et al., 1998; Saeed & Bruce, 1998), which is probably linked to their action on norepinephrine receptors. The therapeutic effects of TCAs usually occur after 3 to 4 weeks, but effects as early as 2 weeks after initiation of drug treatment have been observed.

Monitoring and Administration of Medications. The TCAs have a relatively long half-life, and complaints of sedation are common. Therefore, single bedtime doses might be most helpful for patients. TCAs are highly bound to plasma proteins and metabolized in the liver. These medications should be used with extreme caution in patients at risk for suicide. TCAs affect cardiac conduction, and overdose may lead to death. An electrocardiogram is indicated before initiating therapy because of the cardiovascular effects. In cross-tapering to different medications, note that sudden discontinuation of TCAs leads to flu-like symptoms of nausea, headache, and malaise, owing to cholinergic rebound phenomenon. Assure patients that these effects do not symbolize addiction to the medication.

TCAs may complicate underlying glaucoma, urinary retention, cardiovascular disorders, hepatic disease, and thyroid dysregulation because of their systemic effects. They also lower the seizure threshold in patients. Monitor closely if the patient has a seizure disorder.

The maximum daily dose of imipramine is 200 mg for outpatient treatment and 300 mg daily for inpatients. The maximum dose of clomipramine is 250 mg daily. These medications have narrow therapeutic indexes and therefore require monitoring for toxicity at high doses.

Side-Effect Monitoring. Adverse side effects of TCAs may compromise patients' willingness to continue their use, but this problem can be reduced by starting with a small dose and increasing slowly (see Drug Profile: Imipramine). Lower initial doses and slower increases can also lessen the possibility of these side effects. It is recommended that treatment with these agents be started at very low doses and increased gradually. Because patients with panic disorder usually require higher doses of antidepressant medication, anticholinergic side effects may be particularly difficult to tolerate. Nurses should actively assess for anticholinergic side effects

---

DRUG PROFILE: Imipramine
(Tricyclic antidepressant)
Trade names: Tofranil, Janimine, Tipramine, and various generic formulations
Tofranil-PM (imipramine pamoate)

Receptor affinity: Mechanism of action is unknown; thought to inhibit presynaptic reuptake of norepinephrine and serotonin. Also displays anticholinergic action at central nervous system and peripheral receptors.
Indications: Treatment of symptoms of depression (endogenous depression most responsive); sedative effects may be helpful in patients with depression associated with anxiety and sleep disturbances. Treatment of enuresis in children 6 years of age or older. Unlabeled uses for chronic pain control (such as intractable cancer pain, peripheral neuropathies, posttherapeutic neuralgia, tic douloureux, and central pain syndromes).
Routes and dosages: Available in 10-, 25-, and 50-mg tablets; 12.5 mg/mL solution for injection; 75-, 100-, 125-, and 150-mg capsules (pamoate).
Adults: For hospitalized patients with depression: 100 to 150 mg/d PO in divided doses, gradually increasing to 200 mg/d as needed; increased to 250 to 300 mg/d if no response after 2 weeks. For outpatients with depression: Initially 75 mg/d PO increasing to 150 mg/d. Dosages more than 200 mg/d are not recommended. Total daily dose may be given at bedtime. Maintenance dose is 50 to 150 mg/d. For patients unable or unwilling to take oral form (for depression): Up to 100 mg/d in divided doses; replaced with oral form as soon as possible. For patients with chronic pain: 50 to 200 mg/d PO. Geriatric patients to 40 mg/d PO; doses >100 mg/d usually not needed.
Adolescents: 30 to 40 mg/d PO; doses >100 mg/d usually not needed.
Children 6 years of age and older: For enuresis: Initially, 25 mg/d, 1 hour before bedtime, increasing to 50 mg nightly in children younger than age 12, 75 mg nightly in children over age 12, if unsatisfactory response after 1 week. Not to exceed 2.5 mg/kg/d.
Half-life (peak effect): 8 to 16 h (2–4 h)
Selected adverse reactions: Sedation, dizziness, drowsiness, confusion, disturbed concentration, seizures, blurred vision, dry mouth, nausea, constipation, orthostatic hypotension, photosensitivity. When used for childhood enuresis—nervousness, sleep disorders, and gastrointestinal disturbances.
Warnings: Contraindicated in patients with tartrazine and aspirin hypersensitivity, concomitant therapy with MAOI and electroshock therapy. Avoid use in patients with recent myocardial infarction, myelography within previous 24 h or scheduled within next 48 h, pregnancy, and breast-feeding. Use cautiously in patients with pre-existing cardiovascular disorders, hyperthyroidism, angle closure glaucoma, urine retention, and impaired hepatic or renal function. Use cautiously in patients with schizophrenia or paranoia, which may cause worsening of psychosis; manic-depressive patients may shift to hypomania or manic phase. Drug may increase serum levels and risk for bleeding if taken concurrently with anticoagulants. Concomitant administration with MAOIs may cause hyperpyretic crisis, severe convulsions, hypertensive episodes, and death. Use with caution in patients with seizure disorders because drug may lower seizure threshold.
Specific patient/family education:
* Take drug exactly as prescribed.
* Do not stop taking this drug abruptly or without consent of health care provider.
* Avoid prolonged exposure to sunlight or sun lamps. Use a sunscreen or protective clothing.
* Report any signs and symptoms of adverse reactions.
* Avoid driving a car or performing tasks that require alertness if dizziness, drowsiness, or blurred vision occur.
* Use hard, sugarless candy to relieve dry mouth.
* Notify physician if difficulty urinating, excessive sedation, fever, chills, sore throat, or palpitations occur.

(dry mouth and eyes, blurred vision, photophobia, constipation, urinary hesitancy or retention, mydriasis, and tachycardia) and implement necessary interventions (see Chap. 8). Dry mouth is a common side effect and may be soothed with hard candy.

Acetylcholine is positively linked to cognition, and anticholinergic side effects of TCAs may negatively affect cognition in elderly patients. Additionally, many TCAs have α-adrenergic receptor effects on the body that lead to orthostatic hypotension, placing elderly individuals at increased risk for falls. Lying and standing blood pressure and pulse should be monitored frequently, especially during periods of increasing the dosage. Also observe for signs of dizziness or ataxia. Nortriptyline (Pamelor) has a lower risk for orthostatic hypotension and may therefore be indicated if falls present a substantial risk.

Drug–Drug Interactions. TCAs produce drug interactions with several medications, including MAOIs (severe hypertensive crises) and other CNS depressants (enhanced CNS depression). Concomitant treatment with methylphenidate (Ritalin), cimetidine, and oral contraceptives may increase TCA serum levels.

Teaching Points. Instruct the patient to take the medication exactly as prescribed and to inform the provider of any OTC medications before taking them. Alcohol should be avoided. Warn the patient of the potential for sedation, especially at initiation of treatment, and to avoid operating machinery until the effects of the medication are observed. Additionally, common and serious side effects of the medications should be discussed to minimize treatment noncompliance and to establish knowledge of under what situations that notification of the health care provider is imperative.

Benzodiazepines. High-potency benzodiazepines have produced antipanic effects, and their therapeutic onset is much more rapid than antidepressants (comparing hours to weeks). Therefore, benzodiazepines are tremendously useful in treating intensely distressed patients. Alprazolam (Xanax), lorazepam (Ativan), and clonazepam (Klonopin) are widely used for panic disorder. They are well tolerated but carry the risk for withdrawal symptoms upon discontinuation (see Drug Profile: Alprazolam). Lorazepam, a shorter-acting benzodiazepine, also affects panic symptoms but may produce rebound anxiety as the dose effect quickly wears off. For more information on benzodiazepines, see Table 21-6.

Monitoring and Administration of Medications. Treatment protocols may include the administration of benzodiazepines concurrently with antidepressants for the first 4 weeks, then tapering the benzodiazepine to a maintenance dose. This strategy provides rapid symptom relief but avoids the complications of long-term benzodiazepine use. Benzodiazepines with short half-

---

DRUG PROFILE: Alprazolam
(Antianxiety agent)
Trade name: Xanax

Receptor affinity: Exact mechanism of action is unknown; believed to increase the effects of γ-aminobutyrate.
Indications: Management of anxiety disorders, short-term relief of anxiety symptoms or depression-related anxiety, panic attacks with or without agoraphobia. Unlabeled uses for school phobia, premenstrual syndrome, and depression.
Routes and dosages: Available in 0.25-, 0.5-, 1-, and 2-mg scored tablets.
Adults: For anxiety: Initially, 0.25 to 0.5 mg PO tid titrated to a maximum daily dose of 4 mg/d in divided doses. For panic disorders: Initially, 0.5 mg PO tid increased at 3- to 4-d intervals in increments of no more than 1 mg/d. For school phobia: 2 to 8 mg/d PO. For premenstrual syndrome: 0.25 mg PO tid.
Geriatric patients: Initially, 0.25 mg bid to tid, increased gradually as needed and tolerated.
Half-life (peak effect): 12 to 15 h (1–2 h)
Selected adverse reactions: Transient mild drowsiness, initially; sedation, depression, lethargy, apathy, fatigue, lightheadedness, disorientation, anger, hostility, restlessness, headache, confusion, crying, constipation, diarrhea, dry mouth, nausea, and possible drug dependence.

Warnings: Contraindicated in patients with psychosis, acute narrow angle glaucoma, shock, acute alcoholic intoxication with depressed vital signs, pregnancy, labor and delivery, and breast-feeding. Use cautiously in patients with impaired hepatic or renal function, and severe debilitating conditions. Risk for digitalis toxicity if given concurrently with digoxin. Increased CNS depression if taken with alcohol, other CNS depressants, and propoxyphene (Darvon).
Specific patient/family education:
• Avoid using alcohol, sleep-inducing or other OTC drugs.

• Take drug exactly as prescribed and do not stop taking the drug without consulting health care provider.

• Take drug with food if gastrointestinal upset occurs.

• Avoid driving a car or performing tasks that require alertness if drowsiness or dizziness occurs.

• Report any signs and symptoms of adverse reactions.

• Notify health care provider if severe dizziness, weakness, or drowsiness persists; rash or skin lesions, difficulty voiding, palpitations, or swelling of extremities occur.

TABLE 21.6 Benzodiazepine Pharmacokinetics

Drug	Half-life (h)	Lipid solubility	Important Active Metabolites
Chlordiazepoxide	10–20	Moderate	Desmethylchlordiazepoxide, demoxepam, desmethyldiazepam
Diazepam	20–70	High	Desmethyldiazepam
Clorazepate	40–100	Moderate	Desmethyldiazepam
Prazepam	40–100	Low	Desmethyldiazepam
Temazepam	8–20	Moderate	Desmethyldiazepam
Clonazepam	30–60	Low	None
Alprazolam	8–15	Moderate	None
Lorazepam	10–20	Moderate to low	None
Oxazepam	30–120	Moderate to low	None
Triazolam	1.5–5	—	—

lives do not accumulate in the body, whereas drugs with half-lives between 5 and 24 hours exhibit some accumulation. Long-acting benzodiazepines reach a steady state quickly and are eliminated rapidly when the drug is discontinued. Benzodiazepines with half-lives of longer than 24 hours tend to accumulate with chronic treatment, are removed more slowly, and produce less intense symptoms on discontinuation (see Chap. 21).

Short-acting benzodiazepines are associated with rebound anxiety, or anxiety that increases after the peak effects of the medication have decreased. Medications with short half-lives (alprazolam, lorazepam) should be given in divided doses spaced throughout the day (three or four times daily). Clonazepam is a longer-acting benzodiazepine that requires less frequent dosing and has a lower risk for rebound anxiety. Taking low doses throughout the day with a higher dose at bedtime curtails anxiety symptoms and assists with anxiety-related insomnia.

Benzodiazepines should not be used to treat patients with comorbid sleep apnea because of their depressive CNS effects. In fact, they may actually decrease the rate and depth of respirations. Exercise caution in elderly patients for these reasons. Medication discontinuation requires a slow taper over several weeks to avoid rebound anxiety and serious withdrawal symptoms. Benzodiazepines are not indicated in the chronic treatment of patients with substance abuse but can be useful in quickly treating anxiety symptoms until other medications take effect.

Withdrawal symptoms of benzodiazepine use are more likely to occur after high doses and long-term therapy. They can also occur, however, after short-term therapy. Withdrawal symptoms manifest in several different ways, including psychological (apprehension, irritability, insomnia, and dysphoria), physiologic (tremor, palpitations, vertigo, sweating, muscle spasm, seizures), and perceptual (sensory hypersensitivity, depersonalization, feelings of motion, metallic taste).

Side-Effect Monitoring. The side effects of benzodiazepine medications generally include headache, confusion, dizziness, disorientation, sedation, and visual disturbances. Sedation should be monitored after beginning the medication or increasing the dose. Avoid operating heavy machinery until the sedative effects are known.

Drug–Drug Interactions. Drug–drug interactions with the benzodiazepines include TCAs and digoxin, which may result in increased serum TCA or digoxin levels. Alcohol and other CNS depressants, while used with benzodiazepines, increase CNS depression. Their concomitant use is contraindicated. Histamine-2 blockers (cimetidine) used with benzodiazepines may potentiate sedative effects. Finally, cigarette smoking may increase the clearance of benzodiazepines. Monitor closely for effectiveness in patients who smoke.

Teaching Points. Warn the patient to avoid alcohol products because of the chance of CNS depression. Additionally, warn not to operate heavy machinery until the sedative effects of the medication are known.

Monoamine Oxidase Inhibitors. MAOIs, particularly phenelzine (Nardil), have been used effectively to block panic attacks in some patients. The MAOIs are sometimes used if the individual has not responded to other medications; they are not considered first-line treatment for panic disorder. They are, however, effective in patients refractory to the TCAs and SSRIs in treatment of panic disorder (Saeed & Bruce, 1998). Their side-effect profiles and drug–food and drug–drug interactions have limited their use in the age of newer and safer medications.

Monitoring and Administration of Medications. Although serum medication levels peak about 3 to 4 hours after initial dosing, the onset of therapeutic effects of MAOIs can take between 3 and 8 weeks. The effects of the drugs last for up to 10 days after stopping therapy. MAOIs are known to produce hypotensive effects in patients and care should be taken to minimize associated risks. Care must be taken not to initiate treatment within 14 days of other psychotropic medications or medications containing vasoconstrictors because of the risk for hypertensive crises.

The maximum dose of phenelzine is 90 mg daily. Therapy begins at 15 mg daily and is then increased quickly up to 60 mg. Dosing can be reduced to achieve therapeutic effects at the lowest possible dose. Tranylcypromine (Parnate) requires slower titration. Begin at 10 mg three time daily, increasing by 10 mg a week in 1- to 3-week intervals. The maximum dose is 60 mg daily.

Side-Effect Monitoring. Sedation and weight gain are two side effects that can be minimized by starting at a lower dose with gradual titration. Other side effects include hypertension, hypotension, dizziness, edema, agranulocytosis and thrombocytopenia (Parnate), and various uncomfortable, yet common anticholinergic symptoms.

Drug–Drug Interactions. MAOIs have several drug interactions that carry serious implications. Contraindications to MAOI use include use of dibenzodiazepine derivatives, CNS stimulants, diuretics, antihypertensives, buspirone, ephedrine, levodopa, sympathomimetics, and antihistamines, which can enhance the pressor effects of the drug. Antiparkinsonian medications, CNS depressants (alcohol, narcotics), TCAs, spinal anesthetics, and SSRIs increase adverse CNS effects. Concomitant use of buspirone (BuSpar) can result in hypertension, and oral hypoglycemic agents and insulin can increase episodes of hypoglycemia. Cheeses or foods containing tryptophan (eg, yogurt, wines, beer, bananas) can stimulate hypertensive crises during treatment with MAOIs.

Teaching Points. All patients being treated with MAOIs should be informed of the potential drug–drug and drug–food interactions in foods containing tyramine. Such foods include aged cheeses, wines, beer, avocados, chicken liver, chocolate, bananas, soy sauce, meat tenderizers, and cold cuts. Assist the patient with developing a tyramine-free diet.

Instruct the patient not to stop the medication abruptly and to minimize strenuous exercise. MAOIs have been known to suppress symptoms of angina pain. Instruct the patient to consult with his or her provider before taking additional medications, including over-the-counter drugs, because of the high risk for drug interactions.

Psychological Domain

Psychological Assessment

A complete psychological assessment determining the patterns of panic attacks, characteristic symptoms in attacks, and the patient's emotional, cognitive, or behavioral responses to the attacks is necessary (see Chap. 21). A comprehensive assessment includes overall mental status, suicidal tendencies and thoughts, cognitive thought patterns, and avoidance behavior patterns. Moreover, a complete psychological evaluation provides the health care professional with a picture of the patient's current psychiatric condition at baseline of treatment. The nurse assesses the behavioral responses of the patient during the interview, cuing into topics that elicit behaviors suggesting the patient is uncomfortable or nervous (twisting hair, leg movements). The patient's self-concept is assessed. Additionally, present and past coping strategies are discussed to determine how stress is handled by the individual. Finally, a risk assessment is performed to determine the risk for developing psychiatric disorders, what threatens the patient's well-being, and the risk for symptom deterioration (see Chap. 10).

Rating Scales. Several tools are available to characterize and rate the patient's state of anxiety. Examples of these symptom and behavioral rating scales are provided in Text Box 21-3. All of these tools are self-report measures and as such are limited by the individual's self-awareness and openness. However, the Hamilton Rating Scale for Anxiety (HAM-A) is provided in Table 21-7 as an example of a scale rated by the clinician (Hamilton, 1959). This 14-item scale reflects both psychological and somatic aspects of anxiety.

The State-Trait Anxiety Inventory (STAI) is one of the most tested scales available. It is a brief self-report measure of state and trait anxiety in which there are two sections. First, a series of 20 statements asks patients to rate how they usually feel (trait anxiety). The second series of 20 statements asks patients to rate how they feel at a particular moment (state anxiety). Responses to both are rated on a four-point, Likert-type scale. The STAI can be used as a screening tool and to measure changes occurring during treatment.

Self-evaluation is often made more difficult, especially in panic disorder. Symptoms experienced during the attack are often so overwhelming that memory of the exact thoughts or feelings during the attack is unretrievable. However, use of these tools heightens an individual's awareness of the feelings and events around the attack. This awareness can then serve as a cue to assist the patient in implementing cognitive interventions and regaining some sense of control.

Mental Status Examination. During mental status examination, individuals with panic disorder often ex-

TEXT BOX 21.3

Rating Scales for Assessment of Panic Disorder and Anxiety Disorders

Panic Symptoms

Panic-Associated Symptom Scale (PASS)

Argyle, N., Delito, J., Allerup, P., et al. (1991). The Panic-Associated Symptom Scale: Measuring the severity of panic disorder. *Acta Psychiatrica Scandinavica, 83,* 20–26.

Acute Panic Inventory

Dillon, D. J., Gorman, J. M., Liebowitz, M. R., et al. (1987). Measurement of lactate-induced panic and anxiety. *Psychiatry Research, 20,* 97–105.

National Institute of Mental Health Panic Questionnaire (NIMH PQ)

Scupi, B. S., Maser, J. D., & Uhde, T. W. (1992). The National Institute of Mental Health Panic Questionnaire: An instrument for assessing clinical characteristics of panic disorder. *Journal of Nervous and Mental Disease, 180,* 566–572.

Cognitions

Anxiety Sensitivity Index

Reiss, S., Peterson, R. A., & Gursky, D. M. (1986). Anxiety sensitivity, anxiety frequency, and the prediction of fearfulness. *Behavior Research and Therapy, 24,* 1–8.

Agoraphobia Cognitions Questionnaire

Chambless, D. L., Caputo, G. C., Bright, P., & Gallagher, R. (1984). Assessment of fear in agoraphobics: The Body Sensations Questionnaire and the Agoraphobic Cognitions Questionnaire. *Journal of Consulting and Clinical Psychology, 52,* 1090–1097.

Body Sensations Questionnaire

Chambless, D. L., Caputo, G. C., Bright, P., & Gallagher, R. (1984). Assessment of fear in agoraphobics: The Body Sensations Questionnaire and the Agoraphobic Cognitions Questionnaire. *Journal of Consulting and Clinical Psychology, 52,* 1090–1097.

Phobias

Mobility Inventory for Agoraphobia

Chambless, D. L., Caputo, G. C., Jasin, S. E., et al. (1985). The Mobility Inventory for Agoraphobia. *Behavior Research and Therapy, 23,* 35–44.

Fear Questionnaire

Marks, I. M., & Matthews, A. M. (1979). Brief standard self-rating for phobic patients. *Behavior Research and Therapy, 17,* 263–267.

Anxiety

State-Trait Anxiety Inventory (STAI)

Spielberger, C. D., Gorsuch, R. L., & Luchene, R. E. (1976). *Manual for the State-Trait Anxiety Inventory.* Palo Alto, CA: Consulting Psychologists Press.

Penn State Worry Questionnaire (PSWQ)

16-items developed to assess the trait of worry.

Meyer, T., Miller, M., Metzger, R., & Borkovec, T. (1990). Development and validation of the Penn State Worry Questionnaire. *Behaviour Research and Therapy, 28*(6), 487–495.

Beck Anxiety Inventory

21-items rating severity of symptoms on a four-point scale.

Beck, A., Epstein, N., Brown, G., & Steer, R. (1988). An inventory for measuring clinical anxiety: The Beck Anxiety Inventory. *Journal of Consulting and Clinical Psychology, 56,* 893–897.

---

hibit symptoms of anxiety, including restlessness, irritability, poor concentration, watchful or worried facial expression, decreased attention span, difficulty problem solving or organizing a plan, and apprehensive behavior. Disorganized thinking, irrational fears, and decreased ability to communicate verbally often occur during a panic attack. Assess by direct questioning if the patient is experiencing suicidal thoughts—especially if the person is abusing substances or is taking antidepressant medications.

Assessment of Cognitive Thought Patterns. Catastrophic misinterpretations of trivial physical symptoms can trigger panic symptoms. Once identified, these thoughts should serve as a basis for individualizing patient education to counter such false beliefs. Table 21-8 shows an example of a scale to assess catastrophic misinterpretations of the symptoms of panic.

Assessment of the patient's fears regarding losing control has yielded findings. Several studies have found that individuals who feel a sense of control have de-

creases in the severity of panic attacks. These individuals also tend to show low self-esteem, feelings of helplessness, demoralization, and overwhelming fears of experiencing panic attacks. They may have difficulty with assertiveness or expressing feelings. Individuals who fear loss of control during a panic attack often make the following type of statements:

- "I feel trapped."
- "I'm afraid others will know, or I'll hurt someone."
- "I feel alone. I can't help myself."
- "I'm losing control."

Nursing Diagnoses Related to Psychological Domain

Anxiety is the primary nursing diagnosis applied to patients with any of these disorders, although many diagnoses address the individual areas regarding one's inability to manage the stress of the disorder. Other

TABLE 21.7 Hamilton Rating Scale for Anxiety

Max Hamilton designed this scale to help clinicians gather information about anxiety states. The symptom inventory provides scaled information that classifies anxiety behaviors and assists the clinician in targeting behaviors and achieving outcome measures. Provide a rating for each indicator based on the following scale:

0 = None   1 = Mild   2 = Moderate
3 = Severe   4 = Severe, grossly disabling

Item	Symptoms	Rating
Anxious mood	Worries, anticipation of the worst, fearful anticipation, irritability	
Tension	Feelings of tension, fatigability, startle response, moved to tears easily, trembling, feelings of restlessness, inability to relax	
Fear	Of dark, strangers, being left alone, animals, traffic, crowds	
Insomnia	Difficulty in falling asleep, broken sleep, unsatisfying sleep and fatigue on waking, dreams, nightmares, night terrors	
Intellectual (cognitive)	Difficulty concentrating, poor memory	
Depressed mood	Loss of interest, lack of pleasure in hobbies, depression, early waking, diurnal swings	
Somatic (sensory)	Tinnitus, blurring of vision, hot and cold flushes, feelings of weakness, picking sensation	
Somatic (muscular)	Pains and aches, twitchings, stiffness, myoclonic jerks, grinding of teeth, unsteady voice, increased muscular tone	
Cardiovascular symptoms	Tachycardia, palpitations, pain in chest, throbbing of vessels, fainting feelings, missing beat	
Respiratory symptoms	Pressure or constriction in chest, choking feelings, sighing, dyspnea	
Gastrointestinal symptoms	Difficulty in swallowing, wind, abdominal pain, burning sensations, abdominal fullness, nausea, vomiting, borborygmi, looseness of bowels, loss of weight, constipation	
Genitourinary symptoms	Frequency of micturition, urgency of micturition, amenorrhea, menorrhagic, development of frigidity, premature ejaculation, loss of libido, impotence	
Autonomic symptoms	Dry mouth, flushing, pallor, tendency to sweat, giddiness, tension headache, raising of hair	
Behavior at interview	Fidgeting, restlessness or pacing, tremor of hands, furrowed brow, strained face, sighing or rapid respiration, facial pallor, swallowing, belching, brisk tendon jerks, dilated pupils, exophthalmos	

From Hamilton, M. (1959). The assessment of anxiety states by rating. *British Journal of Medical Psychology, 32*, 54.

diagnoses include Risk for Self-Harm, Social Isolation, Powerlessness, and Ineffective Family Coping. Diagnoses specific to physical panic symptoms such as dizziness, hyperventilation, and so forth are likely. These diagnoses may be applied to all the anxiety disorders covered in this chapter. Outcomes will vary.

Psychological Interventions

Psychological interventions are especially important in the effective treatment of anxiety disorders. Pharmacotherapy treats only the biologic aspects a disorder. If the psychological domain of the disorder goes untreated, anxiety symptoms will certainly resurface and continue to affect the person's life.

Peplau devised a system of general guidelines for the types of nursing interventions that might be used suc-

cessfully in treating patients with varying degrees of anxiety. These interventions deal chiefly with helping the patient attend to and react to input other than the subjective experience of anxiety. These interventions are aimed at helping the patient learn to focus on other stimuli and cope with anxiety in whatever form it appears (Table 21-9). These general interventions apply to all anxiety disorders and therefore will not be reiterated in subsequent sections. Other interventions, both pharmacologic and psychosocial, specific to a particular disorder are covered under the pertinent headings (Fig. 21-1).

Psychological interventions should focus on providing patients with information and skills to minimize some of the emotions and beliefs that contribute to their anxiety. If a behavioral analysis was conducted, the ante-

TABLE 21.8 Panic Attack Cognitions Questionnaire

Rate each of the following thoughts according to the degree to which you believe each thought contributes to your panic attack.

1 = Not at all   3 = Quite a lot
2 = Somewhat   4 = Very much

1. I'm going to die.	1	2	3	4
2. I'm going insane.	1	2	3	4
3. I'm losing control.	1	2	3	4
4. This will never end.	1	2	3	4
5. I'm really scared.	1	2	3	4
6. I'm having a heart attack.	1	2	3	4
7. I'm going to pass out.	1	2	3	4
8. I don't know what people will think.	1	2	3	4
9. I won't be able to get out of here.	1	2	3	4
10. I don't understand what is happening to me.	1	2	3	4
11. People will think I am crazy.	1	2	3	4
12. I'll always be this way.	1	2	3	4
13. I'm going to throw up.	1	2	3	4
14. I must have a brain tumor.	1	2	3	4
15. I'll choke to death.	1	2	3	4
16. I'm going to act foolish.	1	2	3	4
17. I'm going blind.	1	2	3	4
18. I'll hurt someone.	1	2	3	4
19. I'm going to have a stroke.	1	2	3	4
20. I'm going to scream.	1	2	3	4
21. I'm going to babble or talk funny.	1	2	3	4
22. I'll be paralyzed by fear.	1	2	3	4
23. Something is physically wrong with me.	1	2	3	4
24. I won't be able to breathe.	1	2	3	4
25. Something terrible will happen.	1	2	3	4
26. I'm going to make a scene.	1	2	3	4

Adapted from Clum, G. A. (1990). Panic attack cognitions questionnaire. *Coping with panic: A drug-free approach to dealing with anxiety attacks.* Pacific Grove, CA: Brooks/Cole.

cedents, including feelings, thoughts, situations, and behaviors, will have been identified. The nurse can then assist the patient in countering these antecedents with a number of individualized psychological measures, including distraction techniques, positive self-talk, panic control treatment, exposure therapy, implosion therapy, and cognitive-behavioral therapy (CBT). These techniques should be used collectively and in concert with each other for maximum effect.

Whatever the intervention is used, consistent and supportive reassurance should be given to the patient in crisis. Reassure the patient that the panic symptoms are only temporary and that they will quickly disappear. After the crisis, the patient should be encouraged to vent his or her feelings. The feedback received from the patient should be used to revise or tailor the plan of care.

Distraction. When patients have identified the early symptoms of panic, they may learn to implement **distraction** behaviors that take the focus off the physical sensations. Some of these distracting activities include initiating conversation with a nearby person or engaging in physical activity (eg, walking, gardening, or house cleaning). Performing simple repetitive activities like counting backward from 100 by threes or counting objects along the roadway such as signs might wart off an impending attack. Moreover, snapping a rubber band against the wrist may help the person to focus on other sensations that are not anxiety provoking. Distraction techniques are to be tailored to the individual, and breathing exercises should be used along with distraction to minimize anxiety symptoms.

Positive Self-Talk. During states of increased anxiety and panic, individuals can learn to counter fearful or negative thoughts by using preplanned and rehearsed positive coping statements, called **positive self-talk.** "This is only anxiety and it will pass," "I can handle these symptoms," and "I'll get through this" are examples of positive self-talk. These types of positive state-

TABLE 21.9 Nursing Interventions Based on Degrees of Anxiety

Degree of Anxiety	Nursing Interventions
Mild	Learning is possible. Nurse assists patient to use energy anxiety provides to encourage learning.
Moderate	Nurse to check own anxiety so patient does not empathize with it. Encourage patient to talk: to focus on one experience, to describe it fully, then to formulate the patient's generalizations about that experience.
Severe	Learning is less possible. Allow relief behaviors to be used but do not ask about them. Encourage the patient to talk: ventilation of random ideas is likely to reduce anxiety to moderate level. When this is observed by the nurse, proceed as above.
Panic	Learning is impossible. Thereness: Nurse to stay with the patient. Allow pacing and walk with the patient. No content inputs to the patient's thinking should be made by the nurse. (They burden the patient, who will distort them.) Use instrumental inputs only, the fewest possible and with the fewest number of words: eg, "Drink this" (give liquids to replace lost fluids and to relieve dry mouth); "Say what's happening to you," "Talk about yourself," or "Tell what you feel now" (to encourage ventilation and externalization of inner, frightening experience). Pick up on what the patient says, eg, Pt: "What's happening to me—how did I get here?" N: "Say what you notice." Short phrases by the nurse—direct, to the point of the patient's comment, and investigative—match the current attention span of the patient in panic and therefore are more likely to be heard, grasped, and acted on, with the patient's responses gradually reducing the anxiety in a helpful way. Do not touch the patient; patients experiencing panic are very concerned about survival, are experiencing grave threat to self, and usually distort intentions of all invasions of their personal space.

From Peplau, H. (1989). Theoretical constructs: Anxiety, self, and hallucinations. In A. O'Toole & D. Welt (Eds.), *Interpersonal theory in nursing practice: Selected works of Hildegard E. Peplau.* New York: Springer.

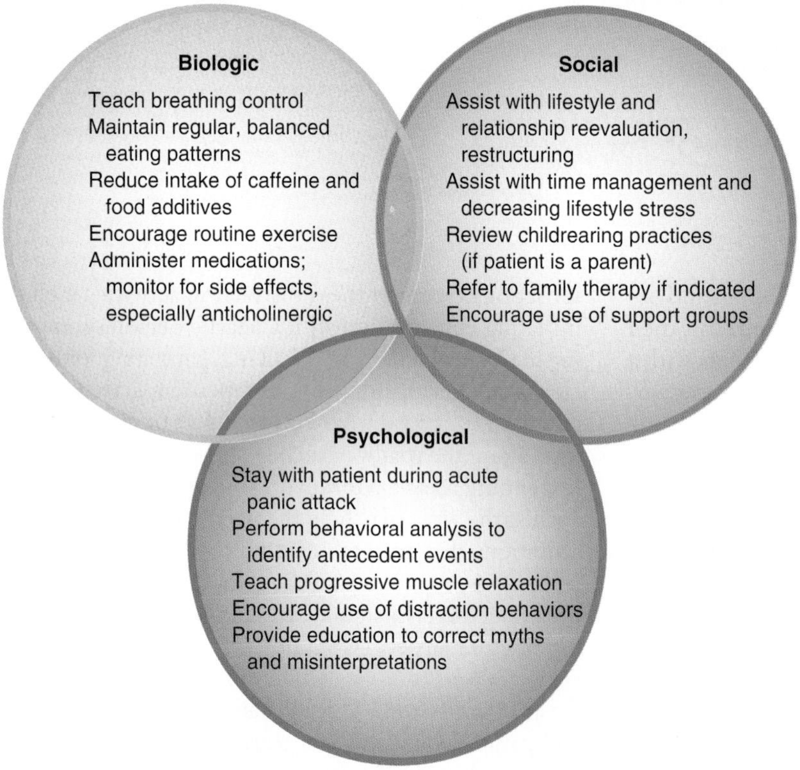

Biologic

Teach breathing control
Maintain regular, balanced
  eating patterns
Reduce intake of caffeine and
  food additives
Encourage routine exercise
Administer medications;
  monitor for side effects,
  especially anticholinergic

Social

Assist with lifestyle and
  relationship reevaluation,
  restructuring
Assist with time management and
  decreasing lifestyle stress
Review childrearing practices
  (if patient is a parent)
Refer to family therapy if indicated
Encourage use of support groups

Psychological

Stay with patient during acute
  panic attack
Perform behavioral analysis to
  identify antecedent events
Teach progressive muscle relaxation
Encourage use of distraction behaviors
Provide education to correct myths
  and misinterpretations

FIGURE 21.1 Biopsychosocial interventions for patients with panic disorder.

ments can give the individual a focal point and reduce fear when panic symptoms begin. Handheld cards that carry positive statements can be carried in a purse or wallet so that the person can retrieve them quickly when panic symptoms are felt (see Therapeutic Dialogue: Panic Disorder With Agoraphobia).

Panic Control Treatment. **Panic control treatment** involves systematic structured exposure to panic-invoking sensations such as dizziness, hyperventilation, tightness in chest, and sweating. The person's patterns of feared sensations are assessed by inducing those sensations through exercise because physical activity produces such sensations. Identified patterns become targets for treatment. Patients are taught to use breathing training and cognitive restructuring to manage their responses. Patients are instructed to practice these tech-

niques between sessions to be able to adapt the skills learned to situations outside therapy sessions.

Exposure Therapy. **Exposure therapy** is the treatment of choice for agoraphobia. The patient is repeatedly exposed to anxiety-provoking situations until he or she becomes desensitized and anxiety subsides. The patient may be exposed to real or simulated situations through visual and auditory imagery.

Systematic Desensitization. **Systematic desensitization** is another exposure method used to desensitize patients to anxiety-provoking situations. This includes exposing the patient to a hierarchy of feared situations that the patient has rated from least to most feared. The patient is taught to use muscle relaxation as levels of anxiety increase through multisituational exposure. Planning

---

THERAPEUTIC DIALOGUE | **Panic Disorder With Agoraphobia**

Nancy is a 27-year-old woman who was admitted to the psychiatric–mental health unit of a general hospital for treatment of panic disorder with agoraphobia. When Janet, her primary nurse, is assigned to her case, Nancy is crying inconsolably in her room.

Ineffective Approach

Nurse: Why are you crying?
Patient: (Stops crying briefly and gives the nurse a frightened look.) Because I'm upset. I don't want to be here.
Nurse: This is the best place you could be in your present condition.
Patient: I'm not crazy, if that's what you mean!
Nurse: Nobody said you were.
Patient: But you think it. Why else would I be here?
Nurse: To learn ways to deal with your disorder.
Patient: I don't have a *disorder.* Nerve problems run in my family. You'd know that if you had bothered to read my chart!
Nurse: (Looks about anxiously.) Maybe I should come back after you've calmed down a little.

Effective Approach

Nurse: Nancy, what's troubling you?
Patient: I feel so nervous all the time that I just don't know what to do.
Nurse: Can you tell me more about what "nervous" feels like for you?
Patient: I feel like I'm going crazy. I worry all the time about having another panic attack. They are so awful and make me scared I'm going to die.
Nurse: It sounds like there are at least two parts to this feeling.
Patient: (Pauses.) I don't understand what you mean.
Nurse: One part is that you wonder what this disorder means in terms of your mental health. And the second part has to do with how scary the panic attacks are.
Patient: (Sobbing loudly.) I'm not crazy! I just have nerve problems like my mother.

Nurse: (Remains silent.)
Patient: I don't know what to think anymore. What do you think is wrong with me?
Nurse: Nancy, what have you learned about the symptoms that you experience?
Patient: Well, I learned in relaxation group that panic symptoms are probably caused by chemicals in my brain that are not working correctly.
Nurse: What else have you learned?
Patient: I learned that medication can help the panics. I need to do my exposure plan and relaxation techniques to deal with my fears of leaving the house and my chronic anxiety.
Nurse: It sounds like you have learned that you have a biologic illness, one that can be treated, so that you don't always have to feel this way.
Patient: This is easier to say right now when I'm here and can get help if I need it. It's hard to remember this when I'm in the middle of a panic attack and think I'm dying.
Nurse: It's harder when you're alone?
Patient: Much harder! And I'm alone so much of the time.
Nurse: Let's talk about some ways you can manage your panics when you're alone. Tell me some of the techniques you've learned.

Critical Thinking Challenge

- What tone is established by the nurse's opening question in the first scenario?
- Which therapeutic communication techniques did the nurse use in the second scenario to avoid the pitfalls encountered in the first scenario?
- What information was uncovered in the second scenario that was not touched on in the first?
- What predictions can you make about the interpersonal relationship likely to develop between the nurse and the patient in each scenario?

and implementation of exposure therapy requires special training. Because of the multitude of outpatients in treatment for agoraphobia, exposure therapy would be a useful tool for home health psychiatric nurses.

Outcomes of home-based exposure treatment are not different from outcomes in clinic-based treatment.

Implosive Therapy. **Implosive therapy** is a provocative technique useful in treating agoraphobia in which the therapist identifies phobic stimuli for the patient and then presents highly anxiety-provoking imagery to the patient. The therapist describes the feared scene as dramatically and vividly as possible. **Flooding** is a technique used to desensitize the patient to the fear associated with a particular stimulus. This is done by repetitively presenting real objects or situations representing the most anxiety-provoking stimulus. There are no session breaks until the anxiety dissipates. For example, an individual who is afraid of snakes might be presented with a real snake repeatedly until his or her anxiety decreases.

Cognitive-Behavioral Therapy. CBT, often combined with pharmacotherapy, is a highly effective tool for the treatment of panic disorder. In fact, it has been considered first-line treatment for panic disorder along with other anxiety disorders. The goals of CBT include assisting the patient in the management of his or her anxiety and correcting anxiety-provoking thoughts. However, psychosocial therapies are not widely used and in fact may be declining because of length of therapy and reimbursement issues (Goisman, Warshaw, & Keller, 1999). Nevertheless, most patients who suffer panic disorder who are exposed to CBT benefit from the therapy (Barlow, 1997; Saeed & Bruce, 1998; Barlow et al., 2000).

Psychoeducation. Psychoeducation programs rebut myths and misinterpretations about the symptoms of panic. Individuals with panic disorder have fixed, legitimate fears of going crazy, of losing control, or that they are in imminent danger because of their physical symptoms. Arguing with or attempting to convince these patients to the contrary will heighten anxiety and impede therapeutic rapport. Information and physical evidence, such as electrocardiogram results, laboratory test results, and so forth should be presented in a caring and open manner demonstrating acceptance and understanding of their situation.

The accompanying Psychoeducation Checklist: Panic Disorder provides suggested topics for discussion that may be conducted individually or in a small group. It is especially important to cover such topics as the differences between panic attacks and heart attacks, the difference between panic disorder and other psychiatric disorders, and the effectiveness of various treatment methods.

PSYCHOEDUCATION CHECKLIST
Panic Disorder

When caring for the patient with panic disorder, be sure to include the following topic areas in the teaching plan:

- Psychopharmacologic agents (anxiolytics or antidepressants) if ordered, including drug action, dosage, frequency, and possible adverse effects
- Breathing control measures
- Nutrition
- Exercise
- Progressive muscle relaxation
- Distraction behaviors
- Exposure therapy
- Time management
- Positive coping strategies

Social Domain

Individuals with anxiety disorders, especially panic disorder and social phobias, often deteriorate socially. The disorder often takes it's toll on friend and family relationships. If the disorder becomes severe enough, the person may even isolate himself or herself completely from society. Therefore, the social domain must be assessed and treated.

Social Assessment

Marital and parental functioning is adversely affected in patients with panic disorders (Beck, 1998; Mendlowicz & Stein, 2000). During the assessment, the nurse should try to grasp the patient's understanding of how panic disorder with or without severe avoidance behavior has affected his or her life along with that of the family. Pertinent questions include the following:

- How has the disorder affected the social life of the family?
- What limitations has the disorder placed on the patient or family related to travel?
- What coping strategies has the patient used to manage symptoms?
- How has the disorder affected each family member or significant other?

Cultural Factors

Cultural competence calls for the understanding of cultural knowledge, cultural awareness, cultural assessment skills, and cultural practice. Therefore, cultural differences must be considered in the assessment of panic disorder. Different cultures interpret sensations, feelings, or understandings differently. For example, symptoms of anxiety might be seen as witchcraft or magic (APA,

2000). Additionally, some countries restrict women or children from being seen in public without body coverings. It is important that the nurse appreciates and respects the cultural values of the patient because they may differ from his or her own.

Social Interventions

Individuals with panic disorder, especially those with significant anxiety sensitivity, may need assistance in reevaluating their lifestyle. Time management can be a useful tool. Whether in the workplace or completing tasks at home, underestimating the time taken to complete a chore or being overinvolved in several activities at once increases stress and anxiety. Procrastination, lack of assertiveness, and difficulties with prioritizing or delegating tasks intensifies these problems.

Writing a list of chores to be completed, including estimated time to complete and actual time to complete, provides concrete feedback to the individual. Crossing out each activity as it is completed helps the patient to regain a sense of control and accomplishment. Large tasks should be broken into a series of smaller tasks to minimize stress and maximize sense of achievement. In completing a daily schedule, rest time, relaxation time, and family time are frequently omitted but must be included.

Family Response to Disorder

Families inflicted with panic disorder have difficulty with overall communication. Parents with agoraphobia may become critical of their childrearing abilities, which may cause their children to be overly dependent. Mothers with panic disorder often worry that their disorders will cause their children to develop excessive fears or phobic attitudes or to be excessive worriers (Beck, 1998). Individuals will need a tremendous amount of support and encouragement from significant others.

Indicated pharmacologic treatment for panic disorder also affects the family in other ways. Medications used to treat panic disorder readily cross the placenta and are excreted in breast milk, which may restrict treatment approaches (Beck, 1998; Altshuler et al., 1998). Although pregnancy may actually protect against certain anxiety disorders, postpartum onset is not uncommon. Decisions about taking medications during pregnancy and postdelivery child feeding may lead to guilt, anxiety, and an exacerbation of symptoms.

Evaluation and Treatment Outcomes

Patients can be assisted to keep a daily log of the severity of anxiety and the frequency, duration, and severity of episodes of panic. This will be a basic tool for monitoring progress as symptoms decrease over time. Rating scales may also be helpful to monitor changes in misinterpretations or other symptoms related to panic. Medications alone provide significant improvement for many individuals, but the effects appear to be only temporary. In the age of health care, when hard, measurable data are required for reimbursement for treatment, individuals with panic disorder often receive short-term improvement from medication. Symptom recurrence is common after the medication is discontinued. Long-term combined psychosocial and pharmacologic treatment is usually necessary.

Although many researchers consider panic disorder a chronic, long-term condition, the positive results from outcome studies should be shared with patients to provide encouragement and optimism that individuals can learn to manage these symptoms. Successful outcome studies have been produced for panic control treatment, CBT therapy, exposure therapy, and various medications specific to certain symptoms. Figure 21-2 illustrates a number of examples of biopsychosocial treatment outcomes for individuals with panic disorder.

Continuum of Care

As with any disorder, continuum of patient care across multiple settings is crucial. Patients are treated in the least restrictive environment that will meet their safety needs. As the patient progresses through treatment, the environment of care changes from an emergency or inpatient setting to outpatient clinics or individual therapy sessions.

Inpatient-Focused Care

Inpatient settings provide control for the stabilization of the acute panic symptoms. Often, medications are initiated here because patients who show initial panic symptoms require in-depth assessment to determine the etiology. The patient is formally introduced to the disorder after the diagnosis is made. As crisis stabilization begins, medication management, milieu, and psychotherapies are introduced, and discharge linkage appointments with outpatient health care providers are set at a level that will meet the patient's physical and emotional safety needs.

Emergency Care

Because individuals with panic disorder are more likely to first present for treatment in an emergency room or primary care setting, nurses working in these settings should be involved in early recognition and referral. Several interventions may be useful both in assisting the patient after the emergency care is given and in reducing the number of emergency room visits related to panic symptoms. Pamphlets on common psychiatric disorders, brief sessions with a psychiatric representative,

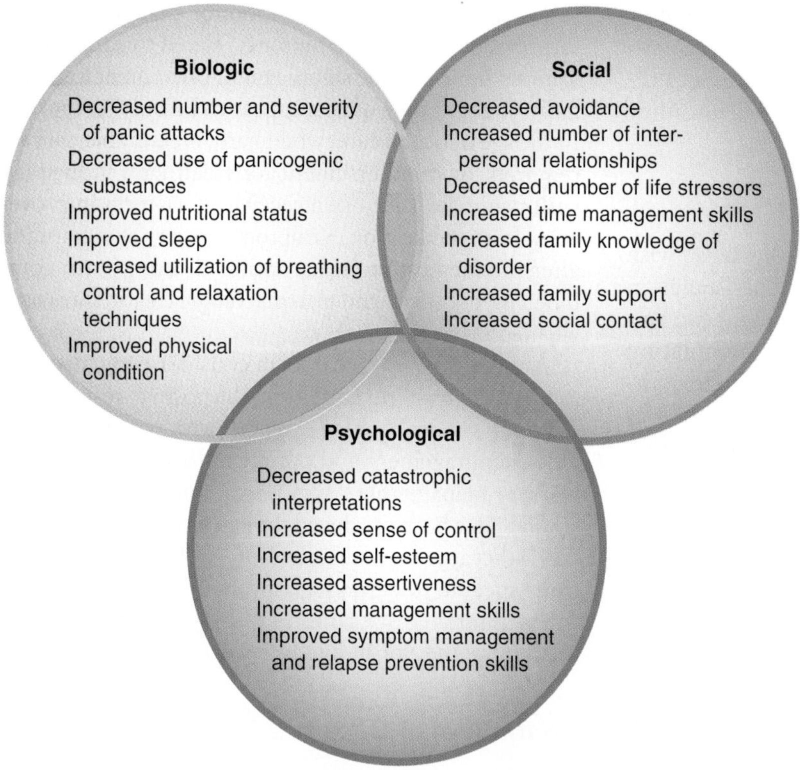

Biologic

Decreased number and severity
  of panic attacks
Decreased use of panicogenic
  substances
Improved nutritional status
Improved sleep
Increased utilization of breathing
  control and relaxation
  techniques
Improved physical
  condition

Social

Decreased avoidance
Increased number of inter-
  personal relationships
Decreased number of life stressors
Increased time management skills
Increased family knowledge of
  disorder
Increased family support
Increased social contact

Psychological

Decreased catastrophic
  interpretations
Increased sense of control
Increased self-esteem
Increased assertiveness
Increased management skills
Improved symptom management
  and relapse prevention skills

FIGURE 21.2 Biopsychosocial outcomes for patients with panic disorder.

and follow-up referrals to a mental health clinic may encourage the patients to exercise other options than the emergency room (Dyckman et al., 1999). Because of unnecessary emergency room visits and other services, it is estimated that effective treatment of panic disorder can result in a 90% reduction in the patient's medical costs (Rosenfeld, 1998).

Remembering that the patient experiencing a panic attack is in crisis, nurses can take several measures to help alleviate symptoms, including the following:

- Stay with the patient and maintain a calm demeanor. (Anxiety often produces more anxiety, and a calm presence will help calm the patient.)
- Reassure the patient that you will not leave, that this episode will pass, and that he or she is in a safe place. (The patient often fears dying and cannot see beyond the panic attack.)
- Give clear, concise directions, using short sentences. Do not use medical jargon.
- Assist the patient to an environment with minimal stimulation. Walk or pace with the patient. (The patient in panic has excessive energy.)
- Administer PRN anxiolytic medications as ordered and appropriate. (Pharmacotherapy is effective in treating acute panic.)

After the panic attack has resolved, allow the patient to vent his or her feelings. This often helps the patient in clarifying his or her feelings.

Family Interventions

In addition to becoming knowledgeable concerning the symptoms of panic disorder, nurses in these settings should have information sheets or pamphlets available concerning the disorder and any medications prescribed. Parents, especially single parents, will need assistance in childrearing practices and may benefit from services designed to provide some respite. Moreover, the entire family will need support in adjusting to the disorder. A referral for family therapy may be indicated. Involving the entire family in the therapy process is imperative. Families experience the symptoms, treatments, clinical setbacks, and recovery from chronic mental illnesses as a unit. Misunderstandings, misconceptions, false information, and stigma of mental illness singly or collectively impede recovery efforts.

Community Treatment

Most individuals with panic disorder will be treated on an outpatient basis. Referral lists of community resources and support groups are also useful. Nurses in these settings are more directly involved in treatment by conducting psychoeducation groups on relaxation and breathing techniques, symptom management, and anger management. Advanced practice nurses are involved in conducting CBT and individual and family psychotherapy. Additionally, medication monitoring groups re-emphasize the role of the medications, monitor for side effects, and enhance treatment compliance overall. See Nursing Care Plan 21-1 and the Interdisciplinary Treatment Plan that follows it.

OBSESSIVE-COMPULSIVE DISORDER

Obsessive-compulsive disorder (OCD) is a relatively rare psychiatric disorder characterized by severe obsessions or compulsions that interfere with normal daily routines. The impact of the obsessions and compulsions has devastating consequences for the individual.

Obsessions are characterized by excessive, unwanted, and thoughts or impulses that occur repetitively causing severe anxiety and distress. Common obsessions include fears of contamination, pathologic doubt, the need for symmetry and completion, thoughts of hurting someone, and thoughts of sexual images (APA, 2000). Compulsions are employed in an attempt to neutralize the anxiety felt from the obsession. Compulsions therefore are repetitive actions or behaviors. For example, people with obsessive thoughts of becoming contaminated with dirt may begin to wash their hands repeatedly to keep from becoming contaminated.

KEY CONCEPT Obsessions. **Obsessions** are unwanted, intrusive, and persistent thoughts, impulses, or images that cause anxiety and distress. Obsessions are considered ego-dystonic because they are not under the patient's control and are incongruent with the patient's usual thought patterns.

KEY CONCEPT Compulsions. **Compulsions** are behaviors that are performed repeatedly, in a ritualistic fashion, with the goal of preventing or relieving anxiety and distress caused by obsessions.

Obsessions and compulsions are also not necessarily signs of a psychiatric disorder if they are short lived and do not persistently interfere with the person's ability to function. However, obsessions consume the judgment of a person to the degree that most of his or her day is spent performing actions in attempt to minimize severe anxiety.

Clinical Course of Disorder

The typical age of onset of OCD is in the early to late 20s in females and between 6 and 15 years of age in males. Males are affected most often in the childhood years (Castle & Groves, 2000). Males are most commonly affected by ruminations, and women have a higher incidence of checking and cleaning rituals (Castle & Groves, 2000). Even though many patients have symptoms of OCD beginning in childhood, many

receive treatment only after the disorder has significantly affected their lives. In childhood, the astute parent may notice that the child spends great amounts of time on trivial tasks or has falling grades owing to poor concentration. Symptom onset of the disorder is gradual, and 15% of inflicted people show progressive decline in social and occupational functioning (APA, 2000). This chronic disorder is characterized by episodes of symptom amelioration and exacerbation during its course.

During the course of the disorder, the patient begins to realize that the obsessive thought and compulsive actions are excessive and unnecessary but continues to have thoughts and feels compelled to perform compulsions. The obsessions are determined to be ego-dystonic. This means that they are alien to the person, are not able to be controlled by the person, and are not the kind of thoughts that the person would tend to have (APA, 2000).

Comorbidity

Tourette's syndrome has an interesting relationship with OCD. There are estimates that up to 50% of patients with Tourette's syndrome also have OCD. Other psychiatric disorders co-occur as well. Two thirds of individuals with OCD subsequently experience depression because of the impact of the disorder on their lifestyle. A significant number of older depressed patients have OCD (Beekman et al., 2000). Additionally, up to 60% of people with OCD experience panic attacks. The lifetime risk for panic disorder, social phobia, specific phobias, and eating disorders is significantly greater in patients with OCD than in the general population.

Because the stress to perform compulsions resulting from obsessions is untenable, many patients attempt to self-medicate to relieve the anxiety produced by obsessive thoughts. About one third will suffer from substance abuse or dependence in their lifetime. Additionally, some patients may abuse the use of benzodiazepines and other anxiolytics, hypnotic, and sedative drugs.

Personality disorders are also prevalent in OCD, occurring in more than 80% of patients. Most prevalent are cluster C disorders (see Chap. 22). It was once thought that obsessive-compulsive personality disorder predisposed an individual to the development of OCD and would, therefore, be the most commonly diagnosed. However, dependent personality disorder is the most frequent coexisting disorder, diagnosed in about half of patients with OCD. Other personality disorders occurring at rates higher than for the general population, in descending order of frequency, include obsessive-compulsive, avoidant, borderline, schizotypal, and paranoid personality disorders (Black et al., 1993).

(text continues on page 483)

NURSING CARE PLAN 21.1
Patient With Panic Disorder

RW is a 78-year-old Asian American man who began having his first panic attacks shortly after his wife died 2 years ago. He has been able to live alone until recently, when his daughter became concerned that there was not food in the house. He admitted to being fearful of leaving because of extreme nervousness and fear of a panic attack. His daughter convinced him to seek help, and he is now in a day treatment program at a local facility. He is able to attend the program most days.

SETTING: DAY TREATMENT PROGRAM, GERIATRIC PSYCHIATRIC SERVICES

Baseline Assessment: RW averages three or four panic attacks per week. His mental status is normal, with no cognitive impairment. MMSE within normal limits. He is slightly depressed but does not meet criteria for depressive disorder. He misses his wife, but is relieved that she is no longer suffering. Vital signs are normal. He has a history of slight cardiac arrhythmias that are being treated with medications. He would like to "get rid of the feeling of nervousness" and be able to enjoy what is left of his life.

Associated Psychiatric Diagnosis	Medications

Axis I: Panic disorder with agoraphobia
Axis II: None
Axis III: History of cardiac arrhythmias
Axis IV: Social problems (unable to leave home)
  GAF = Current 60
        Potential 90
	Sertraline (Zoloft) 25 mg qd
	Procainamide (Pronestyl, Procan-SR) 750 mg bid
	Lorazepam (Ativan) 0.5 mg PRN for extreme anxiety

NURSING DIAGNOSIS 1: ANXIETY

Defining Characteristics	Related Factors
Trembling, increased pulse Fearful, irritable, scared, worried Apprehensive	Impending panic attacks Panic attacks

OUTCOMES

Initial	Long-term
Develop skills to decrease impact of panic attack	Carry-out normal daily living and social activities outside of the house.

INTERVENTIONS

Interventions	Rationale	Ongoing Assessment
Meet daily with RW to assess if he has had a panic attack within the last 24 hours.	Asking RW to monitor panic attacks will provide data regarding potential antecedents to attacks.	Determine whether RW has had a panic attack. Explore the antecedents and whether or not he was able to practice techniques from education programs.
Using a calm, reassuring approach, encourage verbalization of feelings, perceptions, and fears. Identify periods of time when anxiety is at its highest.	Discussion of the experience of anxiety will help the patient identify when his anxiety increases.	Determine his commitment to living a more normal life.
Instruct RW on the use of relaxation techniques.	Having strategies to deal with impending panic attack will decrease the intensity of the experience.	Observe effectiveness of his technique and changes in anxiety/panic episodes.
Teach patient about the actions and side effects of sertraline. Explain the purposes of the medication. Track the number of PRN medications that are used for anxiety. Also, monitor for use of alcohol and herbal supplements.	Panic attacks are neurobiologic occurrences that respond to medications.	Determine whether panic attacks decrease over time and whether there are side effects.

(continued)

NURSING CARE PLAN 21.1 (Continued)

EVALUATION

Outcomes	Revised Outcomes	Interventions
RW's panic attacks decreased to once a week. Attended day treatment program everyday. Able to go to grocery store.	Increase social activity outside of house.	Meet with RW twice a week to monitor progress. Continue to reinforce the use of strategies in managing anticipatory anxiety.

INTERDISCIPLINARY TREATMENT PLAN 21.1
Patient With Panic Disorder

GERIATRIC PSYCHIATRIC CENTER DAY TREATMENT PROGRAM FOR RW, A 78-YEAR-OLD MALE

Admission Date:	Date of This Plan:	Type of Plan: Check Appropriate Box					
1/5/01	1/6/01	☒ Initial	☐ Master	☐ 30	☐ 60	☐ 90	☐ Other

Treatment Team Present:
Smith, M., MD; S. Jones, RNC; G. Stevens, LCSW (social worker); V. Bond (Music Therapist)

DIAGNOSIS (*DSM-IV-TR*):

AXIS I: Panic disorder with agoraphobia
AXIS II: None
AXIS III: History of cardiac arrhythmias
AXIS IV: Social Problems (unable to leave home)
AXIS V: Current GAF: 60
              Highest level GAF this past year: 90

ASSETS (MEDICAL, PSYCHOLOGICAL, SOCIAL, EDUCATIONAL, VOCATIONAL, RECREATIONAL):

1. No physical illness evident
2. Cognitive abilities intact, normal MMSE, wants to get better
3. Family supportive. Daughter is primary support and helps with cleaning and shopping. Able to live alone. Has a few old friends. Is able to drive.
4. Now retired. Worked as an accountant for many years. Enjoys card games with friends. Able to maintain his own home.

MASTER PROBLEM LIST

Prob. No.	Date	Problem	Code	Change Code	Change Date
1.	1/5/01	Recurring panic attacks interfere with his ability to engage in social activities and maintain independence.	T		
2.					
3.					
4.					
5.					
6.					
7.					
8.					

CODE T = Problem must be addressed in treatment.
       N = Problem noted and will be monitored.
       X = Problem noted, but deferred/inactive/no action necessary.
       O = Problem to be addressed in aftercare/continuing care.
       I = Problem incorporated into another problem.
       R = Resolved.

INDIVIDUAL TREATMENT PLAN PROBLEM SHEET

# Problem/Need:	Date Identified	Problem Resolved/Discontinuation Date
Recurring panic attacks interfere with his ability to engage in social activities and maintain independence.	1/5/01	

Objective(s)/Short-Term Goals:	Target Date	Achievement Date
1. Patient reports that there is no more than 2 panic attacks per week (down from 2–3 daily)	2/05/01	
2. Patient begins to go places outside of home.	3/5/01	

Treatment Interventions:	Frequency	Person Responsible
Attend day treatment program.	Daily	RN monitor attendance
Relaxation group	Daily	AT
Panic Disorders Education Group	Daily	SW, RN
Individual counseling for monitoring anxiety and panic attacks	Daily	RN
Medications for anxiety and prevention of panic attacks	Daily	MD/RN
Family support group (patient's family)	Weekly	SW

Describe Patient Participation (and/or family, guardian, other agencies, significant others):

Responsible QMHP   **Patient or Guardian**   **Staff Physician**

Signature   Date   Signature   Date   Signature   Date

Cluster A personality disorders may predict poorer treatment outcomes.

Diagnostic Criteria

The APA (2000) described five diagnostic criteria for OCD:

Criterion A. The presence of obsessions or compulsions. Obsessions are defined as (1) persistent thoughts, images, or impulses that are intrusive and inappropriate causing marked anxiety and (2) are not simply excessive fretting over real-life situations; (3) the person tries to ignore or suppress the thoughts, or tries to neutralize them by employing compulsions; and (4) the person understands that the thoughts are a product of his or her own mind. Compulsions are defined as (1) repetitive behaviors that the person feels he or she must perform because of the thoughts or because of rules that must be rigidly followed, and (2) actions performed to reduce stress or to prevent a catastrophe from occurring. The actions and thoughts are not realistically connected and are excessive to the situation.

Criterion B. At some point in the disorder, the patient recognizes that the thoughts and actions are excessive. This does not apply to children.

Criterion C. The presence of the thoughts and rituals cause severe disturbance in performing daily routines or are time-consuming, taking longer than 1 hour a day to complete.

Criterion D. The thoughts or behaviors are not a result of another Axis 1 disorder.

Criterion E. The thoughts or behaviors are not a result of the presence of a substance or a medical condition.

The specifier With Poor Insight is added if the patient does not see that the thoughts or behaviors are excessive or unreasonable.

Obsessive-Compulsive Disorder in Special Populations

OCD affects people across the life span. Proper identification, diagnosis, and treatment of OCD is imperative for the recovery of the patient and to bring him or her to an optimal level of functioning.

Children

OCD affects between 1% and 2.3% of the child and adolescent population, but may affect more. As children subscribe to myths, superstition, and magical thinking in childhood, obsessive and ritualistic behaviors may go unnoticed. Behaviors such as touching every third tree, avoiding cracks in the sidewalk, or consistently verbalizing fears of losing a parent in an accident may have some underlying pathology, but are common behaviors in childhood. Typically, parents begin to notice that a child's grades begin to fall as a result of decrease concentration and spending great amounts of time performing rituals.

Elderly People

OCD is a disorder that typically manifests in childhood and the second decade of life. It can be a lifelong illness that can last more than 30 years. Predictors of poor outcomes during lifelong treatment include an initial onset of symptoms during childhood, low social functioning, and the prevalence of both obsessions and compulsions (Castle & Groves, 2000).

Epidemiology

OCD has a 2.5% lifetime prevalence and a 1-year prevalence rate of 0.5% to 2.1% in the adult population. Rates of OCD are similar among women and men. A familial trait must exist because first-degree relatives with OCD have a higher prevalence rate than the general population.

Many obsessive thoughts and compulsive acts are common in OCD. Checking rituals are common in this disorder, and those who perform these rituals are usually considered perfectionists. These patients must have objects in a certain order, perform motor activities in a rigid fashion, or have things perfectly symmetric. They may take a great deal of time to complete even the simplest task. These individuals tend to experience discontent, rather than anxiety, when things are not symmetric or perfect. Other patients have magical thinking and perform compulsive rituals to ward off an imagined disaster. They use counting rituals to perform doing-and-undoing rituals (eg, repeatedly turning on and off the alarm clock) to help them feel that a disaster will not occur. Hoarders feel compelled to check their belongings repeatedly to see that all is accounted for, and they may check the garbage to ensure that nothing of value was cast out.

Some patients have obsessions surrounding aggressive acts of hurting someone or themselves. After hitting a bump in the road, for example, these patients may obsess for hours over whether or not they hit a person.

Patients with religious obsessions obsess over the meaning of sins and whether they have followed the letter of the law. They tend to be hypermoral and have the need to confess. They may view their obsessions as a form of religious suffering. Often, these patients are resistant to treatment. The frequency of religious obsessions is higher in areas of the world where severe religious restrictions exist. Diagnosis is not made unless the thoughts or rituals are clearly in excess of cultural or religious norms, occur at inappropriate times as described by members of the same religion or culture, or interfere with social obligations (APA, 2000).

People with OCD are highly somatic and frequently seek medical treatment for physical symptoms, often just to get reassurance. AIDS, cancer, heart attacks, and venereal diseases are some of the most common obsessional fears.

Etiology

During the 1990s, research evidence from neuroimaging studies, neurochemical studies, and treatment advances have substantiated a predominantly neurobiologic basis for OCD. The following sections provide a brief overview of these research findings as well as evidence for a genetic vulnerability. Psychological factors are also discussed because of their contributions to the disorder. Because no one explanation accounts for all aspects of OCD, it is likely that a combination of explanations will be found to produce the disorder.

Biologic Theories

Research suggests that OCD has a biologic basis involving several neuroanatomic structures. Genetic, neuropathologic, and biochemical research is reviewed in this section.

Genetic. OCD occurs more often in people who have first-degree relatives with OCD or with Tourette's disorder than it does in the general population. Some studies have also shown an increased prevalence of anxiety and mood disorders in relatives of individuals who have OCD. Studies of twins have indicated that OCD occurs more frequently in both siblings of monozygotic twins than in dizygotic twins. Furthermore, Mundo and colleagues (2000) discovered a link between the pathogenesis of OCD and the 5-HT (β_{1D}) receptor gene. This may lead to breakthroughs in pharmacologic treatments of OCD.

Neuropathologic. Structural neuroimaging studies using computed tomography and magnetic resonance imaging of patients with OCD have been performed to find total-volume differences in brain structures in people with OCD. Specifically, affected individuals have enlarged basal ganglia (caudate, putamen, and globus pallidus) (Giedd et al., 2000).

Positron emission tomography and single-photon emission computed tomography reveal differences in cerebral glucose metabolism between patients with OCD and controls (see Chap. 18, Figure 18-3). Variation in methods of measurement produces some inconsistencies in the research findings. However, the most replicated

results demonstrate increased glucose metabolism in the caudate nuclei (part of the basal ganglia), the orbitofrontal gyri (the gyri directly above the orbit of the eye), and the cingulate gyri (considered to be part of the limbic system). Studies measuring cerebral blood flow and glucose metabolism in OCD patients during exposure to feared stimuli and during relaxation have further implicated these regions of the brain (Baxter, 1992; Rauch et al., 1994).

Biochemical. Serotonin does play a role in OCD. It has been studied through challenge tests in which serotonin agonists was administered to OCD patients and controls. The most convincing evidence for serotonin's role in OCD comes from the fact that antidepressants acting more specifically on serotonin relieve the symptoms of OCD for most patients. It is unlikely that one particular neurotransmitter is responsible for OCD, but to date, serotonin is the only neurotransmitter to have been implicated in the disorder. Antipsychotic medications have been used in conjunction with serotonin-targeting medications to treat refractory symptoms, indicating that another biochemical process may exist.

Psychological Theories

Psychological theories of OCD have not been scientifically tested, yet a rich literature exists describing clinical examples and case histories. These theories may still provide a basis for understanding the symptoms and behaviors related to OCD. Additionally, behavioral treatment of individuals with severe compulsions has resulted in symptom improvement.

Psychodynamic. The psychodynamic theory hypothesizes that OCD symptoms and character traits arise from implementation of three unconscious defense mechanisms: isolation (separation of affect from a thought or impulse), undoing (an act performed with the goal of preventing consequences of a thought or impulse), and reaction formation (behavior and consciously stated attitudes that are opposite to underlying impulses). Classic psychoanalytic theory describes OCD as regression from the oedipal phase to the anal phase of development (see Chap. 6). This regression occurs when the patient becomes anxious about retaliation or loss of love from a significant other. The anal phase is ambivalent, sadistic, and preoccupied with anger and dirt, hence the frequent occurrence of aggression and cleanliness obsessions.

Behavioral. Behavioral explanations for OCD stem from learning theory. From this viewpoint, obsessions are seen as conditioned stimuli. Through a process of being associated with noxious events, stimuli that are usually thought of as neutral become anxiety provoking. The individual then engages in activities to escape or avoid the anxiety. Compulsions then develop as the individual discovers behaviors that successfully reduce the obsessional anxiety. As the principles of operant conditioning indicate, the more successful the individual is at decreasing the anxiety, the more likely the compulsions will continue to be used. However, the rituals or compulsions preserve the fear response because the person avoids the initial stimuli and thus never extinguishes the behavior. Interrupting this cycle is the focus of behavioral therapy in treating an individual with OCD.

Risk Factors

Studies have found a link between infection with β-hemolytic streptococci and OCD (Giedd et al., 2000; Castle & Groves, 2000). Additionally, higher rates of OCD have been found among individuals who are young, divorced or separated, and unemployed. OCD appears to be less common among African Americans than among non-Hispanic whites.

Interdisciplinary Treatment

Patients with OCD can be difficult to treat because of the symptoms and the pathology of the disease. The obsessions and compulsions consistently interfere with recovery efforts during the treatment course. Staff may have differing opinions about the amount of control the patient has over the behavior, but it is extremely important that these differences of opinion be resolved within the multidisciplinary treatment plan and that all staff be consistent in their expectations and acceptance of the patient's behaviors. Consistency in treatment is essential so that these patients do not become confused regarding treatment expectations (Text Box 21-4).

Priority Care Issues

As with any patient with a psychiatric disorder, a suicide assessment must be completed. OCD causes great distress to the patient, who realizes the frustration and absurdness of the behaviors. Often, the patient has tolerated symptoms for quite some time before seeking treatment. The patient may feel a sense of hopelessness and helplessness and may contemplate suicide to end the suffering. An additional risk for suicide is created by the high probability of comorbid major depression, which often accompanies OCD.

Patient who are at risk for self-harm require personal and environmental protective measures. Some patients have aggressive obsessions, and it may be necessary to provide external limits for protection of others (see Chap. 36).

TEXT BOX 21.4

Critical Thinking Dilemma: Obsessive-Compulsive Disorder

Sarah is primary nurse for Joan, a patient with OCD. Joan's obsessions relate to cleanliness and are followed by compulsions to bathe five times per day. Joan insists that the tub be cleaned before and after each use and is unable to do this for herself, fearing contamination. The nursing assistants are assigned to help Joan with baths and are angry. Their statements include, "Joan is doing this just to get our attention away from other patients. She doesn't really need all these baths. We should lock her out of the bathroom."

Critical Thinking Questions
1. How might the beliefs of the nursing assistants affect Joan's care?
2. How might Sarah's interventions be altered at different points in time during Joan's hospital stay?
3. How can Sarah explain Joan's unusual behaviors to the nursing assistants? How can she develop a consistent team approach to Joan's care?

Nursing Diagnoses and Outcome Identification

Patients with OCD may present with any number of symptoms, depending on the particular obsession and the compulsions that have evolved to cope with that obsession. As a result, the nursing diagnoses applied to patients with this disorder can run the gamut from the primary diagnosis of Anxiety to other physiologic disturbances of the compulsion, such as Skin Integrity, Impaired, which may result from continuous hand washing. Outcomes depend on the selected nursing diagnoses and treatment modalities.

NURSING MANAGEMENT: HUMAN RESPONSE TO DISORDER

Obsessions create tremendous anxiety in the individual with OCD, and the person performs compulsions, or rituals, to relieved the anxiety temporarily. If the compensatory ritual is not performed, the person feels increased anxiety and distress. Common compulsions include washing, cleaning, checking, counting, repeating actions, ordering (eg, insisting items be stored in a particular manner), making confessions (eg, repeatedly confessing to past misconduct), and requesting assurances.

Individuals with OCD do not consider their compulsions to derive pleasure. They simply act on the obsessions to minimize anxiety and tension, and often they recognize them as odd and may initially try to resist them. Resistance in performing compulsions eventually fail, and repetitive behaviors are incorporated into daily routines. The routines tend to develop into a ritual of performing activities daily in a specific order. If the sequence is disturbed, the person experiences extreme anxiety until the process can be repeated in the correct sequence (Table 21-10).

The most commonly seen obsession is focused on fear of contamination and a resulting compulsion toward hand washing. These fears of contamination are usually focused on dirt or germs, but other materials may be feared as well, such as toxic chemicals, poison, radiation, an heavy metals. Patients with contamination obsessions report anxiety as their most common effect, but shame and disgust, which are in turn linked with embarrassment and guilt, are experienced as well.

Patients with OCD may become incapacitated by the extensiveness of their symptoms. They may spend most of their waking hours locked in a cycle of obsessions and compulsions. They may reach the point of being unable to complete as simple a task as walking through a door without becoming involved in rituals surrounding this activity. Interpersonal relationships suffer, and the patient may become isolative as he or she becomes a prisoner of the symptoms of OCD and of the embarrassment of having to perform rituals in public.

Patients with OCD may employ dissociation as a defense mechanism. (see Table 6-2 in Chap. 6). **Depersonalization** is a dissociative-type symptom that can be particularly predominant. It is a nonspecific experience in which the individual loses the sense of personal identity and feels strange or unreal. The repetitive acts or compulsions of OCD are sometimes experienced by the individual in a depersonalized manner, as if their body is performing these acts without their intention or will. OCD patients who have dissociative symptoms tend to have more severe OCD symptoms and more depression and are more likely to have a coexisting personality disorder.

Biologic Domain

Biologic Assessment

Patients with OCD do not have a higher prevalence of physical disease. However, they may complain of multiple physical symptoms. With late-onset OCD (after 35 years of age) and with symptoms that occur with a febrile illness, cerebral pathology should be ruled out. Each patient with OCD should be assessed for derma-

TABLE 21.10 Key Diagnostic Characteristics of Obsessive-Compulsive Disorder 300.3	
Diagnostic Criteria and Target Symptoms	**Associated Findings**

• Recurrent obsession or compulsions
  Obsessions: inappropriate and intrusive recurrent and persistent thoughts, impulses, or images causing marked anxiety or distress that are not simply excessive worries
  Attempts to ignore, suppress, or neutralize obsessions with some other thought or action
  Recognizes them as a product of his or her own mind
  Compulsions: repetitive behaviors (such as hand-washing, ordering, checking) or mental acts (such as praying, counting) person feels driven to perform in response to obsession or according to rigid rules
  Acts aimed at preventing or reducing the distress or preventing some dreaded event or situation
  Compulsions not connected realistically with what they are designed to neutralize or prevent or are clearly excessive
• Recognition by person that obsessions or compulsions are excessive or unrealistic (if not, specify with poor insight)
• Obsessions or compulsions are excessive or unrealistic
• Marked distress that is time-consuming or significantly interfering with normal routine and functioning
• If another psychiatric disorder present, content of obsessions or compulsions not restricted to it
• Not a direct physiologic effect of substance use or medical condition
	Associated Behavioral Findings
	• Avoidance of situations involving the content of the obsession or compulsion
	• Hypochondriacal concerns with frequent physician visits
	• Guilt
	• Sleep disturbances
	• Excessive use of alcohol or sedative, hypnotic, or anxiolytic medications
	• Compulsion performance a major life activity; may lead to serious marital, occupational, or social disability
	
	Associated Physical Examination Findings
	• Possible dermatologic problems caused by excessive washing with water or caustic cleaning agents
	
	Associated Laboratory Findings
	• Increase autonomic activity when confronted with circumstances that trigger obsession

tologic lesions secondary to repetitive hand washing, excessive cleaning with caustic agents, or bathing. Osteoarthritic joint damage secondary to cleaning rituals may be observed.

Other conditions that have a high comorbidity with OCD include head trauma, Economo's encephalitis (commonly known as *sleeping sickness*), abnormalities in the birth process, diabetes insipidus, Huntington's and Sydenham's chorea, and possibly some seizure disorders (Taylor & Gorman, 1992).

Biologic Interventions

Electroconvulsive Therapy. ECT has not been effective in reducing obsessions or compulsions in OCD, but it is helpful in treating obsessional symptoms that occur in depression. It also may be used in the treatment of depressive symptoms in patients who have not responded to other treatments and who are at risk for suicide. Nursing's role in caring for the patient undergoing ECT is outlined in Chapter 20.

Psychosurgery. Psychosurgery has been used to treat extremely severe OCD that has not responded to prolonged and intensive drug treatment, behavioral therapy, or a combination of the two. Modern stereotactic surgical techniques that produce lesions of the cingulum bundle or anterior limb of the internal capsule may bring about substantial clinical benefit in some patients without causing significant morbidity (Gelder, 1992; Goodman et al., 1993). There is some indication that other types of treatments, such as pharmacotherapy and behavior therapy, are more likely to be effective in the treatment-resistant OCD patient after psychosurgery (Mindus & Jenike, 1992).

Maintaining Skin Integrity. For the patient with cleaning or hand-washing compulsions, attention to skin condition is necessary. Encourage the patient to use tepid water when washing and hand cream after washing. Remove harsh, abrasive soaps and replace with moisturizing soaps. Attempt to decrease the frequency of washing by agreeing on a time schedule and time-limited washing.

Psychopharmacologic Treatment. The SSRIs and TCAs are considered to be the most effective treatment agents used for OCD. Clomipramine was the first drug to produce significant advances in the treatment of OCD. Other medications have proved effective in the treatment, including sertraline, fluoxetine, fluvoxamine, and paroxetine.

Other drugs may be used to treat refractory OCD symptoms, including MAOIs, lithium, and some anticonvulsants. Risperidone (Risperdal) and haloperidol (Haldol), both neuroleptics, have also been used to augment the SSRIs, but their use is limited.

Monitoring and Administration of Medications. Antidepressants used to treat OCD are often given in higher doses than what is usually used for the treatment of depression. Aggressive treatment may be indicated to bring the symptoms under control. Medication effects therefore must be closely monitored, including signs of toxicity, to provide safe and adequate care. These medications often take several weeks and even months to relieve the compulsions, and even longer to decrease obsessions.

Clomipramine pharmacotherapy should begin at 25 mg daily, with subsequent titration to 100 mg daily in divided doses within 2 weeks. The dosage can be increased to 250 mg in divided doses if symptoms persist. The maximum dose set for children is 200 mg daily in divided doses.

Sertraline and fluvoxamine are indicated for OCD and should be initiated at 50 mg daily. Sertraline can be titrated to a maximum dose of 200 mg daily, but in increments not to exceed 1 week. Fluvoxamine can be titrated 50 mg daily every 4 to 7 days to a maximum daily dose of 300 mg. Doses over 100 mg should be in divided doses.

Paroxetine or fluoxetine should be started at 20 mg daily, usually in the morning. Paroxetine is to be titrated 10 mg per week in weekly intervals to a maximum of 50 mg daily. Fluoxetine dose is titrated according to patient response to a maximum of 100 mg daily.

Side-Effect Monitoring. Side effects pose a particular problem for some individuals who are preoccupied with somatic concerns. Unwanted physical symptoms from the medications can become the focus of obsessions. These individuals particularly need frequent reassurance that the side effects are a common response to medication and that they are not becoming physically ill. To ignore or minimize these concerns will only heighten the patient's anxiety and potentially interfere with the desire to continue treatment.

Common side effects of clomipramine include significant sedation, anticholinergic side effects, and an increased risk for seizures. Dizziness, tremulousness, and headache are frequent complaints. The medication can be given at night to minimize the complaints of sedation and fatigue.

SSRIs also share side effects of sedation, dizziness, somnolence, and headache as well. Additionally, sexual dysfunction is a frequent complaint in patients being treated with fluvoxamine, sertraline, paroxetine, and fluoxetine. The SSRIs can cause excitability in patients when first started on the medications. Monitor for insomnia and adjust the dose time if needed.

Drug–Drug Interactions. All antidepressant medications interact with other CNS depressants including alcohol by producing CNS depression, and with MAOIs, causing hypertensive crises. Therefore, concomitant use should be avoided. Additionally, sertraline interacts with diazepam and tolbutamide. Clomipramine interacts with histamine-2 blockers, methylphenidate, oral contraceptives, clonidine, epinephrine, and norepinephrine. Paroxetine has documented interactions with histamine-2 blockers (cimetidine), digoxin, anticonvulsants, procyclidine, and warfarin. Fluoxetine interacts with flecainide, carbamazepine, vinblastine, insulin, and oral antidiabetic agents, lithium and other TCAs, Dilantin, tryptophan, and warfarin.

Drug–drug interactions with fluvoxamine include astemizole, terfenadine, benzodiazepines, theophylline, and warfarin. Additionally, carbamazepine, clozapine, methadone, metopranol, propanolol (Inderal), TCAs, diltiazem, lithium, and tryptophan create potential interactions.

Because of the extensive list of drug–drug interactions associated with these medications, a prudent nurse would consult a drug reference handbook before administering medications. The quick recognition of signs and symptoms of interactions or toxic symptoms are imperative for safe care.

Teaching Points. Nurses play an important interdisciplinary role in medication management for the patient with OCD. That role includes patient and family medication education. All patients should be warned not to stop the prescribed medications abruptly. Because patients may become discontent with the perceived lack of effect from the medications, they should be informed that these medications may take several weeks before their effects are felt.

Patients should be instructed not to operate heavy machinery while taking these medications until the sedative effects are known to the patient. Alcohol should be avoided. Finally, instruct the patient to inform his or her provider about any over-the-counter medications that he or she wishes to take because some will interact with these medications to produce serious effects.

Psychological Domain

Psychological Assessment

The nurse should assess the type and severity of the patient's obsessions and compulsions. If the assessment is occurring in a hospital, the nurse should remember that some OCD patients experience a transient decrease in symptoms when admitted to a hospital; therefore, it is important to allow enough time for an accurate assessment. Because this may not be possible, family members or significant others may provide an important source of information, with the patient's permission.

Most often, the individual will appear neatly dressed and groomed, cooperative, and ready to answer questions. Orientation and memory are not usually impaired, but at times they may be distracted by obsessional thoughts. For individuals with severe symptoms,

thought content may be preoccupied with fears or discussion of their obsessions, but in most instances, direct questions must be asked to reveal symptoms of the disorder. For example, the nurse may begin indirectly by asking how long it takes the individual to dress in the morning or leave the house, but usually follow-up questions are needed, such as: Do you find yourself frequently returning to the house to make sure that you have turned off the lights or the stove, even when you know that you have already checked this? Does this happen every day? Are you ever late for work or for important appointments?

Speech will be of normal rate and volume, but often, individuals with an obsessional style of thinking will exhibit circumferential speech. This speech is loaded with irrelevant details but eventually addresses the question. It may be frustrating and require considerable patience, but it is important to remember that it is part of the disorder and may be beyond the patient's awareness. Continually interrupting and redirecting them can interfere with the establishment of a therapeutic relationship, especially in the initial assessment. Redirection should be done in a gentle and noncritical manner to allow the patient to refocus.

It is important to identify the degree to which the OCD symptoms interfere with the patient's daily functioning. Therefore, several rating scales exist to assist in identifying symptoms and monitoring improvement. Examples of these scales are provided in Text Box 21-5. Some of these scales are to be used by the nurse; others are self-rating scales. The (Yale-Brown Obsessive Compulsive Scale (Y-BOCS) is a highly used, clinician-rated 16-item scale that obtains separate subtotals for severity of obsessions and compulsions. The Maudsley Obsessive-Compulsive Inventory is a 30-item, true–false, self-assessment tool that may be helpful in

TEXT BOX 21.5

Rating Scales for the Assessment of Obsessive-Compulsive Symptoms

Yale-Brown Obsessive Compulsive Scale (Y-BOCS)
Goodman, W., Price, L., Rasmussen, S., et al. (1989). The Yale-Brown obsessive compulsive scale (Y-BOCS): Part I. Development, use and reliability. *Archives of General Psychiatry, 46,* 1006–1011.

The Maudsley Obsessional-Compulsive Inventory (MOC)
Rachman, S., & Hodgson, R. (1980). *Obsessions and compulsions.* New York: Prentice-Hall.

The Leyton Obsessional Inventory
Cooper, J. (1970). The Leyton obsessional inventory. *Psychiatric Medicine, 1,* 48.

assisting the individual in recognizing individual target symptoms.

Psychological Interventions

The nurse's interpersonal skills are crucial to successful intervention with the patient who has OCD. Nurses must control their own anxiety. The nurse should interact with the patient in a calm, nonauthoritarian fashion while demonstrating empathy. It is important that the patient know that the nurse is concerned about the life distress that the disorder has caused and that the nurse does not disapprove of the patient or the patient's behaviors. The ability to acknowledge the patient's distress without focusing solely on the ritualistic behaviors is one of the most effective means available for communicating an appreciation for the individual as separate from the illness.

Response Prevention. A behavioral intervention for patients with OCD is exposure with response prevention. This technique is used for OCD patients with rituals. The patient is exposed to situations or objects that are known to induce anxiety. At the same time, the patient is asked to refrain from performing the ritualistic behaviors that have been developed to cope with the anxiety. One goal of this procedure is to help the patient understand that exposure to the feared object while resisting the accompanying rituals is less stressful and time-consuming than performing the compulsive behaviors employed to minimize the anxiety. Another goal is to disconfirm the expectation of distressing outcomes and eventually extinguish the compulsive behaviors. Between 60% and 70% of patients improve with exposure and response prevention, but few are completely symptom free (Gelder, 1992).

Thought Stopping. Thought stopping is used with patients who have obsessional thoughts. The patient is taught to interrupt obsessional thoughts by saying "Stop!" either aloud or subvocally. This activity interrupts and delays the uncontrollable spiral of obsessional thoughts. There is little research support for this technique; however, practitioners have found it useful in multimodal treatment with exposure and response prevention, relaxation, and cognitive restructuring.

Relaxation Techniques. Patients with OCD suffer from insomnia because of their heightened anxiety levels. Relaxation exercises may be helpful in improving sleep patterns. These exercises do not affect OCD symptoms, but they may be used to decrease anxiety associated with the disorder. The nurse may also teach the patient other relaxation measures, such as deep breathing, taking warm baths, meditation, music therapy, or other quiet activities.

Cognitive Restructuring. Cognitive restructuring is a method of teaching the patient to restructure dysfunc-

tional thought processes through a system of defining and testing the patient's distorted thought patterns. It is based on the work of Beck (Beck & Emery, 1985) and aimed at altering the patient's immediate dysfunctional appraisal of a situation and perception of long-term consequences. The patient is taught to monitor automatic thoughts, then to recognize the connection between thoughts, emotional response, and behaviors. The distorted thoughts are examined and tested by for-or-against evidence presented by the therapist. In this way, the therapist helps the patient to doubt the real likelihood that the feared event will happen even if the compulsive behavior is not performed. The patient begins to analyze his or her thoughts as being distorted with reality. In other words, and for example, even if the alarm clock is not checked 30 times before going to bed, it will still go off in the morning, and being disciplined for tardiness at work will not happen. Maybe it only needs to be checked once or twice.

Cue Cards. Cue cards are tools used to help the patient restructure thought patterns and contain statements that are positively oriented and pertain to the patient's specific obsessions and compulsions. Cue cards use information from the patient's symptom hierarchy, which is an organizational system that breaks down the obsessions and compulsions from least to most anxiety provoking. These cards can help reinforce in patients the belief that they are safe and can tolerate the anxiety caused by delaying or controlling compulsive rituals. Examples of cue cards are in Text Box 21-6.

Psychoeducation. Psychoeducation is a crucial nursing intervention for the OCD patient. Knowledge is power, and the more the patient knows about his or her

---

TEXT BOX 21.6

Examples of Cue Card Statements

- It's the OCD, not me.
- These are only OC thoughts; OC thoughts don't mean action; I will not act on the thoughts.
- My anxiety level goes up but will always go down. I never sat with the anxiety long enough to see that it would not harm me.
- Trust myself.
- I did it right the first time.
- Checking the locks again won't keep me safe. I really am safe in the world.

From Boyarsky, B., Perone, L., Lee, N., & Goodman, W. (1991). Current treatment approaches to obsessive-compulsive disorder. *Archives of Psychiatric Nursing, V*(5), 299–306.

disorder, the more control that the patient will have over his or her symptoms. The patient should be instructed not only about the biologic components of OCD but also about its treatments and disease course. Treatment is a shared responsibility between the patient and the provider, and the patient should be included in the medication and treatment decision-making processes. If local support groups are available, the patient should be referred, in an effort to reduce feelings of uniqueness and embarrassment about the disease. Family education is also important, so that the patient will have help in practicing behavioral homework. See Psychoeducation Checklist: Obsessive-Compulsive Disorder.

Social Domain

Social Assessment

Nurses must consider sociocultural factors when evaluating OCD. At times, cultural or religious beliefs may be misunderstood and mistaken for obsessions or compulsions. These beliefs and actions must be evaluated in the context of the individual's culture. If these beliefs are consistent with their social or cultural environment, not harmful to themselves or others, and do not interfere with their functioning in that environment, they are not considered symptoms of the disorder.

For the hospitalized patient, unit routines must be carefully and clearly explained to decrease the patient's fear of the unknown. At least initially, it is important not to prevent the patient from engaging in rituals because of the increasing levels of anxiety that will follow. It is important that the nurse recognize the significance of the rituals to the person and empathize with the patient's need to perform them. The nurse can assist the patient in arranging a schedule of activities that allows for some private time but also integrates the patient into normal unit activities.

PSYCHOEDUCATION CHECKLIST
Obsessive-Compulsive Disorder

When caring for the patient with OCD, be sure to include the patient's caregiver, if appropriate, and address the following topic areas in the teaching plan:

- Psychopharmacologic agents (SSRIs, MAOIs, lithium, or anxiolytics) if ordered, including drug action, dosage, frequency, and possible adverse effects
- Skin care measures
- Ritualistic behaviors and alternative activities
- Thought stopping
- Relaxation techniques
- Cognitive restructuring
- Community resources

Family Response to Disorder

Marital status appears to be affected by OCD. Patients with OCD tend to remain single more often than people without the disorder. They also have higher rates of celibacy, possibly because of the thought of being dirty or becoming contaminated. The divorce rate is lower than would be expected given the stress of living with this disorder, and patients with OCD are able to draw their families gradually into accommodating abnormal behavior. For example, the families of patients with cleaning compulsions may forego normal family and social activities to "help" the patient complete compulsive cleaning of the family home. They may become involved in the patient's rituals to decrease the anxiety level in the household. Evaluate the family's understanding of the disorder and of proposed treatments. Are they able and willing to help the patient practice cognitive and behavioral techniques? Are they knowledgeable about prescribed medicines? These questions offer a wonderful opportunity for patient and family education.

Family members offer a perspective on the severity of the patient's illness. Family members are experts in the patient's rituals and may observe subtle changes of which caregivers are unaware. Family assessment will reveal the amount of education and support needed and will begin the partnership among the patient, family, and treatment team. Evaluate the family's response to changes in the patient's behavior as treatment progresses. It may be necessary to discuss how the family will manage the changes brought about by a decrease in rituals.

If obsessions and compulsions make it difficult for the individual to leave the home or function at work, financial difficulties may result and add to the stress or the concerns of the family. These factors should be assessed and appropriate assistance obtained through social services when necessary.

Evaluation and Treatment Outcomes

Several methods can be used to measure the response to treatment. Response to treatment, including nursing care, can be measured through changes in Y-BOCS scores or other rating scales, remission of presenting symptoms, and the ability to complete activities of daily living without interference from obsessions or compulsions. The patient should be able to participate in social or group activities with a degree of comfort as well as feel free of suicidal or aggressive intent. He or she should also be able to demonstrate common knowledge of OCD by describing its symptoms, biologic basis, and treatments.

Continuum of Care

The symptoms of OCD can become debilitating. The obsessive and compulsive symptoms wax and wane throughout treatment. As the focus of treatment shifts from inpatient to outpatient environments, the patient must continually be assessed to ensure favorable patient outcomes through early intervention should symptoms resurface.

Inpatient-Focused Care

In an inpatient setting, the presence of a patient with severe OCD may present a nursing management challenge. These patients require a significant amount of staff time. They may monopolize bathrooms or showers or have disruptive rituals involving eating. Nurses play an integral role in treating the patient with OCD. The nurse should assist with the performance of activities of daily living to ensure that they are completed. Monitoring medication effects, teaching psychoeducation groups, ensuring adequate caloric intake, and providing individual patient counseling are additional inpatient interventions.

Emergency Care

Individuals with OCD frequently use medical services long before they seek psychiatric treatment. Therefore, early recognition of symptoms and referral are important concerns for nurses working in primary care and other medical settings. Once referred, most psychiatric treatment of individuals with OCD occurs on an outpatient basis. Only those individuals with severely debilitating symptoms will be hospitalized to maintain safety. Patients, however, may develop intense anxiety symptoms to the point of panic. Benzodiazepines and other anxiolytics can be used on an emergency basis during episodes of panic.

Family Interventions

The families of patients with OCD need to be educated about the etiology of the disorder. Understanding the biologic basis of the disorder should decrease some of the stigma and embarrassment they may feel related to the bizarre nature of the patient's obsessions and compulsions. The family needs to be educated about both biologic and psychological treatment approaches.

Family assistance in monitoring symptom remission and medication side effects is invaluable. Family members can also assist the patient with behavioral and cognitive interventions.

When caring for the patient with OCD, be sure to include the patient's caregiver, if appropriate, and address the following topic areas in the teaching plan:

- Psychopharmacologic agents (SSRIs, MAOIs, lithium, or anxiolytics) if ordered, including drug action, dosage, frequency, and possible adverse effects

- Skin care measures
- Ritualistic behaviors and alternative activities
- Thought stopping
- Relaxation techniques
- Cognitive restructuring
- Community resources

Community Treatment

Partial hospitalization programs and day treatment programs treat most patients with OCD. They allow individuals to maintain significant independence while beginning medications and behavioral therapies. The intensity of the required outpatient treatment is discussed by the multidisciplinary treatment team during inpatient treatment. Some patients require outpatient treatment on a daily basis during times of increased symptoms. Maintenance outpatient therapy may be scheduled weekly or twice weekly for several weeks until the symptoms are well controlled. Community agency visits are still recommended for medication monitoring.

GENERALIZED ANXIETY DISORDER

Generalized anxiety disorder (GAD) is an anxiety disorder that is characterized by excessive worry and anxiety (apprehensive expectation). Individuals with this disorder experience excessive worry and anxiety almost daily for weeks to months on end. Moreover, the worry and anxiety is disproportionate to the situation that is concerning them. The anxiety does not usually pertaining to a specific situation; rather, it concerns a number of activities or events. Ultimately, the excessive worry and anxiety cause great distress and interfere with the patient's daily personal or social life.

Clinical Course of Disorder

The onset of GAD is insidious. Many patients complain of being chronic worriers. About half the individuals presenting for treatment report onset in childhood or adolescence, although onset after 20 years of age is also common. GAD affects individuals across the life span. Adults with GAD often worry about matters such as their job, health of family members, or minor matters, such as household chores or being late for appointments. The intensity of the worry tends to fluctuate. Any stress tends to intensify the worry and anxiety symptoms (APA, 2000).

Patients with GAD may exhibit mild depressive symptoms such as dysphoria. They are also highly somatic with complaints of multiple clusters of physical symptoms, including muscle aches, soreness, and gastrointestinal ailments (APA, 2000). In addition to physical complaints, patients with GAD often experience trembling, twitching, muscle aches, and soreness and exhibit an exaggerated startle response. When at rest, patients with GAD appear to be physiologically similar to nonanxious people.

Generally speaking, patients with GAD feel frustrated, disgusted with life, demoralized, and hopeless. They may go further to state that they cannot remember a time that they did not feel anxious. There is a sense of ill-being and uneasiness and a fear of imminent disaster. Over time, they may recognize that their chronic tension and anxiety is unreasonable.

Comorbidity

Patients with GAD often suffer from other psychiatric disorders. In fact, up to 74% of patients with GAD have at least one additional current or lifetime psychiatric diagnosis. The most common comorbid disorders are major depressive disorder, social phobia, specific phobia, panic disorder, and dysthymia. GAD has many symptoms suggestive of an underlying mood disorder; thus, it is not surprising that many any patients with GAD have a history of major depression. Lenze and associates (2000) found that 27.5% of depressed elderly patients have a comorbid anxiety disorder. Beekman and coworkers (2000) reached similar results on comorbidity, finding that 30.3% of patients with GAD also had major depressive disorder.

Alcoholism is a significant problem associated with GAD; it is thought that alcohol is used to self-medicate anxiety symptoms. Anxiolytics and barbiturates may also be used by the GAD patient in an effort to relieve symptoms, but these potentially lead to dependency.

Diagnostic Criteria

The APA (2000) discusses the diagnostic features of GAD, which include excessive worry and anxiety about several issues that occurs more days than not for a period of at least 6 months (Criterion A). The patient has little or no control over the worry (Criterion B). The anxiety and worry are accompanied by at least three of the following symptoms for at least 6 months: difficulty sleep, becoming easily fatigued, restlessness, poor concentration, irritability, and muscle tension (Criterion C). The worry and anxiety focuses are not limited to the qualities of another psychiatric diagnosis, including panic disorder, social phobia, OCD, anorexia nervosa, or hypochondriasis, and do not exclusively occur with PTSD (Criterion D). The worry and anxiety cause significant impairment in social, occupational, or another significant area of functioning (Criterion E). Finally, the disturbance is not substance-induced or due to a general medical condition (Criterion F) (see Table 21-11).

Generalized Anxiety Disorder in Special Populations

GAD may be overdiagnosed in children because of the overlap of symptoms with other psychiatric disorders (APA, 2000). Additionally, children only have to meet one (rather than three) of the additional symptoms outlined previously in Criterion C. Children with GAD manifest their symptoms through worry about their performance in school or sports and often excel in these areas (Castellanos & Hunter, 1999). Somatic complaints in children with GAD are heightened. Children may

---

TABLE 21.11   Key Diagnostic Characteristics of General Anxiety Disorder

Diagnostic Criteria and Target Symptoms	Associated Findings

• Excessive anxiety and worry (apprehensive expectation) occurring for more days than not for at least 6 months involving a number of events or activities
    Restlessness or feeling keyed up or on edge
    Being easily fatigued
    Difficulty concentrating or mind going blank
    Irritability
    Muscle tension
    Sleep disturbance
• Difficulty controlling the worry
• Focus of anxiety and worry not confined to another psychiatric disorder
• Clinically significant distress or impairment of functioning resulting from anxiety, worry, or physical symptoms
• Not a direct physiologic effect of a substance or medical condition
• Does not occur exclusively during a mood disorder, psychotic disorder, or pervasive developmental disorder
	Associated Behavioral Findings
	• Possible depressive symptoms
	
	Associated Physical Examination Findings
	• Muscle tension with twitching, trembling, feeling shaky, and muscle aches and soreness
	• Clammy cold hands, dry mouth, sweating, nausea or diarrhea, "lump in the throat"

also worry about trivial issues, such as what clothes to wear, or about physical appearance or social interactions. Children with the disorder tend to be perfectionistic and conforming, seeking frequent approval from parents or authority figures.

Elderly people also suffer from GAD, although anxiety in old age has not received much attention. Many prescribe to the myth that old people do not have anxiety. On the contrary, a significant number of elderly patients in depression and anxiety studies meet criteria for GAD or have significant anxiety symptoms (Beekman et al., 2000; Lenze et al., 2000; Wang et al., 2000).

Epidemiology

Because of the high prevalence of comorbid psychiatric diagnoses, it is difficult to assess the true prevalence of this disorder. However, generalized anxiety disorder is a common psychiatric disorder affecting nearly 3% of the population at any given time (Kessler et al., 1999). The lifetime prevalence rate nears 5%. Of those presenting at anxiety disorder clinics, 25% have GAD and a primary or comorbid diagnosis (APA, 2000). In clinical settings, women and men are fairly equally distributed. In wider studies, roughly 66% of patients with GAD are female (APA, 2000).

Etiology

Biologic theories of causation for GAD have not been extensively studied. It has been postulated that GAD is not a true disease in itself, but rather a phase of other psychiatric disorders. Nonetheless, the symptoms of GAD and the control of these symptoms with a number of medications have led investigators to consider several biologic possibilities.

Neurochemical Theories

Although symptoms of activation of the sympathetic nervous system are common to both GAD and panic disorder, studies have found only limited evidence of norepinephrine system dysregulation in GAD. Medications that act on serotonin, such as the SSRIs, have been effective in the treatment of GAD. This has led to more promising investigations of serotonin dysfunction related to GAD. The effects of benzodiazepines in reducing the symptoms of anxiety have been well documented, yet little research has been done to clarify the function of GABA and the benzodiazepine receptors in GAD.

Genetic Theories

Few studies have examined genetic and familial factors in the etiology of GAD. One study of twins revealed that GAD is a moderately inheritable disorder. The tendency for GAD to be familial appears to be a result of genetic factors. Individuals with GAD may have a genetic vulnerability that predisposes them to anxiety sensitivity. Biologic foundations involved in development of anxiety disorders might be the same responsible for depression (APA, 2000). The family environment might also play an important role as one may become anxious through learned behavior.

Psychological Theories

Cognitive-behavioral theory regarding the etiology of GAD proposes that the disorder results from inaccurate assessment of perceived environmental dangers. These inaccuracies result from selective focus on negative details, distorted information processing, and overly pessimistic view of one's coping ability. Psychoanalytic theory postulates that anxiety represents unresolved unconscious conflicts. Sources of anxiety change in different developmental stages and include such conflicts as fear of separation from a source of love or fear of loss of love from important others.

Sociologic Theories

Although there are no specific sociocultural theories related to the development of GAD, a high-stress lifestyle and multiple stressful life events may be contributors. Kindling results from overstimulation or repeated stimulation of nerve cells through environmental stressors. Individuals with GAD have a hypersensitivity to stress and anxiety-provoking events. Although more research is needed to understand the underlying pathophysiology, serotonin and the GABA–benzodiazepine receptor complex appear to be most implicated.

Risk Factors

Unresolved conflicts, cognitive misinterpretations, and life stressors are examples of potential contributors to the development of the disorder. Patients may have a genetic predisposition to anxiety sensitivity. Behavioral inhibition, characterized by shyness, fear, or becoming withdrawn in unfamiliar situations, may be a risk factor for GAD and other anxiety disorders (Castellanos & Hunter, 1999).

NURSING MANAGEMENT: HUMAN RESPONSE TO DISORDER

Nursing assessment and intervention for individuals with GAD include many of the same biopsychosocial considerations as discussed with panic disorder. Assessment of the patient's anxiety symptoms should include the following questions, and their answers are used to tailor individual approaches:

- How does the patient experience anxiety symptoms?
- Are the patient's symptoms primarily physical, psychological, or both?
- Is the patient aware when he or she is becoming anxious?
- Is the patient aware that anxiety induces the physical symptoms?
- What coping mechanisms does the patient routinely use to deal with anxiety?
- What life stressors add to these symptoms? What changes can be made to reduce these stressors?

Biologic Domain

Biologic Assessment

Diet and Nutrition. It is accepted that some ordinary food stimulants induce anxiety symptoms, and patients with GAD may be hypersensitive to caffeine. A concrete step that patients with GAD can take to reduce anxiety is to eliminate caffeine from their diets. Nurses can help patients achieve a caffeine-free state through education and dietary management, while assisting with pain relief in response to the headache that often accompanies caffeine withdrawal.

Sleep Patterns. Sleep disturbance is also a common symptom for individuals with GAD. Therefore, close assessment of the patient's sleep pattern is important. Alcohol should be avoided because it disturbs the sleep cycle. Assistance with implementing sleep hygiene measures can promote sleep (see Chap. 23). Timing the last meal of the day to be in the early evening, avoiding fluids after 8 PM, and taking a warm bath before bedtime may promote sleep.

Biologic Interventions: Pharmacologic Treatment

The involved neurotransmitter systems and physical symptoms of anxiety suggest that several medications are effective in the treatment of GAD. Benzodiazepines are most commonly used, but antidepressants (imipramine and venlafaxine), buspirone, and β-blockers have all produced effective results.

Monitoring and Administration of Medications. Although widely used in the treatment of GAD, benzodiazepine treatment remains somewhat controversial. With high comorbid substance abuse, benzodiazepines may complicate treatment because of their addictive qualities. Many people with GAD are reluctant to take prescribed medications, and most patients who request benzodiazepines are not those looking for quick relief

from slight discomfort. Most patients with GAD do not seek treatment until their level of suffering is substantial. If there is a significant potential for dependence on a benzodiazepine, antidepressants may be a better choice. Benzodiazepines offer quicker relief from anxiety symptoms, but the therapeutic effects of antidepressants are equal to those of benzodiazepines at 4 weeks (Roerig, 1999).

Buspirone. Buspirone is an azapirone agent and acts by inhibiting spontaneous firing of serotonergic neurons in the dorsal raphe and by antagonism of 5-HT1a receptors located in the dorsal raphe, hippocampus, and parts of the frontal cortex. Buspirone does not interact with benzodiazepine receptors and may increase brain noradrenergic and dopaminergic activity (see Chap. 8 for additional information).

Buspirone must be taken for 2 to 4 weeks before its anxiolytic effects are felt. This delay may be difficult for patients to tolerate, particularly if they have used benzodiazepines in the past and are familiar with their rapid onset of action. When compared with the benzodiazepines, buspirone is equally effective in the treatment. It is also less effective in individuals with a history of substance abuse. More treatment dropouts have been found with the use of buspirone than with benzodiazepines, presumably because of the lag in effect.

Antidepressants. Venlafaxine and imipramine are effective treatment options for GAD because they have serotonergic and noradrenergic effects, which are implicated in the reduction of anxiety symptoms (Rickels et al., 2000a, 2000b).

Side-Effect Monitoring. TCAs (imipramine) and benzodiazepines have significant side effects, drug interactions, and teaching points that require ongoing monitoring. (See the discussions of these medications in the section on treatment of panic disorder.)

Buspirone side effects include dizziness, insomnia, drowsiness, and nervousness. Dry mouth, blurred vision, and abdominal distress can occur but are uncommon.

Venlafaxine is an SSRI that has a relatively safe side-effect profile. Anticholinergic effects, including dry mouth and constipation, are common. Additionally, this drug causes dizziness, nervousness, and insomnia. Transient hypertension occurs in some patients; therefore, blood pressure should be monitored. Gastrointestinal effects of nausea and vomiting can occur as well.

Drug–Drug Interactions. Venlafaxine and buspirone both interact with MAOIs. Neither should be initiated within 14 days of treatment with an MAOI. Alcohol should be avoided while taking buspirone because of the effects of CNS depression.

Teaching Points. Teaching points for venlafaxine and buspirone include informing the patient that the anxiolytic effects of the medication will not be felt for several weeks. Patients should be warned against operating heavy machinery until the effects of the medication are known to the patient. If the patient is being tapered off of benzodiazepines and being placed on buspirone, instruct him or her not to discontinue the benzodiazepine suddenly because of the risks of withdrawal, including rebound anxiety and seizures.

Psychological and Social Domains

Psychological and social assessment and intervention strategies for GAD and panic disorder are similar (see the psychological and social assessments and interventions in the section on panic disorder).

Cognitive psychotherapy is an effective treatment of GAD. Outcome studies of cognitive treatments of GAD indicate that on average, there is a 50% reduction in the severity of somatic symptoms and a 25% reduction in trait anxiety, with about 50% of patients regaining normal function. These results are inclined to be maintained at the 6-month follow-up (Durham & Allan, 1993). Another study reported that gains made with relaxation, cognitive therapy, or a combination of the two lasted for up to 2 years (Zinbarg et al., 1992). Applied relaxation, CBT, and nondirective psychotherapy have been compared in patients with GAD. Both applied relaxation and CBT produced equal symptom relief, whereas nondirective psychotherapy produced little lasting relief (Borkovec & Costello, 1993). Roerig (1999) states that dynamic and supportive psychotherapies and CBT are effective in treating GAD, especially when combined with other treatments. Goisman and colleagues (1999) discovered that although CBT has been proved effective in the treatment of GAD, it is underutilized in treating anxiety disorders.

Evaluation and Treatment Outcomes

Nursing diagnoses that apply to GAD are the same as for panic disorder, including Anxiety, Powerlessness, Sleep Pattern, Low Self-Esteem, and Disturbed, Ineffective Family Coping. Interventions are individualized and are focused on the patient and the family in controlling or coping with the anxiety. The individual- and family-centered interventions for panic disorder apply to controlling the symptoms of GAD.

Treatment outcomes for patients with GAD include reducing frequency and intensity of anxiety and controlling the factors that stimulate or provoke this uncomfortable state. Specifically, evaluation can focus on the individual's ability and skills in using techniques that control anxiety, such as relaxation, positive self-talk, and stress management. Reducing personal and environmental stress, eliminating foods and drinks such as caffeine in the diet, and developing strategies to deal with stressful family situations are outcome successes.

Continuum of Care

Like patients with panic disorder, patients with GAD often seek treatment in emergency rooms or from medical internists because of the physical symptoms associated with the illness. It is estimated that only one third of patients with GAD seek psychiatric treatment, and many patients do not seek any treatment for their symptoms. Of those patients with GAD who do seek treatment, many consult internists, cardiologists, or neurologists for the physiologic symptoms they experience. It is essential that nurses in these settings be aware of the disorder and provide necessary assessment and intervention. Nurses in home health settings have an excellent opportunity to identify symptoms of undiagnosed GAD and make appropriate referrals.

Inpatient and outpatient management of GAD is very similar to the treatments detailed in the section on panic disorder. Because anxiety produces more anxiety, a calm, reassuring and nonjudgmental approach is necessary. Whether treatment is home or clinic based, both the patient and the provider must actively participate in monitoring and managing environmental stress levels. For patients to relax and reduce stress, they need a relaxing and unstimulating environment. Reduction of noise and lighting induces relaxation. Relaxation methods such as breathing control exercises, progressive muscle relaxation, and other interventions discussed previously in this chapter may also be helpful (see Psychoeducation Checklist: Generalized Anxiety Disorder).

OTHER ANXIETY AND RELATED DISORDERS

Specific Phobia

Specific phobia is a disorder marked by persistent fear of clearly discernible, circumscribed objects or situations, which often leads to avoidance behaviors. The lifetime

---

PSYCHOEDUCATION CHECKLIST
Generalized Anxiety Disorder

When caring for the patient with generalized anxiety disorder, be sure to include the following topic areas in the teaching plan:

- Psychopharmacologic agents (benzodiazepines, antidepressants, nonbenzodiazepine anxiolytics, and/or β-blockers) if ordered, including drug action, dosage, frequency, and possible adverse effects
- Breathing control
- Nutrition and diet restriction
- Sleep measures
- Progressive muscle relaxation
- Time management
- Positive coping strategies

prevalence rates range from 7% to 11%, and the disorder generally affects women twice that of men. It has a bimodal distribution, peaking in childhood and then again in the 20s. The focus of the fear in specific phobia may result from the anticipation of being harmed by the phobic object. For example, dogs are feared because of the chance of being bitten or automobiles are feared because of the potential of crashing. The focus of fear may likewise be associated with concerns about losing control, panicking, or fainting on exposure to the phobic object.

Anxiety is usually felt immediately on exposure to the phobic object, and the level of anxiety is usually related to both the proximity of the object and the degree to which escape is possible. Anxiety heightens as a cat comes closer to a person fearing cats, and reduces when the cat moves away. At times, the level of anxiety escalates to a full panic attack, particularly when the person must remain in a situation from which escape is deemed to be impossible. Fight-or-flight responses become heightened when faced with the phobic object and when escape is difficult.

Fear of specific objects is fairly common, and the diagnosis of specific phobia is not made unless the fear significantly interferes with functioning or causes marked distress. Assessment differentiates simple phobia from other diagnoses with overlapping symptoms. Table 21-3 lists a number of specific phobias. Among adult patients who are seen in clinical settings, the most to least common phobias are situational phobia, natural environment phobias, blood–injection–injury phobia, and animal phobia. The most common phobias among community samples are of heights, mice, spiders, and insects (APA, 2000).

Blood–injection–injury phobias merit special consideration as the phobia surrounds medical treatments. The physiologic processes that are exhibited during phobic exposure include a strong vasovagal response, which significantly increases blood pressure and pulse, followed by deceleration of the pulse and lowering of blood pressure in the patient. Monitor closely when giving required injections or medical treatments.

About 75% of patients with blood–injection–injury phobias report fainting on exposure. Factors that may predispose individuals to specific phobias may include traumatic events, unexpected panic attacks in the presence of the phobic object or situation, observation of others experiencing a trauma, or repeated exposure to information warning of dangers. For example, parents repeatedly warning young children that dogs bite.

Phobic content must be evaluated from an ethnic or cultural background. In many cultures, fears of spirits or magic are common. They should only be considered part of a disorder if the fear is excessive in the context of the culture, causes the individual significant distress, or impairs the ability to function.

Psychotropic drugs have not been effective in treatment of specific phobia. Anxiolytics may give short-term relief of phobic anxiety, but there is no evidence that they affect the course of the disorder. The treatment of choice for specific phobia is exposure therapy.

Social Phobia

Social phobia involves a persistent fear of social or performance situations in which embarrassment may occur. Exposure to a feared social or performance situation nearly always provokes immediate anxiety and may trigger panic attacks. People with social phobias fear that others will scrutinize their behavior and judge them negatively. They often do not speak up in crowds out of fear of embarrassment. They will go to great lengths to avoid feared situations. If avoidance is not possible, they will suffer through the situation with visible anxiety.

People with social phobia appear to be highly sensitive to disapproval or criticism, tend to evaluate themselves negatively, and have poor self-esteem and a distorted view of personal strengths and weaknesses. They may magnify personal flaws and underrate any talents. They often believe others would act with more assertiveness in a given social situation. Children tend to underachieve in school because of test-taking anxiety.

Social phobias can be specific or generalized. Generalized social phobia is diagnosed when the individual experiences fears related to most social situations, including public performances and social interactions. These individuals are more likely to demonstrate deficiencies in social skills and interference with their ability to function. Generalized social phobia may be linked to low dopamine receptor binding, as discovered in recent research (Schneier et al., 2000).

People with specific social phobias fear and avoid only one or two social situations. Classic examples of such situations are eating, writing, or speaking in public or using public bathrooms. The most common fears for individuals with social phobia are public speaking, fear of meeting strangers, eating in public, writing in public, using public restrooms, and being stared at or being the center of attention.

A unique difference exists between the person with a specific versus a generalized social phobia. When a person with generalized social phobia experiences stressors unrelated to the phobia, the response to unsolicited support from friends or family exacerbates anxiety because it is interpreted as scrutiny. When in the same situation, the person with specific social phobia benefits from the support of others.

Pharmacotherapy is a relatively new area of research for treatment approaches to social phobia. SSRIs are used in treatment of social phobia. In open clinical trials, paroxetine and fluvoxamine significantly reduced social

TABLE 21.12 Key Diagnostic Characteristics of Other Anxiety Disorders

Disorder	Diagnostic Characteristics and Target Symptoms
Phobias	• Marked, persistent, excessive, or unreasonable fear response • Exposure causes immediate anxiety • Recognition by person that fear is excessive or unreasonable • Situation avoided or endured with extreme anxiety and distress • Impairment of normal routine, functioning, social activities, or relationships resulting from avoidance, anxious anticipation, or distress in feared situation; marked distress with having phobia • Duration of at least 6 months in individuals younger than age 18 y • Fear not a direct physiologic effect of substance or general medical condition; not better accounted for by another mental disorder

Specific phobia	• Characteristics as above
	• Fear in response to presence or anticipation of specific object or event
	    Animal (eg, dogs, cats)
	    Natural environment (eg, height)
	    Blood–injection–injury (eg, seeing blood)
	    Situation (eg, flying)
	    Other

Social phobia	• Characteristics as above • Fear in response to one or more social or performance situations in which person is exposed to unfamiliar persons or possible scrutiny Fear of acting in an embarrassing or humiliating way or showing symptoms of anxiety

Posttraumatic stress disorder	• Exposure to traumatic event
	    Witnessed, experienced, or confronted with event(s) involving actual or threatened death or serious injury or threat to physical integrity of self or others
	    Response involving intense fear, helplessness, or horror
	• Persistent re-experiencing of traumatic event
	    Recurrent and intrusive distressing recollections
	    Recurrent distressing dreams
	    Acting or feeling like traumatic event was recurring
	    Intense psychological distress and physiologic reactions when exposed to cues symbolizing or resembling the event
	• Persistent avoidance of stimuli associated with trauma with numbing of general responsiveness
	    Thoughts, feeling, or conversations associated with the trauma avoided
	    Activities, places, or people who arouse recollection of trauma avoided
	    Inability to recall important aspects of trauma
	    Insignificant decreased interest or participation in activities
	    Detachment and estrangement from others
	    Restricted range of affect
	    Sense of a shortened future
	• Persistent symptoms of arousal
	    Difficulty falling or staying asleep
	    Irritability and anger outbursts
	    Difficulty concentrating
	    Hypervigilance
	    Exaggerated startle response
	• Duration of symptoms greater than 1 month (acute: duration less than 3 months; chronic: duration longer than 3 months; with delayed onset: if symptoms appear 6 months or more after event)
	• Significant distress or impairment of social, occupational, or other important areas of functioning

Acute stress disorder	• Exposure to traumatic event
	    Witnessed, experienced, or confronted with event(s) involving actual or threatened death or serious injury or threat to physical integrity of self or others
	    Response involving intense fear, helplessness, or horror
	• Dissociative symptoms during or after the event
	    Sense of numbing, detachment or absence of emotional response

(continued)

TABLE 21.12 Key Diagnostic Characteristics of Other Anxiety Disorders (Continued)

Disorder	Diagnostic Characteristics and Target Symptoms
	Reduced awareness of surroundings Derealization Depersonalization Inability to recall important aspects of trauma (dissociative amnesia) • Persistent re-experiencing of traumatic event through recurrent images, thoughts, dreams, illusions, flashbacks, or a sense of reliving the experience or distress on exposure to reminders of the trauma • Marked avoidance of stimuli that arouse recollection of event • Marked anxiety or increased arousal • Significant distress or impairment of social, occupational, or other important areas of functioning or inability to pursue necessary tasks • Duration of at least 2 days up to a maximum of 4 weeks; occurring within 4 weeks of trauma • Not a direct physiologic effect of a substance or general medical condition; not better accounted for by other mental disorder
Dissociative identity disorder	• Two or more distinct identities or personality states—each with own pattern of perceiving, relating to, and thinking about the environment and the self • Control of person's behavior by at least two of the identities • Inability to recall important personal information; too extensive to be due to forgetfulness • Not a direct physiologic effect of a substance or general medical condition

anxiety and phobic avoidance (Mancini & Ameringen, 1996; Stein et al., 1999). Alprazolam has also been effective in treating social phobia when combined with exposure therapy (Van-Ameringen et al., 1993; Versiani et al., 1992). It is estimated that fewer than 23% of Americans with a phobia have received treatment because of factors such as misdiagnosis, ignorance, stigma, and lack of affordable treatment. Providing referrals for appropriate psychiatric treatment is one of the most critical nursing interventions.

Posttraumatic Stress Disorder

PTSD affects roughly 8% of the general population, and women are more likely than men to be afflicted. PTSD is defined by characteristic symptoms that develop after a traumatic event. This traumatic event involves a personal experience of threatened death, injury, or threat to physical integrity. It may also include witnessing such an event happening to another person or learning that a family member or close friend has experienced such an event. Examples of traumatic events are violent personal assault, military combat, natural disasters, terrorist attack, being taken hostage, incarceration as a prisoner of war, torture, automobile accident, or being diagnosed with a life-threatening illness.

Risk factors for PTSD include a prior diagnosis of acute stress disorder (Brewin, 1999). Pre-existing personality; extent, duration, and intensity of trauma involved; environmental issues; higher levels of anxiety; lower self-esteem; and existing personality difficulties may increase the likelihood of developing PTSD.

Acute Stress Disorder

Acute stress disorder involves the development of anxiety, dissociation, and other symptoms within 1 month of an exposure to a traumatic stressor. Stressors include those specified in PTSD. The patient must have three dissociative symptoms, including numbing, detachment, a reduction of awareness to one's surroundings, derealization, depersonalization, or dissociative amnesia (APA, 2000). Additionally, for at least 2 days, the patient continually re-experiences the event, avoids situations that remind him or her of the event, and has increased anxiety and excitation that negatively affect his or her lifestyle. After 1 month, the diagnosis is changed to PTSD if symptoms persist.

Dissociative Disorders

Dissociative disorders are thought to be responses to extreme external or internal events or stressors. Roughly 10% of people experience dissociative disorders, and they are highest among those who suffer childhood physical or sexual abuse. The onset of these disorders may be sudden or occur gradually, and the course of each may be long-term or transient.

Dissociation, or a splitting from self, may occur as a form of coping with severe anxiety. The essential feature of the five disorders in this class involves a failure to integrate identity, memory, and consciousness. This class of disorders includes dissociative amnesia, the inability to recall important, yet stressful information; dissociative fugue, unexpected travel away from home with the inability to recall one's past and confusion about personal identity or the assumption of a new identity; depersonalization disorder, the feeling of being detached from one's mental processes; dissociative identity disorder, formally multiple personality disorder (see Chap. 37); and dissociate disorder not otherwise specified. See Table 21-12 for diagnostic criteria and assessment findings.

Summary of Key Points

➤ Anxiety-related disorders are the most common of all psychiatric disorders and comprise a wide range of disorders, including panic disorder, obsessive-compulsive disorder, generalized anxiety disorder, phobias, acute stress disorder, posttraumatic stress disorder, and dissociative disorder.

➤ The anxiety disorders share the common symptom of recurring anxiety but differ in symptom profiles. Panic attacks occur in many of the disorders.

➤ Those experiencing anxiety disorders have a high level of physical and emotional illness and often suffer dual diagnoses with other anxiety disorders, substance abuse, or depression. These disorders often render individuals unable to function effectively at home or at a job.

➤ Patients with panic disorder are often seen in a number of health care settings, frequently in hospital emergency rooms or clinics, presenting with a confusing array of physical and emotional symptoms. Skillful assessment is required to eliminate possible life-threatening causes.

➤ Current research points to a combination of biologic and psychosocial factors that cause persistent anxiety. The initial stage of panic attack seems to be biologically generated by neural activity in the brain stem. There is also biologic evidence that anticipatory anxiety is linked to the kindling phenomenon occurring in the limbic system, which lowers one's biologic threshold for response to stressors. The last stage of phobic avoidance is a learned phenomenon that involves considerable cognitive activity, occurring in the prefrontal cortex. Other research demonstrates that there are also personality traits that predispose individuals to anxiety disorders, including low-self esteem, external locus of control, some negative family influences, and some traumatic or stressful precipitating event. These biologic and psychosocial components combine to yield a true biopsychosocial theory of causation.

➤ Treatment approaches for all anxiety-related disorders are somewhat similar, including pharmacotherapy, psychological treatments, or often a combination of both.

➤ Nurses at the generalist level use interventions from each of the dimensions—biologic, psychological, and social. Approaching these patients with knowledge of the disorder, understanding, and calmness is crucial. Nurses can be instrumental in crisis intervention, medication management, and psychoeducation.

➤ Psychoeducation is crucial in the management of anxiety disorders and includes methods to help patients control and cope with the anxiety reactions (ie, control of breathing, stress reduction, and relaxation techniques), education regarding medication side effects and management, and education of family members to understand these disorders.

➤ Obsessive-compulsive disorder is a rather rare disorder but is often difficult to diagnose because patients do not often seek help. It is characterized by unwanted, intrusive, and persistent thoughts (ie, fear of germ contamination) that cause so much anxiety and distress that the individual feels compelled to perform ritualistic, repetitive actions (excessive hand washing and cleaning) to reduce the agonizing anxiety.

Critical Thinking Challenges

1. How is normal anxiety differentiated from pathologic anxiety?
2. What features are common to the anxiety disorders? What features are unique to each disorder?
3. What factors might contribute to the high comorbidity rate found in the anxiety disorders?
4. Are the anatomic abnormalities found in certain anxiety disorders (eg, obsessive-compulsive disorder) causes or effects of the disorders?
5. How can nurses be involved in prevention with regard to anxiety disorders?
6. How can nurses integrate therapeutic use of self with biologic treatment approaches?
7. What is the importance of the nurse's self-awareness and self-management of her or his own anxiety?
8. What are the ethical issues involved in treating anxiety disorders?
9. Diverse groups of psychopharmacologic agents are used successfully to treat anxiety disorders. How is this explained? What does this fact mean about the relationship between different types of disorders?

 WEB LINKS

www.nimh.nih.gov/anxiety This is the National Institute of Mental Health's anxiety disorder website. An anxiety disorders education program available.

www.algy.com   This Anxiety Panic Internet Resource site has self-help resources for those with panic disorder.

www.panicdisordersabout.com   This site provides a guide to more than 700 other sites and also contains recent articles and resources.

www.mcpamd.com/anxiety   This website on anxiety disorders in children and adults focuses on the diagnosis and treatment of anxiety disorder in children and adolescents.

MOVIES

As Good As It Gets: 1997. Novelist Melvin Udall, played by Jack Nicholson, lives in his own world of obsessive-compulsive behavior patterns, avoiding cracks in sidewalks and rigidly adhering to a regime of daily breakfasts in the café, where single mom Carol Connelly, played by Helen Hunt, works. Udall's world is changed when he unwillingly becomes a sitter for his next-door neighbor's dog. A friendship leading to a romance develops between Udall and Connelly.
Viewing Points: Identify the behaviors that indicate that Udall has an anxiety disorder. Observe feelings that are generated in you by Udall's behavior. How are Udall's friends able to tolerate his behavior?

REFERENCES

Altshuler, L., Hendrick, V., & Cohen, L. (1998). Course of mood and anxiety disorders during pregnancy. *Journal of Clinical Psychiatry, 157*(Suppl. 2), 29–33.

American Psychiatric Association. (2000). *Diagnostic and statistical manual of mental disorders* (4th ed., Text revision). Washington, DC: Author.

Ballenger, J., Wheadon, D., Steiner, M., et al. (1998). Double-blind, fixed-dose, placebo-controlled study of paroxetine in the treatment of panic disorder. *American Journal of Psychiatry, 155*(1), 36–42.

Bandelow, B., Wedekind, D., Pauls, J., Brooks, A., Hajak, G., & Ruther, E. (2000). Salivary cortisol in panic attacks. *American Journal of Psychiatry, 157,* 454–456.

Barlow, D. (1997). Cognitive-behavioral therapy for panic disorder: current status. *Journal of Clinical Psychiatry, 58*(Suppl. 2), 32–36.

Barlow, D., Gorman, J., Shear, M., & Woods, S. (2000). Cognitive-behavioral therapy, imipramine, or their combination for panic disorder: A randomized controlled trial. *Journal of the American Medical Association, 283*(19), 2529–2536.

Baxter, L. (1992). Neuroimaging studies of obsessive compulsive disorder. *Psychiatric Clinics of North America, 15*(4), 871–883.

Beck, A., & Emery, G. (1985). *Anxiety disorders and phobias: A cognitive perspective.* New York: Basic Books.

Beck, C. (1998). Postpartum onset of panic disorder. *Image— The Journal of Nursing Scholarship, 30*(2), 131–134.

Beekman, A., de Beurs, E., von Balkom, A., et al. (2000). Anxiety and depression in later life: Co-occurrence and communality of risk factors. *American Journal of Psychiatry, 157,* 89–95.

Ben-Zion, I., Meiri, G., Greenberg, B., et al. (1999). Enhancement of CO_2-induced anxiety in healthy volunteers with the serotonin agonist metergoline. *American Journal of Psychiatry, 156,* 1635–1637.

Borkovec, T., & Costello, E. (1993). Efficacy of applied relaxation and cognitive-behavioral therapy in the treatment of generalized anxiety disorder. *Journal of Consulting and Clinical Psychology, 61*(4), 611—619.

Bradwejn, J., Koszycki, D., du Tertre, A., et al. (1992). The cholecystokinin hypothesis of panic and anxiety disorders: A review. *Journal of Psychopharmacology, 6,* 345–351.

Brewin, C., Andrews, B., Rose, S., & Kirk, M. (1999). Acute stress disorder and posttraumatic stress disorder in victims of violent crime. *American Journal of Psychiatry, 156*(3), 360–366.

Broocks, A., Bandelow, B., Pekrun, G., et al. (1998). Comparison of aerobic exercise, clomipramine, and placebo in the treatment of panic disorder. *American Journal of Psychiatry, 155*(5), 603–609.

Castle, D., & Groves, A. (2000). The internal and external boundaries of obsessive-compulsive disorder. *Australian and New Zealand Journal of Psychiatry, 34,* 249–255.

Castellanos, D., & Hunter, T. (2000). Anxiety disorders in children and adolescents. *Southern Medical Journal, 92*(10), 946–954.

Dickstein, L. (2000). Gender differences in mood and anxiety disorders. From bench to bedside: American psychiatric press review of psychiatry, (vol. 18). *American Journal of Psychiatry, 157*(7), 1186–1187.

Durham, R., & Allan, T. C. (1993). Psychological treatment of generalized anxiety disorder: A review of clinical significance of results in outcome studies since 1980. *British Journal of Psychiatry, 163,* 19–26.

Dyckman, J., Rosenbaum, R., Hartmeyer, R., & Walter, L. (1999). Effects of psychological interventions of panic attack patients in the emergency department. *Psychosomatics, 40*(5), 422–427.

Fleet, R., Marchand, A., Dupuis, G., et al. (1998). Comparing emergency department and psychiatric setting patients with panic disorder. *Psychosomatics, 39*(6), 512–518.

Gardos, G. (2000). Long-term treatment of panic disorder with agoraphobia in private practice. *Journal of Psychiatric Practice, 6,* 140–146.

Gelder, M. (1992). Treatment of the neuroses. *International Journal of Mental Health, 21*(3), 3–42.

Giedd, J., Rapaport, J., Garvey, M., et al. (2000). MRI assessment of children with obsessive compulsive disorder or tics associated with streptococcal infection. *American Journal of Psychiatry, 157*(2), 281–283.

Goisman, R., Warshaw, M., & Keller, M. (1999). Psychosocial treatment for generalized anxiety disorder, panic disorder, and social phobia, 1991–1996. *American Journal of Psychiatry, 156,* 1819–1821.

Gorman, J., Kent, J., Sullivan, G., & Coplan, J. (2000). Neuroanatomical hypothesis of panic disorder, revised. *American Journal of Psychiatry, 157*(4), 493–505.

Gorman, J., Liebowitz, M., Fyer, A., & Stein, J. (1989). A neuroanatomical hypothesis for panic disorder. *American Journal of Psychiatry, 146,* 148–161.

Grove, C., Coplan, J., & Hollander, E. (1997). The neuro-anatomy of 5-HT dysregulation and panic disorder. *Journal of Neuropsychiatry and Clinical Neuroscience, 9*(2), 198–207.

Hamilton, M. (1959). The assessment of anxiety states by rating. *British Journal of Medical Psychology, 32,* 54.

Hayward, C., Killen, J., & Kraemer, H. (2000). Predictors of panic attacks in adolescents. *Journal of the American Academy of Child and Adolescent Psychiatry, 39*(2), 207–214.

Hoyer, D., & Martin, G. (1997). 5-HT receptor classification and nomenclature: Toward a harmonization with the human genome. *Neuropharmacology, 36,* 419–428.

Johnson, M., & Lydiard, R. (1995). The neurobiology of anxiety disorders. *Psychiatric Clinics of North America, 18,* 681–725.

Kessler, R., DuPont, R., Berglund, P., & Wittchen, H-U. (1999). Impairment in pure and comorbid generalized anxiety disorder and major depression at 12 months in two national surveys. *American Journal of Psychiatry, 156*(12), 1915–1923.

Kessler, R., McGonagle, K., Zhao, S., et al. (1994). Lifetime and 12-month prevalence of *DSM-III-R* psychiatric disorders in the United States. *Archives of General Psychiatry, 51,* 8–19.

Kunovac, J. L., & Stahl, S. M. (1995). Future directions in anxiolytic pharmacotherapy. *Psychiatric Clinics of North America, 18,* 895–909.

Lenze, E., Mulsant, B., Shear, M., et al. (2000). Comorbid anxiety disorders in depressed elderly patients. *American Journal of Psychiatry, 157*(5), 722–728.

Mancini, C., & Ameringen, M. (1996). Paroxetine in social phobia. *Journal of Clinical Psychiatry, 57*(14), 519–522.

Marshall, R., Schneier, F., Lin, S. H., et al. (2000). Childhood trauma and dissociative symptoms in panic disorder. *American Journal of Psychiatry, 157*(3), 451–453.

Mendlowicz, M., & Stein, M. (2000). Quality of life in individuals with anxiety disorders. *American Journal of Psychiatry, 157*(5), 669–682.

Mindus, P., & Jenike, M. (1992). Neurosurgical treatment of malignant obsessive compulsive disorder. *Psychiatric Clinics of North America, 15*(4), 921–937.

Modestin, J. (1992). Multiple personality disorder in Switzerland. *American Journal of Psychiatry, 149*(1), 88–92.

Mundo, E., Ritcher, M., Sam, F., et al. (2000). Is the 5-HT (1D beta) receptor gene implicated in the pathogenesis of obsessive-compulsive disorder? *American Journal of Psychiatry, 157*(7), 1160–1161.

Owens, M., & Nemeroff, C. (1993). *The role of corticotropin-releasing factor in the pathophysiology of affective and anxiety disorders: Laboratory and clinical studies.* Corticotropin-releasing factor, Ciba Foundation symposium 172. New York: John Wiley & Sons.

Peplau, H. (1989). Theoretic constructs: Anxiety, self, and hallucinations. In A. O'Toole & S. Welt (Eds.), *Interpersonal theory in nursing practice: Selected works of Hildegard E. Peplau.* New York: Springer.

Pilowsky, D., Wu, L-T., & Anthony, J. (1999). Panic attacks and suicide attempts in mid-adolescence. *American Journal of Psychiatry, 156*(10), 1545–1549.

Pohl, R., Wolkow, R., & Clary, C. (1998). Sertraline in the treatment of panic disorder: A double-blind multicenter trial. *American Journal of Psychiatry, 155*(9), 1189–1195.

Rauch, S., Jenike, M., Alpert, N., et al. (1994). Regional cerebral blood flow measured during symptom provocation in obsessive-compulsive disorder using oxygen 15-labeled carbon dioxide and positron emission tomography. *Archives of General Psychiatry, 51,* 62–70.

Rickels, K., DeMartinis, N., Garcia-Espana, F., et al. (2000a). Imipramine and buspirone in treatment of patients with generalized anxiety disorder who are discontinuing long-term benzodiazepine therapy. *American Journal of Psychiatry, 157*(12), 1973–1979.

Rickels, K., Pollack, M., Sheehan, D., & Haskins, J. (2000b). Efficacy of extended-release venlafaxine in non-depressed outpatients with generalized anxiety disorder. *American Journal of Psychiatry, 157*(6), 968–974.

Roerig, J. (1999). Diagnosis and management of generalized anxiety disorder. *Journal of the American Pharmacological Association, 39*(6), 811–821.

Rosenfeld, I. (1998). When chest pain, shortness of breath, and palpitations are not due to cardiopulmonary pathology (epitomes: important advances in clinical medicine). *Western Journal of Medicine, 169*(1), 41–42.

Roy-Byrne, P., Stein, M., Russo, J., et al. (1999). Panic disorder in the primary care setting: Comorbidity, disability, service utilization, and treatment. *Journal of Clinical Psychiatry, 60*(7), 492–499.

Saeed, S., & Bruce, T. (1998). Panic disorder: Effective treatment options. *American Family Physician, 57*(10), 2405–2412.

Sallee, F., Sethuraman, G., Sine, L., & Liu, H. (2000). Yohimbine challenge in children with anxiety disorders. *American Journal of Psychiatry, 157,* 1236–1242.

Schneier, F., Liebowitz, M., Abi-Dargham, A., et al. (2000). Low dopamine D2 receptor binding potential in social phobia. *American Journal of Psychiatry, 157*(3), 457–459.

Shear, M. K., Cooper, A. M., Klerman, G. L., et al. (1993). A psychodynamic model of panic disorder. *American Journal of Psychiatry, 150,* 859–866.

Stein, M., Fryer, A., Davidson, J., et al. (1999). Fluvoxamine treatment of social phobia (social anxiety disorder): A double-blind, placebo-controlled trial. *American Journal of Psychiatry, 156*(5), 756–760.

Taylor, L., & Gorman, J. (1992). Theoretical and therapeutic considerations for the anxiety disorders. *Psychiatric Quarterly, 63*(4), 319–342.

Van-Ameringen, M., Mancini, C., & Streiner, D. (1993). Fluoxetine efficacy in social phobia. *Journal of Clinical Psychiatry, 54,* 27–32.

Versiani, M., Nardi, A., Mundim, F., et al. (1992). Pharmacotherapy of social phobia: A controlled study with moclobemide and phenelzine. *British Journal of Psychiatry, 161,* 353–360.

Wang, P., Berglund, P., & Kessler, R. (2000). Recent care of common mental disorders in the United States: Prevalence and conformance with evidenced-based recommendations. *Journal of General Internal Medicine, 15,* 284–292.

Yonkers, K., Zlotnick, C., Allsworth, J., et al. (1998). Is the course of panic disorder the same in women and men? *American Journal of Psychiatry, 155*(5), 596–602.

Personality and Impulse-Control Disorders

Barbara J. Limandri and Mary Ann Boyd

LEARNING OBJECTIVES

After studying this chapter, you will be able to:

➤ Identify the common features of personality disorders.

➤ Distinguish between the concepts of personality and personality disorder.

➤ Analyze the prevailing biologic, psychological, and social theories explaining the development of personality disorders.

➤ Discuss the epidemiology of each personality disorder.

➤ Distinguish among the three clusters of personality disorders.

➤ Formulate nursing diagnoses and plan interventions for patients with specific personality disorders.

➤ Compare the psychoanalytic explanation of the borderline personality disorder with biosocial theory.

➤ Apply the nursing process to individuals with a diagnosis of borderline personality disorder.

➤ Analyze special concerns within the nurse–patient relationship common to treating those with personality disorders.

➤ Compare and contrast the impulse-control disorders.

KEY TERMS

adaptive inflexibility
affective instability
attachment
cognitive schema
communication triad
Dialectical Behavior
   Therapy (DBT)
dichotomous thinking
dissociation
emotional
   dysregulation
emotional vulnerability
emotions
identity diffusion
impulsivity
inhibited grieving
invalidating
   environment

kleptomania
parasuicidal behavior
projective identification
psychopathy
pyromania
self-identity
separation-
   individuation
skills groups
temperament
tenuous stability
thought stopping
trichotillomania
vicious circles
   of behavior

KEY CONCEPTS

personality
personality disorder
personality traits

The concept personality seems deceivingly simple but is very complex. Historically, the term personality was derived from the Greek term, *persona*, the theatrical mask used by dramatic players. Originally, the term had the connotation of a projected pretense or allusion. Over time, the connotation changed from being an external surface representation to the internal traits of the individual.

KEY CONCEPT   Personality. Personality is a complex pattern of characteristics, largely outside of the person's awareness, that comprise the individual's distinctive pattern of perceiving, feeling, thinking, coping, and behaving. The personality emerges from a complicated interaction of biologic dispositions, psychological experiences, and environmental situations.

Today, personality is conceptualized as a complex pattern of psychological characteristics, largely outside of the person's awareness, that are not easily altered. These characteristics or traits include the individual's specific style of perceiving, thinking, and feeling about the self, others, and the environment in which the individual lives. These styles or traits are similar across many different social or personal situations and are expressed in almost every facet of functioning. Intrinsic and pervasive, they emerge from a complicated interaction of biologic dispositions, psychological experiences, and environmental situations that ultimately comprise the individual's distinctive personality (Millon & Davis, 1999).

PERSONALITY DISORDERS

No sharp division exists between normal and abnormal personality functioning. Instead, personalities are viewed on a continuum from normal at one end to abnormal at the other. Many of the same processes involved in the development of a "normal" personality are responsible for the development of a personality disorder.

KEY CONCEPT   Personality Disorder. A **personality disorder** is an enduring pattern of inner experience and behavior that deviates markedly from the expectations of the individual's culture, is pervasive and inflexible, has an onset in adolescence or early adulthood, is stable over time, and leads to distress or impairment (American Psychiatric Association [APA], 2000, p. 685).

Personality disorders are classified on Axis II of the *Diagnostic and Statistical Manual of Mental Disorders (DSM-IV-TR)* multiaxial system for diagnoses, separate from the other mental disorders presented thus far, which are classified under Axis I (APA, 2000). Separate classification under Axis II was intended to focus attention on manifestations of behavior patterns that might

be overlooked in the light of more pronounced disorders of Axis I; it does not imply difference in pathogenesis nor treatment interventions. Frequently, an Axis II diagnosis coexists with an Axis I diagnosis, in which case the Axis II diagnosis may serve as the background through which the person experiences the other diagnosis. For example, a person who has a dependent personality disorder might also have symptoms of generalized anxiety disorder when faced with demands to function autonomously.

Ten personality disorders are recognized as psychiatric diagnoses and are organized into three clusters based on the dimensions of *odd-eccentric, dramatic-emotional,* and *anxious-fearful* behaviors or symptoms. Cluster A consists of the disorders that are most broadly characterized as odd, eccentric misfits and include paranoid personality disorder, schizoid personality disorder, and schizotypal personality disorder. Cluster B disorders show great **impulsivity** (acting without considering the consequences of the act or alternate actions) and emotionality and consist of antisocial personality disorder, borderline personality disorder (BPD), histrionic personality disorder, and narcissistic personality disorder. Dramatic and erratic behavior best characterizes people with cluster B disorders. Cluster C disorders include a predominant sense of anxiety and fearfulness and include avoidant personality disorder, dependent personality disorder, and obsessive-compulsive personality disorder.

BPD is highlighted in this chapter because it is severely incapacitating and difficult to treat. Even though it is not a highlighted disorder, antisocial personality disorder is also emphasized. Symptoms from both of these disorders often provoke negative reactions on the part of the clinician, which interfere with the ability to provide effective care. Impulse-control disorders are summarized at the end of the chapter. It is outside the scope of this text to cover them in detail. These disorders commonly coexist with other mental disorders.

Personality Disorder Versus Personality Traits

To be diagnosed with a personality disorder, the individual must demonstrate the criteria behaviors persistently and to such an extent that they impair her or his ability to function socially and occupationally. In some people, the underlying feelings and behaviors may be intermittent and interfere interpersonally without impairment. Instead of having a personality disorder, the individual is said to have personality traits of the disorder, which also can be noted on Axis II without a formal diagnosis.

KEY CONCEPT   Personality Traits. Personality traits are prominent aspects of personality that are exhibited in a wide range of important social and personal contexts (APA, 2000, p. 770).

Students learning about personality disorders and traits for the first time will probably question whether or not these personality patterns are truly mental disorders. These questions are shared by much of the general public. Even within the psychiatric community, there is much debate regarding the status of personality disorders. Students may also feel frustrated in caring for individuals with these disorders or traits because sometimes problems may seem to be patterns of behaviors over which the individual could gain control and because the patient may seem otherwise emotionally healthy. Unfortunately, that is not the case. These patterns of thinking and behavior are not easily changed, and these individuals need a great amount of help and understanding from mental health providers. Changing lifelong personality patterns is difficult and requires much understanding and support.

Common Features and Diagnostic Criteria

The diagnosis of personality disorder is based on manifestation of abnormal, inflexible behavior patterns of long duration, traced back to adolescence or early adulthood. These behaviors are pervasive across a broad range of personal and social situations and cause significant distress or impairment to social or occupational functioning. These abnormal behavior patterns must deviate markedly from expectations of the individual's culture and must manifest in two or more of the following areas: cognition, or ways of perceiving and interpreting self, other people, and events; affectivity, or the range, intensity, lability, and appropriateness of emotional responses; interpersonal functioning; and impulse control.

Maladaptive Cognitive Schema

Cognitive schema are patterns of thoughts that determine how a person interprets events. Each person's cognitive schema screen, code, and evaluate incoming stimuli. In personality disorders, maladaptive cognitive schema cause misinterpretation of other people's actions or reactions and of events that result in dysfunctional ways of responding (Young, 1994). For example, if a person thinks that no one can be trusted, an innocent, friendly gesture can be interpreted as an suspicious behavior provoking a hostile response instead of a reciprocal friendly greeting.

Affectivity and Emotional Instability

Emotions are psychophysiologic reactions that define a person's mood and can be categorized as negative (anger,

fright, anxiety, guilt, shame, sadness, envy, jealousy, and disgust), positive (happiness, pride, relief, and love), and neutral (hope, compassion, empathy, sympathy, and contentment) (see Chap. 35). Emotions can affect one's ability to learn and function by affecting one's memory and how one accesses and stores information. Emotional arousal, particularly increased negative emotional arousal characteristic of people with personality disorders, can decrease one's ability to remember new information and accurately perceive the environment (Herpertz et al., 1999).

Impaired Self-Identity and Interpersonal Functioning

Self-identity is central to the normal development of one's personality. Self-identity includes an integration of social and occupational roles and affiliations, self-attributed personality traits, attitudes about gender roles, beliefs about sexuality and intimacy, long-term goals, political ideology, and religious beliefs. Without an adequately formed identity, goal-directed behavior is impaired, and interpersonal relationships are disrupted. Each individual's abilities, limitations, and goals are shaped by one's identity. In personality disorders, self-identity is often minimal or absent.

Impulsivity and Destructive Behavior

People with personality disorders often come to the attention of the mental health clinician because their impulsive behavior results in negative consequences to others or themselves. They seem not to be able to consider the consequences of their actions before acting on their impulses. For example, an individual may experience intense anger toward another and then lack skills to resist an impulse to attack that person physically, even though this action may be punished.

Cultural Considerations

For a diagnosis to be made, the behaviors are assessed to be outside the individual's cultural norm. For immigrants who may be having difficulty learning new acceptable social and cultural behavior patterns and adjusting to a new culture, the diagnosis of a personality disorder must be delayed beyond this difficult adjustment period.

Severity of Disorder

There are three generally agreed-on essential and interdependent criteria used for determining the *severity* of personality pathology: tenuous stability, adaptive inflexibility, and tendency to become trapped in rigid and inflexible patterns of behavior that are self-defeating.

Tenuous stability refers to fragile personality patterns that lack resiliency under subjective stress. These individuals may have exaggerated emotional reactions to stressful situations and are unable to cope emotionally with normal stressful situations. They do not easily learn coping skills and are susceptible to being overwhelmed when new difficulties arise.

Adaptive inflexibility describes rigidity in interactions with others, achievement of goals, and coping with stress. In the normal course of daily living, people learn when to take the initiative and modify environmental factors as well as when to adapt to the situation. They learn to be flexible in interactions with other people and their environment. Socially appropriate reactions that are proportional to the situation are the norm. Personalities become pathologic when individuals are unable to adapt effectively to new circumstances and, instead, begin arranging their lives to avoid stressful situations. They become inflexible because of their view of the world and expectations of people within in it. Consequently, there are no opportunities to learn and practice new coping skills.

The tendency to become trapped in rigid and inflexible patterns of behavior creates **vicious circles of behavior** that are self-defeating. These individuals become so rigid and inflexible in their interactions and role functioning that they generate and perpetuate dilemmas, provoke new predicaments, and set into motion self-defeating sequences with others. They restrict opportunities for new learning, misconstrue benign events, and provoke reactions in others that reactivate earlier problems (Millon & Davis, 1999). For example, a normal reaction of being angry at receiving a parking ticket usually subsides, and the person decides either to pay the fine or appeal the case before a judge. The person with a personality disorder may get angry about receiving the ticket, but the anger controls his actions. He is likely to lash out verbally at the police officer who gave the ticket, get another citation, and when appearing in court, may scream at the judge in the courtroom and end up receiving a contempt charge and having to serve time in jail. What begins as a normal stressful daily life event becomes a series of disastrous interpersonal conflicts and ends in a tragic situation for the person with personality disorder. Modulating their emotions and behavior require both psychoneurologic resources and learned coping skills. The individual with a normal reaction of anger may count to 10 before responding to the ticket or complain to a companion in seeking empathy and commiseration. The person with a personality disorder, however, lacks cognitive modulation of the emotion and may intimidate others with an irrational angry outburst.

CLUSTER A DISORDERS: ODD-ECCENTRIC

PARANOID PERSONALITY DISORDER: SUSPICIOUS PATTERN

The most prominent features of paranoid personality disorder are mistrust of others and the desire to avoid relationships in which they are not in control or lose power. These individuals are suspicious, guarded, and hostile. They are consistently mistrustful of others' motives, even relatives and close friends. Actions of others are often misinterpreted as deception, deprecation, and betrayal, especially regarding fidelity or trustworthiness of a spouse or friend (Millon & Davis, 1999). Minor innocuous incidents are often misinterpreted as having sinister or hidden meaning, and suspicions are magnified into major distortions of reality. They are unforgiving and hold grudges; typical emotional responses are anger and hostility. They distance themselves from others, and when meeting new acquaintances, they are often argumentative and abrasive. Paranoid people presents as frightening and dangerous, yet their internal experience is that of powerlessness and fearful vulnerability (Bodner & Mikulincer, 1998).

Other hallmark features of paranoid personality disorder are persistent ideas of self-importance and the tendency to be rigid and controlled. These people are blind to their own unattractive behaviors and characteristics; they often attribute these traits to others and are hypercritical of others. Outward demeanor often appears cold, sullen, and humorless. They want to appear controlled and objective, yet often they react emotionally, displaying signs of nervousness, anger, envy, and jealousy. Orderly by nature, they are hypervigilant to any environmental changes that may loosen their control on the world. Because people with this disorder are extremely sensitive about appearing "strange" or "bizarre," they will not seek mental health care until they decompensate into a psychotic state (Table 22-1).

Epidemiology

The prevalence of paranoid personality disorder is reported to be 0.5% to 2.5% in the general population. In inpatient settings, 10% to 30% of patients have this disorder, and in outpatient settings, 2% to 10% have the disorder (APA, 2000). This disorder is more often reported in men (Lyons, 1995). Axis I disorders, such as general anxiety disorder, mood disorders, and schizophrenia, can coexist with paranoid personality disorder, but minor Axis I symptoms are not usually seen. Other Axis II disorders can also coexist, such as narcissistic, avoidant, and obsessive-compulsive personality disorders (Millon & Davis, 1999).

TABLE 22.1	Summary of Diagnostic Characteristics of Cluster A Disorders: Diagnostic Criteria and Target Symptoms

Paranoid Personality Disorder 301.0	• Pervasive distrust and suspiciousness of others interpreted as malevolent (often with little or no justification or evidence to support it)
	    Assumption of exploitation, harm, or deception; feelings that others are plotting against him or her with possible sudden attacks (associated with feelings of deep or irreversible injury) at any time for no reason
	    Preoccupation with doubts of loyalty or untrustworthiness of friends and associates; deviation from doubts viewed as support for assumptions
	    Reluctance to confide in others or become close in fear that information will be used against him or her
	    Interpretation of hidden meanings into remarks or events, believing them to be demeaning and threatening
	    Holding of grudges with unwillingness to forgive; minor intrusions arouse major hostility, persisting for long periods of time
	    Quick to react and counterattack to perceived insults—possible pathologic jealousy with recurrent suspiciousness about fidelity of spouse or sexual partner
	• Not occurring exclusively during course of another psychiatric disorder; not a direct physiologic effect of a general medical condition

Schizoid Personality Disorder 301.20	• Pervasive pattern of detachment from social relating
	• Restricted range for emotional expression
	    Lacking desire for intimacy
	    Indifference to opportunities for close relationships
	    Little satisfaction from being part of family or social group
	    Preference for alone time rather than being with others; choosing solitary activities or hobbies
	    Little if any interest in having sexual experiences with others
	    Reduced pleasure from sensory, bodily, or interpersonal experiences
	    No close friends or relatives
	    Indifference to approval or criticism from others
	    Emotional coldness, detachment, or flattened activity
	• Not occurring exclusively during course of another psychiatric disorder; not a direct physiologic effect of a general medical condition

Schizotypal Personality Disorder 301.22	• Pervasive pattern of social and interpersonal deficits evidenced by acute discomfort and reduced capacity for close relationships and cognitive and perceptual distortions and eccentric behavior
	    Ideas of reference
	    Odd beliefs or magical thinking influencing behavior, such as superstitions, and preoccupation with paranormal phenomena, special powers
	    Perceptual alterations
	    Odd thinking and speech
	    Suspiciousness or paranoid ideation
	    Stiff, inappropriate, or constricted interactions
	    Odd or eccentric behavior or appearance
	    Few close friends or confidants (other than first-degree relative)
	    Anxiety in social situation, especially unfamiliar ones; no decrease in anxiety with increasing familiarity
	• Not occurring exclusively during course of another psychiatric disorder

Etiology

The etiologic factors of paranoid personality disorder are unclear. Experts speculate that there may be a genetic predisposition for an irregular maturation. An underlying excess in limbic and sympathetic system reactivity or a neurochemical acceleration of synaptic transmission may exist. These dysfunctions can give rise to the hypersensitivity, cognitive autism, and social isolation that characterize these patients. As children, these individu-

als tend to be active and intrusive, have frequent temper outbursts, are difficult to manage, and are hyperactive and irritable. Often, they had mothers who were seriously depressed or unavailable because of substance abuse (Beckwith et al., 1999).

Nursing Management

Nurses most likely see these patients for other health problems, but will formulate nursing diagnoses based on the patient's underlying suspiciousness. Assessment of these individuals will reveal disturbed or illogical thoughts that demonstrate misinterpretation of environmental stimuli. For example, a man was convinced that his wife was having an affair with the neighbor because his wife and the neighbor left home for work at the same time each morning. Even though his beliefs were illogical, he never once considered that he was wrong. He frequently followed them but would never catch them together. He continued to believe they were having an affair. The nursing diagnosis of Disturbed Thought Processes is usually supported by the assessment data.

Because of their inability to develop relationships, these patients are often socially isolated and lack social support systems, yet they do recognize their need for or lack of social support. Thus, the nursing diagnosis of Social Isolation is not appropriate for paranoid personality disorder because the person does not meet the defining characteristics of feelings of aloneness, rejection, desire for contact with people, and insecurity in social situations.

Nursing interventions based on the establishment of a nurse–patient relationship are difficult to implement because of the patient's mistrust. If a trusting relationship is established, the nurse helps the patient identify problematic areas, such as getting along with others or keeping a job. Through therapeutic techniques such as acceptance, confrontation, and reflection, the nurse and patient examine a problematic area to gain another view of the situation. Changing thought patterns takes time. Patient outcomes are evaluated in terms of small changes in thinking and behavior.

SCHIZOID PERSONALITY DISORDER: ASOCIAL PATTERN

People with schizoid personality disorder are expressively impassive and interpersonally unengaged (Millon & Davis, 1999). These individuals seem to lack the ability to experience the joyful and pleasurable aspects of life. They are introverted and seclusive and clinically appear distant, aloof, apathetic, and emotionally detached. They have difficulties making friends, seem uninterested in social activities, and appear to gain little satisfaction in personal relationships. In fact, they appear to be incapable of forming social relationships. Interests are directed at objects, things, and abstractions. As children, they engage primarily in solitary activities, such as stamp collecting, computer games, electronic equipment, or academic pursuits such as mathematics or engineering.

There seems to be a cognitive deficit characterized by obscure thought processes, particularly about social matters. Communication with others is confused and often lacks focus. These individuals reveal minimum introspection and self-awareness, and interpersonal experiences are described in a very mechanical way (see Table 22-1).

Epidemiology

Schizoid personality disorder is rarely diagnosed in clinical settings (Lyons, 1995). It is estimated that the prevalence of schizoid disorder ranges from 0% to 8%, with a median prevalence of 1% (Widiger, 1991). The most prevalent comorbid disorder is avoidant personality disorder, which occurs in 30% to 35% of the cases. Dependent and obsessive-compulsive disorders have been shown to coexist with schizoid personality disorder (Lyons, 1995).

Etiology

The etiologic processes are speculative. There may be defects in either the limbic or reticular regions of the brain that may result in the development of the schizoid pattern (Millon & Davis, 1999). The defects of this personality may stem from an adrenergic–cholinergic imbalance in which the parasympathetic division of the autonomic nervous system is functionally dominant. Excesses or deficiencies in acetylcholine and norepinephrine may result in the proliferation and scattering of neural impulses that may be responsible for the cognitive "slippage" or affectivity deficits.

Nursing Management

Impaired Social Interactions and Chronic Low Self-Esteem are typical diagnoses of patients with schizoid personality disorder. Major treatment goals are to enhance the experience of pleasure, prevent social isolation, and increase emotional responsiveness to others. Because these individuals often lack customary social skills, social skills training is useful in enhancing their ability to relate in interpersonal situations. The primary focus is to increase the patient's ability to feel pleasure. The nurse balances interventions between encouraging enough social activity that prevents the individual from retreating to a fantasy world and too much social activity that becomes intolerable.

The nurse may find working with these individuals unrewarding and become frustrated, feel helpless, or feel bored during the interactions. It is difficult to establish a therapeutic relationship with these individuals because they tend to shy away from interactions. Evaluation of outcomes should be in terms of increasing the patient's feelings of satisfaction with solitary activities.

SCHIZOTYPAL PERSONALITY DISORDER: ECCENTRIC PATTERN

Persons with the schizotypal personality disorder are characterized by a pattern of social and interpersonal deficits. They are void of any close friends other than first-degree relatives. They have odd beliefs about their world that are inconsistent with their cultural norms. Ideas of reference (incorrect interpretations of events as having special, personal meaning) are often present, as well as unusual perceptual delusions and odd, circumstantial, and metaphorical thinking and speech. Their mood is constricted or inappropriate and they have excessive social anxieties of a paranoid character that do not diminish with familiarity. Their appearance and behavior are characterized as odd, eccentric, or peculiar. They usually exhibit an avoidant behavior pattern (see Table 22-1).

If these individuals do become psychotic, they seem totally disoriented and confused. Many will exhibit posturing, grimacing, inappropriate giggling, and peculiar mannerisms. Speech tends to ramble. Fantasy, hallucinations, and bizarre, fragmented delusions may be present. Regressive acts such as soiling and wetting the bed may occur. These individuals may consume food in an infantile or ravenous manner. These symptoms mirror but fall short of features that would justify the diagnosis of schizophrenia. Their tendency is to remain socially isolated, dependent on family members or institutions. Well intentioned relatives or institutional staff will protect these individuals, reinforcing their dependency. These patients avoid social interaction that can keep them functional. People with this disorder are particularly prone to developing disorganized schizophrenia.

Epidemiology

The prevalence of schizotypal personality disorder is estimated to range from 0.7% to 5.1%, with a median rate of about 3% of the nonclinical population. In a clinical sample (of psychiatric patients), the prevalence ranged from 2.0% to 64%, with a median prevalence of 17.5% (Lyons, 1995). This wide variation in prevalence rates may reflect the controversy surrounding the classification of schizotypal disorder as a separate personality disorder instead of a component of schizophrenia.

Etiology

The etiology of schizotypal personality disorder is unknown. The neurodevelopmental explanation posits that schizotypy can be explained by insults to the nervous system at critical developmental periods. In a study of 499 undergraduates, an excess of pregnancy and birth complications were related to the development of schizotypal disorder. The pregnancy and birth complications that were most predictive of schizotypy were breathing problems or need for oxygen, artificial induction of labor, and breech birth (Bakan & Peterson, 1994). There is considerable speculation that this disorder is part of a continuum of schizophrenia-related disorders and is really closely related to chronic schizophrenia (Mata et al., 2000). When the genetics of personality disorders are considered, there is evidence of a link of schizotypal personality disorder to schizophrenia (Mata et al., 2000). Additional research is needed to determine whether this disorder is a milder form of schizophrenia. The person with schizotypal personality disorder has widespread cognitive deficits involving the left hemisphere more than the right. They therefore have difficulty with short term memory retention and verbal learning (Voglmaier et al., 2000; Cadenhead et al., 1999). They also show visual perceptual and working memory deficits (Farmer et al., 2000).

Nursing Management

Depending on the amount of decompensation (deterioration of functioning and exacerbation of symptoms), the assessment of a patient with a schizotypal personality disorder can generate a range of nursing diagnoses. If a person is symptomatic with severe symptoms such as delusional thinking or perceptual disturbances, the nursing diagnoses are similar to those for a person with schizophrenia (see Chap. 18). If symptoms are mild, the typical nursing diagnoses include Social Isolation, Ineffective Coping, Low Self-Esteem, and Impaired Social Interactions.

People with schizotypal personality disorder need help in increasing their self-worth and recognizing their positive attributes. They can benefit from interventions such as social skills training and environmental management that increases their psychosocial functioning. Their odd, eccentric thoughts and behaviors alienate them from others. Reinforcing socially appropriate dress and behavior can improve their overall appearance and ability to relate in the environment. Because they have a hard time generalizing from one situation to another, attention to cognitive skills is important (Waldeck & Miller, 2000).

Continuum of Care

People with cluster A personality disorders are rarely seen in mental health clinics because they often do not admit to mental health problems. They can improve their quality of life through psychotherapy, but their suspiciousness, lack of trust, or impaired social interactions make it difficult to establish a therapeutic relationship. They do not usually seek out treatment unless more serious symptoms appear, such as depression or anxiety. Medications are not generally used unless there is coexisting anxiety or depression. Even patients with schizotypal personality disorder have a relatively stable course. Few actually develop schizophrenia or another psychotic disorder (APA, 2000). They too seek out health care for other problems and come to the attention of mental health professionals when their odd behavior interferes with their daily activities. At these times, brief interventions are needed, such as self-care assistance, reality orientation, and role enhancement (McCloskey & Bulechek, 1996).

Nursing care is often provided in a home or clinic setting, with the personality disorder being secondary to the purpose of the care. This means that nurses are focusing on other aspects of patient care and may miss the underlying psychiatric disorder. A psychiatric nursing consult may be needed for these patients to help identify the disorder.

CLUSTER B DISORDERS: DRAMATIC-EMOTIONAL

BORDERLINE PERSONALITY DISORDER: UNSTABLE PATTERN

Clinical Course of Disorder

BPD has been described in the literature for several years but has only recently been recognized as a formal mental disorder. In 1938, the term borderline was first used to refer to a group of disorders that did not quite fit the definition of either neurosis or psychosis (Stern, 1938). The term evolved from the psychoanalytic conceptualization of the disorder as a dysfunctional personality structure. In 1980, BPD was formally recognized as a distinct disorder in the *DSM-III.* Many believe that the term borderline should be replaced with a word that more accurately describes the disorder's clinical characteristics rather than denoting one specific theoretic perspective. Despite the controversy, the term borderline continues to be used. In the *DSM-IV-TR,* BPD is defined as "a pervasive pattern of instability of interpersonal relationships, self-image, and affects, and marked impulsivity that begins by early adulthood and is present in a variety of contexts" (APA, 2000, p. 706). Table 22-2 outlines the diagnostic characteristics of BPD.

> Borderline personality disorder is defined as "a pervasive pattern of instability of interpersonal relationships, self-image, and affects, and marked impulsivity that begins by early adulthood and is present in a variety of contexts" (APA, 2000, p. 706).

People with BPD have problems in regulating their moods, developing a sense of self, maintaining interpersonal relationships, maintaining reality-based cognitive processes, and avoiding impulsive or destructive behavior. They appear more competent than they actually are and often set unrealistically high expectations for themselves. When these expectations are not met, they experience intense shame, self-hate, and self-directed anger. Their lives often are like soap operas—one crisis after another. Some of the crises are caused by the individual's dysfunctional lifestyle or inadequate social milieu, but many are caused by fate—a death of a spouse or a diagnosis of an illness. They react emotionally with minimal coping skills for mood and behavior. The intensity of their dysregulation is often frightening to themselves and others. Friends, family members, and coworkers limit their contact with the person, which furthers their sense of aloneness, abandonment, and self-hatred. It also diminishes the opportunity for learning self-corrective measures.

TABLE 22.2   Key Diagnostic Characteristics of Borderline Personality Disorder 301.83

Diagnostic Criteria and Target Symptoms	Associated Findings
Diagnostic Criteria and Target Symptoms	*Associated Findings*
• Pervasive pattern of unstable interpersonal relationships, self-image, and affects	*Associated Behavioral Findings*
Frantic efforts to avoid real or imagined abandonment	• Pattern of undermining self at the moment a goal is to be realized
Pattern of unstable and intense interpersonal relationships (alternating between extremes of idealization and devaluation)	• Possible psychotic-like symptoms during times of stress
Identity disturbance (markedly and persistently unstable self-image or sense of self)	• Recurrent job losses, interrupted education, and broken marriages
Impulsivity in at least two areas that are potentially self-damaging (spending, sex, substance abuse, reckless driving, or binge eating)	• History of physical and sexual abuse, neglect, hostile conflict, and early parental loss or separation
Recurrent suicidal behavior, gestures, or threats, or self-mutilating behavior	
Affective instability due to a marked reactivity of mood (intense episodes lasting a few hours and only rarely more than a few days)	
Chronic feelings of emptiness	
Inappropriate, intense anger or difficulty controlling anger	
Transient, stress-related paranoid ideation or severe dissociative symptoms	
• Beginning by early adulthood and presenting in a variety of contexts	

Affective Instability

Affective instability, rapid and extreme shifts in moods, is one of the core characteristics of BPD and is evident by sudden shifts in moods, erratic emotional responses to situations, and intense sensitivity to criticism or perceived slights. For example, a person may greet a casual acquaintance with intense affections as if they were very close friends. Yet later, the person may treat that same friend with aloofness. Friends describe individuals with BPD as moody, irresponsible, or intense. These individuals fail to recognize their own emotional responses, thoughts, beliefs, and behaviors. Clinically, when a stressful situation is encountered, these individuals react with shifts in emotions. They seem to have limited ability to develop emotional buffers to the impact of stressful situations. Regulating anger, anxiety, and sadness is particularly problematic (Kernberg, 1994; Stein, 1996).

Identity Disturbances

Identity diffusion occurs when a person lacks aspects of personal identity or when personal identity is poorly developed (Erikson, 1968). Four factors of identity are most commonly disturbed: role absorption (narrowly defining self within a single role), painful incoherence (distressed sense of internal disharmony), inconsistency (lack of coherence in thoughts, feelings, and actions), and lack of commitment (Wilkinson-Ryan & Western, 2000). Other factors of the personality identity (religious ideology, moral value systems, sexual attitudes) appear to be less important in identity diffusion. Clinically, these patients appear to have no sense of their own identity and direction; this becomes a source of great distress to these patients and is often manifested by chronic feelings of emptiness and boredom. Not surprisingly, adolescent immaturity (especially in girls) is a predictor of cluster B disorders (Bernstein et al., 1996).

It is not unusual for people with BPD to view themselves and direct their actions toward the wishes of other people. For example, this is a woman with BPD describing herself: "I am a singer because my mother wanted me to be. I live in the city because my manager thought that I should. I become whatever anyone tells me to be. Whenever someone recommends a song, I wonder why I didn't think of that. My boyfriend tells me what to wear."

Unstable Interpersonal Relationships

People with BPD have an extreme fear of abandonment as well as a history of unstable, insecure attachments (Sack et al., 1996). This abandonment stems from ambivalent early childhood attachment. Consequently, these individuals are intolerant of being alone, as evident by clinging behavior and attention seeking (Gunderson,

1996). Most never experienced a consistently secure, nurturing relationship and are constantly seeking reassurance and validation. In an attempt to meet their interpersonal needs, they overidealize others and establish intense relationships that violate others' interpersonal boundaries, which leads to rejection. When these relationships do not live up to their expectations, they devalue the person. Continually disappointed in relationships, these individuals, who already are intensely emotional and have a poor sense of self, feel estranged from others and feel inadequate in the face of perceived social standards (Miller, 1994). Intense shame and self-hate follow. These feelings often result in self-injurious behaviors, such as cutting the wrist, self-burnings, or head banging.

In social situations, these patients use elaborate strategies to structure interactions. That is, they restrict their relationships to ones in which they feel in control. They distance themselves from groups when feeling anxious (which is most of the time) and rarely use their social support system. Even if they are married or have a supportive extended family, they are reluctant to share their feelings. They do not want to burden anyone; they fear rejection and also assume that people are tired of hearing them repeat the same issues (Miller, 1994).

A controversial area of BPD is separating early childhood abuse and trauma from pathologic development. In fact, people with confirmed childhood abuse and neglect histories showed a fourfold likelihood of having a personality disorder even when such factors as age, parental education, and parental psychiatric disorders were controlled (Johnson et al., 1999). However, trauma and childhood sexual abuse do not seem to cause BPD but rather sufficiently disturb identity and affect regulation to contribute to pathologic personality development (Zanarini et al., 1997; Sansone et al., 1998).

Cognitive Dysfunctions

The thinking of people with BPD is dichotomous. Cognitively, they evaluate experiences, people, and objects in terms of mutually exclusive categories (eg, good or bad, success or failure, trustworthy or deceitful). The effect of this type of thinking is to force extreme interpretations of events that would normally be viewed as incorporating both positive and negatives. They are not able to tolerate inconsistencies in others. There are also times when their thinking becomes disorganized. Losing the focus of a conversation or expressing generalities may occur during periods of stress. Irrelevant, bizarre notions and vague or scattered thought connections are sometimes present as well as delusions and hallucinations.

Dissociation, both a normal mechanism and a psychopathologic phenomenon, is defined as splitting or separating closely connected behaviors, thoughts, or feelings (Leichsenring, 1999). Dissociation can be conceptualized as lying on a continuum from minor dissociations of daily life, such as daydreaming, to a breakdown in the usually integrated functions of consciousness, memory, perception of self or the environment, and sensory-motor behavior. During dissociation, there are disturbances in memory about events that happen. For example, in driving familiar roads, people often get lost in their thoughts or dissociate and suddenly do not remember what happened during that part of the trip. Environmental stimuli are ignored, and there are changes in the perception of reality. The individual is physically present but mentally in another place. Dissociation serves a useful purpose. In the case of driving a familiar road, dissociation alleviates the boredom of driving. It is also a way of handling traumatic events. The person does not have to be aware of traumatic events and does not have to remember them. Dissociation becomes a coping strategy, a way of dealing with unpleasant thoughts or events. There is a strong correlation between dissociation and self-injurious behavior (Golynkina & Ryle, 1999; Zanarini et al., 2000).

In BPD, dissociation is a common experience in both men and women. In one study of 150 women, the 78 women with BPD scored significantly higher on the Dissociative Experiences Scale, which measures components of dissociative experiences, than the 72 without the diagnosis (Zweig-Frank et al., 1994a). Similar findings indicated that men with BPD (n = 32) who experienced significantly more dissociation than men without BPD (n = 60). One of the causes of dissociation was generally thought to be sexual and physical abuse. These researchers were unable to show any relationship between dissociation and childhood sexual or physical abuse (Zweig-Frank et al., 1994a). They hypothesized that dissociation in the person with BPD may be accounted for by intrinsic, constitutional factors. Zanarini and colleagues, however, found that those with BPD and posttraumatic stress disorder (PTSD) had a higher range of dissociative experiences than controls who had some other Axis II disorder (Zanarini et al., 2000).

Dysfunctional Behaviors

Impaired Problem Solving. In BPD, there is often failure to engage in active problem solving. Instead, problem solving is attempted by soliciting help from others in a helpless, hopeless manner (Linehan, 1993). Suggestions are rarely taken.

Impulsivity. Impulsivity is also characteristic of people with BPD. Impulse-driven people have difficulty delaying gratification or thinking through the consequences before acting on their feelings. Their actions are often

unpredictable. Essentially, they act in the moment and clean up the mess afterward. Gambling, spending money irresponsibly, binge eating, engaging in unsafe sex, and abusing substances are typical of these individuals. They can also be physically or verbally aggressive. Job losses, interrupted education, and unsuccessful relationships are common.

Self-Injurious Behaviors. This disorder is damaging to individuals, who are generally miserable because of unsuccessful interpersonal relationships and social experiences. Going from crisis to crisis, they live in a state of constant turmoil. They have a tendency to undermine themselves when a goal is about to be reached. On the most serious side, these individuals frequently attempt suicide or engage in **parasuicidal behavior** (deliberate self-injurious behavior accompanied by an intent to harm self), one of the most distressing aspects of this disorder. For example, in one study of a burn unit from 1980 to 1991, of the 31 patients who were admitted with self-inflicted burns, 16 inflicted nonlethal injuries and the other 15 lethal injuries (Tuohig et al., 1995). The prevalence of self-injurious behavior is estimated to be 43% to 67% of the patients with BPD (Soloff et al., 1994). Physical disability following injury is common. Suicidal behavior among those with BPD differs from that in patients with other personality disorders or with Axis I disorders in that the latter patients almost always had concurrent substance use disorders and depressive syndromes (Isometsa et al., 1996), anger (Fava, 1998), and impulsive aggression (Coccaro & Kavoussi, 1997).

Self-injurious behavior is more likely to occur when the individual with BPD (1) is depressed, (2) has highly unstable interpersonal relationships, especially problems with intimacy and sociability, and (3) is paranoid, hypervigilant (alert, watchful), and resentful (Yeomans et al., 1994). Self-injury is directly related to dissociation and unstable interpersonal relationships, but research has failed to support the long-held belief that parasuicidal behavior is directly related to childhood abuse. It is hypothesized that early childhood physical or sexual abuse is one of many of the traumatic events that contributes to the development of BPD (Zweig-Frank et al., 1994c). Self-injurious behaviors can be compulsive, episodic, or repetitive.

Compulsive self-injurious behaviors occur many times daily and are repetitive and ritualistic. For example, hair-pulling can either be a separate disorder (**trichotillomania**) or a behavior of other personality disorders, such as BPD. It involves pulling out hair from anywhere on the body, especially from the scalp, eyebrows, and eyelashes. Hair is plucked, examined, and sometimes eaten. Hairs may be piled before being discarded. Hair-pulling sessions may take several hours (Favazza, 1996). Most of these individuals do not seek help unless the symptoms are severe and, then, usually, from dermatologists or family practitioners.

Episodic self-injurious behaviors occur every so often. These are especially common in people with BPD and develop into habitual coping behavior patterns. During periods of stress, a state of progressive tension manifested by feelings of anger, depression, or anxiety rises to an intolerable level. The patient reports being numb or empty and ends this dissociated state with self-injurious behavior such as cutting wrists, arms, or other body parts with sharp objects such as razor blades, glass, or knives. One half to two thirds of BPD patients with self-injurious behaviors experience little or no associated pain (Links et al., 1998). In fact, endogenous endorphins (opioids) are released, which dampen pain perception and activate the brain's pleasure center.

Tension may be relieved and a sense of calmness or even pleasure may follow. These feelings are believed to be reinforcing, and the person learns to relieve stress and anxiety by mutilating acts. The individuals harm themselves to feel better, get rapid relief from distressing thoughts and emotions, and gain a sense of control. The following are some of the reasons patients give for injuring themselves (Favazza, 1996):

- Tension release—relieves anxiety, stress
- Return to reality—decreases sense of emptiness, makes the world real
- Establishing control—when out of control, injury helps return to normal
- Security and uniqueness—knows that pain is there when all else fails
- Influencing others—shows others how deeply they are being hurt
- Negative perceptions—hates self and deserves to be hurt
- Sexuality—enhances sexual feelings or eliminates memories of abuse
- Euphoria—feels good, gets a high feeling
- Venting anger—hurts self instead of others
- Relief from alienation—injury provides relief from profound sense of loneliness

When the occasional self-injury turns into an overwhelming preoccupation, it becomes *repetitive self-mutilation*. These people develop an identity as a "cutter" or "burner" and describe themselves as being addicted to their self-harm. In an interpretive phenomenologic study with people with BPD, Nehls (1999) described the emotional conflict these patients experience when their perceived efforts to comfort self are interpreted by others as manipulation, resulting in their being denied care.

Sometimes, patients and nurses determine risk for suicide by whether the intended outcome of a parasuicidal episode is death or injury. The underlying assumption is that those who attempt to kill themselves are at higher risk than those who self-injure. In reality, there should be no distinction between self-damaging behaviors and suicide attempts. In fact, studies show patients with a history of self-injuries have more serious suicidal tendencies (Soloff et al., 1994). The prevalence of suicide attempts in patients with BPD may exceed 70%. In a study of 81 people with BPD, 45 patients (55.6%) had both self-injured and attempted suicide. Only a small minority (8% or 10%) had neither behavior. Completed suicides are estimated to occur in 3% to 9% of patients with BPD (Soloff et al., 1994). All self-injurious behavior should be considered potentially life-threatening and taken seriously.

Borderline Personality Disorder in Special Populations

Many children and adolescents show symptoms similar to those of BPD, such as moodiness, self-destruction, impulsiveness, lack of temper control, and rejection sensitivity. If a family member has BPD, the adolescent should be carefully assessed for this disorder. Because symptoms of BPD begin in adolescents, it makes sense that some of the children and adolescents would meet the criteria for BPD, even though it is not diagnosed before young adulthood. More likely, there are personality traits, such as impulsivity and mood instability, in many adolescents that that should be recognized and treated whether or not BPD actually develops.

Epidemiology

The estimated prevalence of BPD in the general population ranges from 0.4% to 2.0%, with a median rate of 1.6%. In clinical populations, BPD is the most frequently diagnosed personality disorder; its prevalence ranges from 11% to 70%, with a median of 31%. The reasons for the high representation of the BPD diagnosis in the clinical populations are unclear, especially because it was not a formal psychiatric diagnosis until 1980. The average prevalence of outpatients is 8% to 27%, and among inpatients, 15% to 51% (Lyons, 1995; Widiger & Weissman, 1991).

Gender

More than three fourths (77%) of the patients diagnosed with BPD are women, who tend to be young, with a mean age in the mid-20s (Lyons, 1995). There is controversy about what this increased rate of BPD in women actually means, and a variety of explanations are offered for the high diagnosis rate. One theory is that it is more socially acceptable for women to seek help from the health care system than men (see Chap. 23). Another reason is that childhood sexual abuse, which has been shown to be more common in girls, is one of the strongest risk factors for BPD. Others believe that the evidence of gender bias in diagnosing could also account for the overrepresentation of women. In general, however, people who live with the diagnosis of BPD are often marginalized and not taken seriously when they present for mental health care (Nehls, 1998), which is more a problem of the institutions than of the patient.

Comorbidity

There are ample clinical reports of the coexistence of personality disorders with Axis I disorders, but epidemiologic research is scant. BPD is associated with mood, substance abuse, eating, dissociative, and anxiety disorders (Grilo et al., 1996; Comtois et al., 1999; Oldham et al., 1995).

Risk Factors

Physical and Sexual Abuse

Physical and sexual abuse appear to be significant risk factors for BPD. Several traumatic childhood experiences were examined in a study in Canada of 751 psychiatric records of female patients aged 16 to 45 years of age; 366 were diagnosed with BPD and 385 with other personality disorders. These patients had been seen in the psychiatric services in general hospitals in the greater Montreal area serving people of all socioeconomic levels. The categories of traumatic childhood experiences that were identified from the chart information included major abuse (verbal, physical, and sexual abuse; witnessing domestic violence), major losses (adoption placement, divorce, desertion, leaving home before the age of 16 years, death of mother or father), and parental drug or alcohol abuse. Significantly more of the women with BPD (83%) had a history of childhood abuse when compared with the patients with other personality disorders (52%; $P = 0.001$). The women with BPD also had a higher frequency of major losses (69%) when compared with the control group (48%; $P = 0.001$). There were no differences between the groups in drug problems reported for the fathers, but fathers of women with BPD are more likely to abuse alcohol (38% versus 28%; $P = 0.008$). There was no difference in the use of drugs for the mothers (Laporte & Guttman, 1996). This study has been substantiated by other studies with very similar results (1997; Johnson et al., 1999; Sansone et al., 1998).

Parental Loss or Separation

Separation or loss of parent at an early age appears to be a risk factor for BPD, and it appears that loss of same-sex parent could have some significance. For men, separation or loss of the father during childhood appears to be an especially important risk factor. In one study, 61 men with BPD were compared with 60 men who did not have BPD. Results showed 42.6% of the BPD group had a parental separation or loss, compared with 23.3% of the non-BPD group, and 80% of the parental separation or loss involved their fathers (Zweig-Frank et al., 1994b). In another study of psychological risk factors, childhood sexual abuse, early separation or loss, and abnormal parental bonding were studied in 78 women with BPD and 72 women with other, non-BPD personality disorders. Childhood sexual abuse was common in both samples, but the rate was significantly higher in the BPD sample (70.5%) than in the non-BPD sample (45.8%; $P = 0.002$). Results were different in this study than in the previously discussed chart review study in the area of major loss. In this study, there were no differences in separation or loss of a parent between these groups (51.3% in BPD group versus 45.8% in non-BPD group), but the maternal affection scores on the Parental Bonding Index were lower for the BPD group (Zweig-Frank et al., 1994a). Clearly, more studies are needed to identify risk factors for the development of the personality disorders.

Etiology

Biologic Theories

There is no consensus regarding a biologic etiology of BPD, and studies are lacking to show whether or not a genetic component exits. The underlying assumption of the biologic explanations of BPD is that personality disorders develop within the context of the normal personality, which is on a continuum from normal to abnormal. Some even argue that personality and Axis I disorders actually exist on a continuum and that personality traits and mood episodes are derived from the same underlying neurotransmitter dysfunctions and genetic constitution. These genetically determined traits become the organizing principle for the entire personality.

Magnetic resonance imaging studies of 21 female patients with both BPD and PTSD, compared with a matched healthy control sample, showed that women with BPD had a 16% smaller amygdala than the healthy controls (Driessen et al., 2000) These findings are consistent with neurologic effects of prolonged exposure to cortisol.

Biologic abnormalities are associated with three BPD characteristics: affective instability, transient psychotic episodes, and impulsive, aggressive, and suicidal behavior. Impulsivity and emotional instability are unusually intense in these patients, and these traits are known to be heritable. Associated brain dysfunction occurs in the limbic system and frontal lobe and increases the behaviors of impulsiveness, parasuicide, and mood disturbance. A decrease in serotonin activity and an increase in α_2-noradrenergic receptor sites may be related to the irritability and impulsiveness common in people with this disorder (Coccaro et al., 1998; Oquendo & Mann, 2000). It has also been hypothesized that an increase in dopamine may be responsible for transient psychotic states. These dysfunctions could be caused by a number of events, including trauma, epilepsy, and attention deficit hyperactivity disorder (ADHD) (Greene & Ugarriza, 1995; van Reekum, 1993).

Psychological Theories

Psychoanalytic Theories. The psychoanalytic views of BPD focus on two important psychoanalytic concepts: separation-individuation and projective identification. Psychoanalytic theory says that in BPD, the person has not achieved the normal and healthy developmental stage of **separation-individuation,** during which a child develops a sense of self, a permanent sense of significant others (object constancy), and an integration of seeing both bad and good components of self (Mahler et al., 1975). Those with BPD lack the ability to separate from primary caregiver or nurturer and develop a separate and distinct personality or self-identity. Psychoanalytic theory suggests that these difficulties in separating from the primary caregiver or nurturer and developing an autonomous self occur because the primary caregivers' behaviors have been inconsistent or insensitive to the needs of the child during childhood. The child develops ambivalent feelings regarding interpersonal relationships and has no basis on which to establish trusting and secure relationships in the future. Children experience feelings of intense fear and anger in separating themselves from others. This problem continues into adulthood, and they continue to experience difficulties in maintaining personal boundaries and in interpersonal interactions and relationships. This lack of self-identity continues, and they may idolize significant others for a time. When those with whom they form relationships show any weakness or seem inattentive to them, they immediately devalue and reject them. There is no negotiation or expression of one's feelings regarding the other person's actions; it is just immediate rejection and withdrawal. They become ingrained in a pattern of anticipating rejection from those they love, so they quickly reject others first at the least sign of conflict.

Often, these patients falsely attribute to others their own unacceptable feelings, impulses, or thoughts, termed **projective identification.** Projective identification is believed to play an important role in the development of BPD and is a defense mechanism by which these patients hope to protect their fragile self-image. For example, when these patients feel overwhelmingly anx-

ious or angry at being disregarded by another, they cannot tolerate the intensity of their feelings, and to defend against these feelings, they unconsciously blame others for what happens to them. They project their feelings onto a significant other with the unconscious hope that the other knows how to deal with it. Projective identification becomes a defensive way of interacting with the world, which leads to more rejection.

Maladaptive Cognitive Processes. Cognitive schemas are important in understanding the borderline disorder as well as antisocial personality disorder. The individual with personality disorders develops maladaptive schemas that cause them to misinterpret environmental stimuli continuously and result in rigid and inflexible behavior patterns in response to new situations and people. Because those with BPD have been conditioned to anticipate rejection and disappointment in the past, they become entrenched in a pattern of fear and anxiety regarding encountering new people or situations. They have fears that disaster is going to strike any minute. Early in life, patients with BPD and other personality disorders develop maladaptive schemas or dysfunctional ways of interpreting people and events. Table 22-3 explains 15 major maladaptive schemas within four major domains (autonomy, connectedness, worthiness, and expectations and limits) that are at work in those with personality disorders. Autonomy is the sense that the individual can function independently in the world and express needs, interests, preferences, opinions, and feelings. The connectedness domain is the sense that an individual is connected to others in a stable, enduring, and trusting way. Connectedness includes intimacy (close emotional ties to another) and social integration (sense of belonging and fitting into a group of friends, family, and community). Worthiness is believing that one is lovable, competent, acceptable, and desirable to others and worthy of attention and respect. Having the capacity to set realistic, achievable standards for self and others describes the domain of reasonable expectations and realistic limits. The work of cognitive therapists is to challenge these distortions in thinking patterns and replace them with realistic ones.

Social Theories: Biosocial Theories

Theodore Millon. The biosocial learning theory was developed by Theodore Millon, who viewed BPD as a distinct disorder that develops as a result of both biologic and psychological factors (Millon & Davis, 1996). Although he believed one's personality was biologically determined, he believed that a child's interaction with the environment and learning and experience could greatly affect biologic predisposition. He argued that each individual possesses a biologically based pattern of sensitivities and behavioral dispositions that shape

TABLE 22.3 Maladaptive Schemas	
Domain	**Schemas With Definitions**

I. Autonomy	1. Dependence
	   Belief that one is unable to function on one's own
	2. Subjugation/lack of individuation
	   The voluntary or involuntary sacrifice of one's own needs to satisfy others' needs, often with an accompanying failure to recognize one's own needs
	3. Vulnerability to harm and illness
	   The fear that disaster is about to strike at any time (natural, criminal, medical, or financial)
	4. Fear of losing self-control
	   The fear that one will involuntarily lose control of one's own behavior, impulses, emotions, mind, body, and so on
	5. Emotional deprivation
	   The expectation that one's needs for nurturance, empathy, affection, and caring will never be adequately met by others
	6. Abandonment/loss
	   Fear that one will imminently lose significant others and then be emotionally isolated forever

II. Connectedness	7. Mistrust
	   The expectation that others will fully hurt, abuse, cheat, lie, manipulate, or take advantage
	8. Social isolation/alienation
	   The feeling that one is isolated from the rest of the world, different from other people, or not a part of any group or community
	9. Defectiveness/unlovability
	   The feeling that one is inwardly defective and flawed, or that one would be fundamentally unlovable to significant others if exposed
	10. Social undesirability
	   The belief that one is outwardly undesirable to others (eg, ugly, sexually undesirable, low in status, poor in conversational skills, dull)

III. Worthiness	11. Incompetence/failure
	   The belief that one cannot perform competently in areas of achievement (school, career), daily responsibilities to self or others, or decision making
	12. Guilt/punishment
	   The belief that one is morally or ethically bad or irresponsible, and deserving of harsh criticism or punishment
	13. Shame/embarrassment
	   Recurrent feelings of shame or self-consciousness, experienced because one believes that one's inadequacies (as reflected in any of the other schemas) are totally unacceptable to others and are exposed
	14. Unrelenting standards
	   The relentless striving to meet extremely high expectations of self, at the expense of happiness, pleasure, health, sense of accomplishment, or satisfying relationships

IV. Expectations and limits	15. Entitlement/sufficient limits Insistence that one should be able to do, say, or have whatever one wants immediately; disregard for what others consider reasonable, what is actually feasible, the time or patience usually required, or the costs to others; may include difficulty with self-discipline

Young, J. E. (1994). *Cognitive therapy for personality disorders: A schema-focused approach* (pp. 13–14). Sarasota, FL: Professional Resource Press.

his or her experiences, including active-passive behavior or tendency to take initiative versus reacting to events; sensitivity to pleasure or pain; and sensitivity behavior to self and others. Millon believed that BPD is a particular cycloid personality pattern representing a moderately dysfunctional dependent or ambivalent orientation, often expressed in intense endogenous moods, described as patterns of recurring dejection and apathy interspersed with spells of anger, anxiety, or euphoria.

A further elaboration of Millon's multidimensional model incorporates biologic explanations into the behavior. Cloninger and colleagues (1998) described personality disorder behaviors based on temperament and character dimensions derived from a factor analysis design. Cluster A disorders are associated with low reward dependence and social attachment mediated by norepinephrine and serotonin. Cluster C disorders are associated with high harm avoidance mediated by γ-aminobutyric acid (GABA) and serotonin. Cluster B disorders are associated with high novelty seeking mediated by dopamine. Novelty seeking behavior includes exhilaration, exploration, impulsivity, extravagance, and irritability.

Marsha Linehan. The current biosocial theory of BPD proposed by Marsha Linehan and colleagues at the University of Washington is similar to Millon's theory, with a focus on the interaction of both biologic and social learning influences. Her primary focus is on the particular behavioral patterns observed in BPD, including emotional vulnerability, self-invalidation, unrelenting crises, inhibited grieving, active passivity, and apparent competence (Linehan, 1993) (Text Box 22-1).

This biosocial viewpoint sees BPD as a multifaceted problem, a combination of a person's innate emotional vulnerability, and their inability to control that emotion in social interactions (**emotional dysregulation**) and the environment (Linehan, 1993). People with this disorder appear to have an **emotional vulnerability,** and they have difficulty regulating their moods within their social environment. They are extremely sensitive to environmental stress and experience extreme emotional reactions. What might be viewed as a minor inconvenience to others will evoke an emotional outburst in a person with BPD.

The emotional dysregulation and aggressive impulsivity entails both social learning and biologic regulation. Much of the neurobiologic research is directed at neurotransmitter functions involving serotonin, norepinephrine, dopamine, acetylcholine, GABA, and vasopressin (Coccaro et al., 1998; Silk, 2000). In fact, restoring balance in these systems permits smother, more consistent neural firing between the limbic system, and the frontal and prefrontal cortex. When these pathways are functional, the person has greater capacity to think about their emotions and modulate their behavior more responsibly.

The biosocial viewpoint supports the notion that the ability to control one's emotion is in part a learning process, learned from one's private experiences and encounters with their social environment. BPD is believed to develop when these emotionally vulnerable individuals interact with an **invalidating environment,** a social situation that negates the individual's private emotional responses and communication. In other words, when the person's core emotional responses and communications

TEXT BOX 22.1

Behavioral Patterns in Borderline Personality Disorder

1. *Emotional vulnerability.* Person experiences a pattern of pervasive difficulties in regulating negative emotions, including high sensitivity to negative emotional stimuli, high emotional intensity, and slow return to emotional baseline.

2. *Self-invalidation.* Person fails to recognize one's own emotional responses, thoughts, beliefs, and behaviors and sets unrealistically high standards and expectations for self. May include intense shame, self-hate, and self-directed anger. Person has no personal awareness and tends to blame social environment for unrealistic expectations and demands.

3. *Unrelenting crises.* Person experiences pattern of frequent, stressful, negative environmental events, disruptions, and roadblocks—some caused by the individual's dysfunctional lifestyle, others by an inadequate social milieu, and many by fate or chance.

4. *Inhibited grieving.* Person tries to inhibit and overcontrol negative emotional responses, especially those associated with grief and loss, including sadness, anger, guilt, shame, anxiety, and panic.

5. *Active passivity.* Person fails to engage actively in solving of own life problems but will actively seek problem-solving from others in the environment; learned helplessness, hopelessness.

6. *Apparent competence.* Tendency for the individual to appear deceptively more competent than he or she actually is; usually due to failure of competencies to generalize across expected moods, situations, and time, and failure to display adequate nonverbal cues of emotional distress.

Linehan, M. (1993). *Cognitive-behavioral treatment of borderline personality disorder* (p. 10). New York: Guilford Press.

are continuously dismissed, trivialized, devalued, punished, and discredited (invalidated) by others whom the person respects or values, the person receives confused messages about expressing his or her own feelings. The person's experience of painful emotions is disregarded; the individual's interpretation of his or her own behavior is dismissed (Fig. 22-1).

The following is a minor example of invalidating environment or response: A preschool-aged child has been told by her parents that the family is going to grandmother's house for a family meal. The child responds: "I am not going to Gramma's. I hate Stevie (cousin)." Parents' reaction: "You don't hate Stevie. He is a wonderful child. He is your cousin, and only a spoiled, selfish little girl would say such a thing." The parents have devalued and discredited her feelings and comments and

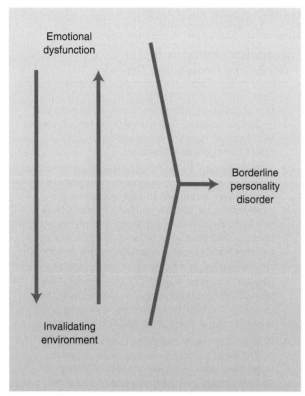

FIGURE 22.1 Biosocial theory of borderline personality disorder. (Courtesy of Marsha M. Linehan, Ph.D., Dept. of Psychology, Box 351525, University of Washington, Seattle, WA 98195. © 1993 by Marsha M. Linehan.)

undermined her own feelings. The child's feelings and personal worth are invalidated by her parents' denigration and contradiction of her.

The most severe form of invalidation occurs in situations of child sexual abuse. Often, the abusing adult has told the child that this is a "special secret" between them, that the child should feel guilty if she tells anyone, and that telling someone would end their trust and special relationship. The child is experiencing feelings of fear, pain, and sadness, yet this trusted adult is continuously dismissing her true feelings and telling what she should feel. In patterns of sexual abuse, children often learn to endure sexual abuse for years, suppressing their true feelings. If she does disclose to a nonoffending adult, there is a risk that she will not be believed or attended to.

In reality, all children, not just those who are emotionally vulnerable, learn to trust their own feelings and learn when and how to express them by interacting with their environments, including parents, family, friends, and social situations. If they constantly meet with an invalidating environment, they cannot learn to trust their own feelings—when to be angry, sad, or happy—or how to regulate their emotions. They are emotionally dysregulated. This emotional dysregula-

tion leads to further difficulties in identity disturbances, interpersonal relationships, and the development of impulsive, parasuicidal behavior.

Interdisciplinary Treatment

BPD is a very complex disorder that requires the whole mental health care team. The symptoms of the disorder usually require a variety of medications, including mood stabilizers, antidepressants, and at times, anxiolytics. Careful monitoring of medication is necessary, which involves both nurses and physicians. Psychotherapy is needed to help the individual manage the dysfunctional moods, impulsive behavior, and self-injurious behaviors. Specially trained therapists who are comfortable with the many demands of these patients are needed. These therapists represent a variety of mental health disciplines, including psychology, social work, and advanced practice nursing. This is a life-long disorder requiring ongoing treatment as the individual copes with multiple interpersonal crises.

Dialectical Behavior Therapy

Dialectical Behavior Therapy (DBT), developed by Linehan, is an important biosocial approach to treatment that combines numerous cognitive and behavior therapy strategies. It requires patients to understand their disorder by actively participating in formulating treatment goals by collecting data about their own behavior, identifying treatment targets in individual therapy, and working with the therapists in changing these target behaviors. The core treatment procedures include problem solving, exposure techniques (gradual exposure to cues that set off aversive emotions), skill training, contingency management (reinforcement of positive behavior), and cognitive modification. **Skills groups** are an integral part of DBT and are taught in group settings in which patients practice emotional regulation, interpersonal effectiveness, distress tolerance, core mindfulness, and self-management skills. Mindfulness skills are the psychological and behavioral versions of meditation skills usually taught in Eastern spiritual practice and are used to help the person improve observation, description, and participation skills by learning to focus the mind and awareness on the current moment's activity. Interpersonal effectiveness skills include the development of assertiveness and problem-solving skills within an interpersonal context. Emotion regulation skills are taught to manage the intense, labile moods and involve helping the patient label and analyze the context of the emotion and develop strategies to reduce emotional vulnerability. Teaching individuals to observe and describe emotions without judging them or blocking them helps patients experience emotions without stimulating secondary feelings that cause more distress. For example, describing the emotion of anger without judging it as being "bad" can eliminate feelings of guilt that lead to self-injury. Distress tolerance skills involve helping the individual tolerate and accept distress as a part of normal life. Self-management skills are focused on helping patients learn how to control, manage, or change behavior, thoughts, or emotional responses to events (Linehan, 1993).

The DBT model has been the most researched of any single treatment strategy and consistently demonstrates clinical effectiveness. When used on an inpatient basis, it requires total staff commitment and reinforcement and has shown significant improvement in depression, anxiety, and dissociation symptoms and a highly significant decrease in parasuicidal behavior (Bohus et al., 2000). DBT is more often incorporated into a long-term partial hospitalization and outpatient treatment approach because the greatest effectiveness occurs when skills are reinforced over time and practiced in a variety of daily living settings (Bateman & Fanagy, 1999). Key to DBT is that staff maintain a positive approach and assume a skills coach role with patients. Probably the most significant interference in treatment with people with BPD is a pessimistic and oppositional attitude of health care professionals (Horsfall, 1999; Nehls, 1998, 1999).

Priority Care Issues

The priority for these individuals is safety. Because these patients use self-injurious behavior, the nurse should always assess for thoughts of self-injury.

 Family Response to Disorder

Individuals with BPD are typically part of a chaotic family system but usually add to the chaos. Their family often feels captive to these patients. Family members are afraid to disagree with them or refuse to meet their multiple needs, fearing that self-destructive behavior will follow. Over the course of the disorder, family members often get "burned out" and withdraw from the patient, only adding to the patient's fear of abandonment.

NURSING MANAGEMENT: HUMAN RESPONSE TO DISORDER

People with BPD are unstable in a variety of areas, including mood, interpersonal relationships, self-esteem, and self-identity, and they often exhibit behavioral and cognitive dysregulation. These manifest in a number of ways, the most prominent of which are listed in Text Box 22-2. These people have problems in daily living—maintaining intimate relationships, keeping a job, living within the law (Text Box 22-3).

TEXT BOX 22.2

Response Patterns of Persons With Borderline Personality Disorder

Affective (mood) dysregulation

Mood lability

Problems with anger

Interpersonal dysregulation

Chaotic relationships

Fears of abandonment

Self-dysregulation

Identity disturbance or difficulties with sense of self

Sense of emptiness

Behavioral dysregulation

Parasuicidal behavior or threats

Impulsive behavior

Cognitive dysregulation

Dissociative responses

Paranoid ideation

Courtesy of M. Linehan, Department of Psychology, Box 351525, University of Washington, Seattle, WA 98195-1525, 1993.

They often enter the mental health system early (young adulthood or before), but because of their chaotic lifestyle, they do not receive consistent treatment. They drop in and out of treatment as it suits their mood and usually do not remain with one clinician over time. People with BPD usually seek help from health care workers because of consequences of their numerous life crises, medical conditions, other psychiatric disorders (ie, depression), or for physical treatment of self-injury. Thus, other problems often need attention before the patient's underlying personality disorder can be addressed. Sometimes, the nurse will not know that the person has BPD. However, during an assessment, it becomes clear that these individuals let things bother them more than others or have an inflexible view of the world. They also seem to have great difficulty changing behavior, no matter the consequences. Because they see the world so differently than the average person, they have difficulty in successfully relating to other people and living a quality life.

Biologic Domain

Assessment of Biologic Domain

Systems Review and Physical Functioning. People with BPD are usually able to maintain personal hygiene and physical functioning. Because of the comorbidity of BPD and eating disorders and substance abuse,

TEXT BOX 22.3

Clinical Vignette: Joanne Smith (Borderline Personality Disorder)

Joanne Smith is a 22-year-old single woman who was recently fired from her job as a data entry clerk. She is living with her mother and stepfather, who brought her to the emergency room after finding her crouched in a fetal position in the bathroom, her wrists bleeding. She seemed to be in a daze. This is her first psychiatric admission, although her mother and stepfather have suspected that she has "needed help" for a long time. In high school, she received brief treatment for a potential eating disorder. She remains very thin but is able to eat at least one meal per day. During periods of stress, she will go for days without eating. Joanne is the second of three children. Her parents divorced when she was 3-years-old. She has not seen her father since he left. Although she has pleasant memories of her father, her mother has told her that he beat Joanne and her sisters when he was drinking. When Joanne was 6-years-old, her older sister died following an automobile accident. Joanne was in the car, but uninjured. As a child, Joanne was seen as a potential singing star. Her natural musical talent attracted her teachers' support, who encouraged her to develop her talent. She received singing lessons and entered state-wide competitions in high school. Although she enjoyed the attention, she was never really comfortable in the limelight and felt "guilty" about having a talent that she sometimes resented. She was able to make friends but found that she was unable to keep them. They

described her as "too intense" and emotional. She had one boyfriend in high school, but she was very uncomfortable with any physical closeness. After ending the relationship with the boyfriend, she concentrated on dieting to have a "perfect body." When her dieting attracted her parents' attention, she vowed to eat just enough to keep them "off her back about it." She spent much of her leisure time with her grandmother. She attended college briefly but was unable to concentrate. It was during college and after her grandmother's death that Joanne began cutting her wrists during periods of stress. It seemed to calm her.

After leaving college, Joanne returned home. She had several jobs and short-lived friendships. She was usually fired from her job because of "moodiness," and it would take her several months before she would again find another. She would spend days in her room listening to music. Her recent episode followed being fired from work and spending 3 days in her bedroom.

Critical Thinking Questions
- How would you describe Joanne's mood?
- Are Joanne's losses (father, sister) really severe enough to affect her ability to relate to others now? Do the losses seem to relate to the self-injury?
- What behaviors indicate that there are problems with self-esteem and self-identity?

---

a nutritional assessment may be needed. Either overeating, bulimia, or undereating may be present. The assessment should also include exploring the use of caffeinated beverages, such as coffee, tea, and soda. Use of alcohol can also be assessed during the nutritional assessment. With patients who do engage in binging or purging, assessment should include examining the teeth for pitting and discoloration as well as the hands and fingers for redness and callouses due to inducing vomiting. The patient should be queried about physiologic responses of emotion.

Sleep patterns should be assessed because there are indications that sleep patterns of people with BPD are different from those of people with no mental disorder. In one study of male veterans, those with BPD had less total sleep, more stage 1 sleep, and less stage 4 sleep than normal subjects. Sleep alteration may also result from a coexisting disorder such as depression or mania.

Physical Indicators of Self-Injurious Behaviors. Patients with BPD should be carefully assessed for any evidence of self-injurious behavior or suicide attempts. It is important to ask the patient about specific self-abusive behaviors, such as cutting, scratching, or swallowing. The patient may wear long sleeves to hide injury on the arms. Specifically asking about thoughts of

hurting oneself when experiencing a major upset provides an opportunity for prevention and for coaching the patient toward alternative self-soothing measures.

Pharmacologic Assessment. Patients with BPD may be taking several medications, which often vary from individual to individual. For example, one patient may be taking a small dose of an antipsychotic and a mood stabilizer such as carbamazepine. Another may be taking a selective serotonin reuptake inhibitor (SSRI). Initially, patients may be reluctant to disclose all of the medications they are taking because, for many, there has been a period of trial and error. They are fearful of having medication taken away from them. Development of rapport with special attention to a nonjudgmental approach is especially important when eliciting current medication practices. The effectiveness of the medication in relieving the target symptom needs to be determined. Use of alcohol and street drugs should be carefully assessed to determine drug interactions.

Nursing Diagnoses Related to Biologic Domain

Nursing diagnoses focusing on the biologic domain include Self-Mutilation, Risk for Self-Mutilation, Disturbed Sleep Pattern, and Ineffective Therapeutic Regimen Management.

Interventions for Biologic Domain

The interventions focusing on the biologic dimensions could include the whole spectrum of problems. Usually, the patients are managing hydration, self-care, and pain well. This section focuses on those areas most likely to be problematic: sleep, nutrition, management of self-mutilation, and pharmacologic management.

Sleep Enhancement. Facilitation of regular sleep–wake cycles may be needed because of disturbed sleep patterns. Conservative approaches should be exhausted before recommending medication. Establishing a regular bedtime routine, monitoring bedtime snacks and drinks, and avoiding foods and drinks that interfere with sleep should be tried. If relaxation exercises are used, they should be adapted to the tolerance of the individual (see Chap. 14).

Moderate exercises (eg, brisk walking) 3 to 4 hours before bedtime activates both serotonin and endorphins, thereby enhancing calmness and a sense of well-being before bedtime. For patients who have difficulty falling asleep and interrupted sleep, it helps to establish some basic sleeping routines. The bedroom should be reserved for only two activities: sleeping and sex. Therefore, the patient should remove the television, computer, and exercise equipment from the bedroom. If not asleep within 15 minutes, get out of bed and go to another room to read, watch TV, or listen to soft music. Return to bed when sleepy. If not asleep in 15 minutes, repeat the same process.

Special consideration must be made for patients who have been physically and sexually abused and who may be unable to put themselves in a vulnerable position (such as lying down in a room with other people or closing their eyes). These patients may need additional safeguards to help sleep, such as a nightlight, reposition furniture to afford easy exit, or other, based on patient's needs.

Nutritional Enhancement. The nutritional status of the person with BPD can quickly become a priority, particularly if the patient has coexisting eating disorders or substance abuse. Food and eating are often used as responses to stress, and patients can quickly become overweight. This is especially a problem when the patient has also been taking medications that promote weight gain, such as antipsychotics, antidepressants, or mood stabilizers. Helping the patient to learn the basics of nutrition, make reasonable choices, and develop other coping strategies are useful interventions. If patients are engaging in purging or severe dieting prac-

tices, teaching the patient about the danger of both of these practices is important (see Chap. 24). Referral to an eating disorders specialist may be needed.

Prevention and Treatment of Self-Injury. Patients with BPD are usually admitted to the inpatient setting because of threats of self-injury. Observing for antecedents of self-injurious behavior and intervening before an episode is an important safety intervention. Patients can be taught to identify situations that lead to self-destructive behavior and develop strategies to prevent self-injurious behavior. Because these patients are impulsive and may respond to a stressful situation by injuring themselves, observation of the patient's interactions and assessment of the mood, level of distress, and agitation are important indicators of impending self-injury.

Remembering that self-injury is an effort to self-soothe by activating endogenous endorphins, the nurse can assist the patient to find more productive and enduring ways to find comfort. Linehan (1993) suggests using the Five Senses Exercise:

- Vision (eg, go outside and look at the stars or flowers or autumn leaves)
- Hearing (eg, listen to beautiful or invigorating music or the sounds of nature)
- Smell (eg, light a scented candle, boil a cinnamon stick in water)
- Taste (eg, drink a soothing, warm, nonalcoholic beverage)
- Touch (eg, take a hot bubble bath, pet your dog or cat, get a massage)

Pharmacologic Interventions. Less medication is better for people with BPD. No specific drug is available for the treatment of BPD and its learned dynamics. These patients should take medications only for target symptoms for a short period of time (eg, an antidepressant for a bout with depression) because they may be taking many medications, particularly if they have a comorbid disorder such as a mood disorder or substance abuse. Pharmacotherapy is used to control emotional dysregulation, impulsive aggression, cognitive disturbances, and anxiety so that these patients can be amenable to psychotherapy.

Controlling Emotional Dysregulation. In the area of emotional dysregulation, target symptoms include instability of mood, marked shifts from or to depression, stress-related and transient mood crashes, rejection sensitivity, and inappropriate and intense outbursts of anger. Clinical trials have shown the efficacy of the monoamine oxidase inhibitors (phenelzine) in treating depression in people with BPD. Because decreased central serotonin neurotransmission has been implicated in the emotional dysregulation and impulsive-aggressive behaviors, the SSRIs have been tried, with some efficacy shown. Improvement in depressed mood and lability, rejection sensitivity, impulsive behavior, self-injury, psychosis, and hostility have been shown with fluoxetine in BPD. Most commonly, SSRIs and serotonin-norepinephrine reuptake inhibitors have been most extensively studied and used clinically to treat depression, aggression, and emotional dysregulation. Sertraline, paroxetine, citalopram are most often used, and venlafaxine and mirtazapine have been similarly effective, especially with attentional disturbance and agitation symptoms (Stahl, 2000).

Reducing Impulsivity. There is also evidence that the medications used in mania and hypomania, lithium carbonate and carbamazepine, are also useful in mood lability and behavioral impulsivity. Impulsivity, anger outbursts, and mood lability may be treated effectively with the newer GABA-ergic anticonvulsants such as lamotrigine, gabapentine, and topiramate (Pinto & Akiskal, 1998; Coccaro, 1998). These appear to act by regulating neural firing in the mesolimbic area. Carbamazepine, divalproex, and lithium have also been used, but these have a slightly less favorable side-effect profile.

Managing Transient Psychotic Episodes. Antipsychotic medications may be useful when the patient demonstrates thought disorganization, misinterpretation of reality, and high levels of emotional instability. Low doses of antipsychotics are most often used (Soloff, 2000).

Reducing Self-Injurious Behavior. In some patients who injure themselves repeatedly and feel no pain, but instead experience emotional release after the injury, medication that blocks the endogenous opioids system or reward system may help control the behavior. Blocking the endogenous opiate system has proved useful in stopping other repetitive self-destructive behaviors. Preliminary studies have shown that naltrexone has reduced the incidence of self-injurious behavior, such as cutting and self-burning. Naltrexone has been studied and used to treat dissociative symptoms with some success (Bohus et al., 1999), as have low doses of serotonin-dopamine antagonists, such as clozapine, olanzapine, and risperdone (Chengappa et al., 1999; Links et al., 1998; McDougle, 2000).

Decreasing Anxiety. If a patient is experiencing anxiety, a nonbenzodiazepine such as buspirone may be used (see Drug Profile: Buspirone). Buspirone appears to be an ideal antianxiety drug. Unlike the benzodiazepines, it does not have the sedation, ataxia, tolerance, and withdrawal symptoms. It does not lead to abuse. Buspirone does take longer to act than the benzodiazepines. However, if a patient has been taking benzodiazepines for years, buspirone may not lead to much improvement. When switching from a benzodiazepine to buspirone, the withdrawal symptoms may be unpleasant (or even dangerous), and buspirone will not have any effect on the distress. Because buspirone is a serotonin (5-HT1A) agonist, its use with an SSRI enhances the benefits of both drugs to reduce anxiety and depression symptoms (Stahl, 2000) but exposes the patient to serotonin syndrome risk.

Monitoring and Administration of Medications. In an inpatient setting, it is relatively easy to control medications, but in the other settings, patients must be aware that it is their responsibility to take their medication and

---

DRUG PROFILE: Buspirone
(Antianxiety Agent)
Trade Name: BuSpar

Receptor affinity: Binds to serotonin receptors and acts as an agonist to 5-HT$_{1B}$. Clinical significance unclear. Exact mechanism of action unknown.

Indications: Management of anxiety disorders or short-term relief of symptoms of anxiety.

Routes and dosage: Available in 5- and 10-mg tablets.

Adults: Initially, 15 mg/d (5 mg tid). Increased at 5 mg/d at intervals of 2–3 d to achieve optimal therapeutic response. Not to exceed 60 mg/d.

Children: Safety and efficacy under 18 years of age not established.

Half-life (peak effect): 3–11 h (40–90 min).

Select adverse reactions: Dizziness, headache, nervousness, insomnia, light-headedness, nausea, dry mouth, vomiting, gastric distress, diarrhea, tachycardia, and palpitations.

Warning: Contraindicated in patients with hypersensitivity to buspirone, marked liver or renal impairment and during lactation. Alcohol and other CNS depressants can cause increased sedation. Decreased effects seen if given with fluoxetine.

Specific patient/family education:

• Take drug exactly as prescribed; may take with foods or meals if gastrointestinal upset occurs.

• Avoid alcohol and other CNS depressants.

• Notify prescriber before taking any over-the-counter or prescription medications.

• Avoid driving or performing hazardous activities that require alertness and concentration.

• Use ice chips or sugarless candies to alleviate dry mouth.

• Notify prescriber of any abnormal involuntary movements of facial or neck muscles, abnormal posture, or yellowing of skin or eyes.

• Continue medical follow-up and do not discontinue abruptly.

monitor the number and type of drugs being taken. Patients who rely on medication to help them deal with stress or those who are periodically suicidal are at high risk for abuse of medications. Patients who have unusual side effects are also at high risk for noncompliance. The nurse determines whether the patient is actually taking medication, whether the medication is being taken as prescribed, the effect on target symptoms, and the use of any over-the-counter drugs, such as antihistamines, sleeping pills, and so on.

The patient cannot rely just on the medication, however. Assuming responsibility for taking the medication regularly, understanding the effects of the medication, and augmenting the medication with other strategies is the most effective approach. The nurse helps the patient assume this responsibility and provides guidance that supports self-efficacy and competence. It is also important for the nurse to emphasize that the medications provide the physiologic balance, but it is the patient's effort and skills that provide the social and behavioral balance. By stressing this, the patient does not overinvest in the medication and feels more confident of her or his own skills.

Side-Effect Monitoring and Management. The side effects of these medications are discussed throughout this text. Patients with BPD appear to be sensitive to many of the medications and often dose the medication according their understanding of the side effects. Listen carefully to the patient's description of the side effects. Any unusual side effects should be accurately documented and reported to the prescriber.

Drug–Drug Interactions. Clinically, these individuals appear to be prone to drug interactions. They need to be carefully assessed for the use of over-the-counter medications and herbal supplements.

Teaching Points. Patients should be educated about the medications and their interactions with other drugs and substances. Interventions include teaching the patient about the medication and how and where it acts in the brain, helping the patient establish a routine for taking prescribed medication, reporting side effects, and facilitating the development of positive coping strategies to deal with daily stresses rather than relying on medications.

Psychological Domain

Assessment of Psychological Domain

Appearance and Activity Level. Appearance and activity level generally reflect the person's mood and psychomotor activity. Depression is often experienced by those who have been victims of physical and sexual abuse, and many of those with BPD have been physically or sexually abused and thus should be assessed for depression (Hall et al., 1993). A disheveled appearance can re-

flect depression or an agitated state. When feeling good, these patients can be very engaging; they tend to be dramatic in their style of dress and attract attention, such as by wearing an unusual hairstyle or heavy makeup. Because physical appearance reflects identity, patients may experiment with their appearance and seek affirmation and acceptance from others. Body piercing, tattoos, and other body adornments provide a mechanism to define self as different from others.

Moods. People with BPD have usually experienced significant losses in their lives that shape their view of the world. They experience **inhibited grieving**, "a pattern of repetitive, significant trauma and loss, together with an inability to fully experience and personally integrate or resolve these events" (Linehan, 1993, p. 89). They have unresolved grief that can last for years and avoid situations that evoke those feelings of separation and loss. During the assessment, the nurse can identify the losses (real or perceived) and explore the patient's experience during these losses, paying particular attention to whether the patient has reached resolution. History of physical or sexual abuse and early separation from significant caregivers may provide important clues to the severity of the disturbances.

Mood fluctuations are common and can be assessed by any number of the depression and anxiety screening scales or by asking the following questions:

What things or events bother you and make you feel happy, sad, angry?
Do these things or events trouble you more than other people?
Do friends and family tell you that you are moody?
Do you get angry easily?
Do you have trouble with your temper?
Do you think you were born with these feelings or did something happen to make you feel this way?

Impulsivity. Impulsivity can be identified by asking the patient if he or she does things impulsively or spur of the moment. Have there been times when you were hurt by your actions or were sorry later that you did it? Direct questions about gambling, choices in sexual partners, sexual activities, fights, arguments, arrests, and alcohol drinking habits can also help in identifying areas of impulsive behavior.

Cognitive Disturbances. The mental status examination of those with BPD usually reveals normal thought processes that are not disorganized or confused except under periods of stress.

Those with BPD usually exhibit **dichotomous thinking** or a tendency to view things as absolute, either black or white, good or bad, with no perception of compromise. In dichotomous thinking, the patient tends to fixate on one extreme perception or alternate between two extremes. Dichotomous thinking can be assessed by asking patients how they view other people. Evidence of dichotomous thinking is indicated with responses of "good" or "bad," "wonderful" or "terrible."

Dissociation and Transient Psychotic Episodes. There may be periods of dissociation and transient psychotic episodes. Dissociation can be assessed by asking if there is ever a time when the patient does not remember events or has the feeling of being separate from his or her body. Some patients refer to this as "spacing out." By asking specific information about how often, how long, and when first dissociation was used, the nurse can get an idea of how important dissociation is as a coping skill. It is important to ask the person what is happening in the environment when dissociation occurs. Frequent dissociation indicates that it is a highly habitual coping mechanism that will be difficult to change. Because transient psychotic states occur, it is also important to elicit data regarding the presence of hallucinations or delusions, their frequency and circumstances.

Interpersonal Skills. Assessment of the person's ability to relate to others is important because interpersonal problems are linked to dissociation and self-injurious behavior. Information about friendships, frequency of contacts, and intimate relationships will provide data about the person's ability to relate to others. These patients are often sexually active and may have numerous sexual partners. Their need for closeness clouds their judgment about sexual partners, and it is not unusual to find these patients in abusive, destructive relationships with people with antisocial personality disorder. Because many women with BPD also have childhood sexual abuse histories, their relationship and sexual behaviors are often laced with distrust and control conflicts.

During the assessment, nurses should use their own self-awareness skills to examine their personal response to the patient. How the nurse responds to the patient can often be a clue to how others perceive and respond to this person. For example, if the nurse becomes irritated or impatient during the interview, that is a sign that others respond to this person in the same way; on the other hand, if the nurse feels empathy or closeness, chances are this patient can provoke these same feelings in others.

Self-Esteem and Coping Skills. Coping with stressful situations is one of the major problems of people with BPD. Assessment of their coping skills and their ability to deal with stressful situations is important (see Chap. 35). Their self-esteem is usually very low. Assessment of self-esteem can be done with a self-esteem assessment tool or by interviewing the patient and analyzing the assessment data for evidence of personal self-worth and confidence. Self-esteem is highly related to

identifying with health care workers. They perceive their families and friends as being weary of their numerous crises and seeming unwillingness to break the vicious self-destructive cycle. Feeling rejected by their natural support system, these individuals create one within the existing health system. During periods of crises or affective instability, they call or visit various psychiatric units—especially late evening, early morning, or on weekends—asking to speak to specific personnel who formerly cared for them. They even know different nurses' scheduled days off and make the rounds to several hospitals and clinics. Sometimes, they bring gifts to nurses and will call them at home. Because their newly created social support system cannot provide the support that is needed, the patient continues to feel rejected. One of the goals of treatment is to help the individual establish a natural support network.

Risk Assessment: Suicide or Self-Injury. It is critical that patients with BPD be assessed for suicidality and self-damaging behavior, including alcohol and drug abuse. (Suicide assessment is discussed in Chap. 38.) An assessment should include direct questions, asking if the patient thinks about or engages in self-injurious behaviors. If so, the nurse should continue to explore the behaviors: what is done, how it is done, its frequency, and the circumstances surrounding the self-injurious behavior. It is helpful to explain briefly to the patient that sometimes people cut, scratch, or pick at themselves as a way of bringing some relief and comfort. Although the behavior brings temporary relief, it also places the person at risk for infection. Approaching the assessment in this way is more likely to invite the patient to disclose honestly and conveys a sense of understanding.

Nursing Diagnoses Related to Psychological Domain

One of the first diagnoses to consider is Risk for Self-Mutilation because protection of the patient from self-injury is always a priority. If cognitive changes are present (dissociation and transient psychosis), two other diagnoses may be appropriate—Disturbed Thought Process and Ineffective Coping. The Disturbed Thought Process diagnosis is used if dissociative and psychotic episodes actually interfere with daily living. A secretary could not complete typing letters because she was unable to differentiate whether the voices on the dictating machine were being transmitted by the machine or her hallucinations. The nurse helped her learn to differentiate the hallucinations from dictation. If the individual copes with stressful situations by dissociating or hallucinating, the diagnosis Ineffective Coping is used. The outcome in this instance would be the substitution of positive coping skills for the dissociations or hallucinations. Other nursing diagnoses that are typically supported by assessment data include Personal Identity Disturbance, Anxiety, Grieving, Low Self-Esteem, Powerlessness, Social Isolation, Post-Trauma Response, Defensive Coping, and Spiritual Distress. Identification of outcomes will depend on the nursing diagnoses (Fig. 22-2).

Interventions for Psychological Domain

Special Issues in the Nurse–Patient Relationship. The challenge of working with people with BPD is engaging the patient in a therapeutic relationship that will survive its emotional ups and downs. It is important to convey to the patient that the nurse is there to coach her or him in developing skills in self-modulation. Developing a relationship based on mutual respect and consistency is crucial in helping the patient with those skills. Self-awareness skills are needed by the nurse along with access to supervision. Because patients with BPD are frequently hospitalized, even nurses in acute care settings have an opportunity to develop a long-term relationship (Fig. 22-3).

Establishing a Trusting Relationship. Difficulty in interpersonal relationships is a major problem, and establishing therapeutic relationships requires patience and planning. Generalist psychiatric–mental health nurses do not function as the patient's primary therapists, but they do need to establish a trusting, therapeutic relationship that enhances self-esteem, aids in patient self-validation, strengthens the patient's coping skills, and supports individual psychotherapy. The purpose of the therapeutic relationship is for the patient to experience a model of healthy interaction. In developing a trusting relationship with the patient, the nurse shows consistency, limit setting, caring, and respect for others (both self-respect and respect for the patient). Patients who have low self-esteem need help in recognizing genuine respect from others and reciprocating with respect for others. Through this exchange, they improve their self-esteem. In the therapeutic relationship, the nurse models self-respect by observing personal limits, being assertive, and clearly communicating expectations. Consistency is critical in building self-esteem.

Abandonment and Intimacy Fears. A key to helping patients with BPD is recognizing their conflicting fears of abandonment and intimacy. Informing the patient of the length of the relationship as much as possible allows the patient to both engage in and prepare for termination with the least pain of abandonment. If the patient's hospitalization is time limited, the nurse overtly acknowledges the limit and reminds the patient with each contact how many sessions remain (see Therapeutic Dialogue: Borderline Personality Disorder).

In day-treatment and outpatient settings, the duration of treatment may be indeterminate, but the nurse may not be available that entire time. The termination process cannot be casual; this would stimulate abandonment fears. However, some patients end prematurely when the nurse informs them of the impending end as a way to leave before being rejected. Anticipating

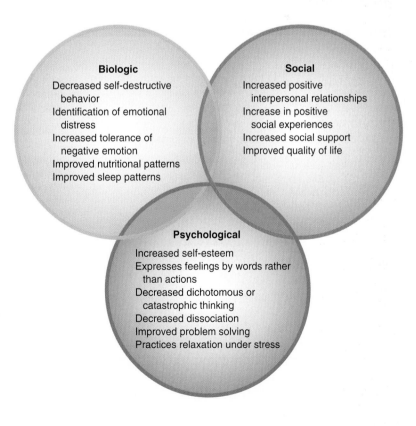

Biologic
Decreased self-destructive behavior
Identification of emotional distress
Increased tolerance of negative emotion
Improved nutritional patterns
Improved sleep patterns

Social
Increased positive interpersonal relationships
Increase in positive social experiences
Increased social support
Improved quality of life

Psychological
Increased self-esteem
Expresses feelings by words rather than actions
Decreased dichotomous or catastrophic thinking
Decreased dissociation
Improved problem solving
Practices relaxation under stress

FIGURE 22.2 Biopsychosocial outcomes for patients with borderline personality disorder.

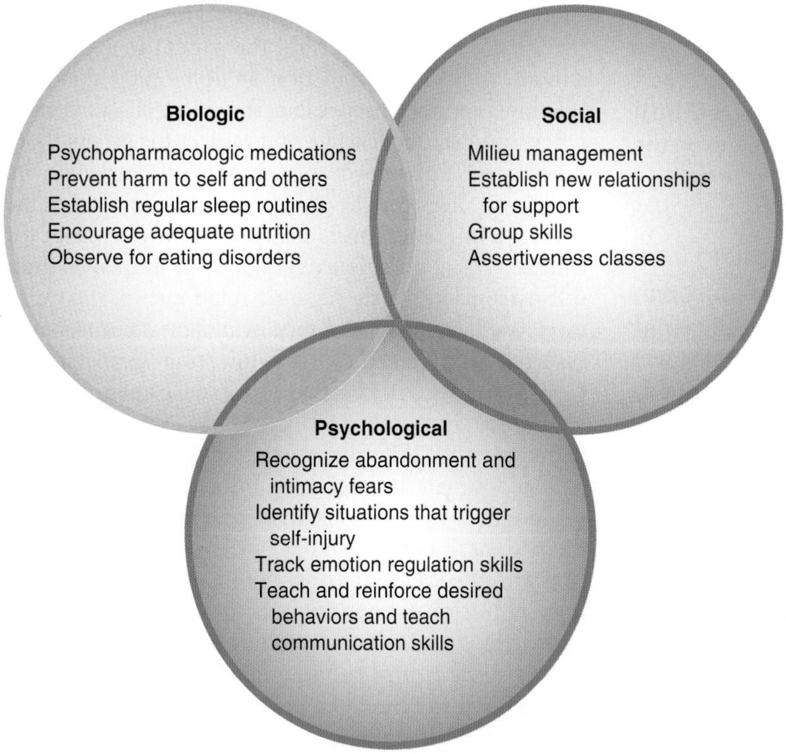

Biologic

Psychopharmacologic medications
Prevent harm to self and others
Establish regular sleep routines
Encourage adequate nutrition
Observe for eating disorders

Social

Milieu management
Establish new relationships
  for support
Group skills
Assertiveness classes

Psychological

Recognize abandonment and
  intimacy fears
Identify situations that trigger
  self-injury
Track emotion regulation skills
Teach and reinforce desired
  behaviors and teach
  communication skills

FIGURE 22.3 Biopsychosocial interventions for patients with borderline personality disorder.

THERAPEUTIC DIALOGUE   Borderline Personality Disorder

Ineffective Approach

Patient: Hey, you know what? You are my favorite nurse. That night nurse sure doesn't understand me the way you do.

Nurse: Oh, I'm glad you are comfortable with me. Which night nurse?

Patient: You know, Sue.

Nurse: Did you have problems with her?

Patient: She is terrible. She sleeps all night or she is on the telephone.

Nurse: Oh, that doesn't sound very professional to me. Anything else?

Patient: Yeah, she said that you didn't know what you were doing. She said that you couldn't nurse your way out of a paper bag (smiling).

Nurse: She did, did she. (Getting angry.) She should talk.

Patient: Well, I gotta go to group. Where will you be? I feel so much better if I know where you are. I don't know how I can possibly be discharged tomorrow.

Effective Approach

Patient: Hey, you know what? You are my favorite nurse. That night nurse sure doesn't understand me the way you do.

Nurse: I really like you, Sara. Tomorrow you will be discharged, and I'm glad that you will be able to return home.

(Nurse avoided responding to "favorite nurse" statement. Redirected interaction to impending discharge.)

Patient: That night nurse slept all night.

Nurse: What was your night like? (Redirecting the interaction to Sara's experience.)

Patient: It was terrible. Couldn't sleep all night. I'm not sure that I'm ready to go home.

Nurse: Oh, so you are not quite sure about discharge? (Reflection.)

Patient: I get so, so lonely. Then, I want to hurt myself.

Nurse: Lonely feelings have started that chain of events that led to cutting, haven't they? (Validation.)

Patient: Yes, I'm very scared. I haven't cut myself for 1 week now.

Nurse: Do you have a plan for dealing with your lonely feelings when they occur?

Patient: I'm supposed to start thinking about something that is pleasant—like spring flowers in the meadow.

Nurse: Does that work for you?

Patient: Yes, sometimes.

Critical Thinking Questions

- How did the nurse in the first scenario get side-tracked?

- How was the nurse in the second scenario able to keep the patient focused on herself and her impending discharge?

premature closure, the nurse explores with the patient anticipated feelings, including the wish to run away. After careful planning, the nurse anticipates, in advance, the patient's feelings, discusses how to cope with them, reviews the progress the patient has made, and summarizes what the patient has learned from the relationship that can be generalized to future encounters.

Establishing Personal Boundaries and Limitations. Personal boundaries are highly context specific; for example, stroking the hair of a stranger on the bus would be inappropriate, but stroking the hair and face of one's intimate partner while sitting together would be appropriate. Our personal physical space needs (ie, boundaries) are distinct from behavioral and emotional limits we have. These concepts apply both to the patient and the nurse as well as the organization in which we function. Furthermore, limits may be temporary (eg, "I can't talk with you right now, but after the change of shift, I can be available for thirty minutes").

Pushing limits is a natural way of identifying where the boundaries are and how strong they are. Therefore, it is necessary to state clearly the enduring limits (eg, the written rules or contract) and the consequences of violating them. The limits must then be consistently maintained. Clarifying limits requires making explicit what is usually implicit. Despite the clinical setting (eg, hospital, day-treatment setting, outpatient clinic), the nurse must clearly state the day, time, and duration of each contact with the patient and remain consistent in those expectations. This may mean having a standing appointment in day treatment or the mental health clinic or noting the time during each shift the nurse will talk individually with the hospitalized patient. The nurse should refrain from offering personal information, which is frequently confusing to the person with BPD. At times, the person may present in a somewhat arrogant and entitled way. It is important for the nurse to recognize such a presentation as reflective of internal confusion and dissonance. Responding in a very neutral manner avoids confrontation and a power struggle, which might also unwittingly reinforce the patient's internal sense of inferiority.

Some additional strategies for establishing the boundaries of the relationship include the following:

- Documenting in the patient chart the agreed-on appointment expectations
- Sharing the treatment plan with the patient
- Confronting violations of the agreement in a non-punitive way
- Discussing the purpose of limits in the therapeutic relationship and applicability to other relationships

Management of Dissociative States. The desired outcome for someone who dissociates is to reduce or eliminate the dissociative experiences. The natural ten-

dency is to want to "fix it." Unfortunately, there are limited medications for dissociation, but because the SSRIs and the dopamine antagonists and serotonin-dopamine antagonists affect other target symptoms, the dissociative experiences decrease. Because dissociation occurs during periods of stress, the best approach is to help the patient develop other strategies to deal with stress. Once the nurse understands when the patient dissociates and under what circumstances, it is possible to focus on the stressful situation. If the patient cannot identify any triggers, the nurse can focus on other aspects of care.

The nurse can teach the patient how to identify when he or she is dissociating and then to use some ground strategies in the moment. Basic to grounding is planting both feet firmly on the floor or ground, then taking a deep abdominal breath to the count of 4, holding it to the count of 4, exhaling to the count of 4, then holding it to the count of 4. This is called the four-square method of breathing. After the ground exercise, the patient uses one or more senses to make contact with the environment, such as touching the fabric of a nearby chair or listening to the traffic noise. As the patient improves in self-esteem and ability to relate to others, along with a decrease in parasuicidal behavior, the frequency of dissociation should decrease.

Behavioral Interventions. The goal of behavioral interventions is to replace dysfunctional behaviors with positive ones using the behavioral models discussed in Chapters 6 and 14. The nurse has an important role in helping patients control emotions and behaviors by acknowledging and validating desired behaviors and ignoring or confronting undesired behaviors. Patients often test the nurse for a response, and nurses must decide how to respond to particular behaviors. This can be tricky because even negative responses can be viewed as a positive reinforcer for the patient. In some instances, if the behavior is irritating but not harmful or demeaning, it is best to ignore the behavior rather than focusing on it. Grossly inappropriate and disrespectful behaviors, however, require confrontation. For example, if a patient throws a glass of water on a nurse's aide because she is angry at the treatment team for refusing to increase her hospital privileges, an appropriate intervention would include confronting the patient with her behavior and issuing the consequences, such as losing her privileges. However, this incident can be used to help the patient understand why such behavior is inappropriate and how it can be changed. The nurse should explore with the patient what happened, what events led up to the behavior, what were the consequences, and what feelings were aroused. Advanced practice nurses or other therapists will explore the origins of the patient's behaviors and responses, but the generalist nurse needs to help the patient explore ways to change behaviors involved in the present situation. Assistance with coping skills, such as learning stress management techniques, seeking out others for support, and improving self-concept, can help patients deal with the multitude of daily stresses in their lives.

Cognitive Interventions

Emotional Regulation. One of the major goals of cognitive therapeutic interventions is emotional regulation, that is, being able to recognize and control the expression of feelings. Patients often fail even to recognize their feelings; instead, they respond quickly without thinking about the consequences. The nurse can help the patient identify feelings and gain control over expressions such as anger, disappointment, or frustration. The goal is for patients to tolerate their feelings without acting on them. They learn to experience intense feelings without feeling compelled to act out those feelings on another person or on themselves.

Communication Triad. One technique that is helpful in managing feelings is using the **communication triad.** The triad provides a specific syntax and order for patients to identify and express their feelings and seek relief. The "sentence" consists of three parts:

- An "I" statement to identify the prevailing feeling
- A nonjudgmental statement of the emotional trigger
- What the patient would like differently or what would restore comfort to the situation

The nurse must emphasize with patients that they begin with the "I" statement and the identification of feelings, although many want to begin with the condition. If the patient begins with the condition, the statement becomes accusatory and likely to evoke defensiveness (eg, "When you interrupt me, I get mad."). Beginning with "I" allows the patient to identify and express the feeling first and take full ownership. For example, the patient who is angry with another patient in the group might say, "Joe, I feel angry ("I" statement with ownership of feeling) when you interrupt me (the trigger or conditions of the emotion), and I would like you to apologize and try not to do that with me (what the patient wants and the remedy)." This simple skill is easy to teach, is easy to reinforce and to encourage others to reinforce, and is a surprisingly effective way of moderating the emotional tone.

Distraction or Thought Stopping. Another element of emotional regulation is learning to delay gratification. When the patient wants something that is not immediately available, the nurse can teach patients to distract themselves, find alternate ways of meeting the need, and think about what would happen if they have to wait to meet the need.

The practice of **thought stopping** might also help the patient to control the inappropriate expression of feelings. In thought stopping, the person identifies what

feelings and thoughts exist together. For example, when the person is ruminating about a perceived hurt, the individual might say "Stop that" (referring to the ruminative thought) and engage in a distracting activity. Thought stopping is more effective when the following are included: taking a quick deep breath when the person notices the behavior (this also stimulates relaxation); subvocalizing the "stop" when possible, which allows the person to hear externally and internally; and deliberately replacing the behavior with a positive alternative (eg, instead of ruminating about an angry situation, thinking about a neutral or positive self-affirmation). The sequencing and combining of the steps puts the person back in control.

Challenging Dysfunctional Thinking. The nurse can often challenge the patient's dysfunctional ways of thinking and challenge the person to think about the event in a different way. When a patient engages in catastrophic thinking, the nurse can challenge by asking: "What is the worst that could happen?" and "How likely would that occur?" Or, in dichotomous thinking, when the patient fixates on one extreme perception or alternates between the extremes only, the nurse can challenge such dichotomous thinking patterns by asking the patient to think about any examples of exceptions to the extreme. By helping patients rethink and look at an event in a different manner, they can begin to alter their way of viewing things in the extreme. The point of the challenge is not to debate the point or argue with the patient but to provide different perspectives to consider. Encouraging patients to keep journals of real interactions is another effective way of testing the reality of their thinking and anticipations, affording more choices and flexibility (Text Box 22-4).

In problem solving, the nurse might encourage the patient to debate both sides of the problem and then search for common ground. Practicing communication and negotiation skills through role playing helps the patient make mistakes and correct them without harm to the self-esteem. The nurse also encourages patients to use these skills in their everyday life and report back on the results, asking patients how they feel applying the skills and how doing so affects their self-perceptions. Success, even partial success, builds a sense of competence and self-esteem (Text Box 22-5).

Management of Transient Psychotic Episodes.
During psychotic episodes, the patient should be protected from self-harm and from hurting other people. In an inpatient setting, the patient should be monitored more closely and determination made whether the voices are telling the patient to engage in self-harm (command hallucinations). The patient may be placed on closer observation. Antipsychotic medication may be initiated. In the community setting, the nurse should help the patient develop a plan for managing the voices. For example, if

TEXT BOX 22.4

Challenging Dysfunctional Thinking

Ms. S had worked for the same company for 20 years with a good job record. Following an accident, she made some minor mistakes in her work that she quickly corrected. She informed her company nurse that her work was "really slipping" and that she was fearful of her coworkers' disapproval and getting fired from her job. The nurse asked her to keep a journal of coworkers' comments for the next week. At the next visit, the following dialogue occurred:

Nurse: I noticed that you received several compliments on your work. Even a close friend of your boss expressed appreciation for your work.

Ms. S: It was a light week at work. I really don't believe they meant what they said.

Nurse: I can see how you can believe that one or two comments are not genuine, but how do you account for four and five good reports on your work?

Ms. S: Well, I don't know.

Nurse: It looks like your beliefs are not supported by your journal entries. Now, what makes you think that your boss wants to fire you after 20 years of service?

the voices return, the patient contacts the clinic and returns for evaluation. There may be a friend or relative who should be contacted or a case manager who can help the patient get the necessary protection if it is needed. In some instances, hearing the voices is a prelude to self-

injury. Another person can help the patient resist the voices. Once other aspects of the disorder are managed, the episodes of psychosis decrease or disappear.

Teaching and practicing distress tolerance skills helps the patient have power over the voices and control intense emotions. When not experiencing hallucinations, the nurse teaches the patient deep abdominal breathing, which calms the autonomic nervous system. Using brainstorming techniques, the patient identifies early internal cues of rising distress while the nurse writes them on an index card for the patient to refer to later. Next, the nurse teaches some skills for tolerating painful feelings or events. To help the patient remember, suggest the mnemonic "Wise mind ACCEPTS" with the following actions:

- **A**ctivities to distract from stress
- **C**ontributing to others such as volunteering or visiting a sick neighbor
- **C**omparing yourself to people less fortunate than you
- **E**motions that are opposite what you are experiencing
- **P**ushing away from the situation for a while
- **T**houghts other than you are currently experiencing
- **S**ensations that are intense, such as holding ice in your hand (Linehan, 1993, pp. 165–166)

Patient Education. Patient education within the context of a therapeutic relationship is one of the most important, empowering interventions for the generalist

TEXT BOX 22.5

Thought Distortions and Corrective Statements

Thought Distortion	**Corrective Statement**
Catastrophizing	
"This is the most awful thing that has ever happened to me."	"This is a sad thing, but not the most awful."
"If I fail this course, my life is over."	"If you fail the course, you can take the course again. You can change your major."
Dichotomizing	
"No one ever listens to me."	"Your husband listened to you last night when you told him . . . "
"I never get what I want."	"You didn't get the promotion this year, but you did get a merit raise."
"I can't understand why everyone is so kind at first, then always dumps me when I need them the most."	"It is hard to remember those kind things at times when your friends have stayed with you when you needed them."
Self-Attribution Errors	
"If I had just found the right thing to say, she wouldn't have left me."	"There is not a single right thing to say; and she left you because she chose to."
"If I had not made him mad, he wouldn't have hit me."	"He has a lot of choices in how to respond, and he chose hitting. You are responsible for your feelings and actions."

psychiatric–mental health nurse to use. Teaching patients skills to resist parasuicidal urges, improve emotional regulation, enhance interpersonal relationships, tolerate stress, and enhance overall quality of life provides the foundation for long-term behavioral changes. These skills can be taught in any treatment setting as a part of the overall facility program (see Psychoeducation Checklist: Borderline Personality Disorder). If nurses are practicing in a facility where DBT is the treatment model, they can serve as group skills leaders.

Another important area of patient education is teaching communication skills. Patients lack interpersonal skill in relating because they often had inadequate modeling and few opportunities to practice. The goals of relationship skill development are to identify problematic behavior that interferes with relationships and to use appropriate behaviors in improving relationships. The starting point is with communication. The nurse teaches the patient basic communication approaches, such as making "I" statements, paraphrasing what the other party says before responding, checking the accuracy of perceptions with the other, compromising and seeking common ground, listening actively, and offering and accepting reactions. Besides modeling the behaviors, the nurse guides patients in practicing a variety of communication approaches for common situations. When role playing, the nurse needs to discuss not only what and how to do the skills but also the feelings patients have before, during, and after the role play. In day treatment and outpatient settings, the nurse can give the patient homework, such as keeping a journal, applying role-playing skills to actual situations, and observing behaviors in others. In the hospital, the patient can experience the same process, and the nurse is available to offer immediate feedback. Whatever the setting, or even the specific problems addressed, the nurse must keep in mind and remind the patient that change occurs slowly. Working on the problems, therefore, occurs gradually, with severity of symptoms as the guide in deciding how fast and how much change to expect.

Social Domain

Assessment of Social Domain

Functional Status. Individuals with BPD can function very well except during periods when symptoms erupt. They hold jobs, are active in communities, and are able to perform well. During periods of stress, symptoms often appear. On the other hand, in severe cases, these individuals do not function well at all, and they are always in a crisis, which they have often created.

Social Support Systems. Identification of social support is the purpose in assessing resources. Family, friends, and religious organizations are examples of some of the possible support resources. Knowing how the patient obtains social support is important in understanding the quality of interpersonal relationships. For example, some patients consider their "best friends" nurses, doctors, and other health care personnel.

Family Assessment. Family members may or may not be involved with the patient. These individuals have chaotic lives and are often estranged from their families. In some instances, they are dependent on them, which is also a source of stress. Because childhood abuse is so common in these families, the perpetrator may be a family member. Ideally, family members are interviewed for their perspectives on the patient's problem. Assessment of any mental disorder in the patient's family and of the current level of functioning is useful in understanding the patient and identifying potential resources for support.

Interventions for Social Domain

Milieu Management. Environmental management becomes critical in caring for a patient with BPD. Because the unit can be structured to represent a microcosm of the patient's community, patients have an opportunity to identify relationship problems, boundary violations, and stressful situations. When these situations occur, the nurse can intervene by helping the patient provide alternative explanations for the situation and practice new skills. Individual sessions help the patient to try out some skills, such as putting feelings into words without actions. Role playing may help patients experience different degrees of effectively relating feelings without the burden of hurting someone they care about. Day treatment and group settings are excellent places for patients to learn more effective feeling management

---

PSYCHOEDUCATION CHECKLIST
Borderline Personality Disorder

When caring for the patient with borderline personality disorder, be sure to include the following topic areas in the teaching plan:

- Management of medication, if used, including drug action, dosage, frequency, and possible adverse effects
- Regular sleep routines
- Nutrition
- Safety measures
- Functional versus dysfunctional behaviors
- Cognitive strategies (distraction, communication skills, thought-stopping)
- Structure and limit setting
- Social relationships
- Community resources

and practice these techniques with each other. The group helps develop members' empathic abilities and diffuses attachment to any one person or therapist that may become too dependent and regressive.

Group Interventions. In the hospital, the nurse can use groups to discuss feelings and ways to cope with them. Women with BPD benefit from assertiveness class and women's health issues classes. Many of the women are involved in abusive relationships and lack the ability to leave these relationships because of their extreme fears and anxiety regarding separating from those they love and their extreme need to feel connected. These women verbalize desires to leave, but they do not have the strength and self-confidence needed to leave. Exposing them to a different style of interaction as well as validation from other people increases their self-esteem and ability to separate from negative influences.

Family and Social Support. Dependency on family members is a problem for many people with BPD. One 35-year-old patient received a new hairstyle and new clothes before discharge from the hospital. When she first appeared on the unit, she was very proud of her "new look." When she called her older sister to tell her about the clothes, the sister told her that hairstyle would be unsuitable and the clothes unnecessary. Her mood immediately changed, and she removed the clothes. Her mood was regulated by her sister's response. This patient needs help in maintaining a separate identity while staying connected to family members for social support. Family support groups sometimes help. Usually, the nurse helps the patient explore new relationships that can provide additional social contacts.

Evaluation and Treatment Outcomes

Evaluation and treatment outcomes vary depending on the severity of the disorder, the presence of comorbid disorders, and the availability of resources. For a patient with severe symptoms or continual self-injury, keeping the patient safe and alive may be a realistic outcome. Helping the patient resist parasuicidal urges may take years. In contrast, individuals who rarely need hospitalization and have adequate resources can expect to recover from the self-destructive impulses and learn positive interaction skills that promote a qualitative lifestyle. Most patients fall somewhere in between, with periods of symptom exacerbation and remission. In these patients, increasing the symptom-free time may be the best indicator of outcomes.

Continuum of Care

Treatment of BPD involves long-term therapy. Hospitalization is sometimes necessary during acute episodes involving parasuicidal behavior, but once this behavior is controlled, patients are discharged. It is important for these individuals to continue with treatment in the outpatient or day treatment setting. They often appear more competent and in control than they are, and nurses must not be deceived by these outward appearances. They need continued follow-up and long-term therapy, including individual therapy, psychoeducation, and positive role models. See Nursing Care Plan 22-1.

Mental Health Promotion

The ultimate aim of many of the interventions is to promote mental health. These individuals are constantly struggling to overcome their intense feelings and urges to stay mentally healthy. When not symptomatic, these patients are excellent candidates for activities promoting positive mental health, such as wellness activities, assertiveness training, and supportive women's groups.

ANTISOCIAL PERSONALITY DISORDER: AGGRANDIZING PATTERN

Clinical Course of Disorder

In the *DSM-IV,* antisocial personality disorder (APD) is defined as "a pervasive pattern of disregard for, and violation of, the rights of others that begins in childhood or early adolescence and continues into adulthood" (APA, 2000, p. 701).

The term **psychopathy,** which originated in Germany in the late 19th century, initially referred to all personality disorders (Dolan, 1994) but has gradually became equated with only APD. People with this disorder are behaviorally impulsive and interpersonally irresponsible and fail to adapt to the ethical and social standards of the community. They act hastily and spontaneously, are shortsighted, and fail to plan ahead or consider alternatives. They lack a sense of personal obligation to fulfill social and financial responsibilities, including those involved with being a spouse, a parent, an employee, or a friend or member of the community. Disdainful of traditional values, they fail to conform to social norms and values. They enjoy a sense of freedom and relish being unencumbered and unconfined by people, places, or responsibilities. They can be interpersonally engaging, which is often mistaken for a genuine sense of concern for other people. In reality, they lack empathy, are unable to express human compassion, and tend to be insensitive, callous, and contemptuous of others. Easily irritated, they often become aggressive, disregarding the safety of themselves or others. They lack remorse for transgressions. No matter what the consequences, they are rarely able to delay gratification (APA, 2000).

(text continues on page 534)

NURSING CARE PLAN 22.1
Patient With Borderline Personality Disorder

YJ, a 28-year-old, single woman, was brought to the Emergency Department of a hospital by police officers after finding her in a Burger Chef with superficial self-inflicted laceration on both forearms. She pleaded with the police not to take her to the hospital. The police report noted that she fluctuated between intense crying and pleading to fighting physically and using foul language. By the time she arrived in the emergency department, however, she was calm, cooperative, pleasant, and charming. When asked why she cut herself, YJ reported she wasn't sure but added that her therapist was leaving today for a 4-week trip to Europe. YJ specifically asked the staff not to call her therapist because "she will be angry with me."

After the emergency physician examined Yolanda, the advanced practice mental health nurse assessed her developmental and psychiatric history and a summary of recent events, before she reached a provisional diagnosis of borderline personality disorder with a primary nursing diagnosis of risk for self-mutilation related to abandonment anticipation. She has had several previous self-destructive episodes with minor injuries, only one requiring sutures, and two hospitalizations. She lives with her boyfriend, who

is currently on a business trip, and works part-time at a bookstore. Her invalid mother lives with her younger sister. There are no other relatives. YJ's father died traumatically in an automobile accident when she was 3-years-old. YJ was in the car when it crashed; she received minor injuries.

Because YJ refused to agree not to harm herself, the nurse admitted YJ to the psychiatric unit with suicide precautions. Once on the unit, YJ was assessed by a staff nurse as having a basically normal mental status examination except that her mood was very tearful at times but charming and joking at other times. She said, "Don't mind me, I cry at the drop of a hat sometimes." Toward the middle of the interview she said, "I feel safer here than I ever felt before. It must be you. Are you sure you're just a staff nurse?" YJ agreed to contract for safety just for today, but added, "Are you going to be my nurse tomorrow? I feel safest with you." When the nurse had completed her assessment, she showed YJ around the unit. As the nurse left her in the day room, YJ said, "My therapist doesn't understand me very well. I don't care she is going out of town. After 4 years, she hasn't helped at all. If I had you as a therapist, I wouldn't be here now."

SETTING: INPATIENT PSYCHIATRIC UNIT IN A GENERAL HOSPITAL

Baseline Assessment: YJ, a 28-year-old woman, came into the emergency department with superficial self-inflicted wounds on both forearms. There was a marked discrepancy in her behavior at the scene of the incident reported by emergency medical technicians from her presentation in the emergency department and now on the inpatient unit. She was admitted this time because she refused to agree not to harm herself further if released. She is angry and sad that her therapist is leaving for 4 weeks for a vacation and doesn't know how she will cope while the therapist is gone. She fears the therapist will not return.

Psychiatric Diagnosis	*Medications*
Axis I: Adjustment disorder with depressed mood Axis II: Borderline personality disorder Axis III: Superficial wounds to both forearms Axis IV: Social support (inadequate social support) Axis V: GAF current = 60; GAF past year = 75	Sertraline (Zoloft) 150 mg qd for anxiety and depression

NURSING DIAGNOSIS 1: SELF-MUTILATION

Defining Characteristics	*Related Factors*
Cuts and scratches on body Self-inflicted wounds	Fears of abandonment secondary to therapist's vacation Inability to handle stress

OUTCOMES

Initial	*Discharge*
1. Remain safe and not harm herself. 2. Identify feelings before and after cutting herself. 3. Agree not to harm herself over the next 24 h.	4. Identify ways of dealing with self-harming impulses if they return. 5. Verbalize alternate thinking with more realistic base. 6. Identify community resources to provide structure and support while therapist is gone.

(continued)

NURSING CARE PLAN 22.1 (Continued)

INTERVENTIONS

Intervention	Rationale	Ongoing Assessment
Monitor patient for changes in mood or behavior that might lead to self-injurious behavior. Discuss with patient need for close observation and rationale to keep her safe.	Close observation establishes safety and protection of patient from self-harm and impulsive behaviors. Explanation to patient for purpose of nursing interventions helps her cooperate with the nursing activity.	Document according to facility policy. Continue to observe for mood and behavior changes. Assess her response to increasing level of observation.
Administer medication as prescribed and evaluate medication effectiveness in reducing depression, anxiety, and cognitive disorganization.	Allows for adjustment of medication dosage based on target behaviors and outcomes.	Observe for side effects.
After 6–8 h, present written agreement to not harm herself.	Permits patient time to return to more thoughtful ways of responding rather than her previous reactive response. Also permits her to save face and avoid embarrassment of a losing power struggle if presented much earlier.	Observe for her willingness to agree to not harm herself.
Communicate information about patient's risk to other nursing staff.	The close observation should be continued throughout all shifts until patient agrees to resist self-harm urges.	Review documentation of close observation for all shifts.

EVALUATION

Outcomes	Revised Outcomes	Interventions
Remained safe without further harming self. Identified fears of abandonment before cutting herself and relief of anxiety afterward. She identified friends to call when fears return and hotlines to use if necessary.	Use hotlines or call friends if fears to harm self return.	Give patient hotline number and ask her to record friend's numbers in an accessible place.
Agreed to not harm herself over the next 3 d.	Does not harm self for 3 d.	Remind her to call someone if urges return.
Enrolled in a day hospital program for 4 wk.	Attend day hospital program.	Follow-up on enrollment.

NURSING DIAGNOSIS 2: RISK FOR LONELINESS

Defining Characteristics	Related Factors
Social isolation	Fear of abandonment secondary to therapist's impending vacation

OUTCOMES

Initial	Discharge
1. Discuss being lonely. 2. Identify previous ways of coping with loneliness.	3. Identify strategies to deal with loneliness while therapist is away.

INTERVENTIONS

Intervention	Rationale	Ongoing Assessment
Develop a therapeutic relationship	People with BPD are able to examine loneliness within the structure of a therapeutic relationship.	Assess her ability to relate and nurse's response to the relationship.

(continued)

NURSING CARE PLAN 22.1 (Continued)

INTERVENTIONS

Intervention	Rationale	Ongoing Assessment
Discuss past experience with therapist being gone with emphasis on how she was able to survive it.	She has survived therapist's absences before. By identifying the strategies she used, she can build on those strengths.	Assess her ability to assume any responsibility for "living through it." This will become a strength.
Acknowledge that it is normal to feel angry when therapist is gone, but there are other strategies that may help the patient deal with the loneliness besides cutting.	Acknowledging feelings is important. Helping patient focus on the possibility of other strategies for dealing with the anger helps her regain a sense of control over her behavior.	Assess whether she is willing to acknowledge that there are other behavioral strategies of handling anger.
Begin immediate disposition planning with focus on day hospitalization or day treatment for skills training and management of loneliness.	While patient is in hospital, she is out of stressful environment in which she can learn more effective behaviors and use therapy. Moving out of the hospital and back into outpatient therapy decreases possibility of regression and lost learning (Linehan, 1993).	Assess her willingness to learn new skills within a day treatment setting.
Teach her about stress management techniques. Assign her to anger management group while she is in the hospital.	Learning about ways of dealing with feelings and stressful situations helps the patient with BPD choose positive strategies rather than self-destructive ones.	Monitor whether she actually attends the groups. She should be encouraged to attend.

EVALUATION

Outcomes	Revised Outcomes	Interventions
YJ was able to verbalize her anger about her therapist leaving and fears of abandonment. The last two times her therapist went on vacation, the patient became self-injurious and was hospitalized for 2 wk.	None.	
YJ was willing to be discharged the next day if she could attend day treatment while her therapist was gone.	Identify other strategies of dealing with therapist vacations besides cutting.	Attend stress management, communication, and self-comforting classes.

*McCloskey, J., & Bulechek, G. (1996). *Nursing interventions classification (NIC)* (p. 182). St. Louis: Mosby–Year Book.

These individuals have faith only in themselves and are secure only when they are independent from those whom they fear will harm or humiliate them. Their need for independence is based on their mistrust of others rather than an inherent belief in their own self-worth. They are driven by a need to prove their superiority and see themselves as the center of the universe. Some of these individuals openly and flagrantly violate laws, ending up in jail. But most people with APD never come in conflict with the law and, instead, find a niche in society such as in business, the military, or politics that rewards their competitive, tough behavior (Millon & Davis, 1999). Most common social problems statistically associated with APD include substance abuse (Lejoyeux et al., 2000; Bucholz et al., 2000), sexual assault and other criminal behavior (Smallbone & Dadds, 2000; Hare, 1999; Gatz et al., 1999), and family violence (Hanson et al., 1997) (Table 22-4). This disorder has a chronic course, but the antisocial behaviors tend to diminish later in life, particularly after 40 years of age (APA, 2000).

Epidemiology and Risk Factors

APD was the only personality disorder included in the Epidemiological Catchment Area (ECA) study (see Chap. 3). The prevalence in nonclinical studies ranges from 2% to 3% of the population, with a median value

TABLE 22.4 Key Diagnostic Characteristics of Antisocial Personality Disorder 301.7

Diagnostic Criteria and Target Symptoms	*Associated Findings* *Associated Behavioral Findings*

• Pervasive pattern of disregard for and violation of the rights of others
   Failure to conform to social norms with respect to lawful behaviors (repeatedly performing acts that are grounds for arrest)
   Deceitfulness (repeated lying, use of aliases, or conning others for personal profit or pleasure)
   Impulsivity or failure to plan ahead
   Irritability and aggressiveness (repeated physical fights or assaults)
   Reckless disregard for safety of self or others
   Consistent irresponsibility (repeated failure to sustain consistent work behavior or honor financial obligations)
   Lack of remorse (being indifferent to or rationalizing having hurt, mistreated, or stolen from another)
• Occurring since 15 years of age
• At least 18 years of age
• Evidence of conduct disorder with onset before 15 years of age
• Not exclusive during the course of schizophrenia or manic episode
	• Lacking empathy
	• Callous, cynical, and contemptuous of the feelings, rights, and sufferings of others
	• Inflated and arrogant self-appraisal
	• Excessively opinionated, self-assured, or cocky
	• Glib, superficial charm; impressive verbal ability
	• Irresponsible and exploitative in sexual relationships; history of multiple sexual partners and lack of a sustained monogamous relationship
	• Possible dysphoria, including complaints of tension, inability to tolerate boredom, and depressed mood

of about 2% (Moran, 1999). In prison populations, the prevalence of antisocial disorder rises to 60%. In clinical samples, the prevalence ranges from 0% to 37%, with a median value of 7% (Widiger, 1991).

Age of Onset

To be diagnosed with APD, the individual must have exhibited one or more childhood behavioral characteristics of conduct disorder and ADHD, such as aggression to people or animals, destruction of property, deceitfulness or theft, or serious violation of rules. This requirement of exhibiting antisocial behavior before 15 years of age is based on older studies of adults with APD (Barry et al., 2000; Faraone et al. 1998; Myers et al., 1998).

Gender

Men are more often diagnosed with APD than are women (Marcus, 1999; Eley et al., 1999). The best estimate for lifetime prevalence of APD from the ECA data is 7.3% for men and 1% for women (Robins et al., 1991). The cause for this discrepancy between men and women has received considerable speculation. It is generally believed that APD is underdiagnosed in women or manifested differently in men than in women, who are usually diagnosed with somatization (see Chap. 19) or histrionic disorders (discussed later in this chapter). Results from one study of 180 undergraduate students (90 men, 90 women) support the hypothesis that psychopathy (antisocial personality traits such as fearlessness, guilessness, and egocentricity) is manifested differently in men and women. In this study, men with antisocial personality traits were more likely to exhibit

behaviors associated with APD, and women with psychopathy exhibit those of histrionic personality disorders (Hamburger et al., 1996). Another study examined gender differences in the childhood behaviors of 106 male and 34 female drug abusers with APD enrolled in a relapse program. In childhood, the women had more often run away but less often used weapons in fights, been cruel to animals, and set fires. Women also reported less vandalism. In adulthood, women had more often been irresponsible as parents and in financial matters, engaged in prostitution, been physically violent against sex partners and children, failed to plan ahead, and lacked remorse (Goldstein et al., 1996). Some imply that males have early-onset and adolescent-onset disorder, whereas females primarily have an adolescent-onset disorder (Silverthorn & Frick, 1999) contributing to less severe symptoms and deficits. Similarly, APD development in females entails more affect dysregulation, resulting in a competing diagnosis of BPD, even though they meet the overall criteria for APD (Zlotnick, 1999) (Text Box 22-6).

Cultural and Ethnic Differences

People with APD or psychopathic personalities are found in many cultures, including industrialized and nonindustrialized societies (Cooke, 1996). In an analysis of the Inuit of Northwest Alaska, individuals who break the rules when they are known are called *kunlangeta*, meaning "his mind knows what to do but he does not do it" (Murphy, 1976, p. 1026). This term is used for someone who repeatedly lies, cheats, and steals. He is described as someone who does not go hunting and, when the other men are out of the village, takes sexual

TEXT BOX 22.6

Clinical Vignette: Antisocial Personality Disorder: Male Versus Female

Stasia (female) and Jackson (male) are fraternal twins, 22-years-old, who were diagnosed with antisocial personality disorder. The following are their clinical profiles.

Jackson

Jackson is currently in the county jail for the third time. Although his juvenile records begin at age 9 years and include a variety of misdemeanors and class B felonies, this burglary conviction is his first adult crime. His school teachers thought Jackson was very bright but that he had significant difficulty with peers and authority figures. He fought regularly, was described as a bully, and seemed always to be scamming. At 16 years of age, Jackson dropped out of school and joined a gang.

Jackson's juvenile probation officer explained that Jackson came from a very violent family and neighborhood and described the situation by saying, "If gangs hadn't gotten him, his father would have." His lawyer described him as "a likeable guy, but I wouldn't turn my back on him."

The jail nurse described Jackson as "a real charmer, but nothing is ever his fault." Oddly, he is the only person in the jail with an adequate supply of cigarettes and music tapes. "We get along fine. I don't understand why guards have such difficulty with him." Sometimes, the guards send Jackson to the dispensary for injuries, and Jackson plaintively explains to the nurse, "Those guards beat me up again, I don't know why."

Stasia

Stasia was recently hospitalized for the sixth time when one of her male friends beat her. She has been working as a prostitute for 5 years. Her physical examination noted not only multiple bruises but also the presence of body tattoos that cover 50% of her body. In addition, she has piercings of her tongue, ears, brow, lips, and nipples. She is emotionally volatile, manipulative, and angry. Stasia has many acquaintances and sexual partners, but none are truly intimate. She has periods when she uses drugs regularly.

Their mother was jailed when Stasia and Jackson were 18-months-old and didn't return until they were 6-years-old. They were raised mostly by their paternal grandmother, who hated their mother and reminded Stasia frequently of how much she looked like her mother. Their father, when present, was violent toward Jackson and sexually abused Stasia.

Critical Thinking Questions

- How might gender influence the development of symptoms?
- How might culture influence early recognition of problems and provision of early intervention to prevent future serious mental disorders?
- What might be some possible outcomes in this situation?
- How does this case demonstrate the interaction between socialization, biology, and culture?

---

advantage of the women. In another culture in rural southwest Nigeria, the Yorubas use the word *arankan* to mean a "person who always goes his own way regardless of others, who is uncooperative, full of malice and bullheaded" (Murphy, 1976, p. 1026). In both cultures, the healers and shamans do not consider them treatable.

The number of people within a culture who actually have APD appears to depend on whether the society is individualistic, where competitiveness and independence are encouraged and temporary relationships the norm, or collectivistic, such as China, where group loyalties and responsibilities are more important than self-expression (Cooke, 1996). Cultural distribution variation may have more to do with economic conditions, legal structures, social tolerance, and co-occurring conditions than specific diagnostic factors. Poverty and academic failure were significantly related to delinquency in boys (Pagani et al., 1999), and gang entry was seen as a developmental step in boys with conduct disorder (Lahey et al., 1999). A study comparing male prisoners in North America and Scotland showed a lower prevalence of APD among Scots than North Americans, but Scots had higher levels of antisocial traits (Cooke & Michie, 1999).

Comorbidity

APD is strongly associated with alcohol and drug abuse. Substance-related disorders are common (Lejoyeux et al., 2000; Waldman & Slutske, 2000). The association between substance abuse and APD is stronger in women than in men. It is rare for APD to be the only disorder present. In the ECA study, less than 10% of patients with APD had no other diagnoses. In the ECA data, men with active APD were three times more likely to abuse alcohol and five times more likely to abuse drugs as those without APD. Women with APD were 13 times more likely to use alcohol and 12 times more likely to use drugs (Robins et al., 1991). Other disorders that typically occur with APD include ADHD (Schubiner et al., 2000), depression, and schizophrenia (Nolan et al., 1999).

Etiology

Biologic Theories

Genetic. There appears to be a genetic component in APD, which is five times more common in first-degree biologic relatives of men with the disorder than among the general population. There is nearly 10 times greater risk to women who are first-degrees biologic relatives.

Pooled data of 229 pairs of identical twins from seven twin studies conducted in North America, Japan, Norway, Germany, and Denmark showed a concordance rate of 51.5% for APD, whereas data from the 316 fraternal twins yielded a corresponding rate of 23.1% (Gottesman & Goldsmith, 1994).

Biochemical. The biochemical basis of antisocial disorder is not clearly understood. Some curious biologic markers have been identified, however. Gotz and colleagues (1999) found significantly higher antisocial behavior in adolescent and adult men with XYY sex chromosome abnormality than controls. Another study found higher concentration of serum testosterone and sex hormone–binding globulin in incarcerated men who met the criteria for APD (Stalenheim et al., 1998). In another direction, several studies have found 5-HT1B autoreceptor polymorphism among two large samples of alcoholic patients with APD (Lappalaimer et al., 1998) and other evidence of serotonin deficiency (Dolan, 1994). Low dopamine levels have also been implicated in APD. In a study of 21 hospitalized boys ranging in ages from 8 to 16 years who had diagnoses of conduct disorder, oppositional deviant disorder, and ADHD, low levels of dopamine activity were found in those who had been abused or neglected before 3 years of age (Galvin et al., 1991). These researchers suggested that low levels of dopamine may reflect an attachment disruption that occurs at critical times in the lives of these abused and neglected boys. This disruption causes the child to be biologically vulnerable, resulting in low levels of dopamine and less effective regulation of the noradrenergic system when activated by stressors.

Psychological Theories

Attachment. Learning, social behavior, empathy, emotional awareness, and regulation are all directly influenced by the nature of the relationship between the caregiver and child. One of the leading explanations of APD is that these individuals had unsatisfactory attachments in early relationships that led to antisocial behavior in later life. Normal relationships begin with **attachment** that can be defined as:

Behavior that results in a person attaining or retaining proximity to some other differentiated and preferred individual. During the course of healthy development, attachment behavior leads to the development of affectional bonds or attachments, initially between child and parent and later between adult and adult. The forms of behavior and the bonds to which they lead are present and active throughout the life cycle (Bowlby, 1980, p. 39).

An attachment relationship between the child and caregivers depends on the response of both parties. The sense of security in any relationship depends on the quality of the responsiveness experienced with the

attachment figure (Smallbone & Dadds, 2000). If the parental figures are overanxious or avoidant, the child does not develop a sense of security with others and instead experiences self as an island. Secure attachments facilitate a balance between connection to another and the ability to go out into the world autonomously. In a secure attachment, a child feels safe, loved, and valued but also develops the self-confidence to interact with the rest of the world (see Chap. 28). Experiences in successive relationships interact with prior experiences to determine an individual's trust in others.

Insecure attachments are formed as a result of faulty interaction between the caregiver and the child and are expressed in relationships as ambivalence, avoidance, or disorganization (Ainsworth, 1989). In APD, a failure to make or sustain stable attachments in early childhood can lead to avoidance of future attachments. Studies have found several childhood situations to be risk factors for developing dysfunctional attachments, such as parental abandonment or neglect, loss of parent or primary caregiver, and physical or sexual abuse. However, evidence supports the theory that ability to foster secure emotional attachments may be a learned parenting skill and that parents who lacked secure attachment relationship in their own childhood may lack the ability to form secure attachment relationships with their own children (see Research Box 22-1).

Temperament. Children are born with a particular **temperament,** a recognizable and distinctive way of behavior that is evident in the first few months of life. Some infants are more relaxed or calm and sleep a lot, whereas others are extremely alert, startled by the slightest noise, cry more, and sleep less. Scientists believe temperament is neurobiologically determined, and many believe that it is central to understanding personality disorders. Children seem to be born with certain temperaments that remain fairly stable throughout development.

Temperament consists of the interaction of two behavioral dimensions—activity and adaptability. Activity patterns vary along a spectrum from active or intense children whose actions display decisiveness and vigor as they continuously relate to their environment to passive children are more cautious and slow to relate to their environment—a "wait-and-see" pattern of behavior. Adaptability includes a spectrum, with the extreme at one end being the child who is regular in biologic functions such as eating or sleeping, has a positive approach to new stimuli, and maintains a high degree of flexibility in response to changing conditions. At the other end of the adaptability dimension are children who display irregularity in biologic functions, withdrawal reactions to new stimuli, and minimal flexibility in response to change (see Chap. 28).

Some studies seem to indicate that extreme temperaments make one vulnerable to antisocial behavior

RESEARCH BOX 22.1

*Attachment Theory
and Aggression*

Secure attachment relationships early in life are associated with a lower rate of aggression later in childhood. The quality of attachment in relationships can be predicted by the parent's "representations" of their own early childhood experience. In this study, single parents of abnormally aggressive preschoolers were compared with single parents of nonaggressive children. The parents (n = 10) were matched according to age, sex, and race, and the children all attended low-income day centers. The mothers' attachment relationships with their own parents were measured by the Adult Attachment Interview, which measures secure and insecure attachments. Results indicated that all the parents of the aggressive children had insecure attachment relationships and only one parent of the nonaggressive group did.

Utilization in Clinical Setting: This study supports the idea that parents who have a secure attachment with their own parents are more likely to form a secure attachment with their children, who in turn become less aggressive. Parents who have had insecure attachments may need help in developing attachment skills.

Constantino, J. (1996). Intergenerational aspects of the development of aggression: A preliminary report. *Journal of Developmental and Behavioral Pediatrics, 17*(3), 176–182.

patterns. A difficult temperament is characterized by withdrawal from novel stimuli, low adaptability, and intense emotional reactions. Four key behaviors are present in a difficult temperament: aggression, inattention, hyperactivity, and impulsivity. There is a strong relationship between difficult temperament and problem behaviors such as those of ADHD, oppositional behavior, and conduct disorder (Jansen et al., 1995).

Hyperactivity alone is not related to the development of antisocial personality in adults; whereas hyperactivity occurring with aggression and the other behaviors is related to APD (Barry et al., 2000; Giancola, 2000; Schubiner et al., 2000). Temperament and problem behaviors are generally consistent over time. There is a strong relationship between conduct disorder in childhood and antisocial behavior in adulthood with substance abuse (Myers et al., 1998). In a longitudinal study of 961 children whose temperament related to the development of psychiatric problems in childhood, those children with a difficult temperament were more likely to be diagnosed in adulthood with APD, be a recidivistic offender, and be convicted for a violent offense (Hare, 1999; Grann et al., 1999).

Social Theories

Social factors are important in the development of APD. These individuals often come from chaotic families in which alcoholism and violence are the norm. Individuals who have been victims of abuse or neglect, live in a foster home, or had several primary caretakers are more likely to develop antisocial behaviors, especially aggression (Andrews et al., 2000; Pagani et al., 1999; Kim et al., 1999). It is difficult, however, to separate the influence of social factors on the development of the disorder because the symptoms of APD are social manifestations—unemployment, marital divorces and separations, and violence.

Interdisciplinary Treatment of Disorder

People with APD rarely seek mental health care because of the disorder itself but rather for treatment of depression, substance abuse, or uncontrolled anger or for forensic evaluation (Black et al., 1995). Patients who are admitted through the forensic system (see Chap. 4) often have a comorbid diagnosis of APD. Treatment is difficult and involves helping the patient alter his or her cognitive schema. The overall treatment goals are to develop empathy for other people and situations and to live within the norms of society.

Priority Care Issues

Even though they can be interpersonally charming, these patients can become verbally and physically abusive if their expectations are not met. Protection of other patients and staff from manipulative and sometimes abusive behavior is a priority.

Family Response to Disorder

If there are family members, they have probably been abused, mistreated, or intimidated by these patients. For example, one patient sold his mother's possessions while she was at work. Another would abuse his wife after drinking. However, family members may be fiercely loyal to the patient and blame themselves for his or her shortcomings.

NURSING MANAGEMENT: HUMAN RESPONSE TO DISORDER

Assessment of Biopsychosocial Domains

The nursing assessment usually focuses on other problems in addition to the response to the personality disorder. In fact, eliciting data may be difficult because of the basic mistrust these individuals have toward authority figures. Patients may not give an accurate history or may embellish aspects to project themselves in a more positive light. Often, they deny any criminal activity, even if they are admitted in police custody. Key areas of assessment are determining quality of relationships, impulsivity, and the extent of aggression. These individuals do not assume responsibility for their own actions and often blame others for their misfortune. Their disregard for others is manifested in their interactions. For example, one patient with human immunodeficiency virus was engaging in unprotected sex with several different women because he wanted to "have fun as long as I can." He was completely unconcerned about the possibility of transmitting the virus. These individuals often make good first impressions. Self-awareness is especially important for the nurse because of the initial charming quality of many of these individuals. Once these patients realize that the nurse cannot be used or manipulated, they lose interest in the nurse and revert to their normal, egocentric behaviors.

Nursing Diagnoses and Outcome Identification

Nursing diagnoses for patients with APD are related to their interpersonal detachment, lack of awareness of others, avoidance of feelings, impulsiveness, and discrepancy between their perception of themselves and others' perception of them. Typical diagnoses are Ineffective Role Performance (unemployment), Ineffective Individual Coping, Impaired Communication, Impaired Social Interactions, Low Self-Esteem, and Risk for Violence. Outcomes should be short-term and relevant to a specific problem. For example, if a patient has been chronically unemployed, a reasonable short-term outcome would be to set up job interviews rather than obtaining a job.

Planning and Implementing Nursing Interventions

Biologic Interventions

Antisocial personality disorder does not significantly impair the biologic dimension unless there are coexisting substance abuse or Axis I disorders. In instances in which there are coexisting disorders, the personality disorder may actually interfere with nursing interventions aimed at improving physical functioning. For example, a patient with schizophrenia and APD may not develop enough trust within a relationship to examine his or her delusional thoughts. Because substance abuse is a major problem with this population, the physical effects of chronic use of addictive substances must be considered (see Chap. 33).

Psychological Interventions

Therapeutic relationships are difficult to establish because these individuals do not attach to others and are often unable to use the relationship to change behavior. After the first few meetings with these patients, the nurse may feel that the relationship has a good start, but in reality, a superficial alliance is usually formed. Additional sessions reveal the lack of patient commitment to the relationship. These patients begin to revisit topics discussed in sessions or lose interest in trying to work on problems. By using self-awareness skills and accessing supervision regularly, the nurse can identify blocks in the development of a therapeutic relationship (or lack of) and his or her response to the relationship. The goal of the therapeutic relationship is to identify dysfunctional thinking patterns and develop new problem-solving behaviors.

These patients have a long-standing history of difficulty in interpersonal relationships. In an inpatient unit, interventions can be more intense and focus on helping the patient develop positive interaction skills and experience a consistent environment. For example, the focus of nursing interventions may be the patient's continual disregard of the rights of others. On one unit, a patient continually placed orders for pizzas in the name of another patient who had limited intelligence and was genuinely afraid of the person with APD. The victimized patient always paid for the pizza and gave it to the other patient. When the nursing staff realized what was happening, they confronted the patient with APD about the behavior and revoked his unit privileges.

The nursing intervention, self-responsibility facilitation (encouraging a patient to assume more responsibility for personal behavior), is useful with patients with APD (McCloskey & Bulechek, 1996). The nursing activities that are particularly helpful include holding the patient responsible for his or her behavior, monitoring the extent that self-responsibility is assumed, and discussing the consequences of not dealing with responsibilities. The nurse needs to refrain from arguing or bargaining about the unit rules such as time for meals, use of the television room, smoking, and so forth. Instead, positive feedback is given to patient for accepting additional responsibility or changing behavior.

Self-awareness enhancement (exploring and understanding personal thoughts, feelings, motivation, and behaviors) is another nursing intervention that is important in helping these individuals develop a sense of understanding about relating to the rest of the world (McCloskey & Bulechek, 1996). Encouraging patients to recognize and discuss thoughts and feelings helps the nurse understand how the patient views the world. The nurse can then use many of the same communication techniques discussed in the section on BPD.

Patient education efforts have to be creative and thought provoking. In teaching a person with APD, a direct approach is best, but the nurse must avoid "lecturing," which the patient will resent. In teaching the patient about positive health care practices, impulse control, and anger management, the best approach is to engage the patient in a discussion about the issue and then direct the topic to the major teaching points. These patients often take great delight in arguing or showing how the rules of life do not apply to them. A sense of humor is important, as are clear teaching goals and avoiding being sidetracked (see Psychoeducation Checklist: Antisocial Personality Disorder).

Social Interventions

Group interventions are more effective than individual modalities because other patients and staff can validate or challenge the patient's view of a situation (Messina et al., 1999). Problem-solving groups that focus on identifying a problem and developing a variety of alternative solutions are particular helpful because patient self-responsibility is reinforced when patients remind each other of the better alternatives. Patients are likely to confront each other with dysfunctional schemas or thinking patterns. Teaching patients with APD the same communication techniques as those with BPD will also encourage self-responsibility. These patients often attend groups that focus on the development of empathy.

Milieu interventions, such as providing a structured environment with rules that are consistently applied to patients who are responsible for their own behavior, are important. While living in close proximity to others, the individual with APD will demonstrate dysfunctional social patterns that can be identified and targeted for correction. For example, these patients often violate ward rules, such as no smoking or limitations on the number of visitors, and may bring contraband, such as illegal drugs, to the unit.

PSYCHOEDUCATION CHECKLIST
Antisocial Personality Disorder

When caring for the patient with antisocial personality disorder, be sure to include the following topic areas in the teaching plan:

- Positive health care practices, including substance abuse control
- Effective communication and interaction skills
- Impulse control
- Anger management
- Group experience to help develop self-awareness and impact of behavior on others
- Analyzing an issue from the other person's viewpoint
- Maintenance of employment
- Interpersonal relationships and social interactions

Aggressive behavior is often a problem for these individuals and their family members. Like patients with BPD, people with APD tend to be impulsive. Instead of self-injury, these individuals are more likely to strike out at those who are perceived to be interfering with their immediate gratification. Anger control assistance (helping to express anger in an adaptive, nonviolent manner) becomes a priority intervention. Because the expression of anger and aggression develops over a lifetime, these individuals can benefit from anger management techniques and taking responsibility for expression (see Chap. 36).

Social support for these individuals is often minimal, just as it is for individuals with BPD, but the reasons are different. These individuals have often taken advantage of friends and relatives who in turn no longer trust them. Helping the patient build a new support system once new skills are learned is usually the only option. For these individuals to develop friends and reengage family members, they must learn to interact in new ways, develop empathy, and risk an attachment. For many, this truly never becomes a reality.

Family Interventions

Family members of patients with APD usually need help in establishing boundaries. Because there is a long-term pattern of interaction in which family members are responsible for patient's antisocial behavior, these patterns need to be interrupted. Families need help in recognizing the patient's responsibility for his or her actions.

Evaluation and Treatment Outcomes

The antisocial personality patterns developed over a lifetime. The outcomes need to be evaluated in terms of management of specific problems, such as maintaining employment or developing a meaningful interpersonal relationship. The nurse will most likely see these patients for other health care problems, so that adherence to treatment recommendations and development of health care practices (eg, reduce smoking and alcohol consumption) can also be factored into the evaluation of outcomes.

Continuum of Care

People with APD rarely seek mental health care. In the ECA study, only 14.5% of those with a diagnosis of APD had ever discussed any of its symptoms with a physician. Only 4% had visited a mental health provider in the last 6 months (Robins et al., 1991). Nurses will most likely see these patients in medical-surgical settings for comorbid conditions. Consistency in interventions is necessary in treating the patient throughout the whole continuum of care.

HISTRIONIC PERSONALITY DISORDER: GREGARIOUS PATTERN

"Attention seeking" and "emotional" describe people with histrionic personality disorders. These individuals are lively and dramatic and draw attention to themselves by their enthusiasm, dress, and apparent openness. They are the "life of the party" and, on the surface, seem interested in others. Their insatiable need for attention and approval quickly becomes obvious. These needs are inflexible and persistent even after others attempt to meet them. They are moody and often experience a sense of helplessness when others are disinterested in them. They are sexually seductive in their attempts to

gain attention and often are uncomfortable within a single relationship. They are highly suggestible and have a tendency to change opinions often. Their appearance is provocative and their speech dramatic. They express strong opinions without supporting facts. Loyalty and fidelity are lacking (APA, 2000) (Table 22-5).

Gender influences the manifestations of this disorder. Women dress seductively, may express dependency on selected men, and may "play" a submissive role. Men may dress in a very masculine manner and seek attention by bragging about athletic skills or successes in the job. Individuals with this disorder have difficulty achieving any true intimacy in interpersonal relationships. They seem to possess an innate sensitivity to the moods and thought of those they wish to please. This hyperalertness enables them to maneuver quickly to gain their attention. Then, they attempt to control relationships by their seductiveness at one level but become extremely

TABLE 22.5 Key Diagnostic Characteristics of Histrionic and Narcissistic Personality Disorders 301.50

Diagnostic Criteria and Target Symptoms for Histrionic Disorders	*Associated Findings* *Associated Behavioral Findings*
• Pervasive and excessive emotionality and attention-seeking behavior Feelings of being uncomfortable and unappreciated when not the center of attention (lively and dramatic in drawing attention to self) Inappropriately sexually seductive or provocative Shallow and rapidly shifting emotional expression Use of physical appearance to draw attention to self Impressionistic and vague style of speech Exaggerated expression of emotion, theatricality, and self-dramatization Highly suggestible Viewing of relationships as more intimate than they really are	• Difficulty achieving emotional intimacy in romantic and sexual relationships • Use of emotional manipulation and seductiveness coupled with marked dependency • Impaired relationships with same-sex friends • Constant demanding of attention, leading to alienation of friends • Craving novelty, excitement, and stimulation; easily bored with routines • Difficulty in situations involving delayed gratification • Increased risk for suicidal gestures and threats for attention
Diagnostic Criteria and Target Symptoms for Narcissistic Disorders	*Associated Findings* *Associated Behavioral Findings*
• Pervasive pattern of grandiosity; need for admiration; lack of empathy Grandiose sense of self-importance Preoccupation with fantasies of unlimited success, power or vigilance, beauty, or ideal love Belief of own superiority, specialness, and uniqueness; association with individuals of higher or special status Need for excessive admiration and constant attention Sense of entitlement (unreasonable expectation of highly favorable treatment) Exploitation and taking advantage of others Lack of empathy; difficulty recognizing desires, experiences, and feelings of others Envious of others; feeling that others are envious of him or her Arrogant, haughty behavior or attitudes	• Sensitive to injury from criticism or deficit • Criticism causes inward feelings of humiliation, degradation, hollowness, and emptiness • Social withdrawal • Impaired interpersonal relationships • Impaired performance because of intolerance to criticism • Unwilling to take risk in competitive situation when defeat is possible

dependent on their friends at another level. Their demand for constant attention quickly alienates their friends. They become depressed when they are not the center of attention.

Epidemiology

The prevalence of histrionic personality disorder is estimated at 2% to 3% of the general population. In the mental health settings, the prevalence rate is reported to be 10% to 15% (APA, 2000). In the reappraisal of the ECA Baltimore data, there were no differences in prevalence by sex, race, or education. In men, but not in women, the prevalence declined with age. There was a higher rate of this disorder among separated and divorced subjects than among married subjects (Nestadt et al., 1990). This disorder co-occurs with borderline, dependent, and antisocial personality disorders. It also exists with anxiety disorders, substance abuse, and mood disorders (Millon & Davis, 1999). Men with histrionic disorders are more likely to also have substance abuse problems, and women are more likely to experience depressive episodes, suicide attempts, and two or more unexplained medical symptoms (Nestadt et al., 1990).

Etiology

There is a need for research in determining the etiologic factors of histrionic personality disorder. There is speculation that this disorder has a biologic component and that heredity may play a role, but that the biologic influence is less than in some of the previously discussed personality disorders. In infancy and early childhood, these individuals are extremely alert and emotionally responsive. The tendencies for sensory alertness may be traced to responses of the limbic and reticular systems. They demonstrate a high degree of dependence on others and a type of dissociation in which they have reduced awareness of their behavior in relation to others (Bornstein, 1998). It is believed these highly alert and responsive infants seek more gratification from external stimulation in their first few months of life. Depending on the responsiveness of caregivers to them, they develop behavior patterns in response to their caregivers. It is believed that these children experience brief, highly charged, and irregular reinforcement from multiple caretakers (parents, siblings, grandparents, foster parent) who are unable to provide consistent experiences. They learn to receive gratification from short, concentrated reinforcement or attention from different sources rather than learning to establish a secure attachment to one or two parents. The adult histrionic behavior is observed in one who shifts from one person to another, continuously seeks new situations and adventures, and is unable to tolerate boredom.

Parental behavior and role modeling are also believed to contribute to the development of histrionic personality disorder. Many of the women with this disorder reported that they are just like their mother, who is emotionally labile, bored with the routines of home life, flirtatious with men, and clever in dealing with people. It is believed that through role modeling, these children learn and mimic the behaviors observed in caregivers or adults. When these children have siblings with whom they compete for parental attention, they try to be cute, attractive, and seductive to secure attention (Sigmund et al., 1998).

Nursing Management

The ultimate treatment goal for patients with histrionic personality disorder is to correct the tendency to fulfill all their needs by focusing on others to the exclusion of themselves. When these individuals seek mental health care, they have usually experienced a period of social disapproval or deprivation. Their hope is that the mental health providers will help fulfill their needs. Specific goals are needed to protect the person from becoming dependent on a mental health system. In the nursing assessment, the nurse focuses on the quality of the individual's interpersonal relationships. It is common that the person is dissatisfied with his or her partner, and sexual relations may be nonexistent. During the assessment, the patient will make statements that indicate a low self-esteem. Because these individuals believe that they are incapable of handling life's demands and have been waiting for a truly competent person to take care of them, they have not developed a positive self-concept or adequate problem-solving abilities. Nursing diagnoses that are usually generated include Chronic Low Self-Esteem, Ineffective Individual Coping, and Ineffective Sexual Patterns. Outcomes focus on helping the patient develop autonomy, a positive self-concept, and mature problem-solving skills.

A variety of interventions support the outcomes. A nurse–patient relationship that allows the patient to explore positive personality characteristics and develop independent decision-making skills forms the basis of the interventions. Reinforcing personal strengths, conveying confidence in the patient's ability to handle situations, and examining negative perceptions of self can be done within the therapeutic relationship. Encouraging the patient to act autonomously can also improve the individual's sense of self-worth (McCloskey & Bulechek, 1996). Attending assertiveness groups can help increase the individual's self-confidence and improve self-esteem.

NARCISSISTIC PERSONALITY DISORDER: EGOTISTIC PATTERN

People with a narcissistic personality disorder are grandiose, have an inexhaustible need for admiration, and lack empathy. Beginning in childhood, these individuals believe that they are superior, special, or unique and that others should recognize them in this way (APA, 2000). They are often preoccupied with fantasies of unlimited success, power, beauty, or ideal love. They overvalue their personal worth, direct their affections toward themselves, and expect others to hold them in high esteem. They define the world through their own self-centered view. They are concerned with power, prestige, status, and superiority. People with narcissistic personality disorder are benignly arrogant and feel themselves above the conventions of their cultural group. They believe they are entitled to be served and that it is their inalienable right to receive special considerations. These individuals are often successful in their jobs but may alienate their significant others, who grow tired of their narcissism (see Table 22-5).

Epidemiology

The prevalence of narcissistic personality disorder in the general population is estimated to be less than 1%. In the mental health clinical population, the prevalence ranges from 2% to 16% (APA, 2000). In nonclinical samples, the prevalence rate ranges from 0.0% to 0.4% (Lyons, 1995). Narcissistic personality disorder is found more frequently in men than in women (Millon & Davis, 1999). It also commonly occurs in only children and among first-born boys in cultural groups in which males have special privileges. This disorder can coexist with other Axis II disorders such as antisocial, histrionic, and paranoid disorders and Axis I disorders of mood, anxiety, and substance abuse.

Etiology

There is little evidence of any biologic factors that contribute to the development of this disorder. One notion about its development is that it is the result of parents' overvaluation and overindulgence of a child. These children are overly pampered and indulged, with every whim catered to. They learn to view themselves as special beings and to expect special treatment and subservience from others. They do not learn how to cooperate, share, or consider others' desires and interests. An alternate explanation is that the child never truly separated emotionally from his or her primary caregiver and, therefore, cannot envision functioning independently. The underlying basis of the outward aggrandizement is one of profound self-hatred and inferiority (Bushman & Baumeister, 1998). To avoid feeling this self-hatred, the person develops a defensive need for power over others (Joubert, 1998; Paulhus, 1998).

Nursing Management

The nurse will encounter these patients in medical settings and in psychiatric settings with a coexisting psychiatric disorder. They are difficult patients. They are often snobbish, condescending, and patronizing in their attitudes. It is unlikely that these individuals are motivated to develop sensitivity to others and socially cooperative attitudes and behaviors. Nurses are often alienated from these individuals and need to use their self-awareness skills in interacting with them. The nursing process focuses on the coexisting responses to other health care problems.

Continuum of Care

Patients with histrionic and narcissistic personality disorders do not seek mental health care unless they have a coexisting medical or mental disorder. They are likely to be treated within the community for most of their lives, with the exception of short hospitalizations for nonpsychiatric problems.

CLUSTER C DISORDERS: ANXIOUS-FEARFUL

AVOIDANT PERSONALITY DISORDER: WITHDRAWN PATTERN

Avoidant personality disorder is characterized by avoiding social situations in which there is interpersonal contact with others. This avoidance is purposeful and deliberate because of fears of criticism and feelings of inadequacy. These individuals are extremely sensitive to negative comments and disapproval. They engage in interpersonal relationships only when they receive unconditional approval. The behavior becomes problematic when they restrict their social activities and work opportunities because of their extreme fear of rejection. They appear timid, shy, and hesitant. In childhood, they are shy, but instead of growing out of the shyness, it becomes worse in adulthood. They distance themselves from activities that involve personal contact with others. They perceive themselves as socially inept, inadequate, and inferior, which in turn justifies their isolation and rejection by others. They rely on fantasy for gratification of needs, confidence, and conflict resolution. These individuals withdraw into their fantasies as a means of dealing with frustration and anger. They also have underlying feelings of tension, sadness, and anger that vacillate between desire for affection, fear of rebuff, embarrassment, and numbness of feeling (APA, 2000; Millon & Davis, 1999) (Table 22-6).

Epidemiology

The prevalence estimates in nonclinical samples range from 0.0% to 1.3%, with a median value of about 1.1% (Lyons, 1995). Lifetime prevalence of avoidant personality disorder was estimated at 3.6% (Faravelli et al., 2000). Avoidant personality disorder has been reported in about 10% of outpatients in mental health clinics.

The problem with examining the epidemiology of avoidant personality disorder is its potential overlap with the Axis I disorder, generalized social phobia. Several studies found that a significant portion of the patients diagnosed with social phobia also met criteria for avoidant personality disorder. Social phobia was found to be more pervasive and characterized by a higher level of interpersonal sensitivity (Perugi et al., 1999). Avoidant personality disorder, on the other hand, involves greater overall psychopathology (Boone et al., 1999). Not surprisingly, social phobia frequently co-occurs with avoidant personality disorder (Moutier & Stein, 1999). Patients with avoidant personality disorder differ from those with generalized social phobia only in the severity of the anxiety symptoms (less than those with social phobia) and in the depressive symptomatology. Avoidant personality disorder may actually be a more severe from of social phobia (Boone et al., 1999).

Etiology

No data support the relationship of biologic factors to the development of avoidant personality disorder. Experts have speculated that these individuals experience

---

TABLE 22.6 Key Diagnostic Characteristics of Cluster C Disorders

Diagnostic Criteria and Target Symptoms

Avoidant Personality Disorder 301.82	• Pervasive pattern of social inhibition with feelings of inadequacy and hypersensitivity to negative evaluation
	  Avoidance of activities involving significant personal contact because of fear of criticism, disapproval, or rejection
	  Lack of willingness for involvement unless certainty of being liked
	  Restraint within intimate relationships for fear of shame or ridicule
	  Preoccupation with criticism or rejection in social situations
	  Inhibition in new interpersonal situations
	  Viewing self as socially inept, personally unappealing, or inferior
	  Unusual reluctance to take personal risks or engage in new activities

Dependent Personality Disorder 301.6	• Pervasive and excessive need for being taken care of, resulting in submission and clinging with fears of separation
	  Advice and reassurance needed from others for decision making
	  Responsibility for major areas of life assumed by others
	  Difficulty expressing disagreement with others for fear of loss of support or approval
	  Difficulty initiating things by self
	  Excessive methods used to obtain support and nurturance from others
	  Uncomfortable and helpless when alone
	  Urgent seeking of another relationship if previous one ends
	  Unrealistic preoccupation with fears of having to take care of self

Obsessive-Compulsive Personality Disorder 301.4	• Pervasive pattern of preoccupation with orderliness, perfectionism, mental and interpersonal control at the expense of flexibility, openness, and efficiency
	  Major point of activity lost because of preoccupation
	  Task completion interfered with because of perfectionism
	  Excessive devotion to work and productivity, excluding friends and leisure
	  Overly conscientious, scrupulous, and inflexible about morality, ethics, or values
	  Difficulty discarding worn-out or worthless objects
	  Reluctance to delegate tasks or work with others
	  Miserly spending attitude
	  Rigidity and stubbornness

aversive stimuli more intensely and more frequently than others because they may possess and overabundance of neurons in the aversive center of the limbic system (Millon & Davis, 1999). A general biologic vulnerability may be inherited and interact with environmental factors. The evidence for this biologic influence is the impact of pharmacotherapies on these individuals. When taking medications (benzodiazepines, β-blockers, and monoamine oxidase inhibitors), symptoms are reduced, but they return once medication is stopped (Mattick & Newman, 1991). Research indicates that those with avoidant personality disorder demonstrate significantly less curiosity and novelty seeking than healthy controls. The research postulated that those with avoidant personality disorder had a more tenuous early attachment (Johnston, 1999). In adulthood, they maintain an ambivalent connection with others, wishing deeply for close enduring relationships but fearing rejection and loss. A history of child abuse may be an early experience.

Nursing Management

Assessment of these individuals will reveal a lack of social contacts, a fear of being criticized, and evidence of chronic low self-esteem. The nursing diagnoses Chronic Low Self-Esteem, Social Isolation, and Ineffective Coping can be used. The establishment of a therapeutic relationship is necessary to be able to help these individuals meet their treatment outcomes. The development of the nurse–patient relationship is a slow process and requires an extreme amount of patience on the part of the nurse. These individuals have not had positive interpersonal relationships and need time to be able to trust that the nurse will not criticize and demean them. Interventions should focus on refraining from any negative criticism, assisting the patient to identify positive responses from others, exploring previous achievements of success, and exploring reasons for self-criticism. The patient's social dimension should be examined for the presence of activities that increase self-esteem. Interventions are focused on gradually increasing these self-esteem–enhancing activities. Social skills training is effective in reducing symptomatology (Stravynski et al., 1994).

DEPENDENT PERSONALITY DISORDER: SUBMISSIVE PATTERN

People with dependent personality disorder cling to others in a desperate attempt to keep them close. Their need to be taken care of is so great that it leads to doing anything to maintain the closeness, including total submission and disregard for self. Because of their dependency on others, they do not learn to make decisions, even

everyday choices such as what clothes to wear. They adapt their behavior to please those to whom they are attached. They lean on others to guide their lives. They ingratiate themselves to others and denigrate themselves and their accomplishments. Their self-esteem is determined by others. Behaviorally, these individuals withdraw from adult responsibilities by acting helpless and seeking nurturance from others. In interpersonal relationships, they need excessive advice and reassurance. They are compliant, conciliatory, and placating. They rarely disagree with others and are easily persuaded. Friends describe them as gullible. They are warm, tender, and noncompetitive. They timidly avoid social tension and interpersonal conflicts (APA, 2000) (see Table 22-6). Dependent personality disorder bears a great deal of resemblance to histrionic personality disorder. People with dependent personality disorder demonstrate high levels of self-attributed dependency needs, whereas those with histrionic personality disorder have greater implicit dependency and will even argue against needing others (Bornstein, 1998).

Epidemiology

Dependent personality disorder is one of the most frequently reported disorders in mental health clinics (APA, 2000). The prevalence in nonclinical samples ranges from 1.5% to 5.1%, with a median value of about 1.8% (Lyons, 1995). In clinical samples, the prevalence of this disorder ranges from 2% to 55%, with a median of 20% (Widiger, 1991). The diagnosis is made more frequently in women than in men. This gender difference may represent a sex bias by clinicians because when standardized instruments are used, men and women are diagnosed equally. This disorder often coexists with other personality disorders, including borderline, avoidant, histrionic, and schizotypal disorders (Lyons, 1995).

Etiology

It is likely that there is a biologic predisposition to develop the dependency attachments of this disorder. However, no research studies support a biologic hypothesis. Dependent personality disorder is most often explained as a result of parents' genuine affection, extreme attachment, and overprotection. Children then learn to rely on others to meet basic needs but do not learn the necessary skills for autonomous behavior.

Nursing Management

Nurses can determine the extent of dependency by assessment of self-worth, interpersonal relationships, and social behavior. They should determine whether there is currently someone on whom the person relies (parent, spouse) or if there has been a separation from a significant relationship by death or divorce. Nursing diagnoses that are usually generated from the assessment data are Ineffective Individual Coping, Low Self-Esteem, Impaired Social Interaction, and Impaired Home Maintenance Management. Home management skills may be a problem if the patient does not have the useful skills and now has to make decisions related to finances, shopping, cooking, and cleaning. The challenge of caring for these patients is to help them recognize their dependent patterns, motivate them to want to change, and teach them adult skills that have not been developed, such as balancing a checkbook, planning a weekly menu, and paying bills. Occasionally, if a patient is extremely fatigued, lethargic, or anxious and the disorder interferes with efforts at developing more independence, antidepressants or antianxiety agents may be used.

These patients readily engage in a nurse–patient relationship and initially will look to the nurse to make all decisions. The nurse can support patients to make their own decisions by resisting the urge to tell them what to do. Ideally, these patients are in individual psychotherapy and working toward long-term personality changes. The nurse can encourage patients to stay in therapy and to practice the new skills that are being learned. Assertiveness training is helpful.

CHAPTER 22

OBSESSIVE-COMPULSIVE PERSONALITY DISORDER: CONFORMING PATTERN

Obsessive-compulsive disorder stands out in Axis II because it bears close resemblance to obsessive-compulsive anxiety disorder (Axis I). A distinguishing difference is that those with the anxiety disorder tend to use obsessive thoughts and compulsions when anxious but less so when anxiety decreases. With this personality disorder, the person does not demonstrate obsessions and compulsions as much as an overall rigidity, perfectionism, and control. Individuals with this disorder attempt to maintain control by careful attention to rules, trivial details, procedures, and lists (APA, 2000). These people are not fun. They may be completely devoted to work, which typically has a rigid character, such as maintaining financial records or tracking inventory. They are uncomfortable with unstructured leisure time, especially vacations. Leisure activities are likely to be formalized (season tickets to sports, organized tour groups). Hobbies are approached seriously.

Behaviorally, these individuals are perfectionists, maintaining a regulated, highly structured, strictly organized life. A need to control others and situations is common in personal and in work life. They are prone to repetition and have difficulty making decisions and completing tasks because they become so involved in the details. They can be overly conscientious about morality and ethics and value polite, formal, and correct interpersonal relationships. They also tend to be rigid, stubborn, and indecisive and are unable to accept new ideas and customs. Their mood is tense and joyless. Warm feelings are restrained, and they tightly control the expression of emotions (APA, 2000; Slade, 1998) (see Table 22-6).

Epidemiology

The prevalence of obsessive-compulsive personality disorder is 1% in the general population and 3% to 10% in individuals being treated in mental health clinics (APA, 2000). In a reappraisal of the Baltimore ECA data, men had a significantly higher prevalence (3.0%) than women (0.6%). Whites had a higher rate than African Americans. This disorder is associated with higher education, employment, and being married. Subjects with the disorder had a higher income than those without the disorder. This disorder is associated with a greater risk for generalized anxiety disorder and simple phobia and lowered risk for alcohol abuse (Nestadt et al., 1990).

Etiology

As with some of the other personality disorders, there is little evidence for a biologic formulation. The basis of the compulsive patterns that characterize obsessive-compulsive personality disorder is parental overcontrol and overprotection that is consistently restrictive and sets distinct limits on the child's behavior. Parents teach these children a deep sense of responsibility to others and to feel guilty when these responsibilities are not met. Play is viewed as shameful, sinful, and irresponsible, leading to dire consequences. They are encouraged to resist the natural inclinations toward play and impulse gratification, and parents try to impose guilt on the child to control behavior.

Nursing Management

These individuals seek mental health care when they have attacks of anxiety, spells of immobilization, sexual impotence, and excessive fatigue. To change the compulsive pattern, psychotherapy is needed. There may be short-term pharmacologic intervention with an antidepressant or anxiolytic as an adjunct. The assessment of the generalist psychiatric–mental health nurse will focus on the patient's physical symptoms (sleep, eating, sexual), interpersonal relationships, and social problems. The nursing diagnoses include Anxiety, Risk for Loneliness, Decisional Conflict, Sexual Dysfunction, Disturbed Sleep Pattern, and Impaired Social Interactions. Development of outcomes will be easier to establish than realized. These individuals realize that they could improve their quality of life, but they will find it extremely anxiety provoking to make the necessary changes. A supportive nurse–patient relationship based on acceptance of the patient's need for order and rigidity will help the person have enough confidence to try new behaviors. Examining the patient's belief that underlies the dysfunctional behaviors can set the stage for challenging the childhood thinking. Because the compulsive pattern was established in childhood, it will take a long time to modify the behavior.

Continuum of Care

Long-term therapy is ideal for patients with avoidant personality disorder because it takes time to make the changes. Generalist psychiatric–mental health nurses may see these individuals for other health problems. Encouraging the patient to continue with therapy and contacting the therapist when necessary are important in maintaining continuity of care. These patients are hospitalized only for a coexisting disorder.

People with dependent and obsessive-compulsive personality disorders are treated primarily in the community. If there is a coexisting disorder or the person experiences periods of depression, hospitalization may be useful for a short period of time.

IMPULSE-CONTROL DISORDERS

A group of mental disorders has as an essential feature: irresistible impulsivity. These disorders are not part of other disorders but often coexist with them. The following impulse-control disorders have been identified:

- Intermittent explosive disorder
- Kleptomania
- Pyromania
- Pathologic gambling
- Trichotillomania

These disorders are characterized by an inability to resist an impulse or temptation to complete an activity that is considered harmful to self or others, an increase in tension before the individual commits the act, and excitement or gratification at the time the act is committed. The release of tension is perceived as pleasurable, but remorse and regret usually follow the act (Gallop et al., 1992) (Table 22-7).

Intermittent Explosive Disorder

Episodes of aggressiveness that result in assault or destruction of property characterize people with intermittent explosive disorder. The severity of aggressiveness is out of proportion to the provocation. The episodes can have serious psychosocial consequences, including job loss, interpersonal relationship problems, school expulsion, divorce, automobile accidents, or jail. This diagnosis is given only after all other disorders with aggressive components (delirium, dementia, head injury, BPD, APD, substance abuse) have been ruled out. Little is known about this rare disorder. It is more common in men than in women (APA, 2000).

The treatment of this disorder is multifaceted. Psychopharmacologic agents are sometimes used as an adjunct to psychotherapeutic, behavioral, and social interventions. GABA-ergic mood stabilizers have been used. Anxiolytics are used for obsessive patients who develop tension states and explosive outbursts. Medication alone is not sufficient. The nursing management of the aggressive patient is presented in Chapter 36.

Kleptomania

In **kleptomania,** individuals cannot resist the urge to steal, and they independently steal items that they could easily afford. These items are not particularly useful or wanted. The underlying issue is the act of stealing. The term kleptomania was first used in 1838 to describe the behavior of several kings who stole worthless objects (Goldman, 1992). These individuals experience an increase in tension and then pleasure and relief at the time of the theft. It is a rare condition that occurs in fewer than 5% of shoplifters (APA, 2000). There is little information about this disorder, but it is believed to last for years, despite numerous convictions for shoplifting. It appears to be more common in women. About 81% of reported cases of kleptomania involve women (Goldman, 1991) (see Table 22-7).

Some shoplifting appears to have symptoms of anxiety and stress, but it has also served as symptom relief. In a few instances, brain damage has been associated with kleptomania. Depression is the most common symptom identified in a compulsive shoplifter. Kleptomania is difficult to detect and treat. There are few accounts of treatment. It appears that behavior therapy is frequently used. Antidepressant medication that helps relieve the depression has been successful in some cases. More investigation is needed (Schatzberg, 2000).

Pyromania

Irresistible impulses to start fires characterizes **pyromania.** These individuals are aroused before setting a fire and are fascinated with fires. They are attracted to fires, often becoming regular "fire watchers" or even firefighters. These arsonists, people who intentionally set fires or make an effort at fire setting, are not motivated

TABLE 22.7 Summary of Diagnostic Characteristics for Impulse-Control Disorders

Diagnostic Criteria and Target Symptoms

Kleptomania 312.32	• Recurrent failure to resist impulse to steal object that is not needed • Increased tension before theft • Pleasure, gratification, or relief at time of theft • Theft not related to anger or vengeance; not in response to delusion or hallucination • Not better accounted for by another psychiatric disorder

Pyromania 312.23	• Multiple episodes of deliberate and purposeful fire setting
	• Tension or affective arousal before act
	• Fascination with, interest in, curiosity about, or attraction to fires
	    Regular fire watchers
	    False alarm setters
	    Pleasure with institution, equipment, and personnel associated with fires
	• Pleasure, gratification or tension relief with fire starting, watching its effects or participating in aftermath
	• Not done for monetary gain; expression of ideology, anger, or vengeance; concealing criminal activity; improving living conditions; or as a response to hallucination or delusion
	• Not better accounted for by another psychiatric disorder

Pathologic gambling 312.31	• Persistent and recurrent maladaptive gambling behavior
	• Disruption of personal, family, or vocational pursuits
	    Preoccupation with gambling
	    Increased amounts of money needed to achieve excitement
	    Unsuccessful efforts to stop, cut back, or control
	    Restlessness and irritability with attempts to control or cut back
	    Means of escape from problems or mood
	    Chasing of losses; attempts to get even
	    Lying to family and others to conceal involvement
	    Commission of illegal acts to finance behavior
	    Significant relationships, job, or opportunities jeopardized or lost
	    Reliance on others for relief of poor financial situation
	• Not better accounted for by manic episode

Trichotillomania 312.39	• Recurrent pulling of one's hair with subsequent hair loss
	    Brief episodes throughout day or sustained periods of hours
	    Increased during stress and relaxation periods
	• Increased tension immediately before act and with attempts to resist urge
	• Gratification, pleasure, or relief with act
	• Not better accounted for by another psychiatric disorder; not the effect of a general medical condition

Intermittent Explosive Episodes 312.34	• Significant distress and impairment of functioning • Discrete episodes of failing to resist aggressive impulses, resulting in serious assaultive acts or property destruction • Degree of aggressiveness grossly out of proportion to provocation or stressor • Not better accounted for by another psychiatric disorder; not a direct physiologic effect of a substance or general medical condition

by aggression, anger, suicidal ideation, or political ideology. They may make advanced preparation for the fire. Little is known about this disorder. Most of the fire setting is not by people with this disorder. This disorder occurs infrequently, mostly in men (APA, 2000) (see Table 22-7).

Low serotonin and norepinephrine levels are associated with arson (Virkkunen et al., 1989). Little is known

about the treatment, and as with the other impulse-control disorders, no one approach is uniformly effective. A treatment plan should reflect the special needs of the individual (Soltys, 1992). Education, parenting training, behavior contracting with token reinforcement, problem-solving skills training, and relaxation exercises may all be used in the management of the patient's responses.

Pathologic Gambling

Social gambling becomes pathologic when it becomes recurrent and disrupts personal, family, or vocational pursuits. These individuals are preoccupied with gambling and experience an aroused, euphoric state during the actual betting. They are drawn to the games and begin making bigger and bigger bets. Characteristically, they relentlessly chase their losses in an attempt to win them back. They are unable to control their gaming and may lie to family, friends, and employers to hide their gambling. These individuals are highly competitive, energetic, restless, and easily bored. The prevalence is estimated at 1% to 3% of the population (APA, 2000); another study found a 3.9% lifetime prevalence (Shaffer et al., 1999). Of those individuals in treatment for pathologic gambling, 20% have reported attempting suicide (see Table 22-7).

This disorder is conceptualized as similar to alcohol and other substances of dependence. Pathologic gambling is associated with alcohol and drug dependence (Slutskey, 2000; Hall et al., 2000). When substances are used in conjunction with gambling, they cause a deterioration in play and accelerate the progression of the gambling disorder. Other comorbid disorders include depression, ADHD, Tourette's syndrome, and personality disorders, especially obsessive-compulsive, avoidant, schizoid, paranoid, and antisocial (Black & Moyer, 1998; Crockford & el-Guebaly, 1998). The disorder has four phases: winning, losing, desperation, and hopelessness. Pathologic gambling can be treated by psychotherapists experienced in disorder; for many, Gamblers Anonymous is sufficient (Petry & Armentano, 1999). People with this disorder feel omnipotent in their ability to win back what was lost. This omnipotence serves as self-deception that leads to denial. In managing these patients, their omnipotent beliefs are confronted. These individuals quickly irritate staff by their self-assurance and overbearing attitude. Staff education about the disorder is important. Family involvement is also crucial. Families have often been dealing with the patient in a dysfunctional manner. Relapse prevention involves learning about specific cues that trigger the gambling behavior (Selzer, 1992).

With the rise in pathologic gambling and its social consequences, there have been greater efforts to identify supportive pharmacotherapy. Because the underlying mechanisms are anxiety and impulsivity, the first line of drugs are SSRIs. These have shown moderate effectiveness in drug studies (Hollander et al., 1998, 2000), especially when combined with cognitive-behavioral approaches (Oakley-Browne et al., 2000).

Trichotillomania

Trichotillomania is chronic, self-destructive hair pulling that results in noticeable hair loss, usually in the crown, occipital, or parietal areas, although sometimes of the eyebrows and eyelashes. The patient has an increase in tension immediately before pulling out the hair or when attempting to resist the behavior. After the hair is pulled, the person feels a sense of relief. Some would classify this disorder as one of self-mutilation. It becomes a problem when there is a significant distress or an impairment in other areas of function. A hair-pulling session can last several hours, and the individual may ritualistically eat the hairs or discard them. Hair ingestion may result in the development of a hair ball, which can lead to anorexia, stomach pain, anemia, obstruction, and peritonitis. Other medical complications include infection at the hair-pulling site. Hair pulling is done alone, and usually patients deny it. Instead of pain, these persons experience pleasure and tension release (APA, 2000; Warmbrodt et al., 1996) (see Table 22-7).

The onset of trichotillomania occurs among children before the age of 5 years and in adolescence. For the young child, distraction or redirection may successfully eliminate the behavior. The behavior in adolescents may begin a chronic course that may last well into adulthood. This disorder is poorly understood. Its prevalence is estimated at 2% to 4% of the population (APA, 2000). The cause is unknown (APA, 2000). SSRIs, such as clomipramine and fluoxetine, have shown some success in diminishing the hair-pulling behavior, as have dopamine antagonists, such as haloperidol (Van Ameringen et al., 1999), and opioid antagonists (Kim, 1998).

The assessment includes any current problems, developmental history (especially school conflicts, learning difficulties), family history, social history, identification of support systems, previous psychiatric treatment, and health history. Hair-pulling history and pattern is also solicited to determine the duration and severity of the disorders. The typical nursing diagnoses include Risk for Self-Mutilation, Low Self-Esteem, Hopelessness, Impaired Skin Integrity, and Ineffective Denial. Within the therapeutic relationship, a cognitive behavioral approach can be used to help the patient identify when hair-pulling occurs, what are the precipitating events, and what are the details of the episode. Teaching about the disorder will help patients understand that they are not alone and that others have also suffered with this problem. The goal of treatment is to help the patient learn to substitute positive behaviors for the hair-pulling behavior through self-monitoring of events that precipitate the episodes.

Continuum of Care

Impulse-control disorders require long-term treatment, usually in an outpatient setting. Hospitalization is rare, except when there are comorbid psychiatric or medical disorders.

Summary of Key Points

➤ Personality is a complex pattern of characteristics, largely outside of the person's awareness, that comprise the individual's distinctive pattern of perceiving, feeling, thinking, coping, and behaving. The personality emerges from a complicated interaction of biologic dispositions, psychological experiences, and environmental situations.

➤ Personality disorder is an enduring pattern of inner experience and behavior that deviates markedly from the expectations of the individual's culture, is pervasive and inflexible, has an onset in adolescence or early adulthood, is stable over time, and leads to distress or impairment.

➤ Severity of personality disorder can be determined by the characteristics of tenuous stability, adaptive inflexibility, and vicious circles of rigid and inflexible behavior that result in serious interpersonal problems and social dysfunction.

➤ In the *DSM-IV*, personality disorders are on Axis II and are organized around three clusters or dimensions: cluster A, odd-eccentric disorders; cluster B, dramatic-emotional disorders; and cluster C, anxious-fearful disorders. Any of the personality disorders can coexist with Axis I disorders.

➤ People with cluster A personality disorders whose odd, eccentric behaviors often alienate them from others can benefit from interventions such as social skills training, environmental management, and cognitive skill building. Changing patterns of thinking and behaving are difficult and take time; hence, patient outcomes must be evaluated in terms of small changes in thinking and behavior.

➤ In cluster A, paranoid personality disorder is characterized by a suspicious pattern, schizoid personality disorder by an asocial pattern, and schizotypal personality disorder by an eccentric pattern.

➤ People with borderline personality disorder (Cluster B) have difficulties regulating emotion and have extreme fears of abandonment, leading to dysfunctional relationships; they often engage in self-injury.

➤ Antisocial personality disorder (Cluster B), often synonymous with psychopathy, includes people who have no regard for and refuse to conform to social rules.

➤ Patients with Cluster B personality disorders often have difficulties with emotional regulation or being able to recognize and control the expression of their feelings, such as anger, disappointment, and frustration. The nurse can help these patients identify feelings and gain control over their feelings and actions by teaching communication skills and techniques, thought-stopping techniques, distraction, or problem-solving techniques.

➤ Cluster C personality disorders are characterized by anxieties and fears and include avoidant, dependent, and obsessive-compulsive disorders. The obsessive-compulsive personality disorder differs from the obsessive-compulsive anxiety disorder because the individual demonstrates an overall rigidity, perfectionism, and need for control.

➤ For many patients with personality disorders, maintaining a therapeutic nurse–patient relationship can be one of the most helpful interventions. Through this therapeutic relationship, the patient experiences a model of healthy interaction, establishing trust, consistency, caring, boundaries, and limitations and helping to build the patient's self-esteem and respect for self and others. In some personality disorders, nurses will find it more difficult to engage the patient in a true therapeutic relationship because of the patient's avoidance of interpersonal and emotional attachment (ie, antisocial personality disorder or paranoid personality disorder).

➤ Patients with personality disorders are rarely treated in an inpatient facility except during periods of destructive behavior or self-injury. Treatment is delivered in the community and over time. Continuity of care is important in helping the individual change lifelong personality patterns.

➤ Although not classified as personality disorders, the impulse-control disorders share one of the primary characteristics of impulsivity, which leads to inappropriate social behaviors that are considered harmful to self or others and that give the patient excitement or gratification at the time the act is committed.

Critical Thinking Challenges

1. Compare and contrast the three common features of personality disorders: tenuous stability, adaptive inflexibility, and vicious circles of behavior.

2. Define the concepts personality and personality disorder. When does a normal personality become a personality disorder?

3. Karen is a 36-year-old inpatient admitted for depression who also has a diagnosis of borderline personality disorder. Following an earlier telephone argument with her husband, she approaches the nurse's station with her wrist dripping with blood from cutting. What nursing diagnosis best fits this behavior? What interventions should the nurse use with the patient once the self-injury is treated?

4. A 22-year-old man with borderline personality disorder is being discharged from the psychiatric–mental health unit after a severe suicide attempt. As his primary psychiatric nurse, you have been able to establish a therapeutic relationship with

him but are now terminating the relationship. He asks you to meet with him "for just a few sessions" after his discharge because his therapist will be on vacation. What are the issues underlying this request? What should you do? Explain and justify.

5. Compare the psychoanalytic explanation of the development of borderline personality disorder with Linehan's biosocial theory.

6. Compare the characteristics, epidemiology, and etiologic theories of antisocial and borderline personality disorders.

7. Discuss the differences between histrionic and borderline personality disorders.

8. Compare and contrast antisocial and narcissistic personality disorders.

9. Define and summarize the three personality disorders of cluster A. Compare the following among the three disorders:
   a. Defining characteristics
   b. Epidemiology
   c. Biologic, psychological, and social theories
   d. Key nursing assessment data
   e. Nursing diagnoses and outcomes
   f. Specific issues related to a therapeutic relationship
   g. Interventions

10. Define and summarize the three personality disorders of cluster C. Compare the following among the three disorders:
    a. Defining characteristics
    b. Epidemiology
    c. Biologic, psychological, and social theories
    d. Key nursing assessment data
    e. Nursing diagnoses and outcomes
    f. Specific issues related to a therapeutic relationship
    g. Interventions

11. Define and summarize the impulse-control disorders. Compare the following among the three disorders:
    a. Defining characteristics
    b. Epidemiology
    c. Biologic, psychological, and social theories
    d. Key nursing assessment data
    e. Nursing diagnoses and outcomes
    f. Interventions

 WEB LINKS

www.mhsanctuary.com/borderline   A website for consumers, the Borderline Personality Sanctuary offers a chat room and books.

www.palace.net~llama/psych/bpd.html   This site provides an overview of theories on borderline personality disorder.

www.bpdcentral.com   This website of Borderline Personality Disorder Central provides consumer and professional information and resources.

www.borderlineresearch.org   The Borderline Research Organization is a research foundation that supports research on borderline personality disorder.

www.mentalhealth.com   Internet Mental Health is a website for mental health disorders.

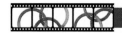 **MOVIES**

Fatal Attraction: 1987. The award winning film portrays the relationship between a married attorney, Dan Gallagher, (played by Michael Douglas) and Alex Forest, a single woman (played by Glenn Close). Their one-night affair turns into a nightmare for the attorney and his family as Alex becomes increasingly possessive and aggressive, demonstrating behaviors characteristic of borderline personality disorder: anger, impulsivity, emotional lability, fear of rejection and abandonment, vacillation between adulation and disgust, and self-mutilation.

Viewing Points: Identify the behaviors of Alex that are characteristics of borderline personality disorder. Identify the feelings that are generated by the movies. With which characters do you identify? For which characters do you feel sympathy? If Alex had lived and been admitted to your hospital, what would be your first priority?

References

Ainsworth, M. (1989). Attachments beyond infancy. *American Psychologist, 44*(4), 709–716.

American Psychiatric Association. (2000). *Diagnostic and statistical manual of mental disorders* (4th ed., Text revision). Washington, DC: Author.

Andrews, J. A., Foster, S. L., Capaldi, D., & Hop, H. (2000). Adolescent and family predictors of physical aggression, communication, and satisfaction in young adult couples: A prospective analysis. *Journal of Consulting Clinical Psychology, 68*(2), 195–208.

Bakan, P., & Peterson, K. (1994). Pregnancy and birth complications: A risk factor for schizotypy. *Journal of Personality Disorders, 8*(4), 299–306.

Barry, C. T., Frick, P. J., DeShazo, T. M., McCoy, M. G., Ellis, M., & Loney, B. R. (2000). The importance of callous-unemotional traits for extending the concept of psychopathy to children. *Journal of Abnormal Psychology, 109*(2), 335–340.

Bateman, A., & Fonagy, P. (1999). Effectiveness of partial hospitalization in the treatment of borderline personality disorder: A randomized controlled trial. *American Journal of Psychiatry, 156*(10), 1563–1569.

Beckwith, L., Howard, J., Espinosa, M., & Tyler, R. (1999). Psychopathology, mother-child interaction, and infant development: Substance-abusing mothers and their offspring. *Development & Psychopathology, 11*(4), 715–725.

Bernstein, G. A., Borchardt, C. M., & Perwien, A. R. (1996). Anxiety disorders in children and adolescents: A review of the past 10 years. *Journal of the American Academy of Child & Adolescent Psychiatry, 35*(9), 1110–1119.

Black, D., Baumgard, C., & Bell, S. (1995). The long-term outcome of antisocial personality disorder compared with depression, schizophrenia, and surgical conditions. *Bulletin of the American Academy of Psychiatry and Law, 23*(1), 43–52.

Black, D. W., Baumgard, C. H., & Bell, S. E. (1995). A 16- to 45-year follow-up of 71 men with antisocial personality disorder. *Comprehensive Psychiatry, 36*(2), 130–140.

Black, D. W., & Moyer, T. (1998). Clinical features and psychiatric comorbidity of subjects with pathological gambling behavior. *Psychiatric Services, 49*(11), 1434–1439.

Bodner, E., & Mikulincer, M. (1998). Learned helplessness and the occurrence of depressive-like and paranoid-like responses: The role of attentional focus. *Journal of Personality & Social Psychology, 74*(4), 1010–1023.

Bohus, M., Haaf, B., Stiglmary, C., Pohl, U., Bohme, R., & Linehan, M. (2000). Evaluation of inpatient dialectical-behavioral therapy for borderline personality disorder—a prospective study. *Behavior Research Therapy, 38*(9), 875–887.

Bohus, M. F., Landwehrmeyer, G. B., Stiglmayr, C. E., Limberger, M. F., Bohme, R., & Schmahl, C. G. (1999). Naltrexone in the treatment of dissociative symptoms in patients with borderline personality disorder: An open-label trail. *Journal of Clinical Psychiatry, 60*(9), 598–603.

Boone, M. L., McNeil, D. W., Masia, C. L., Turk, C. L., Carter, L. E., Ries, B. J., & Lewin, M. R. (1999). Multimodal comparisons of social phobia subtypes and avoidant personality disorder. *Journal of Anxiety Disorders, 13*(3), 271–292.

Bornstein, R. F. (1998). Implicit and self-attributed dependency needs in dependent and histrionic personality disorders. *Journal of Personality Assessment, 71*(1), 1–14.

Bowlby, J. (1980). *Loss: Sadness and depression.* New York: Basic Books.

Bucholz, K. K., Heath, A. C., & Madden, P. A. (2000). Transitions in drinking adolescent females: Evidence from the Missouri adolescent female twin study. *Alcohol Clinical Experimental Research, 24*(6), 914–923.

Bushman, B. J., & Baumeister, R. F. (1998). Threatened egotism, narcissism, self-esteem, and direct and displaced aggression: Does self-love or self-hate lead to violence? *Journal of Personality Social Psychology, 75*(1), 219–229.

Cadenhead, K. S., Perry, W., Shafer, K., & Braff, D. L. (1999). Cognitive functions in schizotypal personality disorder. *Schizophrenia Research, 37*(2), 123–132.

Chengappa, K. N., Ebeling, T., Kang, J. S., Levine, J., & Parepally, H. (1999). Clozapine reduces severe self-mutilation and aggression in psychotic patients with borderline personality disorder. *Journal of Clinical Psychiatry, 60*(7), 477–484.

Cloninger, C. R., Bayon, C., & Svrakic, D. M., (1998). Measurement of temperament and character in mood disorders: A model of fundamental states as personality types. *Journal of Affective Disorders, 51*(1), 21–32.

Coccaro, E. F. (1998). Clinical outcome of psychopharmacologic treatment of borderline and schizotypal personality disordered subjects. *Journal Clinical Psychiatry, 59*(Suppl 1), 30–35.

Coccaro, E. F., & Kavoussi, R. J. (1997). Fluoxetine and impulsive aggressive behavior in personality-disordered subjects. *Archives of General Psychiatry, 54*(12), 1081–1088.

Coccaro, E. F., Kavoussi, R. J., Hauger, R. L., Cooper, T. B., & Ferris, C. F. (1998). Cerebrospinal fluid vasopressin levels: Correlates with aggression and serotonin function in personality-disordered subjects. *Archives of General Psychiatry, 55*(8), 708–714.

Comtois, K. A., Cowley, D. S., Dunner, D. L., & Roy-Byrne, P. P. (1999). Relationship between borderline personality disorder and Axis I diagnosis in severity of depression and anxiety. *Journal of Clinical Psychiatry, 60*(11), 752–758.

Constantino, J. (1996). Intergenerational aspects of the development of aggression: A preliminary report. *Journal of Developmental and Behavioral Pediatrics, 17*(3), 176–182.

Cooke, D. (1996). Psychopathic personality in different culture: What do we know? What do we need to find out? *Journal of Personality Disorders, 10*(1), 23–40.

Cooke, D. J., & Michie, C. (1999). Psychopathy across cultures: North America and Scotland compared. *Journal of abnormal Psychology,* 58–68.

Crockford, D. N., & el-Guebaly, M. (1998). Psychiatric comorbidity in pathological gambling: A critical review. *Canadian Journal of Psychiatry, 43*(1), 43–50.

Dolan, M. (1994). Psychopathy: A neurobiological perspective. *British Journal of Psychiatry, 165*(2), 151–159.

Driessen, M., Herrmann, J., Stahl, K., Zwaan, M., Meier, S., Hill, A., Osterheider, M., & Petersen, D. (2000). Magnetic resonance imaging volumes of the hippocampus and the amygdala in women with borderline personality disorder and early traumatization, *Archives of General Psychiatry, 57*(12), 1115–1122.

Eley, T. C., Lichtenstein, P., & Stevenson, J. (1999). Sex differences in the etiology of aggressive and nonaggressive antisocial behavior: Results from two twin studies. *Child Development, 70*(1), 155–168.

Erikson, E. (1968). *Identity: Youth and crisis.* New York: Norton.

Faraone, S. V., Biederman, J., Mennin, D., & Russell, R. (1998). Bipolar and antisocial disorders among relatives of ADHD children: Parsing familial subtypes of illness. *American Journal of Medical Genetics, 81*(1), 108–116.

Faravelli, C., Zucchi, T., Viviani, B., salmoria, R., Perone, A., Paionni, A., Scarpato, A., Vigliaturo, D., Rosi, S., D'adamo, D., Bartolozzi, D., Cecchi, C., & Abrardi, L. (2000). Epidemiology of social phobia: A clinical approach. *European Psychiatry, 15*(1), 17–24.

Farmer, C. M., O'Donnell, B. F., Niznikiewicz, M. A., Voglmaier, M. M., McCarley, r. W., & Shenton, M. E.

(2000). Visual perception and working memory in schizotypal personality disorder. *American Journal of Psychiatry, 157*(5), 781–788.

Fava, M. (1998). Depression with anger attacks. *Journal of Clinical Psychiatry, 59*(Suppl 18), 18–22.

Favazza, A. (1996). *Bodies under siege: Self-mutilation and body modification in culture and psychiatry.* Baltimore: Johns Hopkins University Press.

Gallop, R., McCay, E., & Esplen, J. (1992). The conceptualization of impulsivity for psychiatric nursing practice. *Archives of Psychiatric Nursing, 6*(6), 366–373.

Galvin, M., Shekhar, A., Simon, J., et al. (1991). Low dopamine-beta-hydroxylase: A biological sequela of abuse and neglect? *Psychiatry Research, 39*(1), 1–11.

Gatz, Johnstone, Ratcliffe, 1999

Giancola, P. R. (2000). temperament and antisocial behavior in preadolescent boys with or without a family history of a substance use disorder. *Psychological Addictive Behaviors, 14*(1), 56–68.

Goldman, M. (1991). Kleptomania: Making sense of the nonsensical. *American Journal of Psychiatry, 148*(8), 986–999.

Goldman, M. (1992). Kleptomania: An overview. *Psychiatric Annals, 22*(2) 68–71.

Goldstein, R. B., Powers, S. I., McCusker, J., Mundt, K. A., Lewis, B. F., & Bigelow, C. (1996). gender differences in manifestations of antisocial personality disorder among residential drug abuse treatment clients. *Drug & Alcohol Dependency, 41*(1), 35–45.

Golynkina, K., & Ryle, A. (1999). The identification and characteristics of the partially dissociated states of patients with borderline personality disorder. *British Journal of Medicine & Psychology, 72*(Pt 4), 429–445.

Gottesman, I., & Goldsmith, H. (1994). Developmental psychopathology of antisocial behavior: Inserting genes into its ontogenesis and epigenesis. In C. Nelson (Ed.), *Threats to optimal development: Integrating biological, social, and psychological risk factors* (Vol. 27, pp. 69–104). Hillsdale, NJ: Erlbaum.

Gotz, M. J., Johnstone, E. D., & Ratcliffe, S. G. (1999). Criminality and antisocial behaviour in unselected men with sex chromosome abnormalities. *Psychology & Medicine, 29*(4), 953–962.

Grann, M., Lanstrom, N., Tengstrom, A., Kullgren, G. (1999). Psychopathy (PCL-R) predicts violent recidivism among criminal offenders with personality disorders in Sweden. *Law & Human Behavior, 23*(2), 205–217.

Greene, H., & Ugarriza, D. (1995). The "stably unstable" borderline personality disorder: History, theory, and nursing intervention. *Journal of Psychosocial Nursing, 33*(12), 26–30.

Grilo, C., Becker, D., Fehon, D., et al. (1996). Gender differences in personality disorders in psychiatrically hospitalized adolescents. *American Journal of Psychiatry, 153*(8), 1089–1091.

Gunderson, J. G. (1996). The borderline patient's intolerance of aloneness: Insecure attachments and therapist availability. *American Journal of Psychiatry, 153*(6), 752–758.

Hall, G. W., Carriero, N. J., Takushi, R. Y., Montoya, I. D., Preston, K. L., & Gorelick, D. A. (2000). Pathological gambling among cocaine-dependent outpatients. *American Journal of Psychiatry, 157*(7), 1127–1133.

Hall, L., Sachs, B., Rayens, M., & Lutenbacher, J. (1993). Childhood physical and sexual abuse: Their relationship with depressive symptoms in adulthood. *Image—The Journal of Nursing Scholarship, 25*(4), 317–323.

Hamburger, M., Lilienfeld, S., & Hogben, M. (1996). Psychopathy, gender, and gender roles: Implications for antisocial and histrionic personality disorders. *Journal of Personality Disorders, 19*(1), 41–55.

Hansen, R. K., Cadsky, O., Harris, A., & Lalond, C. (1997). Correlates of battering among 997 men: Family history, adjustment, and attitudinal difference. *Violence Vict, 12*(3), 191–208.

Hare, R. D. (1999). Psychopathy as a risk factor for violence. *Psychiatric Quarterly, 70*(3), 181–197.

Herpertz, S. C., Kunnert, H. J., Schwenger, U. B., & Sass, H. (1999). Affective responsiveness in borderline personality disorder: A psychophysiological approach. *American Journal of Psychiatry, 156*(10), 1550–1556.

Hollander, E., DeCaria, C. M., Finkell, J. N., Begaz, R., Wong, C. M., & Carwight, C. (2000). A randomized double-blind fluvoxamine/placebo crossover trial in pathologic gambling. *Biological Psychiatry, 47*(9), 813–817.

Horsfall, J. (1999). Towards understanding some complex borderline behaviours. *Journal of Psychiatric Mental Health Nursing, 6*(6), 425–432.

Isometsa, E. T., Henriksson, M. M., Heikkinen, M. E., Aro, H. M., Marttunen, M. J., Kuoppasalmi, K. I., & Lonnqvist, J. K. (1996). Suicide among subjects with personality disorders. *American Journal of Psychiatry, 153*(5), 667–673.

Jansen, R., Fitzgerald, H., Ham, H., & Zucker, R. (1995). Pathways into risk: Temperament and behavior problems in three-to five-year-old sons of alcoholics. *Alcoholism: Clinical and Experimental Research, 19*(2), 501–509.

Johnson, J. G., Cohen, P., Brown, J., Smailes, E. M., & Bernstein, D. P. (1999). Childhood maltreatment increases risk for personality disorders during early adulthood. *Archives of General Psychiatry, 56*(7), 607–608.

Johnston, M. A. (1999). Influences of adult attachment in exploration. *Psychological Reports, 84*(1), 31–34.

Joubert, C. E. (1998). Narcissism, need for power, and social interest. *Psychological Report, 82*(2), 701–702.

Kernberg, O. (1994). Aggression, trauma, and hatred in the treatment of borderline patients. *Psychiatric Clinics of North America, 17*(4), 701–714.

Kim, J. E., Hetherington, E. M., & Reiss, D. (1999). Associations among family relationships, antisocial peers, and adolescents' externalizing behaviors: Gender and family type differences. *Child Development, 70*(5), 1209–1230.

Kim, S. W. (1998). Opioid antagonists in the treatment of impulse-control disorders. *Journal of Clinical Psychiatry, 59*(4), 159–164.

Lahey, B. B., Gordon, R. A., Loeber, R., Stouthamer-Loeber, M., & Farrington, D. P. (1999). Boys who join gangs: A prospective study of predictors of first gang entry. *Journal of Abnormal Child Psychology, 27*(4), 261–276.

Laporte, L., & Guttman, H. (1996). Traumatic childhood experiences as risk factors for borderline and other personality disorders. *Journal of Personality Disorders, 10*(3), 247–259.

Leichsenring, F. (1999). Splitting: An empirical study. *Bulletin Menninger Clinic, 63*(4), 520–537.

Lejoyeux, M., Boulenguiez, S., Fichelle, A., McLoughlin, M., Claudon, M., & Ades, J. (2000). Alcohol dependence among patients admitted to psychiatric emergency services. *General Hospital Psychiatry, 22*(3), 206–212.

Linehan, M. (1993). *Cognitive-behavioral treatment of borderline personality disorder.* New York: The Guilford Press.

Links, P. S., Heslegrave, R., & van Reekum R. (1998). Prospective follow-up study of borderline personality disorder: Prognosis, prediction of outcome, and Axis II comorbidity. *Canadian Journal of Psychiatry, 43*(3), 265–270.

Lyons, M. (1995). Epidemiology of personality disorders. In M. Tsuang, M. Tohen, & G. Zahner (Eds.), *Textbook in psychiatric epidemiology.* New York: Wiley-Liss.

Mahler, M., Pine, F., & Bergman, A. (1975). *The psychological birth of human infant: Symbiosis and individuation.* New York: Basic Books.

Marcus, R. F. (1999). A gender-linked exploratory factor analysis of antisocial behavior in young adolescents. *Adolescence, 34*(133), 33–46.

Matta, I., Sham, P. C., Gilvarry, C. M., Jones, P. B., Lewis, S. W., & Murray, R. M. (2000). Childhood schizotypy and positive symptoms in schizophrenic patients predict schizotypy in relatives. *Schizophrenia Research, 44*(2), 129–136.

Mattick, R., & Newman, C. (1991). Social phobia and avoidant personality disorder. *International Review of Psychiatry, 3*(2), 163–173.

McCloskey, J., & Bulechek, G. (1996). *Nursing interventions classification (NIC).* St. Louis: Mosby–Year Book.

McDougle, C. J., Kresch, L. E., & Posey, D. J. (2000). Repetitive thoughts and behavior in pervasive developmental disorders: Treatment with serotonin reuptake inhibitors. *Journal of Autism & Development Disorders, 30*(5), 427–435.

Messina, N. P., Wish, E. D., & Nemes, S. (1999). Therapeutic community treatment for substance abusers with antisocial personality disorder. *Journal of Substance Abuse Treatment, 17*(1–2), 121–128.

Miller, S. (1994). Borderline personality disorder from a patient's perspective. *Hospital and Community Psychiatry, 45*(12), 1215–1219.

Millon, T., & Davis, R. (1999). *Personality disorders in modern life.* New York: John Wiley & Sons.

Moran, P. (1999). The epidemiology of antisocial personality disorder. *Social Psychiatry & Psychiatric Epidemiology, 34*(5), 231–242.

Moutier, C. Y., & Stein, M. B. (1999). The history, epidemiology, and differential diagnosis of social anxiety disorder. *Journal of Clinical Psychiatry, 60*(Suppl 9), 4–8.

Murphy, J. (1976). Psychiatric labeling in cross-cultural perspective: Similar kinds of disturbed behavior appear to be labeled abnormal in diverse cultures. *Science, 191*(4231), 1019–1028.

Murray, J. (1992). Kleptomania: A review of the research. *Journal of Psychology, 126*(2), 131–137.

Myers, M. G., Stewart, D. G., & Brown, S. A. (1998). Progression from conduct disorder to antisocial personality disorder following treatment for adolescent substance abuse. *American Journal of Psychiatry, 155*(4), 479–485.

Nehls, N. (1998). Borderline personality disorder: Gender stereotypes, stigma and limited system of care. *Issues in Mental Health Nursing, 19*(2), 97–112.

Nehls, N. (1999). Borderline personality disorder: The voice of patients. *Research in Nursing & Health, 22*(4), 285–293.

Nestadt, G., Romanoski, A., Chahal, R., et al. (1990). An epidemiological study of histrionic personality disorder. *Psychological Medicine, 20*(2), 413–422.

Nolan, K. A., Volavka, J., Mohr, P., & Czobor, P. (1999). Psychopathy and violent behavior among patients with schizophrenia or schizoaffective disorder. *Psychiatric Services, 50*(6), 787–792.

Oakley-Browne, Adams, P., & Mobberly, P. M. (2000). Interventions for pathological gambling. *Cochrane Database System Review*, (2), CD001521.

Oldham, J., Skodol, A., Kellman, H., et al. (1995). Comorbidity of Axis I and Axis II disorders. *American Journal of Psychiatry, 152*(4), 571–578.

Oquendo, J. A., & Mann, J. J. (2000). The biology of impulsivity and suicidality. *Psychiatric Clinics of North America, 23*(1), 11–25.

Oquendo, M. A., & Mann, J. J. (2000). The biology of impulsivity and suicidality. *Psychiatric Clinics of North America, 32*(4), 353–360.

Pagani, L., Boulerice, B., Vitaro, F., & Tremblay, R. E. (1999). Effects of poverty on academic failure and delinquency in boys: A change and process model approach. *Journal of Child Psychology & Psychiatry, 40*(8), 119–120.

Paulhus, D. L. (1998). Interpersonal and intrapsychic adaptiveness of trait self-enhancement: A mixed blessing? *Journal of Personality Social Psychology, 74*(5), 1197.

Perugi, G., Nassini, S., Socci, C., Lenzi, M., Toni, C., Simonini, E., & Akiskal, H. S. (1999). Avoidant personality in social phobia and panic-agoraphobia disorder: A comparison. *Journal of Affective Disorders, 54*(3), 277–282.

Petry, N. M., & Armentano, C. (1999). Prevalcene, assessment, and treatment of pathological gambling: A review. *Psychiatric Services, 50*(8), 1021–1027.

Pinto, O. C., & Akiskal, H. S. (1998). Lamotrigine as a promising approach to borderline personality: An open case series without concurrent DSM-IV major mood disorder. *Journal of Affective Disorder, 51*(3), 333–343.

Robins, L, Tipp, J., & Przybeck, T. (1991). Antisocial personality. In L. N. Robins & D. Reiger (Eds.), *Psychiatric disorders in America: The epidemiological catchment area study* (pp. 258–291). New York: Free Press.

Sack, A., Sperling, M., Fagen, G., & Foelsch, P. (1996). Attachment style, history, and behavioral contrasts for a borderline and normal sample. *Journal of Personality Disorders, 10*(1), 88–102.

Sansone, R. A., Wiederman, M. W., & Sansone, L. A. (1998). Borderline personality symptomatology, experience of multiple types of trauma, and health care utilization among women in a primary care setting. *Journal of Clinical Psychiatry, 59*(3), 108–111.

Schatzbert, A. F. (2000). New indications of antidepressants. *Journal of Clinical Psychiatry, 61*(Suppl 11), 9–17.

Schubiner, H., Tzelepis, A., Milberger, S., Lockhart, N., Kruger, M., Kelley, B. J., & Schoener, E. P. (2000). Prevalence of attention-deficit/hyperactivity disorder and conduct disorder among substance abusers. *Journal of Clinical Psychiatry, 61*(4), 244–251.

Selzer, J. (1992). Borderline omnipotence in pathological gambling. *Archives of Psychiatric Nursing, 6*(4), 215–218.

Shaffer, H. J., Hall, M. N., & Vander Bilt, J. (1999). Estimating the prevalence of disordered gambling behavior in the United States and Canada: A research synthesis. *American Journal of Public Health, 89*(9), 1369–1376.

Sigmund, D., Barnett, W., & Mundt, C. (1998). The hysterical personality disorder: A phenomenological approach. *Psychopathology, 31*(6), 318–330.

Silk, K. R. (2000). Borderline personality disorder. Overview of biologic factors. *Psychiatric Clinical North America, 23*(1), 61–75.

Silverthorn, P., & Frick, P. J. (1999). Developmental pathways to antisocial behavior: The delayed-onset pathway in girls. *Developmental Psychopathology, 11*(1), 101–126.

Smallbone, S. W., & Dadds, M. R. (2000). Attachment and coercive sexual behavior. *Sex Abuse 12*(1), 3–15.

Soloff, H., Lis, J. A., Kelly, T., Cornelius, J., & Ulrich, R. (1994). Risk factors for suicidal behavior in borderline personality disorder. *American Journal of Psychiatry, 151*(9), 1316–1323.

Soloff, P. H. (2000). Psychopharmacology of borderline personality disorder. *Psychiatric Clinics of North America, 23*(1), 169–192.

Soloff, P., Lis, J., Kelly, T., et al. (1994). Self-mutilation and suicidal behavior in borderline personality disorder. *Journal of Personality Disorders, 8*(4), 257–267.

Soltys, S. (1992). Pyromania and firesetting behaviors. *Psychiatric Annals, 22*(2), 79–83.

Stahl, S. (2000). *Essential psychopharmacology.* (2nd ed.). Cambridge: Cambridge University Press.

Stalenheim, E. G., von Knorring, L., & wide, L. (1998). Serum levels of thyroid hormones as biological markers in a Swedish forensic psychiatric population. *Biological Psychiatry, 43*(10), 755–761.

Stein, K. (1996). Affect instability in adults with a borderline personality disorder. *Archives of Psychiatric Nursing, 10*(1), 32–40.

Stern, A. (1938). A psychoanalytic investigation and therapy in the borderline group of neuroses. *Psychoanalytic Quarterly, 7,* 467–489.

Stravynski, A., Belisle, M., Marcouiller, M., et al. (1994). The treatment of avoidant personality disorder by social skills training in the clinic or in real-life setting. *Canadian Journal of Psychiatry, 39*(8), 377–383.

Tuohig, G., Saffle, J., Sullivan, J., et al. (1995). Self-inflicted patient burns: Suicide versus mutilation. *Journal of Burn Care and Rehabilitation, 16*(4), 429–436.

Van Ameringen, M., Mancini, C., Oakman, J. M., & Farvolden, P. (1999). The potential role of haloperidol in the treatment of trichotillomania. *Journal of Affective Disorders, 56*(2–3), 219–226.

van Reekum, R. (1993). Acquired and developmental brain dysfunction in borderline personality disorder. *Canadian Journal of Psychiatry, 38*(1), 54–58.

Virkkunen, M, Dejong, J., Bartko, J., et al. (1989). Relationship of psychobiological variables to recidivism in violent offenders and impulsive fire setters. *Archives of General Psychiatry, 46*(7), 600–603.

Voglmaier, M. M., Seidman, L. J., Niznikiewicz, M. A., Dickey, C. C., Shenton, M. E., & McCarley, R. W. (2000). Verbal and nonverbal neuropsychological test performance in subjects with schizotypal personality disorder. *American Journal of Psychiatry, 157*(5), 787–793.

Waldeck, T. L., & Miller, L. S. (2000). Social skills deficits in schizotypal personality disorder. *Psychiatry Research, 93*(3), 237–246.

Waldman, I. D., & Slutske, W. S. (2000). Antisocial behavior and alcoholism: A behavioral genetic perspective on comorbidity. *Clinical Psychological Review, 20*(2), 255–287.

Warmbrodt, L., Hardy, E., & Chrisman, S., (1996). Understanding trichotillomania. *Journal of Psychosocial Nursing, 34*(12), 11–15.

Widiger, T. (1991). *DSM-IV* reviews of the personality disorders: Introduction to special series. *Journal of Personality Disorders, 5*(2), 122–134.

Widiger, T., & Weissman, M. (1991). Epidemiology of borderline personality disorder. *Hospital & Community Psychiatry, 42*(10), 1015–1021.

Wilkinson-Ryan, T., & Westen, D. (2000). Identity disturbance in borderline personality disorder: An empirical investigation. *American Journal of Psychiatry, 157*(4), 528–541.

Yeomans, F., Hull, J., & Clarkin, J. (1994). Risk factors for self-damaging acts in a borderline population. *Journal of Personality Disorders, 8*(1), 10–16.

Young, J. E. (1994). *Cognitive therapy for personality disorders: A schema-focused approach* (revised edition). Sarasota, FL: Professional Resource Press.

Zanarini, M. C., Williams, A. A., Lewis, R. E., Reich, R. B., Vera, S. C., Marino, M. F., Levin, A., Yong, L., & Frankenburg, F. R. (1997). Reported pathological childhood experiences associated with the development of borderline personality disorder. *American Journal of Psychiatry, 154*(8), 1101–1106.

Zanarini, M. C., Ruser, T., Frankenburg, F. R., & Hennen, J. (2000). The dissociative experiences of borderline patients. *Comprehensive Psychiatry, 41*(3), 223–227.

Zlotnick, C. (1999). Antisocial personality disorder, affect dysregulation and childhood abuse among incarcerated women. *Journal of Personality Disorders, 13*(1), 90–95.

Zweig-Frank, F., Paris, J., & Guzder, J. (1994a). Dissociation in female patients with borderline and non-borderline personality disorders. *Journal of Personality Disorders, 8*(3), 203–209.

Zweig-Frank, F., Paris, J., & Guzder, J. (1994b). Psychological risk factors for dissociation and self-mutilation in female patients with borderline personality disorder. *Canadian Journal of Psychiatry, 39*(5), 259–264.

Zweig-Frank, F., Paris, J., & Guzder, J. (1994c). Psychological risk factors for dissociation and self-mutilation in female patients with borderline personality disorder. *Canadian Journal of Psychiatry, 39*(5), 259–264.

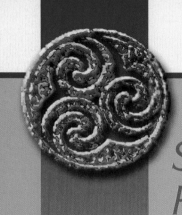

Somatoform and Related Disorders

Mary Ann Boyd

LEARNING OBJECTIVES

After studying this chapter, you will be able to:

➤ Explain the concept of somatization and its occurrence in people with mental health problems.

➤ Discuss the epidemiologic factors related to somatic problems.

➤ Compare the etiologic theories of somatization disorder from a biopsychosocial perspective.

➤ Contrast the major differences between somatoform and factitious disorders.

➤ Discuss human responses to somatization disorder.

➤ Apply the elements of nursing management to a patient with somatization disorder.

factitious disorders
malingering
pseudologia fantastica
pseudoneurologic
  symptoms

psychosomatic
somatization disorder
somatoform disorders

somatization

*The connection between the "mind" and "body" has been hypothesized and described for centuries. The term **psychosomatic** describes conditions in which a psychological state contributes to the development of a physical illnesses. For example, the connection between stress and heart disease is well documented and serves as the rationale for stress management interventions for heart attack victims. The term somatization is used when unexplained physical symptoms are present that are related to psychological distress. This chapter explores the concept of somatization and explains the care of patients whose psychiatric disorder has as its primary characteristic the manifestation of unexplained physical symptoms related to psychological distress.*

KEY CONCEPT Somatization. **Somatization** is the term used when unexplained physical symptoms are present that are related to psychological distress.

Although somatization is common in many psychiatric disorders, including depression, anxiety, and psychosis, it is the primary symptom of somatoform and factitious disorders. A **somatoform disorder** is one in which the patient suffers physical symptoms as a result of psychological stress. A **factitious disorder** is one in which the patient self-inflicts injury as a result of psychological stress to seek out medical treatment. The major difference between the two diagnostic categories is that in the somatoform disorders, the physical symptoms are not deliberately produced by the patient. The somatoform disorders are clustered into six different clinical syndromes:

1. Somatization disorder
2. Undifferentiated somatoform disorder
3. Conversion disorder
4. Pain disorder
5. Hypochondriasis
6. Body dysmorphic disorder

The factitious disorders include (1) factitious disorder and (2) factitious disorder not specified. This chapter reviews these disorders using selected examples of somatization disorder and factitious disorder. A person with somatization disorder can have symptoms of all the other somatoform disorders, including conversion, pain, hypochondriasis, and preoccupation with a physical defect. However, a person with just one of the other disorders does not meet the criteria for somatization disorder.

SOMATIZATION

Anyone who feels the pain of a sore throat or the ache of the flu has a somatic symptom (from *soma*, meaning body), but it is not considered to be somatization unless the physical symptoms are an expression of emotional stress. There may or may not be an identifiable physiologic cause for the medical problems, but chronic stress is obvious. In somatization, physical sensations are amplified, and the individual seeks medical care for the symptoms. People who somatize view their personal problems in physical terms rather than in psychosocial terms. For example, a woman quits her job complaining of chronic fatigue rather than recognizing that she is emotionally stressed from the constant harassment of a coworker. These individuals internalize their stress or cope with life problems and stressors by expressing anxiety, stress, and frustration through their own physical symptoms.

Cultural Differences in Somatization

Because norms, values, and expectations about illness are culturally based, physical sensations are experienced according to culturally defined expectations. In cultures in which the expression of physical discomfort is more acceptable than psychological distress, the disruption of routine body cycles, such as digestive or menstrual cycles, sleep, physical balance, and orientation, are commonly the focus of patient concern instead of problems in interpersonal relationships, economic crises, death of a spouse, adjustment to marriage, and inability to become pregnant, for example.

Gender and Somatization

Somatization has long been associated with women. In 1900 BC, the ancient Egyptians described a "woman aching in all her limbs with pain to the sockets of her eyes" (Smith, 1990). Both the Egyptians and the Greeks attributed unexplained female pains to hysteria, which in Greek means the "wandering uterus." They believed that the multiple symptoms were caused by the migration of the uterus throughout the body. Treatment involved attracting the uterus to proper alignment by placing sweet-smelling balms and herbs at the vagina and noxious potions at the nostrils. Gynecologist Thomas Syndenham dispelled the wandering womb myth in the 17th century and associated somatization with a psychological disturbance. He also was the first to recognize it in men (Guggenheim, 2000). In the 19th century, somatization was blamed on constipation, masturbation, and nervous exhaustion (Stewart, 1990).

Today, scientific support for gender differences is contradictory. In some early studies, women clearly had more somatic symptoms than men and reported more disabilities, even after adjusting for the presence of gynecologic problems (Nathanson, 1975; Verbrugge, 1985; Verbrugge & Steiner, 1981). Other studies reported no differences in somatic complaints between men and women (Pennebaker & Roberts, 1992; Phillips & Segal, 1969). In a recent study of 225 college students, women who encountered frequent sexism had more somatic symptoms than women who were not subject to that kind of discrimination (Klonoff et al., 2000). These findings suggest that gender-specific stressors may account for gender differences in symptoms.

Some studies implicated culture, age, and social status. Mexican American women were found to somatize more than non-Hispanic women (Escobar et al., 1987), and urban female residents were more likely to experience somatization than their rural counterparts (Swartz et al., 1989). Being older, separated, widowed, or divorced was related to having more somatic complaints. Less educated women also had more somatic complaints (Wool & Barsky, 1995).

The actual somatic experience appears to be different in men than in women. One group of researchers was able to show that women were more likely to be diversified somatizers who have frequent, brief sickness with a variety of complaints. Men were more likely to be asthenic somatizers with less diverse complaints, but were more chronically disabled by fatigue, weakness, or common minor illnesses (Cloninger et al., 1986a; Cloninger et al., 1986b).

Generally, most studies conclude that women somatize more often than men. Wool and Barsky (1994) offer five possible explanations for this gender difference:

1. In the United States, boys are taught not to cry and to "be a man." Thus, as grown men, they are more reluctant than women to report somatic distress.
2. It is more socially acceptable for women to seek medical treatment than men. Women use internists and psychiatrists more often than men.
3. Women have a higher incidence of psychiatric disorders that have prominent somatic symptoms (eg, depression). Somatization may be related to an underlying psychiatric disorder that occurs more often in women.
4. Strong evidence suggests that trauma such as childhood sexual abuse is related to the somatization. Because girls are more likely to be victims of sexual abuse, the higher prevalence of somatization in women may be related to childhood sexual victimization (Kinzl et al., 1995; Wool & Barsky, 1994).
5. Women are more likely than men to have relationships in which they can express their fears and suspicions to others who, in turn, give treatment and resource information (Wool & Barsky, 1994).

SOMATIZATION DISORDER

Somatization disorder is a chronic relapsing condition characterized by multiple physical symptoms that typically develop during times of emotional distress. The disorder can change over time and can vary from person to person (American Psychiatric Association [APA], 2000; Gureje & Simon, 1999).

Somatization disorder can be defined as "a polysymptomatic disorder that begins before age 30 years, extends over a period of several years, and is characterized by a combination of pain, gastrointestinal, sexual, and psychoneurological symptoms" (APA, 2000).

Clinical Course

In somatization disorder, there are recurring, multiple, and clinically significant somatic problems that involve several body systems, in contrast to other somatoform disorders that are characterized by only one set of complaints, such as conversion disorder (see later discussion) or pain disorder. Physical problems in somatization disorder cut across all body systems, such as gastrointestinal (nausea, vomiting, diarrhea), neurologic (headache, backache), or musculoskeletal (aching legs). The episode of physical illness may last 6 to 9 months. These individuals perceive themselves as being "sicker than the sick" and report all aspects of their health as poor. It is unusual for these individuals to go for more than a year without visiting a health care provider. They are often disabled and cannot work. They quickly become frustrated with their primary health care providers, who do not seem to appreciate the seriousness of their symptoms and who are unable to verify a particular problem that accounts for their extreme discomfort. Consequently, they shop for providers until they find one who will either give them new medication, hospitalize them, or perform surgery. Characteristically, these individuals have multiple surgeries. People with somatization disorder evoke negative subjective responses in the health care provider, who usually wishes that the patient would go to someone else Text Box 23-1).

Because a psychiatric diagnosis of somatization disorder is made only after numerous unexplained physical problems, psychiatric–mental health nurses do not usually care for these individuals early in the disorder. Instead, nurses in primary care and medical-surgical settings are more likely to encounter these patients.

Diagnostic Criteria

The diagnosis is made when there is a pattern of multiple, recurring, "significant" somatic complaints. Table 23-1 lists the key diagnostic criteria and target symptoms. A significant complaint is one that received medical treatment or for which the symptoms cause impairment in social, occupational, or other areas of functioning (APA, 2000).

TEXT BOX 23.1

Clinical Vignette: Somatization Disorder

Mrs. A is a 47-year-old white woman who comes to a managed care office, newly eligible to be seen under a provider plan that has just become available at the steel mill where her husband is employed as a laborer. She states that she would rather be seen by a nurse because nurses really understand people and she is tired of being seen by "careless" physicians. She is not pleased that she is in the mental health clinic, but has been told to come here to get her diazepam prescription refilled.

Her real problems are chest pain and bloating that have bothered her for the past 6 months. Her chest pain is constant throughout the day. It keeps her from doing many of her usual activities, such as housekeeping; however, it does not keep her from bowling in her league. She describes her pain as sharp in quality and at times accompanied by a throbbing sensation.

On her new patient information sheet, she has indicated that she is bothered frequently or occasionally by 42 of the 67 possible symptoms of your review of systems. Under history of family medical problems, she writes that she is the last child of six children and that she has been sickly since birth.

She reports that she has had eight operations. These included a cholecystectomy; an exploratory laparotomy where adhesions were found; breast biopsy surgery; a hemorrhoidectomy; three D & Cs, one of which followed a miscarriage during which, she reports, she almost bled to death; and a total abdominal hysterectomy at age 26 for pain and fibroids.

She takes four medications on a daily basis—one for low energy, quinine tablets for leg cramps, a nonsteroidal anti-inflammatory agent for arthritis, and diazepam for nerves. The primary provider has been unable to find anything causing the chest pain. Her physical examination is normal except for mild obesity and abdominal scars from her surgeries. Her electrocardiogram is normal.

Mrs. A is vague about her use of diazepam, which she started taking intermittently 25 years ago during her first marriage, shortly after the birth of her first child. She described her first husband as an unemployed alcoholic who abused her. He was killed in an automobile accident after a night of drinking 20 years ago, but she confessed that he was the only one she would ever love. She reports that her current husband is a nice man who has not been drinking since his release from jail 10 years ago for tax evasion. He has maintained steady employment at the steel mill. She does report that her chest pain is worse when he works double shift and is gone a lot.

After reading Mrs. A's case history, what emotions are evoked in you?

Adapted from Smith, G. (1990). *Somatization disorder in the medical setting.* (DHHS Publication No. ADM 90-1631, p. 5). Washington, DC: U.S. Government Printing Office.

TABLE 23.1 Key Diagnostic Characteristics of Somatization Disorder 300.81

Diagnostic Criteria and Target Symptoms	Associated Findings

• History of many physical complaints beginning before age 30 and occurring over a period of several years
• Complaints requiring treatment or causing significant impairment in social, occupational, or other important area of functioning
   History of pain related to at least four different sites or functions, such as head, abdomen, back, joints, extremities, chest, rectum, during menstruation, during sexual intercourse, or during urination
   History of at least two gastrointestinal symptoms, such as nausea, bloating, vomiting (other than during pregnancy), diarrhea, or intolerance of several different foods
   History of at least one sexual or reproductive symptom, such as sexual indifference, erectile or ejaculatory dysfunction, irregular menses, excessive menstrual bleeding, vomiting throughout pregnancy
   History of one pseudoneurologic symptom or deficit suggesting a neurologic condition not limited to pain, such as conversion symptoms (impaired coordination or balance, paralysis or localized weakness, difficulty swallowing or lump in throat, aphonia, urinary retention, hallucinations, loss of touch or pain sensation, double vision, blindness, deafness, seizures; dissociative symptoms, for example, amnesia, or loss of consciousness other than fainting)
• Symptoms cannot be explained by a known general medical condition or direct effects of a substance
   Symptoms unexplainable or excessive
   When a general medical condition exists, the physical complaints or resulting impairments are in excess of what would be expected from the history, physical examination, or laboratory findings
• Symptoms are not intentionally produced or feigned
	Associated Behavioral Findings
	• Colorful, exaggerated complaints lacking specific factual information
	• Inconsistent historians
	• Treatment sought from several physicians with numerous medical examinations, diagnostic procedures, surgeries, and hospitalizations
	• Anxiety and depressed mood
	• Impulsive with antisocial behavior, suicide threats and attempts, and marital discord
	Associated Physical Findings
	• Absence of objective findings to fully explain subjective complaints
	• Possible diagnosis of functional disorders, such as irritable bowel syndrome

Somatization Disorder in Special Populations

Evidence suggests that this disorder occurs in all populations and cultures. The type and frequency of somatic symptoms may differ across cultures.

Children

Somatization disorder is not usually diagnosed in children but typically begins in adolescence. However, many children experience unexplained medical symptoms. Menstrual difficulties may be one of the first symptoms. More research is needed to identify risk factors and treatment outcomes (Lieb et al., 2000).

Elderly People

Somatization disorder occurs in the elderly, but there is little research specific to this population. One of the nursing challenges is to differentiate the somatic symptoms of this disorder from other medical problems that should be diagnosed and treated. In the elderly, somatic symptoms can represent many things, such as depression, bereavement, and so forth. It is important to recognize the complexity of physical manifestations and to assess the symptom pattern.

Epidemiology

The estimated prevalence of somatization disorder ranges from 0.2% to 2% of the general population (APA, 2000). Because these individuals see themselves as medically sick and may never see a mental health provider, these estimates are believed to underrepresent the true prevalence of the disorder. Individuals with somatization disorder tend to congregate in medical offices rather than mental health settings. It is estimated that as many as 2 or 3 of every 50 patients seen in a primary care practice have somatization disorder. Thus, many people who have somatization disorder are often unrecognized, undiagnosed, and mismanaged in primary care settings. The real prevalence of somatization disorder is probably closer to 4 to 5 patients per 1,000 (Smith, 1990).

Age of Onset

Somatization disorder, by definition, has an onset before the age of 30 years, usually during adolescence. This does not mean that the individual is diagnosed before the age of 30 years, but that the patient must have one unexplained somatic symptom before this age. In the Epidemiologic Catchment Area study, the age of onset was under 10 years for 40% of the patients and under 15 years for 55%. In women, the age of onset is usually at the time of menarche, when they experience dysmenorrhea and excessive bleeding (Swartz et al., 1990).

Getting older does not increase the likelihood of being diagnosed with somatization disorder because epidemiologic data indicate that the prevalence rate for somatization disorder is just as great for those younger than 45 years of age as for those older than 45 years. However, patients who begin to have symptoms after the age of 30 years are not likely to have the number of symptoms to meet the *Diagnostic and Statistical Manual of Mental Disorder*, 4th ed., Text revision (*DSM-IV-TR*) criteria for somatization disorder and are more likely to have a diagnosable medical problem.

Gender, Ethnic, and Cultural Differences

Somatization disorder occurs primarily in women but can also occur in men. The prevalence in men is less than 0.2%, but there are higher reports of somatization disorder in men from Greece and Puerto Rico. This variation in prevalence rates suggests that cultural factors contribute to the appearance of the disorder.

Somatization disorder appears to be inversely related to socioeconomic status, with the disorder occurring more often among those who are less well educated and in the lower occupational classes. In a large World Health Organization study of more than 25,000 primary care patients representing 14 countries (Turkey, Greece, Germany, India, Nigeria, the Netherlands, United Kingdom, Japan, France, Brazil, Chile, United Stated, China, and Italy), the rates of somatization disorder were higher in South America. There were also high levels of somatization among Mexican Americans and Puerto Ricans (Gureje et al., 1997).

Comorbidity

Somatization disorder frequently coexists with other psychiatric disorders. Depression is the most common coexisting psychiatric disorder, but others include panic disorder, mania, phobic disorder, obsessive-compulsive disorder, psychotic disorders, and personality disorders (Garyfallos et al., 1999). It is rare that nurses would see patients who have only this disorder. Usually, other psychiatric disorders are present.

Ultimately, numerous unexplained medical problems also coexist with somatization disorder. Because many have received medical and surgical treatments, these individuals are constantly plagued with the side effects of previous, often unnecessary treatment. A disproportionately high number of women who are eventually diagnosed with somatization disorder have been treated for irritable bowel syndrome, polycystic ovary disease, and chronic pain (Smith, 1990). Many also have

had non–cancer-related hysterectomies. Even after the patient is treated by mental health providers and develops some understanding of the disorder, the physical problems do not disappear.

Etiology

The cause of somatization disorder is unknown. The following discussion centers on theories that are thought to contribute to the development of the disorder.

Biologic Theories

Neuropathologic. Evidence suggests a left hemisphere dysfunction related to this disorder (Flor-Henry et al., 1981). Also, the results of electroencephalographic studies suggest that abnormalities in cortical function may be present, especially in the right frontal region (Drake et al., 1988; Gordon et al., 1986). In these studies, individuals with somatization disorder responded with equal intensity to both relevant and irrelevant stimuli, whereas the normal response is to only relevant stimuli. Thus, the ability to discriminate between significant and insignificant stimuli may be compromised in these individuals. These results may explain why these individuals appear to have intense reactions to everything.

Genetic. Although it has been demonstrated that somatization disorder runs in families, the exact transmission is unclear. Strong evidence suggests an increased risk for somatization disorder in first-degree family relatives, indicating a familial or genetic effect (APA, 2000). Because many of the women with somatization disorder live in chaotic families, the environmental influence could also explain the higher prevalence in first-degree relatives. The male relatives in these families show a higher risk for antisocial personality disorder and substance abuse.

Biochemical Changes. Research is as yet insufficient to identify specific biochemical changes. However, because these patients develop other psychiatric problems, such as depression or panic, clearly many neurobiologic changes occur. Women with this disorder often have numerous menstrual problems and frequently have hysterectomies. Because of these symptoms, research studies are needed to determine the involvement of the hypothalamic–pituitary–gonadal axis, which regulates estrogen and testosterone secretion.

Psychological Theories

Somatization has been explained as a form of social or emotional communication, meaning the bodily symptoms express an emotion that cannot be verbalized. The adolescent who develops a severe abdominal pain after her parents' argument or the wife who receives nurturing from her husband only when she has back pain are two examples (Smith, 1990). From this perspective, somatization may be a way of maintaining relationships. Following this line of reasoning, as an individual's physical problems become a way of controlling relationships, somatization becomes a learned behavior pattern. Over time, physical symptoms develop automatically in response to perceived threats. Finally, somatization disorder develops when somatizing becomes a way of life.

During the Freudian period, classic psychoanalytic theory was used to explain the appearance of some somatic symptoms. It was believed that the development of unexplained medical problems was actually a substitute for repressed impulses related to anal and oedipal conflicts. Some of Freud's more interesting case studies involved people who were depicted as having unconscious psychic conflicts related to a particular physical problem.

Social Theories

Even though somatization disorders occur cross-culturally, the symptoms may vary from culture to culture. Also, the conceptualization of somatization disorder is primarily used by Western society. In non-Western societies where the mind–body distinction is not made and symptoms have different meanings and explanations, these physical manifestations are not labeled as a psychiatric disorder. Moreover, in some Asian cultures, symptoms of depression or anxiety are believed to be caused by a weakness in some parts of the body, such as the kidney, heart, bones, lung, or nerve, or by a vitamin deficiency (Ganesan et al., 1989). In these cultures, the health provider treats the weak part of the body, not the mind (Text Box 23-2).

Risk Factors

This disorder tends to run in families, and children of mothers with multiple unexplained somatic complaints are more likely to have somatic problems. Adults are at higher risk for unexplained medical symptoms if as children they experienced unexplained symptoms or if their parents were in poor health when the children were about 15 years of age (Hotopt et al., 1999). There are also indications that women with somatization disorder are more likely to have been sexually abused as children than those with other psychiatric conditions, such as mood disorders (Smith, 1990). Individuals with depression are more likely to develop new episodes of somatization (Gureje & Simon, 1999).

Somatization disorder is also associated with antisocial personality disorder or alcoholism in family members. It is hypothesized that women with somatization disorder selectively choose men with antisocial personality disorder. Other evidence suggests that hyperactivity in children is more common in families with mothers who

TEXT BOX 23.2

Somatization in Chinese Culture

In Chinese tradition, the health of the individual is seen as a reflection of the balance between positive and negative forces within the body. There are five elements at work both in nature and in the body that control conditions (fire, water, wood, earth, metal), five viscera (liver, heart, spleen, kidneys, lungs), five emotions (anger, joy, worry, sorrow, fear), and five climatic conditions (wind, heat, humidity, dryness, cold). All illness is explained by imbalances among these elements. Because emotion is related to the circulation of vital air within the body, anger is believed to result from an adverse current of vital air to the liver. Rather than attributing the behavior to the person who has individual responsibility, emotional outbursts are seen as results of imbalances between the natural elements.

The stigma of mental illness in the Chinese culture is so great that it can have an adverse effect on a family for many generations. If problems can be attributed to these natural causes, the individual and family are less responsible, and less of a stigma is attached. The Chinese have a culturally acceptable term for symptoms of mental distress—neurasthenia—which is often experienced through somatic complaints of headaches, insomnia, dizziness, aches and pains, poor memory, anxiety, weakness, and loss of energy.

Adapted from Tabora, B., & Flaskerud, J. (1994). Depression among Chinese Americans: A review of the literature. *Issues in Mental Health Nursing, 15*(6), 569–584.

have somatization disorder and with fathers who have antisocial personality disorder (Biederman et al., 1992).

Interdisciplinary Treatment

The general consensus is that the overall management of patients with these disorders involves three approaches:

1. Providing long-term general management of the chronic condition
2. Conservatively treating comorbid psychiatric and physical problems symptomatically
3. Providing care in special settings, including group treatment (Smith, 1990)

The cornerstone of management is the establishment of a trusting relationship. Ideally, the patient sees only one health care provider at regularly scheduled visits. During each visit in the primary care setting, a partial physical examination of the organ system in which the patient has complaints should be conducted. However, these physical symptoms are treated conservatively using the least intrusive approach. In the mental health setting, the use of cognitive-behavior therapy (CBT) is promising. In a review of clinical trials ($n = 31$) of CBT, patients treated with CBT improved more than control subjects in 71% of the studies. Benefits can occur whether or not psychological distress is ameliorated (Kroenke & Swindle, 2000).

NURSING MANAGEMENT: HUMAN RESPONSE TO DISORDER

Somatization is the major response to this disorder. Even though somatization has not been established by the North American Nursing Diagnosis Association (NANDA) as a nursing diagnosis, studies are underway to validate the diagnosis of somatization (Whitney et al., 1988). The defining characteristics are depicted in the biopsychosocial model (Fig. 23-1). In fact, the characteristics are so well integrated that it is difficult to separate the psychological and social dimensions. The most commonly occurring characteristics are as follows:

- Reporting the same symptoms repeatedly
- Receiving support from the environment that otherwise might not be forthcoming (such as gaining a spouse's attention because of severe back pain)
- Expressing concern about the physical problems inconsistent with the severity of the illness (being "sicker than the sick")

Biologic Domain

During the assessment interview, the nurse needs to allow enough time for the patient to explain all medical problems because a rushed assessment interview blocks communication. Past medical treatment has been ineffective because the management regimen did not address the underlying psychiatric disorder. However, psychiatric–mental health nurses typically see these patients for problems related to the coexisting psychiatric disorder, such as depression, not because of the somatization disorder. While taking the patient's history, the nurse will realize that the individual has had multiple surgeries or medical problems and that somatization disorder is a strong possibility. If the patient has not already been diagnosed with somatization disorder, the nurse should screen for it by determining the presence of the most commonly reported problems associated with this disorder, which include dysmenorrhea, lump in throat, vomiting, shortness of breath, burning in sex organs, painful extremities, and amnesia (Othmer & DeSouza, 1985). If the patient has these symptoms, he or she should be seen by a mental health provider qualified to make the diagnosis. Text Box 23-3 presents the Health Attitude Survey, which can be used as a screening test for somatization.

Review of Systems

Even though these patients' symptoms have usually received considerable attention from the medical community, a careful review of systems is important because the appearance of physical problems is usually related to psychosocial problems. Even as the nurse continues to see the patient for mental health problems,

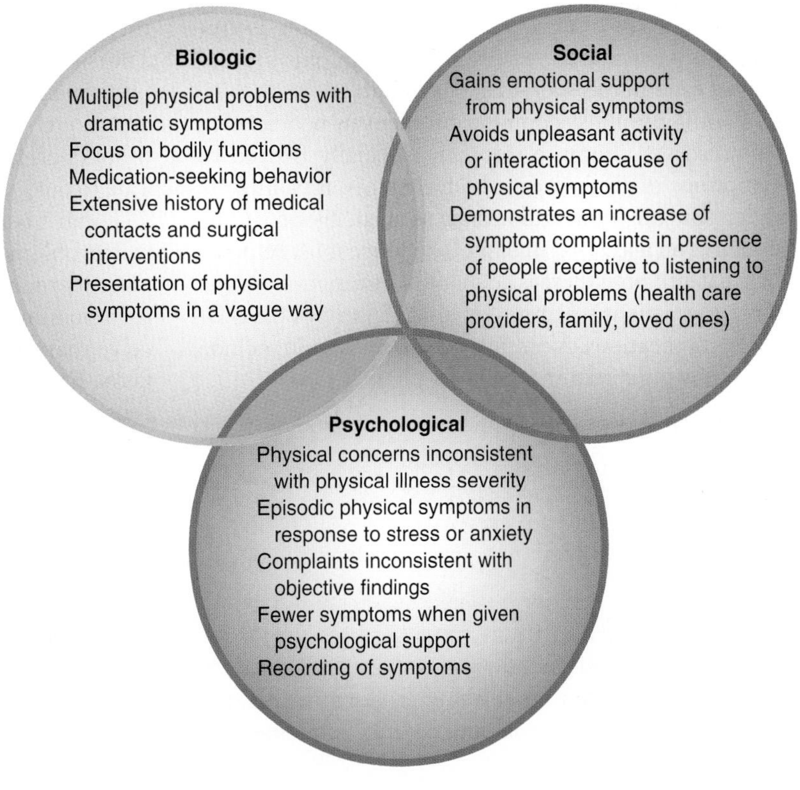

Biologic

Multiple physical problems with dramatic symptoms
Focus on bodily functions
Medication-seeking behavior
Extensive history of medical contacts and surgical interventions
Presentation of physical symptoms in a vague way

Social

Gains emotional support from physical symptoms
Avoids unpleasant activity or interaction because of physical symptoms
Demonstrates an increase of symptom complaints in presence of people receptive to listening to physical problems (health care providers, family, loved ones)

Psychological

Physical concerns inconsistent with physical illness severity
Episodic physical symptoms in response to stress or anxiety
Complaints inconsistent with objective findings
Fewer symptoms when given psychological support
Recording of symptoms

FIGURE 23.1 Biopsychosocial characteristics of patients with somatization disorder.

TEXT BOX 23.3   Health Attitude Survey

On a scale of 1 to 5, please indicate the extent to which you agree (5) or disagree (1).

Dissatisfaction With Care

1. I have been satisfied with the medical care I have received. (R)
2. Doctors have done the best they could to diagnose and treat my health problems. (R)
3. Doctors have taken my health problems seriously.
4. My health problems have been thoroughly evaluated. (R)
5. Doctors do not seem to know much about the health problems I have had.
6. My health problems have been completely explained. (R)
7. Doctors seem to think I am exaggerating my health problems.
8. My response to treatment has not been satisfactory.
9. My response to treatment is usually excellent. (R)

Frustration With Ill Health

10. I am tired of feeling sick and would like to get to the bottom of my health problems.
11. I have felt ill for quite a while now.
12. I am going to keep searching for an answer to my health problems.
13. I do not think there is anything seriously wrong with my body. (R)

High Utilization of Care

14. I have seen many different doctors over the years.
15. I have taken a lot of medicine recently.
16. I do not go to the doctor often. (R)
17. I have had relatively good health over the years.

Excessive Health Worry

18. I sometimes worry too much about my health.
19. I often fear the worst when I develop symptoms.
20. I have trouble getting my mind off my health.

Psychological Distress

21. Sometimes I feel depressed and cannot seem to shake it off.
22. I have sought help for emotional or stress-related problems.
23. It is easy to relax and stay calm. (R)
24. I believe the stress I am under may be affecting my health.

Discordant Communication of Distress

25. Some people think that I am capable of more work than I feel able to do.
26. Some people think that I have been sick just to gain attention.
27. It is difficult for me to find the right words for my feelings.

(R) indicates items reversed for scoring purposes. Scoring—The higher the score, the more likely somatization is a problem.
Noyes, R., Jr., Langbehn, D., Happel, R., et al. (1999). Health Attitude Survey: A scale for assessing somatizing patients. *Psychosomatics, 40*(6), 470–478.

---

an ongoing awareness of biologic symptoms is important, particularly because these symptoms are deemphasized in the overall management.

Pain is the most common problem in people with this disorder. Because the pain is usually related to symptoms of all the major body systems, it is unlikely that a somatic intervention such as an analgesic will be effective on a long-term basis. The nurse must remember that although there is no medical explanation for the pain, the patient's pain is real and has serious psychosocial implications. A careful assessment should include the following questions:

- What is the pain like?
- What is the extent of the pain?
- What helps the pain get better?
- When is it the pain its worst?
- What has worked in the past to relieve the pain?

Physical Functioning

The actual physical functioning of these individuals is often marginal. They usually have problems with sleep, fatigue, activity, and sexual functioning. Assessment of these areas will generate data to be used in establishing a nursing diagnosis. The amount and quality of sleep are important. The actual times that the individual sleeps are also relevant. One individual was sleeping a total of 6 hours each diurnal cycle but could sleep only from 2:00 to 6:00 AM and needed an afternoon nap.

Fatigue is a constant problem, and a variety of physical problems interfere with normal activity. These patients report overwhelming lack of energy, making it impossible to maintain usual routines. They perceive that they need more energy to accomplish daily tasks. Fatigue is accompanied by the inability to concentrate on simple functions, leading to decreased performance and disinterest in surroundings. Patients tend to be lethargic and listless, and often have little energy (Text Box 23-4).

Patients with this disorder usually have had multiple gynecologic problems. The reason for these symptoms is not understood, but the symptomatology of dysmenorrhea, painful intercourse, and pain in the "sex organs" suggests involvement of the hypothalamic–pituitary–gonadal axis. Because the understanding of its role with the limbic system is only rudimentary, biologic indica-

TEXT BOX 23.4

Clinical Vignette: Somatization Disorder

Ms. J is a 42-year-old white woman who has been coming to the mental health clinic for 2 years for her nerves. She has only seen the physician for medication, but has now been referred to the nurse's new stress management group because she has developed side effects to all the medications that have been tried. The psychiatrist has diagnosed her with somatization disorder and wants her to learn to manage her "nerves" without medication.

At the first meeting with the nurse, Ms. J was preoccupied with chest pain and bloating that had lasted for the last 6 months. Her chest pain is constant and sharp at times. The pain does not prevent her from going to her job as a waitress, but does interfere with meal preparation at night for her family and her ability to have sexual intercourse. She has numerous other physical problems, including allergies to certain perfumes, dysmenorrhea, ovarian polycystic disease (presence of cysts in the ovaries), chronic urinary tract infections, and rashes. She is constantly fatigued and has frequent leg cramps. She states that she is too tired to fix dinner for her family and often takes a nap in the afternoon, sleeping until evening. She is unable to fall asleep at night.

She believes that she will soon have to have her gallbladder removed because of occasional referred pain to her back and nausea that occurs a couple hours after eating. She is not excited about a stress management group and does not believe that it will help her problems. She has agreed to consider it as long as the psychiatrist will continue prescribing diazepam.

Critical Thinking Questions

• How should Ms. J's physical symptoms be prioritized?
• Identify possible explanations for Ms. J's fatigue.

---

tors, such as those produced by laboratory tests, are not available. However, a careful assessment of the patient's menstrual history, gynecologic problems, and sexual functioning is important. The physical manifestations of somatization disorder often lead to altered sexual behavior.

Pharmacologic Assessment

A psychopharmacologic assessment of these patients is challenging. Patients with somatization disorder frequently "provider-shop," or move from one provider to another. It is not unusual for them to see seven or eight different providers within a year. Because they often receive medications from each provider, they are usually taking a large number of drugs. They tend to protect their sources and may not be truthful in identifying the actual number of medications they are ingesting. A pharmacologic assessment is needed not only because of the number of medications but also because these individuals have many unusual side effects.

Because of their somatic sensitivity, they often overreact to medication.

These patients spend much of their life trying to find out what is wrong with them. When one provider after another can find little if any explanation for their symptoms, many become anxious. To alleviate their anxiety, they either self-medicate with over-the-counter medications and substances of abuse (eg, alcohol, marijuana) or find a provider who prescribes an anxiolytic. Because the anxiety of their disorder cannot be treated within a few weeks with an anxiolytic, they become dependent on medication that should not have been prescribed in the first place. Although anxiolytics have a place in therapeutics, they are not recommended for long-term use and only complicate the treatment of somatoform disorders. These medications should also be avoided because of their addictive qualities. Unfortunately, by the time these individuals are seen by a mental health provider, they have already begun taking an anxiolytic for anxiety, usually a benzodiazepine. Many times, they only agree to be seen by a mental health provider because the last provider would no longer prescribe an anxiolytic without a psychiatric evaluation.

Nursing Diagnoses Related to Biologic Domain

Because this is a chronic illness, individuals with somatization disorder could have almost any one of the nursing diagnoses at some time in their life. It is likely that there will be at least one nursing diagnosis related to the individual's physical state. Fatigue, pain, and disturbed sleep patterns are usually supported by the assessment data. The challenge in devising outcomes for these problems is to avoid focusing on the biologic aspects and instead help the patient overcome the fatigue, pain, or sleep problem through biopsychosocial approaches.

Biologic Interventions

Nursing interventions that focus on the biologic dimension become especially important because of the conservative medical treatment and the avoidance of aggressive pharmacologic treatment. Each time a nurse sees the patient, a limited amount of time should be spent on the physical complaints. Several biologic interventions may be useful in caring for patients with somatization disorder. Pain management, activity enhancement, nutrition regulation, relaxation, and pharmacologic interventions have all been useful.

Pain Management. In establishing pain management interventions, rarely does only one approach work (see Chap. 14). Pain is a primary issue. After a careful assessment of the pain, the nurse should develop nonpharmacologic strategies to reduce the pain. If gastrointestinal pain is frequent, eating and bowel habits should be explored and modified. For back pain, exercises and consultation from physical therapist may be useful. Headaches are a challenge. Self-monitoring of when headaches appear engages the patient in the therapeutic process and helps in identifying psychosocial triggers.

Activity Enhancement. Helping the patient establish a daily routine may alleviate some of the difficulty with sleeping. Because most of these patients do not work, a daily routine is not easily established. Encouraging the patient to get up in the morning and retire at a specific time at night helps to establish a routine. Ideally, these patients should engage in regular exercise to improve their overall physical state. These patients often have all sorts of reasons why they cannot carry out these recommendations. This is where the nurse's patience is tested.

Nutrition Regulation. Patients with somatization disorder often have gastrointestinal problems and may have special nutritional needs. The nurse discusses with the patient the nutritional value of food choices. Because these individuals often have been taking medications that promote weight gain, weight control strategies may be discussed (see Chap. 14). For overweight individuals, healthy, low-calorie food choices should be suggested. Teaching patients about balancing dietary intake with activity levels helps them begin to increase awareness of food choices.

Relaxation. If the patient is taking anxiety-relieving medication, relaxation techniques can be taught to alleviate stress. It will be a challenge to help these patients really use these strategies. The nurse should consider a variety of techniques, including simple relaxation techniques, distraction, and guided imagery (see Chap. 14).

Psychopharmacologic Interventions

No medication is particularly recommended for somatization disorder. Psychiatric symptoms of the other comorbid disorders, such as depression and anxiety, are treated pharmacologically as appropriate. Usually, these patients are depressed and are prescribed an antidepressant. Depressed mood itself is not an indication for initiation of antidepressant treatment. If the symptoms of insomnia, decreased appetite, decreased libido, and anhedonia are present along with a persistently depressed mood, aggressive psychopharmacologic management is indicated (Smith, 1990). A wide variety of drugs are available, including the selective serotonin reuptake inhibitors (SSRIs), tricyclic antidepressants, and the monoamine oxidase inhibitors (MAOIs) (see Chap. 20). Patients with somatization disorder usually have experience with several different antidepressants throughout the course of the disorder. Antidepressants are used only when the depressive disorder is present, but there should be evidence that the depressive symp-

toms are cleared before discontinuing the medication (see Drug Profile: Phenelzine, which is one of the MAOIs (trade name, Nardil). The MAOIs not only are effective in treating depression but also are useful in treating chronic pain and headaches, common in people with somatization disorder. Depression is usually successfully treated with antidepressants (see Chap. 20).

Side effects of MAOIs are generally more severe or frequent than those with other antidepressants. The most frequent side effects are dizziness, headache, dry mouth, insomnia, constipation, blurred vision, nausea, peripheral edema, forgetfulness, fainting spells, trauma, hesitancy of urination, weakness, and myoclonic jerks (Krishnan, 1995). Orthostatic hypotension is common with MAOIs. Elevated liver enzymes are found in 3% to 5% of patients, but liver function tests are indicated only if the patient has symptoms of malaise, jaundice, or excessive fatigue. Some side effects first emerge during maintenance treatment. These include weight gain (in about half of patients), edema, muscle cramps, carbohydrate craving, sexual dysfunction, pyridoxine (vitamin B_6) deficiency, hypoglycemia, hypomania, urinary retention, and disorientation. Edema and weight gain are a particular problem with phenelzine. These side effects are treated symptomatically (Krishnan, 1995).

Food and food interactions are the most serious side effects. While taking the MAOIs, patients should avoid foods high in tyramine (see Chap. 8). A mild tyramine interaction can produce hypertension, occipital headache, palpitations, nausea, vomiting, apprehension, occasional chills, sweating, and restlessness. Physical findings include stiff neck, pallor, mild pyrexia (fever), dilated pupils, and motor agitation. The reaction develops within 20 to 60 minutes after ingesting food. A severe reaction could lead to altered consciousness, hyperpyrexia, and cerebral hemorrhage. Although death can occur, it is rare. The treatment of the hypertensive crisis is intravenous administration of phentolamine (Regitine), an α-adrenergic receptor blocking agent that dilates blood vessels and lowers arterial blood pressure. A calcium-channel blocker, nifedipine (Procardia), is also effective. The advantage of nifedipine is that it is administered orally or sublingually and can be carried by the patient. Anxiety is more difficult to treat pharmacologically than depression. Nonpharmacologic approaches such as biofeedback or relaxation should be used. Benzodiazepines should be avoided because of the psychological dependence associated with these medications. Although symptomatic relief is immediate, patients are reluctant to give them up. Buspirone (BuSpar), a nonbenzodiazepine, does not lead to tolerance or withdrawal and may be useful for relief of anxiety. If panic disorder is present, it should be treated aggressively.

Monitoring and Administration of Medications. In somatization disorder, patients are usually treated

DRUG PROFILE: Phenelzine
(Monoamine Oxidase Inhibitor Antidepressant)
Trade Name: Nardil

Receptor affinity: Inhibits MAO, an enzyme responsible for breaking down biogenic amines, such as epinephrine, norepinephrine, and serotonin, allowing them to accumulate in neuronal storage sites throughout the central and peripheral nervous systems.

Indications: Treatment of depression characterized as "atypical, nonendogenous," or "neurotic" or nonresponsive to other antidepressant therapy or in situations in which other antidepressant therapy is contraindicated.

Route and dosage: Available as 15-mg tablets.

Adults: Initially, 15 mg PO tid, increasing to at least 60 mg/d at a fairly rapid pace consistent with patient tolerance. Therapy at 60 mg/d may be necessary for at least 4 weeks before response occurs. After maximum benefit achieved, dosage reduced gradually over several weeks. Maintenance dose may be 15 mg/d or every other day.

Geriatric: Adjust dosage accordingly because patients over 60 years of age are more prone to develop adverse effects.

Pediatric: Not recommended for children under 16 years of age.

Half-life (peak effects): Unknown (48–96 h).

Selected adverse reactions: Dizziness, vertigo, headache, overactivity, hyperreflexia, tremors, muscle twitching, mania, hypomania, jitteriness, confusion, memory impairment, insomnia, weakness, fatigue, overstimulation, restlessness, increased anxiety, agitation, blurred vision, sweating, constipation, diarrhea, nausea, abdominal pain, edema, dry mouth, anorexia, weight changes, hypertensive crisis, orthostatic hypotension, and disturbed cardiac rate and rhythm.

Warnings: Contraindicated in patients with pheochromocytoma congestive heart failure, hepatic dysfunction, severe renal impairment, cardiovascular disease, history of headache, and myelography within previous 24 h or scheduled within next 48 h. Use cautiously in patients with seizure disorders, hyperthyroidism, pregnancy, lactation, and those scheduled for elective surgery. Possible hypertensive crisis, coma, and severe convulsions may occur if administered with tricyclic antidepressants; possible hypertensive crisis when taken with foods containing tyramine. Increased risk for adverse interaction is possible when given with meperidine. Additive hypoglycemic effect can occur when taken with insulin and oral sulfonylureas.

Specific patient/family education:
- Take drug exactly as prescribed; do not stop taking abruptly or without consulting your health care provider.
- Avoid consuming any foods containing tyramine while taking this drug and for 2 weeks afterward.
- Avoid alcohol, sleep-inducing drugs, over-the-counter drugs such as cold and hay fever remedies and appetite suppressants—all of which may cause serious or life-threatening problems.
- Report any signs and symptoms of adverse reactions.
- Maintain appointments for follow-up blood tests.
- Report any complaints of unusual or severe headache or yellowing of eyes or skin.
- Avoid driving a car or performing any activities that require alertness.
- Change position slowly when going from a lying to sitting or standing position to minimize dizziness or weakness.

in the community and self-medicated. The nurse should carefully question patients about the actual self-administration of medicine and ask specific questions about which medicines are now currently taken (including over-the-counter and herbal supplements). The nurse should listen carefully to determine effects the patient attributes to the medication. This information should be documented and reported to the rest of the team. The patient should be encouraged to continue taking only prescribed medication.

Side-Effect Monitoring and Management. These individuals often have idiosyncratic reactions to their medications. Side effects should be assessed, but the patient should be encouraged to compare the benefits of the medication with any problems related to side effects.

Drug–Drug Interaction. In working with patients with somatization disorder, the nurse always needs to be on the lookout for drug–drug interactions. These patients are most likely taking several medications for physical problems, and these medications could interact with psychiatric medications. It is not unusual for

patients to be taking alternative medicines, such as herbal supplements, but they usually willingly disclose their experiments (Garcia-Campayo & Sanz-Carrillo, 2000). The patient should be encouraged to use the same pharmacy for filling prescriptions so that possible reactions can be checked.

Psychological Domain

The mental status of individuals with somatization disorder is usually within normal limits. What is most noticeable is the flamboyant appearance and exaggerated speech. They are often dressed in attention-getting clothes such as bright colors, flashy shoes, or an outrageous hairstyle. Their language is colorful and can be entertaining. Generally, cognition is not impaired. However, these individuals seem preoccupied with personal illnesses and may even keep a record of symptoms. They have a constant focus on bodily functions, and "living with diseases" truly becomes a way a life.

Individuals with somatization disorder usually have intense emotional reactions to life stressors. These patients usually have a series of personal crises beginning at an early age. Typically, a new symptom or medical problem develops during times of emotional stress. It is critical that the physical assessment data be linked to psychological and social events that are occurring in the patient's life. A life history of the major psychological events should be compared to the chronology of physical problems. Special attention should be paid to any history of sexual abuse or trauma in the patients' younger years. Early sexual abuse also has implications for sexual functioning and may prevent the individual from being able to perform sexually.

The individual's mood is usually labile, often shifting from extremely excited to depressed. Response to the physical symptoms is usually exaggerated, such as interpreting a simple cold as pneumonia or a brief chest pain as a heart attack. Family members may not believe the physical symptoms are real and view them as attention-getting behavior because symptoms often improve when the patient receives the attention. For example, a woman who has been in bed for 3 weeks with severe back pain may suddenly feel much better once her children visit her.

Nursing Diagnoses Related to Psychological Domain

Nursing diagnoses targeting responses to somatization disorder typical to the psychological domain include the following:

- Anxiety
- Ineffective Sexuality Patterns
- Impaired Social Interactions
- Ineffective Coping
- Ineffective Management of Therapeutic Regimen

Psychological Interventions

The choice of psychological intervention depends on the specific problem that the patient is experiencing. The most important and ongoing intervention is the maintenance of a therapeutic relationship.

Development of a Therapeutic Nurse–Patient Relationship. The most difficult aspect of the nursing care is the development of a positive nurse–patient relationship. It is crucial that a sound relationship develop between the patient and the nurse. Without the relationship, the nurse is just one more provider who fails to meet the patient's expectations. Developing a relationship requires time and patience. Therapeutic communication techniques should be used to redirect the patient to psychosocial problems that are related to the physical manifestations (see Therapeutic Dialogue: Establishing a Relationship).

During periods when other psychiatric disorders become symptomatic, additional interventions for the new problems is needed. For example, if depression occurs, additional supportive or cognitive approaches may be needed.

| **THERAPEUTIC DIALOGUE** | **Establishing a Relationship** |

Ineffective Approach

Nurse: Good morning Ms. C.
Patient: I'm in so much pain. Take that breakfast away.
Nurse: You don't want your breakfast?
Patient: Can't you see? I hurt! When I hurt, I can't eat!
Nurse: If you don't eat now, you probably won't be able to have anything until lunch.
Patient: Who cares. I have no intention of being here at lunchtime. I don't belong here.
Nurse: Ms. C, I don't think that your doctor would have admitted you unless there is a problem. I would like to talk to you about why you are here.
Patient: Nurse, I'm just here. It's none of your business.
Nurse: Oh.
Patient: Please leave me alone.
Nurse: Sure, I will see you later.

Effective Approach

Nurse: Good morning, Ms. C.
Patient: I'm in so much pain. Take that breakfast away.
Nurse: (Silently removes tray. Pulls up chair and sits down.)
Patient: My back hurts.
Nurse: Oh, when did the back pain start?
Patient: Last night. It's this bed. I couldn't get comfortable.

Nurse: These beds can be pretty uncomfortable.
Patient: My back pain is shooting down my leg.
Nurse: Does anything help it?
Patient: Sometimes if I straighten out my leg it helps.
Nurse: Can I help you straighten out your leg?
Patient: Oh, it's OK. The pain is going away. What did you say your name is?
Nurse: I'm Susan Miller, your nurse while you are here.
Patient: I won't be here long. I don't belong in a psychiatric unit.
Nurse: While you are here, I would like to spend time with you.
Patient: OK, but you understand, I do not have any psychiatric problems.
Nurse: We can talk about whatever you want. But, since you want to get out of here, we might want to focus on what it will take to get you ready for discharge.

Critical Thinking Challenge

- What communication mistakes did the nurse in the first scenario make?
- What communication strategies helped the patient feel comfortable with the nurse in the second scenario? How is the first scenario different from the second?

Counseling. Counseling with a focus on problem solving is needed from time to time. These patients have chaotic lives and need support through the multitude of crises. Although they sometimes appear flamboyant and self-assured, they easily irritate others because of their constant complaints. Their consequences of impaired social interaction with others needs to be examined within a counseling framework. It will become evident to the nurse that the patient's problem-solving and decision-making skills could be improved. Identifying stresses and strengthening positive coping responses helps the patient deal with a chaotic lifestyle.

Health Teaching. Health teaching is useful throughout the nurse–patient relationship. These patients have many questions about different illnesses, symptoms, and treatment. Health teaching should emphasize positive health care practices and minimize the effects of serious illness. Because of problems in managing medications and treatment, the recommended therapeutic regime needs constant monitoring, thus resulting in ample opportunities for teaching. One area that might require special health teaching is in the area of impaired sexuality. Because of their long history of physical problems related to reproductive tract, these patients may have difficulty carrying out normal sexual activity, such as intercourse, reaching orgasm, and so forth. Basic teaching about normal sexual function is often needed (see Psychoeducation Checklist: Somatization Disorder).

Social Domain

People with this disorder spend excessive time seeking medical care and treating their multiple illnesses. Because they believe themselves to be very sick, they also believe that they are disabled and cannot work. Most of the people with this disorder are unemployed. Because their symptoms are often inconsistent with an identifiable medical diagnosis, these individuals are rarely satisfied with health care providers who can find nothing wrong. However, even though they change providers frequently, their social network often consists of a series of providers instead of peers. Identification of a support network requires sorting out the health care providers from family and friends.

Family members become weary of the individual's constant complaints of physical problems. These individuals live in chaotic families with multiple problems. In assessing the family structure, other members with psychiatric disorders need to be identified. Women may be married to abusive men who have antisocial personality disorders. Alcoholism is common in these families. It is important to identify the positive and negative relationships within the family.

Somatization disorder is particularly problematic because it disrupts the family's social aspects of living. Changes in routine or major life events often seem to precipitate the appearance of a symptom. For example, a patient may be planning a vacation with the family, but at the last minute decides she cannot go because her back pain has returned and she will not be able to sit in the car. These types of family disruptions are common.

Nursing Diagnoses Related to Social Domain

Some of the nursing diagnoses related to the social domain that are typical of people with somatization disorder include the following:

- Caregiver Role Strain, Risk for
- Ineffective Community Coping
- Disabled Family Coping
- Social Isolation

Social Interventions

Patients with somatic disorders are usually isolated from their families and communities. Strengthening social relationships and activities often becomes the focus of the nursing care. The nurse should help the patient identify individuals with whom contact is desired, ask for a commitment to contact them, and encourage them to reinitiate a relationship. The nurse should counsel the patient about talking too much about their symptoms with these individuals, pointing out to the patient that medical information needs to be shared with the nurse. The nurse must also ensure that the patient knows when the next appointment is scheduled.

Group Interventions. Even though these patients are not candidates for insight group psychotherapy,

---

PSYCHOEDUCATION CHECKLIST
Somatization Disorder

When caring for the patient with somatization disorder, be sure to include the following topic areas in the teaching plan:

- Psychopharmacologic agents (anxiolytics) if ordered, including drug, action, dosage, frequency, and possible adverse effects
- Nonpharmacologic pain relief measures
- Exercise
- Nutrition
- Social interaction
- Appropriate health care practices
- Problem-solving
- Relaxation and anxiety reduction techniques

they do benefit from problem-solving groups that focus on developing coping skills for everyday life. Because most of the patients are women, participation in groups that address feminist issues should be encouraged to strengthen their assertiveness skills and improve their generally low self-esteem (Fig. 23-2).

When leading a group that has members with this disorder, redirection can keep the group from giving too much attention to a person's illness. However, these individuals need reassurance and support while in a group. They may verbalize that they do not fit in or belong in the group. In reality, they are feeling insecure and threatened in the situation. The group leader needs to show patience and understanding in order to engage the individual effectively in meaningful group interaction.

Family Interventions. The results of a family assessment often reveal that families of these individuals need education about the disorder, helpful strategies for dealing with the multiple complaints of the patient, and usually help in developing more effective communication patterns. Because of the chaotic nature of their families and the lack of healthy problem solving, physical and psychological abuse may be evident in the family. The nurse should be particularly sensitive to any evidence of physical or sexual abuse (see Chap. 37).

Evaluation and Treatment Outcomes

The outcomes for patients with somatization disorder should be realistic. Because this is a lifelong disorder, small successes should be expected. Specific outcomes should be identified, such as gradually increasing social contact. Over time, there should be a gradual reduction in the number of health care providers that the individual contacts and a slight improvement in the ability to cope with stresses (Fig. 23-3).

Continuum of Care

Inpatient Care

Hopefully, these individuals will spend minimal time in the hospital. Inpatient stays occur at the times when their comorbid disorders become symptomatic. While in the inpatient unit, the patient should be assigned to one primary nurse who is responsible for providing or overseeing all of the nursing care. The inpatient nurse has the responsibility of establishing a relationship with the patient (and family) as well as teaching other nursing staff members about this disorder.

Emergency Care

The emergencies these individuals experience may be physical (eg, chest pain, back pain, gastrointestinal symp-

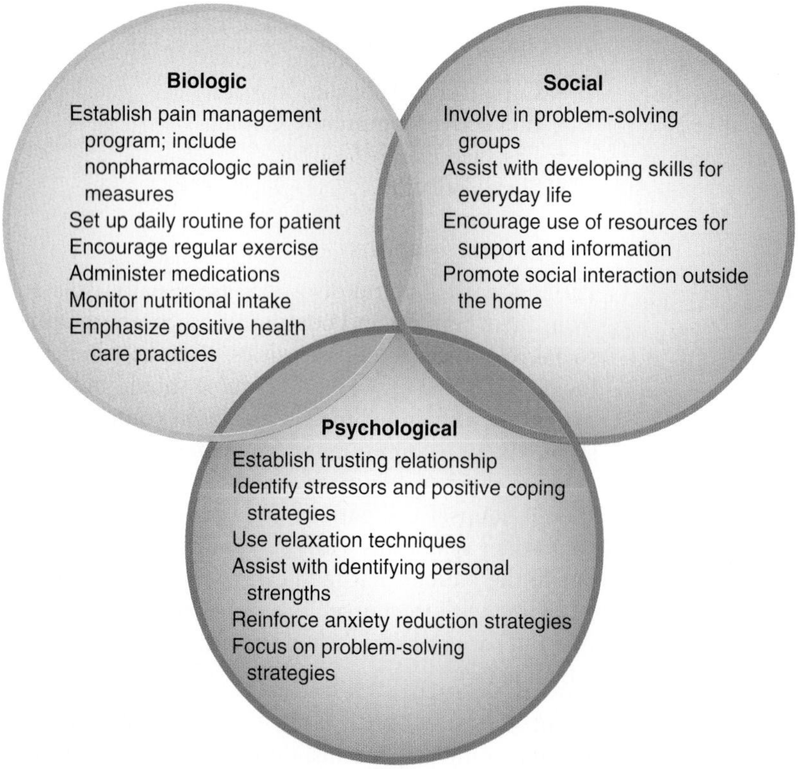

Biologic

Establish pain management program; include nonpharmacologic pain relief measures
Set up daily routine for patient
Encourage regular exercise
Administer medications
Monitor nutritional intake
Emphasize positive health care practices

Social

Involve in problem-solving groups
Assist with developing skills for everyday life
Encourage use of resources for support and information
Promote social interaction outside the home

Psychological

Establish trusting relationship
Identify stressors and positive coping strategies
Use relaxation techniques
Assist with identifying personal strengths
Reinforce anxiety reduction strategies
Focus on problem-solving strategies

FIGURE 23.2 Biopsychosocial interventions for patients with somatization disorder.

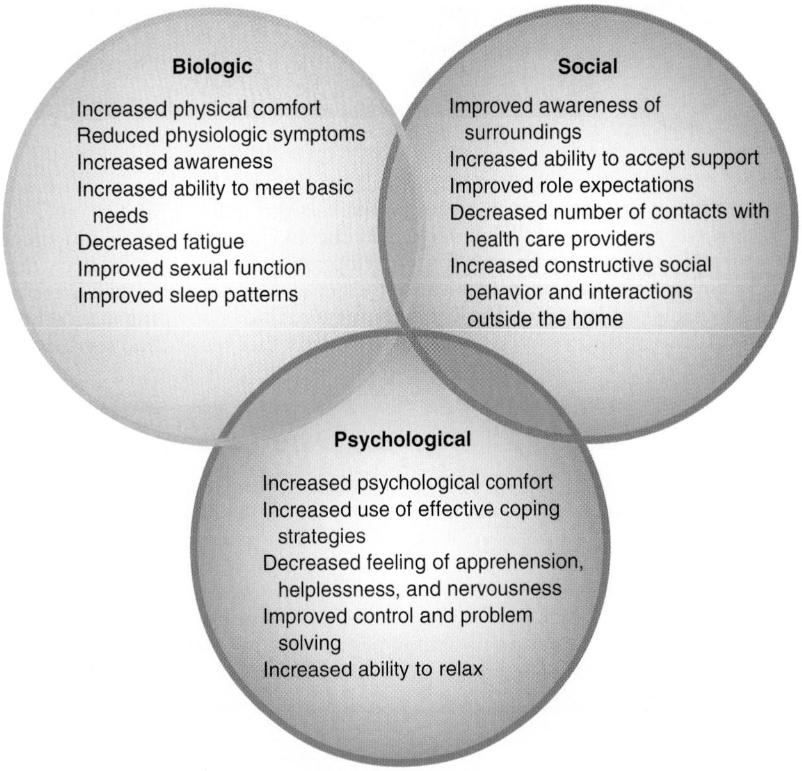

Biologic
Increased physical comfort
Reduced physiologic symptoms
Increased awareness
Increased ability to meet basic needs
Decreased fatigue
Improved sexual function
Improved sleep patterns

Social
Improved awareness of surroundings
Increased ability to accept support
Improved role expectations
Decreased number of contacts with health care providers
Increased constructive social behavior and interactions outside the home

Psychological
Increased psychological comfort
Increased use of effective coping strategies
Decreased feeling of apprehension, helplessness, and nervousness
Improved control and problem solving
Increased ability to relax

FIGURE 23.3 Biopsychosocial outcomes for patients with somatization disorder.

toms) or stress responses related to a psychosocial crisis. Occasionally, these individuals become suicidal and require a more intensive level of care. Generally speaking, nonpharmacologic interventions should be tried first, with very conservative use of antianxiety medications. All attempts should be made to retrieve records from other facilities.

Community Treatment

These patients can spend a lifetime in the health care system and still have little continuity of care. Switching from provider to provider is characteristic of patients with this disorder and detrimental to their long-term management. Most care is delivered within outpatient settings. When hospitalized, it is usually for evaluation of medical problems. When their comorbid psychiatric disorders such as depression become symptomatic, these patients may also be hospitalized for a short period of time. See Nursing Care Plan 23-1.

Mental Health Promotion

Patients with somatization disorder need to focus on "staying healthy" instead of focusing on their illness. For these individuals, approaching the topic of promotion usually has to be within the context of preventing further problems. Setting aside time for them-

selves and identifying activities that meet their psychological and spiritual needs, such as going to church or synagogue, are important in maintaining a healthy balance.

OTHER SOMATOFORM DISORDERS

The other somatoform disorders have many symptoms that are similar to those of somatization disorder but are often not as debilitating. The following discussion summarizes the other somatoform disorders and highlights the primary focus of nursing management.

Undifferentiated Somatoform Disorder

Patients who have unexplained physical problems for at least 6 months are diagnosed with undifferentiated somatoform disorder. This disorder is different from somatization disorder in that these patients do not have multiple, unexplained physical problems before 30 years of age, but instead may have just one. Fatigue, loss of appetite, and gastrointestinal or genitourinary problems are the most common complaints. This disorder is most frequently seen in women of lower socioeconomic status. The course of the disorder is unpredictable, and often another mental or physical disorder

(text continues on page 574)

NURSING CARE PLAN 23.1
Nursing Care Plan for a Patient
With Somatization Disorder

SC is a 48-year-old woman who is making her weekly visit to her primary care physician for unexplained multiple somatic problems. This week, her concern is reoccurring abdominal pain that fits no symptom pattern. Upon physical examination, a cause for her abdominal pain could not be found. She is requesting a refill of alprazolam (Xanax) which is the only medication that re-lieves her pain. She is in the process of applying for dis-ability income because of being completely disabled by neck and shoulder pain. The physician and office staff avoid her whenever possible. The physician will not re-fill the prescription until SC is evaluated by the consult-ing mental health team that provides weekly evaluations and services.

SETTING: PRIMARY CARE OFFICE

Baseline Assessment: 48-year-old Caucasian, obese woman who appears very angry. She resents being forced to see a psychiatric clinician for the only medication that works. She denies any psychiatric problems or emotional distress. SC is wearing a short, black top and too tight slacks. Her hair is in curlers and she says that it is too much trouble to comb her hair. Her mental status is normal, but she admits to being slightly depressed and takes the alprazolam for her nerves. She says she has nothing to live for, but denies any thoughts of suicide. She is dependent on her children for everything and feels very guilty about it. She spends most of her waking hours going to various doctors and taking combinations of medications to relieve her pains. She has no friends or nonfamily social contacts because they would not be able to stand her.

Associated Psychiatric Diagnosis	*Medications*
Axis I: R/O depression	Premarin, 1.2 mg qd
Axis II: Somatization disorder	Hydroxynie HCL (Atarax), 25 mg tid
Axis III: S/P hysterectomy	Ranitidine HCL (Zantac), 150 mg with meals
S/P gastric bypass	Simethicone, 1,235 mg qid with meals
S/P carpel tunnel release	Calcium carbonate, 1,200 mg qd
Chronic shoulder, neck pain, vertigo	Multiple vitamin, qd
Axis IV: Social problems (father died 6 months ago, divorced 9 months)	Zolpidem tartrate (Ambien), 10 mg at hs PRN
Economic problems (small pension)	Ibuprofen, 600 mg q4h PRN pain
Occupational problems (potential disability)	Maalox, PRN
GAF = Current, 60	Preparation H suppositories
Potential, 75	

NURSING DIAGNOSIS 1: CHRONIC LOW SELF-ESTEEM

Defining Characteristics	*Related Factors*
Self-negating verbalizations (long-standing)	Feeling unimportant to family
Hesitant to try new things	Feeling rejected by husband
Expresses guilt	Constant physical problems interfering with
Evaluates self as being unable to deal with events	normal social activities

OUTCOMES

Initial	*Long-term*
Identify need to increase self-esteem	Participate in individual or group therapy for esteem building

INTERVENTIONS

Interventions	*Rationale*	*Ongoing Assessment*
Establish rapport with patient	Individuals with low self-esteem are reluctant to discuss true feelings	Self-exam feelings provoked by pa-tient (discuss with supervisor if interfering with care). Determine if patient is beginning to engage in a relationship.

(continued)

NURSING CARE PLAN 23.1 (Continued)

Encourage patient to spend time dressing and grooming appropriately.	Confidence and self-esteem improve when a person looks well-groomed.	Monitor response to suggestions.
Encourage patient to discuss various somatic problems, but allow some time to discuss psychological & interpersonal issues.	Patients with somatization disorder need time to express their physical problems. It helps them feel valued. The best way to build a relationship is to acknowledge physical symptoms.	Monitor time that patient spends explaining physical symptoms.
Explore opportunities for SC to meet other people with similar, nonmedical interests.	Focus SC on meeting others will improve the possibilities of increasing contacts.	Observe willingness to identify other interests besides physical problems.

EVALUATION

Outcomes	Revised Outcomes	Interventions
SC admitted to having low self-esteem, but was very reluctant to consider meeting new people.	Focus on building self-esteem.	Identify activities that will enhance personal self-esteem.

NURSING DIAGNOSIS 2: INEFFECTIVE THERAPEUTIC REGIMEN MANAGEMENT

Defining Characteristics	Related Factors
Choices of daily living ineffective for meeting health care goal. Verbalizes difficulty with prescribed regimens.	Inappropriate use of benzodiazepines for nerves.

OUTCOMES

Initial	Long-term
Honestly discuss the use of medications.	Use nonpharmacologic means to for stress reduction, especially antianxiety medications.

INTERVENTIONS

Interventions	Rationale	Ongoing Assessment
Clarify the frequency and purpose of taking alprazolam.	Unsupervised polypharmacy is very common with these patients. Further clarification is usually needed.	Carefully track self-report of medication use; determine if patient is disclosing the use of all medications.
Educate patient about the effects of combining medications, emphasizing negative effects.	Education about combining medication is the beginning of helping patient become effective in medication regimen.	Observe patient's ability and willingness to consider negative effects.
Recommend that patient gradually reduce number of medications and problem-solve other means of managing physical symptoms.	Giving patients clear directions about managing health care regimens needs to be followed up with specific strategies to change behavior.	Evaluate patient's ability to problem solve.

EVALUATION

Outcomes	Revised Outcomes	Interventions
Patient disclosed use of medications, but was unwilling to consider changing ineffective use of medication.	Identify next step if primary care physician does not refill prescription.	Discuss the possibility of not being able to obtain alprazolam. Refer patient to mental health clinic for further evaluation.

is diagnosed. For this disorder, nursing care is similar to that for somatization disorder.

In many other parts of the world, the term *neurasthenia* is used to describe a syndrome of chronic fatigue and weaknesses. In the United States, these individuals would be diagnosed as having undifferentiated somatoform disorder if it has lasted for 6 months.

Conversion Disorder

In conversion disorder, the somatic symptoms pertain specifically to neurologic conditions affecting voluntary motor or sensory function, called **pseudoneurologic symptoms**. Patients with conversion disorder patient present with symptoms of impaired coordination or balance, paralysis, aphonia (inability to produce sound), difficulty swallowing, or a sensation of a lump in the throat and urinary retention. They also may have loss of touch, vision problems, blindness, deafness, and hallucinations. In some instances, they may have seizures (APA, 2000). These symptoms do not follow neurologic paths, but rather follow the individual's conceptualization of the problem. If only the pseudoneurologic symptoms are present, the patient is diagnosed with conversion disorder. It is important for the nurse to realize that the physical sensation is real for the patient. In approaching this patient, the nurse treats the conversion symptom as a real symptom and focuses on helping the patient deal with it. As trust develops within the nurse–patient relationship, the nurse can help the patient develop problem-solving approaches to everyday problems.

Pain Disorder

In pain disorder, pain severe enough to seek medical attention interferes with social and occupational functioning. The onset of the pain is associated with psychological factors, such a traumatic or humiliating experience. Because of the pain, the individual cannot return to work or school. Unemployment, disability, and family problems frequently follow. Pain disorder is believed to be relatively common. It is estimated that 10% to 15% of adults in the United States within a given year have disability from back pain (APA, 2000). Pain disorder may occur at any age. Women experience headaches and musculoskeletal pain more often than men. Acute pain tends to be resolved within a short period of time. Chronic pain may be present for many years. Pain medication should be conservatively prescribed. If mood disorders are also present, mood stabilizers not only may treat the depression but also may treat the pain (Maurer et al., 1999). Nursing care fo-

cuses on helping patients identify strategies to relieve pain and to examine stressors in their lives.

Hypochondriasis

The difference between hypochondriasis and the other somatoform disorders is that patients with hypochondriasis are preoccupied with their fears about developing a serious illness based on their misinterpretation of body sensations. In hypochondriasis, the fear of having an illness continues despite medical reassurance and interferes with the psychosocial functioning. These individuals spend time and money on repeated examinations looking for feared illnesses. For example, an occasional cough or the appearance of a small sore results in the person making an appointment with a oncologist. Hypochondriasis sometimes appears if the patient had a serious childhood illness or if a family member has a serious illness. The prevalence of hypochondriasis in the general medical practice is estimated to be between 2% and 7% (APA, 1994). These patients are most likely seen in medical-surgical settings unless they have a coexisting psychiatric disorder.

Several interventions have been effective in reducing patients' fears of developing serious illnesses. CBT, stress management, and group interventions lead to a decrease in intensity and increase in control of symptoms (Fava et al., 2000; Walker et al., 1999). It is unclear whether the positive outcomes are a result of the intervention itself or the symptom validation and increased attention that is given to the patient. However, based on these studies, nursing management should include listening to the patient's report of symptoms and fears, validating that the fears may be real, asking the patient to monitor symptoms in a journal, and encouraging the patient to bring the journal to the next visit. By actually seeing the symptom pattern, the nurse can continue to educate the patient and assess for significant symptoms. The outcome of this approach should be a decrease in fears and better control of the symptoms.

Body Dysmorphic Disorder

Patients with body dysmorphic disorder (BDD) focus on real (but slight) or imagined defects in appearance, such as a large nose, thinning hair, or small genitals. Preoccupation with the defect causes significant distress and interferes with their ability to function socially. They feel so self-conscious that they avoid work or public situations. Some are fearful that their "ugly" body part will malfunction. It occurs equally in men and women, but little epidemiologic data are available. In anxiety disorders and depression, BDD is estimated to occur in 5% to 40% of patients (APA, 2000). BDD may be present in 25% of patients with anorexia nervosa (Rabe-Jablonska et al., 2000). In the field of dermatology and cosmetic surgery, the estimate is 6% to 15% (Phillips et al., 1995, 2000).

BDD usually begins in adolescence and continues throughout adulthood. These individuals are not usually seen in psychiatric settings unless they have a co-existing psychiatric disorder or a family member insists on psychiatric attention. BDD is an extremely debilitating disorder and can significantly impair an individual's quality of life (Text Box 23-5). The obvious nursing diagnosis is Impaired Body Image. While focusing on developing a therapeutic relationship, the nurse should respect these patients' preoccupation and avoid challenging beliefs. However, the nurse should also assess the extent of preoccupation with the body part associated with BDD. If the patient is actually disfigured, the preoccupation may take on a phobic quality (Newell, 1999). If so, referral to a mental health specialist should be considered. The generalist nurse can help the patient by developing interventions for other nursing diagnoses that may be present, such as Social Isolation, Low Self-Esteem, and Ineffective Coping.

TEXT BOX 23.5

Clinical Vignette: Body Dysmorphic Disorder

Joan is a 16-year-old white girl who has been suffering for about 6 months from the belief that her pubic bone was becoming increasingly dislocated and prominent. She believed that everyone would stare at and talk about it. She did not remember a particular event that was related to the appearance of the symptom, but was absolutely convinced that she could only be helped by a surgical correction of her pubic bone. She had recently been treated for anorexia nervosa with marginal success. Although her weight was close to normal, she continued to be preoccupied with the looks of her body. She spent almost the entire day in her bedroom, wearing excessively large pajamas, and she refused to leave the house. Once or twice a day, she lowered herself to the ground and measured, with her fingers, the distance between her pelvic girdle and the ground in order to check the position of the pubic bone. Her parents were desperate and called the clinic for help. The family was referred to a home health agency and a psychiatric–home health nurse who arranged for an assessment visit.

Critical Thinking Questions

- How should the nurse approach Joan? Should she begin an assessment immediately?

- From the vignette, identify nursing diagnoses, outcomes, and interventions.

Adapted from Sobanski, E., & Schmidt, M. H. (2000). "Everybody looks at my pubic bone"—a case report of an adolescent patient with body dysmorphic disorder. *Acta Psychiatric Scandinavia, 101*(1), 80–82.

FACTITIOUS DISORDERS

The other type of psychiatric disorders characterized by somatization is factitious disorders; patients with these disorders intentionally cause an illness or injury to receive the attention of health care workers. These individuals are motivated solely by the desire to become a patient and develop a dependent relationship with a health care provider. There are two classes of factitious disorders: factitious disorder and factitious disorder, not otherwise specified.

FACTITIOUS DISORDER

Even though feigned illnesses have been described for centuries, it was not until 1951 that the term *Münchausen's syndrome* was used to describe the most severe form of this disorder, which was characterized by fabricating a physical illness, having recurrent hospitalizations, and going from one provider to another (Asher, 1951). Today, this disorder is called factitious disorder and is differentiated from **malingering**, in which the individual who intentionally produces illness symptoms is motivated by another specific self-serving goal, such as being classified as disabled or avoiding work.

Unlike the overt self-injury typical of people with borderline personality disorder, who readily admit to self-harm, patients with factitious disorder injure themselves covertly. The illnesses are produced in such a manner that the health care provider is tricked into believing that a true physical or psychiatric disorder is present. The *DSM-IV-TR* identifies three subtypes of factitious disorder: (1) one that has predominantly psychological symptoms, (2) one that has predominately physical symptoms (Münchausen's syndrome), and (3) one that has a combination of physical and psychological manifestations, with neither one predominating (APA, 2000).

The self-produced physical symptoms appear as medical illnesses and cut across all body systems. They include seizure disorders, wound-healing disorders, the abscess processes (introduction of infectious material below the skin surface), and feigned fever (rubbing the thermometer). These patients are extremely creative in simulating illnesses and tell fascinating, but false, stories of personal triumph. These tales are referred to as **pseudologia fantastica** and are a core symptom of the disorder. Pseudologia fantastica are stories that are not entirely improbable and often contain a matrix of truth and falsehood. These patients falsify blood, urine, and other samples by contaminating them with protein or fecal material. They self-inject anticoagulants to be diagnosed with "bleeding of undetermined origin" or ingest thyroid hormones to produce thyrotoxicosis. They also inflict injury on themselves by inserting objects or feces into body orifices, such as the urinary tract and open wounds. They produce their own surgical scars, especially abdominal, and when treated surgically, they delay wound healing through scratching, rubbing, or manipulating the wound and introducing bacteria into the wound. These patients put themselves in life-threatening situations through actions such as ingesting allergens known to produce an anaphylactic reaction. Individuals who produce physical illnesses are often members of the health care field who have the knowledge to create an illness. For example, one nurse developed hypoglycemia after a miscarriage. The hypoglycemia was eventually diagnosed as being induced with insulin injections (Eisendrath, 1996).

Patients who manifest primarily psychological symptoms produce psychotic symptoms such as hallucinations and delusions, cognitive deficits such as memory loss, dissociative symptoms such as amnesia, and conversion symptoms such as pseudoblindness or pseudoparalysis. These individuals often become psychotic, depressed, or suicidal after an unconfirmed tragedy. When questioned about details, they become defensive and uncooperative. Sometimes, these individuals have a combination of both physical and psychiatric symptoms.

Epidemiology

The prevalence of this disorder is unknown because of the difficulty in diagnosing it and obtaining reliable data. It has had a higher prevalence when researchers were actually looking for the disorder in specific populations. Within large general hospitals, factitious disorders are diagnosed in about 1% of patients with whom mental health professionals consult. The age range of patients with the disorder is between 19 and 64 years. The median age of onset is the early 20s. Once thought to occur predominantly in men, now a preponderance of women are being described with the disorder. No genetic pattern has been implicated, but it does seem to run in families. Many of these people have comorbid psychiatric disorders, such as mood disorders, personality disorders, and substance-related disorders.

Etiology

The etiology of factitious disorders is believed to have a psychodynamic basis. The theory is that these individuals, who were often abused as children, received nurturance only during times of illness; hence, they try to re-create illness or injury in a desperate attempt to receive love and attention. During the actual self-injury, the individual is reported to be in a trance-like, dissociative state. Many patients report having an intimate relationship with a health care provider, either as a child or as an adult, and then experiencing rejection when the relationship ended. The self-injury and subsequent attention is an attempt by the individual to reenact those experiences and gain control over the situation and other person. Often, the patient exhibits aggression after being discovered, allowing them to express revenge on their perceived tormenter (Feldman & Ford, 2000).

These patients are usually discovered in medical-surgical settings. They are hostile and distance themselves from others. Their network is void of friends and family and usually consists only of health care providers, who change at regular intervals. In factitious disorder, the patients fabricate a detailed and exaggerated medical history. When the interventions do not work and the fabrication is discovered, the health care team feels manipulated and angry. When the patient is confronted with the evidence, he or she becomes enraged and often leaves that health care system, only to enter another. Eventually, the person is referred for mental health treatment. The course of the disorder usually consists of intermittent episodes (APA, 2000).

NURSING MANAGEMENT: HUMAN RESPONSE TO DISORDER

The overall goal of treatment is for the patient to replace the dysfunctional, attention-seeking behaviors with positive behaviors. To begin treatment, the deception needs to be acknowledged by the patient. The mental health team needs to be able to accept and value the patient as a human being who needs help. The pattern of self-injury is well established and meets overwhelming psychological needs. Giving up the behaviors is difficult. The treatment is long-term psychotherapy. The generalist psychiatric–mental health nurse will most likely care for the patient during or after periods of feigned illnesses. More is known about the treatment of individuals with factitious physical disorders than psychological disorders.

A nursing assessment should focus on obtaining a chronicle history of medical and psychological illnesses. Physical disabilities should be identified. Early childhood experiences focusing on instances of abuse, neglect, or abandonment should be identified to understand the underlying psychological dynamics of the individual and the role of self-injury. Family relationships become strained as the members become aware of the self-inflicted nature of this disorder. Family assessment is important. The nursing diagnoses could include almost any diagnosis, including Risk for Trauma, Risk for Self-Mutilation, Ineffective Individual Coping, or Low Self-Esteem. Outcomes target decreasing self-injurious behaviors and supporting positive coping behaviors. Any nursing intervention needs to be implemented within the context of a strong nurse–patient relationship.

Nurses are continually faced with examining their own feelings about these patients. The fabrications and deceits of these individuals provoke anger and a sense of betrayal in the nurse. To be effective with these patients, the nurse must be aware of these feelings and resolve them by developing a better understanding of the underlying psychodynamic issues. Confronting the patient has been reported effective if the patient feels supported and accepted and if there is clear communication among the patient, mental health care team, and family members. All care for patients should be centralized within one facility, and the patient should be seen regularly by providers, even when the individual has no active crisis. Offering the patient a face-saving way of giving up the factitious disorder is often crucial. The treatment goal is recovery, not confession. Behavioral techniques that shape new behaviors help the patient move forward toward a new life (Eisendrath & Feder, 1996).

Continuum of Care

The goal is for care to be given within the context of one system. A team that knows the patient, agrees on a treatment approach, and follows through is crucial to the patient's eventual recovery. For this to happen, the medical, psychiatric, inpatient, and outpatient teams need to communicate with each other on a regular basis. Family members must be aware of the need for consistency in treatment.

FACTITIOUS DISORDERS, NOT OTHERWISE SPECIFIED

This diagnosis, factitious disorder, not otherwise specified, is reserved for those people who do not quite meet the all the diagnostic criteria of factitious disorder (Table 23-2). Within the category of factitious disorder, not otherwise specified, the *DSM-IV* (APA, 2000) includes a rare, but dramatic disorder, factitious disorder by proxy, or Münchausen's by proxy, which involves another person, usually the mother, who inflicts injuries on her child to gain the attention of the health care provider through her child's injuries. These actions include inducing seizures, poisoning, or smothering. This most severe form of child abuse is usually identified in the emergency room. The mother rarely admits injuring the child and, therefore, is not amenable to treatment and the child is removed from the care of the

---

TABLE 23.2 **Key Diagnostic Characteristics of Factitious Disorder**
300.16 With predominantly psychological signs and symptoms
300.19 With predominantly physical signs and symptoms
300.19 With combined psychological and physical signs and symptoms

Diagnostic Criteria and Target Symptoms	Associated Findings

• Intentionally producing psychological or physical signs and symptoms
   Subjective complaints, such as pain in absence of pain
   Self-inflicted conditions
   Exaggeration or exacerbation of preexisting medical conditions
   Any combination or variation
• Motivated by need to assume sick role
• Absence of external incentives for behavior
	Associated Behavioral Findings
	• Very dramatic, but vague, inconsistent history
	• Pathologic lying about history to intrigue listener
	• Extensive knowledge of medical terminology and hospital routines
	• Repeated hospitalizations in numerous hospitals, in many locations
	• Complaints of pain and requests for analgesics common
	• Eagerly undergo extensive workups with invasive procedures and operations
	• Deny allegations that symptoms are factitious once revealed, usually followed by rapid discharge against medical advice
	(With predominantly psychological signs and symptoms)
	• Claims of depression, suicidal ideation, auditory and visual hallucinations, recent and remote memory loss, and dissociative symptoms
	• Extremely suggestible
	• Negativistic and uncooperative when questioned
	
	Associated Physical Examination
	• Severe right lower quadrant pain with nausea and vomiting, massive hemoptysis, generalized rashes and abscesses, fever of unknown origin, bleeding secondary to ingestion of anticoagulants, and "lupus-like" syndromes
	• Symptoms limited to person's knowledge, sophistication, and imagination

mother. This form of child abuse is distinguished from other forms by the routine involvement (unknowingly) of health care workers who subject the child to physical harm and emotional distress through tests, procedures, and medication trials (Rand, 1996).

Summary of Key Points

➤ Somatization is psychological stress that is manifested in physical symptoms and is the chief characteristic of somatoform disorders and factitious disorders. The difference between these two types of disorders is that in somatoform disorders, the individuals suffer unexplained physical symptoms but do not self-inflict injuries, whereas in factitious disorders, the individual self-inflicts injuries to gain medical attention.

➤ Somatization has been shown to be affected by sociocultural and gender factors. It occurs more frequently in women than men; more frequently in those less educated; those living in urban areas, those who are older, separated, widowed, divorced; and in Mexican American women more than non-Hispanic women.

➤ The somatoform disorders are clustered into six different clinical syndromes: (1) somatization disorder, (2) undifferentiated somatoform disorder, (3) conversion disorder, (4) pain disorder, (5) hypochondriasis, and (6) body dysmorphic disorder. The person with somatization disorder suffers multiple physical problems and symptoms, in contrast to the other clinical subtypes, in which one major symptom recurs.

➤ Somatization disorder, the most complex of the somatoform disorders, is a chronic relapsing condition characterized by multiple physical symptoms that develop during times of emotional distress and occurs primarily in women.

➤ Factitious disorders include two subtypes: (1) factitious disorder and (2) factitious disorder, not otherwise specified. In factitious disorder, physical or psychological symptoms (or both) are fabricated to assume the sick role. Factitious disorder, not otherwise specified includes factitious disorder by proxy, the intentional productions of symptoms in others, usually children.

➤ There are many complexities in identifying and diagnosing patients with somatoform and factitious disorders because they refuse to accept any psychiatric basis to their problems and often go for years moving from one health care provider to another to receive medical attention and avoid psychiatric assessment.

➤ These patients are often seen on the medical-surgical units of hospitals and go years without being properly diagnosed. In most cases, they finally receive mental health treatment because of comorbid conditions, such as depression and panic.

➤ The development of the nurse–patient relationship is crucial to assessing these patients and identifying appropriate nursing diagnoses and interventions. Because these patients deny any psychiatric basis to their problem and continue to focus on their symptoms as being medically based, the nurse must take a flexible, relaxed, and nonjudgmental approach that acknowledges the symptoms, but focuses on new ways of coping with stress and avoiding recurrence of symptoms.

➤ Health teaching is important in helping the individual develop positive lifestyle changes in place of somatization responses. Identifying personal strengths and supporting the development of positive skills improve self-esteem and personal confidence. Teaching the use of biofeedback and relaxation provides the patient with positive coping skills.

Critical Thinking Challenges

1. A depressed young white woman is admitted to a psychiatric unit in a state of agitation. She reports extreme abdominal pain. Her admitting provider tells you that she has a classic case of somatization disorder and to deemphasize her physical symptoms. Under no circumstances is she to have any pain medication. Conceptualize the assessment process and how you would approach this patient.

2. Compare and contrast somatoform disorders with factitious disorders.

3. Develop a continuum of "self-injury" for patients with borderline personality disorder, somatization disorder, factitious disorder, and factitious disorder by proxy.

4. Develop a teaching plan for an individual who has a long history of somatization disorder, but who was also recently diagnosed with breast cancer. How will the patient be able to differentiate the physical symptoms of somatization disorder from those associated with the treatment of her breast cancer?

5. A Chinese American patient was admitted for panic attacks and numerous somatic problems, ranging from dysmenorrhea to painful joints. All medical examinations have been negative. She truly believes that her panic attacks are caused by a weak heart. What approaches should the nurse use in providing culturally sensitive nursing care?

6. A person with depression is started on Nardil, 15 mg tid. She believes that she is allergic to most foods, but insists on having wine in the evenings because it helps digest her food. Develop a teaching plan that provides the knowledge that she needs to prevent a hypertensive crisis caused by excessive tyramine but that is sensitive to the patient's food preferences.

WEB LINKS

www.athealth.com   Somatization and somatoform disorders. Friday's Progress Notes, July 14, 2000, Mental Health Information, Volume 4, Issue 21.

www.intelihealth.com   InteliHealth provides health information. Somatization disorder can be found through a search on this website.

MOVIES

Freud: 1962. This is an account of Sigmund Freud's life and the development of his early psychiatric theories and treatment. The film focuses on his struggle for acceptance in the Viennese medical community, rather than on the development of his actual theories. However, conversion disorder is depicted in his patients throughout this movie.

Significance: Somatoform disorders are rarely clearly depicted in films. This movie has examples of people with somatoform disorders.

Viewing Points: Identify the symptoms of somatoform disorder.

Fatal Attraction: 1987. This award-winning film portrays the relationship between a married attorney, played by Michael Douglas, and Alex Forest, a single woman played by Glenn Close. Their one night affair turns into a nightmare for Douglas' character and his family as Alex becomes increasingly possessive and aggressive.

Significance: The main character demonstrates behaviors characteristic of borderline personality disorder: anger, impulsivity, emotional liability, fear of rejection and abandonment, vacillation between adulation and disgust, and self-mutilation.

Viewing Points: Indentify the behaviors of Alex that are characteristics of borderline personality disorder. Identify the feelings that are generated by the movies. With which characters do you identify? For which characters do you feel sympathy? If Alex has lived and had been admitted to your hospital, what would be your first priority?

REFERENCES

American Psychiatric Association. (2000). *Diagnostic and statistical manual of mental disorders* (4th ed., Text revision). Washington, DC: Author.

Asher, R. (1951). Münchausen's syndrome. *Lancet, 1,* 339–341.

Biederman, J., Farone, S., Keenan, K., et al. (1992). Further evidence for family-genetic risk factors in attention deficit hyperactivity disorder. *Archives of General Psychiatry, 49*(9), 728–738.

Cloninger, C., Martin, R., Guze, S., & Clayton, P. (1986a). A prospective follow-up and family study of somatization in men and women. *American Journal of Psychiatry, 143*(7), 873–878.

Cloninger, C., von Knorring, A., Sigvardsson, S., et al. (1986b). Symptoms patterns and causes of somatization in men. II. Genetic and environmental independence from somatization in women. *General Epidemiology, 3*(3), 171–185.

Drake, M., Padamadan, H., & Pakainis, A. (1988). EEG frequency analysis in conversion and somatoform disorder. *Clinical Electroencephalography, 19*(3), 123–128.

Eisendrath, S. (1996). Current overview of factitious physical disorders. In M. Feldman & S. Eisendrath (Eds.), *The spectrum of factitious disorders* (pp. 21–36). Washington, DC: American Psychiatric Press.

Eisendrath, S., & Feder, A. (1996). Management of factitious disorders. In M. Feldman & S. Eisendrath (Eds.), *The spectrum of factitious disorders* (pp. 195–231). Washington, DC: American Psychiatric Press.

Escobar, J., Burnman, A., Karno, M., et al. (1987). Somatization in the community. *Archives of General Psychiatry, 44*(8), 713–718.

Fava, G., Grandi, S., Rafanelli, C., et al. (2000). Explanatory therapy in hypochondriasis. *Journal of Clinical Psychiatry, 61*(4), 317–323.

Flor-Henry, P., Fromm-Auch, D., Tapper, M., & Schopflocher, D. (1981). A neuro-psychological study of the stable syndrome of hysteria. *Biological Psychiatry, 16*(7), 601–626.

Ganesan, S., Fine, S., & Lin, T. (1989). Psychiatric symptoms in refugee families from South East Asia: Therapeutic challenges. *American Journal of Psychotherapy, 43*(2), 218–228.

Garcia-Campayo, J., & Sanz-Carrillo, C. (2000). The use of alternative medicines by somatoform disorder patients in Spain. *British Journal of General Practice, 50*(455), 487–488.

Garyfallos, G., Adamopoulou, A., Karastergious, A., et al. (1999). Somatoform disorder: Comorbidity with other DSM-III-R psychiatric diagnoses in Greece. *Comprehensive Psychiatry, 40*(4), 299–307.

Gordon, E., Kraiuhin, C., Meares, R., & Howson, A. (1986). Auditory evoked response potentials in somatization disorder. *Journal of Psychiatric Research, 20*(3), 237–248.

Guggenheim, F. (2000). Somatoform disorders. In B. Sadock & V. Sadock (Eds.), *Kaplan & Sadock's comprehensive textbook of psychiatry* (7th ed., pp. 1504–1532). Philadelphia: Lippincott Williams & Wilkins.

Gureje, O., & Simon, G. E. (1999). The natural history of somatization in primary care. *Psychological Medicine, 29*(3), 669–676.

Gureje, O., Simon, G. E., Ustun, T. B., et al. (1997). Somatization in cross-cultural perspective: A World Health Organization study in primary care. *American Journal of Psychiatry, 154*(7), 989–995.

Hotopt, M., Mayou, R. W., & Michael Wessely, S. (1999). Childhood risk factors for adults with medically unexplained symptoms: Results from a national birth cohort study. *American Journal of Psychiatry, 156*(11), 1796–1800.

Feldman, M., & Ford, C. (2000). Factitious disorders. In B. Sadock & V. Sadock (Eds.), *Kaplan & Sadock's comprehensive textbook of psychiatry* (7th ed., pp. 1533–1543). Philadelphia: Lippincott Williams & Wilkins.

Kinzl, J., Traweger, C., & Bieble, W. (1995). Family background and sexual abuse associated with somatization. *Psychotherapy and Psychosomatics, 64*(2), 82–87.

Klonoff, E., Landrine, H., & Campbell, R. (2000). *Psychology of Women Quarterly, 24*(1), 93–99.

Krishnan, K. (1995). Monoamine oxidase inhibitors. In A. Schatzberg & C. Nemeroff (Eds.), *The American Psychiatric Press textbook of psychopharmacology* (pp. 183–194). Washington, DC: American Psychiatric Press.

Kroenke, K., & Swindle, R. (2000). Cognitive-behavioral therapy for somatization and symptom syndromes: A critical review of controlled clinical trials. *Psychotherapy Psychosomatics, 69*(4), 205–215.

Lieb, R., Pfister, H., Mastaler, M., & Wittchen, H. U. (2000). Somatoform syndromes and disorders in a representative population sample of adolescents and young adults: Prevalence, comorbidity and impairments. *Acta Psychiatr Scand, 101*(3), 194–208.

Maurer, I., Volz, H. P., & Sauer, H. (1999). Gabapentin leads to remission of somatoform pain disorder with major depression. *Pharmacopsychiatry, 32*(6), 255–257.

Nathanson, C. (1975). Illness and the feminine role: A theoretical review. *Social Science Medicine, 9*, 57–63.

Newell, R. J. (1999). Altered body image: A fear-avoidance model of psycho-social difficulties following disfigurement. *Journal of Advanced Nursing, 30*(5), 1230–1238.

Noyes R., Jr., Langbehn, D., Happel, R., et al. (1999). Health Attitude Survey: A scale for assessing somatizing patients. *Psychosomatics, 40*(6), 470–478.

Othmer, E., & DeSouza, C. (1985). A screening test for somatization disorder (hysteria). *American Journal of Psychiatry, 142*(10), 1146–1149.

Pennebaker, J., & Roberts, R. (1992). Toward a his and her theory of emotion: Gender differences in visceral perception. *Journal of Social and Clinical Psychology, 3*, 199–212.

Phillips, D., & Segal, B. (1969). Sexual status and psychiatric symptoms. *American Sociological Review, 34*(1), 58–72.

Phillips, K. A., Dufresne, R. J., Wilkel, C. S., & Vittorio, C. C. (2000). Rate of body dysmorphic disorder in dermatology patients. *Journal of American Academy of Dermatology, 42*(3), 436–441.

Phillips, K., Kim, J., & Hudson, J. (1995). Body image disturbance in body dysmorphic disorder and eating disorder: Obsessions or delusions? *Psychiatric Clinics of North America, 18*(2), 317–334.

Rabe-Jablonska, J. J., & Tomasz, M. (2000). The links between body dysmorphic disorder and eating disorders. *European Psychiatry, 15*(5), 302–305.

Rand, D. (1996). Comprehensive psychosocial assessment in factitious disorder by proxy. In M. Feldman & S. Eisendrath (Eds.), *The spectrum of factitious disorders* (p. 133). Washington, DC: American Psychiatric Press.

Sobanski, E., & Schmidt, M. H. (2000). "Everybody looks at my pubic bone"—a case report of an adolescent patient with body dysmorphic disorder. *Acta Psychiatric Scandinavia, 101*, 80–82.

Smith, F. (1990). *Somatization disorder in the medical setting.* (DHHS Publication No. ADM-90-1931). Rockville, MD: U.S. Government Printing Office.

Stewart, D. (1990). The changing faces of somatization. *Psychosomatics, 31*(2), 153–158.

Swartz, M., Landerman, R., Blazer, D., et al. (1989). Somatization in the community: A rural/urban comparison. *Psychosomatics, 30*(1), 44–53.

Swartz, M., Landerman, R., George, L., et al. (1990). Somatization disorder. In L. Robins & D. Regier (Eds.), *Psychiatric disorders in America.* New York: Free Press.

Verbrugge, L. (1985). Gender and health: An update on hypotheses and evidence. *Journal of Health and Social Behavior, 26*(3), 157–177.

Verbrugge, L., & Steiner, R. (1981). Physical treatment of men and women patients-sex bias or appropriate care? *Medical Care, 19*, 609–632.

Walker, J., Vincent, N., Furer, P., et al. (1999). Treatment preference in hypochondriasis. *Journal of Behavior Therapy & Experimental Psychiatry, 30*(4), 251–258.

Whitney, F., Sanger, E., Thomas, M., & Wolf-Wilets, V. (1988). A validation study of the nursing diagnosis "Somatization." *Archives of Psychiatric Nursing, 2*(6), 345–349.

Wool, C., & Barsky, A. (1994). Do women somatize more than men? *Psychosomatics, 35*(5), 445–452.

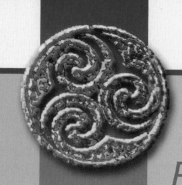

Eating Disorders

Jane H. White and Lyn Marshall

LEARNING OBJECTIVES

After studying this chapter, you will be able to:

➤ Distinguish the signs and symptoms of anorexia nervosa from those of bulimia nervosa.

➤ Describe two etiologic theories of both anorexia nervosa and bulimia nervosa.

➤ Explain the importance of body image, body dissatisfaction, and gender identity in developmental theories that explain etiology of eating disorders.

➤ Explain the impact of sociocultural norms on the development of eating disorders.

➤ Describe the risk factors and protective factors associated with the development of eating disorders.

CHAPTER 24

➤ Formulate the nursing diagnoses for individuals with eating disorders.

➤ Describe the nursing interventions for individuals with anorexia nervosa and bulimia nervosa.

➤ Differentiate binge eating disorder from bulimia nervosa.

➤ Analyze special concerns within the nurse–patient relationship for the nursing management of individuals with eating disorders.

➤ Identify strategies for prevention and early detection of eating disorders.

KEY TERMS

anorexia nervosa
binge eating
binge eating disorder
body image

bulimia nervosa
cue elimination
self-monitoring

KEY CONCEPTS

body dissatisfaction
body image distortion
dietary restraint
drive for thinness
enmeshment
interoceptive awareness
sexuality fears

*O*nly since the 1970s, have eating disorders have received national attention, primarily because several high-profile personalities and athletes with these disorders have received front-page news coverage. Since the 1960s, the increased incidence of anorexia nervosa and bulimia nervosa has prompted mental health professionals to address their cause and effective treatment. Moreover, there has been a concomitant increase in research studies addressing this intense obsession with being thin and the dissatisfaction with one's body that underlie these potentially life-threatening disorders. Thus, mental health professionals are crucial to prevention, early diagnosis, and treatment of both anorexia nervosa and bulimia nervosa.

This chapter focuses on anorexia nervosa and bulimia nervosa. In addition, binge eating disorder (BED), a newly identified eating disorder in its infancy relative to research, is briefly considered in this chapter. There is a significant overlap of symptoms in these disorders, such as dieting, binge eating, and preoccupation with weight and shape. Experts view the symptoms of these overlapping disorders along a continuum of normal to pathologic eating behaviors (White, 2000a) (Fig. 24-1). Viewing symptoms on a continuum assists in the identification of subclinical or subthreshold cases.

Many individuals with anorexia nervosa have bulimic symptoms, and many with bulimia nervosa have anorexic symptoms. For this reason, types of anorexia, such as the purging type, and types of bulimia, such as the restricting type, are differentiated based on the predominant symptom the individual uses to restrict food and weight. The definition and clinical course of both of these disorders, as well as their etiologies and interventions, differ and will be considered separately in this chapter. However, because the risk factors and prevention strategies for the development of anorexia nervosa and bulimia nervosa are similar, they will be discussed together, under one heading.

ANOREXIA NERVOSA

Clinical Course of Disorder

The onset of **anorexia nervosa** is usually early adolescence. The disorder can have a slow onset in that serious dieting can be present long before an emaciated body—the result of starvation—is noticed. A diagnosis is often made following this discovery. Because there is a higher incidence of subclinical or partial-syndrome cases, in which the symptoms are not severe enough to establish a diagnosis, many young women may not receive early treatment for their symptoms, or in some cases, they receive no treatment (see Fig. 24-1). Partial-syndrome cases are diagnosed in the American Psychiatric Association (APA's) *Diagnostic and Statistical Manual for Eating Disorders*, 4th ed., Text revision (*DSM-IV-TR*) *Eating*

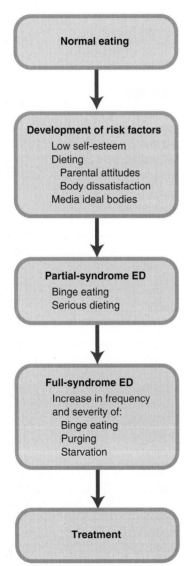

Normal eating

Development of risk factors
Low self-esteem
Dieting
Parental attitudes
Body dissatisfaction
Media ideal bodies

Partial-syndrome ED
Binge eating
Serious dieting

Full-syndrome ED
Increase in frequency
and severity of:
Binge eating
Purging
Starvation

Treatment

FIGURE 24.1 Continuum of dieting disorders with symptoms. ED, eating disorder.

Disorder Not Otherwise Specified (APA, 2000). The patient's refusal to maintain a normal weight because of a distorted body image and an intense fear of becoming fat makes this disorder difficult to identify and treat.

The long-term outcome of anorexia nervosa has improved in the last 15 to 20 years, because of an awareness of the disease and resulting early detection. It can, however, be a chronic condition, with relapses that are usually characterized by significant weight loss. The difficulty in reporting conclusive outcomes for anorexia nervosa is the result of the variety of definitions used to determine recovery. Even though patients determined to be recovered have restored weight and menses, some continue to be preoccupied with weight and food, many develop bulimia nervosa, and many continue to have symptoms of other psychiatric illnesses. In follow-up studies of patients 5 to 10 years after hospitalization for anorexia nervosa, 55% to 75% were considered fully recovered. Recovery time was lengthy and ranged from 57 to 79 months (Fichter & Quadflieg, 1999; Strober et al., 1997). In these and other studies, about 10% to 25% of patients go on to develop bulimia nervosa (White, 2000b). A poor outcome has been related to an initial lower minimum weight, the presence of purging (vomiting), and a later age of onset. Adolescents have better outcomes than adults, and younger adolescents have better outcomes than older adolescents (Fichter & Quadflieg, 1999).

Diagnostic Criteria

The diagnostic criteria for anorexia nervosa have been refined in each edition of the *Diagnostic and Statistical Manual for Mental Disorders* (APA, 2000). Research on core symptomatology has resulted in very specific criteria for a diagnosis of anorexia nervosa (Table 24-1). Originally, the most central feature of the disorder was thought to be a distorted body image (Bruch, 1973). However, whereas body image distortion remains an important criterion, recent investigators have highlighted the importance of a drive for thinness and fear of becoming fat as most essential to diagnosing anorexia nervosa (Wiederman & Pryor, 2000). Table 24-2 lists the common psychological characteristics of eating disorders. Recent diagnostic criteria have included a criterion for weight loss that is quite specific and necessary for a diagnosis—weight loss of 25 pounds. Refinement has also resulted in specific criteria for the absence of menses of at least three consecutive months or periods (APA, 2000).

Anorexia nervosa is further categorized into two major types: restricting and purging. Therefore, as noted earlier, there are some overlapping symptoms of anorexia nervosa and bulimia nervosa.

It is now more clearly understood that many of the clinical features associated with anorexia nervosa may re-

TABLE 24.1   Key Diagnostic Characteristics for Anorexia Nervosa

Diagnostic Criteria	Target Symptoms and Associated Findings
• Refusal to maintain body weight at or above a minimally normal weight for age and height • Intense fear of gaining weight or becoming fat, even though underweight • Disturbance in way person experiences body shape or weight • Undue influence of body weight or shape on self-evaluation or denial of seriousness of current low body weight • Absence of at least three consecutive menstrual cycles (in postmenarchal females) • Restricting type: not regularly engaged in binge eating or purging behavior (such as self-induced vomiting or misuse of laxatives, diuretics, or enemas) • Binge eating and purging type: regularly engaging in binge eating or purging behavior	• Depressive symptoms such as depressed mood, social withdrawal, irritability, insomnia, and diminished interest in sex. • Obsessive-compulsive features related and unrelated to food • Preoccupation with thought of food • Concerns about eating in public • Feelings of ineffectiveness • Strong need to control one's environment • Inflexible thinking • Limited social spontaneity and overly restrained initiative and emotional expression ***Associated Physical Examination Findings*** • Complaints of constipation, abdominal pain • Cold intolerance • Lethargy and excess energy • Emaciation • Significant hypotension, hypothermia, and skin dryness • Bradycardia and possible peripheral edema • Hypertrophy of salivary glands, particularly the parotid gland • Dental enamel erosion related to induced vomiting • Scars or calluses on dorsum of hand from contact with teeth for inducting vomiting ***Associated Laboratory Findings*** • Leukopenia and mild anemia • Elevated blood urea nitrogen • Hypercholesterolemia • Elevated liver function studies • Electrolyte imbalances, metabolic alkalosis, or metabolic acidosis • Low normal serum thyroxine levels; decreased serum triiodothyronine levels • Low serum estrogen levels • Sinus bradycardia • Metabolic encephalopathy • Significantly reduced resting energy expenditure • Increased ventricular/brain ratio secondary to starvation

TABLE 24.2   Psychological Characteristics Related to Eating Disorders

Anorexia Nervosa	*Anorexia Nervosa and Bulimia Nervosa*
Decreased interoceptive awareness Sexuality conflict/fears Maturity fears Ritualistic behaviors	Difficulty expressing anger Low self-esteem Body dissatisfaction Powerlessness Ineffectiveness Perfectionism Dietary restraint Obsessiveness Compulsiveness Nonassertiveness Cognitive distortions
Bulimia Nervosa Impulsivity Boundary problems Limit-setting difficulties	

sult from malnutrition or semistarvation. For example, classic research on volunteers who have been semi-starved and the result of observations of prisoners of war and conscientious objectors has demonstrated that, during these states, symptoms of food preoccupation, binge eating, depression, obsessionality, and apathy are present. Drastic measures to resist overeating persist long after the semistarvation experience, even when food is plentiful. The medical complications and well-established signs and symptoms of eating disorders that result from starving or binge eating and purging are presented in Table 24-3. Many somatic systems are compromised in individuals with eating disorders.

KEY CONCEPT Body image distortion. **Body image distortion** is how each individual perceives his or her body disparately from how the world or society views the individual.

For adolescents, body image is important because it has a complex psychological impact on the overall self-concept of this age group. It is a crucial factor in determining how adolescents interacts with others and think society will respond to them. For most individuals, body image is consistent with how others view the individual. Those with anorexia nervosa have a body image severely distorted from reality. They see themselves as fat, obese, and undesirable because of this perceived distortion, even when they are emaciated. They are unable to accept the reality and perceptions of the outside world. Perceptions, attitudes, and behaviors are all part of this disturbance. **Body image** in its simplest form refers to a mental picture of one's own body. Body image disturbance occurs when there is extreme discrepancy between one's own mental picture of his or her body and the perception of the outside world.

TABLE 24.3   Medical Complications of Eating Disorders

Body System	Symptoms
From Starvation to Weight Loss	
Musculoskeletal	Loss of muscle mass, loss of fat (emaciation) Osteoporosis
Metabolic	Hypothyroidism (symptoms include lack of energy, weakness, intolerance to cold, and bradycardia) Hypoglycemia, decreased insulin sensitivity
Cardiac	Bradycardia, hypotension, loss of cardiac muscle, small heart, cardiac arrhythmias including atrial and ventricular premature contractions, prolonged QT interval, ventricular tachycardia, sudden death
Gastrointestinal	Delayed gastric emptying, bloating, constipation, abdominal pain, gas, diarrhea
Reproductive	Amenorrhea, low levels of luteinizing hormone and follicle-stimulating hormone, irregular periods
Dermatologic	Dry, cracking skin and brittle nails due to dehydration, lanugo (fine baby-like hair over body), edema, acrocyanosis (bluish hands and feet); hair thinning
Hematologic	Leukopenia, anemia, thrombocytopenia, hypercholesterolemia, hypercarotenemia
Neuropsychiatric	Abnormal taste sensation (possible zinc deficiency) Apathetic depression, mild organic mental symptoms, sleep disturbances, fatigue
Related to Purging (Vomiting and Laxative Abuse)	
Metabolic	Electrolyte abnormalities, particularly hypokalemia, hypochloremic alkalosis; hypomagnesemia; increase blood urea nitrogen
Gastrointestinal	Salivary gland and pancreatic inflammation and enlargement with increase in serum amylase; esophageal and gastric erosion (esophagitis) rupture; dysfunctional bowel with haustral dilation; superior mesenteric artery syndrome
Dental	Erosion of dental enamel (perimyolysis), particularly frontal teeth with decreased decay
Neuropsychiatric	Seizures (related to large fluid shifts and electrolyte disturbances), mild neuropathies, fatigue, weakness, mild organic mental symptoms
Cardiac	Ipecac cardiomyopathy arrhythmias

Adapted from Yager, J. (1990). Eating disorders. In A. Stoudemire (Ed.), *Clinical psychiatry for medical students* (p. 324). Philadelphia: J. B. Lippincott; Litovitz, G., & White, J. (1994). Detecting eating disorders in your patients. *Internal Medicine, 15* (4), 54–63.

Because of this distortion, individuals with anorexia nervosa have an intense drive for thinness. Closely related to this is also a fear of fat. Thus, they see themselves as fat, fear becoming fatter, and are "driven" to work toward "undoing" this fear.

KEY CONCEPT **Drive for thinness. Drive for thinness** is an intense physical and emotional process that overrides all physiologic body cues, such as hunger and weakness.

The individual with anorexia nervosa ignores these body cues and concentrates all efforts on controlling food intake. The entire mental focus of the young patient with anorexia nervosa begins to narrow to only one goal: weight loss. Typical thought patterns are: "If I gain a pound, I'll keep gaining." This all-or-nothing thinking keeps these patients on rigid regimens for weight loss.

The behavior of patients with anorexia nervosa becomes organized around food-related activities, such as preparing food, counting calories, and reading cookbooks. Much of their behavior is ritualistic, such as what, when, and how they eat. Some food combinations and the order in which foods may be eaten, and under which circumstances, can seem almost bizarre. One anorexic patient, for example, would only eat cantaloupe, carrying it with her to all meals outside of her home, and consuming it only if it were cut-up in smaller than bite-sized pieces and only if she could use chopsticks, which she also carried with her.

Feelings of inadequacy and a fear of maturity are also characteristic of the clinical picture of the individual with anorexia nervosa. The weight loss becomes a way for these individuals to experience some sense of control and combat feelings of inadequacy and ineffectiveness. Every lost pound is viewed as a success. They often compare their feelings of weight loss to a feeling of virtuousness. Because they feel inadequate, they fear emotional maturation and the unknown of the next developmental stages they must encounter. For some of these individuals, remaining physically small is believed to symbolize remaining child-like.

Patients with anorexia nervosa also have difficulty defining feelings because they are confused about or unsure of emotions and visceral cues, such as hunger. This is called a lack of interoceptive awareness.

KEY CONCEPT **Interoceptive awareness. Interoceptive awareness** is a term used to describe the sensory response to emotional and visceral cues, such as hunger.

Patients with anorexia nervosa are confused about sensations; therefore, their responses to cues are inaccurate and inappropriate. This profound lack of interoceptive awareness is thought to be partially responsible for the development and maintenance of this disorder and, in some instances, in the development and maintenance of bulimia nervosa.

In addition, patients with anorexia nervosa avoid conflict and have difficulty expressing negative emotions, especially anger (Geller et al., 2000). These traits are also common in families of those who develop this disorder.

Because of the ritualistic behaviors accompanying anorexia nervosa, an all-encompassing focus on food and weight, and feelings of inadequacy, social contacts are gradually reduced, and the patient with anorexia nervosa becomes isolated from others. With more severe weight loss comes others symptoms, such as apathy, depression, and even mistrust of others.

Epidemiology

In this country, lifetime prevalence of anorexia nervosa is reported to be from 0.5% to 1%. The occurrence of anorexia nervosa is less common than that of bulimia nervosa. A similar prevalence is found in most Western countries. However, in non-Western countries such as Japan, the incidence is increasing and has been attributed to westernization (Nadoaka et al., 1996). Eating disorders among Chinese women in Hong Kong exposed to Western views of ideal body types have also increased. Chinese-American men and women living in the United States have higher rates of eating disorders than those living in their native country (Davis & Katzman 1999).

Age of Onset

The age of onset is typically between 14 and 16 years. Some experts have reported an even earlier age of onset. The vulnerability of adolescents is known to be the result of stressors associated with their development, especially body image concerns, autonomy, peer pressure, and the susceptibility to such influences as the media, which extols an ideal body type.

Gender Differences

Females are more likely than males to develop anorexia nervosa. The ratio of female to male prevalence is 10:1. The disparity in incidence and prevalence rates has been accounted for by society's influence on females to achieve an ideal body type. Text Box 24-1 highlights some of the findings about eating disorders in males. Many of these findings are preliminary because samples of males with eating disorders are generally limited.

Ethnic and Cultural Differences

In United States, eating disorders are as common or slightly more common among Hispanic and white populations and less common in African Americans and Asians (Fitzgibbon et al., 1998). In the last 15 to

TEXT BOX 24.1

Boys and Men With Eating Disorders

Eating disorders in boys and men are becoming more prevalent. Men are more likely to have a later onset than women, and at around age 20.5 years. Boys and men are also more likely to be involved in an occupation or sport in which weight control influences performance, such as wrestling (Braun et al., 1999).

Men with anorexia nervosa of the restricting type were found to have lower testosterone levels. In studies comparing men and women on psychological characteristics, men had lower drive for thinness and body dissatisfaction scores, but higher perfectionism scores (Joiner et al., 2000).

In another investigation, predictors of binge eating were different for men compared with women. Anger and depression preceded binges in men, whereas dieting failure was the most significant predictor of a binge in women (Costanzo et al., 1999).

20 years, the incidence among these other ethnic groups has increased.

Familial Predisposition

First-degree relatives of those with anorexia nervosa have higher rates of this disorder. When partial syndrome or subthreshold cases are considered, there are even higher rates in female family members of individuals with anorexia nervosa (Strober et al., 2000). Female relatives also have high rates of depression, leading researchers to hypothesize that there may be a shared genetic factor that influences the development of both disorders.

Comorbidity

Comorbid major depression and dysthymia are prevalent in individuals with anorexia nervosa (North & Gowers, 1999). Obsessive-compulsive disorder (OCD) and anxiety disorders are also prevalent comorbid conditions. It has been estimated that OCD is found in about 66% of women with anorexia nervosa (Thornton & Russell, 1997). In a large percentage of these individuals, OCD predated the anorexia nervosa diagnosis by about 5 years, leading many to see it as a causative factor in its development. Anxiety disorders such as phobias and panic disorder are also prevalent at high rates. Cluster C personality disorders are well-established comorbid conditions associated with anorexia nervosa (Kaye et al., 2000b). In most instances, these comorbid conditions may resolve when anorexia nervosa has been treated successfully. In other cases, symptoms of a premorbid condition, such as OCD, remain, even though

an individual has recovered from anorexia nervosa. This finding has influenced many experts to believe that many of the characteristics of anorexia nervosa, such as perfectionism, are trait rather than state characteristics and may actually influence the development of the disorder.

Etiology

There is an overlap between some of the risk factors for eating disorders and the etiologic factors. For example, dieting is a risk factor for the development of anorexia nervosa. It is also a biologic etiologic factor in its development, and in its most serious form—starving—it is a symptom as well. In considering etiologic factors, this overlap of risk factors, causes, and symptoms must be kept in mind. Viewing them along a continuum from less to more severe helps with this conceptualization (see Fig. 24-1). Most experts agree that anorexia nervosa (as well as bulimia nervosa) is multidimensional and multidetermined. Figure 24-2 depicts the biopsychosocial etiologic factors for anorexia nervosa.

Biologic Theories

Most of what is known about the etiology of anorexia nervosa is focused on psychological factors. There is little conclusive evidence regarding biologic theories of causation. Part of this difficulty is because of the many comorbid conditions associated with a diagnosis of anorexia nervosa. Some researchers view its development as a shared etiology with such comorbid conditions as depression and OCD. In addition, many of the biologic changes noted in anorexia nervosa have been determined to be the result of starvation and are considered state rather than trait or causative factors. Little evidence exists to substantiate that there are dysregulations in appetite-satiety systems causing anorexia nervosa. Appetite dysregulation is best viewed as the end product or result of an interaction between the environment and physiology. The biopsychosocial model of this interaction best explains the etiology (see Fig. 24-2).

Neuropathologic. Magnetic resonance imaging (MRI) and computed tomography (CT) have revealed a variety of changes in the brain of individuals with anorexia nervosa who have significant weight loss. For example, changes such as cerebral ventricular enlargement, in particular dilation of the third and lateral ventricles, and enlargement of the cortical sulci and the interhemispheric fusion have been found. All of these changes, however, were reversed in investigations in which individuals regained a normal body weight (Addolorato et al., 1997; Golden et al., 1996). To date, there is no evidence that brain structure changes cause anorexia nervosa.

Genetic. Research on the genetic influence in the development of eating disorders is in its infancy. There is

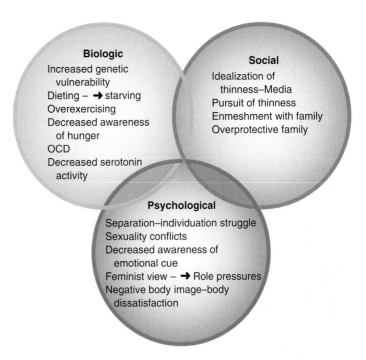

FIGURE 24.2 Biopsychosocial etiologies for patients with anorexia nervosa. OCD, obsessive-compulsive disorder.

little precise evidence supporting a specific gene influencing anorexia nervosa (Bulik et al., 2000). It is difficult to separate genetic influences from environmental influences when twins share a similar family environment. However, recently, investigators reviewing research on twin studies demonstrated that the concordance rate for monozygotic twins is higher (44%) than for dizygotic twins (12.5%), showing that there may be a genetic factor involved in the etiology of anorexia nervosa (Bulik et al., 2000). Most patients with anorexia nervosa have a comorbid condition or conditions, and this makes it difficult to determine the influence of genetics on the development of anorexia nervosa.

Biochemical. Studies of neurendocrine, neuropeptide, and neurotransmitter functioning in patients with eating disorders indicate that these systems may be related to the maintenance of the disorder. Endogenous opioids may contribute to the denial of hunger in patients with anorexia nervosa. Some studies have shown weight gain after opiate antagonists. Thyroid function is decreased as well. However, most of the research reported has established that these neurotransmitter and neuroendocrine abnormalities, such as serotonergic function seen in low-weight anorexic patients, must be viewed with caution as causative factors because these disturbances are state related and tend to normalize after symptom remission. At best, these changes may be viewed as the result of points of vulnerability for some individuals, who then, under certain psychological and environmental conditions, such as cultural pressures, starve themselves. In these individuals, central serotonergic function may be affected as a result (Ward et al., 2000).

Psychological Theories

The most widely accepted psychological theory explaining anorexia nervosa is psychoanalytic in origin. In this theory, separation-individuation and autonomy are interrupted key tasks. Struggles around identity and role, body image formation, and sexuality fears predominate as a result of developmental arrests.

Because anorexia nervosa is usually diagnosed between 14 and 18 years of age, developmental struggles of adolescence have long been an acceptable theory of causation (Bruch, 1973) Two key conflicts for this age group are autonomy and separation-individuation.

During early adolescence when individuals begin to establish their independence and autonomy, a conflict may develop for some girls who feel inadequate or ineffective. They may grow up in families in which they have not had an opportunity to "try out" independence. Thus, dieting and weight control are viewed as a means to defend against this conflict In later adolescence, when separation-individuation is a developmental task, similar conflicts arise when the adolescent is ill prepared for this stage and feels inadequate and ineffective in going forward emotionally.

Gender identity has been hypothesized to explain the significant difference in the number of girls versus boys who develop anorexia nervosa and bulimia nervosa. Studies have shown that girls and boys do not differ dramatically in self-esteem until just before adolescence. At the time self-doubt increases in girls, pubertal weight gain can also occur, resulting in a more rounded shape. Thus, normal occurrences can add to confusion about one's identity. Others believe that confusion and self-doubt are aided by conflicting messages young women receive from society about their roles in life. Expectations young girls may interpret about how they should look, what roles they should perform, and what they should achieve in society can pressure them into assuming they have to achieve "all." Young women who aspire to their interpretation of these expectations often try to please others to avoid conflicts around perceived expectations. Feminists have focused on this role pressure as one part of an explanation for the significant increase in eating disorders and for the prevalence in females versus males. Text Box 24-2 outlines some feminist assumptions regarding role, feminism, and the development of eating disorders.

KEY CONCEPT Sexuality fears. **Sexuality fears** are often underlying issues for patients with anorexia nervosa. Starvation is viewed as a response to these fears.

Onset of anorexia nervosa usually occurs during adolescence. This is a time when girls begin to date. Girls usually experience dating as more stressful than boys because intimacy is more of an emphasis for girls. Relationships are more important to girls, and they tend to attribute the failure of a relationship to an inadequacy in themselves (Streigel-Moore, 1993). A major trend over

the past several years is the involvement of girls sexually at increasingly younger ages. They are often ill prepared and can experience a great deal of pressure from peers to become sexually active. Parents may be unprepared to address sexual activity with daughters at younger ages than expected. The unavailability of parents to help with decisions can increase anxiety about them. Bruch (1973) has described self-starvation as the adolescent girl's response to her fear of adult sexuality. Sexual anxieties may promote binge eating as well, as a way of coping with this conflict.

Social Theories

More than any other psychiatric condition, society plays a significant role in the development of eating disorders. Sociologic theories about norms and expectations in a society explain some of the causes of eating disorders (Brumberg, 1988). As noted earlier, societal factors such as the media, the fashion industry, and peer pressure are significant influences. Magazines and television shows depict young girls and adolescents with thin and often emaciated bodies (Tiggerman & Pickering, 1996). Wanting to be like these models both in character and appearance influences girls to diet. For young girls, dolls such as Barbie® have been found to influence negatively their views of normal body types (Brownell & Napolitano, 1995) (see Research Box 24-1). In addition, many types of media discuss dieting and exercise as ways to achieve success, popularity, power, and the like. Comparing one's own body to the bodies of models produces significant body dissatisfaction. Body dissatisfaction has been a key characteristic associated with dieting, low self-esteem, and the development of an eating disorder.

KEY CONCEPT Body dissatisfaction. Particularly for women with bulimia nervosa, **body dissatisfaction** has been related to low self-esteem, depression, dieting, bingeing, and purging. The body becomes overvalued as a way of determining one's worth.

Once the body has been established as all-important, the individual begins to compare her body with others, such as celebrities. These images from television and fashion magazines are particularly powerful for young girls and adolescents struggling with the tasks of identity and body image formation. The dissatisfaction is the result of this comparison, perceiving to fall short of an ideal, and may be dissatisfaction about one's weight, shape, size, or even a certain body part. Even in the absence of overweight, dissatisfaction was present in most adolescents surveyed in numerous studies. Many adolescents act to overcome this dissatisfaction through dieting and overexercising. In those who have other risk factors and are thus more vulnerable, eating disorder symptoms develop.

TEXT BOX 24.2

Feminist Ideology and Eating Disorders

Since the 1970s, proponents of the feminist cultural model of eating disorders have advanced a position to explain the higher prevalence of these disorders in women. Feminists believe there is a struggle women have today similar to ones they believe women have had in history. They believe that during the Victorian era, "hysteria," a well-known emotional illness, developed as a result of oppression when women were not allowed to express their feelings and opinions and were "silenced" by a male-dominated society. Feminist scholars claim that women today are socialized to avoid self-expression in the face of conflict, seek attachment through putting others first, judge self by external standards, and present an outward compliant self while the inner self grows angry. They believe that the development of an eating disorder is a reaction against these expectations and norms of society (Gutwill, 1994).

Feminists have taken issue with what they call the biomedical model of explanation for the development of eating disorders, seeing it as limiting and patriarchal. It is the recovery of society that must take place to decrease the prevalence of eating disorders. Feminists believe that this will only occur when women are emancipated, given a voice, and socialized differently. They call for more research in which women are coresearchers as well as "subjects," helping to provide the investigators with their own stories and perspectives.

RESEARCH BOX 24.1

Barbie® and Ken® Dolls

A great deal of research has focused on ideal body types and how these affect American women such as Miss America contestants. This study was designed to examine body proportions in popular dolls, Barbie® and Ken®, to determine the extent to which they vary from the proportions of young, healthy adults. Measurements on young adult subjects, men and women, aged 22 to 32 years, who were of normal weight and average height, were taken. Hips, waist, chest, neck length, and neck circumference were recorded. The same measurements were made on Barbie and Ken dolls, and a ratio of the measurements of the real subjects to doll figures was calculated. The ratio was then applied to estimate changes needed for the subjects to have the same proportional measurements as the dolls.

The researchers found that for the female subject to attain Barbie's proportions, there would have to be an increase in 24 inches in height, 5 inches in the chest, and 2 to 3 inches in neck length and a decrease of 6 inches in the waist and 0.2 inches in the neck circumference. For the male subject to attain Ken's proportions, he would require increases in height by 20 inches, waist by 10 inches, chest by 11 inches, and neck length by 0.85 inches. The neck circumference for the male would need to increase 7.9 inches.

The results of this study provide more evidence that individuals are exposed to highly unrealistic models for shape and weight. Although Barbie and Ken dolls are not meant to show ideal proportions, the discrepancies are obvious. Healthy, normal-weight children use such models as standards for comparison, leading logically to an outcome of body dissatisfaction.

Utilization in the Clinical Setting: The findings from this study can be used to assist parents in choosing appropriate models for dolls for children. Also, this research provides a basis for helping women with eating disorders understand how subtle environmental cues influence the formulation of their ideal body types at an early age.

Brownell, K., & Napolitano, M. A. (1995). Distorting reality for children: Body size proportions for Barbie and Ken dolls. *International Journal of Eating Disorders, 18,* 295–298.

Family Responses

The family of the anorexic patient has classically been labeled as overprotective, enmeshed, being unable to resolve conflicts, and being rigid regarding boundaries.

KEY CONCEPT   **Enmeshment. Enmeshment** refers to an extreme form of intensity in family interactions.

Changes between two family members reverberate through the whole family system. Direct communication between members is blocked, and one member relays communication from another to a third. In an enmeshed family, the individual gets lost in the system. The boundaries that define individual autonomy are weak. This excessive togetherness intrudes on privacy (Minuchin et al., 1978).

Overprotectiveness is defined a high degree of concern for one another. The parent's overprotectiveness retards the child's development of autonomy and competence (Minuchin et al., 1978). *Rigidity* refers to families who are heavily committed to maintain the status quo and find change difficult. Conflict is avoided, and it is usually a strong ethical code or religious orientation that is the rationale. Today, more is known to amplify this original understanding of the family's impact on the development of anorexia nervosa (see Research Box 24-2).

In summary, no one etiologic factor is predominant in the development of anorexia nervosa. Biopsychosocial factors converge to contribute to its development.

Risk Factors

Risk factors in the development of eating disorders are well known. Similar factors put women at risk for both anorexia nervosa and bulimia nervosa. Risk factors are often classified in the same way as the etiologic categories: biologic, psychological, sociocultural, and family (Fig. 24-3).

Biologic

Dieting and weight gain or an increase in basal metabolic index (BMI) are the most significant biologic risk factors studied. Overexercising is also a risk factor. Girls at an early age begin to diet because of body dissatisfaction, a need for control, or prepubertal weight increase, making both actual weight gain and the fear of weight gain risk factors (Taylor et al., 1998). Sociocultural risk factors influence dieting. Ideal body type images prevalent in the media lead to dieting whether or not weight gain is present. This restriction of food can lead to starvation in the case of anorexia nervosa or to binge eating and purging for others. It is believed that this dieting and starvation lead to many of the physiologic, neuorologic, and metabolic symptoms in both anorexia nervosa and bulimia nervosa. High-level exercise and compulsive physical activity can precipitate and maintain such eating disorder symptoms as food obsessing, poor concentration, and binge eating (Davis et al, 1997).

Psychological

Low self-esteem, body dissatisfaction, and feelings of ineffectiveness also put individuals at risk for the development of an eating disorder. For example, investigators

RESEARCH BOX 24.2

Role of Mother–Daughter Relationship and Weight Concerns

The literature highlights two different possible roles for the mother–daughter relationship and how these roles influence the development of weight concerns measured by dietary restraint and body dissatisfaction. The first role is simply the mother's own modeling of her concerns about her weight; the second model influencing weight concerns that was tested is the actual interaction between mothers and daughters. *Interaction* was defined as how autonomous the mother was perceived to be by the daughter, and vice versa, how enmeshed they were emotionally, and the overall view of the mother's role. This study compared the two models of explanation and found no support for the first model, mothers simply being concerned about their own weight and dieting. The results showed that high body dissatisfaction and dietary restraint for the daughters were related to the mother's own belief as well as the daughter's

view of the mother's low autonomy. When both believed in factors that related to high enmeshment and unclear boundaries, more restraint and body dissatisfaction were found. This study lends support to a complex picture of risk factors in the families of girls who develop eating disorders. Whereas parental attitudes about weight shape and size have been shown to be important influences on body dissatisfaction for girls, modeling autonomy, clear boundaries, and valuing differentiation of family members (nonenmeshment) are also important family functions and tasks.

Utilization in the Clinical Setting: Assessment of parents and the family before providing psychoeducation should include questions related to whether boundaries are clear and whether members are autonomous or enmeshed.

Ogden, J., & Steward, J. (2000). The role of the mother–daughter relationship in explaining weight concern. *International Journal of Eating Disorders, 28*(11), 78–83.

have demonstrated that self-esteem regardless of body size influences eating disorder behavior. In numerous studies, dissatisfaction with one's body, influenced by culture, has been reported to influence dieting in adolescents, even if they did not have low self-esteem. Feeling ineffective in social situations has been predictive of eating disorder symptom development. Much of the recent research on these factors has demonstrated that in the presence of resilience or protective factors, such as ath-

letic achievement and family support, these risk factors can be mediated and the development of an eating disorder prevented (Fulkerson et al., 1999; Taylor et al., 1998).

Sociocultural

The media, fashion industry, and society's focus on the ideal body type are risk factors for eating disorders. In addition, peer pressure and peer attitudes influence eating behaviors. Some adolescents have reported that di-

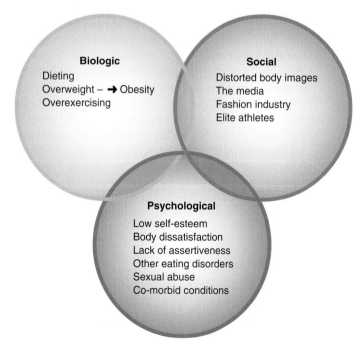

FIGURE 24.3 Biopsychosocial risk factors for anorexia and bulimia nervosa.

eting, binge eating, and purging were learned behaviors, resulting from peer pressure and a need to conform.

Athletes are at greater risk for the development of eating disorders because excessive exercise and perfectionism are thought to precipitate symptoms (Davis et al., 1999). Pressure from coaches and parents, along with the actual physical demands of a sport, can contribute to the development of these disorders as well. In particular, elite athletes, those who train for national and international competition, are more at risk (Garner et al., 1998). Ballet dancers are at high risk for developing eating disorders because of the need to maintain a particular appearance (see Research Box 24-3).

 ## Family

The family can transmit attitudes about weight, shape, and size that are unrealistic, often unwittingly. Adoles-

cents in particular are sensitive to comments about their bodies because this is the stage for body image formation. Thus, parental comments about weight or shape, or even parents' worrying about their own weight, can influence adolescents in similar ways as the does media (Smolak et al., 1999). Parental attitudes about weight have been found to influence body dissatisfaction and dieting. In investigations on attitudes, parents of individuals with eating disorders were found to have often teased girls about their weight, and mothers were found to overestimate their daughters' weight as opposed to their sons' (Schwartz et al., 1999). See Research Box 24-2 for further information about the role of mother–daughter relationships and body dissatisfaction.

Concurrent Disorders

Comorbidity has been discussed as an etiologic issue for eating disorders. Anorexia nervosa puts women at risk for developing bulimia nervosa. It has been estimated that 25% to 30% of women with anorexia nervosa go on to develop binge eating and purging (White, 2000b). This relationship has been explained as the result of anorexic patients never truly recovering and eventually turning to purging when restricting is no longer effective.

Sexual Abuse

Childhood sexual abuse has been suggested as a risk factor for eating disorders. Many investigations have supported the notion that, although childhood sexual abuse is seen in a larger percentage of women with bulimia nervosa than in the general population, the occurrence may not be more significant than the percentage found in women with other psychiatric disorders (Perkins & Luster, 1999). In both community and clinical samples of women with eating disorders and reported sexual abuse, other comorbid conditions, such as borderline personality disorder and substance abuse disorder, are also present (Casper & Lyubomorisky, 1997). Therefore, when a concurrent history of sexual abuse and an eating disorder is assessed, several other factors must be taken into account to clarify the nature of this relationship. Sequencing of events and the development of eating disorder symptoms need further research before this relationship can be conclusively established.

Interdisciplinary Treatment

The goals of treatment for the patient with anorexia nervosa focus on initiating nutritional rehabilitation, resolving conflicts around body image disturbance, increasing effective coping, addressing the underlying conflicts related to maturity fears and role conflict, and assisting the family with healthy functioning and communication. A variety of treatment modalities are used to accomplish these goals during the different stages of illness and recovery.

When selecting the type of treatment (ie, inpatient or outpatient) for anorexia nervosa and bulimia nervosa, clinicians rely on criteria that have been developed to assist them. Typically, the medical complications presented in Table 24-3 influence a decision to hospitalize an individual with an eating disorder. Suicidality is another reason for hospitalization. These specific established criteria for admission are outlined in Table 24-4.

In most instances, hospitalization of the anorexic patient will be necessary to restore weight. Individuals are admitted to a specialized eating disorder unit or program or to a general psychiatric unit. If somatic systems are significantly compromised, a medical unit might be the choice for this initial intensive refeeding phase. On most psychiatric units, a protocol for weight gain is established in which all members of the team participate. Dietitians plan the weight-increasing program. Physicians, nurses, psychologists, and social workers participate in care directed at monitoring the refeeding process and its effects on the patient and establishing the intensive therapies that must be instituted after the refeeding phase.

A significant amount of monitoring of the individual's systems is necessary because at the time of admission, most anorexic patients are severely malnourished (see Table 24-3 for Medical Complications). Patients are usually placed on a privilege-earning program, a type of behavior program in which privileges such as having visitors and receiving passes for outside the hospital are earned based on a schedule of pounds gained (see Chap. 14 for a discussion of these types of programs).

The course of hospitalization does not usually go smoothly at first for individuals with anorexia nervosa because of the resistance of the patient to gaining weight. After the establishment of an acceptable weight (at least 85% of ideal), the patient is discharged to either a partial hospitalization program or an intensive outpatient pro-

gram. It is well accepted that the intensive therapies needed to help anorexic patients with their underlying issues (eg, body distortion and maturity fears) and to help families with communication and enmeshment are usually recommended for after the refeeding process. This is because concentration for the severely undernourished individual with anorexia is usually impaired. Family therapy is typically begun during the hospital phase of treatment.

Pharmacologic Interventions

Research has demonstrated that selective serotonin reuptake inhibitors (SSRIs) are not effective for individuals who are in the acute phase of this disorder or hospitalized, as was initially believed (Strober et al., 1999). One explanation for this is that the low body weights of these individuals cause low protein stores, and protein is needed for SSRI metabolism. Other experts claim that the symptoms of anorexia nervosa, such as body distortion, hyperkinesis, and apathy, are, for the most part, the result of starvation. The starvation causes changes in the brain chemistry; thus, restoration of weight, rather than psychopharmacology, influences more significantly symptom remission. Of course, comorbid conditions such as depression should be treated with appropriate antidepressant medication (see Chap. 20). Some clinical experts who work with anorexic patients have used the SSRIs with some effectiveness later during outpatient treatment and after weight restoration. Target symptoms such as obsessiveness, ritualistic behaviors, and perfectionism can remit with these medications. The SSRIs need to be used with caution and the patient's weight constantly monitored because during the initiation phase, some of the SSRIs may cause weight loss. Recently, olanzapine has been used for severe

TABLE 24.4   Criteria for Hospitalization of Patients With Eating Disorders

Medical	Psychiatric
• Weight loss, <75% below ideal	• Risk for suicide
• Heart rate, <40 beats/min; children <20 beats/min	• Severe depression
• Temperature, <36°C	• Failure to comply with treatment
• Blood pressure, <90/60mmHg; children, 80/50 mmHg	• Inadequate response to treatment at another level of care (outpatient)
• Glucose, <60 mg/dL	
• Serum potassium, <3 mEq/L	
• Severe dehydration	
• Electrolyte imbalance	

Adapted from Yoel, J., & Workgroup in Eating Disorders. (2000). Practice guidelines for the treatment of patients with eating disorders. *American Journal of Psychiatry, 157*(1), 1–35.

anorexia with a resulting weight gain, less resistance to treatment, and reduced agitation (LaVia et al., 2000). However, further exploration of the use of this drug and others in this category is needed.

Priority Care Issues

Mortality is a significant factor for patients with anorexia nervosa. The crude mortality rate has been determined to be between 5% and 7% (Crow et al., 1999). Factors that correlate with fatal outcome are a longer duration of illness, bingeing and purging, comorbid substance abuse, and comorbid depression. (Herzog et al., 2000).

Another issue to consider with this population is stigma. Many young girls are "avoided," especially in their emaciated state. Peers do not know how to approach them because they may appear both frightening and fragile (Gowers & Shore, 1999). A recent university study supported this theory and found that most men would feel uncomfortable dating a woman with an eating disorder. Those in the study who had experienced dating someone with an eating disorder were found to express even stronger uncomfortable feelings about them, stating that conflict was the predominant issue in the dating relationship (Sobol & Bursztyn, 1998).

NURSING MANAGEMENT: HUMAN RESPONSE TO DISORDER

Anorexia nervosa is a complex, serious disorder, often involving many bodily systems and comorbid conditions. The primary nursing diagnoses are Imbalanced Nutrition: Less Than Body Requirement, Anxiety, Ineffective Coping, and Disturbed Body Image. Nursing management involves biopsychosocial assessment and interventions.

Therapeutic Nurse–Patient Relationship

It may be difficult to establish an immediate therapeutic relationship with individuals with anorexia nervosa because they are suspicious and mistrustful. They often express fear of all adults, and especially health care professionals, whom they believe want to "make them fat." By the time they are hospitalized, mistrust can almost reach a state of paranoia. Because of their low body weight and starvation, they are often impatient and irritable. A firm, accepting, and patient approach is important in working with these individuals. Providing a rationale for all interventions helps build trust, as does a consistent nonreactive approach. Power struggles over eating are common, and remaining nonreactive is a challenge for the nurse. The nurse should always think about her own feelings of frustration and her need to control during such power struggles (see Therapeutic Dialogue: Eating Disorder).

Biologic Domain

A thorough evaluation of systems is important because many systems can be compromised because of starvation. A careful history from both the patient with anorexia nervosa and the family are necessary to assess altered nutrition. Therefore, the length and duration of symptoms,

---

THERAPEUTIC DIALOGUE | Eating Disorder

Ineffective Approach

Nurse: You haven't eaten your lunch yet.
Patient: I can't, I'm already fat.
Nurse: Look at you, you're skin and bones.
Patient: I'll eat when I go out this afternoon on pass.
Nurse: You can't go on pass. You have to start realizing that you are sick. Because you can't take care of yourself, we are in charge.
Patient: You're trying to control me.
Nurse: We are trying to be responsible.
Patient: I won't eat!
Nurse: We have set up punishments for not eating.
Patient: Then I won't go out! At least I won't get fatter.

Effective Approach

Nurse: You haven't eaten your lunch.
Patient: I can't, I'm already fat.
Nurse: Seeing yourself as fat is part of your eating disorder. We are here to help you.
Patient: I'll eat when I go out on pass.

Nurse: We wrote your behavioral plan together, and you know you will not be able to go out because your pass is dependent on eating both breakfast and lunch. Here!
Patient: You're trying to control me.
Nurse: We are worried about you. That's why we set up this plan. How can I help you now with this meal?
Patient: What if I eat half?
Nurse: No, you must eat all of it. Why don't I sit here while you eat? Eating is scary for you. We can talk about other choices you have on the unit; tonight, you can choose the movie or board games.
Patient: Okay, at least I have some choices.

Critical Thinking Challenge

- What effect did the first interaction have on the patient's behavior? Why?

- In the second interaction, what theories and interventions regarding eating disorders did the nurse use in her approach to the patient?

such as fasting, avoiding meals, and overexercising, are critical assessment information to collect. Patients with longer duration of these maladaptive behaviors will typically have more difficult and longer recovery periods.

The patient's weight is determined by using the BMI and a scale. Currently, criteria for discharge are based on height and weight tables requiring patients to be 85% of ideal according to these tables. BMI, thought to be more accurately reflective of weight status because exact height is used, is calculated by dividing current weight in kilograms squared by height in meters. An acceptable BMI is between about 19 and 25.

Refeeding is the most important intervention for the hospital or initial stage of treatment (Fig. 24-4). It is also the most challenging. The nurse will find that resistance to weight gain and refusal to eat are the usual attitudes of this patient. Strict monitoring and recording of all intake are important as part of the weight gain protocol.

The refeeding protocol typically starts with 1,500 calories a day and is increased slowly until the patient is consuming about 3,500 calories a day in several meals. The usual plan for anorexic patients with very low weights is a weight gain of between 1 to 2 pounds a week. Again, the goal during hospitalization is to reach at least 85% of ideal weight before discharge can be considered.

Weight-increasing protocols usually take the form of a behavioral plan. Privileges are earned (positive reinforcement), such as leaving with a pass, or negative reinforcements (eg, returning to bed rest) are used to increase weight. It is important to help patients understand that these actions are not punitive. When there is a clear protocol agreed on by all staff members for behaviors related to eating and weight gain, reactivity on the part of the staff to the patient is greatly reduced. These protocols provide a ready-made, consistent response to food-refusal behaviors. The protocol should be carried out in a caring and supportive context. On rare occasions when the patient is unable to recognize or accept her illness and may be in denial, nasogastric tube feedings may be necessary.

Menses history also needs to be explored. Most anorexic patients have reached menarche but have experienced amenorrhea for some months because of starvation. A return to regular menses is a sign of significant body fat restoration. Sleep disturbance is also common, and these individuals are viewed as hyperkinetic. They sleep little, but usually awake in an energized state. A structured, healthy sleep routine will need to be established immediately to conserve energy. To further conserve energy and calorie expenditure, because of low weights, anorexic patients are often placed on bed rest until a certain amount of weight is regained. Exercise is generally not permitted during the refeeding period and only with caution after this phase. Patients need to be closely supervised in the hospital because they are often found exercising in their rooms, running in place and doing calisthenics.

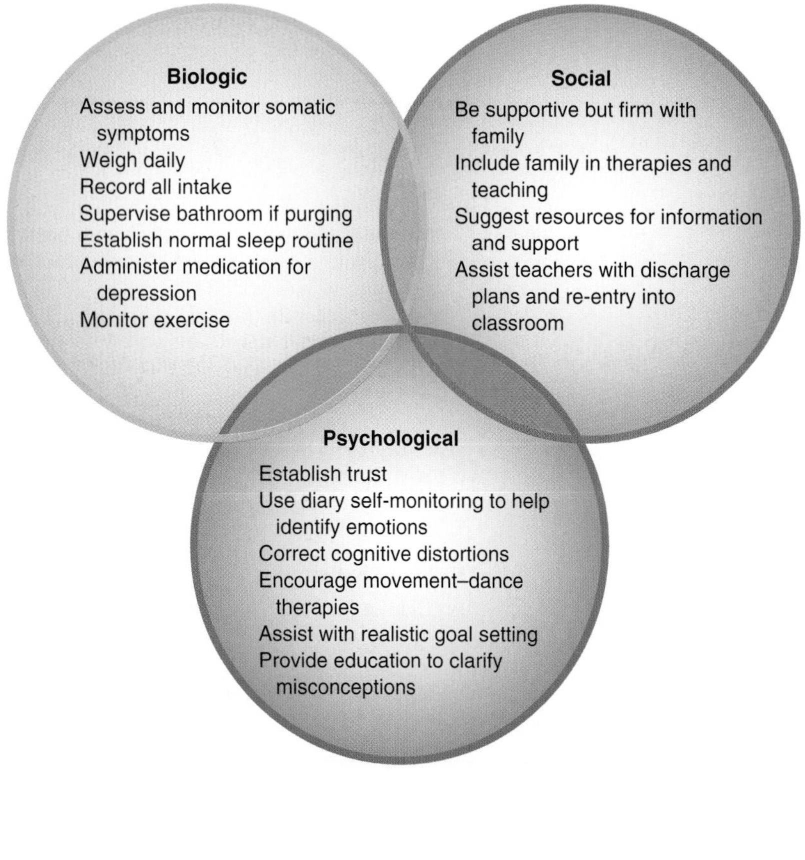

Biologic
Assess and monitor somatic symptoms
Weigh daily
Record all intake
Supervise bathroom if purging
Establish normal sleep routine
Administer medication for depression
Monitor exercise

Social
Be supportive but firm with family
Include family in therapies and teaching
Suggest resources for information and support
Assist teachers with discharge plans and re-entry into classroom

Psychological
Establish trust
Use diary self-monitoring to help identify emotions
Correct cognitive distortions
Encourage movement–dance therapies
Assist with realistic goal setting
Provide education to clarify misconceptions

FIGURE 24.4 Biopsychosocial interventions for patients with anorexia nervosa.

Psychological Domain

The psychological symptoms that anorexic patients experience are listed in Table 24-2. The classic symptoms of body distortion, fear of weight gain, unrealistic expectations and thinking, and ritualistic behaviors are easily noted during a clinical interview. Often, people with anorexia nervosa avoid conflict and have difficulty expressing negative emotions, such as anger. There may also be other conflicts underlying this disorder, such as sexuality fears and ineffectiveness. These symptoms may not be apparent during a clinical interview; however, there are a variety of instruments that both clinicians and researchers use to determine the presence and severity of these and other psychological or cognitive symptoms such. Text Box 24-3 lists the well-known instruments used to assess various psychological symptoms associated with eating disorders. The Eating Attitudes Test is frequently used in community and clinical samples (Text Box 24-4). There is also a child version of this test, the CHEAT. The results of these paper and pencil tests can help target the most significant symptoms for the individual patient. Interventions, especially in the form of therapy, can thus focus on these particular problems.

For interoceptive awareness problems, the lack of ability to experience visceral cues and emotions, patients can benefit from keeping a journal. Most anorexic patients use a somatic complaint like "I feel bloated" or "fat" to replace a negative emotion such as guilt or anger. Whereas in some cases the bloating may be due to the refeeding process following a state of starvation, it is often imagined and part of body image distortion. Assisting the patient in identifying these feelings can be accomplished by having the patient write down the "fat feeling" and list possible underlying emotions and troublesome situations next to this maladaptive feeling. Identifying feelings, especially negative emotions such as anger, is the first step in helping patients to decrease conflict avoidance and develop effective coping strategies for these feelings.

It is best not to attempt to change distorted body image by merely pointing out to that the patient is ac-

TEXT BOX 24.3

Assessment Instruments

1. Tests for Disordered Eating (Symptoms)
Compulsive Eating Scale
Dunn, P. K., & Ondercin, P. (1981). Personality variables related to compulsive eating in college women. *Journal of Clinical Psychology, 31*, 43–49.

Eating Attitudes Test
Garner, D. M., & Garfinkel, P. E. (1979). The eating attitudes test: An index of the symptoms of anorexia nervosa. *Psychosomatic Medicine, 10*, 647–656.

Children's Eating Attitude Test (CHEAT)
Maloney, M. McGuire, J., & Daniels, S. R. (1988). Reliability testing of 6 children's version of the FAT. *Journal of the American Academy of Child and Adolescent Psychiatry, 27*, 541–543.

Eating Disorder Examination-Questionnaire (EDE-O)
Carolyn Black, Rutgers University Eating Disorders Clinic, 41C Gordon Road, Piscataway, NJ 08854.

Eating Disorder Inventory-2 (EDI-2) and EDI-2 Symptom Checklist (EDI-2-SC).
Psychological Assessment Resources, P.O. Box 998, Odessa, FL 33556 (800-331-8378).

Eating Habits Questionnaire (Restraint Scale)
Herman, C. P., & Mack, D. (1975). Restrained and unrestrained eating. *Journal of Personality, 43*, 647–660.

Yale-Brown-Cornell Eating Disorder Scale (YBC-EDS)
Mazure, C. M., Haimi, K. A., Sunday, S. R., et al. (1994). Yale-Brown-Cornell Eating Disorder Scale: Development, use, reliability, and validity. *Journal of Psychiatric Research, 28*, 425–445.

2. Tests of Body Dissatisfaction/Body Image
Body Shape Questionnaire (BSQ)
Cooper, P., Taylor, M., Cooper, Z., & Fairburn, C. (1987). The development and validation of the BSQ. *International Journal of Eating Disorders, 6*, 485–494.

Color-a-Person Test
Wooley, S. C., & Kearney-Cooke, A. (1986). Intensive treatment of bulimia and body image disturbance. In K. D. Brownell & J. P. Foreyt (Eds.), *Handbook of eating disorders: Physiology, psychology and treatment of obesity anorexia and bulimia* (pp. 476–502). New York: Basic Books.

3. Tests of Emotional and Cognitive Components
Cognitive Behavioral Dieting Scale
Martz, D. M., Sturgis, E. T., & Gustafson, S. B. (1996). Development and preliminary validation of the cognitive behavioral dieting scale. *International Journal of Eating Disorders, 19*, 297–309.

Emotional Eating Scale
Arrow, B., Kenardy, J., & Agras, W. S. (1995). The emotional eating scale: The development of a measure to assess coping with negative affect by eating. *International Journal of Eating Disorders, 18*, 79–90.

4. Risk Factors Identification
The McKnight Risk Factor Survey
Shisslak, C. M., Renger, R., Sharpe, T., et al. (1999). Development and evaluation of the McKnight Risk Factor Survey for assessing potential risk and protective factors for disordered eating in preadolescent and adolescent girls. *International Journal of Eating Disorders, 25*, 195–214 (versions available for younger and older children).

TEXT BOX 24.4

Eating Attitudes Test

Please place an (x) under the column that applies best to each of the numbered statements. All of the results will be strictly confidential. Most of the questions relate to food or eating, although other types of questions have been included. Please answer each question carefully. Thank you.

	Always	Very Often	Often	Sometimes	Rarely	Never
1. Like eating with other people						x
2. Prepare foods for others but do not eat what I cook	x					
3. Become anxious before eating	x					
4. Am terrified about being overweight	x					
5. Avoid eating when I am hungry	x					
6. Find myself preoccupied with food	x					
7. Have gone on eating binges in which I feel that I may not be able to stop	x					
8. Cut my food into small pieces	x					
9. Am aware of the calorie content of foods that I eat	x					
10. Particularly avoid foods with a high carbohydrate content (eg, bread, potatoes, rice)	x					
11. Feel bloated after meals	x					
12. Feel that others would prefer I ate more	x					
13. Vomit after I have eaten	x					
14. Feel extremely guilty after eating	x					
15. Am occupied with a desire to be thinner	x					
16. Exercise strenuously to burn off calories	x					
17. Weigh myself several times a day	x					
18. Like my clothes to fit tightly						x
19. Enjoy eating meat						x
20. Wake up early in the morning	x					
21. Eat the same foods day after day	x					
22. Think about burning up calories when I exercise	x					
23. Have regular menstrual periods						x
24. Am aware that other people think I am too thin	x					
25. Am preoccupied with the thought of having fat on my body	x					
26. Take longer than others to eat	x					
27. Enjoy eating at restaurants						x
28. Take laxatives	x					
29. Avoid foods with sugar in them	x					
30. Eat diet foods	x					
31. Feel that food controls my life	x					
32. Display self-control around food	x					
33. Feel that others pressure me to eat	x					

TEXT BOX 24.4 (*Continued*)

	Always	Very Often	Often	Sometimes	Rarely	Never
34. Give too much time and thought to food	x	—	—	—	—	—
35. Suffer from constipation	—	x	—	—	—	—
36. Feel uncomfortable after eating sweets	x	—	—	—	—	—
37. Engage in dieting behavior	x	—	—	—	—	—
38. Like my stomach to be empty	x	—	—	—	—	x
39. Enjoy trying new rich foods	—	—	—	—	—	x
40. Have the impulse to vomit after meals	x	—	—	—	—	—

Scoring: The patient is given the questionnaire without the X's, just blank. 3 points are assigned to endorsements that coincide with the X's; the adjacent alternatives are weighted as 2 points and 1 point, respectively. A total score of more than 30 indicates significant concerns with eating behavior.

tually too thin. This symptom is often the last to resolve itself, and it may take years for some individuals to see their bodies realistically. However, even though this symptom is difficult to abate, patients can continue to fear becoming fat but not be driven to act on the distortion by starving. The fear of becoming fat related to the distortion does lessen overtime.

The nurse can help individuals with cognitive distortions and unrealistic assumptions in the way they view the world, especially relative to food, eating, weight, and shape. Ineffective coping is the result of faulty ways of viewing situations. Table 24-5 lists some distortions commonly experienced by individuals with eating disorders and some typical restructuring responses or statements that challenge the distortion. In communicating with patients with anorexia nervosa, the nurse will hear many of these statements from the patient. During therapeutic communication, more realistic ways of perceiving a situation can be presented. Other therapies, such as movement and dance therapy, can be useful in helping the patient experience pleasure from her body. Caution regarding the use of dance is recommended during the refeeding phase because of energy-expenditure concerns. Imagery and relaxation are often used to

TABLE 24.5   Cognitive Distortions Typical of Patients With Eating Disorders, With Restructuring Statements

Distortion	Clarification or Restructuring
Dichotomous or all-or-nothing thinking "I've gained 2 pounds, so I'll be up by 100 pounds soon."	"You have never gained 100 pounds, but I understand that gaining 2 pounds is scary."
Magnification "I binged last night, so I can't go out with anyone."	"Feeling bad and guilty about a binge are difficult feelings, but you are in treatment and you have been monitoring and changing your eating."
Selective abstraction "I can only be happy 10 pounds lighter."	"When you were 10 pounds lighter, you were hospitalized. You can choose to be happy about many things in your life."
Overgeneralization "I didn't eat anything yesterday and did okay, so I don't think *not* eating for a week or two will harm me."	"Any starvation harms the body, whether or not outward signs were apparent to you. The more you starve, the more problems your body will encounter."
Catastrophizing "I purged last night for the first time in 4 months— I'll never recover."	"Recovery includes up and downs, and it is expected you will still have some mild but infrequent symptoms."

overcome distortions and to decrease anxiety related to a distorted body image.

While in the hospital, patients are usually evaluated for discharge to partial hospitalization or intensive outpatient therapy, depending on the resources available, the extent of family support, and comorbidity. In both instances, the patient and family will be seen for a combination of individual and family therapy.

Interpersonal therapy (IPT) is a type of treatment that focuses on uncovering and resolving the developmental and psychological issues underlying the disorder, such as ineffectiveness. Role transitions, control, and ineffective feelings are typically the focus (McIntosh et al., 2000). Cognitive therapy may also be incorporated to continue to address and change distortions about food and interactions with others.

Family therapy is usually initiated in the hospital and continued more intensively after discharge. The section on Etiology: Family discusses some of the family symptoms, such as enmeshment, which are the focus of the therapy.

Patient Education

When weight is restored and concentration is improved, patients with anorexia nervosa can benefit from psychoeducation. Although these individuals have a wealth of knowledge about food and calories, they also have misinformation that needs clarifying. For example, they are often unclear about the role of "fats" in a healthy diet and try to be as "fat free" as possible. A thorough assessment of their knowledge base is important because they seem to be "walking calorie books" with little information on the role of all of the nutrients and the importance of including them in a healthy diet.

One of the most helpful teaching points is the setting of realistic goals around food and also around other activities or tasks. Because of perfectionism, anorexic patients often set up unrealistic goals that end up frustrating them. The nurse can assist with establishing smaller, more realistic, attainable goals. (See Psychoeducation Checklist: Anorexia Nervosa.)

Families and friends are eager to help the patient with anorexia but often need some direction about how to best help. Text Box 24-5 provides a list of strategies and suggested readings that may assist these family members and friends.

Social Domain

The patient with anorexia will have lost some school time because of hospitalization. Integrating back into a school and classroom setting is a difficulty for most. Shame and guilt over having an eating disorder and being hospitalized need to be addressed. Because these

---

PSYCHOEDUCATION CHECKLIST
Anorexia Nervosa

When caring for the patient with anorexia nervosa, be sure to include the following topic areas in the teaching plan:

- Psychopharmacologic agents, if used, including drug, action, dosage, frequency, and possible adverse effects
- Nutrition and eating patterns
- Effect of restrictive eating or dieting
- Weight monitoring
- Safety and comfort measures
- Avoidance of triggers
- Self-monitoring techniques
- Trust
- Realistic goal setting
- Resources

TEXT BOX 24.5

What Family and Friends Can Do to Help Those With Eating Disorders

- Tell the person you are concerned, that you care, and would like to help. Suggest that the person seek professional help from a physician or the therapist.

- If the person refuses to seek professional help, encourage reaching out to an adult, such as a teacher, school nurse, or counselor.

- Do not discuss weight, the number of calories being consumed, or particular eating habits. Do try to talk about things other than food, weight, counting calories, and exercise.

- Avoid making comments about a person's appearance. Concern about weight loss may be interpreted as a compliment; comments regarding weight gain may be felt as criticism.

- It will not help to become involved in a power struggle. You cannot force the person to eat.

- You can offer support. Ultimately, however, the responsibility and the decision to accept help and to change rest with the person.

- Read and educate yourself regarding these disorders (good sources listed below).

  - *Surviving an Eating Disorder: Strategies for Family and Friends* by Michelle Siegel, New York, Harper Perennial, 1997.

  - *A Parent's Guide to Eating Disorders* by Brett Valette, New York: Avon Book, (1990).

  - *A Parent's Guide to Anorexia and Bulimia* by Katherine Byrne, New York, Henry Holt (An "Owl" Publication), 1989.

individuals have isolated themselves for periods before hospitalization and treatment, renewing friendships and relationships with peers may be anxiety provoking. It is helpful to involve school nurses and teachers in the reentry process.

Denial, guilt, and subsequent greater overprotectiveness are common reactions of the family with a member who has anorexia nervosa, especially when hospitalization has been necessary. Family therapy is important for every family if the patient still lives at home. Skilled therapists are able to help family members with their feelings and increase effective communication, decrease protectiveness, and resolve guilt. Often, siblings become resentful of the patient with an eating disorder because of the significant amount of attention the parents place on the child or adolescent. It is helpful to have siblings attend family sessions to discuss these feelings and the effect the illness has had on them.

Evaluation and Treatment Outcomes

There are several factors that influence the outcome of treatment for anorexia nervosa. As noted earlier, longer duration of symptoms and lower weight at initiation of treatment have been related to poorer outcomes. Fam-

ily support and involvement have been demonstrated to affect the outcome of treatment positively. As with any disorder, comorbid conditions and their severity will also influence recovery. Today, individuals are discharged from the hospital when their weight has reached 85% of what is considered ideal. However, restoration of healthy eating and change in maladaptive thinking may not have yet occurred. Individuals often continue to try to restrict foods. Therefore, without intensive outpatient treatment, including nutritional counseling and support, it is unlikely that they will fully recover. Distorted thinking and eating patterns can set the stage for a relapse and later for the possible development of bulimia nervosa. Many of the instruments used to assess eating disorder symptoms can be used throughout the patient's treatment to evaluate attitudes and thinking processes specifically that continue to prevent full recovery (see Text Box 24-3).

Continuum of Care

Hospitalization

Hospitalization is required based on criteria noted in Table 24-4. It is unlikely that anorexia nervosa can be managed in its acute stage in outpatient settings.

NURSING CARE PLAN 24.1
Nursing Care Plan for a Patient With Anorexia Nervosa

JS is a 16-year-old girl who appears much younger. She is 5'5' and weighs 92 pounds. She has been treated unsuccessfully in an outpatient clinic and now is being admitted to stabilize her weight. She does not believe that she is too thin and resents being forced to be hospitalized. Hospitalization precipitated by being asked to leave gymnastics team because of low body weight.

SETTING: INPATIENT PSYCHIATRIC UNIT

Baseline assessment: JS appears frail, pale, and dressed in oversized clothes. She tearful, states that she is depressed and angry, and that she has no friends. Physical examination results: bradycardia– pulse = 58, hypotension, 88/60, constipation, amenorrhea, dry skin patches, and cold intolerance. Hypokalemia (K+ = 3.5); leukopenia (WBCs<5,000). Dehydration, temperature elevation, 99°F, elevated BUN, abnormal thyroid functioning.

Associated Psychiatric Diagnosis	*Medications*

Axis I: Anorexia nervosa
        Binge–eating/purging type
Axis II: None
Axis III: None
Axis IV: Social support (social withdrawal)
GAF = Current 55
        Potential 75
	Fluoxetine (Prozac), 20 mg in AM

(continued)

NURSING CARE PLAN 24.1 (Continued)

NURSING DIAGNOSIS 1: IMBALANCED NUTRITION: LESS THAN BODY REQUIREMENTS

Defining Characteristics	*Related Factors*
Unable to increase food intake Weight more than 20% below ideal weight	Believes she cannot eat most foods Purges by vomiting "occasionally" Exercises 6–8 h daily Sleep pattern disturbed by exercise

OUTCOMES

Initial	*Long-term*
Maintains daily intake of 1200 calories Eliminates exercising while in hospital Ceases purging for 1 week.	Gains 1–3 pounds Develop strategies to maintain weight.

INTERVENTIONS

Interventions	*Rationale*	*Ongoing Assessment*
Allow patient to verbalize feelings such as anxiety related to food and weight gain—develop a therapeutic relationship.	Through a relationship and examining her feelings, she may be more likely to cooperate with nutritional regimen.	Determine anxiety level when discussing food and weight gain.
Monitor meals and snacks, record amount eaten.	Severe anorexia is life-threatening. Aggressive interventions are needed to ensure adequate intake.	Monitor intake. Assess JS's ability to complete meals on time and without supplements.
Do not substitute other foods for food on patient tray. Limit caffeine intake to 1 cup coffee (soda) daily.	People with anorexia usually "play games" with food. By prohibiting substitution, a more positive approach is encouraged. Caffeine is an appetite suppressant and has a diuretic effect.	Determine how willing JS is to follow nutritional regimen.
Monitor 1 h after meals for purging. Weigh daily in hospital gown after patient has voided. Monitor vital sign daily; electrolytes.	Physical signs of impending complications include evidence of purging, decreasing body weight, hypotension, hyperthermia, and hypokalemia.	Monitor vital signs, weight, and electrolytes, especially potassium.

EVALUATION

Outcomes	*Revised Outcomes*	*Interventions*
JS gains 5 pounds at the end of 1½ weeks. Has been cooperative with meal regimen.	Ceases binge–purge episodes for 1 week. Continues to increase her weight (1–3 pounds/week).	Daily weights while on unsupervised meals. Praise her for her successes. Arrange or discharge to outpatient clinic.
She has begun to acknowledge the seriousness of her illness and the life-threatening aspects of severe dieting and purging.	Establish and maintain regular, adequate nutritional eating habits.	Participation in relapse–prevention classes.

NURSING DIAGNOSIS 2: DISTURBED BODY IMAGE

Defining Characteristics	*Related Factors*
Verbalizes that she is too fat Perceives herself as unattractive Hides body in large, baggy clothing	Inaccurate perceptions of physical appearance secondary to anorexia nervosa Believes that one can never be too rich or too thin Equates physical fitness and attractiveness with thinness

(continued)

NURSING CARE PLAN 24.1 (Continued)

OUTCOMES

Initial	Long-term
Verbalizes feeling related to changing body shape and weight. Identifies beliefs about controlling body size.	Acknowledges negative consequences of too little fat on body. Identifies positive aspects of her body and its ability to function.

INTERVENTIONS

Interventions	Rationale	Ongoing Assessment
Explore JS's beliefs and feelings about body. Maintain a nonjudgmental approach.	To help patient gain a more positive body image, an understanding of her own views is important.	Monitor for statements that identify perceptions of her body. Is her view *distorted* or *dissatisfied*?
Assist patient in identifying positive physical characteristics.	In anorexia, the body is viewed negatively. By focusing on parts of the body that are positive, such as eyes or hands, the patient can begin to experience a positive image of her body.	Observe for patient's reaction to her body. Which areas are viewed positively? Observe for negative statements related to body size and self-esteem.
Clarify patient's views about an ideal body.	Many societal cues idealize an unrealistically thin female body.	Monitor for statements indicating external pressures to lose weight, experiences of teasing about body changes, or evidence of sexual abuse from others.
Provide education related to normal growth of women's bodies, role of fat in protection of body.	Providing education will help in reinforcing a broader view of the importance of a healthy body.	Assess patient's willingness to learn information.

EVALUATION

Outcomes	Revised Outcomes	Interventions
JS revealed that she believes that she is too fat, but does have positive physical traits—eyes. She believes that those who are overweight have lost control of their lives. She knows some models who are 6' and weigh barely 100 lbs.	Accept alternative beliefs related to her own body.	Gradually, focus on other positive physical aspects of JS's body. Discuss grooming that encourages a more attractive look. Challenge her beliefs about body weights of models.
Willing to read information about normal body functioning.	Accept a new view of body functioning as a complex phenomenon.	Discuss the biologic aspect of the development of body weight. Emphasize multiple factors determine body weight.

Emergency Care

Emergency care is not usually needed for individuals with anorexia nervosa. Before systems are compromised to the degree that individuals will require emergency treatment, the patient has usually come to the attention of family members and peers because of weight loss and emaciation. If systems are compromised to the extent that emergency treatment is warranted, patients are usually immediately admitted for inpatient care.

Family Assessment and Intervention

The family of the individual will need a significant amount of treatment and follow-up. The therapist,

psychologist, advanced practice nurse, or social worker meets on a regular basis, at least once a week, with the individual *and* the family. This method has been demonstrated to be more effective than family therapy without the patient present or individual therapy alone (Robin et al., 1999). The family therapy focuses on such issues as separation-individuation, autonomy, ineffective communication, and practical issues, such as how parents can effectively monitor food intake. Many family theorists believe that the eating disorder has developed because of family dysfunction and therefore has some unrealized meaning for each family. For example, in some instances, the patient may be attempting to keep a splitting, divorcing, or estranged family together with her illness. In other instances, parents may be avoiding allowing a daughter to separate and individuate because they are emotionally unprepared for this process. The development of an eating disorder may be a reaction to these situations. The therapy helps to uncover these meanings and to improve effective parenting.

Outpatient Treatment

After refeeding, treatment of anorexia nervosa takes place on an outpatient basis. This type of intervention involves individual and family therapy, nutrition counseling to reinforce healthy eating patterns and attitudes, and physician visits to monitor weight and evaluate somatic recovery. Often, support groups are suggested, but these should not be a substitution for therapy. In fact, some support groups, because they are often not led by professionals but are self-directed by the members, can actually delay or prevent needed professional treatment. However, after full recovery, support groups are useful in maintaining recovery.

Prevention

Eating disorders, both bulimia nervosa and anorexia nervosa, are two of the most preventable disorders. Instruments such as the McKnight Risk Factor Survey (Shisslak et al., 1999) are available to measure the presence and degree of risk factors. These instruments can be used to plan for prevention or treatment after early detection (see Text Box 24-3). On a national level, eating disorder awareness and advocacy groups work toward educating the general public, those at risk, and those who work with groups at risk, such as teachers and coaches. They also work toward monitoring the media and removing unhealthy advertisements and articles that appear in magazines appealing to young girls. A list of on-line resources and some programs and their purposes are found in the Web Links at the end of this chapter.

Prevention and early detection strategies for parents and schoolteachers are often the focus of school nurses and mental health nurses who work in the community. Some of these strategies appear in Table 24-6 and are based on the research on risk factors and protective factors. These protective factors, such as confidence and healthy competition in athletics, have been shown to prevent the development of an eating disorder for individuals who were at risk (Fulkerson et al., 1999; Taylor et al., 1998). Dieting, being overweight, and body dissatisfaction are examples of risk factors underlying the development of eating disorders that can be reversed with early identification and intervention.

BULIMIA NERVOSA

Bulimia nervosa is a relatively new disorder and until about 25 years ago was thought to be a type of anorexia nervosa. However, findings from extensive investigations have identified its characteristics as a separate entity. It is a more prevalent disorder than anorexia nervosa. Individuals with bulimia nervosa are usually older at onset than those with anorexia nervosa. The disorder is generally not as life-threatening as anorexia nervosa. The usual treatment is outpatient therapy. Outcomes are better for bulimia nervosa than for anorexia nervosa, and mortality rates are lower.

Definition and Clinical Course

There are few outward signs associated with bulimia nervosa. Individuals binge and purge in secret and are typically of normal weight; therefore, it does not come

TABLE 24.6 Prevention Strategies for Parents and Children	
Parents	**Children**
Education	**Education**
Real vs. ideal weight	Peer pressure regarding eating, weight
Influence of attitudes, behaviors, teasing	Menses, puberty, normal weight gain
Ways to increase self-esteem	Strategies for obesity
Role of media: TV, magazines	Ways to develop or improve self-esteem
Signs and symptoms	Body image traps: media, retail clothing
Interventions for obesity	Adapting and coping with problems
Boys at risk also	Reporting friends with signs of eating disorders
Observe for rituals	**Screening** for risk factors
Supervision of eating and exercise	**Assessment** for treatment
	Follow-up: monitor for relapse

to the attention of parents and peers as readily as does anorexia nervosa. Treatment consequently can be delayed for years as individuals attempt on their own to get their eating under control. Individuals therefore usually initiate their own treatment when control of their eating becomes impossible. Once treatment is undertaken and completed, patients typically recover completely, except in cases in which personality disorders and comorbid serious depression are also present.

Patients with bulimia nervosa present as overwhelmed and overly committed individuals who have difficulty with setting limits and establishing appropriate boundaries. They appear to be "social butterflies," involved in too many activities. They have an enormous amount of rules regarding food and food restrictions. They relate shame, guilt, and disgust around their binge eating and purging. They may also be impulsive in other areas of their lives such, as spending.

Diagnostic Criteria

The key characteristics for the diagnosis of bulimia nervosa appear in Table 24-7 (also see Table 24-2). There are two types of bulimia nervosa: purging type and restricting type. Patients with the restricting type are similar to those with anorexia nervosa. However, in bulimia, restricting is followed by binge eating, which is then followed by another period of restricting. In the purging type, binge eating is followed by purging. The difference between the purging anorexic and the purging bulimic is the severe weight loss and amenorrhea that accompanies anorexia nervosa. Bulimia nervosa is an eating disorder that involves engaging in recurrent episodes of binge eating and compensatory behavior such as purging in the form of vomiting or using laxatives, diuretics, or emetics, or in nonpurging compensatory behaviors, such as fasting or overexercising in order to avoid weight gain. These episodes must occur at least twice a week for a period of at least 3 months in order to meet the *DSM-IV-TR* criteria (APA, 2000). People with this disorder may binge and purge up to several times a day.

Binge eating is defined as rapid, episodic, impulsive, and uncontrollable ingestion of what would be considered a large amount of food over a short period of time, usually 1 to 2 hours. Eating is followed by feelings of guilt, remorse, and often self-contempt, leading to purging. To assuage the out-of-control feeling, severe dieting is instituted, and these restrictions, referred to as dietary restraint, precipitate the next binge. The restrictions are viewed as "rules," such as

---

TABLE 24.7 Key Diagnostic Characteristics for Bulimia Nervosa

Diagnostic Criteria	Target Symptoms and Associated Findings
• Recurrent episodes of binge eating • Characterized by both of the following: eating in a discrete period of time an amount larger than most people would eat during a similar period of time and under similar circumstances; sense of lack of control over eating during the episode • Recurrent inappropriate compensatory behavior to prevent weight gain, such as self-induced vomiting, misuse of laxatives, diuretics, enemas, or other medications; fasting; or excessive exercise • Binge eating and inappropriate compensatory behaviors occurring on average at least twice a week for 3 months • Self-evaluation unduly influenced by body shape and weight • Not occurring exclusively during episodes of anorexia nervosa • *Purging type*: regular engagement in self-induced vomiting or misuse of diuretics, laxatives, or enemas • *Nonpurging type*: use of other inappropriate compensatory behaviors, such as fasting or excessive exercise without regular engagement in self-induced vomiting, or misuse of laxatives, diuretics, or enemas	• Usually within normal weight range, possible overweight or underweight • Restriction of total calorie consumption between binges, selecting low-calorie foods while avoiding foods perceived to be fattening or likely to trigger a binge • Increased frequency of depressive symptoms and anxiety symptoms • Possible substance abuse or dependence, involving alcohol or stimulants *Associated Physical Examination Findings* • Loss of dental enamel • Chipped, ragged, or moth-eaten teeth appearance • Increased incidence of dental caries • Scars on dorsum of hand from manually inducing vomiting • Cardiac and skeletal myopathies from use of syrup of ipecac for vomiting • Menstrual irregularities • Dependence on laxatives • Esophageal tears *Associate Laboratory Findings* • Fluid and electrolyte abnormalities • Metabolic alkalosis (from vomiting) or metabolic acidosis (from diarrhea) • Mildly elevated serum amylase levels

no sweets, no fats, and so forth. Each binge seems to influence stricter and stricter rules about what cannot be consumed, leading to more frequent binge eating. This cycle has prompted clinicians to focus treatment primarily on interventions related to dietary restraint. When dietary restraint is resolved, binge eating is decreased, and generally the purging that follows binge eating is also decreased.

KEY CONCEPT **Dietary restraint.** The concept of **dietary restraint** has been described by researchers in the field of eating disorders as a way to explain the relationship between dieting and binge eating (Polivy & Herman, 1993).

Dieters' deprivation, or restraint, whether real or imagined, has been identified as contributing to overeating and bingeing. Deprivation may operate in a straightforward fashion by instigating a drive toward repletion. Another possibility is that deprivation alters one's perceptual reactivation to attractive food cues, making them more irresistible. The attempted deprivation may make dieters more prone to feel distress over their dietary "failures," especially if dieting has become a way to overcome body dissatisfaction. This feeling of distress may be compensated for through binge eating. Whether the eating is influenced by the attraction of forbidden foods or by internal needs to assuage failure, there is significant evidence that restraining one's intake is a precondition for bouts of overeating.

A number of studies have uncovered a group of individuals who binge in the same way as those with bulimia nervosa, but who do not purge or compensate for binges through other behaviors. This disorder is now classified in a temporary way in the *DSM-IV-TR* as binge eating disorder (BED). These individuals also differ in that most of them are also obese. Text Box 24-6 describes BED and the current understanding about this disorder. Because this is a newly recognized disorder, until further research clarifies its symptoms, etiology, and treatment, it is now described in the Appendix of the *DSM-IV-TR* (APA, 2000). Clinicians classify BED as an "eating disorder not otherwise specified" until it has been researched further for inclusion as a separate diagnosis in the *DSM-IV-TR*. Its etiology is believed to be similar to that of bulimia nervosa. The treatment of binge eating disorder is still in the investigative stages, and most experts use similar interventions as those for bulimia nervosa.

Bulimia Nervosa in Special Populations

Bulimia nervosa occurs in all age groups. It is not as common in children as in adolescents and adults. More often, binge eating without purging (binge eating disorder) is prevalent in children. This finding has only recently

TEXT BOX 24.6

Binge Eating Disorder

Binge eating disorder (BED), although still in the research stage to refine its characteristics for inclusion in the *DSM-IV-TR* (APA, 2000) as a separate entity, is estimated to affect 3% to 4% of the population. The criteria for BED consist of binge eating, which includes both the ingestion of a large amount of food in a short period of time and a sense of loss of control during the binge; distress regarding the binge; and eating until uncomfortably full; and feelings of guilt or depression following the binge. Purging does not occur with BED, and this differentiates it from bulimia nervosa. In addition, investigators have shown that individuals with BED have lower dietary restraint and are higher in weight, even though many are not obese, than those with bulimia nervosa. It has been estimated that 10% to 30% of obese individuals have BED. Some women with bulimia nervosa have reported that they binged without purging for several years before developing bulimia nervosa and as young as age 10 years (Bulik et al., 1998).

Cognitive behavior therapy has not been as effective for BED as it is for bulimia nervosa. Investigations have shown that sertraline has been effective in reducing binges. Topiramate, used for epilepsy, has been studied for use for BED and was found to decrease binge eating and appetite. Some weight loss was also a result of treatment with this medication. More studies are needed to confirm its effectiveness (Shapira, Goldsmith, & McElroy, 2000).

been reported, and more data are needed to substantiate this theory.

Epidemiology

Lifetime prevalence of bulimia nervosa is reported to be from 3% to 8%, depending on whether clinical or community populations are sampled. Stricter criteria are used when clinical groups are studied, making the prevalence rate lower. The occurrence is more common than that of anorexia nervosa.

Age of Onset

Typically, the age of onset is between 18 and 24 years. The incidence of bulimia nervosa is increasing among women between 25 and 45 but has been relatively stable in the typical age group (Pawluck & Gorey, 1998).

Gender Differences

As with anorexia nervosa, females are more likely than males to develop bulimia nervosa; the ratio is 10:1. Text Box 24-1 highlights differences in males with eating disorders.

Ethnic and Cultural Differences

Bulimia nervosa is related to culture in the same way as anorexia nervosa. In Western cultures and those becoming westernized in their norms, the focus on achieving a thin body ideal underlies the dieting and dietary restraint that sets up the trajectory toward a diagnosable eating disorder. Hispanic and white women have higher rates than Asian and African American women.

Familial Differences

There is some support for a familial link for bulimia nervosa. First-degree relatives of women with bulimia nervosa were more likely than controls and women with other psychiatric disorders to have bulimia nervosa. In addition, when subclinical symptoms were considered, the prevalence in first-degree relatives was even higher (Lilenfeld et al., 1998).

Comorbidity

The most significant comorbid conditions are substance abuse and dependence, depression, and OCD. In one study, women were found to continue having OCD after remission of their bulimic symptoms, again stressing the notion that some comorbid conditions may occur before the eating disorder, are trait-related features and may actually have a role in precipitating the disorder (von Ranson et al., 1999).

Cluster B, Axis II disorders, such as borderline personality disorder, are also found in high rates in these individuals (Matsunaga et al., 2000). In addition, a significant number of women with bulimia nervosa have had prior anorexia nervosa.

Etiology

Some of the predisposing or risk factors for both anorexia nervosa and bulimia nervosa overlap with theories of causality (see Fig. 24-3). For example, dieting puts an individual at risk for the development of bulimia nervosa. The dieting can turn into dietary restraint, a symptom that leads to binge eating and purging. However, not all individuals who diet develop bulimia nervosa. It is the interplay of other risk factors (eg, body dissatisfaction and separation individuation issues) that most likely explain the development of this disorder.

Biologic Theories

Some progress has been made in understanding the biologic causes of bulimia nervosa, although it is a fairly new conceptualized condition. Dieting, one of the most important causative factors, has been found to occur in this country in girls as young as 8 years of age (Hill & Pallin, 1998). Girls, adolescents, and women diet because of body dissatisfaction, which can occur whether or not they are overweight. It is believed that dieting affects serotonergic regulation. As in anorexia nervosa, overexercising has also contributed to some of the symptoms of bulimia nervosa, especially in individuals with the restricting type of this disorder.

Neuropathologic. The changes noted in the brain by MRI are the result of eating dysregulation, rather than the cause. As with anorexia nervosa, these changes disappear when symptoms such as dietary restraint, binge eating, and purging remit.

Genetic. A specific gene responsible for bulimia nervosa has not been identified. Recently, twin studies have been reviewed to determine the role genetics might play in the development of bulimia nervosa. Whereas it has been widely recognized that environment also plays a role, in several twin studies, genetic influences outweighed environmental ones (Bulik et al., 2000). Findings continue to be treated with caution because it is difficult to sort out environmental and genetic influences when twins live in the same environment.

Biochemical. The most frequently studied biochemical theory in bulimia nervosa relates to lowered brain serotonin neurotransmission. It is believed that women with bulimia nervosa may have altered modulation of central serotonin neuronal systems (Kaye et al., 2000a).

Studies have typically looked to tryptophan, an amino acid and serotonin precursor, to explain this mechanism. Findings from several studies have demonstrated that women with bulimia nervosa experience symptoms of depressed mood, a desire to binge, and an increase in weight and shape concerns when tryptophan is depleted through dieting (Smith et al., 1999). To further advance these findings, in another study, women who had recovered from bulimia nervosa (ie, symptoms had remitted) were examined after ingestion of a formula to deplete tryptophan. They returned to symptoms of a desire to binge, preoccupation with shape, and a decrease in mood (Wolfe et al., 2000). Chronic depletion of plasma tryptophan is thought to be one of the major mechanisms whereby persistent dieting can lead to the development of eating disorders in vulnerable individuals.

Psychological and Social Theories

Psychological factors in the etiology of bulimia nervosa have been studied extensively, and most experts believe that these factors converge with environmental or sociocultural factors within individuals with a biologic predisposition, causing symptoms to develop. As with anorexia nervosa, psychoanalytic developmental theories that explain separation-individuation are important in causality. Because the age of onset for bulimia nervosa is late adolescence, going away to college, for example, may represent the first physical separation for some adolescents, who are unprepared for the emotional separation. In addition, an inability to set limits and develop healthy boundaries leads to a sense of being overwhelmed and "drained." In most instances, women with bulimia nervosa are not assertive and have difficulty saying no, fearing that they will not be liked. Overwhelming feelings often lead to binge eating, either to avoid or to distract oneself from feelings such as resentment; or binge eating can serve to assuage emptiness, or as a filling up of a "drained" self with food.

Cognitive Theory.   Many experts view cognitive theory as influential in eating disorder symptoms. It explains the distorted thinking present in those with bulimia nervosa. This explanation is similar for depression, in which a particular thought pattern is learned (see Chaps. 6, 14, and 20 for an explanation of cognitive theory). Many experts view bulimia as a disorder of thinking in that the distortions are foundational to behaviors such as binge eating and purging. Psychological triggering mechanism models explain that cues such as stress, negative emotions, and even environmental cues (eg, the presence of attractive food) play a role in the etiology of bulimia nervosa. However, today, these cognitive and triggering theories are viewed as an explanation for maintaining the binge eating once it has been established, rather than an explanation of causality.

The same sociocultural factors that underlie anorexia nervosa, such as striving for a thin body ideal, an image perpetuated through the media, play a significant role in the development of bulimia nervosa.

Family.   The families of individuals who develop bulimia nervosa are reported to be chaotic, with few rules and unclear boundaries. Often, there is an overly close or enmeshed relationship between the daughter and mother. Daughters may relate that their mother is their "best friend." The boundaries are blurred in that the mother may interact with the daughter as a confidante, and this unhealthy relating further impedes the separation-individuation process. The daughters often feel guilty about separation and responsible for their mother's happiness and emotional well-being (see Research Box 24-3). Some research on families of individuals with bulimia nervosa has found them to be unempathic and unavailable.

In summary, as with anorexia nervosa, theories of causation do not individually explain the development of bulimia nervosa. Rather, it is the convergence of many of these factors at a vulnerable stage of development for the adolescent or young girl that best explains causality.

Risk Factors

The risk or predisposing factors for bulimia nervosa are similar to those for anorexia nervosa (see Fig. 24-3). Society's influences, such as the media and peer pressure, underlie the desire to achieve an ideal thin body type. Comparing oneself to these ideal body types leads to body dissatisfaction. These factors influence behaviors such as dietary restraint and overexercising. Dietary restraint leads to binge eating, and purging ensues because of a fear of becoming fat.

Interdisciplinary Treatment

Individuals with bulimia nervosa benefit from a comprehensive multifaceted treatment approach. The goals for treatment for individuals with bulimia nervosa focus on stabilizing and then normalizing eating, which means stopping the binge–purge cycles; restructuring dysfunctional thought patterns and attitudes, especially about eating, weight, and shape; teaching healthy boundary setting; and resolving conflicts about separation-individuation. Treatment usually takes place in an outpatient setting, except when the patient is suicidal or when past outpatient treatment has failed (Table 24-4).

In addition to intensive psychotherapy, usually cognitive behavioral therapy (CBT) or IPT, pharmacologic interventions are also necessary. The SSRIs have been demonstrated in numerous studies to be effective for the treatment of binge eating and purging, even without comorbid depression. Nutrition counseling is an important part of the outpatient treatment to stabilize and normalize eating. A number of mental health professionals, psychologists, advanced practice psychiatric nurses, and social workers specialize in the treatment of eating disorders and often work in collaboration with nutritionists who also have expertise in working with this population. Family therapy is not usually a part of the treatment because many women with bulimia nervosa live on college campuses away from home, or are older and on their own. Group psychotherapy and support groups are also used to treat individuals with this disorder. Usually, treatment becomes less intensive as symptoms remit and therapy sessions may be less frequent. Many of the psychological issues, such as boundary setting and separation-individuation conflicts, are the focus of the therapy, as well as changing problematic behaviors and dysfunctional thinking using CBT.

Priority Care Issues

Because of the comorbid conditions of depression and borderline personality disorder, some individuals with bulimia nervosa may become suicidal. They are also often at risk for self-mutilation. Because they display high levels of impulsivity, shoplifting, and overspending, financial and legal difficulties have been associated with bulimia nervosa.

NURSING MANAGEMENT: HUMAN RESPONSE TO DISORDER

The primary nursing diagnoses for patients with bulimia nervosa are Imbalanced Nutrition: Less Than Body Requirements, Powerlessness, Anxiety, and Ineffective Coping. Establishing a therapeutic relationship precedes biopsychosocial assessment and interventions.

Therapeutic Nurse–Patient Relationship

Individuals with bulimia nervosa experience a great deal of shame and guilt. They also often have an intense need to please and be liked and may approach the nurse–patient relationship in a superficial manner. They are too ashamed to discuss their symptoms, but do not want to disappoint others, so they may discuss more social or unrelated issues in an attempt to engage the nurse. A nonjudgmental, accepting approach stressing the importance of the relationship and outlining its purpose are important at the outset of the relationship. Explaining the nature of the relationship and the goals will help clarify the boundaries.

Biologic Domain

Despite the fact that most individuals with bulimia nervosa maintain normal weights, the physical ramifications of this disorder may be similar to those of anorexia nervosa. Hypokalemia can contribute to muscle weakness and fatigability as well as to the development of cardiac arrhythmias, palpitations, and cardiac conduction defects. Patients who purge risk fluid and electrolyte abnormalities that can further compromise cardiac status. Neuropsychiatric disturbances, such as poor concentration and attention, and sleep disturbances are common.

Current eating patterns need to be assessed, along with the number of times a day the individual binges and purges. Dietary restraint practices need to be noted. Sleep patterns and exercise habits are also important to assess.

If the patient is admitted to the hospital, strict monitoring of meals and all intake is necessary to accomplish the goal of normalized eating. Bathroom privileges should also be supervised; patients will be accompanied to the bathroom to prevent purging. In outpatient settings, patients are asked to record their intake, binges, and purges. These records form the foundation for changing behaviors and are incorporated into CBT. Regular sleep patterns are also encouraged, and often patients are asked to go to bed and rise at about the same time every day. Individuals with bulimia nervosa have chaotic lifestyles, as mentioned, and are often overcommitted, making sleep less of a priority. Disturbed sleep can influence binge eating in that individuals can assume, when they are tired, that food would be helpful. They begin to eat, triggering a binge, when, in fact, it is actually sleep that they require.

Pharmacologic Interventions

Experts agree that, whereas pharmacologic intervention is effective for symptom remission in bulimia nervosa, the combination of CBT and medication has had the best results (Wilson et al., 1999). Fluoxetine has been the most studied for bulimia nervosa in clinical trials (see Drug Profile: Fluoxetine Hydrochloride). Effective doses are usually 60 mg per day. This is more than the dosage used to treat depression. For some individuals, sertraline has also been used effectively. These medications are prescribed for the target symptoms of binge eating and purging and are effective even when depression is not present (Goldstein et al., 1999). The most important concern in using these medications is weight loss. Typically, over the first few weeks of administration, patients may have a decrease in appetite and concomitant weight loss. Weight should be monitored, especially during this period.

Monitoring and Administration of Medication. It is important in individuals with bulimia nervosa to monitor the intake of medication for possible purging after administration. The effect of the medication will depend on whether it has had time to absorb.

Teaching Points. Patients should be instructed to take medication as prescribed. It is important that SSRIs be taken in the morning because of their well-known side effect of insomnia, potentially creating further sleep deprivation in patients who have poor sleep habits to begin with because of their chaotic and overextended lifestyles. Patients should be informed that the weight loss they initially experience is temporary and is usually regained after a few weeks, when the medication dosage has stabilized.

Psychosocial Domain

For the individual with bulimia nervosa, psychological assessment focuses on cognitive distortions—cues or stimuli that lead to dysfunctional behavior affecting symptom development—and knowledge deficits. The psychological characteristics typical of patients with bulimia nervosa are presented in Table 24-2.

Individuals with bulimia nervosa display a significant number of cognitive distortions; examples of these are found in Table 24-5. These thought patterns are im-

DRUG PROFILE: Fluoxetine Hydrochloride
(A Selective Serotonin Reuptake Inhibitor)
Trade Name: Prozac

Receptor affinity: Inhibits central nervous system neuronal uptake of serotonin with little effect on norepinephrine; thought to antagonize muscarinic, histaminergic, and α adrenergic receptors.

Indications: Treatment of depressive disorders, most effective in major depression, obesity, bulimia, and obsessive-compulsive disorder

Routes and dosage: Available in 10- and 20-mg pulvules and 20 mg/5 mL oral solution

Adults: 20 mg/d in the morning, do not exceed 80 mg/d. Full antidepressant effect may not be seen for up to 4 weeks. If no improvement, dosage is increased after several weeks. Dosages >20 mg/d are administered twice daily. **For eating disorders: typically 40 to 60 mg/d recommended.**

Geriatric: Administer at lower or less frequent doses; monitor responses to guide dosage.

Children: Safety and efficacy have not been established.

Half-life (peak effect): 2 to 3 d (6–8 h)

Selected adverse reactions: Headache, nervousness, insomnia, drowsiness, anxiety, tremors, dizziness, light-headedness, nausea, vomiting, diarrhea, dry mouth, anorexia, dyspepsia, constipation, taste changes, upper respiratory infections, pharyngitis, painful menstruation, sexual dysfunction, urinary frequency, sweating, rash, pruritus, weight loss, asthenia, and fever

Warnings: Avoid use in pregnancy and while nursing. Use with caution in patients with impaired hepatic or renal function and diabetes mellitus. Possible risk for toxicity if taken with tricyclic antidepressants.

Special patient and family education:
- Be aware that drug may take up to 4 weeks to get full antidepressant effect.
- Take drug in the morning or divided doses, if necessary.
- Report any adverse reactions.
- Avoid driving a car or performing hazardous activities because the drug may cause drowsiness or dizziness.
- Eat small, frequent meals to help with complaints of nausea and vomiting.

---

portant to identify because they form the basis for "rules" and lead the way for destructive eating patterns, such as dietary restraint and bingeing. During routine history taking, patients relate many of these erroneous assumptions. Situations that produce feelings of being overwhelmed and powerless need to be explored, as does the patient's ability to set boundaries, control impulsivity, and maintain quality relationships. These factors are underlying issues precipitating binge eating. Body dissatisfaction should be openly explored. There are a number of assessment tools available to gauge such characteristics as body dissatisfaction and impulsivity (see Text Box 24-3). Mood is an important area for evaluation because a large percentage of women with bulimia nervosa also have depression. Symptoms of depression, especially the vegetative signs, should be thoroughly explored (see Chap. 20).

Treatment Therapies

Both CBT and IPT have been used for individuals with bulimia nervosa. The combination of CBT and pharmacologic interventions has had the best outcomes for the initial decrease in symptoms (Leung et al., 2000; Keel & Mitchell 1997). IPT has been demonstrated to have positive outcomes but may take longer to change binge eating and purging symptoms. Behavioral therapy alone has not been as effective as CBT for symptom reduction. When binge eating and purging are present, little work on underlying interpersonal issues, such boundary setting, can take place because the attention of the patient is on feelings of being out of control with eating. Therefore, cognitive therapy, which addresses the distorted thinking processes influencing dietary restraint, binge eating, and purging, is begun first. Decreasing symptoms will eliminate the out-of-control feelings.

CBT is usually conducted in a group with one or two sessions a week. A series of sessions are instituted, in which a trained therapist works toward changing dysfunctional thinking, rigid rules about eating, and impulsive behaviors. The cognitive interventions focus on distorted or dysfunctional thought patterns.

Behavioral Intervention. The behavioral techniques, such as **cue elimination** and response prevention, require self-monitoring to individualize the therapy. **Self-monitoring** is accomplished using a diary format, in which binges and purges and the precipitating emotions and environmental cues are recorded. Emotional and environmental cues to behavior such as binge eating are identified, and alternative responses are suggested, tried, and reinforced. When a cue or stimuli leads to a response that is dysfunctional or unhealthy, it can be eliminated, or, if this is not possible, an alternate response to the cue, one that is healthier, is substituted, tried, and then reinforced. Figure 24-5 gives two examples of behavioral interventions. In example 1, for the patient with anorexia nervosa, the response is modified or altered to a healthier one; in example 2, for the patient with bulimia nervosa, the cue is changed to produce a different, healthier response. Other techniques, such as postponing binges and purges through distraction, a technique to interrupt the cycle, are also effective.

Psychoeducation. In addition to cognitive and behavioral techniques, educational strategies are also incorpo-

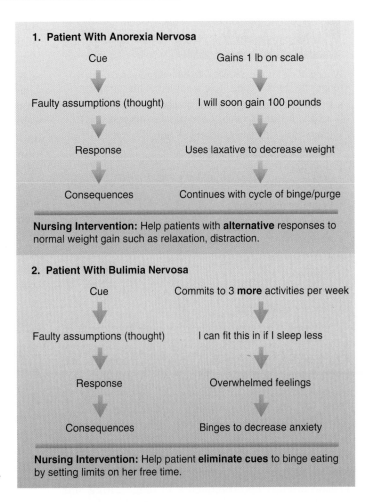

1. Patient With Anorexia Nervosa

Cue   Gains 1 lb on scale

Faulty assumptions (thought)   I will soon gain 100 pounds

Response   Uses laxative to decrease weight

Consequences   Continues with cycle of binge/purge

Nursing Intervention: Help patients with **alternative** responses to normal weight gain such as relaxation, distraction.

2. Patient With Bulimia Nervosa

Cue   Commits to 3 **more** activities per week

Faulty assumptions (thought)   I can fit this in if I sleep less

Response   Overwhelmed feelings

Consequences   Binges to decrease anxiety

Nursing Intervention: Help patient **eliminate cues** to binge eating by setting limits on her free time.

FIGURE 24.5 Examples of the relationship of cues, thoughts, responses: behavioral interventions.

rated into the CBT framework during weekly sessions. For individuals with bulimia nervosa, psychoeducation focuses on teaching boundary setting and healthy limit setting, assertiveness, nutritional concepts related to healthy eating, and clarification of misconceptions about food (White, 1999). Rules that are the result of dichotomous thinking also need to be addressed because of their role in dietary restraint and resulting binge eating.

A group format is cost-effective and increases learning more effectively than an individual model because patients learn from each other as well as from the nurse, therapist, or leader. Some experts have recommended 12-step programs for the treatment of bulimia nervosa. One important problem that many clinicians who work in this specialty have noted is that these programs can be counterproductive for patients with bulimia nervosa. Individuals with this disorder have rigid rules and are already "abstinent" in many ways that lead to binge eating. Broad parameters regarding food choices (eg, all foods allowed in moderation), in combination with knowledge about healthy eating, rather than strict rules, are to be encouraged.

After symptom remission, patients can concentrate on interpersonal issues in therapy, such as a fused re-lationship with their mother, or feelings of inadequacy and low self-esteem, often underlying their lack of assertiveness.

The nurse can assist patients in outpatient and inpatient settings to understand the binge–purge cycle and the role of rigid rules in contributing to the cycle. The value of regularly eaten meals to ward off hunger and reduce the possibility of a binge is another significant area for teaching. Patients who use laxatives will need to know how ineffective they are for actual weight loss. Many individuals who abuse laxatives believe the drop in weight on the scale is actually real weight, rather than water weight. Patients also need information about potassium depletion, electrolyte imbalances, dehydration, and the medical consequences of binge eating and purging. Other topics for psychoeducation are included in the Psychoeducation Checklist: Bulimia Nervosa.

Evaluation and Treatment Outcomes

Patients with bulimia nervosa have better recovery outcomes than those with anorexia nervosa. The outcomes for patients with bulimia nervosa have improved since the early 1990s. This improvement is partially because

---

PSYCHOEDUCATION CHECKLIST
Bulimia Nervosa

When caring for the patient with bulimia nervosa, be sure to include the following topic areas in the teaching plan:

- Psychopharmacologic agents, if used, including drug, action, dosage, frequency, and possible adverse effects
- Binge–purge cycle and effects on body
- Nutrition and eating patterns
- Hydration
- Avoidance of cues
- Cognitive distortions
- Limit setting
- Appropriate boundary setting
- Assertiveness
- Resources
- Self-monitoring and behavioral interventions
- Realistic goal setting

---

of earlier detection, research on what treatments are most effective, and neuropharmacologic research and advances. Experts in the field of eating disorders report a 69% to 70% recovery with a combination of CBT and medication (Keel et al., 1999). Other studies have investigated various methods and their effects, again demonstrating that CBT, when compared with other methods such as supportive therapy, has the best results (Wilson et al., 1999). Frequency of binge eating and purging and severity of dietary restraint at initial treatment, depression, and borderline personality disorder predict a poorer outcome after treatment (Bulik et al., 1998; Keel et al., 1999). Good outcome has been associated with a shorter duration of illness; receiving treatment within the first few years of illness is associated with an 80% recovery rate (Reas et al., 2000).

Continuum of Care

Although patients with bulimia nervosa are less likely than those with anorexia nervosa to require hospitalization, those with extreme dehydration and electrolyte imbalance, depression and suicidality, or symptoms that have not remitted with outpatient treatment need hospitalization.

Most treatment, however, takes place in outpatient settings. After treatment, referrals to recovery groups and support groups are important to prevent relapse. Rarely do patients with bulimia nervosa require emergency care.

Prevention

As with anorexia nervosa, the prevention of bulimia nervosa requires effort on the part of teachers, school nurses, parents, and society as a whole. Because many of the risk factors are seen early in children attending elementary school, educating school nurses and teachers is an important focus for psychiatric–mental health nurses working in the community. Protective factors that mediate between risk factors and the development of an eating disorder need to be stressed and developed. Table 24-6 covers important prevention interventions for parents and their children or adolescents.

Society has begun to engage in an effort to help young girls. The federal government has developed a website called "girl power" devoted to self-confidence in such areas as body image (see Text Box 24-5). Many of the advocacy groups listed in this table have on-line help and web pages with resources for girls, families, teachers, and health care professionals.

Summary of Key Points

➤ Anorexia nervosa and bulimia nervosa have some common symptoms but are classified as discreet disorders in the *DSM-IV-TR*.

➤ Eating disorders are best viewed along a continuum in which subclinical or partial-syndrome disorders are described; because these occur more frequently than full syndromes, they are often missed in detection but, when identified, can be prevented.

➤ There are a number of similar predisposing factors for the development of anorexia nervosa and bulimia nervosa, and these represent a biopsychosocial model of risk. These disorders are preventable, and identifying risk factors assists with prevention strategies.

➤ Etiologic factors in the development of eating disorders are considered to contribute to their development in combination; no one factor provides an explanation.

➤ Treatment of anorexia nervosa almost always includes hospitalization for refeeding; bulimia nervosa is primarily treated on an outpatient basis.

➤ Cognitive behavioral therapy has been shown to improve symptoms sooner than interpersonal therapy for bulimia nervosa. For bulimic patients, the combination of medication and cognitive behavioral therapy is the most effective. For anorexic patients, family therapy in combination with individual interpersonal therapy is the most effective.

➤ Pharmacotherapy has been demonstrated to be effective for bulimia nervosa but not for anorexia nervosa, especially at acute stages during malnourishment.

➤ The outcomes for bulimia nervosa are better than for anorexia nervosa. The type and severity of comorbid conditions and the length of the illness influence poorer outcomes.

Critical Thinking Challenges

1. Discuss the potential difficulties and risks in attempting to treat a patient with anorexia nervosa in an outpatient setting.
2. A patient in the clinic is seen for bulimia nervosa and placed on fluoxetine. She reports great success immediately and attributes this to weight lost. What are your concerns and interventions?
3. Parents are often in need of support and suggestions for how to help in the prevention of eating disorders. Develop a teaching program and include the topics and rationale for those chosen.
4. In establishing a refeeding program for a hospitalized patient with anorexia nervosa, identify the important nursing management components of such a program.
5. Bulimia nervosa is often described as a closet disorder with secretive binge eating and purging. Identify the signs and symptoms of each system involved for someone with this disorder.
6. Positive outcomes for the recovery of bulimia nervosa and anorexia nervosa are dependent on many factors. Identify the factors that promote positive outcomes and those related to poorer outcomes and prognosis.

 WEB LINKS

www.members@aol.com/edapinc   Eating Disorder Awareness and Prevention, Inc. (EDAP), 603 Stewart Street, Seattle, WA 98108. This site provides prevention and self-esteem materials for girls at "Go Girls."

www.anred.com   Anorexia Nervosa and Related Eating Disorders (ANRED), P.O. Box 5102, Eugene, OR 97405. The ANRED site has professional and lay information on eating disorders.

www.members@aol.com/anad20/index.html   National Association of AN and Associated Disorders (ANAD), P.O. Box 7, Highland Park, IL 60035. This site provides professional and lay information on anorexia nervosa.

www.gov.org/gpower   Department of Health and Human Services. This site has information on issues related to girls' self-esteem.

www.mirror-mirror.org/eatdis.htm   Eating Disorders Shared Awareness. This site gives information on how to get help with an eating disorder.

REFERENCES

American Psychiatric Association. (2000). *Diagnostic and statistical manual for mental disorders,* (4th edition, Text revision). Washington, DC: Author.

Addolorato, G., Taranto, C., DeRossi, G., & Gasbarinni, G. (1997). Neuroimaging of cerebral and cerebella atrophy in anorexia nervosa. *Psychiatry Research, 76*(2–3), 105–110.

Braun, D. L., Sunday, S. R., Huang, A., & Halmi. K. A. (1999). More males seek treatment for eating disorders. *International Journal of Eating Disorders, 25*(4), 415–424.

Brownell, K., & Napolitano, M. A. (1995). Distorting reality for children: Body size proportions of Barbie and Ken dolls. *International Journal of Eating Disorders, 18,* 295–298.

Bruch, H. (1973). *Eating disorders: Obesity, anorexia nervosa and the person within.* New York: Basic Books.

Brumberg, J. (1988). *Fasting girls: The emergence of anorexia nervosa as a modern disease.* Cambridge: Harvard University Press.

Bulik, C. M., Sullivan, P. F., Joyce, P. M., et al. (1998). Prediction of one-year outcome in bulimia nervosa. *Comprehensive Psychiatry, 39*(4), 206–254.

Bulik, C. M., Sullivan, P., Wade, T., & Kendler, K. (2000). Twin studies of eating disorders: A review. *International Journal of Eating Disorders, 27,* 1–20.

Casper, R. C., & Lyubomorisky, S. (1997). Individual psychopathology relative to reports of unwanted sexual experiences as predictors of a bulimic eating pattern. *International Journal of Eating Disorders, 21,* 229–236.

Costanzo, P. R., Musante, G. J., Friedman, K. E., et al. (1999). The gender specificity of emotional, situational, and behavioral indicators of binge eating in a diet-seeking obese population. *International Journal of eating disorders, 26*(2), 205–210.

Crow, S., Praus, B., & Thuras, P. (1999). Mortality from eating disorders: A 5-10 year record limiting study. *International Journal of Eating Disorders, 26,* 97–101.

Davis, C., & Katzman, M. A. (1999). Perfection as acculturation: Psychological correlates of eating problems in Chinese male and female students living in the United States. *International Journal of Eating Disorders, 25,* 65–70.

Davis, C., Katzman, D. K., Kaptein, S., et al. (1997). The prevalence of high-level exercise in the eating disorders: Etiological implications. *Comprehensive Psychiatry, 38*(6), 321–326.

Davis, C., Katzman, D. K., & Kirsch C. (1999). Compulsive physical activity with anorexia nervosa: A psychobehavioral spiral of pathology. *Journal of Nervous and Mental Diseases 187*(6), 336–342.

Fichter, M. M., & Quadflieg, N. (1999). Six-year course and outcome of anorexia nervosa. *International Journal of eating Disorders, 26,* 359–385.

Fitzgibbon, M. L., Spring, B., Avellone, M. E., et al. (1998). Correlates of binge eating in Hispanic black and white women. *International Journal of Eating Disorders, 24,* 43–52.

Fulkerson, J., Keel, P., Leon, G., & Dorr, T. (1999). Eating disordered behaviors and personality characteristics of high school athletes and non-athletes. *International Journal of Eating Disorders, 26,* 73–79.

Garner, D. M., Rosen, L. W., & Barry, D. (1998). Eating disorders among athletes: Research and recommendations. *Child and Adolescent Psychiatric Clinics of North America, 7,* 839–857.

Geller, J., Cockell, S., & Goldner, E. (2000). Inhibited expression of negative emotions and interpersonal orientation in anorexia nervosa. *International Journal of Eating Disorders, 28,* 8–19.

Golden, N. H., Ashtari, M., Kohn, M. R., et al. (1996). Reversibility of cerebral ventricular enlargement in anorexia nervosa, demonstrated by quantitative magnetic resonance imaging. *Journal of Pediatrics, 128*(2), 296–301.

Goldstein, D. J., Wilson, M. G., Arscroft, R. C., & Al-Banna, M. (1999). Effectiveness of fluoxetine therapy in bulimia nervosa regardless of comorbid depression. *International Journal of Eating Disorders, 25,* 19–28.

Gowers, S. G., & Shore, A. (1999). The stigma of eating disorders. *International Journal of Clinical Practice, 53*(5), 386–388.

Gutwill, S. (1994). Women's eating problems: Social context and the internalization of culture. In C. Bloom, A. Gitter, S. Gutwill, et al. (Eds.), *Eating problems: A feminist psychoanalytic treatment model* (pp. 1–27). New York: Basic Books.

Herzog, D. B., Greenwood, D. N., Dorer, D. J., et al. (2000). Mortality in eating disorders: A descriptive study. *International Journal of Eating Disorders, 28,* 20–26.

Hill, A., & Pallin, V. (1998). Dieting awareness and low self-worth: Related issues in 8-year-old girls. *International Journal of Eating Disorders, 24,* 405–413.

Joiner, T. E., Katz, J., & Heatherton, T. F. (2000). Personality factors differentiate late adolescent females and males with chronic bulimic symptoms. *International Journal of Eating Disorders, 27,* 191–197.

Kaye, W. H., Gendall, K. A., Fernstrom, M. H., et al. (2000a). Effects of acute tryptophan depletion on mood in bulimia nervosa. *Biological Psychiatry, 47*(2), 151–157.

Kaye, W. H., Klump, K. L., Frank, G. K., & Strober, M. (2000b). Anorexia and bulimia. *Annual Review of Medicine, 51,* 299–313.

Keel, P. K., & Mitchell, J. E. (1997). Outcome in bulimia nervosa. *American Journal of Psychiatry, 154*(3), 313–321.

Keel, P. K., Mitchell, J. E., Milre, K. B., et al. (1999). Long-term outcome of bulimia nervosa. *Archives of General Psychiatry, 56,* 63–69.

LaVia, M. C., Gray, M., & Kaye W. H. (2000). Case reports of olanzapine treatment of anorexia nervosa. *International Journal of Eating Disorders, 27,* 363–366.

Leung, N., Waller, G., & Thomas, G. (2000). Outcome of group cognitive-behavioral therapy for bulimia nervosa: The role of core beliefs. *Behavior Research and Therapy, 38*(2), 15–146.

Lilenfeld, L. R., Kaye, W. H., Greeno, C. G., et al. (1998). A controlled family study of anorexia nervosa and bulimia nervosa: Psychiatric disorders in first-degree relatives and effects of proband comorbidity. *Archives of General Psychiatry, 55*(7), 603–610.

Matsunaga, H., Kaye, W. H., McConaha, C., et al. (2000). Personality disorders among subjects recovered from eating disorders. *International Journal of Eating Disorders, 27,* 353–357.

McIntosh, V. V., Bulik, C. M., McKenzie, J. M., et al. (2000). Interpersonal psychotherapy for anorexia nervosa. *International Journal of Eating Disorders, 27,* 125–139.

Minuchin, S., Rossman, B. L., & Baker, L. (1978). *Psychosomatic families.* Cambridge: Harvard University Press.

Nadoaka, T., Oiiji, A., Takahashi, S., et al. (1996). An epidemiological study of eating disorders in a northern area of Japan. *Acta Psychiatrica Scandinavica, 93,* 305–310.

North, C., & Gowers, S. (1999). Anorexia nervosa, psychopathology and outcome. *International Journal of Eating Disorders, 26,* 386–391.

Ogden, J., & Steward, J. (2000). The role of the mother–daughter relationship in explaining weight concern. *International Journal of Eating Disorders, 28*(11), 78–83.

Pawluck, D. E., & Gorey, K. M. (1998). Secular trends in the incidence of anorexia nervosa: Integrative review of population based studies. *International Journal of Eating Disorders, 23,* 347–352.

Perkins, D. F., & Luster, T. (1999). The relationship between sexual abuse and purging: Findings from a community wide survey of female adolescents. *Child Abuse and Neglect, 23,* 371–382.

Polivy, J., & Herman, C. P. (1993). Etiology of binge eating: Psychological mechanisms. In C. G. Fairburn & G. T. Wilson (Eds.), *Binge eating: Nature, assessment and treatment* (pp. 173–205). New York: Guilford.

Reas, D. L., Williamson, D. A., Martin, C. K., & Zucker, N. L. (2000). Duration of illness predicts outcome for bulimia nervosa: A long term follow up study. *International Journal of Eating Disorders, 27,* 428–434.

Robin, A. L., Siegel, P. T., Moye, A. W., et al. (1999). A controlled comparison of family versus individual therapy for adolescents with anorexia nervosa. *Journal of the American Academy of Child and Adolescent Psychiatry, 38*(12), 1482–1489.

Schwartz, D., Phares, V., Tantleff-Dunn, S., & Thompson, J. K. (1999). Body image, psychological functioning, and parental feedback regarding physical appearance. *International Journal of Eating Disorders, 18,* 339–344.

Shisslak, C., Renger, R., Sharpe, T., et al. (1999). Development and evaluation of the McKnight risk factor survey for assessing potential risk and protective factors for disordered eating in preadolescent and adolescent girls. *International Journal of Eating Disorders, 25,* 195–214.

Shapira, N. A., Goldsmith, T. D., & McElroy, S. L. (2000). Treatment of binge eating disorder with topiramate: A clinical case series. *Journal of Clinical Psychiatry, 61*(5), 368–372.

Smith, K. A., Fairburn, C. G., Cowen, P. J. (1999). Symptomatic relapse in bulimia nervosa following acute tryptophan depletion. *Archives of General Psychiatry, 56*(2), 171–176.

Smolak, L., Levine, M. P., & Schermer, F. (1999). Parental input and weight concern among elementary school children. *International Journal of Eating Disorders, 25,* 263–271.

Smolak, L., Murnen, S. K., & Ruble, A. (2000). Female athletes and eating problems: A meta analysis. *International Journal of Eating Disorders, 27*(4), 371–380.

Sobol, J., & Bursztyn, M. (1998). Dating people with anorexia nervosa and bulimia nervosa: Attitudes and beliefs of university students. *Women & Health, 27*(3), 73–85.

Streigel-Moore, R. (1993). Etiology of binge eating: A developmental perspective. In C. G. Fairburn & G. T.

Wilson (Eds.), *Binge eating, nature, assessment and treatment* (pp. 144–172). New York: Guilford.

Strober, M., Freeman, R., Lampert, C., et al. (2000). Controlled family study of anorexia nervosa and bulimia nervosa: Evidence of shared liability and transmission of partial syndromes. *American Journal of Psychiatry, 157*(3), 393–401.

Strober, M., Freeman, R., & Morrell, W. (1997). The long-term course of severe anorexia in adolescents: Survival, analysis of recovery, relapse and outcome predictors over 10–15 years. *International Journal of Eating Disorders, 23,* 339–360.

Strober, M., Pataki, C., Freeman, R., & DeAntonio, M. (1999). No effect of adjunctive fluoxetine on eating behavior or weight phobia during the impatient treatment of anorexia nervosa: An historical case controlled study. *Journal of Child and Adolescent Psychopharmacology, 9*(3), 195–201.

Taylor, C. B., Sharpe, T., Shisslak, C., et al. (1998). Factors associated with weight loss in adolescent girls. *International Journal of Eating Disorders, 24,* 31–42.

Tiggerman, M., & Pickering, A. (1996). The role of television in adolescent women's body dissatisfaction and drive for thinness. *International Journal of Eating Disorders, 20,* 199–203.

Thornton, C., & Russell, S. (1997). Obsessive-compulsive comorbidity in the dieting disorders. *International Journal of Eating Disorders, 21,* 83–87.

von Ranson, K. M., Kaye, W. H., Weltzin, T. E., Rao, R., & Matsunaga, H. (1999). Obsessive-compulsive disorder

symptoms before and after recovery from bulimia nervosa. *American Journal of Psychiatry, 156*(11), 1703–1708.

Ward, A., Tiller, J., Treasure, J., & Russell, G. (2000). Eating disorders: Psyche or soma. *International Journal of Eating Disorders, 27,* 279–287.

White, J. H. (1999). The development and clinical testing of an outpatient program for women with bulimia nervosa. *Archives of Psychiatric Nursing, 13*(4), 179–191.

White, J. H. (2000a). Eating disorders in elementary and middle school children: Risk factors, early detection and prevention. *The Journal of School Nursing, 16*(2), 26–35.

White, J. H. (2000b). Symptom development in bulimia nervosa: A comparison of women with and without a history of anorexia nervosa. *Archives of Psychiatric Nursing, 14*(2), 81–92.

Wiederman, M., & Pryor, T. (2000). Body dissatisfaction, bulimia, and depression among women: The mediating role of drive for thinness. *International Journal of Eating Disorders, 27,* 90–95.

Wilson, G. T., Loeb, K. L., Walsh, B. T., et al. (1999). Psychological versus pharmacological treatments of bulimia nervosa: Predictors and processes of change. *Journal of Consulting and Clinical Psychology, 67*(4), 451–459.

Wolfe, B. E., Metzger, E. D., Levine, J. M., et al. (2000). Serotonin function following remission from bulimia nervosa. *Neuropsychopharmacology, 22*(3), 257–263.

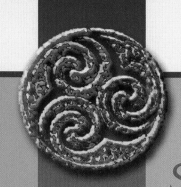

Substance Abuse Disorders

Barbara G. Faltz and Mary K. Skinner

LEARNING OBJECTIVES

After completing this chapter, you will be able to:

➤ Distinguish among the actions, effects, and withdrawal symptoms (if any) of alcohol, marijuana, stimulants, sedatives, hallucinogens, phencyclidine, opiates, nicotine, solvents, and caffeine.

➤ Explain the biologic, psychological, and social theories that attempt to explain substance abuse, dependence, and addiction.

➤ Compare the advantages and disadvantages of several intervention approaches to substance abuse and chemical dependence.

CHAPTER 25

➤ Describe the effects of alcohol and other drug classifications on pregnancy and infants.

➤ Describe appropriate nursing diagnoses and treatment interventions for patients who deny a substance abuse problem.

➤ Formulate nursing diagnoses based on a biopsychosocial assessment of people with substance use disorders.

➤ Formulate nursing interventions that address specific diagnoses related to substance abuse.

KEY TERMS

abuse

addiction

alcohol withdrawal
 syndrome

Alcoholics Anonymous

anhedonia

anxiolytic

codependence

countertransference

craving

delirium tremens

denial

dependence

detoxification

hallucinogen

harm reduction

inhalants

Korsakoff's psychosis

methadone
 maintenance

narcotics

opiates

reality confrontation

relapse

sedative-hypnotic
 drugs

substance-related
 disorders

tolerance

use

Wernicke's syndrome

withdrawal

*A*ncient and modern history chronicles the negative impact of alcohol and drug abuse on various cultures and civilizations. The human use and abuse of alcohol and other drugs has been around since the beginning of history; so too have the subsequent social and emotional problems that accompany substance abuse. Today, alcohol and substance abuse problems have reached epidemic proportions in the United States, with incidence rising in younger age groups, particularly among adolescents and young adults. What used to be a problem primarily of older adolescents and young adults now appears to be a

problem effecting younger and younger children. Exposure to illegal drugs, which 25 years ago was primarily an issue only in certain areas of major cities, is now a threat to children in almost every local neighborhood, community, and school.

Substance abuse has been identified as one of the major health issues in our nation and is the focus of much social and political concern. The connection between substance dependence and addiction and related social and health issues is documented in the literature and includes issues such as the rise of illegal and criminal activities and violence associated with *the sale and distribution of illegal drugs in neighborhoods and schools that jeopardize the health and well-being of communities. Statistics show that younger age groups are being exposed to drugs and that many are experimenting with drugs at early ages. Other major health issues include the increased risk for spread of human immunodeficiency virus (HIV) infection, hepatitis B and C, and other communicable diseases among alcohol and other drug users; the number of premature deaths or traumatic injury due to drug overdoses or other unsafe activities or practices engaged in while under the influence of alcohol or drugs (eg, car accidents); and the enormous increase in domestic violence and child abuse and neglect that has resulted from substance abuse. The medical and social implications are profound as we face a new generation of children who are at risk for the serious medical, developmental, learning, and psychological problems associated with perinatal and childhood exposure to drugs and alcohol. In a recent study Huang and colleagues (1998) estimated that more than 74 million children in the United States lived in a household in which one or more parent was dependent on alcohol or illicit drugs.*

Substance abuse takes a heavy toll in terms of the social, medical, and emotional health of individuals and communities. In fact, it is arguably the primary social health issue facing the United States in the 21st century. It threatens to affect the overall welfare of our nation and our health care system. Nurses and mental health professionals in the next decade can be crucial to implementing assessment techniques, early diagnosis, and early implementation of treatment. They have a vital role in helping to educate individuals and communities, establishing much needed prevention programs, and participating in support groups.

This chapter reviews types of substance abuse, biologic and psychological effects on an individual, current theories regarding the etiology of substance abuse, and intervention programs available to treat substance abuse. The role of the nurse is discussed in assessment and planning interventions to help meet the needs of patients and family members who seek treatment. Professional issues regarding chemical dependency within the nursing profession are examined.

Definitions and Terms

The following different terms are used to describe behavior patterns regarding substance use:

- **Use** is when a person drinks alcohol or swallows, smokes, sniffs, or injects a mind-altering substance.
- **Abuse** is when a person is using alcohol or drugs for the purpose of intoxication or, in the case of prescription drugs, for purposes beyond their intended use.
- **Dependence** is the continuing use of alcohol or drugs despite adverse consequences to one's physical, social, and psychological well-being.

- **Addiction** describes that state when the person experiences severe psychological and behavioral dependence on drugs or alcohol.
- **Withdrawal** is the adverse physical and psychological symptoms that occur when a person ceases using a substance.
- **Detoxification** is the process of safely and effectively withdrawing a person from an addictive substance, usually under medical supervision.
- **Relapse** is the recurrence of alcohol- or drug-dependent behavior in an individual who has previously achieved and maintained abstinence for a significant time beyond the period of detoxification.

Diagnostic Criteria

The American Psychiatric Association's (APA's) *Diagnostic and Statistical Manual of Mental Disorders*, 4th edition, Text revision (*DSM-IV-TR*) classifies **substance-related disorders** as disorders related to the taking of a drug of abuse, including alcohol, amphetamines, cannabis (marijuana), cocaine, hallucinogens, inhalants, nicotine, opioids, phencyclidine, sedatives-hypnotics, anxiolytics, caffeine, and other unknown substances (APA, 2000). These disorders are further categorized as those related to the abuse of a substance, those related to dependence on a substance, or those induced by intoxication or withdrawal. The *DSM-IV-TR* outlines diagnostic criteria for both substance abuse and dependence (Table 25-1).

Epidemiology and Cultural Issues

Epidemiologic data on alcohol and other drug dependence come from several sources. Surveys such as the National Household Survey on Drug Abuse (NHSDA), the National Comorbidity Survey (NCS), and the National Longitudinal Alcohol Epidemiologic Survey (NLAES) examine prevalence in selected populations during a given time period or over a period of years. The Drug Abuse Warning Network (DAWN) collects data on the number of episodes of abuse reported during an emergency room visit by medical examiners, coroners, and crisis centers in key metropolitan areas (Winick, 1997). Estimates of the extent of alcohol dependence range from 5 million to 14 million Americans (Goodwin & Gabrielli, 1997). The NLAES indicated that prevalence of lifetime drinking was highest for men in the age range of 30 to 44 years, with 23.4% of U.S. adults reporting a positive lifetime history of heavy alcohol use and 15.6% drug abuse. Cannabis (marijuana) is the most commonly abused drug, followed by illicit use of prescription drugs (Grant & Dawson, 1999). There has been a general downward

TABLE 25.1 *DSM-IV* Substance Related Disorders

Substance Disorder	Diagnostic Criteria
Substance Dependence Alcohol dependence Amphetamine dependence Cannabis dependence Cocaine dependence Hallucinogen dependence Inhalant dependence Nicotine dependence Opioid dependence Phencyclidine dependence Sedative, hypnotic, or anxiolytic dependence Polysubstance dependence	Maladaptive pattern of substance use leading to clinically significant impairment or distress • Impairment manifested by three or more of the following: tolerance (need for markedly increased amounts of the substance to reach intoxication or desired effect), withdrawal, substance often taken in large amounts or over a longer period than was intended, persistent desire or unsuccessful efforts to cut down or control use, much time spent in activities necessary to obtain the substance or use it, reduction or cessation of important social, occupational, or recreational activities, use continued despite knowledge of having persistent or recurrent physical or psychological problem likely to have been caused or exacerbated by the substance

Substance Abuse
Alcohol abuse
Amphetamine abuse
Cannabis abuse
Cocaine abuse
Hallucinogen abuse
Inhalant abuse
Opioid abuse
Phencyclidine abuse
Sedative, hypnotic, or anxiolytic abuse
	• Maladaptive pattern of substance use leading to clinically significant impairment or distress
	• Impairment manifested by three or more of the following occurring within a 12-month period:
	  Recurrent use, resulting in failure to fulfill major role obligations at work, school, or home
	  Recurrent use in situations that are physically hazardous
	  Recurrent substance-related legal problems
	  Continued use despite feeling persistent or recurrent effects of the substance
	• Symptoms never met criteria for substance dependence

Substance Intoxication Alcohol intoxication Alcohol intoxication delirium Amphetamine intoxication Amphetamine intoxication delirium Caffeine intoxication Cannabis intoxication Cannabis intoxication delirium Cocaine intoxication Cocaine intoxication delirium Hallucinogen intoxication Hallucinogen intoxication delirium Opioid intoxication Opioid intoxication delirium Inhalant intoxication Inhalant intoxication delirium Phencyclidine intoxication, delirium Sedative, hypnotic, or anxiolytic intoxication	• Reversible substance-specific syndrome due to recent ingestion or exposure to a substance • Clinically significant maladaptive behavioral or psychological changes due to effect of substance on central nervous system, developing during or shortly after use of substance • Symptoms not due to general medical condition, nor better accounted for by another mental disorder
Substance Withdrawal Alcohol withdrawal, delirium Amphetamine withdrawal Cocaine withdrawal Opioid withdrawal Sedative, hypnotic, or anxiolytic withdrawal, delirium	• Development of substance-specific syndrome due to cessation or reduction in substance use, previously heavy and prolonged • Syndrome causing significant distress or impairment in social, occupational, or other important areas of functioning

trend in overall per capita alcohol consumption that began in the early 1980s and continues. Studies suggest that contributing factors are a less tolerant national attitude toward drinking, increased legal and social pressures and actions against drinking and driving, and a general increase in health concerns among Americans (U.S. Department of Health and Human Services [U.S. DHHS], 1997b).

Recent studies that report national trends in alcohol and drug consumption among racial and ethnic minorities found that between 1985 and 1995 in all groups, there was a reduction in heavy drinking or the rate remained stable. Despite the reduction in per capita alcohol consumption, minorities, particularly African Americans and Hispanics, are more at risk for drug and alcohol abuse and, ultimately, more at risk for associated negative social and health consequences (National Institute on Drug Abuse [NIDA], 1998).

African Americans

There is serious consideration of the association of race and social disadvantage in the Western world, where most drug dependence studies have been conducted. Traditional studies of drug dependency have centered on populations in public treatment programs or those arrested or incarcerated for drug-related crimes. Often, these are inner-city populations, which have traditionally reflected a disproportionate representation of African Americans, promoting a biased view that perhaps some genetic or biologic predisposition might make African Americans more vulnerable to drug abuse. Studies are just beginning to consider the influences of social disadvantage and high-risk environmental factors associated with these study populations that greatly effect the high rate of substance abuse found in African Americans. Although African American youth have lower rates of both licit and illicit substance use compared with whites, they have experienced more health and legal problems than other ethnic groups (NIDA, 1998). Likewise, alcohol-related consequences for African American males is higher than for white males, although rates of heavy drinking were similar (U.S. DHHS, 1997b). Substance abuse has had a serious impact on the African American community, with one-quarter million African American men in prison serving drug-related sentences (Abramsky, 1997). This can be attributed to the higher rate of crack-cocaine related crimes, which tend to result in more severe sentencing (Abramsky, 1997). African Americans are also more often victims of violence because of their population concentration population in poor neighborhoods, often with higher rates of drug-related crime (Center for Substance Abuse Treatment [CSAT], 1999).

Latino Americans

Latino Americans compose one of the youngest segments of the U.S. population. Data from the NHSDA (U.S. DHHS, 1997) indicated that 1.1 million Hispanics (8%) were illicit drug users in 1996. Studies of prevalence of drug use in this group are alarmingly high among adolescents. Hispanic high school seniors have the highest rates of crack-cocaine and heroin use (NIDA, 1998; CSAT, 1999). Primary substances of abuse are alcohol and heroin (Castro et al., 1999). Stress related to the level of acculturation, poverty, discrimination, and racism have been factors for the high rates of substance abuse among Hispanics (Gloria & Peregoy, 1996). It is important to note that the term Hispanic covers several distinct groups with varying cultures. Nielson (2000) found that there are significant differences in alcohol consumption between different Hispanic groups. Among men, Mexican Americans report the most frequent and heavy drinking and alcohol-related problems. Cuban Americans report the lowest percentages of problems. For women, fewer differences existed than with men (Nielsen, 2000).

Asians and Pacific Islanders

Despite recent increases in studies focused on Asians and Pacific Islanders, epidemiologic data are often limited and are not often differentiated by population subgroup (CSAT, 1999). The substance abuse problems of each group may be influenced by the way in which cultural, economic, social, political, and migratory factors fuse (CSAT, 1999). As a general pattern, Asian and Pacific Islanders have a lower prevalence rate of substance abuse than any other group (NIDA, 1998). Several cultural patterns and attitudes have been suggested as influencing factors:

1. Public drunkenness is viewed as unacceptable and disgraceful behavior.
2. Drinking is viewed as primarily a male activity, and many Asian women do not drink.
3. Seeking professional help is viewed as a sign of character weakness, particularly in Asian men.
4. Asian flushing syndrome, a physiologic reaction that occurs in 30% to 50% of Asian Americans, resulting in a red cutaneous flush or rash that appears on the face and body after drinking alcohol, may serve as deterrent to drinking excessively. The Asian flushing syndrome has been associated with the lack of the liver enzyme acetaldehyde dehydrogenase, which results in an initial rapid rate of alcohol metabolism and sudden buildup of acetaldehyde, a toxic by-product of alcohol metabolism (Kitano, 1989).

Native Americans

Studies indicate that alcohol and other drug use rates are high among members of American Indian and Alaska Native groups (U.S. DHHS, 1998). It is significant that there are about 400 recognized American Indian tribes—all with tribally specific differences in beliefs, ceremonies, cultures, governments, practices, and traditions (CSAT, 1999). Alcohol plays a significant role in the health problems of this group. Cirrhosis of the liver and alcoholism account for more than one third of all American Indian deaths (Westermeyer, 1997).

Empiric studies have mostly focused on alcohol abuse problems on the reservations (278 reservations and 209 Alaska Native villages). Suggestions that there is a biologic predisposition to alcoholism among Native Americans have not been proved scientifically (Westermeyer, 1997). Many believe destructive patterns of alcohol abuse emerged as a result of restrictive liquor laws that prevented these communities from developing acceptable cultural norms and behaviors regarding drinking alcohol (Westermeyer, 1997).

Gender Differences

In the early years of studying drug abuse in the United States, studies centered on men who were incarcerated for drug-related federal offenses. However, recent study results revealed that substance abuse and dependence occurs slightly more in men than women. Incidence rates for men were close to 1.7% per year and were 0.7% per year for women (Anthony & Helzer, 1995). Some interesting differences were found between men and women in their patterns of drug abuse and dependence. Women were marketed as consumers of legal opiate and cocaine preparations before the 1900s and were seen as weak and needing these "medications" to cope with stress and pain (Kendall, 1998). Recent studies showed that men are more likely to abuse drugs and alcohol than women but that women still outnumber men in the frequency of misuse and abuse of prescribed psychoactive medications and are at the same level of abuse of nicotine as men (Gomberg, 1999). Drug and alcohol abuse patterns in women vary with age, education, marital status, employment, race and ethnicity, and the alcohol or drug usage of spouse or significant other (Gomberg, 1999). Many women seeking treatment for alcohol and other drug abuse have multiple issues that impinge on their recovery (Marion, 1995), including the following:

- Functioning as a single parent
- Lack of employment skills
- Living in abusive or unstable living environments
- Lack of transportation, child care, and finances needed for treatment-related activities

Gender-specific services that are ethnically and culturally sensitive, along with a comprehensive array of related services, are essential for successful treatment of women who abuse alcohol or other drugs.

Comorbidity

A high number of substance abusers have comorbid mental disorders. Many mental disorders are in part a by-product of long-term substance abuse; for others, the mental disorder itself predisposes to alcohol or drug abuse. Whatever the reason, nurses should be aware that substance abusers often have coexisting mental disorders, particularly anxiety disorders, phobias, and obsessive-compulsive and affective disorders, such as major depression and dysthymia. Other coexisting mental disorders include attention deficit hyperactivity disorder and personality disorders (Rosenthal & Westreich, 1999). These are discussed in detail in Chapter 33.

Mortality rates for drug-dependent individuals exceed those of the normal population. These people are at high risk for death from drug overdose but are also at increased risk for death from other causes, including homicide, suicide, and opportunistic infections secondary to drug injection practices such as HIV (Selwyn & Merino, 1997). Studies have documented the connection between alcohol abuse and increased risk for diabetes mellitus, gastrointestinal problems, hypertension, liver disease, stroke (U.S. DHHS, 1997b); increased risk for cardiovascular complications in young cocaine users; and risk for traumatic injury from car accidents or other injuries while intoxicated (Caulker-Burnett, 1994).

Etiology

Researchers have long been asking the questions of what causes addictive behavior and why some people feel compelled to keep abusing substances they know are harmful and detrimental to themselves. Growing evidence suggests both the psychological and the biologic bases of addiction, which may explain this apparently self-destructive behavior. Although genetic evidence indicates that there is a familial predisposition toward addiction, a common genetic marker for addiction or dependence has not been found. Evidence of neurochemical, neurophysiologic, and psychopharmacologic mechanisms common to alcohol and other drug addiction has been found (Fig. 25-1).

Genetic Factors

Most of the data regarding the genetic influence of substance abuse are from the alcoholism studies and suggest the influence of genetic factors in its development. Genetic studies primarily focus on family studies, twin studies, adoption studies, and studies seeking a baseline trait marker of alcoholism. The reported prevalence of substance abuse among biologic family members differs from study to study. However, there is a positive association of addiction among family members. This rate decreases as biologic distance increases (Hesselbrock et al., 1999). Other important studies in determining genetic predisposition are adoptive studies in which rates of alcoholism are evaluated in children of alcoholic parents when they are raised in different environments by adoptive parents. One landmark study evaluated individuals

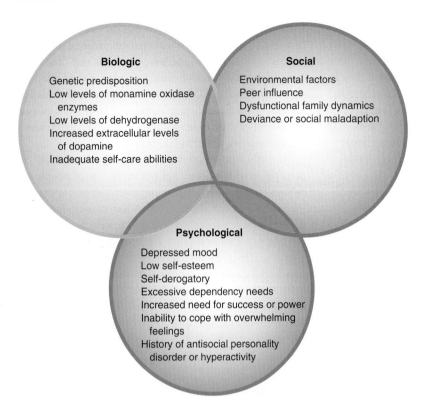

Biologic

Genetic predisposition
Low levels of monamine oxidase
enzymes
Low levels of dehydrogenase
Increased extracellular levels
of dopamine
Inadequate self-care abilities

Social

Environmental factors
Peer influence
Dysfunctional family dynamics
Deviance or social maladaption

Psychological

Depressed mood
Low self-esteem
Self-derogatory
Excessive dependency needs
Increased need for success or power
Inability to cope with overwhelming
feelings
History of antisocial personality
disorder or hyperactivity

FIGURE 25.1 Biopsychosocial etiologies for patients with substance abuse.

raised apart from their biologic parents, comparing those who had a biologic alcoholic parent with those who were raised by an adoptive alcoholic parent. Those who had a biologic parent with severe alcoholism were significantly more likely to develop alcoholism than those being raised by an adoptive alcoholic parent (Schuckit et al., 1972). Another early adoption study in Denmark found that sons of alcoholics (when compared with controls) were about four times more likely to be alcoholic than were sons of nonalcoholics, regardless of whether they were raised by nonalcoholic foster parents or by their own biologic parents (Goodwin, 1979). Recently, Bierut and colleagues (1998) found in data from six sites that the lifetime prevalence of alcohol, marijuana, and cocaine dependence was higher in the biologic siblings of alcohol-dependent people than in control subjects.

Controversy surrounds the search for a specific gene that could cause alcoholism and other drug dependencies. The debate centers around an allele of dopamine receptor D2 that appeared to be implicated in severe cases of alcoholism and some other substance use disorders (Anthenelli & Schuckit, 1997). Until confirming genetic analysis is completed, this finding is theoretic.

Neurobiologic Theories

Some studies suggest that drugs of abuse reinforce dependence by stimulating future use through a biologic brain reward mechanism, whereby the regions in the brain that primarily are stimulated are responsible for

the positive drug dependencies. Often, there is a compelling urge to use alcohol or other drugs that dominates an addict's thoughts and effects the addict's mood and behavior. This is defined as **craving** (Halikas, 1997).

Intoxication with drugs such as cocaine, phencyclidine, alcohol, nicotine, and various opiates produces an increase in extracellular levels of dopamine. This dopamine-related "high" produced by these drugs becomes the reinforcement mechanism in the brain. The neurochemical status in the brain readjusts to these increased levels of dopamine as being the "normal" neurochemical state and then begins to seek or "crave" increased amounts of a substance to produce the same dopamine-related effects (Halikas, 1997; Gold, 1994). This need for increased amounts of a substance to achieve the same results is termed **tolerance** and is what ultimately drives substance abusers to crave more and more of the abused substance. This readjustment of the "normal" neurochemical homeostasis could possibly explain the feelings of diminished enjoyment of life, or **anhedonia,** that occurs in long-term cocaine abusers when they discontinue use.

These neurobiologic theories are further substantiated by animal behavioral studies indicating that both animals and humans self-administer substances in similar patterns, producing addictive behavior. Animals prefer to self-administer drugs rather than eat, drink water, or rest, even to the point of death (Gardner, 1997). Another study showed that animals will work for injections of alcohol and other drugs that are administered to specific areas in the brain that cause craving but not to areas of the brain unrelated to craving (Miller & Gold, 1994). This commonality of drug use patterns across species appears to add validity to the biologic basis of alcohol and substance abuse (Halikas, 1997).

Psychological Theories

The psychological theories support the notion that some individuals are born with personality traits that make them more susceptible to substance abuse; some call it an "addictive personality." One researcher identified five psychosocial needs common to those who become addicted: need to feel self-worth, need to have control over the environment, need to feel intimate contact with others, need to accomplish something valuable, and need to eliminate pain or other powerful negative feelings (Peele, 1985). Kaufman (1994) identified six psychodynamic issues that often lead to substance abuse: excessive dependency needs, need for success or power, inability to care for self adequately, gender identity problems, inability to cope with overwhelming painful feelings, and dysfunctional family dynamics (Table 25-2).

Behavioral Theories

Many investigators have turned their attention to the behavioral characteristics of childhood and adolescence that might predispose a person to substance abuse. Some have postulated that conduct problems of childhood, such as deviance, misbehavior, and aggression, might be important behavioral risk factors for later substance abuse, particularly for boys. A few convincing studies demonstrate a strong connection between childhood conduct problems, hyperactivity, impulsivity, and future substance abuse (Brehm & Khantzian, 1997). A history of general deviance or social maladaption in the form of police trouble or long-standing behavioral problems has been linked to risk for developing drug dependence.

Social Theories

Many studies focused on the areas of peer drug use and affiliation with deviant peers as strong determinants of teenage drug involvement (Chassin et al., 1993; Hawkins et al., 1992). Peer interaction is a crucial influencing factor in determining adolescents' exposure to alcohol and drugs (Hesselbrock et al., 1999). Peers' perceptions of alcohol use as reducing tension and other alleged positive attributes contribute to their increased use (Segal & Stewart, 1996).

Certain neighborhood characteristics may also be factors in increased drug abuse, including high population density, physical deterioration, high levels of crime, and illegal drug trafficking (Hesselbrock et al., 1999). These social factors may increase an individual's feeling of alienation, escapist behavior, and other deviant behavior (Segal & Stewart, 1996).

Summary of Etiologic Theories

The modern disease model of substance abuse is truly a biopsychosocial one—it encompasses the body, the mind, and society's influences in studying the disease and formulating treatment (Wallace, 1990). Recent biologic studies in humans and animals have confirmed that there is a genetic predisposition toward drinking behaviors and significant genetic differences in drug self-administration for several other drugs, yet no precise genetic marker has

---

TABLE 25.2 Psychological Issues Leading to Substance Abuse

Issue	Psychodynamics
Excessive dependence needs	Excessive dependency needs lead to rejection and a sense of failure. Resulting anxiety is relieved by substance abuse.
Need for success or power	Excessive fear of success or failure or appearing weak or challenged. Substance abuse can provide temporary illusion of adequacy and power.
Inadequate self-care abilities	Individual has inadequate abilities to self-regulate or self-soothe, or has low self-esteem. Substance abuse provides temporary resolution of psychological pain.
Gender identity issues	Males more socialized to externalize stress and feelings by drinking alcohol and using drugs. Women are more socialized to "treat" feelings of low self-esteem with alcohol or other drugs.
Affect intolerance	Overwhelming painful feelings from childhood that cannot be tolerated or discussed. Individual may be able to express these feelings when intoxicated.
Family systems	Symbolic fusion with parent, failure to separate from parent and develop own self-identity during adolescence can lead to a too rigid or too flexible bonding with substance-abusing peers, leaving individual vulnerable to peer pressure to drink and use drugs.

Adapted from Kaufman, E. (1994). *Psychotherapy of addicted persons.* New York: Guilford Press.

been established. Recent evidence from genetics, neurochemistry, and pharmacology has revealed the essential biologic component of alcoholism—that it is a disease, a chronic and progressive one that must be treated. But it is a disease influenced not just by the biologic components but also by the individual's temperament and feelings about self (psychological components) and environmental factors, such as parental and family relationships and peer pressure (social components). To understand and treat substance abusers, nurses must understand and treat all facets of this illness.

SUBSTANCES OF ABUSE

ALCOHOL

Definition and Clinical Picture

Most Americans drink alcohol. Reliable surveys indicate that 90% of adult Americans have had a drink of alcohol at some point in their lives. According to the most rigorous study, about 16% of the population suffers from alcoholism. However, 80% or more of the alcohol consumed in the United States is consumed by the alcoholic. (Miller et al., 1997). Alcohol (or ethanol) is a sedative anesthetic found in various proportions in liquor, wine, and beer. Alcohol produces a sedative effect by depressing the central nervous system (CNS). This causes the individual to experience a relaxation of inhibitions, emotions, or mood swings that can range from bouts of gaiety to angry outbursts and cognitive impairments such as reduced concentration or attention span, impaired judgment, and memory. Depending on the amount of alcohol ingested, the effects can range from feelings of mild sedation and relaxation to serious impairment of motor functions and speech and confusion, to severe intoxication that can result in coma, respiratory failure, and death. See Table 25-3 for a summary of the effects of abused substances.

The intensity of CNS impairments depends on how much alcohol is consumed in a given period of time and how rapidly the body metabolizes it. Intoxication is determined by the level of alcohol in the blood, called *blood alcohol level* (BAL). The body can metabolize 1 oz of liquor, a 5-oz glass of wine, or a 12-oz can of beer per hour without intoxication. Table 25-4 shows normal physiologic responses at various BALs.

Excessive or long-term abuse of alcohol can adversely affect all body systems. Table 25-5 lists the major physical complications of alcohol abuse in the major organ systems. Alcohol abuse can have serious and permanent long-term effects. Years of alcohol abuse can cause cerebellar degeneration from increased levels of acetaldehyde, a toxic by-product of alcohol metabolism, and can result in impaired coordination, a broad-based unsteady gait, and fine tremors. Sedative-hypnotic long-term

effects include disturbances in rapid-eye-movement (REM) sleep and chronic sleep disorders. Long-term alcohol abuse can cause specific neurologic complications that lead to organic brain disorders known as alcohol-induced amnestic disorders (discussed later).

People who abuse alcohol can exhibit various patterns of use. Some engage in heavy drinking on a regular or daily basis; others may abstain from drinking during the week and engage in heavy drinking on the weekends; still others can experience longer periods of sobriety interspersed with bouts of binge drinking (several days of intoxication).

Biologic Responses to Alcohol

Alcohol makes the neuronal membranes more permeable to K^+ and Cl^- and closes Na^+ and Ca^{++} channels. This increased permeability causes depression of the CNS; increased adrenergic activity causes elevated blood pressure and heart rate. Alcohol is metabolized in the liver as a carbohydrate into carbon dioxide and water. The breakdown process (oxidation) of the compound ethanol (CH_3CH_2OH) is: ethanol → acetaldehyde + water → acetic acid → carbon dioxide + water. Acetaldehyde is toxic and is usually broken down by acetaldehyde dehydrogenase. Rapid alcohol intake can cause an accumulation of acetaldehyde, which then combines with the neurotransmitters dopamine and serotonin to produce tetrahydroisoquinolines and β-carbolines. Physical dependence on alcohol becomes a problem when central nervous system cells require alcohol to function normally (Moak & Anton, 1999).

People who have abused alcohol for long periods of time often develop alcohol tolerance, a phenomenon producing a more rapid metabolism of alcohol and decreased response to sedating, motor, and **anxiolytic** effects. These individuals may demonstrate higher blood alcohol levels than normal (listed in Table 25-4) before they experience symptoms of intoxication. The locus ceruleus is a brain structure that normally inhibits the action of ethanol and is believed to be instrumental in the development of alcohol tolerance. In alcoholic patients or in those who engage in chronic drinking, the alcohol withdrawal syndrome usually begins within 12 hours after abrupt discontinuation or attempt to cut down. Only 5% of individuals with alcohol dependence ever experience severe complications of withdrawal, such as **delirium tremens** or grand mal (tonic–clonic) seizures (Miller et al., 1997).

Alcohol Withdrawal Syndrome

Alcohol withdrawal syndrome occurs after the reduction of alcohol consumption or when abstaining from alcohol after prolonged use causes changes in vital

TABLE 25.3 Summary of Effects of Abused Substances, Overdose, Withdrawal Syndromes, and Prolonged Use

Substance	Route	Effects (E) and Overdose (O)	Withdrawal Syndrome	Prolonged Use
Alcohol	Oral	E: Sedation, decreased inhibitions, relaxation, decreased coordination, slurred speech, nausea O: Respiratory depression, cardiac arrest	Tremors; seizures; increased temperature, pulse, and blood pressure; delirium tremens	Affects all systems of the body. Can lead to other dependencies.
Stimulants (amphetamines, cocaine)	Oral, IV inhalation, smoking	E: Euphoria, initial CNS stimulation then depression, wakefulness, decreased appetite, insomnia, paranoia, aggressiveness, dilated pupils, tremors O: Cardiac arrhythmias/arrest, increased or lowered blood pressure, respiratory depression, chest pain, vomiting, seizures, psychosis, confusion, seizures, dyskinesias, dystonias, coma	Depression: psychomotor retardation at first, then agitation; fatigue then insomnia; severe dysphoria and anxiety; cravings, vivid, unpleasant dreams; increased appetite. Amphetamine withdrawal is not as pronounced as cocaine withdrawal.	Is often alternated with depressants. Weight loss and resulting malnutrition and increased susceptibility to infectious diseases. May produce schizophrenia-like syndrome with paranoid ideation, thought disturbance, hallucinations, and stereotyped movements.
Cannabis (marijuana, hashish, THC)	Smoking, oral	E: Euphoria or dysphoria, relaxation and drowsiness, heightened perception of color and sound, poor coordination, spatial perception and time distortion, unusual body sensations (weightlessness, tingling, etc.), dry mouth, dysarthria, and food cravings O: Increased heart rate, reddened eyes, dysphoria, lability, disorientation		Can decrease motivation and cause cognitive deficits (inability to concentrate, memory impairment).
Hallucinogens (LSD, MDMA)	Oral	E: Euphoria or dysphoria, altered body image, distorted or sharpened visual and auditory perception, depersonalization, bizarre behavior, confusion, incoordination, impaired judgment and memory, signs of sympathetic and parasympathetic stimulation, palpitations (blurred vision, dilated pupils, sweating) O: Paranoia, ideas of reference, fear of losing one's mind, depersonalization, derealization, illusions, hallucinations, synesthesia, self-destructive/aggressive behavior, tremors		"Flashbacks" or HPPD may occur after termination of use.
Phencyclidine (PCP)	Oral, inhalation, smoking	E: Feeling superhuman, decreased awareness of and detachment from the environment, stimulation of the respiratory and cardiovascular system, ataxia, dysarthria, decreased pain perception O: Hallucinations, paranoia, psychosis, aggression, adrenergic crisis (cardiac failure, CVA, malignant hyperthermia, status epilepticus, severe muscle contractions)		"Flashbacks," HPPD, organic brain syndromes with recurrent psychotic behavior, which can last up to 6 months after not using the drug, numerous psychiatric hospitalizations and police arrests. *(continued)*

TABLE 25.3 Summary of Effects of Abused Substances, Overdose, Withdrawal Syndromes, and Prolonged Use (Continued)

Substance	Route	Effects (E) and Overdose (O)	Withdrawal Syndrome	Prolonged Use
Opiates (heroin, codeine)	Oral, injection, smoking	E: Euphoria, sedation, reduced libido, memory and concentration difficulties, analgesia, constipation, constricted pupils O: Respiratory depression, stupor, coma	Abdominal cramps, rhinorrhea, watery eyes, dilated pupils, yawning, "goose flesh," diaphoresis, nausea, diarrhea, anorexia, insomnia, fever (see Table 25-10)	Can lead to criminal behavior to get money for drugs, risk for infection-related to needle use (eg, HIV, endocarditis, hepatitis).
Sedatives, hypnotics, anxiolytics	Oral, injection	E: Euphoria, sedation, reduced libido, emotional lability, impaired judgment O: Respiratory depression, cardiac arrest	Anxiety rebound and agitation, hypertension, tachycardia, sweating, hyperpyrexia, sensory excitement, motor excitation, insomnia, possible tonic–clonic convulsions, nightmares, delirium, depersonalization, hallucinations	Often alternated with stimulants, use with alcohol enhances chance of overdose, risk for infection related to needle use.
Inhalants (glue, lighter fluid)	Inhalation	E: Euphoria, giddiness, excitation O: CNS depression: ataxia, nystagmus, dysarthria, coma and convulsions	Similar to alcohol but milder, with anxiety, tremors, hallucinations, and sleep disturbance as the primary symptoms	Long-term use can lead to liver and renal failure, blood dyscrasias, damage to the lungs. CNS damage (OBS, peripheral neuropathies, cerebral and optic atrophy, parkinsonism).
Nicotine	Smoking	E: Stimulation, enhanced performance and alertness, and appetite suppression O: Anxiety	Mood changes (craving, anxiety) and physiologic changes (poor concentration, sleep disturbances, headaches, gastric distress, and increased appetite)	Increased chance for cardiac disease and lung disease.
Caffeine	Oral	E: Stimulation, increased mental acuity, inexhaustability O: Restlessness, nervousness, excitement, insomnia, flushing, diuresis, GI distress, muscle twitching, rambling flow of thought and speech, tachycardia or cardiac arrhythmia, agitation	Headache, drowsiness, fatigue, craving, impaired psychomotor performance, difficulty concentrating, yawning, nausea	Physical consequences are under investigation.

CNS, central nervous system; CVA, cerebrovascular accident; GI, gastrointestinal; HPPD, hallucinogen persisting perceptual disorder; OBS, organic brain syndrome.

TABLE 25.4 Behavior and Blood Alcohol Levels

Number of Drinks	Blood Alcohol Levels (mg%)	Behavior
1–2	0.05	Impaired judgment, giddiness, mood changes
5–6	0.10	Difficulty driving and coordinating movements
10–12	0.20	Motor functions severely impaired, resulting in ataxia. There is emotional lability.
15–20	0.30	Stupor, disorientation, and confusion
20–24	0.40	Coma
25+	0.50	Respiratory failure, death

signs, diaphoresis, and other adverse gastrointestinal and CNS side effects. Severity of withdrawal symptoms range from mild to severe, depending on the length and amount of alcohol use. Symptoms include increased heart rate and blood pressure, diaphoresis, mild anxiety, restlessness, and hand tremors (Table 25-6).

Alcohol-Induced Amnestic Disorders

Alcohol is directly toxic to the brain, causing atrophy of the frontal cortex and eventually chronic brain syndrome. Patients with alcohol-induced amnestic disorders usually have a history of many years of heavy alcohol abuse, are generally over the age of 40 years, and can experience sudden onset of symptoms or development of symptoms over many years. Impairment can be severe, and once the disorder is established, it can persist indefinitely.

Wernicke's syndrome is caused by thiamine deficiency and is not exclusive to alcoholism. Wernicke's encephalopathy presents with oculomotor dysfunctions (bilateral abducens nerve palsy), ataxia, and confusion. Glucose administration can precipitate Wernicke's encephalopathy. Encephalopathy often evolves when thiamine deficiency exists, untreated, in a chronic phase. **Korsakoff's psychosis,** also known as alcohol amnestic disorder, is characterized by both retrograde and anterograde amnesia with sparing of intellectual function. Confabulation is a key feature of the psychosis. Up to half of patients with Korsakoff's psychosis do not improve significantly (Miller et al., 1997).

TABLE 25.5 Medical Complications of Alcohol Dependency

Organ System	Effects
Cardiovascular	Cardiomyopathy, congestive heart failure, hypertension
Respiratory	Increased rate of pneumonia and other respiratory infections
Hematologic	Anemias, leukemia, hematomas
Nervous	Withdrawal symptoms, irritability, depression, anxiety disorders, sleep disorders, phobias, paranoid feelings, diminished brain size and functioning, organic brain disorders, blackouts, cerebellar degeneration, neuropathies, palsies, gait disturbances, visual problems
Digestive	Liver diseases (fatty liver, alcoholic hepatitis, cirrhosis), pancreatitis, ulcers, other inflammations of the gastrointestinal (GI) tract, ulcers and GI bleeds, esophageal varices, cancers of the upper GI tract
Nutritional Deficiencies	Pellagra, alcohol amnestic disorder, dermatitis, stomatitis, cheilosis, scurvy
Endocrine and Metabolic	Increased incidence of diabetes, hyperlipidemia, hyperuricemia, and gout
Immune	Impaired immune functioning, higher incidence of infectious diseases, including tuberculosis and other bacterial infections
Skin	Skin lesions, increased incidence of infection, burns, and other traumatic injury
Musculoskeletal	Increased incidence of traumatic injury, myopathy
Genitourinary	Hypogonadism, increased secondary female sexual characteristics in men (hypoandrogenization and hyperestrogenization), impotency in males, electrolyte imbalances due to excess urinary secretion of potassium and magnesium

	Stage I: Mild	**Stage II: Moderate**	**Stage III: Severe**
Vital signs	Heart rate elevated, temperature elevated, normal or slightly elevated systolic blood pressure	Heart rate 100–120; elevated systolic blood pressure and temperature	Heart rate, 120–140; elevated systolic and diastolic blood pressures; elevated temperature
Diaphoresis	Slightly	Usually obvious	Marked
Central nervous system	Oriented, no confusion, no hallucinations	Intermittent confusion; transient visual and auditory hallucinations and illusions, mostly at night	Marked disorientation, confusion, disturbing visual and auditory hallucinations, misidentification of objects, delusions related to the hallucinations, delirium tremens, disturbances in consciousness
	Mild anxiety and restlessness	Painful anxiety and motor restlessness	Agitation, extreme restlessness, and panic states
	Restless sleep	Insomnia and nightmares	Unable to sleep
	Hand tremors, "shakes," no convulsions	Visible tremulousness, rare convulsions	Gross uncontrollable tremors, convulsions common
Gastrointestinal system	Impaired appetite, nausea	Anorexia, nausea and vomiting	Rejecting all fluid and food

TABLE 25.6 Alcohol Withdrawal Syndrome

Psychopharmacology

Several medications can help an individual overcome the symptoms of alcohol withdrawal: benzodiazepines; long-acting CNS depressants, which produce sedation and reduce anxiety symptoms; and neuroleptic drugs, such as haloperidol (Haldol) or other antipsychotic agents, if hallucinations or disorientation should occur. Antianxiety drugs, such benzodiazepines, are useful when they are substituted for the shorter-acting drug, alcohol. They produce sedation and reduce symptoms of anxiety. Benzodiazepines are usually administered based on elevations in heart rate, blood pressure, and temperature and on the presence of tremors. Diazepam (Valium) can be given 5 to 10 mg every 2 to 4 hours, or chlordiazepoxide hydrochloride (Librium) 25 to 100 mg every 4 hours. Medication given early in the course of withdrawal and in sufficient dosages can prevent the development of delirium tremens. Should withdrawal delirium occur, higher doses are used, with careful monitoring of the patient to prevent overdose. They are also extremely effective as anticonvulsants during withdrawal because they act more rapidly than phenytoin (Dilantin), which can take 7 to 10 days to reach therapeutic levels. Seizures, if they occur, usually do so within the first 48 hours of withdrawal.

Disulfiram is not a treatment or cure for alcoholism, but it can be used as adjunct therapy to help deter some individuals from drinking while using other treatment modalities to learn new coping skills to alter abuse behaviors (see Drug Profile: Disulfiram). Disulfiram prevents alcohol use by putting patients at risk for an adverse reaction (including flushing, nausea, vomiting, and diarrhea) to alcohol consumption mediated by the inhibition of acetaldehyde dehydrogenase. In a Veterans Administration multisite study, abstinence rates were no better in the disulfiram group than in controls, although a subgroup of socially stable older patients who relapsed drank less if they were assigned to the disulfiram group (Kristenson, 1995). Because there is other evidence of its efficacy in decreasing alcohol intake, disulfiram may be useful in carefully selected patients provided with appropriate counseling, although adverse effects, such as hepatotoxicity and neuropathy, and potentially severe interactions with alcohol limit its widespread use (O'Connor & Schottenfeld, 1998).

Adequate Nutrition and Supplemental Vitamins

Poor nutrition and vitamin deficiencies are often symptoms of alcohol dependence. Multivitamins and adequate nutrition are essential for patients who are severely malnourished, but other vitamin replacement may be necessary for certain individuals. Thiamine (vitamin B_1) may need to be replaced when a patient is in withdrawal to decrease ataxia and the other symptoms of thiamine deficiency. It is usually given 100 mg four times daily orally. It can be given intramuscularly or by intravenous infusion with glucose. Folic acid deficiency is corrected with administration of 1.0 mg orally four times daily. Magnesium deficiency is another nutritional deficit found in those with long-term alcohol dependence. Magnesium sulfate is given prophylactically if the patient has a

DRUG PROFILE: Disulfiram
(Antialcoholic agent, enzyme inhibitor)
Trade Name: Antabuse

Receptor affinity: Inhibits the enzyme aldehyde dehydrogenase, blocking oxidation of alcohol and allowing acetaldehyde to accumulate to concentrations 5 to 10 times higher than normal in the blood during alcohol metabolism. Believed to inhibit norepinephrine synthesis.
Indications: Management of selected chronic alcohol patients who want to remain in a state of enforced sobriety.
Route and dosage: Available in 250- and 500-mg tablets
Adults: Initially, a maximum dose of 500 mg/d PO in a single dose for 1–2 weeks. Maintenance dosage of 125 to 500 mg/d PO not to exceed 500 mg/d, continued until patient is fully recovered socially and a basis for permanent self-control is established.
Half-life (peak effect): Unclear (12 h)
Selected adverse reactions: Drowsiness, fatigue, headache, metallic or garlic-like aftertaste. If taken with alcohol: flushing, throbbing in head and neck, throbbing headaches, respiratory difficulty, nausea, copious vomiting, sweating, thirst, chest pain, palpitations, dyspnea, hyperventilation, tachycardia, hypotension, syncope, weakness, vertigo, blurred vision, confusion; severe reactions may include arrhythmias, cardiovascular collapse, acute congestive heart failure, and unconsciousness.
Warnings: Never administer to an intoxicated patient or without the patient's knowledge. Do not administer until patient has abstained from alcohol for at least 12 hours.

Contraindicated in patients with severe myocardial disease, coronary occlusion, or psychoses, or in patients receiving current or recent treatment with metronidazole, paraldehyde, alcohol, or alcohol-containing preparations. Use cautiously in patients with diabetes mellitus, hypothyroidism, epilepsy, cerebral damage, chronic and acute nephritis, hepatic cirrhosis or dysfunction.
Possible drug interactions: Concomitant administration of phenytoin, diazepam, or chlordiazepoxide may cause increased serum levels and risk for drug toxicity. Increased prothrombin time caused by disulfiram may lead to a need to adjust dosage of oral anticoagulants.
Specific patient/family education:
• Take the drug daily; take it at bedtime if it makes you dizzy or tired. Crush or mix tablets with liquid if necessary.
• Do not take any form of alcohol (such as beer, wine, liquor, vinegars, cough mixtures, sauces, aftershave lotions, liniments, or cologne); doing so may cause a severe unpleasant reaction.
• Wear or carry medical identification with you at all times to alert any medical emergency personnel that you are taking this drug.
• Keep appointments for follow-up blood tests.
• Avoid driving or performing tasks that require alertness if drowsiness, fatigue, or blurred vision occur.
• Know that the metallic aftertaste is transient and will disappear after the drug is discontinued.

history of withdrawal seizures. It enhances the body's response to thiamine and reduces seizure activity. The usual dose of magnesium sulfate is 1.0 g intramuscularly four times daily for 2 days.

COCAINE

In 1997, it was estimated that 1.5 million Americans used cocaine according to the NHSDA. Men have a higher rate of cocaine use than do women (U.S. DHHS, 1997a). Cocaine is a stimulant, an alkaloid found in the leaves of the *Erythroxylon coca* plant that is native to western South America, where for hundreds of years natives have known the powerful intoxicating effects of chewing the coca leaves. Cocaine is made from the leaves into a coca paste that is refined into cocaine hydrochloride, a crystalline form (white powder appearance), which is commonly inhaled or "snorted" in the nose, injected intravenously (with water), or smoked. The smokable form of cocaine, often called *free-base cocaine*, can be made by mixing the crystalline cocaine with ether or sodium hydroxide.

After cocaine is inhaled or injected, the user experiences a sudden burst of alertness and energy (cocaine "rush") and feelings of self-confidence, being in control,

and sociability, which last 10 to 20 minutes. This high is followed by an intense let-down effect, "cocaine crash," in which the person feels irritable, depressed, and tired, and craves more of the drug. Although it has not been proved that cocaine is physically addictive, it is clear that users experience a serious psychological addiction and pattern of abuse. Users quickly seek more cocaine or other drugs to rid themselves of the terrible after effects of cocaine crashing. Many users also use alcohol, marijuana, or sleeping pills during the crash. Withdrawal causes intense depression, craving, and drug-seeking behavior that may last for weeks. Those who discontinue cocaine use often experience a high rate of relapse. These dramatic effects and easy accessibility to the drug appear to have made it popular among adolescents and young people.

Crack-cocaine, often called "crack," is a form of freebase cocaine produced by mixing the crystal with water and baking soda or sodium bicarbonate and boiling it until a rock precipitant remains. The hardened crystal is then broken into pieces ("cracked") and smoked in cigarettes or water pipes. It is an extremely potent form of cocaine and produces a rapid high and intense euphoria and an even more dramatic crash. It is extremely addictive because of the intense and rapid onset of euphoric effects, which leave users craving more.

Cocaine emerged as the popular drug of the 1990s and was characterized as the drug of the wealthy, the young, upwardly mobile professionals or celebrities, and those in high-profile social circles. It was expensive to use and produced rapid and dramatic effects suited to those of the "nightlife generation" frequenting clubs and social affairs and wanting to feel self-confident and in control. Then crack-cocaine emerged as a cheap street drug, and it became the drug of choice on inner-city streets and available to all socioeconomic circles. Crack quickly became one of the leading problematic addictive drugs of the 1990s, causing serious national health concerns. The media have reported the health concerns of "crack houses" in which addicts congregate to smoke crack and of the huge numbers of "crack babies" who fill the hospitals and who may face serious physical and mental developmental problems and handicaps because of perinatal exposure to cocaine.

Cocaine is absorbed rapidly through the blood–brain barrier and is readily absorbed through the skin and mucous membranes as well. Cocaine can also act as a potent local anesthetic when applied directly to tissue, preventing both the generation and conduction of nerve impulses by inhibiting the rapid influx of sodium ions through the nerve membrane. Rapid peak intoxication occurs with intravenous injection or with inhalation. Injecting releases the drug directly into the bloodstream and heightens the intensity of its effects. Smoking involves the inhalation of cocaine vapor or smoke into the lungs, where absorption into the bloodstream is as rapid as by injection (NIDA, 1999). The resulting increased levels of dopamine in the synaptic cleft cause euphoria and, in excess, psychotic symptoms. Dopamine and dopamine metabolite levels are depleted by prolonged cocaine use. This absence of dopamine (which normally inhibits prolactin secretion) produces increased levels of prolactin in the blood. Drugs of abuse are able to interfere with normal processes and result in the euphoria commonly reported by cocaine abusers (NIDA, 1999). Higher levels of norepinephrine cause tachycardia, hypertension, dilated pupils, and rising body temperatures. Serotonin excess contributes to sleep disturbances and anorexia.

Cocaine Intoxication

Initially, intoxication causes CNS stimulation, followed by depression. The length of the stimulation depends on the dose and route of administration. With steadily increasing doses, restlessness proceeds to tremors and agitation, followed by convulsions and CNS depression. In lethal overdose, death generally results from respiratory failure. A toxic psychosis is also possible and may be accompanied by physical signs of CNS stimulation (tachycardia, hypertension, cardiac arrhythmias, sweating, hyperpyrexia, and convulsions) (NIDA, 1999).

Cocaine Withdrawal

Long-term cocaine use depletes norepinephrine, which results in "crash" states when the drug is discontinued, causing a person to sleep 12 to 18 hours. When an individual awakens, withdrawal symptoms may occur that are characterized by sleep disturbances with rebound REM sleep, anergia, decreased libido, depression with possible suicidality, anhedonia, poor concentration, and cocaine craving (Weaver & Schnoll, 1999). Treatment of cocaine addiction is complex and addresses a variety of problems. Treatment must assess the psychobiological, social, and pharmacologic aspects of the pattern of abuse (NIDA, 1999). Several newly emerging drugs are being investigated for use in cocaine addiction treatment. One of the most promising anticocaine drug medications to date, selegiline, was being taken into multisite phase III clinical trials in 1999 by both transdermal patch and a time-released pill. Disulfiram has shown in clinical studies to reduce cocaine abuse. Antidepressant drugs have shown to be of some benefit. Cocaine overdose results in many deaths every year, and medical treatments are being developed to deal with the acute emergencies resulting from excessive cocaine abuse (NIDA, 1999).

AMPHETAMINES AND OTHER STIMULANTS

Amphetamines were first synthesized for medical use in the 1880s. Amphetamines (Biphetamine, Delcobase, Dexedrine, Obetrol) and other stimulants, such as phenmetrazine (Preludin) and methylphenidate (Ritalin), act on the CNS and peripheral nervous system. They are used to treat attention deficit hyperactivity disorder in children, narcolepsy, depression, and obesity (on a short-term basis). Some people abuse these drugs to achieve the effects of alertness, increased concentration, a sense of increased energy, euphoria, and appetite suppression. Amphetamines are indirect catecholamine agonists and cause the release of newly synthesized norepinephrine. Like cocaine, they block the reuptake of norepinephrine and dopamine but do not have the same strong effect as cocaine on the serotonergic system. They also affect the peripheral nervous system and are powerful sympathomimetics, stimulating both α and β receptors. This results in tachycardia, arrhythmias, increased systolic and diastolic blood pressures, and peripheral hyperthermia (Weaver & Schnoll, 1999). The effects of amphetamine use and the clinical course of an overdose of these drugs are similar to that of cocaine. Amphetamines also have the potential for pharmacologic treatment with similar agents used for cocaine, such as antidepressants and dopaminergic agonists. Amphetamine withdrawal symptoms are not as pronounced as those of cocaine withdrawal.

CANNABIS (MARIJUANA)

Marijuana is often classified as a hallucinogenic drug, but its effects are usually not as dramatic or as intense as those of other hallucinogens. Marijuana is usually smoked and causes relaxation, euphoria, at times dyscoria, spatial misperception, time distortion, and food cravings. It causes relaxation and drowsiness, unlike other hallucinogens, and is often associated with decreased motivation after long-term use.

Marijuana remains the most commonly used illicit drug in the United States. An estimated 2.1 million people started using marijuana in 1998. According to data from the 1998 NHSDA, more than 72 million Americans (33%) 12 years of age and older have tried marijuana at least once in their lifetime, and almost 18.7 million (8.6%) had used marijuana in the past year. In 1985, 56.5 million Americans (29.4%) had tried marijuana at least once in their lifetimes, and 26.1 million (13.6%) had used marijuana within the past year (USDHHS, 1997a). The NIDA-funded Monitoring the Future Study provides an annual assessment of drug use among 12th, 10th, and 8th grade students and young adults nationwide. After decreasing for more than a decade, marijuana use among students began to increase in the early 1990s. From 1998 to 1999, use of marijuana at least once (lifetime use) increased among 12th and 10th graders, continuing the trend seen in recent years. The seniors' rate of lifetime marijuana use is higher than any year since 1987, but all rates remain well below those seen in the late 1970s and early 1980s.

Marijuana use did not change significantly from 1998 to 1999 in any of the three grades, suggesting that the sharp increases of recent years may be slowing. Daily marijuana uses in the past month increased slightly among all three grades as well, according to the 2000 NHSDA (USDHHS, 1997a). A drug is addicting if it causes compulsive, often uncontrollable drug craving, seeking, and use, even in the face of negative health and social consequences. Marijuana meets this criterion. More than 120,000 people enter treatment per year for their primary marijuana addiction. In addition, animal studies suggest marijuana causes physical dependence, and some people report withdrawal symptoms, according to the 2000 NHSDA.

Its active ingredient is D-9-tetrahydrocannabinol (THC). Also known as *hemp, marijuana* is the common name for the plant *Cannabis sativae.* Hashish is the resin found in flowers of the mature *C. sativae* plant and is its strongest form, containing 10% to 30% THC.

Marijuana is fat soluble and is absorbed rapidly after being smoked or taken orally. After ingestion, THC binds with an opioid receptor in the brain—the μ receptor. This action engages endogenous brain opioid receptors, which are associated with enhanced dopamine activity due to THC blockage of dopamine reuptake (Stephens, 1999). THC can be stored for weeks in fat tissue and in the brain and is released extremely slowly. Long-term use leads to the accumulation of cannabinoids in the body. It is concentrated in the frontal cortex, the limbic areas, and the auditory and visual perception centers of the brain. It is found in the pons, exerting cardiovascular effects; in the cerebellum and caudate nucleus, resulting in ataxia; and in the geniculate bodies and the superior and inferior calyculi, resulting in increased psychotropic effects.

Areas of controversy surround the use and effects of marijuana, matters of ongoing debate both in the medical world and in legal circles. Some evidence suggests that marijuana can be successful in the medical treatment of certain disorders. Grinspoon and Bakalar (1997) report that marijuana has been used successfully to treat epilepsy, postsurgery pain, headache and other types of pain, muscle spasms in people with cerebral palsy, asthma, glaucoma, poor appetite in cancer patients with weight loss, or chemotherapy-related nausea and vomiting. Many feel that legitimizing the use of marijuana for medical reasons could possibly legitimize its use for recreational purposes as well. Until published medical research confirms or refutes its use for medical reasons, the controversy will continue. The National Council on Alcoholism and Drug Dependence (NCADD) in 1999, reported in a recent Internet news article that pharmaceutical companies are running trials, believed to be the first of their kind in the world. The goal is to see if marijuana relieves the pain of patients suffering from multiple sclerosis and other forms of severe pain. Other controversy surrounds the issue of long-term effects of marijuana use. Some believe it produces amotivational syndrome, described as changes in personality characterized by diminished drive, decreased ambition, lessened motivation, apathy, shortened attention span, distractibility, poor judgment, impaired communication skills, introversion, magical thinking, derealization, depersonalization, decreased capacity to carry out complex plans or to prepare realistically for the future, a peculiar fragmentation in the flow of thought, habit deterioration, and progressive loss of insight (Gold & Miller, 1992; Miller & Gold, 1989).

It seems unlikely that marijuana directly causes motivational problems: rather, it may interact with predisposing personality characteristics in some individuals to produce this clinical phenomenon (Stephens, 1999). Some researchers attribute this syndrome to long-term effects of THC on the brain and to the slow release of stored THC in fat tissue. Others researchers dispute that there are no effects of heavy marijuana use on motivation, learning, or perception and that these characteristics are not the result of marijuana use but rather part of the causes (Grinspoon & Bakalar, 1997).

HALLUCINOGENS

The term **hallucinogen** refers to a classification of drugs that produces euphoria or dysphoria, altered body image, distorted or sharpened visual and auditory perception, confusion, incoordination, and impaired judgment and memory. Severe reactions may cause paranoia, fear of losing one's mind, depersonalization, illusions, delusions, and hallucinations. Hallucinogens typically have their most immediate effects on the autonomic nervous system and produce an increase in heart rate and body temperature and slightly elevate blood pressure. The individual may experience a dry mouth, dizziness, and subjective feelings of being hot or cold. Gradually, the focus on physiologic changes fades into the background, and perceptual distortions and hallucinations become prominent (Stephens, 1999). There may be intense feelings of closeness to others; whereas, later in the experience or on a different occasion, the user may feel distant and isolated. It is also important to note that the true content of hallucinogenic drugs purchased on the street is always in doubt and has often been misidentified or adulterated with other drugs.

There are more than 100 different hallucinogens with substantially different molecular structures. Psilocybin, D-lysergic acid diethylamide (LSD), mescaline, and numerous amphetamine derivatives are just a few hallucinogens (Stephens, 1999). During the 1960s, LSD became a popular recreational drug associated with the antiestablishment movement of peace, free love, sex, and the use of psychedelic drugs that characterized the "hippies" and the "Woodstock generation." Acute LSD psychological toxicity, so-called bad trips, were often reported or experienced by users in which the users felt extreme anxiety or fears and experienced frightening hallucinations. These are characteristically panic reactions that develop when individuals feel that the hallucinogenic experience will never end or when they have difficulty distinguishing drug effects from reality (Stephens, 1999).

LSD binds to and activates a specific receptor for the neurotransmitter serotonin. Normally, serotonin binds to and activates its receptors and then is taken back up into the neuron that released it. In contrast, LSD binds very tightly to the serotonin receptor, causing a greater than normal activation of the receptor. Because serotonin has a role in many of the brain's functions, activation of its receptors by LSD produces widespread effects, including rapid emotional swings, altered perceptions, and, if taken in a large enough dose, delusions and visual hallucinations.

MDMA, which is similar in structure to methamphetamine, causes serotonin to be released from neurons in greater amounts than normal. Once released, this serotonin can excessively activate serotonin receptors. Scientists have also shown that MDMA causes excess dopamine to be released from dopamine-containing neurons. Particularly alarming is research in animals that has demonstrated that MDMA can damage and destroy serotonin-containing neurons. MDMA can cause hallucinations, confusion, depression, sleep problems, drug craving, severe anxiety, and paranoia.

PCP, which is not a true hallucinogen, can affect many neurotransmitter systems. It interferes with the functioning of the neurotransmitter glutamate, which is found in neurons throughout the brain. Like many other drugs, it also causes dopamine to be released from neurons into the synapse. At low to moderate doses, PCP causes altered perception of body image but rarely produces visual hallucinations. PCP can also cause effects that mimic the primary symptoms of schizophrenia, such as delusions and mental turmoil. People who use PCP for long periods of time have memory loss and speech difficulties (NIDA, 2000).

Nursing interventions depend on presenting behaviors and anticipated complications. Often, patients can present at psychiatric emergency departments in acute states of intoxication or in dissociated states, and they may be combative. Intoxication can last 4 to 6 hours, with an extensive period of de-escalation. The primary goals of intervention are stimulus reduction, maintenance of a safe environment for the patient and others, behavior management, and careful observation for medical and psychiatric complications. Instructions to the patient should be clear, short, and simple and delivered in a firm but nonthreatening tone.

OPIATES

Opiates are powerful drugs derived from the poppy plant that have been used for centuries to relieve pain. They include opium, heroin, morphine, and codeine. Even centuries after their discovery, opiates are still the most effective pain relievers available to physicians for treating pain. Although heroin has no medicinal use, other opiates, such as morphine and codeine, are used in the treatment of pain related to illnesses (eg, cancer) and medical and dental procedures. When used as directed by a physician, opiates are safe and generally do not produce addiction. However, opiates also possess very strong reinforcing properties and can quickly trigger addiction when used improperly (NIDA, 2000).

The term opiate refers to any substance that binds to an opioid receptor in the brain to produce an agonist action. Opiates cause CNS depression, sleep or stupor, and analgesia. Major opiates used today are heroin, codeine, and meperidine. Opiates are commonly referred to as **narcotics,** although in legal terms, narcotics is a catch-all term for all illegal drugs. Recently, a substantial new epidemic of heroin abuse has been developing in the United States and spreading to middle-class users, who were formerly using purer heroin, and the proportion of people inhaling or smoking heroin, as well as the number of people seeking treatment, has continued to increase (Stine & Kosten, 1999).

There are three types of opiate-related drugs: agonists, antagonists, and mixed agonist–antagonists. Opiate agonists increase the CNS effects, and antagonists block these effects. Opiates elicit their powerful effects by activating opiate receptors that are widely distributed throughout the brain and body. Once an opiate reaches the brain, it quickly activates the opiate receptors that are found in many brain regions and produces an effect that correlates with the area of the brain involved. Two important effects produced by opiates, such as morphine, are pleasure (or reward) and pain relief. The brain itself also produces substances known as endorphins that activate the opiate receptors. Research indicates that endorphins are involved in many things, including respiration, nausea, vomiting, pain modulation, and hormonal regulation (NIDA, 2000).

Opiates cause tolerance and physical dependence that appear to be specific for each receptor subtype. Tolerance develops particularly to the analgesic, respiratory depression, and sedative actions of opiates. Often, a 100% increase in dose is used to achieve the same physical effects when tolerance exists. Physical dependence can develop rapidly. When the drug is discontinued, after a period of continuous use, a rebound hyperexcitability withdrawal syndrome usually occurs. Table 25-7 describes the onset, duration, and symptoms of mild, moderate, and severe withdrawal symptoms.

Naltrexone (Trexan)

Naltrexone was originally used as a treatment for heroin abuse, but it has been approved for treatment of alcohol dependence. Naltrexone binds to opiate receptors in the CNS and competitively inhibits the action of opioid drugs, including those with mixed narcotic agonist–antagonist properties. It is contraindicated in pregnant patients and in patients with allergy to narcotic antagonists. Naltrexone has also been used successfully in the treatment of opiate addiction by blocking the intoxicating effects of opiates. If a patient should require analgesia while taking naltrexone, a nonopioid agent is recommended. If opioid analgesia is necessary, such as for surgery or severe pain, it must be administered cautiously because the amount required for analgesia may result in respiratory depression. Patients should be informed that it is extremely dangerous to attempt to take opiates while taking naltrexone because the interaction can cause respiratory depression and death. Should an opiate-dependent individual take naltrexone before he or she is fully detoxified from opiates, withdrawal symptoms may result (see Drug Profile: Naltrexone).

In a recent study, high doses of naltrexone and alcohol interacted to produce the greatest decreases in liking of alcohol. The findings support the role of endogenous opioids as determinants of alcohol's effects and suggest that naltrexone may be particularly clinically useful in those patients who continue to drink heavily (McCaul et al., 2000).

TABLE 25.7 Opiate Withdrawal Syndrome

Initial Onset and Duration	Mild Withdrawal	Moderate Withdrawal	Severe Withdrawal
Onset: 8–12 h after last use of short-acting opiates. 1–3 d after last use for longer-acting opiates, such as methadone	Physical: yawning, rhinorrhea, perspiration, restlessness, lacrimation, sleep disturbance	Physical: dilated pupils, bone and muscle aches, sensation of "goose flesh," hot and cold flashes	Physical: nausea, vomiting, stomach cramps, diarrhea, weight loss, insomnia, twitching of muscles and kicking movements of legs, increased blood pressure, pulse, and respirations
Duration: Severe symptoms peak between 48–72 h. Symptoms abate in 7–10 d for short-acting opiates. Methadone withdrawal symptoms can last several weeks.	Emotional: increased craving, anxiety, dysphoria	Emotional: irritability, increased anxiety, and craving	Emotional: depression, increased anxiety, dysphoria, subjective sense of feeling "wretched"

> **DRUG PROFILE: Naltrexone**
> (Narcotic antagonist)
> Trade Name: Trexan
>
> **Receptor affinity:** Binds to opiate receptors in the CNS and competitively inhibits the action of opioid drugs, including those with mixed narcotic agonist–antagonist properties.
> **Indications:** Adjunctive treatment of alcohol or narcotic dependence as part of a comprehensive treatment program.
> **Route and dosage:** Available in 50-mg tablets
> *Adults:* For alcoholism: 50 mg/d PO; for narcotic dependence: initial dose of 25 mg PO; if no signs or symptoms seen, complete dose with 25 mg. Usual maintenance dose is 50 mg/d PO.
> *Children:* Safety has not been established for use in children under age 18 y.
> **Half-life (peak effect):** 3.9–12.9 h (60 min)
> **Selected adverse reactions:** Difficulty sleeping, anxiety, nervousness, headache, low energy, abdominal pain/cramps, nausea, vomiting, delayed ejaculations, decreased potency, skin rash, chills, increased thirst, joint and muscle pain
> **Warnings:** Contraindicated in pregnancy and patients allergic to narcotic antagonists. Use cautiously in narcotic addiction because may produce withdrawal symptoms. Do not administer unless patient has been opioid free for 7–10 d.
>
> Also, use cautiously in patients with acute hepatitis, liver failure, depression, suicidal tendencies, and breast-feeding. Must make certain patient is opioid free before administering naltrexone. Always give naloxone challenge test before using, except in patients showing clinical signs of opioid withdrawal.
> **Specific patient/family education:**
> * Know that this drug will help facilitate abstinence from alcohol and block the effects of narcotics.
> * Wear a medical identification tag to alert emergency personnel that you are taking this drug.
> * Avoid use of heroin or other opiate drugs; small doses may have no effect, but large doses can cause death, serious injury, or coma.
> * Report any signs and symptoms of adverse effects.
> * Notify other health care providers that you are taking this drug.
> * Keep appointments for follow-up blood tests and treatment program.

Opiate Detoxification

Opiate detoxification is achieved by the gradual reduction of an opiate dose over several days or weeks. Many treatment programs include administering low doses of a substitute drug that can help satisfy the drug craving but not provide the same subjective high, such as methadone.

Methadone Maintenance Treatment

Methadone maintenance is the treatment of opiate addiction with a daily stabilized dose of methadone. Methadone is used because of its long half-life of 15 to 30 hours. Methadone is a potent opiate and is physiologically addicting, but it satisfies the opiate craving without producing the subjective high of heroin (see Drug Profile: Methadone).

Detoxification is accomplished by setting the beginning methadone dose and then slowly reducing it over the next 21 days. Treatment programs determine the dose of methadone that will block subjective feelings of craving and will not cause somnolence or intoxication in patients. The initial dose of methadone is determined by severity of withdrawal symptoms and is usually 20 to 30 mg orally. If, after 1 to 2 hours, symptoms persist, the dosage can be raised and then should be reevaluated daily during the first few days of treatment. Initial doses of greater than 40 mg can cause severe discomfort later as the detoxification proceeds.

Patients receive this dose daily in conjunction with regular drug abuse counseling focused on the elimination of illicit drug use; on lifestyle changes, such as finding friends who do not use drugs or achieving stability in one's living situation; strengthening social supports; and structuring time into non–drug-using pursuits. After illicit drug use ceases for a period of time, major lifestyle changes have been made, and social supports are in place, patients may gradually detoxify from methadone with continuing support through community support groups, such as Narcotics Anonymous.

The length of methadone treatment varies for each patient. When to begin detoxification from methadone varies widely depending on the patient's commitment to abstinence, lifestyle changes that have occurred, and strong peer group support—all of which are needed to sustain the patient during methadone detoxification, when increased cravings often occur.

Methadone treatment has been used effectively and safely to treat opioid addiction for more than 30 years (NIDA, 1997). This is extremely important given concern regarding the spread of HIV infection among intravenous drug abusers. Combined with behavioral therapy and counseling methadone enables patients to stop abusing heroin.

Like methadone, *l*-acetyl-α-methadol (LAAM) is a synthetic opiate that can be used to treat heroin addiction. LAAM can block the effects of heroin for up to 72 hours with minimal side effects when taken orally. The U.S. Food and Drug Administration approved the use of LAAM for treating patients addicted to heroin. It has a longer duration of action, permitting dosing just

---

DRUG PROFILE: Methadone
(Narcotic agonist, analgesic)
Trade Name: Dolophine

Receptor affinity: Binds to opioid receptors in the CNS to produce analgesia, euphoria, sedation; the receptors mediating the effects of the endogenous opioids are thought to be enkaphalins, endorphins.

Indications: Detoxification and temporary maintenance treatment of narcotic addiction; relief of severe pain.

Route and dosage: Available in 5-mg, 10-mg, 40-mg tablets, oral concentrate.

Adults: Detoxification: initially 15–30 mg. Increase to suppress withdrawal signs. 40 mg/d in single or divided dose is usually adequate stabilizing dose; continue stabilizing dose for 2–3 days, then gradually decrease dosage. Usual maintenance dose is 20–120 mg/d in single dosing. Individual dosage as tolerated.

Half-life (peak effect):
PO 90–120 min
IM 1–2 h
SC 1–2 h

Selected adverse reactions: Lightheadedness, dizziness, sedation, nausea, vomiting, facial flushing, peripheral circulatory collapse, arrhythmia, palpitations, urethral spasm, urinary retention, respiratory depression, circulatory depression, respiratory arrest, shock, cardiac arrest

Warnings: Never administer in the presence of hypersensitivity to narcotics, diarrhea caused by poisoning (before toxins are eliminated), bronchial asthma, chronic obstructive pulmonary disease. Use caution in the presence of acute abdominal conditions, cardiovascular disease. Increased effects and toxicity of methadone if taken concurrently with cimetidine, ranitidine.

Specific patient/family education:
- Take drug exactly as prescribed.
- Avoid use of alcohol.
- Take drug with food and lying quietly—should minimize the nausea.
- Eat small, frequent meals to treat nausea and loss of appetite.
- For dizziness and drowsiness, avoid driving a car or performing other tasks that require alertness.
- Administer mild laxative for constipation.
- Report severe nausea, vomiting, constipation, shortness of breath, or difficulty breathing.

---

three times per week and thereby eliminating the need for take home doses over weekends (NIDA, 1997).

Buprenorphine, a mixed agonist–antagonist medication, is being studied by NIDA for usefulness in treating heroin addiction. Discontinuation of buprenorphine does not take the regimen of drug tapering as does methadone, which makes it easier to stop treatment (NIDA, 1997).

SEDATIVE-HYPNOTICS AND ANXIOLYTICS

Sedative-hypnotic drugs and anxiolytic (antianxiety) agents are medications that induce sleep and reduce anxiety. Table 25-8 lists sedative-hypnotic and anxiolytic medications, their generic and trade names, and common indications for use. This classification of substances is essentially one of prescription drugs but can include alcohol and marijuana because of their sedative-hypnotic properties.

The question of sedative-hypnotic and anxiolytic agent abuse is complex. Their use is often controversial because of society's ambivalence regarding the proper or ethical use of medications to treat anxiety and insomnia. Physicians and mental health professionals often face ethical questions regarding how to treat these desperate patients plagued by chronic symptoms of insomnia and anxiety for which they find no medical cure but only medications to relieve symptoms. More pre-

scriptions are written for sedative-hypnotic and anxiolytic drugs than for any other class of drugs in the United States.

Clinicians must take into consideration the risks of prescribing sedative-hypnotics. With careful consideration by both physician and patient concerning the risks of these drugs, they can be a useful, safe, and appropriate treatment for many patients (Brady et al., 1999). Patients who abuse prescription medications are often somnolent, have a clouded mental state, or may feel hyperactive or anxious after use of the medication but then continue to use the medications without reporting their distressing side effects. They often anticipate the next dose ahead of time, may exceed the daily dose of medication prescribed, may lobby their health care provider for a higher dose or a stronger medication, may supplement medication with alcohol or other drugs, or may obtain prescriptions for the same medication from several doctors.

Biologic Reactions to Benzodiazepines

Barbiturates were the first classification of drugs used to treat sleep disturbances and anxiety, but benzodiazepines have largely replaced barbiturates because of their comparative safety with regard to potential toxicity and addictive qualities. Benzodiazepines modulate γ-aminobutyric acid (GABA) transmission and interact with specific receptor sites in the brain. GABA is the

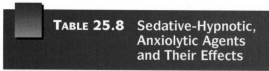

Generic Name	Trade Name	Effects
Benzodiazepines		
alprazolam	Xanax	S, A
chlordiazepoxide	Librium	S, A
clonazepam	Klonopin	anticonvulsant
clorazepate	Tranxene	S, A
diazepam	Valium	S, A, anticonvulsant
estazolam	ProSom	H
flurazepam	Dalmane	H
halazepam	Paxipam	S, A
lorazepam	Ativan	S, A
oxazepam	Serax	S, A
prazepam	Centrax	S, A
quazepam	Doral	H
temazepam	Restoril	H
triazolam	Halcion	H
Barbiturates		
amobarbital	Amytal	S
butabarbital	Butisol	S
butalbital	Fiorinal	S, analgesic
pentobarbital	Nembutal	H
phenobarbital	Barbita, Luminol	S, anticonvulsant
secobarbital	Seconal	H
Others		
buspirone	BuSpar	S, A
chloral hydrate	Noctec, Somnos	H
ethchlorvynol	Placidyl	H
glutethimide	Doriden	H
meprobamate	Miltown, Equanil	S, A
methylprylon	Noludar	H

S, sedative; H, hypnotic; A, antianxiety.

most abundant inhibitor neurotransmitter in the brain. Benzodiazepines enhance GABA function by increasing its affinity for the receptor by displacing an endogenous inhibitor of GABA binding (Brady et al., 1999). Benzodiazepines act in a manner similar to alcohol and other sedative hypnotics by making neuronal membranes more permeable to K^+ and Cl^- and to close Na^+ and Ca^{++} channels, causing depression of the CNS. Benzodiazepines also increase total sleep time and decrease the duration of REM sleep.

Benzodiazepine Withdrawal

The severity of symptoms of benzodiazepine withdrawal depends on the duration and dosage of regular use and include the following:

Anxiety rebound—tension, agitation, tremulousness, insomnia, anorexia

Autonomic rebound—hypertension, tachycardia, sweating, hyperpyrexia

Sensory excitement—paresthesias, photophobia, hyperacusis, illusions

Motor excitation—hyperreflexia, tremors, myoclonus, fasciculation, myalgia, muscle weakness, tonic-clonic convulsions

Cognitive excitation—nightmares, delirium, depersonalization, hallucinations (Cohen, 1991)

Two methods of withdrawal are currently used. The first is to use the same medication in decreasing doses, and the second is to substitute an equivalent dose of phenobarbital and reduce the dose slowly (Brady et al., 1999).

Nursing interventions for withdrawal states are similar to those for alcohol withdrawal. Symptoms may begin to emerge up to 8 days after cessation of a long-acting benzodiazepine. Often, patients combine taking these drugs with alcohol, which is extremely dangerous and can often put patients at risk for overdose, causing coma or death. The combination of benzodiazepines and alcohol also complicates withdrawal treatment because the patient may seem to improve after the alcohol withdrawal syndrome subsides, only to have similar symptoms emerge as the benzodiazepine withdrawal syndrome appears.

INHALANTS

Inhalants are organic solvents, also known as *volatile substances*, which are CNS depressants. When inhaled, they cause euphoria, sedation, emotional lability, and impaired judgment. They can result in respiratory depression, stupor, and coma. Inhalants are used by younger individuals. It is likely that low cost, universal availability, ease of access, and local custom are important factors (Pandina & Hendren, 1999).

Most inhalants are common household products that give off mind-altering chemical fumes when sniffed. These common products include paint thinner, fingernail polish remover, glues, gasoline, cigarette lighter fluid, and nitrous oxide. They also include fluorinated hydrocarbons found in aerosols, such as whipped cream, hair and paint sprays, and computer cleaners. The chemical structure of the various types of inhalants is diverse, making it difficult to generalize about their effects. It is known, however, that the vaporous fumes can change brain chemistry and may be permanently damaging to the brain and CNS (NIDA, 2000). These substances are commonly found in many common products used in the home, including the following:

Adhesives: airplane glue, polyvinyl chloride cement, rubber cement

Aerosols: paint, hair, analgesics, asthma sprays, deodorants, air fresheners

Anesthetics: nitrous oxide, halothane, enflurane, isoflurane, ethyl chloride

Solvents: paint and nail polish removers, paint thinners, typewriter correction fluids, lighter fluid, petroleum

Cleaning agents: dry cleaning fluid, spot removers, degreasers

Food products: whipped cream and cooking oil sprays

Nitrites: amyl, butyl, isopropyl nitrite

Neurotoxicity

Inhalants are easily absorbed through the lungs and are widely distributed in the body, reaching highest concentrations in fat tissue and the nervous system, where the most profound effects are exhibited. Mild intoxication occurs within minutes and can last up to 30 minutes. Often, the drugs are inhaled repeatedly to maintain an intoxicated state for hours. Initially, the person experiences a sense of euphoria, but as the dose increases, confusion, perceptual distortions, and severe CNS depression appear. Inhalant users are also at risk for *sudden sniffing death*, which can occur when the inhaled fumes take the place of oxygen in the lungs and central nervous system. This basically causes the inhalant user to suffocate. Inhalants can also lead to death by disrupting the normal heart rhythm, which can lead to cardiac arrest (NIDA, 2000).

Chronic neurologic syndromes can result from long-term use. Inhalants can also act directly in the brain to cause a variety of neurologic problems. For instance, inhalants can cause abnormalities in brain areas that are involved in movement (eg, the cerebellum) and higher cognitive function (eg, the cerebral cortex) (NIDA, 2000). There is a reported withdrawal syndrome similar to alcohol but milder, with anxiety, tremors, hallucinations, and sleep disturbance as the primary symptoms.

NICOTINE

Nicotine, the addictive chemical primarily responsible for the prevalence of tobacco use, is the primary reason tobacco is named a public health menace (Slade, 1999). A higher prevalence of smoking occurs among alcoholics and polysubstance abusers as well as psychiatric patients (Jarvik & Schneider, 1992). Recent research has shown that the addiction produced by nicotine is extremely powerful and is at least as strong as addictions to other drugs, such as heroin and cocaine (NIDA, 2000).

Nicotine stimulates the central, peripheral, and autonomic nervous systems, causing increased alertness, concentration, attention, and appetite suppression. It is readily absorbed and is carried in the bloodstream to the liver, where it is partially metabolized. It is also metabolized by the kidneys and is excreted in the urine.

Nicotine acts as an agonist of the nicotinic cholinergic receptor sites and stimulates autonomic ganglia in both the parasympathetic and sympathetic nervous systems, resulting in increased release of norepinephrine or acetylcholine. The release of epinephrine by nicotine from the adrenal medulla causes an increase in fatty acids, glycerol, and lactate levels in the blood, thereby increasing the risk for atherosclerosis and cardiac muscle pathology (Slade, 1999).

Other medical complications of nicotine use are numerous. Smoking either cigarettes or cigars can cause respiratory problems, lung cancer, emphysema, heart problems, and peripheral vascular disease. In fact, smoking is the largest preventable cause of premature death and disability. Cigarette smoking kills at least 400,000 people in the United States each year and makes countless others ill, including those who are exposed to secondhand smoke. The use of smokeless tobacco is also associated with serious health problems (NIDA, 2000).

Repeated use of nicotine produces both tolerance and dependence. It is extremely addictive, causing relapse within a year in 70% of those who quit.

Nicotine Withdrawal and Replacement Therapy

Nicotine withdrawal is marked by mood changes (craving, anxiety, irritability, depression) and physiologic changes (difficulty in concentrating, sleep disturbances, headaches, gastric distress, and increased appetite) (Slade, 1999). Nicotine replacements such as transdermal patches, nicotine gum, nasal spray, and inhalers have been used successfully to assist in withdrawal by reducing craving for tobacco. Patches are rotated on skin sites and help maintain a steady blood level of nicotine. Products such as Habitrol, Nicoderm, and ProStep are used daily, with the decrease in strength of nicotine occurring periodically over a period of 6 to 12 weeks.

The use of this medication should be accompanied by social support and education to enhance commitment to abstinence from tobacco. Symptoms of excess of nicotine released by the patches can often resemble withdrawal symptoms. People with cardiovascular disease and peripheral vascular disease may not be candidates for this therapy because of the side effects of increased cardiac stimulation and peripheral vasoconstriction. Patches should not be used for more than 3 months, and if smoking cessation is not successful, their use should not be restarted for a period of time. Smoking while using the patches will enhance the negative cardiovascular side effects. Patients who do smoke during therapy should discontinue use of the transdermal patches.

CAFFEINE

Caffeine is a stimulant found in many drinks (coffee, tea, cocoa, soft drinks), chocolate, and over-the-counter medications, including analgesics, stimulants, appetite suppressants, and cold relief preparations. Twenty to 30% of Americans ingest between 500 and 600 mg of caffeine daily (Greden & Walters, 1997). If caffeine is overused, it can cause physical side effects and precipitate withdrawal syndrome marked by headaches, drowsiness, and craving (APA, 2000).

Symptoms of caffeine intoxication can include five or more of the following: restlessness, nervousness, excitement, insomnia, flushed face, diuresis, gastrointestinal disturbance, muscle twitching, rambling flow of thought and speech, tachycardia or cardiac arrhythmia, periods of inexhaustibility, psychomotor agitation (APA, 2000).

Caffeine is an alkaloid and a xanthine derivative. Doses of less than 200 mg, found in 1 to 2 cups of percolated coffee, stimulate the cerebral cortex and increase mental acuity. Larger doses of greater than 500 mg (more than 5 cups of coffee) increase the heart rate; stimulate respiratory, vasomotor, vagal centers, and cardiac muscles, resulting in increased force of cardiac contraction; dilate pulmonary and coronary blood vessels; and constrict blood flow to the cerebral vascular system.

Psychiatric symptoms such as panic, schizophrenia, or manic-depressive symptoms can be exacerbated by caffeine in higher doses.

Caffeine withdrawal syndrome has been described as headache, drowsiness, and fatigue, with less frequent impaired psychomotor performance, difficulty concentrating, craving, and some psychophysiologic complaints, such as yawning or nausea (Greden & Walters, 1992). Patients with caffeine dependence can be supported in their efforts at withdrawal through education regarding the caffeine content of beverages and medication, using decaffeinated beverages, and managing individual withdrawal symptoms.

NURSING MANAGEMENT: HUMAN RESPONSE TO DISORDER

In psychiatric and substance abuse treatment programs, the assessment process is, in part, a treatment intervention. Often, patients are in denial of the severity of the problem and of the emotional, social, legal, vocational, or other consequences of it. Therefore, the assessment is crucial to understanding level of use, abuse, or dependence and determining the patient's denial or acceptance of treatment. Assessment is often detailed and may involve family members and loved ones. Text Box 25-1

TEXT BOX 25.1

Examples of Behaviors Exhibited in Substance Use, Abuse, Dependence, and Addiction

Substance Use
- Does not have possible danger or potential legal problems
- Engages in use to enhance social situations and interaction
- Is not intended to result in intoxication
- Has control of the amount and frequency of use
- Exhibits socially acceptable behavior while using

Prescription Medication Use
- Use is for the dose, frequency, and indications prescribed
- Use is for the particular episode of the condition for which it was prescribed
- Use is coordinated among prescribing physicians

Substance Abuse
- Use for intoxication or feeling of being "high"
- Use that interferes with normal life functions (eg, producing sleep when inappropriate, excitability or irritability interfering with social interaction)
- Potential harm to self or others (eg, driving while intoxicated, use of injection drug equipment)
- Use that has legal consequences (ie, all use of illicit drugs)
- Use resulting in socially unacceptable behavior (eg, public drunkenness, verbal or physical abuse)

- Use to alter normal feeling states such as sadness or anxiety

Prescription Medication Abuse
- Use is at a higher dose and greater frequency than prescribed
- Use is for indications other than prescribed, or for self-diagnosed condition
- Use results in feeling tired or having a clouded mental state or feeling "hyperactive" or nervous

Substance Dependence
- Supplementing medication with alcohol or drugs
- Soliciting more than one doctor for the same medication
- Inability to control the amount and frequency of use
- Tolerance to larger amounts of the substance
- Withdrawal symptoms when stopping use
- Severe consequences from alcohol or drug use

Substance Addiction
- Drug craving
- Compulsive use
- Presence of aberrant drug-related behaviors
- Repeated relapse into drug use after withdrawal

gives examples of typical behaviors exhibited by individuals in each level of use, abuse, dependence, and addiction, which are helpful to nurses when assessing the severity of patient's use or abuse. Text Box 25-2 is an example of a nursing assessment guide that is helpful in obtaining needed information about an individual's substance use history. Usually, nurses encounter individuals during crisis when they seek professional help. These situations offer an opportunity to explore the denial that keeps their addiction thriving. The nurse's approach should be caring, matter-of-fact, gentle, and direct. Approaches that are punitive or attempt to elicit feelings of guilt or shame are destructive to the therapeutic relationship. See Nursing Care Plan 25-1.

Denial of a Problem

Denial is the patient's inability to accept his or her loss of control over substance use or the severity of the consequences associated with the substance abuse. Denial can be expressed in a variety of behaviors and attitudes and may not be exhibited in an overt denial of the problem. For example, patients may admit to a problem, even thank you for helping them to realize they have a problem, but insist they can overcome the problem on their own and do not need outside help. Often, they blame other people or circumstances for their difficulties, not their drug or alcohol use.

In his classic article on this topic, John Wallace (1990) found the following characteristics typical of a substance abuser who is in denial who will exhibit the following:

- Confusion about severity of drinking history—"I went out drinking with friends last week and didn't have any problems, I don't get drunk all the time."
- Difficulty reconciling early positive experiences of alcohol use with current problems—"I used to drink with my buddies after work to unwind. We had a great time. Those were some good times. . . ."
- Confusion regarding the definition of alcoholic—"Well I don't have withdrawal symptoms, so I can't be an alcoholic."

TEXT BOX 25.2

Substance Abuse Evaluation

Drug/Last Use	Pattern of Use (Amount, route, first use, frequency, and length of use)
Alcohol:	
Stimulants:	
Opiates:	
Sedative-hypnotics and anxiolytic agents:	
Hallucinogens:	
Marijuana:	
Inhalants:	
Nicotine:	
Caffeine:	

Dependency Indicators

1. Tolerance (increasing use of drug or alcohol with the same level of intoxication): _____
2. Withdrawal symptoms: a. Shakes? Tremors? _____ b. Cramps, diarrhea, or rapid pulse? _____
   c. Feeling paranoid, fearful? _____ d. Difficulty sleeping? _____
3. Consequences of use (presenting problems, persistent or recurrent emotional, social, legal, or other problems):
   _____
4. Loss of control of amount, frequency, or duration of use: _____
5. Desire or efforts to decrease use or control use: _____
6. Preoccupation (increasing focus or time spent on use and obtaining substances): _____
7. Social, vocational, recreational activities affected by use: _____
8. Previous alcohol/drug abuse treatment: _____

Nursing Diagnoses:

- Relief when they compare themselves to others and find them in worse condition—"They are the alcoholics, not me!"
- A delusion that drinking can be self-controlled—"If I search hard enough or long enough, I will find a way to control and enjoy drinking."
- Confusion or trouble accepting that behavior is different when intoxicated—"I couldn't have done that, that's just not like me."

This quandary about the nature of their problem has often been met with confrontation by nurses and other professionals in the past. Argumentation, presenting evidence of addiction, and lecturing have all been attempted but often fail to elicit admission of a problem or behavior change.

Enhancing Motivation for Change

Longitudinal studies show that motivation is a key predictor of whether an individual will change their substance use (U.S. DHHS, 1999). Motivation involves recognizing a problem, searching for a way to change, and then beginning and sticking with the change strategy (Miller, 1995). Ambivalence about substance use is normal and can be resolved by working with patient's own concerns about their use of alcohol and other drugs. Motivation is fluid and can be modified. Experiences such as increased distress levels, critical life events, a period of evaluation or appraisal of one's life, the rec-

ognizing of negative consequences of use as well as positive and negative external incentives for change, can influence a patient's commitment to change (U.S. DHHS, 1999). Techniques that enhance motivation are associated with increased success in treatment, higher rates of abstinence, and successful follow-up treatment (U.S. DHHS, 1999). Motivational interviewing is a method of therapeutic intervention that seeks to elicit self-motivational statements from patients, supports behavioral change, and creates a discrepancy between the patient's goals and their continued alcohol and other drug use (Miller & Rollnick, 1991). The acronym FRAMES was coined by Miller and Sanchez in 1994 to summarize elements of brief interventions with patients using motivational interviewing (see Table 25-9).

Reality Confrontation

The issue of confrontation is complex in substance abuse treatment. The term has many different meanings and is often emotionally charged. Moffett (1999) defined **reality confrontation** as "a therapeutic strategy that promotes the person's experience of the natural consequences of one's behavior, ie, thoughts feelings, and actions (Table 25-10). Feedback (from others) is a form of confrontation, ie, information about the impact of one's behavior on oneself or others."

Learning from previous behavior and its consequences is how change occurs. It is helpful for the nurse to be aware of these levels of confrontation and to sup-

TABLE 25.9 F.R.A.M.E.S.—Effective Elements of Brief Intervention

Feedback
Provide patients with personal feedback regarding their individual status, such as personal alcohol and other drug consumption relative to norms, information about elevated liver enzyme values, and so forth.

Responsibility
Emphasize the individual's freedom of choice and personal responsibility for change. General themes are as follows:
1. It's up to you; you're free to decide to change or not.
2. No one else can decide for you or force you to change.
3. You're the one who has to do it if it's going to happen.

Advice
Include a clear recommendation or advice on the need for change, typically in a supportive and concerned rather than in a judgmental manner.

Menu
Provide a menu of treatment options, from which patients may pick those that seem more suitable or appealing.

Empathetic Counseling
Show warmth, support, respect, and understanding in communication with patients.

Self-Efficacy
Reinforce self-efficacy, or an optimistic feeling that he or she can change.

TABLE 25.10   Levels of Reality Confrontation

I. Inform
  A. To inform someone about the general consequences of an anticipated behavior (eg, warning nonsmokers about the health risks of smoking)
  B. To inform someone about the general consequences of their behavior (eg, educating drinkers about the health consequences of drinking)
  C. To inform someone about the personal consequences of their behavior (eg, to give feedback on their liver function tests, other health consequences)
  D. To inform someone emphatically about the consequences of either behavior (eg, attack therapy). This form of confrontation is used much less today in treatment settings because it can have a negative effect on the therapeutic relationship and can be abusive
II. Experience
  A. To experience the consequences of their behavior in their natural environment (eg, loss, job loss, separation, family disaffection, legal fees, and sentences)
  B. To experience the consequences of their behavior in a designed environment that generates those consequences immediately and dramatically (eg, a therapeutic community or interactional group therapy)

Moffett, L. A. (1999). *Reality confrontation*. Unpublished manuscript.

port the patient in using the reality feedback received to grow in the recovery process.

There are several general guidelines for establishing therapeutic interactions (see Therapeutic Dialogue: Alcoholism) with patients in chemical dependence treatment programs:

- Encourage honest expression of feelings.
- Listen to what the individual is really saying.
- Express caring for the individual.
- Hold the individual responsible for behavior.
- Provide consequences for negative behavior that are fair and consistent.

THERAPEUTIC DIALOGUE   Alcoholism

Ineffective Approach

Nurse: I would like to talk with you about your problem with alcoholism.
Patient: Alcoholism! It's not that bad. Everyone gets loaded.
Nurse: You fell while you were drinking. Your wife left you. You drink a quart of vodka a day. Your blood alcohol level was 0.15% when you were admitted.
Patient: So what! I do have some problems, or I wouldn't be here. But, I'm not an alcoholic. (denial)
Nurse: Do you know what an alcoholic is?
Patient: Sure I do. My father was one. He was a useless bum. I'm not anything like him.
Nurse: It sounds like you are a lot like him.
Patient: I think I need to rest now. My back is killing me. (avoidance)

Effective Approach

Nurse: I would like to talk with you about what happens when you drink.
Patient: It's not that bad. Everyone gets loaded!
Nurse: What concerns do you have about your drinking?
Patient: I'm not really concerned. My wife is. She thinks I drink too much. I even quit once for her.
Nurse: What does she tell you about that?
Patient: Well, she nags me a lot, and says it costs too much money but I can stop whenever I want. Her nagging only made me drink again.

Nurse: It sounds as if she is concerned about this, but you have your doubts about how serious it is. Your wife is invited to our family education group so that she can learn about alcohol abuse. Family therapy is also available.
Patient: I have a lot of problems besides alcohol. I never use drugs. I only drink because it relaxes me and makes it easier to deal with stress.
Nurse: Many people drink to help them cope with stress. Sometimes the drinking itself can cause stress. While you are here, do you think it would be useful to look at the stress in your life and how it relates to your drinking?
Patient: Yes. But I only drink when things get too out of hand. My health is pretty good.
Nurse: We can provide information about your health and alcohol use. In order to evaluate what information may be helpful, I would like to get a little more information about your drinking.

Critical Thinking Challenge

- What effect did the nurse have on the patient in using the word *alcoholism* in the first interaction?
- Discuss what communication approaches the nurse used in the second scenario to engage the patient in disclosing problems with alcohol and his relationship with his wife. How does this nurse's approach vary from the one in the first interaction?

- Talk about specific actions that are objectionable.
- Do not compromise your own values or nursing practice.
- Communicate the treatment plan to the patient and to others on the treatment team.
- Monitor your own reactions to the patient.

Countertransference

Countertransference is the total emotional reaction of the treatment provider to the patient (see Chap. 6). Patients with substance abuse disorders can generate strong feelings and reactions in nurses and other health care providers (Table 25-11).

These feelings can be generated by overt unpleasant behaviors of the substance abuser, such as lying, deceit, manipulation, or hostility, or these feelings may be more subconscious and stem from past experiences with alcoholics or addicts or even dealing with situations in their own family.

Codependence

Codependence is a maladaptive coping pattern of family members or others closely related to the abuser that results from prolonged exposure to the behaviors of the alcohol- or drug-dependent person and is characterized by boundary distortions, poor relationship and friendship skills, compulsive and obsessive behaviors, inappropriate anger, sexual maladjustment, and resistance to change (Kitchens, 1991).

Whitfield (1997) listed the following cardinal characteristics of codependence:

1. It is learned and acquired.
2. It is developmental.
3. It is outer focused.
4. It is a disease of lost selfhood.
5. It has personal boundary distortions.
6. It is a feeling disorder.
7. It manifests especially by emptiness, low self-esteem, shame, fear, anger, confusion, and numbness.
8. It produces relationship difficulties with self and with others.
9. It is primary, chronic, progressive, malignant, and treatable.

The development of codependence from childhood to adulthood, characterized by Kitchens (1991), is depicted in Figure 25-2. Over years of coping with the substance abuser's behaviors, family members too become "locked into" certain roles and behaviors and are unable to readjust their behavior patterns for new situations and relationships. They may learn to use some of the same maladaptive behavior patterns and defense mechanisms as the substance abuser, such as denial or

TABLE 25.11   Examples of Patient Behaviors and Countertransference Reactions

Patient Behavior	Common Nursing Reaction
Behaves as a victim	Feels a sense of helplessness, increased need to give advice and "fix" the situation and the patient; shows anger toward the patient for not being able to take care of the situation or himself or herself
Is intrusive, hostile, belittling	Can be frightened, withdraw from patient, express anger overtly, or be passive-aggressive (ie, suggesting discharge to the team or ignoring legitimate requests)
Does everything right, is insightful, pleasant, and so forth	Congratulates self on therapeutic interventions; can become bored or complacent
Relapses into drug or alcohol use	Feels angry, personally betrayed; withdraws from other patients; doubts own abilities
Asks personal question about staff qualifications or prior drug or alcohol abuse	Reveals personal information, resents the intrusion, and may regret divulging information
Is silent, or divulges minimal information	Tries harder, doubts own therapeutic ability, is angered by patient's resistance
Tries to "bend" or ignore milieu and group rules	May permit program rule infractions; may feel pressured, angry, or passive-aggressive
Insists that no one can help him or her	Feels pressure to be the one who can help; may feel angry and inept or helpless

Adapted from Imhoff, J.E. (1991). Countertransference issues in alcoholism and drug addiction. *Psychiatric Annals, 21*(5), 292–306.

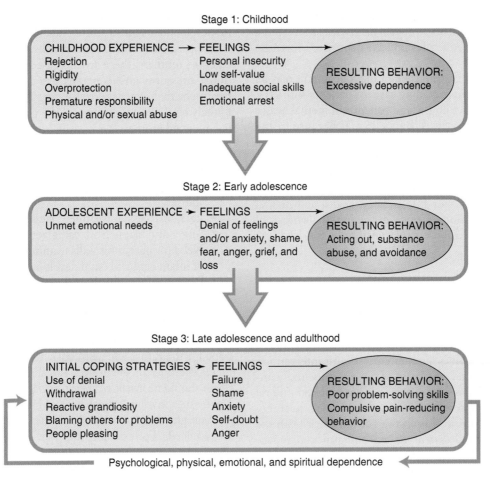

Stage 1: Childhood

CHILDHOOD EXPERIENCE → FEELINGS
Rejection
Rigidity
Overprotection
Premature responsibility
Physical and/or sexual abuse

Personal insecurity
Low self-value
Inadequate social skills
Emotional arrest

RESULTING BEHAVIOR:
Excessive dependence

Stage 2: Early adolescence

ADOLESCENT EXPERIENCE → FEELINGS
Unmet emotional needs

Denial of feelings
and/or anxiety, shame,
fear, anger, grief, and
loss

RESULTING BEHAVIOR:
Acting out, substance
abuse, and avoidance

Stage 3: Late adolescence and adulthood

INITIAL COPING STRATEGIES → FEELINGS
Use of denial
Withdrawal
Reactive grandiosity
Blaming others for problems
People pleasing

Failure
Shame
Anxiety
Self-doubt
Anger

RESULTING BEHAVIOR:
Poor problem-solving skills
Compulsive pain-reducing
behavior

Psychological, physical, emotional, and spiritual dependence

FIGURE 25.2 Psychodynamic stages of codependency.

escape mechanisms, and may even become substance abusers themselves. There has been controversy about using the codependency label as an oversimplification of complex emotions and behaviors of family members. Mental health professionals should be careful not to use it as a catch-all diagnosis and to take special care to assess and plan interventions that address each person's particular situation, problems, and needs.

HIV and Substance Abuse

There is a high risk for HIV among intravenous drug users because of the direct transmission of the HIV through the sharing of hypodermic needles, syringes, and paraphernalia used in injecting drugs and failure to use safe sex practices. Drug-dependent individuals who have financial difficulties or who are experiencing the pain of withdrawal are also more likely to engage in risky sexual encounters when exchanging sex for money or drugs. There is also added risk of infected intravenous drug users transmitting HIV to their sexual partners and pregnant intravenous drug users or pregnant women who are sexual partners of intravenous

drug users, who can transmit the virus to their fetus during the neonatal period and through breast-feeding the infant. Not just intravenous drug users are at risk; other individuals who abuse drugs and alcohol are often at higher risk for sexual transmission not from a lack of knowledge of how to prevent sexual transmission but rather from failure to use adequate precautions and preventive methods while under the influence of alcohol or drugs.

Dual diagnosis of chemical dependency and HIV requires extremely careful assessment and intervention planning. Alcohol and drug abuse can interfere with the medical treatment of acquired immunodeficiency syndrome (AIDS); for example, alcohol, marijuana, cocaine, and amphetamines are immunosuppressants, further compromising the HIV patient's seriously compromised immune system. Other complicating factors include the financial, social, and emotional stressors experienced by substance abusers who must also cope with the devastating diagnosis of HIV disease.

These patients often experience intense feelings of uselessness in trying to overcome substance abuse because they still have to cope with the pain and suffering of a fatal illness and may express desires to "die high" (Faltz, 1993). Patients with dual diagnoses often express anger and are frequently clinically depressed (Sorensen & Batki, 1997).

Alcohol and drug abuse treatment programs play an important role in providing care for patients with HIV disease, substance abuse, and concurrent mental health problems (Sorensen & Batki, 1997). Because of the complex nature of the issues facing these patients, treatment planning and setting treatment priorities are essential. It is important to remember that substance abuse treatment is nearly always necessary for the patient to follow other HIV-related health and mental health interventions. Hence, at the initial diagnosis of AIDS, substance abuse issues need to be resolved first (Faltz, 1993).

Harm-Reduction Strategies

The AIDS epidemic has caused substance abuse treatment professionals to coordinate services with community health and other health care delivery agencies. **Harm reduction** is a community health intervention designed to reduce the harm of substance use to the individual, the family, and society. It has replaced a moral or criminal approach to drug use and addiction. It recognizes that the ideal is abstinence but works with the individual regardless of his or her commitment to reduce use. Marlatt (1998) suggests four general approaches to harm reduction:

- HIV-related interventions, such as needle exchange programs and the distribution of condoms
- More compassionate drug treatment, including both abstinent model and drug substitution treatments
- Drug use management for those who want to continue use
- Changing policy and laws governing drug use and possession of paraphernalia

Interventions for alcohol-related harm reduction are education about the safe use of alcohol, the provision food at bars to reduce the incidence of rapid intoxication, and encouragement of the use of a "designated driver" (Larimer, 1998).

Pregnancy and Substance Abuse

Drug and alcohol use during pregnancy can have serious detrimental effects on the course of pregnancy and on the physiologic status of the fetus and newborn. It is estimated that 11% of infants in the United States have been exposed to illegal drugs in utero (Marion, 1995). Although the severity of problems and complications often depends on amount of substance abuse during pregnancy, studies show that any amount of substance abuse during pregnancy puts the newborn at much higher risk for developmental, neurologic, and behavioral problems.

For pregnant women who are substance abusers and addicted mothers, there are increased social and emotional pressures and concerns associated with their treatment that affect the well-being of their children. Finkelstein (1993) lists some of the clinical issues facing addicted mothers:

- Feelings of guilt and shame
- Difficulties being a single parent (if applicable)
- Care and responsibility of raising children in early sobriety
- Lack of access to treatment facilities
- Anger and blame from caregivers
- Need for parenting skills training and knowledge of infant care and child development
- Potential for child abuse and neglect
- Lack of medical and other supportive services, such as prenatal care, housing, and child care

Finkelstein suggests that service providers convey hope for the future and assist patients in having realistic expectation for themselves and their children. The nurse should be aware of special social, emotional, and legal issues involving treatment of chemically dependent pregnant women and should be sensitive to their special needs. For example, they may fear that by seeking prenatal care, their drug abuse will be detected by urine toxicology tests and cause them to lose custody of their children. Marion (1995) suggested a comprehensive approach to treatment in the perinatal period, including prenatal and perinatal care; pharmacologic interventions, such as methadone maintenance programs; life skills training, such as relapse prevention and social skills training; mother–infant development assessment; and early childhood development programs and social work services, if needed.

Treatment Modalities

Several treatment modalities are used in most substance abuse treatment (pharmacologic modalities were discussed earlier), including 12-step program focused, cognitive or psychoeducational, behavioral, group psychotherapy, and individual and family therapy. Additionally, discharge planning and relapse prevention are essential components of a successful treatment outcome and are incorporated into most treatment programs. See Table 25-12 and Research Box 25-1 for different approaches to chemical dependency treatment.

Twelve-Step Programs

Alcoholics Anonymous was the first 12-step self-help program. (see Table 25-13 for a list of these steps). Al-

TABLE 25.12 Different Approaches to Chemical Dependency Treatment

Approach	Psychiatric	Social	Moral	Learning	Disease	12-Step	Dual Diagnosis	Bio-Psychosocial	Multivariant
Conception of Etiology	Symptom of underlying emotional problem	Society and environment cause dependency	Person is morally weak—can't say "no"	Abuse is a learned, reinforced behavior	Probably caused by genetic or biologic factors	Combination of disease concept and "spiritual bankruptcy"	Both a primary substance dependence and a mental health disorder	Biologic basis, with social and psychological influences	Many different causes; may be different for each individual
Conception of Patient	Emotionally disturbed	Victim of circumstance	"Hustler," morally deficient	Has distorted thinking, poor coping skills	Has a chronic progressive disease	Has an allergy and is powerless over substances	Has both mental and substance abuse disorder	Has deficiencies in all three interacting areas	Has multiple issues to be assessed and addressed
Conception of Treatment Outcome	Emotional conflicts are resolved; there is increased emotional health	Improved social functioning or improved environment	Moral recovery, increased willpower, control, and responsible behavior	Patient learns new ways of thinking and new coping skills	Abstinence, arresting disease progression, and beginning of recovery process	Abstinence, ongoing spiritual recovery	Improvement in both mental health and substance abuse disorders	Improvement in mental and physical health, utilization of social supports	Particular issues for individual addressed, and improvement occurs
Conception of Treatment Process	Psychotherapy, medication to treat "cause" of substance abuse	Removal of environmental influences and increasing coping responses to it	"Street addict" behavior and manipulation confronted	Cognitive therapy techniques and coping skills taught	Is treated as a primary disease, reinforces patient is an addict and has illness	Use 12 steps, seeking spiritual support, making amends, serving others in need	Concurrent treatment of both disorders	Concurrent treatment of all issues	Treatment strategies are matched with individual patient needs
Advantages of Approach	Not punitive, treats co-morbidity	Stresses social supports and coping skills	Holds person responsible for their actions and making amends	Not punitive, teaches new coping skills	Not punitive, stresses support and education	Widespread success, emphasis is on quality of life and spiritual growth	Treats both mental health disorder and dependency, minimizing relapse potential	Utilizes different modalities; is more inclusive	Treatment matched to individual's needs
Disadvantages of Approach	Focus is only on treatment of mental disorder	Blames "ills of society"—the person not responsible for addiction	Punitive, increases low self-esteem and sense of failure	Places emphasis on control of use	Minimizes mental health disorders; discounts return to social use	Self-help group, not a treatment program	Not inclusive enough; does not include social or other issues	Does not match patient and specific interventions	Logistical problems can occur in its implementation

RESEARCH BOX 25.1

Principles of Addiction Treatment

The National Institute on Drug Abuse in 1999 published a review of the research literature that outlined the principles that characterize effective approaches to drug addiction treatment. The following are the summary of these principles:

1. *No single treatment is appropriate for all individuals.*
   - Matching treatment settings, interventions, and services to each individual's particular problems and needs is critical to his or her ultimate success in returning to productive functioning in the family, workplace, and society

2. *Treatment needs to be readily available.*
   - Because individuals who are addicted to drugs may be uncertain about entering treatment, taking advantage of opportunities when they are ready for treatment is crucial. Potential treatment applicants can be lost if treatment is not immediately available or is not readily accessible

3. *Effective treatment attends to multiple needs of the individual, not just his or her drug use.*
   - To be effective, treatment must address the individual's drug use and any associated medical, psychological, social, vocational, and legal problems.

4. *An individual's treatment and services plan must be assessed continually and modified as necessary to ensure that the plan meets the person's changing needs.*
   - A patient may require varying combinations of services and treatment components during the course of treatment and recovery. In addition to counseling or psychotherapy, a patient at times may require medication, other medical services, family therapy parenting instruction, vocational rehabilitation, and social and legal services. It is critical that the treatment approach be appropriate to the individual's age, gender, ethnicity and culture.

5. *Remaining in treatment for an adequate period of time is critical for treatment effectiveness.*
   - The appropriate duration for an individual depends on his or her problems and needs. Research indicates that for most patients, the threshold of significant improvement is reached at about 3 months in treatment. After this threshold is reached, additional treatment can produce further progress toward recovery. Because people often leave treatment prematurely, programs should include strategies to engage and keep patients in treatment.

6. *Counseling (individual and/or group) and other behavioral therapies are critical components of effective treatment for addiction.*
   - In therapy, patients address issues of motivation, building skills to resist drug use, replace drug-using activities with constructive and rewarding non–drug-using activities, and improve problem-solving abilities. Behavioral therapy also facilitates interpersonal relationships and the individual's ability to function in the family and community

7. *Medications are an important element of treatment for many patients, especially when combined with counseling and other behavioral therapies.*
   - Methadone and levo-alpha-acetylmethadol (LAAM) are very effective in helping individuals addicted to heroin or other opiates to stabilize their lives and reduce their illicit drug use. Naltrexone is also an effective medication for some opiate addicts and some patients with co-occurring alcohol dependence. For persons addicted to nicotine, a nicotine replacement product (such as patches or gum) or an oral medication (such as bupropion) can be an effective component of treatment. For patients with mental disorders, both behavioral treatments and medications can be critically important.

8. *Addicted or drug-abusing individuals with coexisting mental disorders should have both disorders treated in an integrated way.*
   - Because addictive disorders and mental disorders often occur in the same individual, patients presenting for either condition should be assessed and treated for the co-occurrence of the other type of disorders

9. *Medical detoxification is only the first stage of addiction treatment and by itself does little to change long-term drug use.*
   - Medical detoxification safely manages the acute physical symptoms of withdrawal associated with stopping drug use. Although detoxification alone is rarely sufficient to help addicts to achieve long-term abstinence, for some individuals, it is a strongly indicated precursor to effective drug addiction treatment.

10. *Treatment does not need to be voluntary to be effective.*
    - Strong motivation can facilitate the treatment process. Sanctions or enticements in the family employment setting or criminal justice system can increase significantly treatment entry, retention rates, and the success of drug treatment interventions.

11. *Possible drug use during treatment must be monitored continuously.*
    - Lapses to drug use can occur during treatment. The objective monitoring of a patient's drug and alcohol use during treatment, such as through urinalysis or other tests, can help the patient withstand urges to use drugs. Such monitoring can also provide early evidence of drug use so that the individual's treatment plan can be adjusted. Feedback to patients who test positive for illicit drug use is an important element of monitoring.

(continued)

RESEARCH BOX 25.1

Principles of Addiction Treatment (Continued)

12. *Treatment programs should provide assessment for HIV/AIDS, Hepatitis b and c, tuberculosis and other infectious diseases, and counseling to help patients modify or change behaviors that place themselves or others at risk for infection.*
    - Counseling can help patients avoid high-risk behavior. Counseling can also help people who are already infected manage their illness.

13. *Recovery from drug addiction can be a long-term process and frequently requires multiple episodes of treatment.*

- As with other chronic illnesses, relapse to drug use can occur during or after successful treatment episodes. Addicted individuals may require prolonged treatment and multiple episodes of treatment to achieve long-term abstinence and fully restored functioning. Participation in self-help support programs during and after treatment is often helpful in maintaining abstinence.

National Institute on Drug Abuse. (1999). *Principles of drug addiction treatment: A research-based guide* (pp.1–3). Rockville, MD: National Institute on Drug Abuse.

coholics Anonymous is a worldwide fellowship of alcoholics who provide support individually and at meetings to others who seek their help. The program steps include spiritual, cognitive, and behavioral components. Many treatment programs discuss concepts from Alcoholics Anonymous, hold meetings at the treatment facilities, and encourage patients to attend community meetings when appropriate. They also encourage continuing use of this and other self-help groups as part of an ongoing plan for continued abstinence. Khantzian & Mack (1994) discuss therapeutic elements of Alcoholics Anonymous, pointing out that it does the following:

- Instills hope through seeing that others are not drinking encourages honesty, openness, and a willingness to listen to others
- Emphasizes shared experiences and the development of a friendship network of sober individuals
- Focuses on abstinence and the loss of control over the ability to drink
- Fosters reliance on others, not on isolation and attempts at control of drinking by the use of willpower
- Adds a spiritual dimension that turns away from ego defense mechanisms such as denial and avoid-

TABLE 25.13 The Twelve Steps

1. We admitted we were powerless over alcohol, that our lives had become unmanageable.
2. We came to believe that a Power greater than ourselves could restore us to sanity.
3. We made a decision to turn our will and our lives over to the care of God *as we understood Him.*
4. We made a searching and fearless moral inventory of ourselves.
5. We admitted to God, to ourselves, and to another human being the exact nature of our wrongs.
6. We were entirely ready to have God remove all these defects of character.
7. We humbly asked Him to remove our shortcomings.
8. We made a list of all persons we had harmed, and became willing to make amends to them all.
9. We made direct amends to such people wherever possible, except when to do so would injure them or others.
10. We continued to take personal inventory and, when we were wrong, promptly admitted it.
11. We sought through prayer and meditation to improve our conscious contact with God as we understood Him, praying only for knowledge of His will for us and the power to carry that out.
12. Having had a spiritual awakening as a result of these steps, we tried to carry this message to alcoholics and to practice these principles in all our affairs.

Alcoholics Anonymous World Services, Inc. (1976). *Alcoholics Anonymous.* New York: Author.

ance toward a better quality of life and the capacity to love and help others

Twelve-step programs do not solicit members, engage in political or religious activities, make medical or psychiatric diagnoses, engage in education about addiction to the general population, or provide mental health, vocational, or legal counseling (Nace, 1997). Alternative peer support groups differ in their approach from these programs. Five groups that are prevalent in the United States are Women for Sobriety, Rational Recovery, Moderation Management, Men for Sobriety, and S.M.A.R.T. Recovery (Horvath, 1997). For an additional discussion of 12-step programs and mental health patients, see Chapter 33.

Cognitive Interventions and Psychoeducation

Cognitive approaches to addiction hypothesize that if a patient can change the way he or she thinks about a situation, both the emotional reaction to it and the behavioral response will change. Psychoeducational materials, groups, and one-on-one interactions with nurses also impart information to reduce knowledge deficits related to alcohol and drug abuse. They enable a patient to make choices regarding behavior and can put emotional reactions into perspective based on knowledge of their problem and the use of alternative coping strategies instead of drug or alcohol use (La Salvia, 1993).

Beck and colleagues (1993) developed a cognitive therapeutic approach to substance abuse in response to their model of a continuing use pattern fueled by distorted thinking. Emphasis is on identifying, understanding, and changing underlying beliefs about the self and the self in relationship to substance abuse (Carroll, 1998). For example, Beck and colleagues (1993) looked at a situation in which a man who has alcoholism goes to a party in which alcohol is served. His automatic thoughts might be, "I can't drink, I wouldn't be any fun, people won't like me, my career would suffer." His underlying belief might be, "I could lose everything." The distortions of thinking, such as predicting other's reactions or his future employment, can lead to increased anxiety and drug and alcohol cravings. Analyzing the situation and the cognitive distortions usually enables a patient to see other ways of thinking that are closer to reality and defuses feelings of anxiety and potential hopelessness. Psychoeducational groups, one-on-one patient education sessions, and reading materials in treatment settings often include the topics that are relevant to substance abuse patients.

Behavioral Interventions

Improvement of coping skills is thought to be one component of preventing relapse into alcohol and drug use. Coping skills include the ability to use thought, emotion, and action effectively to solve interpersonal and intrapersonal problems and to achieve personal goals (Carroll, 1998). Groups in substance abuse treatment programs that also have a relapse prevention component look at coping skills that are needed when drug and alcohol cravings are triggered. The skills listed in Table 25-14 are often taught as coping strategies for dealing with alcohol and drug cravings (Carroll, 1998; Monti et al., 1989). Role-playing new behaviors is utilized and patients learn from the feedback they receive from other group members. They also increase their sense of competency to use these skills in real-life situations. A lengthier discussion of relapse prevention groups will be found in Chapter 33.

Group Therapy and Early Recovery

Isolation and alienation from friends and family are common themes in chemically dependent patients. Additionally, thinking that has become distorted is left unchallenged without contact with others; thus, change is difficult. When a patient enters a group that is working with the goals of continuing recovery, there are nu-

TABLE 25.14 Skills Training Group Topics	
Interpersonal	**Intrapersonal**
Starting conversations	Managing thoughts about alcohol
Giving and receiving compliments	Problem solving
Nonverbal communication	Increasing pleasant activities
Receiving criticism	Relaxation training
Receiving criticism about drinking	Awareness and management of anger
Drink and drug refusal skills	Awareness and management of negative thinking
Refusing requests	Planning for emergencies
Close and intimate relationships	Coping with persistent problems
Enhancing social support networks	
Kadden, et al., 1995; Monti, et al., 1989	

merous healing advantages that can occur. Vanicelli (1989) elaborated the curative elements of a group for alcoholics in early recovery first outlined by Yalom (1995). These groups can accomplish the following:

1. *Reduce the sense of isolation.* Offer a sense of belonging and of being understood.
2. *Instill hope.* Members can see others who are coping and doing well and who have made progress.
3. Help members learn from watching others: they can observe how conflicts are resolved and get a view of successful interactions.
4. *Impart information.* Members learn about group dynamics, how to stay sober, and what works and what does not work in various circumstances.
5. *Alter distorted self-concepts.* Members can examine their own behavior and how their behavior affects others and give feedback to each other.
6. *Provide a reparative family experience.* Members act and react in groups in ways that are similar to their behaviors in their family of origin. Past behaviors are challenged, and the patient has an opportunity to grow and try new behaviors.

Groups in treatment settings focus on immediate goals of maintaining sobriety and not on childhood issues. The emphasis is on the utilization of problem solving and other skills to deal with stressful events that threaten staying abstinent (Yalom, 1995). This type of support group is also extremely effective in outpatient treatment settings. After a period of successful abstinence, group therapy focuses more on traditional psychotherapy work.

Individual Therapy

Often, individual therapy with substance abusers is helpful, particularly in conjunction with group therapy or family therapy. Kaufman (1994) outlines three phases of long-term individual therapy. The first phase is assessment of the problem and its particular emotional and social dynamics, increasing motivation for abstinence, and achieving abstinence. The second phase begins after detoxification and abstinence are established. It involves maintaining abstinence by use of cognitive-behavioral strategies, the emphasis on immediate issues and how they relate to maintaining abstinence, and the encouragement of utilization of community, self-help support groups. Finally, individual therapy focus in the third phase is establishing intimacy with others and achieving autonomy. Often, issues of childhood trauma are examined in this phase. In addiction treatment settings, counselors meet individually to maintain focus on the goals and objections of their individual treatment, to review the individual's fears and anxieties that often arise in early recovery, and to problem solve new and healthy responses and solutions to stressful and difficult situations (Nagy, 1994).

Family Therapy

Family therapy is a vital part of chemical dependency treatment. It can be used in several beneficial ways. It can initiate change and help the family when the substance abuser is unwilling to seek treatment. Behavioral couples therapy with alcoholics has been associated with improved family functioning, reducing stressors, improving marital adjustment, and reducing domestic violence and verbal conflict (O'Farrell, 1999). Family therapy can help stabilize abstinence and relationships when the substance abuser seeks help. Often, inpatient substance abuse treatment programs have family education and group therapy components that help meet these goals (Laundergan & Williams, 1993). Additionally, family therapy can help to maintain long-term recovery and the prevention of relapse (O'Farrell, 1999). Families can often unwittingly support the addiction by continuing to supply money to the individual, allowing adult children to live at home while continuing their substance abuse, and "bailing out" individuals from legal and other difficulties which result from active use (Bale, 1993). Family therapy can bring these behaviors to light and assist family members to set limits on their further support of use (Bale, 1993). Long-term family therapy is often beneficial after the initial stages of detoxification and stabilization of the patient. Stanton and Heath (1997) list six stages of marital and family therapy:

1. Defining the problem and negotiating a treatment contract
2. Establishing the context for a chemical-free life
3. Achieving abstinence
4. Managing the crisis and stabilizing the family
5. Reorganizing the family
6. Termination

Goals of family therapy should be realistic and obtainable. Action plans need to be specific and organized in manageable increments. Target dates should be realistic so that pressure is minimal yet there is motivation to act in a timely manner. Planning for the future is very difficult when there is active alcohol or drug abuse (see Psychoeducational Checklist: Substance Abuse).

Planning and Implementing Nursing Interventions

Because substance abusers differ greatly with respect to both severity of dependence and the biologic, social, and psychological features of their abuse, no one type of treatment program will work for every individual. Often, several approaches can work together for a particular patient, and others may be inappropriate. Treatment programs usually combine many different interventions to

(text continues on page 653)

NURSING CARE PLAN 25.1
Patient With Alcoholism

JG is a 55-year old white, Catholic veteran with a 25-year history of alcohol dependency. He is the youngest of three children born of "blue-collar" parents who valued hard work. His mother is still living with JG's older sister, but his father died of cirrhosis, a complication of years of alcohol abuse. JG has two children who are married with children, living in other states. He rarely sees them. He has been drinking up to 1 quart of vodka per day for 3 years since a work-related back injury. He has a history of binge drinking on weekends. He denies other drug use.

Recently, his wife moved out of the house after 28 years of marriage. An argument about his drinking ended up in a physical fight. She had to be treated in the emergency room for a broken arm. Their relationship had progressively deteriorated over the years. JG was sexually impotent due to excessive drinking, and she had moved into the spare bedroom. He was admitted to the hospital emergency department at a Veteran's Administration Medical Center 2 weeks after his wife left him, with a gash above his right eye from a fall he sustained while intoxicated. His wife returned to care for him.

JG began to have symptoms of alcohol withdrawal and became anxious shortly after admission. He requested hospital admission for alcohol detoxification and was transferred to a detoxification and brief treatment unit.

SETTING: INPATIENT DETOXIFICATION UNIT, VETERANS ADMINISTRATION MEDICAL CENTER

Baseline Assessment: First admission, last drink 7 PM. Admission vital signs: T 99.2°F, HR 98, R 20, BP 140/88 on admission to the ER. He has a history of withdrawal seizures and hallucinosis. He had a blood alcohol level (BAL) of 0.15 mg%, becoming increasingly anxious and restless. He was given diazepam 10 mg PO at that time.

Four hours after admission, vital signs were T 99.8°F, HR 110, R 22, BP 152/100. He continued to be anxious and was tremulous, diaphoretic, and nauseous. Diazepam 20 mg PO stat was given.

Associated Psychiatric Diagnosis	*Medications*
Axis I: Alcohol withdrawal with hallucinations; alcohol abuse	Thiamine
Axis II: None	Folic acid
Axis III: Unspecified back injury	Multivitamins
Axis IV: Social problems (social withdrawal); occupational problems (work-related injury)	Diazepam 10 mg q2h for elevated BP, HR, and tremulousness
Axis V: GAF = Current 60 Potential 75	Haloperidol 5.0 mg IM PRN for hallucinations or agitation

NURSING DIAGNOSIS 1: RISK FOR INJURY

Defining Characteristics	*Related Factors*
Sensory deficits	Altered cerebral function secondary to alcohol withdrawal
Balance and equilibrium deficits	Potential withdrawal seizures resulting from magnesium deficiency or hypoglycemia
Lack of awareness of hazards	Anxiety

OUTCOMES

Initial	*Discharge*
1. Prevent falls and other physical injuries.	2. Relate an intent to practice selected prevention measures such as maintaining sobriety, removing loose throw rugs, using adequate lighting.

(continued)

NURSING CARE PLAN 25.1 (Continued)

INTERVENTIONS

Interventions	Rationale	Ongoing Assessment
Identify stage of alcohol withdrawal and severity of symptoms. Monitor gait and motor coordination, presence of tremors, mental status, electrolyte balance, and seizure activity.	The more severe the reactions, the more likely that disorientation, confusion, and restlessness increase. As the patient moves from stage I to III, he becomes at higher risk for a fall or injury.	Determine whether JG is becoming more disoriented, increasing his risk for injury.
Place patient on seizure precautions (bed in low position, padded side rails).	Withdrawal seizures usually occur within 48 hours after last drink.	Monitor for seizure activity.
Orient patient to surroundings and call light, maintain consistent physical environment.	Disorientation often occurs as blood alcohol level drops. These symptoms can last several days.	Determine JG's level of orientation to surroundings. Determine whether he can use call light.
Avoid sudden moves, loud noises, discussion of patient at bedside, and lighting that casts shadows downward.	Decreased environmental stimulation helps calm the patient, which in turn promotes optimal CNS responses.	Observe reactions to loud noises and monitor room environment.

EVALUATION

Outcomes (at 3 days)	Revised Outcomes	Interventions
Gait steady, patient hydrated. No seizure activities. Patient oriented.	Maintain current level of orientation.	Continue to monitor for any signs of disorientation.

NURSING DIAGNOSIS 2: DISTURBED THOUGHT PROCESSES

Defining Characteristics	Related Factors
Hallucinations (auditory, visual, and tactile) Inaccurate interpretation of stimuli Confusion Disorientation	Physiologic changes secondary to alcohol withdrawal

OUTCOMES

Initial	Discharge
1. Recognize changes in thinking/behavior. 2. Identify situations that occur before hallucinations/delusions.	3. Maintain reality orientation.

INTERVENTIONS

Interventions	Rationale	Ongoing Assessment
Encourage communication that enhances the development of the nurse–patient relationship and promotes JG's sense of integrity.	The therapeutic relationship is important to individuals with alcohol withdrawal because of their fear of withdrawal symptoms and need for reassurance and support.	Monitor the development of the nurse–patient relationship.
Assess for the presence of any hallucinations through observation and interview.	Hallucinations can occur when patients are withdrawing from alcohol. If hallucinations are severe, patient may develop delirium tremens.	Assess patient frequently to determine the presence of hallucinations.
Administer haloperidol 5.0 mg IM PRN for hallucinations or agitation.	Administering an antipsychotic eliminates or reduces the occurrence of hallucinations.	Observe for hypotension. Instruct patient to avoid getting out of bed quickly to prevent falling.

(continued)

NURSING CARE PLAN 25.1 (Continued)

EVALUATION

Outcomes	Revised Outcomes	Interventions
JG had one episode of hallucinations. It occurred 8 h after admission with no identifiable precipitating event.	Continue to maintain reality orientation.	Continue to monitor for hallucinations.

NURSING DIAGNOSIS 3: ANXIETY

Defining Characteristics	Related Factors
Physiologic: increased heart rate, elevated blood pressure, increased respiratory rate, diaphoresis, trembling, nausea Emotional: apprehension about alcohol withdrawal, nervousness, losing control after back injury Cognitive: inability to concentrate, lack of awareness of surroundings	Physiologic changes secondary to alcohol withdrawal

OUTCOMES

Initial	Discharge
1. Identify an increase in physiologic and psychological comfort. 2. Maintain stable vital signs.	3. Describe anxiety as it relates to fear of detoxification process and use of alcohol.

INTERVENTIONS

Interventions	Rationale	Ongoing Assessment
Demonstrate an accepting attitude by being calm and informing JG of any treatments.	A calm attitude of the nurse can help relax a patient.	Observe JG's reaction to the explanations and initiation of any treatments.
Include the patient in decision making regarding his care.	Empowering the patient in decision making helps him gain control over his situation.	Monitor decisions in terms of feasibility.
Administer diazepam 10 mg q2h for elevated BP, HR, and tremulousness PRN.	Diazepam can reduce physiologic impact of alcohol withdrawal.	Monitor vital signs, level of anxiety, and patient's sense of control.
Explain that anxiety is a symptom of withdrawal and is usually time limited.	Knowledge that the anxiety will decrease will help patient deal with the current anxiety.	Monitor whether or not JG understands that his discomfort will disappear.
Observe sleeping behavior.	Sleep is often disturbed. Sleep deprivation contributes to anxiety.	Monitor quality of sleep.

EVALUATION

Outcomes	Revised Outcomes	Interventions
JG was able to refocus and redirect attention when exhibiting mild anxiety. Sleeping about 6 hours.	None.	None.
Identified an increase in apprehension as his BP increased. Given diazepam as ordered.	Relate an increase in apprehension when it occurs.	Assess patient for apprehension and a change in vital signs.
JG discussed his fears of the detoxification process. Expressed mixed feelings about continuing treatment.	Comply with treatment regimen.	Encourage patient to follow up with treatment once he is detoxified.

PSYCHOEDUCATION CHECKLIST
Substance Abuse

When caring for the patient and family with substance abuse, be sure to include the following topic areas in the family's teaching plan:

- Psychopharmacologic agents, if used, including drug action, dosage, frequency, and possible adverse effects
- Manifestations of intoxication, overdose, and withdrawal
- Emergency medical system activation
- Nutrition
- Coping strategies
- Structured planning
- Safety measures
- Available treatment programs
- Family therapy referral
- Self-help groups and other community resources
- Follow-up laboratory testing, if indicated

meet the particular needs of each patient and to provide a comprehensive approach for each patient. Nursing interventions vary depending on the nature of the current problems and their severity. For a patient who is being detoxified, physical interventions (eg, monitoring vital signs and neurologic functioning) are necessary. When the substance abuse problem is secondary to other physical or psychiatric problems, education of patient and family may be a priority. In the home, family interventions may be the priority.

Summary of Key Points

- The *DSM-IV-TR* classifies substance abuse disorders related to the following substances: alcohol, cocaine, amphetamines and other stimulants, cannabis (marijuana), hallucinogens, phencyclidine, opiates, sedative-hypnotics and anxiolytics, inhalants, nicotine, and caffeine.

- Use of a substance is using legal substances within the bounds of sociably acceptable circumstances and behavior that does not pose any harm or risk to the individual or other. Abuse, dependence, and addiction involve risk to the individual and others and are associated with detrimental or harmful psychological and physiologic effects. Dependence and addiction also include symptoms of tolerance and withdrawal syndromes.

- Methadone maintenance treatment is a form of treatment for opiate abusers that includes giving a substitute drug, methadone, in lower, controlled dosages to satisfy the individual's intense drug craving and counteract debilitating withdrawal symptoms while the individual simultaneously receives other rehabilitative therapies (individual and group) to overcome addictive behaviors.

- Opiate intoxication results in sedation, reduced memory and concentration, and euphoria. Withdrawal symptoms are abdominal cramps, runny nose and eyes, diaphoresis, and insomnia.

- Codependence is a maladaptive pattern of coping resulting from prolonged exposure to dysfunctional family dynamics that occur in families of those with active alcohol or drug dependence. Codependence is characterized by boundary distortions, poor relationship and friendship skills, compulsive and obsessive behaviors, inappropriate anger, sexual maladjustment, and resistance to change.

- Several effective modalities are used in substance abuse treatment, and many programs combine several modalities, which can include 12-step programs, social skills groups, psychoeducational groups, group therapy, and individual and family therapies. There is no one best treatment method for all people.

- Denial of a substance abuse problem is the individual's attempt to avoid accepting a diagnoses of substance abuse or dependence and can be exhibited by attempts to rationalize the substance use, minimize the harmful results, deflect attention from one's own problem to society's or someone else's, or blame childhood experiences.

- Nurses should use a nonconfrontational approach when dealing with patients in denial of their problem. Motivational interviewing approaches are most effective using empathy and nonjudgmental approach and helping the patient to realize the discrepancy between life goals and engaging in substance abuse, thus motivating one to change one's own self-destructive behaviors and make personal choices regarding treatment goals.

- Accurate and comprehensive assessment is crucial in planning substance abuse treatment interventions. Substance abuse evaluation should include evaluation of use of all abusable substances for pattern of use, including factors of tolerance; withdrawal symptoms; consequences of use; loss of control of amount, frequency, or duration of use; desire or efforts to cease or control use; social, vocational, and recreational activities affected by use; and history of previous alcohol or drug abuse treatment. Comprehensive evaluation also includes investigating family and social support systems.

- In addressing culturally diverse populations, substance abuse treatment programs need to provide programs that have staff who are knowledgeable about cultural differences and issues and programs that are responsive to those differences and specialized needs of cultural and ethnic groups.

➤ The problem of substance abuse has many social and political ramifications. Even the discipline of nursing is plagued by addiction problems of its members.

Critical Thinking Challenges

1. What is your understanding of the etiology of chemical dependence? Based on this understanding, what would be your priorities for patient education?

2. Jeff H., a 35-year-old cocaine-dependent patient, has entered a rehabilitation program. What goals do you believe would be realistic to achieve by the end of his projected 30-day inpatient stay?

3. You are working in an orthopedic unit, and Mary L. has been admitted for treatment for a fractured femur. She has been drinking recently and has a blood-alcohol level of 0.08 mg%. What further information in the following areas would you need to plan her care?
   a. Medical
   b. Alcohol and drug use related
   c. Other psychosocial issues

4. Medical use of marijuana has been approved in California. What is your opinion of this legislation? What are the pros and cons of this public policy?

5. Normal adolescent behavior is often similar to that associated with substance abuse. How would you differentiate this normal behavior from possible substance abuse?

6. John M. has sought treatment for depression and job stress. He came to your psychiatric assessment unit smelling of alcohol. He does not believe that he has a drinking problem but a job problem. What interventions would you use for possible alcohol abuse?

7. Sylvia G. has been abusing heroin intravenously heavily for 2 years. She has come into the hospital with an abscess on her leg. What symptoms would you expect to observe as she withdraws from opiates? What medications would likely be used to ease these symptoms?

8. After Sylvia G. is free of withdrawal symptoms, she expresses interest in obtaining drug treatment. What are her options? How would you describe them to her?

9. Raymond L. has been treated for hypertension at your clinic. You notice that he complains of peripheral neuropathy and has an unsteady gait. What other medical signs would corroborate alcoholism?

10. What laboratory test results would help confirm a diagnosis of alcoholism?

 WEB LINKS

www.health.org The website of the National Clearinghouse for Alcohol and drug information and PREVline. Included is a catalog of publications which discuss relevant treatment issues and research findings. It is possible to search several databases using this site.

www.nhic.org The National Health Information Center (NHIC). It is consumer focused and has the ability to conduct searches for health-related topics, including alcoholism and addiction issues.

www.os.dhhs.gov U.S. Department of Health and Human Services (DHHS). This website contains important information links to other relevant websites, including the Substance Abuse and Mental Health Services Administration (SAMHSA).

www.al-anon.org The purpose of Al-Anon is to help families and friends of alcoholics recover from the effects of living with the problem drinking of a relative or friend. Similarly, Alateen is the recovery program for young people. The program of recovery is adapted from Alcoholics Anonymous. The only requirement for membership is that there be a problem of alcoholism in a relative or friend.

www.alcoholics-anonymous.org This is the official site for the program of Alcoholics Anonymous. Information about this program and about alcoholism is available.

www.well.com/user/woa Web of Addictions. This site contains fact sheets and in depth information on special topics, links to resources, ways to contact various groups, and to get help with addictions.

www.samhsa.gov The website of the Substance Abuse and Mental Health Services Administration is a federal government site with funding, research, consumer information, and resources.

www.ccsa.ca The Canadian Centre on Substance Abuse is an arms-length, national agency that promotes informed debate on substance abuse; disseminates information on the nature, extent, and consequences of substance abuse; and supports and assists organizations involved in substance abuse treatment, prevention, and educational programming.

www.who.int/dsa/cat98/subs8.htm The World Health Organization website provides access to publications on alcohol and drug abuse.

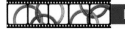 **MOVIES**

Clean and Sober: 1989. Daryl Poynter, played by Michael Keaton, is a real estate broker with a substance-abuse problem that he denies. He embezzled company money and became involved with a woman's death. He decides to hide out in a 21-day detox program that promises total discretion and privacy. He is directly confronted with his addiction. *Viewing Points:* This film is realistic in its portrayal of the detoxification process and the denial that many experience regarding their addictions. Trace Daryl Poynter's thinking process as he struggles with accepting his addiction. What events led up to his relapse?

REFERENCES

Abramsky, S. (1997). Gulag American style. *Toward Freedom, 46*(2).

Alcoholics Anonymous World Services, Inc. (1976). *Alcoholics Anonymous.* New York: Author.

American Psychiatric Association. (2000). *The diagnostic and statistical manual of mental disorders* (4th ed., Text revision). Washington, DC: Author.

Anthenelli, R. M., & Schuckit, M. A. (1997). Genetics. In J. H. Lowinson, P. Ruiz, R. B. Millman, & J. G. Langrod (Eds.), *Substance abuse: A comprehensive textbook* (3rd ed.) (pp. 41–50). Baltimore: Williams & Wilkins.

Anthony, J. C., & Helzer J. E. (1995). Epidemiology and drug dependence. In M. Tsuang, M. Tohen, & G. Zahner (Eds.), *Textbook in psychiatric epidemiology* (pp. 361–407). New York: Wiley-Liss.

Bale, R. (1993). Family treatment in short-term detoxification. In T. O'Farrell (Ed.), *Treating alcohol problems* (pp. 117–144). New York: Guilford Press.

Beck A. A., Wright, F. D., Newman, C. F., & Liese, B. S. (1993). *Cognitive therapy of substance abuse.* New York: Guilford Press.

Bierut, L. J., Dinwiddie, S., Begleiter, H., et al. (1998). Familial transmission of substance dependence: Alcohol, marijuana, and cocaine. *Archives of General Psychiatry, 55,* 982–988.

Brady, K. T., Myrick, H., & Malcolm, R. (1999). Sedative-hypnotic and anxiolytic agents: specific drugs of abuse. Pharmacological and clinical aspects. In B. S. McCrady & E. E. Epstein (Eds.), *Comprehensive guidebook of addictions* (pp. 98–102). New York, Oxford: Oxford University Press.

Brehm, N. M., & Khantzian, E. J. (1997). Psychodynamics. In J. H. Lowinson, P. Ruiz, R. B. Millman, & J. G. Langrod (Eds.), *Substance abuse: A comprehensive textbook* (3rd ed.) (pp. 90–100). Baltimore: Williams & Wilkins.

Carroll, K. M. (1998). *A cognitive-behavioral approach: Treating cocaine addiction* (pp. 8–14). Rockville, MD: National Institute on Drug Abuse.

Castro F. G., Proescholdbell, R. J., Abieta, L., & Rodriguez, D. (1999). Ethnic and cultural minority groups. In B. S. McCrady & E. E. Epstein (Eds.), *Addictions: A comprehensive guide* (pp. 499–505). New York: Oxford University Press.

Caulker-Burnett, I. (1994). Primary care screening for substance abuse. *Nurse Practitioner, 19*(6), 42, 44–48.

Center for Substance Abuse Treatment. (1999). *Cultural issues in substance abuse treatment* (pp. 11–60). Rockville, MD: Author.

Chassin, L., Pillow, D. R., Curran, P. J., et al. (1993). Relation of parental alcoholism to early adolescent substance abuse: A test of three medicating mechanisms. *Journal of Abnormal Psychology, 102,* 3–19.

Cohen, S. (1991). Benzodiazepines in psychotic and related conditions. In P. P. Roy-Byrne, & D. S. Cowley (Eds.), *Benzodiazepines in clinical practice: Risks and benefits* (pp. 59–71). Washington, DC: American Psychiatric Press.

Faltz, B., contributing author. (1993). *Women and HIV: Train the trainer program.* San Francisco: California Nurses Association.

Finkelstein, N. (1993). Treatment programming for alcohol and drug-dependent pregnant women. *International Journal of Addictions, 28*(13), 1275–1309.

Gardner, E. L. (1997). Brain reward mechanisms. In J. H. Lowinson, P. Ruiz, R. B. Millman, & J. G. Langrod (Eds.), *Substance abuse: A comprehensive textbook* (2nd ed.) (pp. 51–85). Baltimore: Williams & Wilkins.

Gloria, A. M., & Peregoy, J. J. (1996). Counseling Latino alcohol and other substance users/abusers: Cultural considerations for counselors. *Journal of Substance Abuse Treatment, 13,* 119–126.

Gold, M. S. (1994). Neurobiology of addiction and recovery: The brain, the drive for the drug, and the 12-step fellowship. *Journal of Substance Abuse Treatment, 11,* 93–97.

Gold, M. S., & Miller, N. S. (1992). Seeking drugs/alcohol and avoiding withdrawal: The neuroanatomy of drive states and withdrawal. *Psychiatric Annals, 22,* 430–435.

Gomberg, E. S. (1999). Women. In B. S. McCrady & E. E. Epstein (Eds.), *Addictions: A comprehensive guide* (pp. 527–541). New York: Oxford University Press.

Goodwin, D. W. (1979). Alcoholism and heredity. *Archives of General Psychiatry, 36*(1), 57–61.

Goodwin, D. W., & Gabrielli, W. F. (1997). In J. H. Lowinson, P. Ruiz, R. B. Millman, & J. G. Langrod (Eds.), *Substance abuse: A comprehensive textbook* (3rd ed.) (pp. 142–148). Baltimore, MD: Williams & Wilkins.

Grant, B. F., & Dawson, D. A. (1999). Alcohol and drug use, abuse and dependence: Classification, prevalence, and comorbidity. In B. S. McCrady & E. E. Epstein (Eds.), *Addictions: A comprehensive guide* (pp. 9–29). New York: Oxford University Press.

Greden, J. F., & Walters, A. (1997). Caffeine. In J. H. Lowinson, P. Ruiz, R. B. Millman, & J. G. Langrod (Eds.), *Substance abuse: A comprehensive textbook* (3rd ed.) (pp. 357–370). Baltimore: Williams & Wilkins.

Grinspoon, L., & Bakalar J. (1997). Marijuana. In J. H. Lowinson, P. Ruiz, R. B. Millman, & J. G. Langrod (Eds.), *Substance abuse: A comprehensive textbook* (3rd ed.) (pp. 236–246). Baltimore: Williams & Wilkins.

Halikas, J. A. (1997). Craving. In J. H. Lowinson, P. Ruiz, R. B. Millman, & J. G. Langrod (Eds.), *Substance abuse: A comprehensive textbook* (3rd ed.) (pp. 85–100). Baltimore, MD: Williams & Wilkins.

Hawkins, J. D., Catalano, R. F., Miller, J. Y. (1992). Risk and protective factors for alcohol and other drug problems in adolescence and early adulthood: Implications for substance abuse prevention. *Psychological Bulletin, 112*, 64–105.

Hesselbrock, M. N., Hesselbrock, V. M., & Epstein, E. E. (1999). Theories of alcohol and other drug use disorders. In B. S. McCrady & E. E. Epstein (Eds.), *Addictions: A comprehensive guide* (pp. 50–71). New York: Oxford University Press.

Horvath, A. T. (1997). Alternative support groups. In J. H. Lowinson, P. Ruiz, R. B. Millman, & J. G. Langrod (Eds.), *Substance abuse: A comprehensive textbook* (3rd ed.) (pp. 393–396). Baltimore: Williams & Wilkins.

Huang, L. X., Cerbone, F. G., & Groerer, J. C. (1998). Children at risk because of parental substance abuse. In Office of Applied Studies, Substance Abuse and Mental Health Services Administration. *Analysis of substance abuse and treatment need issues* (p. 11). Rockville, MD: Substance Abuse and Mental Health Services Administration.

Imhoff, J. E. (1991). Countertransference issues in alcoholism and drug addiction. *Psychiatric Annals, 21*(5), 292–306.

Kaufman, E. (1994). *Psychotherapy of addicted persons.* New York: Guilford Press.

Kendall, R. (1998). The history of drug abuse and women in the United States. In National Institute on Drug Abuse. *Drug addiction research and the health of women: Executive summary* (p. 8). Rockville, MD: U.S. Department of Health and Human Services.

Khantzian, E. J., & Mack, J. E. (1994). How AA works and why it's important for clinicians to understand. *Journal of Substance Abuse Treatment, 11*, 77–92.

Kitano, H. H. L. (1989). Alcohol and the Asian-American. In T. D. Watts & R. Wright (Eds.), *Alcoholism in minority populations* (pp. 143–156). Springfield, IL: Charles C. Thomas.

Kitchens, J. A. (1991). *Understanding and treating codependence.* Englewood Cliffs, NJ: Prentice-Hall.

Kristenson H. (1995). How to get the best out of antabuse. *New England Journal of Medicine, 338*(9), 26.

Larimer, M. E. (1998). Harm reduction for alcohol problems: Expanding access to and acceptability of prevention and treatment services. In G. A. Marlatt (Ed.), *Harm reduction: Pragmatic strategies for managing high-risk behaviors* (pp. 69–121). New York: Guilford Press.

La Salvia, T. A. (1993). Enhancing addiction treatment through psychoeducational groups. *Journal of Substance Abuse Treatment, 10*, 439–444.

Laundergan, J. C., & Williams, T. (1993). The Hazelden residential family program: A combined systems and disease model approach. In T. J. O'Farrell (Ed.), *Treating alcohol problems: Marital and family interventions* (pp. 145–169). New York: Guilford Press.

Lowinson, J. H., Marion, I. J., Joseph, H., & Dole, V. P. Methadone maintenance. (1997). In J. H. Lowinson, P. Ruiz, R. B. Millman, & J. G. Langrod (Eds.), *Substance abuse: A comprehensive textbook* (3rd ed.) (pp. 405–415). Baltimore: Williams & Wilkins.

Marlatt, G. A. (1998). Highlights of harm reduction: A personal report from the first national harm reduction conference in the United States. In G. A. Marlatt (Ed.), *Harm reduction: Pragmatic strategies for managing high-risk behaviors*, pp. 3–29. New York: Guilford Press.

Marion, I. J. (1995). *Pregnant substance abusing women* (pp. 2–11). Rockville, MD: U.S. Department of Health and Human Services.

McCaul, M. E., Wand G. S., Eissenberg T., Rohde C. A., & Cheskin L. J. (2000). Naltrexone alters subjective and psychomotor responses to alcohol in heavy drinking subjects. *Neuropsychopharmacology, 22*(5), 480–492.

Miller, N. S., Gold, M. S., & Smith D. E. (Eds.). (1997). *Manual of therapeutics for addictions* (pp. 23–152). New York, NY: Wiley-Liss, Inc.

Miller, N. S., & Gold, M. S. (1994). A neurochemical basis for alcohol and other drug addiction. *Journal of Psychoactive Drugs, 25*(2), 121–126.

Miller, W. R. (1995). Increasing motivation for change. In R. K. Hester & W. R. Miller (Eds.), *Handbook of alcoholism treatment approaches: Effective alternatives* (2nd ed.) (pp. 89–104). Boston: Allyn & Brown.

Miller, W. R., & Rollnick, S. (1991). *Motivational interviewing: Preparing people to change addictive behavior.* New York: Guilford Press.

Miller, W. R., & Sanchez, V. C. (1994). Motivating young adults for treatment and lifestyle change. In G. Howard & P. E. Nathan (Eds.), *Alcohol use and misuse by young adults.* Notre Dame, IN: University of Notre Dame Press.

Moak, D. H., & Anton, R. F. (1999). Alcohol: specific drugs of abuse: pharmacological and clinical aspects. In B. S. McCrady & E. E. Epstein (Eds.), *Comprehensive guidebook of addictions* (p. 78). New York, Oxford: Oxford University Press.

Moffett, L. A. (1999). *Reality confrontation.* Unpublished manuscript.

Monti, P. M., Abrams, D. B., Kadden, R. M., & Cooney, N. L. (1989). *Treating alcohol dependence.* New York: Guilford Press.

Nace, E. P. (1997). Alcoholics Anonymous. In J. H. Lowinson, P. Ruiz, R. B. Millman, & J. G. Langrod (Eds.), *Substance abuse: A comprehensive textbook* (3rd ed.) (pp. 383–390). Baltimore: Williams & Wilkins.

Nagy, P. D. (1994). *Intensive outpatient treatment for alcohol and other drug abuse* (p. 21). Rockville, MD: U.S. Department of Health and Human Services.

National Council on Alcoholism and Drug Dependence. (1999). NCADD news. ***http://www.ncadd.org.***

National Institute on Drug Abuse, National Institutes of Health. (2000). ***http://www.drugabuse.gov/Infofax.*** (Marijuana 13551).

National Institute on Drug Abuse. (1999). Principles of drug addiction treatment: A research-based guide (pp. 1–3). Rockville, MD: National Institute on Drug Abuse.

National Institute on Drug Abuse. (1998). *Drug use among racial/ethnic minorities* (pp. 5–6). Rockville, MD: National Institute on Drug Abuse.

National Institute on Drug Abuse. (1997). *Research report series: Heroin abuse and addiction* (pp. 1–8). Rockville, MD: National Institute on Drug Abuse.

Nielsen, A. L. (2000). Examining drinking patterns and problems among Hispanic groups: Results from a national survey. *Journal of Studies on Alcohol, 61*(2), 301–310.

O'Connor, P. G., & Schottenfeld, R. S. (1998). Departments of Internal Medicine and Psychiatry Medical Progress:

Patients with alcohol problems. *New England Journal of Medicine, 338*(9), 592–602.

O'Farrell, J. (1999). Alcoholism treatment and the family: Do family and individual treatments for alcoholic adults have preventative effects for children? *Journal of Studies on Alcohol, 13,* 125–129.

Pandina, R., & Hendren, R. (1999). Other drugs of abuse: Inhalants, designer drugs, and steroids. Specific drugs of abuse: Pharmacological and clinical aspects. In B. S. McCrady & E. E. Epstein (Eds.), *Comprehensive guidebook of addictions* (p. 173). New York, Oxford: Oxford University Press.

Peele, S. (1985). What treatment for addiction can do and what it can't; what treatment for addiction should do and what it shouldn't. *Journal of Substance Abuse Treatment, 2,* 225–228.

Rosenthal, R. N., & Westreich, L. (1999). Treatment of persons with dual diagnoses of substance use disorder and other psychological problems. In B. S. McCrady & E. E. Epstein (Eds.), *Addictions: A comprehensive guide* (pp. 439–476). New York: Oxford University Press.

Schuckit, M., Goodwin, D., & Winokur, D. (1972). A study of alcoholism in half-siblings. *American Journal of Psychiatry, 128,* 1132–1136.

Selwyn, P. A., & Merino, F. L. (1997). Medical complications and treatment. In J. H. Lowinson, P. Ruiz, R. B. Millman, & J. G. Langrod (Eds.), *Substance abuse: A comprehensive textbook* (3rd ed.) (pp. 597–619). Baltimore: Williams & Wilkins.

Segal, B. M., & Stewart, J. C. (1996). Substance use and abuse in adolescence: An overview. *Child Psychiatry and Human Development, 26,* 193–210.

Slade, J. (1999). Nicotine. Specific drugs of abuse: Pharmacological and clinical aspects. In B. S. McCrady & E. E. Epstein (Eds.), *Comprehensive guidebook of addictions* (pp. 163–166). New York, Oxford: Oxford University Press.

Sorensen, J. L., & Batki, S. L. (1997). Psychosocial sequelae. In J. H. Lowinson, P. Ruiz, R. B. Millman, & J. G. Langrod (Eds.), *Substance abuse: A comprehensive textbook* (3rd ed.) (pp. 640–644). Baltimore: Williams & Wilkins.

Stanton, M. D., & Heath, A. W. (1997). Family and marital therapy. In J. H. Lowinson, P. Ruiz, R. B. Millman, & J. G. Langrod (Eds.), *Substance abuse: A comprehensive textbook* (3rd ed.) (pp. 448–453). Baltimore: Williams & Wilkins.

Stephens, R. S. (1999). Cannabis and hallucinogens. Specific drugs of abuse: Pharmacological and clinical aspects. In B. S. McCrady & E. E. Epstein (Eds.), *Comprehensive guidebook of addictions* (pp. 122–129). New York Oxford: Oxford University Press.

Stine, S. M., & Kosten, T. R. (1999). Opioids. Specific drugs of abuse: Pharmacological and clinical aspects. In B. S. McCrady & E. E. Epstein (Eds.), *Comprehensive guidebook of addictions* (p. 151). New York, Oxford: Oxford University Press.

U.S. Department of Health and Human Services (DHHS). (1999). *Enhancing motivation for change in substance abuse treatment.* Rockville, MD: Substance Abuse and Mental Health Services Administration.

U.S. Department of Health and Human Services (DHHS). (1998). *Precedence of substance abuse among racial and ethnic subgroup in the United States, 1991–1993.* Rockville MD: Substance Abuse and Mental Health Services Administration.

U.S. Department of Health and Human Services (DHHS). (1997a). *National household survey on drug abuse: highlights 1996.* Rockville, MD: Substance Abuse and Mental Health Administration.

U.S. Department of Health and Human Services (DHHS). (1997b). *Alcohol and health* (pp. 1–31). Rockville, MD: Substance Abuse and Mental Health Administration.

Vanicelli, M. (1989). *Removing the roadblocks: Group psychotherapy with substance abusers and family members.* New York: Guilford Press.

Wallace, J. (1990). The new disease model of alcoholism. *Western Journal of Medicine, 152,* 501–505.

Weaver M. F., & Schnoll, S. H. (1999). Stimulants: Amphetamine and cocaine. Specific drugs of abuse: Pharmacological and clinical aspects. In B. S. McCrady & E. E. Epstein (Eds.), *Comprehensive guidebook of addictions* (p. 115). New York, Oxford: Oxford University Press.

Westermeyer, J. (1997). Cultural perspectives: Native-Americans, Asians, and new immigrants. In J. H. Lowinson, P. Ruiz, R. B. Millman, & J. G. Langrod (Eds.), *Substance abuse: A comprehensive textbook* (3rd ed.) (pp. 712–715). Baltimore: Williams & Wilkins.

Whitfield, C. W. (1997). Co-dependence, addictions, and related disorders. In J. H. Lowinson, P. Ruiz, R. B. Millman, & J. G. Langrod (Eds.), *Substance abuse: A comprehensive textbook* (3rd ed.) (pp. 672–683). Baltimore: Williams & Wilkins.

Winick, C. (1997). Epidemiology. In J. H. Lowinson, P. Ruiz, R. B. Millman, & J. G. Langrod (Eds.), *Substance abuse: A comprehensive textbook* (3rd ed.) (pp. 10–15). Baltimore: Williams & Wilkins.

Yalom, I. (1995). *The theory and practice of group psychotherapy.* New York: Basic Books.

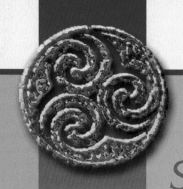

Sleep Disorders

Nancy Anne Hilliker and Mark J. Muehlbach

LEARNING OBJECTIVES

After studying this chapter, you will be able to:

➤ Describe the major features of sleep.

➤ Identify sleep changes in major psychiatric disorders.

➤ Distinguish among primary sleep disorders.

➤ Discuss biopsychosocial aspects of sleep disorders.

➤ Perform a sleep history during a patient's assessment.

➤ Formulate a model nursing care plan for patients with sleep disorders.

cataplexy
circadian rhythm
dyssomnias
hypnagogic
  hallucinations
multiple sleep latency
  test (MSLT)
non–rapid-eye-
  movement sleep
  (NREM)

parasomnias
polysomnography
rapid-eye-movement
  sleep (REM)
sleep architecture
sleep disorders
sleep efficiency
sleep paralysis
slow-wave sleep

insomnia
rhythm

Sleep, an experience that occupies nearly one third of our lives, is a recurrent, altered state of consciousness that occurs for sustained periods, restoring a person's energy and well-being. Sleep is part of a rhythm and pattern that encompasses rest and activity and affects our entire state each and every day and night. Sleep allows the body to restore itself and prepare for the next day.

Sleep is a complex biopsychosocial state. Sleep problems and disorders have a serious impact on an individual's physical and mental health. Sleep disorders have been linked to other mental disorders, such as depression and psychoses. A history of sleep disturbance is associated with increased risk for new-onset depression, substance abuse and anxiety disorders, and nicotine dependence (Breslau et al., 1996).

***Sleep disorders** are ongoing disruptions of normal waking and sleeping patterns. Sleep disorders lead to excessive daytime sleepiness, inappropriate naps, chronic fatigue, and the inability to perform safely or properly at work, school, or home. In a longitudinal epidemiologic study of more than 1,000 young adults ranging in age from 21 to 30 years, lifetime prevalence of insomnia was 16.6% (Breslau et al., 1996). Sleep disturbances are more common in women, and the prevalence of sleep disorders increases with age in both genders (Ganguli et al., 1996).*

Because of these effects, insufficient sleep and sleep disorders have been recognized as public health issues. It has been estimated that 40 million Americans suffer chronically from sleep disorders (National Commission on Sleep Disorders Research, 1993). During the past 100 years, the average nightly total sleep time has been reduced by more than 20%. Many Americans are severely sleep deprived, and the consequences of daytime sleepiness are disastrous.

Accidents owing to sleepiness have been reported since 1929 (Horstmann et al., 2000). About 20% of all drivers have fallen asleep at least once while driving. The Department of Transportation estimates that 200,000 automobile accidents each year are sleep related, and these accidents often result in fatalities. Sleepy drivers are more of a threat to safety than drunken drivers.

There are other, more disastrous effects related to sleepy or sleep-deprived individuals. Three of four night-shift workers report sleepiness every night shift, and at least one of five admits to falling asleep on the job. Short-term adverse effects of shift work include sleep disturbances, psychosomatic troubles, errors, and accidents. In the long-term, there is increased risk for gastrointestinal, psychiatric, neurologic, and cardiovascular disorders (Costo, 1997). Several disasters have demonstrated that our society is vulnerable to the sleepiness of shift workers. Sleepiness and exhaustion were the responsible factors that led to the grounding of the Exxon Valdez *in Prince William Sound in 1989, which resulted in a disastrous oil spill that threatened the environment, killed wildlife, disrupted the ecosystem of that area, cost millions of dollars to clean up, and destroyed the livelihood of many residents and fisherman for years. The nuclear melt down at Chernobyl in Ukraine in 1986 was caused by the poor judgment of sleepy workers in the early morning hours and resulted in radiation contamination to thousands of people, literally causing the surrounding environments to be uninhabitable. In the United States, the near nuclear disaster at Three Mile Island in 1979 was caused by poor judgment of sleepy workers. These incidents are only a few of the prime examples of the disastrous effects of sleep-deprived individuals in the workplace.*

An understanding of sleep and sleep disturbance is crucial for clinicians practicing in the field of mental health today. This chapter discusses normal sleep rhythms and patterns, sleep disorders and their distinguishing characteristics, and nursing diagnoses and interventions appropriate for use in patients with sleep problems.

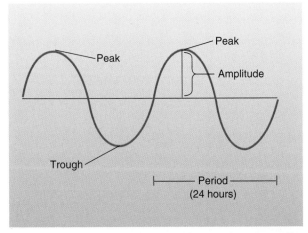

FIGURE 26.1 Circadian body rhythms fluctuate in patterns. The *peak* is the point at which the rhythm reaches its maximum, and the *trough* is the point at which the rhythm reaches its minimum. The *period* is the time it takes to complete a cycle. *Amplitude* is the extent of the peak and is half the distance from peak to trough.

BIOLOGIC BASIS OF SLEEP

All bodily systems have a rhythm and are affected by the environment. These physiologic rhythms occur in time intervals or cycles, such as the cycle of seconds in cardiac rhythms or monthly cycles in a woman's menstrual cycle.

KEY CONCEPT **Rhythm.** **Rhythm** is movement with a cadence, a measured flow that recurs at regular intervals, with a cycle of coming and going, ebbing and rising, to return at the start point and begin again.

Normal Sleep–Wake Circadian Rhythms

The human circadian system is composed of many rhythms that are synchronized to achieve the best physiologic effect, with different body systems reaching maximum and minimum levels at coordinated times. Nearly all physiologic and psychological functions fluctuate in a pattern that repeats itself in a 24-hour cycle, called **circadian rhythm** (Fig. 26-1). Body temperature follows a circadian rhythm, fluctuating in a predictable pattern from lowest, in the early morning hours, to highest, in the mid-evening hours.

Sleep is an integral part of the circadian system. Most physiologic functions reach their lowest levels during the middle of the sleep period. The sleepiness–alertness cycle runs in a circadian rhythm. Other body systems that also follow a circadian rhythm are often interrelated to the sleep–wake cycle and can affect it, such as hormone secretion. The secretions of the hormones melatonin and cortisol also follow a circadian

rhythm and, although the physiologic explanation is complex, the cycle of release of these two hormones promotes wakefulness during the day and induces sleep at night. When rhythms reach their peak at the same time, they are synchronized in phase with each other; if they reach peak at different times, they are desynchronized (Text Box 26-1).

The temporal pattern of sleep and wakefulness affects circadian body rhythms, such as one's alertness and sleepiness rhythms. Manual dexterity, reaction time, and simple recognition appear to coincide with the circadian rhythm of body temperature. For example, body temperature is usually lowest in the early morning hours, coinciding with the time when reaction is slowest. During a conventional 24-hour sleep–wake schedule (asleep at night and awake during the day), the circadian rhythm exhibits a biphasic pattern. The peak of sleepiness occurs during nocturnal hours, from 2 to 6 AM, when people are typically asleep, and a secondary peak of sleepiness occurs during the afternoon (2 to 6 PM), when people usually experience a mid-afternoon slump. The circadian rhythm of sleepiness and alertness is associated with, but not directly dependent on, the sleep–wake cycle (Pollack & Stokes, 1997).

Most circadian rhythms continue even when humans are unaware of what time of day it is. Studies show that individuals in "temporal isolation" (an environment without any time cues) still exhibit natural circadian rhythms, and their body rhythms continue to function in concert with each other. The body's circadian system continues to oscillate, even when external factors are completely constant. When temporal isolation is extended for longer than 24 hours, the circadian system demonstrates a different response. Individual

TEXT BOX 26.1

Melatonin: The Hormone of Darkness

Each evening as dusk falls, the pineal gland goes to work, releasing increasing amounts of melatonin into the bloodstream until it tapers off between 2 and 4 AM. Blood vessels, the gastrointestinal tract, ovaries, and the brain are all equipped to use melatonin, a hormone. Although melatonin may play a large part in many body functions, it's effects are not well understood.

On a larger scale, melatonin is found in all species from microorganisms to humans. In mammals, melatonin provides light-sensitive feedback so that circadian rhythms are synchronized to the changing length of the night in the course of the year (Arendt et al., 1999). In humans, melatonin starts changes through the body that makes people feel sleepy. Melatonin is being investigated as a possible therapeutic agent for insomnia and jet lag.

Currently, melatonin is sold in health food stores as a sleep aid even though the Food and Drug Administration does not regulate the production of this hormone. This means that there is no assurance of the quality of its production. A few years ago, another drug, L-tryptophan, was also a very popular sleep aid sold in health food stores. The process used to make L-tryptophan included a toxin in the product that caused 13 deaths and blood dyscrasias in many others. Further research may demonstrate that melatonin is a safe and natural sleeping pill. At this time, experts are still in the dark regarding timing of administration, best dose, and long-term side effects.

rhythms are no longer synchronized to each other, but fluctuate in their own natural endogenous cycle, called *free-running cycles*. These individual rhythm periods may vary, some running as short as 20 hours, others as long as 28 hours. The sleepiness–alertness rhythm is about 25 hours.

Neurobiologic Basis for Sleep

The location of the biologic clock that regulates our circadian rhythms is an area of the hypothalamus called the *suprachiasmatic nucleus*. This area lies on top of the optic chasm. About the size of the letter "V" on this page, the suprachiasmatic nucleus is a boomerang-shaped cluster of nerve cells.

Neurochemical activity throughout the central nervous system (CNS) controls changes in sleep and wakefulness. Much of the neurochemistry is unknown, but certain neurons and neurotransmitters have been studied. Wakefulness is maintained by the reticular activating system (RAS) in the brain. Neurons in the RAS produce acetylcholine and catecholamine neurotransmitters and other chemicals to maintain wakefulness. As the cycle of the RAS dwindles, neurons that produce chemicals to promote sleep take over. The bulbar synchronizing region is believed to work with the RAS alternately to activate and suppress the brain's higher centers to control sleep. One example of a neurotransmitter involved with sleep is γ-aminobutyric acid (GABA). Most modern prescription hypnotics (benzodiazepines) enhance the effects of GABA.

Stages of Sleep

The electrophysiologic characteristics of sleep show that sleep is a cycle of two phases: **non–rapid-eye-movement sleep** (NREM) and **rapid-eye-movement sleep** (REM). Positron emission tomography (PET) scans of these two phases are shown in Figure 26-2.

The timing, amount, and distribution of REM and NREM stages during a night's sleep follows a predictable pattern referred to as **sleep architecture**. NREM and REM sleep stages have an about 90- to 110-minute cycle. During an 8-hour sleep period, the cycle of NREM and REM sleep repeats itself five or six times. This cycle changes as the night progresses. In the first cycle, the amount of REM sleep is brief. With each succeeding cycle, the amount of time spent in REM sleep lengthens until it seems to dominate at the end of the sleep period. Conversely, slow-wave sleep is most prominent during the initial cycle, but declines throughout the night (Fig. 26-3).

Non–Rapid-Eye-Movement Sleep

After taking an average of about 20 minutes to fall asleep, people enter into about 90 minutes of NREM sleep, which occurs in four substages. Light sleep is characteristic of stages 1 and 2, in which the person is easily arousable. People aroused from stage 1 sleep may even deny having been asleep, such as when one dozes off watching television and arouses minutes later during a loud commercial. In comparison, during stage 4, sleep is much deeper, and arousal from sleep is much more difficult. The characteristics of sleep stages (Rechtschaffen & Kales, 1968) are described as follows.

Stage 1. Sleep is entered through this stage. It is a transition between relaxed wakefulness and sleep. Stage 1 accounts for only 2% to 5% of a night's sleep. Electroencephalographic (EEG) findings show that the drowsy, yet wakeful alpha rhythm is replaced by a theta rhythm.

Stage 2. This stage comprises about 45% to 55% of sleep. EEG findings show the same rhythm as in stage 1; however, stage 2 is marked by the sporadic occurrence of bursts of specific electrical activity identified as "sleep spindles" and "K complexes."

Stages 3 and 4. Also called **slow-wave sleep**, these stages make up 10% to 23% of sleep. EEG findings show high-amplitude waves, slow waves, or delta waves.

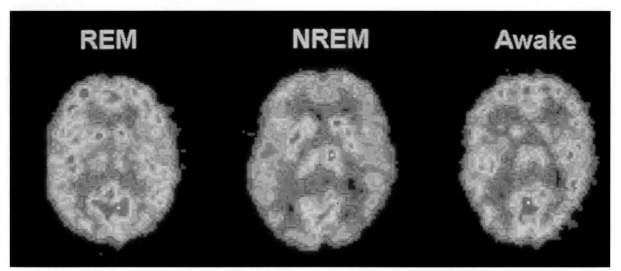

FIGURE 26.2 The brain is as active when awake (right), as in rapid-eye-movement (REM) or dreaming sleep, but is metabolically less active in slow-wave or non–rapid-eye-movement (NREM) sleep. (Courtesy of Monte S. Buchsbaum, M.D. The Mount Sinai Medical Center and School of Medicine, New York, NY.)

The difference between stages 3 and 4 is the amount of delta waves seen, with stage 3 demonstrating 20% to 50% of delta waves and stage 4 showing more than 50% of delta waves.

Slow-wave sleep is often called the "deepest" state of sleep and may be the most important part of sleep. There is little consensus as to why it is so important. Slow-wave sleep may serve a restorative function, although the exact mechanism for this is unclear. It may

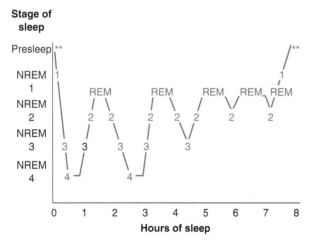

FIGURE 26.3 In typical sleep architecture in normal young adults, non–rapid-eye-movement (NREM) and rapid-eye-movement (REM) sleep stages cycle every 90 to 110 minutes through the night. Wakefulness accounts for less than 5% of the night's sleep pattern (presleep to NREM 1). Slow-wave sleep dominates the first third of the night during NREM stages 3 and 4. REM sleep occurs in four to six separate episodes throughout the night (20%–25% of sleep) and dominates the last third of the night's sleep. (Modified from Biddle, C., & Oaster, T. R. F. (1990) *Journal of the American Association of Anesthetists, 58* [1], 36.)

serve to conserve energy because metabolism and body temperature decrease at this time. Although the function of slow-wave sleep is unknown, it is most likely complex.

Recent studies have suggested that sleep patterns may be different in men and women. Women have more slow-wave sleep and twice as many sleep spindles. Sex hormones appear to influence the physiology (and pathology) of sleep (Manber & Armitage, 1999).

Rapid-Eye-Movement Sleep

REM sleep is a state characterized by bursts of rapid eye movements. REM sleep occurs in four to six separate episodes and makes up about 20% to 25% of a night's sleep. Although REM sleep is a deep sleep, and muscles seem to be at rest, EEG findings demonstrate an active brain. More blood flows to the brain, and brain temperature increases. Brain waves resemble a mixture of waking and drowsy patterns. Although vivid dreaming is the outstanding feature reported by adults when awakened out of REM sleep, people also report dreams when they awaken from NREM sleep (Pivik, 2000).

During REM sleep, nerve impulses are blocked within the spinal cord. Muscle tone diminishes to the point of paralysis of the head and neck, as well as the longer muscle groups. Only stronger impulses are relayed, producing muscular twitches, eye movements, and impulses controlling heart and respiration. Breathing and heart rate become irregular.

This type of sleep also has a circadian rhythm that closely coincides with the body temperature rhythm. The greatest amount of REM sleep is seen when the body temperature cycle is at its lowest. Temperature regulation is impaired; that is, people do not sweat or shiver during REM sleep. Patterns of hormone release, kidney function, and reflexes change. Females have clitoral engorgement and an increase in blood flow to the vagina. Males have penile erections.

The function of REM sleep continues to be debated. Several theories have been put forth, such as that REM sleep may stimulate brain growth or consolidate memory. Only limited evidence supports any of these hypotheses. Furthermore, REM sleep deprivation does not affect personality variables, as popularly believed. The function of REM sleep and dreaming remains a fundamental mystery in the study of sleep.

Normal sleep is sensitive to changes, and the body responds when deprived of certain phases of sleep, particularly REM sleep and slow-wave sleep. Certain activities, such as early rising or alcohol intake before bedtime, or some medications, such as CNS-acting drugs, can suppress REM sleep. When individuals are deprived of REM sleep, there is a subsequent "rebound effect" (making up the lost REM sleep during the next sleep period). The body tends to make up for lost REM sleep by earlier occurrence of REM sleep during the next night. The occurrence of REM at sleep onset implies REM deprivation. If sleep onset is delayed until the peak phase of REM sleep's circadian rhythm, REM sleep will predominate those early sleep hours. Slow-wave sleep does not appear to have a circadian determinant, but is more sensitive to the amount of previous sleep obtained. When one is deprived of both REM sleep and slow-wave sleep, the body prefers to make up the slow-wave sleep first before making up the lost REM sleep.

BIOLOGIC MEASUREMENTS OF SLEEP

A sleep study or polysomnography (meaning multiple parameters that monitor sleep) measures the electrophysiologic variables that define sleep. Polysomnography includes the measurement of brain wave activity with EEG, chin muscle activity with electromyogram (EMG), and eye movement with electrooculogram (EOG). Clinical evaluation of patients for sleep disorders also includes oral and nasal airflow, respiratory effort, oxyhemoglobin saturation, and EMG of limb muscle activity (Fig. 26-4). Polysomnography is conducted continuously during the usual sleep period, typically at night, and results describe sleep architecture and abnormalities. Specific calculations include how long it takes one to fall asleep, or *sleep latency*, the amount of *wakefulness after sleep onset* (WASO), and **sleep efficiency** (expressed as a percentage of the amount of time in bed spent asleep). Results also demonstrate the timing and distribution of sleep stages. In general, abnormalities may indicate breathing-related sleep disturbances, unusual limb movements, bizarre gross motor behaviors, and atypical patterns of sleep architecture.

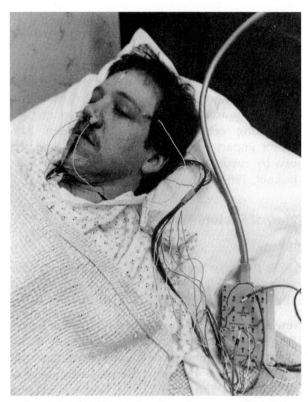

FIGURE 26.4 A patient undergoing polysomnography has electrodes glued or taped to the scalp, face, chest, and legs.

Specific abnormalities found during polysomnography are described in detail in the Primary Sleep Disorders section.

Fragmented sleep interrupts the restorative function that gives individuals the feeling of having had a good night's sleep. Not only does insufficient sleep cause daytime sleepiness, but disturbed sleep affects daytime alertness and performance as well. The restorative biologic processes associated with sleep require an amount of sleep for the completion of these processes. When EEG arousals (during sleep) occur at a rate of once per minute or more, basic restoration does not happen. The devastating effects of fragmented sleep have a greater impact on daytime functioning than is seen by reducing REM sleep or slow-wave sleep.

Subjective symptoms of sleepiness are recognized as heavy eyelids, loss of initiative, reluctance to move, and yawning or slowed speech. Sleepiness can vary from mild to severe. **Polysomnography** objectively measures physiologic sleepiness by measuring sleep latency, or how long it takes a person to fall asleep during a **multiple sleep latency test** (MSLT). The MSLT is a standardized procedure using polysomnography during daytime testing. This test measures sleep variables during a 20-minute period, which is repeated every 2 hours, five times during the day. The faster a person falls asleep during testing, the greater the physiologic sleep tendency.

FACTORS THAT AFFECT SLEEP

Age

Age is the most important factor affecting the normal pattern of sleep. Sleep patterns change dramatically over the course of the life span.

Newborns and Young Children

Neonates need 17 to 18 hours of sleep each day. Their sleep occurs in 3- to 4-hour episodes throughout the day. At about age 3 to 4 months, the circadian organization of sleep and wakefulness becomes evident. More sleep occurs during the night, and daytime sleep organizes into a series of naps. A typical 6-month-old sleeps about 12 hours at night and takes two 1- to 2-hour naps each day. A 2-year-old should sleep about 11 to 12 hours at night, with a 1- to 2-hour nap after lunch. The need for this afternoon nap continues until at least 3 years of age, although some children continue to nap up to 5 years of age (Birkenmeier, 2000a).

School-Aged Children

After 5 years of age, children need gradually less sleep. The preadolescent needs about 10 hours of sleep each night, and napping is rare. A teenager's sleep need is difficult to define. Research indicates that teenagers do not sleep enough. Social schedules and early start times for school compete with the physiologic need for sleep. Higher cognitive functions, such as abstract thinking and verbal ability, are impaired in children who get inadequate sleep (Randazzo et al., 1998).

Young Adults

The matured sleep process may be most restorative for young adults. During this age, people typically need about 8 hours of sleep; napping is arbitrary. Lifestyle choices (eg, irregular sleep schedule, substance abuse) may put the young adult at risk for circadian rhythm disturbances such as delayed sleep phase. The initial symptoms of narcolepsy typically emerge late in adolescence and early adulthood.

Middle-Aged Adults

The amount of sleep needed and sleep architecture typically remain unchanged during the middle-aged years. Poor sleep is associated with menopause; however, sleep improves in women receiving hormone replacement therapy (Montplaisir et al., 1997). Sleep-related breathing disorders and insomnia are prevalent sleep disorders for middle-aged adults.

Elderly Adults

Elderly people obtain less sleep at night and are sleepier during the day. Some sleep requirements are met by day-time napping. Underlying circadian factors may provide some explanation. For many, restricted activity and lack of bright light exposure decreases their rhythm amplitude (Campbell et al., 1995). Further, temperature rhythm in elderly people is phase advanced (peaks earlier); early morning arousals may reflect early rise of body temperature (Bliwise, 2000). Elderly people are at risk for sleep pathologies, particularly periodic leg movements and sleep apnea, which fragment sleep and cause daytime sleepiness. They may also be unable to sleep again after awakening to urinate.

Environmental Stimuli

Environmental cues that entrain circadian rhythms are called *zeitgebers*. A powerful zeitgeber is bright light or sunlight. People can be sleepy, but if in a stimulating environment with bright lights or a lot of activity, they may stay awake. In contrast, if a sleepy person is in a quiet place or engaged in sedentary activity, chances are he or she cannot resist the urge to fall asleep. Sleepiness is a physiologic state, and although a stimulating environment can temporarily forestall it, once these stimuli are removed, the urge to sleep will persist. Even when someone who is chronically sleep deprived does not feel sleepy, the tendency to fall asleep is much greater and may manifest by dozing off while sitting in lectures or during the monotonous operation of machinery or driving.

Lifestyle Factors

Sudden disruption in one' sleep–wake schedule greatly affects one's alertness. Many factors can cause disrupted sleep patterns, such as traveling across time zones, emotional stress or anxiety, or having to change the sleep–wake pattern because of shift work. When traveling across time zones or when working night shifts (and sleeping during the day), one's regular sleepiness–alertness rhythm may persist for several days. Even when daytime sleep is improved with a sedative, which produces longer and less fragmented sleep, sleepiness in the early morning hours usually continues to be profound for the first 2 to 3 nights. This extreme sleepiness significantly decreases after a 4- to 6-day reversal of the sleep–wake cycle, even though daytime sleep remains the same (Van Dongen & Dinges, 2000).

COMORBIDITY

Although most psychiatric disorders have associated sleep disturbances, this section details the known relationship between sleep and three other major types of psychiatric disorders: psychoses, mood disorders, and alcoholism.

Sleep Disorders and Psychoses

Significant sleep disruption, usually sleep-onset insomnia, is often associated with acute psychotic decompensation or the waxing phase of schizophrenia. Preoccupation with delusional material or hallucinations and anxiety cause agitation. The patient eventually falls asleep when exhaustion prevails. A partial or complete reversal of the day–night cycle may be seen.

Sleep disturbance is an important risk factor in the precipitation of the first psychotic episode and of later relapses. During the prodromal period, the patient may complain of insomnia or hypersomnia (sleepiness). The organization of the sleep–wake cycle may break down to the point of frequent, short naps and no long nocturnal sleep episodes.

Sleep Disorders and Mood Disorders

Compared with people who sleep well, individuals who report sleep difficulties are significantly more depressed, lonely, tense, and unhappy. Those who have chronic problems sleeping can attest that more stressful events occurred during the year their insomnia started than in all the previous years. Crisis events appear to have a role in the onset of insomnia for many patients.

Patients with major depression often complain of insomnia. The most common form of insomnia is early morning awakenings, that is, waking up early and not being able to return to sleep. Difficulty falling asleep, frequent nighttime awakenings, and unrefreshing sleep are characteristics of their insomnia complaint.

About 15% to 20% of depressed patients report feeling daytime sleepiness; however, reports of sleepiness may be exaggerated or refer to their lack of energy and fatigue. Measurements of physiologic sleepiness show that depressed individuals are only slightly sleepier than control subjects, but are not nearly as sleepy as individuals with sleep apnea or narcolepsy (Benca, 2000).

Although patients with bipolar disorder report insomnia while depressed, many develop symptoms of excessive sleepiness. They may experience long nocturnal sleep periods, difficulty awakening, and hypersomnia. Their daytime sleepiness measured by the MSLT, however, is relatively normal. During manic periods, patients often report a subjective sense that they need less sleep. Indeed, they have a much reduced total sleep time. Manic episodes are often preceded by periods of sleeplessness.

Sleep Disorders and Alcoholism

Alcohol has significant effects on sleep and wakefulness in normal people and in those who suffer from alcoholism. As a psychoactive substance, however, its effect is somewhat paradoxical. Alcohol acts as a sedative depending on the dose and time of administration. When nonalcoholics drink at bedtime, alcohol shortens sleep latency time and may increase the amount of slow-wave sleep. Effects on sleep are usually limited to the first half of the 8-hour sleep period. After alcohol wears off, a compensatory effect on sleep happens. Sleep is disrupted and more fragmented. The amount of REM sleep is increased. Sometimes, there is an increase in anxiety dreams (Gillin & Drummond, 2000).

During heavy drinking periods, difficulties in falling asleep and maintaining sleep occur even if the alcoholic does not drink at bedtime. As seen in nonalcoholics, ingesting alcohol at bedtime increases slow-wave sleep during the first part of the night, yet fragments and shortens sleep at the end of the night. As alcoholism progresses, REM sleep is profoundly affected. There is a significant fragmentation of REM sleep, and eventually REM sleep becomes markedly suppressed. Abstinence usually produces REM rebound.

Sleep during alcohol withdrawal is a major discomfort for the chronic alcoholic. There is a dramatic loss of sleep. When sleep comes, it is extremely fragmented and often troubled by nightmares and anxiety dreams. For those who develop delirium tremens, a prolonged period of sleep lasting up to 24 hours frequently ends this phase of withdrawal. The recovery of normal sleep is gradual for the alcoholic during long-term abstinence. Patients may continue to complain of fragmented and unrefreshing sleep for as long as 2 years. Certainly, the abstaining alcoholic who complains of insomnia is at risk for renewed drinking.

PRIMARY SLEEP DISORDERS

The *Diagnostic and Statistical Manual of Mental Disorders* (*DSM-IV*) has organized sleep disorders into groups according to their etiology. Primary sleep disorders are those disorders that are not considered the result of another mental or medical disorder or induced by a substance (eg, medication, alcohol). They are subdivided into **dyssomnias**, which are disorders of initiating or maintaining sleep or excessive sleepiness, and **parasomnias**, which are disorders of particular physiologic or behavioral reactions during sleep. There are more than 70 known sleep disorders; the *DSM-IV* describes only the most common ones.

Dyssomnias

Dyssomnias are disorders of initiating or maintaining sleep or of excessive sleepiness and are characterized by disturbances in the amount, quality, or timing of sleep. Our discussion of dyssomnia includes primary insomnia, primary hypersomnia, narcolepsy, breathing-related sleep disorders, and circadian rhythm sleep disorder. Of all sleep-related problems, insomnia is the most prevalent, with estimates ranging from 30% to 35%; the prevalence of chronic or severe insomnia is estimated to range from 10% to 15% (Breslau et al., 1996; Gallup Organization, 1991).

Primary Insomnia

Insomnia refers to difficulty falling asleep, trouble maintaining sleep, or nonrestorative sleep. The word insomnia is used in two different circumstances: as a symptom and a disorder. Insomnia as a symptom can lead to the diagnosis of another disorder (depression, breathing-related sleep disorders). The *DSM-IV* also recognizes that in the absence of these other causes, insomnia is also a free-standing disorder (see the Key Diagnostic Characteristics for Primary Insomnia).

Key Diagnostic Characteristics for Primary Insomnia 307.42

Diagnostic Criteria

- Difficulty initiating or maintaining sleep or non-restorative sleep for at least 1 month
- Clinically significant distress or impairment in social, occupational, or other areas of functioning because of sleep disturbance
- Not occurring exclusively during course of another mental disorder, narcolepsy, breathing-related sleep disorder, circadian rhythm sleep disorder, or a parasomnia
- Not a direct physiologic effect of a substance or a medical condition

Target Symptoms and Associated Findings

- History of light or easily disturbed sleep before development of more persistent sleep problems
- Anxious concern with general health and increased sensitivity to daytime effect of mild sleep loss
- Interpersonal, social, and occupational problems developing because of anxiety about sleep
- Problems with inattention and concentration
- Inappropriate use of medications, such as hypnotics, alcohol, or caffeine

Associated Physical Examination Findings

- Fatigued and haggard appearance

Associated Laboratory Findings

- Poor sleep continuity, increased stage 1 sleep, decreased stages 3 and 4 sleep, increased muscle tension, or increased amounts of electroencephalogram alpha activity during sleep
- Elevated scores on psychological or personality inventories

Definition and Course. Primary insomnia is the diagnosis used when the complaint of insomnia is not an indication of another disorder. The hallmark symptom of primary insomnia is the patient's intense focus and anxiety regarding the inability to fall asleep or maintain sleep. Patients with primary insomnia report daytime fatigue, difficulty with concentration, and poor mood. Although they may report excessive daytime sleepiness, pathologic sleepiness is not demonstrated by the MSLT (Aikens et al., 1999). Complaints of insomnia reflect an increase in sleep latency, increase in wakefulness during the night, and decrease in total sleep time. They usually deny fighting sleep or falling asleep unintentionally during the day.

KEY CONCEPT Insomnia. **Insomnia** is difficulty initiating or maintaining sleep and involves a series of behaviors that perpetuate an abnormal sleep and rest pattern.

Epidemiology. Numerous studies have documented the prevalence of insomnia, but the true prevalence is unknown. It is estimated that insomnia affects 30% to 40% of adults within 1 year and that 15% to 25% of the individuals with chronic insomnia are diagnosed with primary insomnia.

Etiology. Individuals at risk for developing primary insomnia often describe themselves as having been "light sleepers" before persistent sleep problems developed. They have a tendency to be more easily psychologically or physiologically aroused at night. They tend to somatize their feelings and tensions and develop sleep-preventing associations and behaviors. Although initially insomnia may be precipitated by stressful situations and tension, this inability to fall asleep and stay asleep persists after the crisis or stressful situation has passed (Fig. 26-5).

Biologic Measurements. Polysomnography may show poor sleep continuity, increased stage 1 and decreased slow-wave sleep, and an increased amount of EEG alpha activity while asleep. Some patients sleep better in the sleep laboratory than at home, which suggests negative conditioning. The MSLT usually does not demonstrate increased physiologic sleepiness.

Somatic Interventions. Interventions usually involve a combination of approaches (Fig. 26-6). Short-term use of hypnotics may provide immediate relief, but long-term use is detrimental. Interventions focus on teaching patients to develop and maintain good sleep habits (Text Box 26-2). Behavioral interventions, described as follows, include stimulus control, sleep restriction, and relaxation therapy.

- *Stimulus control* is a technique that is used when the bedroom environment no longer provides

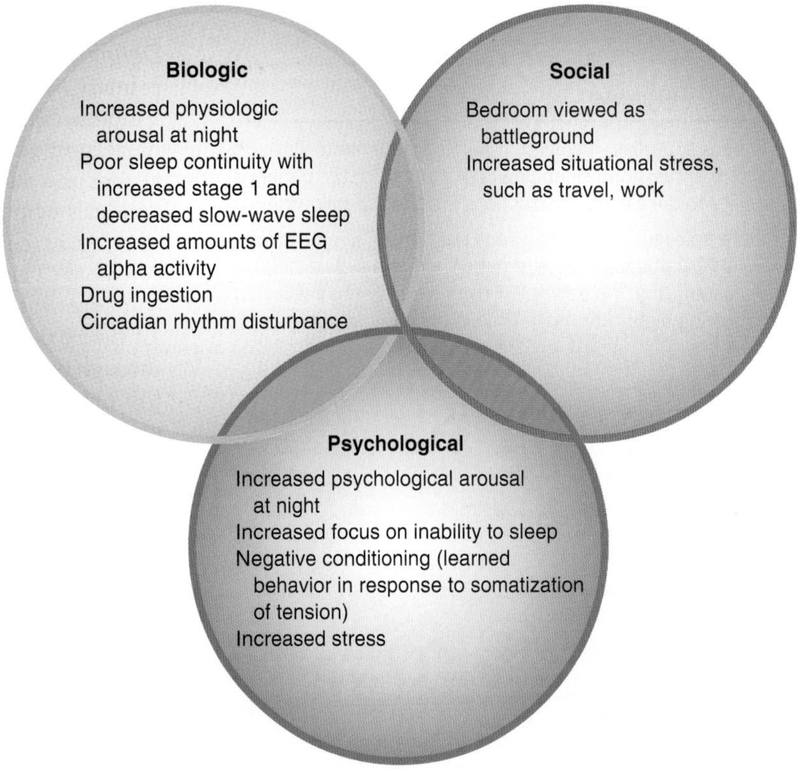

FIGURE 26.5 Biopsychosocial etiologies of primary insomnia. EEG, electroencephalogram.

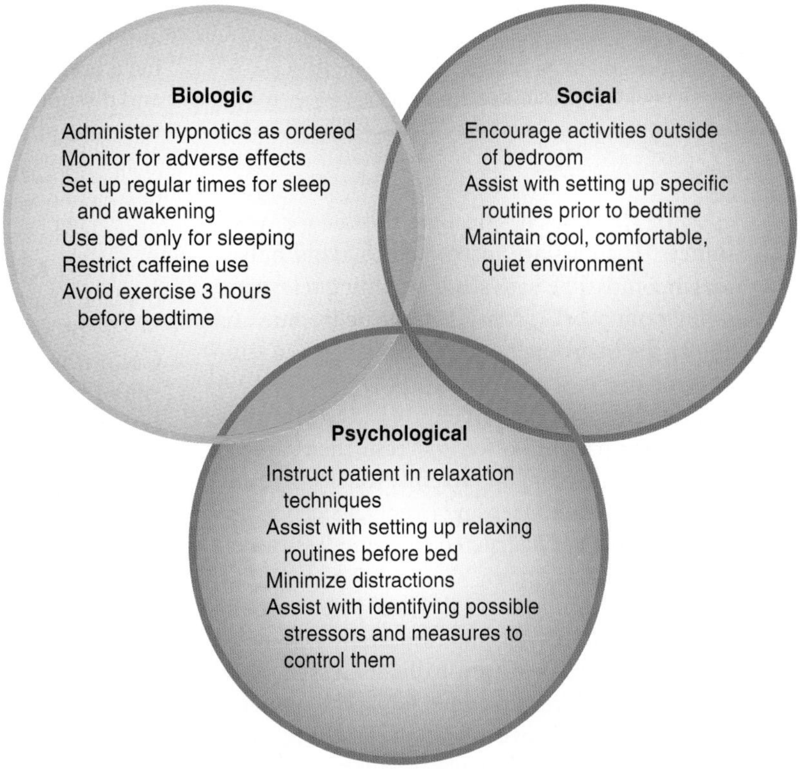

Biologic

Increased physiologic arousal at night
Poor sleep continuity with increased stage 1 and decreased slow-wave sleep
Increased amounts of EEG alpha activity
Drug ingestion
Circadian rhythm disturbance

Social

Bedroom viewed as battleground
Increased situational stress, such as travel, work

Psychological

Increased psychological arousal at night
Increased focus on inability to sleep
Negative conditioning (learned behavior in response to somatization of tension)
Increased stress

FIGURE 26.6 Biopsychosocial interventions for patients with primary insomnia.

Biologic

Administer hypnotics as ordered
Monitor for adverse effects
Set up regular times for sleep and awakening
Use bed only for sleeping
Restrict caffeine use
Avoid exercise 3 hours before bedtime

Social

Encourage activities outside of bedroom
Assist with setting up specific routines prior to bedtime
Maintain cool, comfortable, quiet environment

Psychological

Instruct patient in relaxation techniques
Assist with setting up relaxing routines before bed
Minimize distractions
Assist with identifying possible stressors and measures to control them

Sleep Hygiene

Nurses are often involved in helping patients to develop and maintain good sleep habits that reinforce the patient's ability to fall asleep. Instructions include the following:

1. Keep regular bedtimes and rising times. Even if sleep is very poor, get up and out of bed at a regular, consistent time. "Sleeping in" can disturb sleep the following night. For most, time in bed should not exceed 8 hours.

2. Avoid naps.

3. Abstain from alcohol. Although alcohol may shorten sleep latency, there tends to be an alerting effect when it wears off.

4. Refrain from caffeine after midafternoon. Avoid nicotine before bedtime and during the night. Although many claim that neither affects their sleep, caffeine and nicotine are strong stimulants and fragment sleep.

5. Exercise regularly, but not within 3 hours of bedtime. Exercising 6 hours before bedtime tends to strengthen the circadian rhythms of body temperature and sleepiness.

6. Use the bedroom for sleeping; avoid doing nonsleep activities there. Promote the bedroom as a stimulus for sleep, not for studying, watching television, or socializing on the telephone.

7. Set a relaxing routine to prepare for sleep. Avoid frustrating or provoking activities before bedtime.

8. Provide for a comfortable environment. Slightly cool ambient temperature is better than warm. Reduce the amount of light and noise.

cues for sleep but has become the cue for wakefulness. Patients are instructed to avoid behaviors incompatible with sleep: watching television, doing homework, or eating in the bedroom. This allows the bedroom to be reestablished as a stimulus for sleep.

- Another behavioral intervention is *sleep restriction*. Insomniac patients often increase their time in bed to provide more opportunity for sleep, resulting in fragmented sleep and irregular sleep schedules. Patients are instructed to spend less time in bed and avoid napping.

- *Relaxation training* is used when patients complain of difficulty relaxing, especially if they are physically tense or emotionally distressed. A variety of procedures to reduce somatic arousal can be used—progressive muscle relaxation, autogenic training, and biofeedback. Imagery training, meditation, and thought stopping are attention-focusing techniques that focus on cognitive arousal.

Primary Hypersomnia

Definition and Course. The essential characteristic of primary hypersomnia is excessive sleepiness for at least 1 month, demonstrated by either daytime sleep episodes or sleeping extended periods at night. Sleepiness occurs almost on a daily basis. This diagnosis is reserved for individuals who have had other causes of daytime sleepiness (eg, narcolepsy, obstructive sleep apnea syndrome) ruled out (Table 26-1).

People with primary hypersomnia typically sleep 8 to 12 hours per night. They fall asleep easily and sleep through the night, but often have difficulty awakening in the morning. Sometimes, they are confused or even combative on awakening. This difficulty in making the transition from sleep to wakefulness is sometimes referred to as *sleep drunkenness*. They often have problems meeting morning obligations—students have trouble attending morning classes, or working people are continually late for work. They also exhibit excessive daytime sleepiness, usually demonstrated by taking unintentional or intentional naps, which may last an hour or more, but they usually do not feel refreshed after awakening. Poor concentration and memory are reported as well. People typically report feeling embarrassed by nodding off at work and may even describe dangerous situations that resulted from their falling asleep, such as being sleepy while driving or operating heavy machinery.

Biologic Measurements. Polysomnography shows a short sleep latency, a normal to long sleep duration, and normal sleep architecture. These patients do not have breathing-related sleep disturbances or frequent and disrupting limb movements. The MSLT indicates excessive physiologic sleepiness.

Psychopharmacologic Interventions. Stimulant medications often do not provide relief. In some cases, however, methysergide has been clinically useful. The difficulty in prescribing appropriate treatment comes from the lack of a clear etiology for this disorder.

Sleepy people often self-medicate with caffeine, a CNS stimulant found in a variety of drinks and food. A cup of brewed coffee contains about 100 to 150 mg of caffeine. An ounce of chocolate contains 25 mg of caffeine. Peak plasma concentration is reached 30 to 60 minutes after consumption, and duration of effect is 3 to 5 hours in adults. Caffeine improves psychomotor performance, particularly tasks involving endurance, vigilance, and attention. Alertness significantly increases for 7.5 hours when 300 mg of caffeine is ingested at 11 PM (Bonnet, 2000). High doses, especially in people who are not habitual users, may reduce performance because side effects (irritability, anxiety, jitteriness) interfere.

Narcolepsy

Definition and Course. The overwhelming urge to sleep is the primary symptom of narcolepsy. This ir-

TABLE 26.1 Key Diagnostic Characteristics for Sleep Disorders

Disorder	Diagnostic Characteristics and Target Symptoms
Primary hypersomnia	Excessive sleepiness for at least 1 month occurring almost daily Prolonged sleep episodes Daytime sleep episodes: nodding off unintentionally or napping Significant distress or impairment in social, occupational, or other areas of functioning Not accounted for by insufficient sleep Not a direct physiologic effect of a substance or general medical condition
Narcolepsy	Irresistible attacks of refreshing sleep occurring daily over at least a 3-month period Brief episodes of sudden bilateral loss of muscle tone precipitated by intense emotion (cataplexy) Dream-like hallucinations while falling asleep (hypnagogic hallucinations) Voluntary muscle paralysis at beginning or end of sleep episodes Not a direct physiologic effect of a substance or general medical condition
Breathing-related sleep disorder	Disruption in sleep leading to excessive sleepiness or insomnia Report of loud snoring Report of apparent apneic episodes during sleep
Circadian rhythm sleep disorder	Persistent or recurrent pattern of disrupted sleep leading to excessive sleepiness or insomnia Mismatch between sleep–wake cycle and environment Mismatch between circadian sleep–wake cycle Significant distress or impairment in functioning Not a direct physiologic effect of a substance or general medical condition
Nightmare disorder	Repeated awakenings from major sleep periods Detailed recall of extended and extremely frightening dreams Generally occur during second half of sleep period Rapid orientation and alertness on awakening from the frightening dreams Significant distress or impairment in functioning
Sleep terror disorder	Recurrent episodes of abrupt awakenings Usually occur during the first third of major sleep episode Intense fear and autonomic arousal during episode Onset with a panicked scream Tachycardia, rapid breathing, and sweating Unresponsive to attempts to comfort person during episode Significant distress or impairment in functioning Not a direct physiologic effect of a substance or general medical condition
Sleepwalking disorder	Repeated episodes of rising from the bed during sleep and moving about Usually occur during the first third of sleep episode Blank staring facial expression during episode Relatively unresponsive to attempts to communicate with person Great difficulty to awaken Amnesia for the episode on awakening No impairment of mental activity or behavior within several minutes after awakening Short period of confusion or disorientation Significant distress or impairment in functioning Not a direct physiologic effect of a substance or general medical condition

resistible urge to sleep occurs at any time of the day, regardless of the amount of previous sleep. Falling asleep often occurs in inappropriate situations, such as while driving a car or reading a newspaper. These sleep episodes are usually short, lasting 5 to 20 minutes, or up to an hour if sleep is not interrupted. Typically, people with narcolepsy have two to six sleep attacks a day and frequently report dreaming. They usually feel alert after a sleep attack, only to fall asleep unintentionally again several hours later.

Narcolepsy is distinguished by a group of symptoms known as the narcolepsy tetrad: daytime sleepiness, cataplexy, hypnagogic hallucinations, and sleep paralysis. The symptom of daytime sleepiness is found in all individuals with narcolepsy, but existence of the other three symptoms varies (Text Box 26-3). Only about 15% of individuals with narcolepsy have all four symptoms of the narcolepsy tetrad.

- **Cataplexy** is the bilateral loss of muscle tone triggered by a strong emotion, such as laughter. This

Clinical Vignette: Sleepiness

Jill is a 27-year-old college student and single mother of two young children, ages 10 and 3 years old. Jill had difficulty staying awake during high school classes. She attributed this problem to "boring teachers" and dropped out of school when she was a junior. She has earned her GED and now attends a local community college majoring in computer science. Although she enjoys her studies, she continues to fall asleep during classes. Because of her busy schedule, she gets about 6 hours of sleep each night. Her tendency to nod off is more frequent. She has had a couple of frightening episodes at bedtime, seeing things dance around her bed and not being able to move. She recalls an incident of laughing at a great joke, then feeling her face droop for several seconds.

muscle atonia can range from subtle (drooping eyelids) to dramatic (buckling knees). Eye and respiratory muscles are not affected. Cataplexy usually lasts only seconds. Individuals are fully conscious, oriented, and alert during the episode. Prolonged episodes of cataplexy may lead to sleep episodes. The frequency and severity generally increase with sleep deprivation. Whereas everyone with narcolepsy experiences excessive sleepiness, about 70% of individuals report cataplexy.

- **Hypnagogic hallucinations** are intense dream-like images that occur when an individual is falling asleep and usually involve the immediate environment. For example, individuals report seeing dead relatives standing at their bedside. Most hallucinations are visual, but some can be auditory, such as hearing one's name called or a door slammed; kinetic hallucinations are reported as well, such as "out-of-body" experiences. Hypnagogic hallucinations are reported by 20% to 40% of individuals with narcolepsy.

- **Sleep paralysis,** or being unable to move or speak when falling asleep or waking up, is reported in about 24% to 57% of people with narcolepsy. This muscle atonia is often described as terrifying and is accompanied by a sensation of struggling to move or speak. Although the diaphragm is not involved, patients may also complain of not being able to breathe. These episodes are usually brief, lasting only a few seconds to minutes, and usually terminate spontaneously or when someone touches the individual. Sleep paralysis may also occur in conjunction with a hypnagogic hallucination. These experiences are often cited as accounts of supernatural nocturnal assaults and paranormal experiences (Cheyne et al., 1999). Individuals observed during an episode appear to be sleeping, although there may be occasional twitches or slight moans.

Epidemiology. Narcolepsy is found in about 50 per 100,000 individuals (Partinen & Hublin, 2000). It is more common than other well-known neurologic disorders (eg, multiple sclerosis, myasthenia gravis, or Huntington's chorea). Narcolepsy is a chronic disorder that usually begins in young adulthood, between the ages of 15 and 35 years. Excessive sleepiness is the first symptom to appear, but cataplexy may develop later. Disrupted nocturnal sleep sometimes develops in individuals in their 40s or 50s. The severity of sleepiness remains stable over the lifetime. A secondary sleep disorder, such as sleep apnea, should be considered if sleepiness increases.

Etiology. The cause of narcolepsy is still unknown, but probably involves neuroimmune interactions and genetic factors. There is evidence of a narcolepsy susceptibility gene on chromosome 6, in the class II human leukocyte antigen. Some speculate that individuals who are genetically predisposed develop symptoms after an injury to the CNS (Mignot, 2000).

Biologic Measurement. Narcolepsy is diagnosed by a polysomnographic evaluation, particularly by the MSLT. The MSLT quantifies the severity of daytime sleepiness and documents the presence of sleep-onset REM. Further, the absence of other potential causes of sleepiness and REM sleep onset have been ruled out.

Genetic testing may further support diagnosis in atypical cases, or in patients without definite cataplexy. Narcolepsy is associated with the presence of the human leukocyte antigens DQB1*0602 and DQA1*0102 (DQ1) across all ethnic groups (Mignot, 2000).

Somatic Interventions. Narcolepsy has no cure. Treatment is designed to control symptoms and depends on the clinical presentation and severity. In general, sleepiness is treated with CNS stimulants. Methylphenidate, dextroamphetamine, and pemoline are the most frequently prescribed stimulants. Cataplexy is usually treated with tricyclic antidepressants because of their REM-suppressing effects. Protriptyline is the preferred medication because it is less sedating.

Patient education is another important aspect of treatment. Patients need to understand factors that can make symptoms worse, such as sleep deprivation and alcohol. They need to develop strategies to manage symptom so that naps are integrated into their daily routine. For example, taking naps at lunch or work breaks, scheduling a short nap before the evening meal, or engaging in activities to sustain alertness while driving, such as playing stimulating music or munching on sunflower seeds, may forestall unintentional dozing on the job.

Breathing-Related Sleep Disorders: Obstructive Sleep Apnea Syndrome

Breathing-related sleep disorder is a broad class of sleep disorders identified in the *DSM-IV*. Specifically, obstructive sleep apnea syndrome, central sleep apnea syndrome, and central alveolar hypoventilation syndrome are included in this classification. Obstructive sleep apnea syndrome (OSA) is the most commonly diagnosed breathing-related sleep disorder. Nocturnal polysomnography is used to diagnose these breathing disorders.

Definition and Course. OSA is characterized by excessive snoring during sleep and episodes of sleep apnea (cessation of breathing) that disrupt sleep and cause daytime sleepiness. The hallmark symptoms are snoring and daytime sleepiness. Often, snoring is so loud and disturbing that the partner moves out of the bedroom.

People with OSA are often restless sleepers. Apneic episodes can cause fretful sleep, abrupt awakenings with feelings of choking, falling out of bed, or even leaping out of bed to restore breathing. Esophageal reflux, or heartburn, is a common complaint. Genitourinary symptoms include nocturia (three to seven trips to the bathroom), nocturnal enuresis, and impotence.

Daytime sleepiness, the other hallmark symptom, may reach the same degree of pathologic sleepiness found in narcolepsy. Unlike narcolepsy, naps tend to be unrefreshing. Onset of sleepiness may coincide with weight gain. About two thirds of apnea patients are obese (20% over ideal body weight).

For children with OSA, the symptoms are subtle. They may not snore. Unusual sleep postures (eg, sleeping on hands and knees) and agitated arousals are more common. Nocturnal enuresis in a child who was previously dry at night is often the first symptom. Children may not appear sleepy, but they are noted to have a poor attention span and poor grades. Daytime mouth breathing and poor articulation are other features.

Epidemiology. Conservative estimates give the overall prevalence of OSA as 2.7% of the general population. The incidence of OSA increases however, for older populations, especially those older than 50 years of age (Partinen & Hublin, 2000).

Although it can occur in male or female patients of all age groups, OSA is most common in middle-aged, overweight men. In general, the female-to-male ratio is about 1:8, although women are more likely to develop this syndrome after menopause. Men are twice as likely to snore as women. Snoring occurs in about 60% of men between the ages of 41 and 64 years (American Psychiatric Association, 1994). Obese people with untreated OSA are high risk for developing pulmonary hypertension (Valencia-Flores et al., 2000).

Etiology. An obstruction or collapse of the airway causes apnea or cessation of breathing. In most cases, the site of obstruction is in the pharyngeal area, specifically the supraglottic airway. Vibrations of the soft, pliable tissues found in the pharyngeal airway cause the snoring sounds that occur during breathing. Once breathing stops, the person awakens briefly to restore it. The person does not later recall the awakening. These brief awakenings deprive essential sleep, resulting in excessive daytime sleepiness.

Biologic Measurements. Nocturnal polysomnography is used to diagnose OSA. Apneic episodes last longer than 10 seconds, and rare episodes last up to several minutes. Typically, patients with OSA demonstrate 100 to 600 respiratory events per night during polysomnographic measurement. Other features include frequent, brief awakenings (lasting seconds) and changes in sleep architecture, such as increased amounts of stage 1 sleep and decreased amounts of slow-wave and REM sleep. Bradycardia in association with tachycardia is often seen in association with apneic events. Other cardiac arrhythmias are also seen, specifically, sinus arrhythmias, premature ventricular contractions, atrioventricular block, or sinus arrest.

Somatic Interventions. There are nonsurgical and surgical treatments for OSA. Currently, the most effective nonsurgical treatment is continuous positive airway pressure (CPAP). This treatment during sleep involves wearing a nose mask that is connected by a long tube to an air compressor. Airway patency is maintained with air pressure. Although this method of treatment is highly effective, compliance can be a problem. The most commonly performed surgical procedure to treat OSA is the uvulopalatopharyngoplasty. This procedure involves the removal of redundant soft palate tissue, the uvula, and tonsillar pillars. The surgery usually eliminates snoring and is judged to be about 50% effective in reducing the amount of sleep apnea.

Other, nonsurgical treatments are recommended depending on the severity of OSA. For obese patients with less severe OSA, weight loss may help. For others whose apnea is mild, changing sleeping position from supine to lateral can help control the severity of OSA. There has also been some effort in devising an oral appliance to reduce snoring and the occurrence of apnea.

Circadian Rhythm Sleep Disorder

Definition and Course. The chief feature of a circadian rhythm sleep disorder is the mismatch between the individual's internal sleep–wake circadian rhythm and the timing and duration of sleep. People with these disorders complain of insomnia at particular times during the day and excessive sleepiness at other times. This diagnosis is reserved for those individuals who present with marked sleep disturbance or significant social or occupational impairment. The *DSM-IV* identifies a broad group of subtypes, including delayed sleep phase type, jet lag type, shift work type, and unspecified type.

Delayed Sleep Phase Type. Individuals with delayed sleep phase type tend to be unable to fall asleep before 2 to 6 AM; hence, their whole sleep pattern shifts, and they have difficulty rising in the morning. They are sometimes referred to as "night owls." Often, they devise elaborate strategies to get up in the morning for work, such as setting multiple alarm clocks around the bedroom or enlisting others to awaken them by person or telephone. Many of these individuals are chronically sleep deprived (Text Box 26-4).

Jet Lag Type. Most people have experienced jet lag when they travel across time zones, particularly in coast-to-coast and international travel. This type of circadian disorder occurs when the person's normal endogenous circadian sleep–wake cycle does not match the desired hours of sleep and wakefulness in a new time zone. Individuals traveling eastward are more prone to jet lag because it involves resetting one's circadian clock to an earlier time. It is easier to delay the endogenous clock to a later time period than an earlier one.

Shift Work Type. In this type of disorder, the endogenous sleep–wake cycle is normal but is mismatched to the imposed hours of sleep and wakefulness required by shift work. Rotating shift schedules are disruptive because any consistent adjustment is prevented. Compared with day- and evening-shift workers, night- and rotating-shift workers have a shorter sleep duration and poorer quality of sleep. They may also be sleepier while performing their jobs. This disorder is further exacerbated by insufficient daytime sleep resulting from social and family demands and environmental disturbances (traffic noise, telephone). Because of the job requirements of the professional nurse, nurses often suffer from this disorder.

Morning types (see Text Box 26-4) may be at particular risk for this circadian rhythm disorder. They are sleepier on the night shift, even though they get as much sleep during off-work hours as nonmorning types. Further, they estimate getting less sleep than nonmorning types (Hilliker et al., 1992).

Etiology. Circadian rhythm disorders are caused by the dissociation of the internal circadian pacemaker and conventional time. The cause might be intrinsic, such as delayed sleep phase, or extrinsic, as in jet lag and shift work. Each results in overwhelming daytime sleepiness and overflowing wakefulness at night.

Epidemiology. There are no data regarding the prevalence of circadian rhythm disorders in the general population. Prevalence of circadian rhythm disorders among patients diagnosed at sleep disorder centers accounts for 2% or less of the total patients diagnosed (Roehrs & Roth, 1994). Yet this is a gross underestimate, given that jet lag, a circadian rhythm disorder, occurs for nearly everyone traveling over three time zones. Further, 20% of the U.S. work force is engaged in shift work and thereby at risk for circadian rhythm disorders.

Somatic Interventions

- *Chronotherapy* is frequently used for delayed sleep phase. This treatment manipulates the sleep schedule by progressively delaying bedtime until an acceptable bedtime is attained. A 27-hour day is imposed on successive days by delaying bedtime and rising time 3 hours. Thereafter, strict adherence (within 1 hour) to the final schedule must be maintained.

- *Luminotherapy* is generally a safe treatment for some circadian rhythm disorders when used within standardized guidelines for light intensity and time limits (Chesson et al., 1999). Bright light, a powerful zeitgeber, manipulates the circadian system. Light is measured in lux units of illumination. Indoor light is about 150 lux. Therapeutic light has a potency of 2,500 to 10,000 lux and is produced by commercially prepared light boxes.

- *Chronopharmacotherapy* resets the biologic clock by using short-acting hypnotics to induce sleep. Small amounts of hypnotics can produce high-quality sleep in people who wish to reset their circadian schedule after a long transmeridian flight.

TEXT BOX 26.4

Early Birds ("Larks") Versus "Night Owls"

Aside from the natural age-related changes in circadian sleep rhythms that generally regulate people as they get older more toward regular morning alertness and productivity and sleepiness at night, scientific evidence also suggests that genetic predisposition can result in very different natural tendencies for individual alertness–sleepiness rhythms.

It seems that some individuals are more alert and perform best in the early morning (called "early birds" or "larks"), whereas others are more alert and perform better during the late evening hours (called "night owls"). Night owls may have a slower circadian clock and a natural tendency to stay up late. These natural tendencies can be further reinforced by personal preference or necessity, such as wanting to stay up late to see a particular television show or having a job that requires either early morning or late night alertness. Other external time cues (zeitgebers), such as the absence of daylight exposure, can further reinforce habits of those who have a natural tendency to stay up late. Morning orientation is usually reinforced or imposed when people get a regular daytime job or have young children, requiring morning alertness and function.

Although some people's sleep habits are at an extreme of this sleep–wake spectrum, contributing to sleep difficulties and disorders, most fall somewhere within the normal range of regular hours of sleepiness and wakefulness. Several self-assessment questionnaires are available to measure morningness and eveningness. Horne and Ostberg (1976) developed a questionnaire that has been used most in research for this assessment.

Conversely, for night-shift workers, caffeine taken while working at night improves alertness and performance (Muehlbach & Walsh, 1995). Caffeine should be used judiciously by night-shift workers because they become quickly tolerant to the effects after a few nights.

Recently, melatonin has been promoted as a natural product that resets the circadian clock. When correctly timed, melatonin induces both phase advances and delays in the circadian rhythm system. If incorrectly timed, melatonin has the potential to induce adverse effects. There are no long-term safety data. The optimal dosage and formulation have not been established (Arendt & Deacon, 1997). To date, little research validates the use of this hormone in manipulating biologic rhythms. Further, production of melatonin supplied to health food stores undergoes no quality controls (Culebas, 1996).

Parasomnias

Parasomnias are characterized by abnormal physiologic or behavior events that occur in relationship to sleep or to specific sleep stages, or during transition from sleep to wakefulness. These disorders involve activation of the autonomic nervous system, motor system, or cognitive processes during sleep or sleep–wake transitions. Individuals present with a complaint of unusual behavior during sleep. The *DSM-IV* identifies three types of parasomnias: nightmare disorder, sleep terror disorder, and sleepwalking disorder.

Nightmare Disorder

Definition and Course. The repeated occurrence of frightening dreams that cause an individual to become fully awake is the essential characteristic of nightmare disorder. Typically, the individual is able to recall detailed dream content that involves physical danger (eg, attack or pursuit) or perceived danger (eg, embarrassment or failure). On awakening, the individual is fully alert and experiences a persisting sense of anxiety or fear. Many people have difficulty returning to sleep. Multiple nightmares on the same night may be reported. Some people avoid sleep because of their fear of nightmares. Consequently, people may report that excessive sleepiness, poor concentration, and irritability disrupt their daytime activities.

Epidemiology. The actual prevalence of nightmare disorder is unknown. In adults, at least 50% of the population report occasional nightmares. Women are more likely to report nightmares than men. In children, there is no difference between boys and girls (Partinen & Hublin, 2000). Nightmares often begin in children between the ages of 3 and 6 years. Most children outgrow

them. Nightmares induced by medication would not be considered part of nightmare disorder.

Etiology. The cause of nightmares is unknown. Intriguing evidence provokes a debate as to whether nightmares are a symptom or an adaptive reaction to pathophysiologic factors. Negative emotions, primarily fear, are the most common dream emotions. Brain imaging demonstrates increased metabolic activity during REM sleep in the most primitive regions of the brain, the paralimbic and limbic regions (Paradiso et al., 1997). Many classes of drugs trigger nightmares, including catecholaminergic agents, β-blockers, some antidepressants, barbiturates, and alcohol. Withdrawal from barbiturates and alcohol causes REM rebound and more vivid dreaming.

Biologic Measurements. Nightmares occur in REM sleep almost exclusively. They most often occur during the second half of the night, when REM sleep dominates. Polysomnography demonstrates abrupt awakenings from REM sleep. In most cases, the REM sleep episode has lasted for at least 10 minutes. Tachycardia and tachypnea may be evident.

Somatic Interventions. Traditionally, psychotherapy aimed at conflict resolution has been the treatment of choice. More recent therapies involving cognitive and behavioral interventions, as well as desensitization and relaxation techniques, have gained support. For example, one technique is teaching patients (while awake) to visualize and change their remembered nightmares and rehearse similar scenarios. This technique reduces nightmare distress and frequency.

Sleep Terror Disorder

Definition and Course. The essential characteristic of sleep terror disorder is the repetition of episodes of sleep terrors that cause clinical distress or impairment of social, occupational, or other areas of functioning. Diagnostic considerations may also include the potential for injury to self or others.

Episodes of sleep terrors are frightening to the person and to anyone witnessing them. Screaming, fear, and panic often characterize episodes. These sleep terrors, also called *night terrors* or *pavor nocturnus*, usually occur in the first third of the night and may last 1 to 10 minutes. Often, individuals abruptly sit up in bed screaming; others have been known to jump out of bed and run across the room. Other symptoms include rapid heart rate and breathing, dilated pupils, and flushed skin. Usually, the person having a sleep terror is inconsolable and difficult to awaken completely. Efforts to awaken the individual may prolong the episode. Once awake, most are unable recall a dream or event that precipitated such a response. A few report a fragmentary image. Often, the individual does not fully awaken and is unable to recall the episode the next morning.

Epidemiology. The actual prevalence of this disorder is not known. Episodes of sleep terrors are common in children (up to 6% prevalence) and peak between the ages of 5 and 7 years (Broughton, 2000). This condition usually resolves or diminishes in adolescence. However, sleep terrors can also occur in adults. At any age, the frequency of episodes varies, and it may occur several times a night over several nights.

Etiology. There is little evidence that sleep terrors indicate any significant underlying psychiatric disease or psychological problems. The most important factor is genetic predisposition. Individuals often report a family history of either sleep terrors or sleepwalking. The exact mode of inheritance is not known. Fever and sleep deprivation can increase the frequency of episodes.

Biologic Measurements. Polysomnography shows that sleep terrors usually begin during slow-wave NREM sleep. Although sleep terrors most often occur during the first third of the night, when slow-wave sleep dominates, episodes also occur later during slow-wave sleep.

Sleepwalking Disorder

Definition and Course. Waking up is a neurologic event. Arousal happens through a complex series of processes using several neurotransmitters. An arousal disorder is one that interrupts these processes or does not allow their completion. An arousal disorder occurs when an individual is partially awake, yet partially asleep. Sleepwalking, also called *somnambulism*, is a classic arousal disorder. It is considered to be a milder form of sleep terrors. Repeated episodes of complex motor behavior during sleep are the essential characteristic of sleepwalking disorder.

Sleepwalking involves episodes of mild to complex behaviors during sleep. Mild forms (sometimes called *confusional arousals*) consist of sitting up in bed and mumbling incoherently. More complex behavior may involve getting out of bed, walking around outside the house, even driving an automobile. While sleepwalking, people typically have a blank stare, are relatively unresponsive to conversation, and are difficult to awaken. If individuals do not awaken, they are unable to recall the episode the following morning. Often, they awaken to find themselves in a different place from where they went to sleep. If awakened during the episode, there is a brief period of confusion, followed by a full recovery. Episodes usually happen during the first third of the night. Contrary to popular opinion, sleepwalking (and sleeptalking) are not enactments of the individual's dream.

Sleep-related violence has been documented in people with NREM sleep somnambulism, REM sleep behavior disorder, and epileptic discharges during sleep. Violence during sleep is an area of controversy for the legal system; the jury's willingness to accept sleep disorders as a defense has not always been consistent (Text Box 26-5).

Epidemiology and Etiology. Sleepwalking is common in children. It occurs in 40% of children and peaks at about age 11 to 12 years. There appears to be some genetic predisposition; those patients with relatives who sleepwalk are more likely to sleepwalk themselves (Lecendreux et al., 2000). Sleep deprivation appears to increase dramatically the frequency of sleepwalking episodes (Zadra & Montplaisir, 2000) Internal stimuli (a full bladder) or external stimuli (noise) can precipitate an episode. Sleep deprivation, fever, and stress may increase the likelihood of an episode.

Biologic Measurements. Polysomnography shows EEG elements of both wakefulness and NREM sleep. Because it usually occurs during slow-wave sleep, sleepwalking most often happens during the first third of the night. Sleepwalking rarely occurs during daytime naps.

Somatic Interventions. Patients are instructed to take precautions regarding possible sleepwalking episodes (Text Box 26-6). Treatment might also include medications, such as benzodiazepines. Hypnosis supplemented by psychotherapy has also been useful, at least on a short-term basis (Broughton, 2000).

TEXT BOX 26.5

Clinical Vignette: Violence in Sleepwalking Disorder

On December 26, 1993, a 37-year-old man fatally shot his wife, claiming that he suffered from sleep apnea, which induced a confusional arousal. There was a substantial and apparent motive—spousal abuse and a letter from his wife near the date of the murder describing her intentions to leave. He was convicted of first-degree murder and sentenced to life imprisonment. Two months later, he was admitted to the hospital. His arterial blood gas showed that he was in respiratory distress with severe hypercapnia (pH, 7.31; PCO_2, 75; PO_2, 42 on room air). The clinical impression was sleep apnea syndrome (by history), right ventricular heart failure, and probable hypoxic encephalopathy, for which he was treated with a tracheostomy. Six months after the homicide, he underwent polysomnography while his trachea was plugged. This confirmed that he had severe obstructive sleep apnea. His respiratory disturbance index was 125/h, and the lowest oxyhemoglobin desaturations of 63% occurred in rapid-eye-movement sleep. No evidence of confusional arousals was seen (Nofzinger & Wettstein, 1995).

TEXT BOX 26.6

General Safety Precautions for Sleepwalkers and Their Families

Ensure adequate sleep. The occurrence of sleepwalking dramatically increases after sleep loss. Although a regular sleep schedule is important, making up for lost sleep is more important (Birkenmeier, 2000b).

- Anticipate sleepwalking when there is a significant sleep loss. Alert family members to be aware of the likelihood of sleepwalking for the first 2 hours after the sleepwalker goes to bed.

- Keep a sleep log to identify how much sleep is needed to prevent a sleepwalking event.

- Install noise devices on the sleepwalker's door to alert others that the sleepwalker is up.

- Deadbolt locks should be installed on doors leading outside. Windows should be secured so that they cannot be opened more than 8 inches.

- When spending the night away from home, alert appropriate individuals to the possibility that sleepwalking may occur. Ensure adequate sleep the preceding night.

NURSING MANAGEMENT: HUMAN RESPONSE TO DISORDER

Although polysomnography is used to confirm or diagnose a sleep disorder, the evaluation of a sleep problem also involves a careful sleep history (Rogers, 1997). In taking a sleep history, the nurse's job in assessing this problem is to discover the signs and symptoms. The components of a sleep history include not only the patient's current sleeping patterns but also what the pattern was during health. It is important to identify any medical problems, current medications, current life events, and emotional and mental status that might be affecting sleep (Text Box 26-7).

During the patient interview, the nurse elicits information to provide some well-defined clues. These data enable the nurse to devise a differential diagnosis list. Four clues can help the nurse define possible causes of the sleep disorder. Details of the sleep complaint should include description, duration, stability, and intensity of the problem.

> *Description:* How does the patient describe the problem?
> *Stability:* Does it happen every night (or day)?
> *Intensity:* How bad is the problem?
> *Duration:* When did the problem begin?

Defining the problem is only the beginning step toward understanding the etiology of a sleep complaint. Obviously, a good understanding of the signs and symptoms of different sleep disorders guides the nurse in assessing for further clues to the problem.

The nurse should ask about all medications the patient is taking and consider interactions between certain medications and sleep and wakefulness (see the display, Medications and Other Substances and Their Effects on Sleep). Statements such as, "I fell asleep because I ate a heavy lunch" and "the room was warm" are not valid, and the nurse should probe with further questioning.

Insomnia Assessment

Problems falling asleep or maintaining sleep are the general complaints of insomnia. A careful sleep history is a valuable tool in the final diagnosis and treatment. Remember when assessing the patient that insomnia often begins as a response to stress (eg, loss of a spouse), and a normal rhythm of sleep has not returned. Defining the problem using the four clues previously discussed rapidly narrows the possible causes.

The *description* of the problem involves the timing or pattern of wakefulness. The underlying cause is usually different for those who have trouble falling asleep than for those who are unable to maintain sleep. Several facets to the description of the problem may elicit some useful clues (see Therapeutic Dialogue: Sleep Assessment).

For individuals who have difficulty falling asleep, the estimated amount of time before sleep onset is useful information. Delayed sleep phase is suspected in patients who fall asleep consistently at the same late hour. The emotional state (frustrated, anxious) may provide some indication of primary insomnia. Also, a description of how that interim is spent may point to sleep hygiene problems.

A description of difficulty maintaining sleep should be defined as the number, length, and timing of awakenings. Frequent brief awakenings often indicate a sleep disturbance, such as breathing-related sleep disorders. Depression or alcohol use is implicated in early morning awakenings.

Defining the *duration* of insomnia places it into one of three categories: transient, short-term, or chronic. Although these categories are arbitrary, the duration of the complaint is one of the most helpful clues to defining the problem.

- *Transient insomnia* is identified when the complaint occurs during a period of one to several nights. The cause is often apparent to the patient. Situational stress and travel across several time zones are likely examples.
- *Short-term insomnia* persists for a few days to as long as a month. The cause is often identifiable, such as situational stress or shift work.
- *Chronic insomnia* persists for more than a month. The list of possible causes is longer and more varied. Chronic insomnia may be caused by primary

TEXT BOX 26.7

Sleep Assessment Questions

Patterns and Rhythms

- What time do you go to bed during the work week and on the weekends?
- How long does it take you to fall asleep?
- What time do you get up in the morning?
- Do you awaken spontaneously or depend on an alarm clock?

Insomnia Questions

- What kinds of activities do you engage in during the evening?
- How many times do you wake up during the night?
- What wakes you up?
- How long does it take to return to sleep?
- Do you take daytime naps? How often? At what time?
- Do you just rest your eyes? Doze? Stretch out on the couch for a minute?
- What do you do to aid sleep?
- Do you have problems sleeping when you are away from your home, such as on a vacation?
- Are you aware of any thoughts or worries that prevent sleep? What do you do to cope with these worries?
- Has there been a change in your exercise habits or intake of caffeine?
- Have you suffered a recent loss or change?
- Are their environmental factors that prevent you from going to sleep?

Excessive Daytime Sleepiness

- Have you ever nodded off unintentionally? What is the most unusual situation in which you nodded off?

- When did your sleepiness first begin? Do you recall feeling sleepy in high school, dozing off during classes? Do you nod off every day or sporadically?
- Do you suddenly find yourself awakening feeling refreshed? Or feeling paralyzed for a second?
- Do you know anyone in your family who has or has had unusual sleepiness?
- Have you ever had auditory, tactile, or visual hallucinations when falling asleep or on awakening?

Breathing-Related Sleep Disorder Questions

- Ask the partner if the patient snores. Have him or her describe the noise, frequency, how long it lasts, how long the person does not breathe. What happens when the person starts up again? What position is the person in when snoring?
- How many pillows do you use?
- Do you have difficulty waking up?
- How awake do you feel during the day?
- Do you awaken with a headache?

Circadian Rhythm Sleep Disorder Questions

- What are your working hours?
- How often do they change?
- Does the time you go to bed get later and later?
- Does it get more and more difficult to get up in the morning?
- Does work require you to change time zones, change beginning and ending times, work into the night?
- What results do you notice from your sleep pattern? Any dropping dishes? Any car accidents?

---

insomnia, drug or alcohol use, circadian rhythm disturbances, physiologic disturbances to sleep (breathing-related sleep disorders), or medical or psychiatric illness.

The *stability* of the complaint provides clues to the underlying cause. Fluctuations in the degree of disturbance may coincide with medical or psychiatric illness. Primary insomnia tends to be more consistent; however, some patients may sleep better in locations other than their usual bedroom. A relatively consistent complaint is also an indication of delayed sleep phase syndrome and breathing-related sleep disorders.

The intensity of insomnia is often reflected in the waking hours. Patients should be asked whether their disturbed sleep compromises their daytime function. Irritability, poor performance, and fatigue are often reported. Marked daytime sleepiness suggests an organic cause, which may indicate a need for further polysomnographic testing. The severity of daytime symptoms not

only contributes to making the diagnosis but also indicates the significance of intervention.

Occasionally, patients are unable to provide specific answers to questions, or they give such an extraordinary variability that the information is not useful. Keeping a sleep diary is a helpful tool for these situations. The diary may cover a few days to several weeks. Content of the diary depends on the information being sought. A simple diary is typically a daily record of the patient's bedtimes, rising times, estimated time to fall asleep, number and length of awakenings, and naps. More complicated sleep diaries involve recording the amount and time of alcohol ingestion, ratings of fatigue, medication, and stressful events.

Hypersomnia Assessment

In general, the causes of excessive sleepiness are likely to be the result of a neurologic process induced by alcohol or a CNS depressant, circadian factors, insufficient

Medications and Other Substances and Their Effects on Sleep

Alcohol
- Increases TST during the first half of the night
- Decreases TST during the second half
- Decreases REM sleep during the first half of the night
- Withdrawal from chronic use of alcohol causes a decrease in TST, increased wakefulness after sleep onset, and REM rebound.

Amphetamines
- Disrupt sleep–wake cycle during acute use
- Decrease TST
- Decrease REM sleep
- Withdrawal may cause REM rebound.

Antidepressants (Tricyclics and MAOIs)
- Sleep effects vary with sedative potential
- Increase slow-wave sleep
- Decrease REM sleep

Barbiturates
- Increase TST
- Decrease WASO
- Decrease REM sleep
- Withdrawal may cause decrease in TST and REM rebound.

Benzodiazepines
- Drugs vary in onset and duration of action.
- Decrease SL
- Increase TST
- Decrease WASO

- Decrease REM sleep
- Daytime sedation may occur with long-acting drugs.

β-Adrenergic blockers
- Decrease REM sleep
- Increase WASO, nightmares
- Daytime sedation may occur

Caffeine
- Increases SL
- Decreases TST
- Decreases REM sleep

L-Dopa
- Vivid dreams and nightmares

Lithium
- Increases slow-wave sleep
- Decreases REM sleep

Narcotics
- Effects vary with specific agents
- Increase WASO
- Decrease REM sleep
- Decrease slow-wave sleep

Phenothiazines
- Increase TST
- Increase slow-wave sleep

Steroids
- Increase WASO

MAOI, monoamine oxidase inhibitors; REM, rapid-eye-movement; SL, sleep latency; TST, total sleep time; WASO, wake after sleep onset.

---

sleep, or disturbed sleep. Polysomnography is used to identify factors that disturb sleep, such as OSA. MSLT defines the degree of pathologic sleepiness and identifies circadian factors or neurologic processes, such as narcolepsy. Evaluation of the sleepy patient also involves a detailed sleep history. Assessing subjective daytime sleepiness involves defining the problem using the same four clues previously described.

The *description* of hypersomnolence must distinguishes sleepiness from fatigue, lack of energy, or tiredness. True sleepiness means that the patient fights sleep, falls asleep unintentionally, or needs naps. If a patient says that she is fatigued, but unable to fall asleep for a nap, she would not be judged as hypersomnolent.

Describing daytime sleepiness also involves defining the time of day that sleepiness most likely occurs. Nar-

coleptics report sleepiness throughout the day. Patients with delayed sleep phase syndrome report that sleepiness is most severe in the morning, but improves late in the evening.

The duration of the sleepiness complaint should describe how long the problem has existed and whether the onset was abrupt or gradual. Narcolepsy is suspected in patients who report the onset of sleepiness during their adolescence or 20s. Duration may also suggest other factors, such as weight gain for those with OSA.

The *stability* or consistency of hypersomnolence suggests underlying factors. The amount of total sleep time may suggest that insufficient sleep is a factor. Patients who report that their sleepiness is worse toward the end of the week may be suffering from insufficient sleep. Those who are unable to identify a weekly pattern, but

---

THERAPEUTIC DIALOGUE | **Sleep Assessment**

Ineffective Approach

Nurse: What time do you go to bed at night?
Patient: Oh, my bedtime varies between 10 PM and 2 AM.
Nurse: What time do you get up?
Patient: I get up anywhere between 6 AM and noon.
Nurse: How do you sleep during the night?
Patient: OK.
Nurse: OK?
Patient: Yeah, no problems sleeping.

Effective Approach

Nurse: What time do you go to bed at night and what time do you get up?
Patient: Oh, my bedtime varies between 10 PM and 2 AM. I get up anywhere between 6 AM and noon.
Nurse: Let's be more specific. During a week's time, what time do you go to bed each night?
Patient: Well, this semester I have a morning clinical rotation Monday through Thursday. I'm usually up til midnight writing my care plan. On Friday, I'm usually so exhausted that I go to bed around 10 PM. Saturday nights I go out with my friends and get to bed around 2 AM. On Sunday night, I usually get to bed around 11 PM.
Nurse: What time do you get up each day of the week?

Patient: On the mornings that I have clinicals, I have to get up around 5:30 AM to be at the hospital by 6:45 AM. On Friday I get up at 7 AM for class. Saturday morning, I get up around 8 AM so I can go to my part-time job. On Sunday, I get up at 9 AM so I can get to church.
Nurse: How long do you take to fall asleep?
Patient: That's gotten much better. I fall asleep in 15 minutes or so.
Nurse: Do you take any naps?
Patient: Outside of my lectures, I don't have time to nap. I'm just too busy with my classes and clinicals, homework, job, and social life.
Nurse: Before this semester, how much sleep did you get?
Patient: That was last summer, I had an afternoon job then so I could sleep as much as I wanted. I bet I got 8 or even 9 hours of sleep every night. It was great. I wasn't sleepy back then.

Critical Thinking Challenge

- Compare the quality and quantity of elicited data in the two scenarios.

- What conclusions could be drawn from the first scenario? Are the conclusions different for the second scenario? Explain.

---

report that some days they are more alert, should also define their activity level during their alert days. Patients who have active jobs may not have an opportunity to notice the severity of their sleepiness.

The *intensity* of daytime sleepiness may range from fighting sleep to needing a nap to falling asleep unintentionally. A description of the situation in which hypersomnolence occurs further defines its intensity. Sleepiness could be judged to be more severe when patients fall asleep during social interactions or while standing, in comparison to a relatively more sedentary activity, such as watching a boring television program. Intensity also provides a measure of how immediately diagnosis and treatment should take place. Patients who fall asleep while driving or operating machinery should be immediately referred for polysomnographic evaluation.

The amount of sleep and sleep time schedule should also be assessed in the hypersomnolent patient. When estimating the amount of total sleep time, several factors should be considered. The estimated sleep latency and number and length of awakenings must be subtracted from time spent in bed. Sleep obtained during naps should be calculated. Also, the amount of sleep obtained during unintentional naps (in front of television in the evening) must be considered.

Querying the partner may provide clues about factors that disturb the patient's sleep. Reports of witnessed apneic episodes and snoring are good indications of OSA.

Episodes of parasomnias are often unrealized by the patient but can be described in detail by the partner. Family members may clarify the degree of sleepiness that the patient may want to deny.

Nursing Diagnoses and Outcome Identification

The nursing diagnosis that is usually applied to the patient with a sleep disorder is Sleep Pattern Disturbance. The diagnosis is made when a disruption of sleep time causes discomfort or interferes with lifestyle (see Nursing Care Plan 26-1).

Planning and Implementing Nursing Interventions

Biologic Interventions

Nutrition. What the patient eats and drinks several hours before bedtime can greatly affect sleep. Patients suffering from insomnia should be counseled not to eat anything heavy for several hours before retiring. Spicy foods, alcohol, and caffeine should be avoided. If they insist on a bedtime snack, warm milk is appropriate for most patients.

Milk contains L-tryptophan, an essential amino acid that is a precursor to serotonin, one of the neurotransmitters involved in sleep. L-Tryptophan allows more rapid onset of sleep and lowers the sensitivity to exter-

NURSING CARE PLAN 26.1
Insomnia

Matthew is a 20-year-old student who is majoring in nursing. He presents himself at Student Health Services with a complaint of insomnia. In assessing his problem, the nurse ascertains that Matthew takes 2 to 3 hours to fall asleep. During this interim of wakefulness, he lies in bed, calm but somewhat restless. He has had no prior difficulty with insomnia. His problem falling asleep occurs 3 nights a week—Monday, Wednesday, and Friday. He exercises vigorously during his physical education class (7–9 PM) on these three evenings. He denies any sleep problems during spring break, when he took a trip. The patient drinks 1 cup of coffee in the morning and denies the use of other stimulants. He reports that as a consequence he has had some irritability and difficulty concentrating on the days following a "bad night." He has tried an over-the-counter sleep medication, but does not remember the name of it. When he took these sleeping pills, he was able to fall asleep better, but found them to be costly. He would like a prescription for sleeping medication that would be covered by student health insurance.

Baseline Assessment: A 20-year-old man who presents with difficulty initiating sleep. After vigorous evening exercise, he takes 2–3 hours to fall asleep. Strengths: intelligence, motivated for treatment, adequate insurance coverage, good physical health.

Associated Psychiatric Diagnosis	Medications
Axis I: Primary insomnia	None
Axis II: None	
Axis III: None	
Axis IV: None	
Axis V: GAF = Current 85	
Potential 90	

NURSING DIAGNOSIS 1: SLEEP PATTERN DISTURBANCE

Defining Characteristics	Related Factors
Difficulty falling asleep, estimated sleep latency of 2–3 hours, three nights a week	Changes in usual sleep environment
Mood alterations	Poor sleep hygiene
Poor concentration	

OUTCOMES

Initial	Discharge
1. Describe factors that prevent or inhibit sleep.	3. Report an optimal balance of rest and activity.
2. Identify strategies to improve sleep hygiene.	

INTERVENTIONS

Interventions	Rationale	Ongoing Assessment
Teach patient good sleep hygiene habits	Discussion of good sleep hygiene is the first treatment strategy	Monitor Matthew's reports of estimated sleep latency.
Instruct patient to keep a sleep diary for 1 week—including bedtime, sleep latency, rising time, naps, caffeine intake, time of exercise.	Keeping a sleep diary can give insight into insomnia problems by identifying alerting influences in relation to disturbed sleep.	Exercise before sleep appears to be the primary factor that could be causing insomnia on Monday, Wednesday, and Friday. Monitor other sleep hygiene issues.
Reassure patient that short-term insomnia will resolve when the factors that caused the problem are eliminated.	Anxiety about insomnia is a predisposing factor to the development of primary insomnia.	Determine Matthew's level of anxiety about the insomnia.
Determine whether it is possible to adjust schedule so that vigorous exercise occurs several hours before sleep.	Physical exercise raises basal metabolism, which may interfere with sleep.	Determine whether it is possible to adjust course schedule.

(continued)

NURSING CARE PLAN 26.1 (Continued)

INTERVENTIONS

Interventions	Rationale	Ongoing Assessment
Problem solve with Matthew how to adjust sleep schedule to avoid insomnia.	Problem solving allows the patient to learn how to consider alternative strategies.	Evaluate whether strategies are reasonable.

EVALUATION

Outcomes	Revised Outcomes	Interventions
After readjustment of exercise schedule, Matthew was able to resume normal sleep.	None	None

Summary of Treatment: Within 2 weeks, Matthew's sleep pattern returns to normal. The following October, Matthew presents himself once again to Student Health Services. He no longer has trouble falling asleep. On the contrary, his problem is feeling too sleepy. When the nurse goes to the waiting room to summon Matthew, she observes that Matthew is sitting in a chair, holding a magazine, yet fast asleep. During the assessment interview, the nurse also notes that Matthew has a flat affect and requests several times that the questions be repeated. Matthew reports that he has been sleepy during his afternoon nursing lectures for the past 3 months. He even fell asleep while taking a test. Sleepiness is worse toward the end of the week. He is alert during the weekend if he gets 10 hours of sleep the night before but is rarely able to do so. Matthew is in good health. His weight is appropriate for his height. He denies any reports that he snores or has had witnessed episodes of apnea during his sleep.

nal stimuli during sleep. L-Tryptophan competes with other amino acids for transport into the brain. Therefore, eating an additional snack with milk may diminish the sleep effects of L-tryptophan.

Psychopharmacologic Interventions

Drugs used to treat sleep problems can roughly be grouped as hypnotics or stimulants. The following discussion is on common classes of over-the-counter (OTC) and prescribed medications. Nurses need to be aware that patients often try OTC drugs before they seek help from their doctor.

Sleeping pills bought OTC are usually antihistamines. The most common agents are doxylamine and diphenhydramine. These histamine-1 antagonists have a CNS effect that includes sedation, diminished alertness, and decreased reaction time. These drugs also produce anticholinergic side effects, such as dry mouth, accelerated heart rate, urinary retention, and dilated pupils.

Prescribed hypnotics are often used for short-term treatment of insomnia (see Drug Profile: Zaleplon). Benzodiazepine is a class of drugs whose effects range from short to long acting. With their use, sleep latency is shortened, and total sleep time is increased. Benzodiazepines slightly decrease REM sleep, but greatly sup-

DRUG PROFILE: Zaleplon
(Sedative/Hypnotic)
Trade Name: Sonata

Zaleplon is a pyrazolopyrimidine nonbenzodiazepine hypnotic. It is readily absorbed and metabolized with only about 1% of zaleplon eliminated in the urine.

Receptor affinity: Zaleplon acts at the GABA-benzodiazepine receptor complex.

Indication: Treatment of onset and/or maintenance insomnia

Routes and dosing: Zaleplon is available in 5 mg and 10 mg capsules. It should be taken at bedtime or after a nocturnal awakening with difficulty falling back to sleep (but at least 4 hours prior to the desired rise time).

Adults: The recommended starting dose is 10 mg with 20 mg the maximum. An initial dose of 5 mg should be considered in adults with low body weight. Doses of over 20 mg have not been sufficiently studied.

Geriatric: Initially, 5 mg is recommended as a starting dose. Elderly individuals should not exceed a 10 mg dose.

Half-life (peak plasma concentration): 1 hour (1 hour)

Selected adverse reactions: abdominal pain, headache, dizziness, depression, nervousness, difficulty concentrating, back pain, chest pain, migraine, conjunctivitis, bronchitis, pruritus, rash, arthritis, constipation, dry mouth

Warnings: Zaleplon should not be administered to patients with severe hepatic impairment. Zaleplon potentiates the psychomotor impairments of ethanol.

press slow-wave sleep. Because sleepwalking tends to occur out of slow-wave sleep, benzodiazepines are used to treat patients who show a potential for injury or harm.

Antidepressants have a potent effect on sleep and are used to treat many sleep problems. Most antidepressants decrease REM sleep and are thought to treat depression by depriving REM sleep. These medications are used to control the accessory symptoms of narcolepsy, which include cataplexy, hypnagogic hallucinations, and sleep paralysis. Several antidepressants have sedating effects and are used to treat concurrent complaints of depression and insomnia. Trazodone is often taken at bedtime to improve sleep as well as mood.

Stimulants can be bought OTC. The most common agents are caffeine and those drugs found in cold medications, such as ephedrine and pseudoephedrine. These drugs may cause nervousness and heart palpitations as well.

The most commonly prescribed stimulants used to treat excessive daytime sleepiness in narcolepsy are dextroamphetamine, methylphenidate, and pemoline. These agents increase the patient's ability to stay awake and perform. Amphetamines have a euphoric effect and are an abused drug. As a group, narcoleptics have not shown a tendency toward abuse of stimulant medications; therefore, all three drugs are commonly used.

Psychological Interventions: Patient Education

Psychoeducation interventions are crucial for patients with sleep disorders. An explanation of the sleep cycle and the factors that influence sleep is important for these patients. For those with insomnia, teaching about avoiding food and drink that interfere with sleep should be highlighted. The nurse should emphasize that hypnotics are to be used only for a short period of time and should not become a way of life. See Psychoeducation Checklist: Sleep Disorders.

Family and friends should be instructed on the importance of encouraging the new habits the patient is trying to establish. Patients, spouses, and friends must understand that activities engaged in just before sleep can greatly affect sleep patterns and sleep difficulties, such as socializing, drinking alcohol, or engaging in stimulating activities. Relaxing activities before bedtime are crucial, and family and friends can help create a conducive sleep environment. A gentle massage or stroking offered by a family member may help relax an adult or child. Gentle, soothing sounds or words may provide a sense of safety and help the person drift off to sleep.

Behavioral Interventions

Sleep Hygiene. The nurse can help the patient develop bedtime rituals and good sleep hygiene. Bedtime should

---

PSYCHOEDUCATION CHECKLIST
Sleep Disorders

When teaching patients with sleep disorders, be sure to include the following topics:

- Maintenance of a sleep log
- Foods that are okay to eat before going to bed
- Foods to avoid before going to bed
- Importance of developing a bedtime ritual and good sleep habits (see Text Box 26.3)
- Use of sleep medications for short-term only
- Avoidance of caffeine 6 hours before bedtime
- Avoidance of cigarette smoking during nighttime awakenings and 1 hour before bedtime
- Sleeping 7 to 8 hours per night
- Maintenance of a regular sleep schedule, especially a consistent rising time
- An occasional "bad night" happens to nearly everyone.
- Alcohol disrupts sleep and is a poor hypnotic.
- Daytime sleepiness is a symptom of sleep disorders.
- How to do relaxation exercises
- Bedroom rituals
- Appropriate family support

---

be at a regular time every day, and the bedroom should be conducive to sleep. Preferably, the bedroom should not be where the individual watches television or does work-related activities. The bedroom should be viewed as a room for resting and sleep.

Bedtime routines are important. The patient should engage in a quiet, relaxing activity in preparation for sleep, such as listening to soft music, taking a warm bath, reading for pleasure, or watching television in another room (providing the show is not alarming). Exercise promotes sleep, but regular exercise should be planned for earlier in the day and never within 2 to 3 hours of going to bed.

Cognitive Therapy. Relaxation exercises that begin with slow, deep breathing for several minutes can induce a calm state. Relaxing and contracting muscles in a progressive manner from head to toe can relieve tension and aid falling asleep. Sleep-promoting audiotapes that play gentle instrumentals or nature sounds may help.

Evaluation and Treatment Outcomes

The primary treatment outcome is the establishment of a normal sleep cycle. Change in diet and behavior should be evaluated for its impact on the individual's sleep. Environmental modifications, such as change in lighting, decreased stimulation, or modification in room temperature can be monitored for any changes affecting the sleep cycle.

Summary of Key Points

➤ The normal sleep–wake cycle runs in about a 24-hour pattern called circadian rhythm. Most body systems follow a circadian rhythm and are often associated with the sleep–wake cycle, such as the release of the hormones melatonin and cortisol, which help promote wakefulness during the day and sleepiness at night.

➤ Neurochemical activity throughout the central nervous system is the major mechanism that controls changes in sleep and wakefulness.

➤ Polysomnography is clinical testing used to diagnose or confirm sleep disorders. Results of polysomnography describe a person's sleep architecture (timing and distribution of sleep stages) and any abnormalities occurring during sleep.

➤ Primary sleep disorders are those not considered the result of another mental or medical disorder or induced by a substance (eg, medication, alcohol). Sleep disorders are ongoing disruptions of normal waking and sleeping patterns and are subdivided into dyssomnias and parasomnias.

➤ Primary insomnia is a sleep disorder characterized by difficulty falling asleep or staying asleep. It involves behaviors that perpetuate this abnormal sleep and rest pattern. Although insomnia is often precipitated by feelings of stress or tension, these patients develop sleep-preventing associations and behaviors that persist long after the crisis or stressful situation has passed.

➤ Obstructive sleep apnea syndrome is a commonly diagnosed breathing-related sleep disorder. It is characterized by excessive snoring during sleep and episodes of apnea (cessation of breathing), which disrupt sleep and cause daytime sleepiness.

➤ Parasomnias are characterized by abnormal physiologic or behavioral events that occur during sleep or transition from sleep to wakefulness and include nightmare disorder, sleep terror disorder, and sleepwalking disorder. The etiology of these disorders is unknown, but there appears to be some genetic predisposition. These disorders cause unrestful sleep and can jeopardize daytime activities because of excessive sleepiness, poor concentration, and irritability.

➤ Assessment includes a thorough sleep history, including current sleeping patterns, previous sleep patterns before sleep difficulties, medical problems, current medications, current life events, and emotional and mental status, as well as assessment of the details of the sleep complaint, including description, duration, and stability and intensity of the problem.

➤ Nursing interventions for sleep disorders include educating the patient about good sleep hygiene, instructing patients in relaxation exercises and sleep-inducing activities, providing patients with nutritional counseling regarding foods and substances to avoid, and educating family members and friends regarding the importance of encouraging new sleep habits for the patient.

Critical Thinking Challenges

1. Discuss the relationship of circadian rhythm and sleep.
2. Identify the stages of sleep and briefly describe each one.
3. How does sleep architecture change throughout the life cycle? Highlight the usual sleep pattern of each age group.
4. Identify the sleep changes that occur in the following disorders: mood disorder, schizophrenia, and alcoholism.
5. Compare the sleep problems that occur in primary insomnia with those in primary hypersomnia.
6. How does hypersomnia differ from narcolepsy?
7. Develop nursing interventions for a 24-year-old professional truck driver who experiences insomnia at home.
8. A 55-year-old airline pilot has developed difficulty with sleep and attributes his insomnia to jet lag. Develop a list of assessment questions that could be used in exploring the pilot's sleep patterns.
9. Conduct a sleep history with a child, an adult, and an individual with a major psychiatric illness.

 WEB LINKS

www.users.cloud9.net/~thorpy   This is the Sleep Medicine home page.

www.sleepfoundation.org   This is the website of the National Sleep Foundation.

www.aasmnet.org   This is the site of the American Academy of Sleep Medicine.

www.sleepapnea.org   This is the American Sleep Apnea Association website.

www.narcolepsynetwork.org   This is the site of the Narcolepsy Network.

www.rls.org   This is the website of the Restless Legs Syndrome Foundation.

www.med.stanford.edu/school/psychiatry/coe   This is the site of the Stanford University Center of Excellence for the Diagnosis and Treatment of Sleep Disorders.

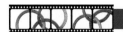 **MOVIES**

The Cabinet of Dr. Caligari (1919)
City of Lost Children (1995)
Dreams (Akira Kurosawa) (1990)
Insomnia (Erik Skjoldbjaerg) (1997)
My Own Private Idaho (1991)
Nightmare on Elm Street collection (beginning 1985)
The Somnambulist (1929)
Spellbound (1945)

REFERENCES

Aikens, J. E., Vanable, P. A., Tadimeti, L., et al. (1999). Overestimation of daytime sleepiness in insomnia: Associations with diagnostic subtype and psychopathology. *Sleep, 21*(Suppl.), 125.

American Psychiatric Association. (1994). *Diagnostic and statistical manual of mental disorders* (4th ed.). Washington, DC: Author.

Arendt, J., & Deacon, S. (1997). Treatment of circadian rhythm disorders—melatonin. *Chronobiology International, 14*(2), 185–204.

Benca, R. M. (2000). Mood disorders. In M. H. Kryger, T. Roth, & W. C. Dement (Eds.), *Principles and practice of sleep medicine* (3rd ed., pp. 1140–1157), Philadelphia: W. B. Saunders.

Birkenmeier, N. (2000a). *Important facts about sleep and young children*. Chesterfield, MO: Unity Sleep Medicine and Research Center.

Birkenmeier, N. (2000b). *General safety precautions for sleepwalkers and their families*. Chesterfield, MO: Unity Sleep Medicine and Research Center.

Bliwise, D. L. (2000). Normal aging. In M. H. Kryger, T. Roth, & W. C. Dement (Eds.), *Principles and practice of sleep medicine* (3rd ed., pp. 26–42), Philadelphia: W. B. Saunders.

Bonnet, M. H. (2000). Sleep deprivation. In M. H. Kryger, T. Roth, & W. C. Dement (Eds.), *Principles and practice of sleep medicine* (3rd ed., pp. 53–71). Philadelphia: W. B. Saunders.

Breslau, N., Roth, T., Rosenthal, L., & Andreski P. (1996). Sleep disturbance and psychiatric disorders: A longitudinal epidemiological study of young adults. *Biological Psychiatry, 39*(6), 411–418.

Broughton, R. J. (2000). NREM arousal parasomnia. In M. H. Kryger, T. Roth, & W. C. Dement (Eds.), *Principles and practice of sleep medicine* (3rd ed., pp. 693–706). Philadelphia: W. B. Saunders.

Campbell, S. S., Terman, M., Lewy, A. J., et al. (1995). Light treatment for sleep disorders: Consensus report. V. Age-related disturbances. *Journal of Biological Rhythms, 10*(2), 151–154.

Chesson, A. L., Jr., Littner, M., Davila, D., et al. (1999). Practice parameters for the use of light therapy in the treatment of sleep disorders. *Sleep, 22*(5), 641–648.

Cheyne, J. A., Rueffer, S. D., & Newby-Clark, J. R. (1999). Hypnagogic and hypnopompic hallucinations during sleep paralysis: Neurological and cultural construction of the nightmare. *Consciousness & Cognition, 8*(3), 319–337.

Costo, G. (1997). The problem: Shiftwork. *Chronobiology International, 14*(2), 89–98.

Culebas, A. (1996). *Clinical handbook of sleep disorders*. Newton MA: Butterworth-Heinemann.

Gallup Organization. (1991). *Sleep in America*. Princeton, NJ: Author.

Ganguli, M., Reynolds, C., & Gilby, J. (1996). Prevalence and persistence of sleep complaints in a rural older community sample: The MoVIES project. *Journal of the American Geriatric Society, 44*(7), 778–784.

Gillin, J. C., & Drummond, S. P. A. (2000). Medication and substance abuse. In M. H. Kryger, T. Roth, & W. C. Dement (Eds.), *Principles and practice of sleep medicine* (3rd ed., pp. 1176–1195), Philadelphia: W. B. Saunders.

Hilliker, N. A. J., Muehlbach, M. J., Schweitzer, P. K., & Walsh J. K. (1992). Sleepiness/alertness on a simulated night shift schedule and morningness-eveningness tendency. *Sleep, 15*(5), 430–433.

Horne, J. A., & Ostberg, O. (1976). A self-assessment questionnaire to determine morningness-eveningness in human circadian rhythms. *International Journal of Chronobiology, 4*, 97–110.

Kahn, A., Mozin, M. J., Rebuffat, E., et al. (1989). Milk intolerance in children with persistent sleeplessness: A prospective double-blind cross-over evaluation. *Pediatrics, 84*, 595–603.

Lecendreux, M., Mayer, G., Bassetti, C., et al. (2000). HLA class II association in sleepwalking. *Sleep, 23* (Suppl. 2), A13.

Manber, R., & Armitage, R. (1999). Sex, steroids and sleep: A review. *Sleep, 22*(5), 540–555.

Mignot, E. (2000). Pathophysiology of sleep. In M. H. Kryger, T. Roth, & W. C. Dement (Eds.), *Principles and practice of sleep medicine* (3rd ed., pp. 663–675), Philadelphia: W. B. Saunders.

Mignot, E., Lin, X., Arrigoni, J., et al. (1994). DQB1*0602 and DQA1*0102(DQ1) are better markers than DR2 for narcolepsy in Caucasian and black Americans. *Sleep, 17*(8), S60–S67.

Montplaisir, J., Lorrain, J., Petit, D., et al. (1997). Emotional activation of limbic circuitry in elderly normal subjects in a PET study. *American Journal of Psychiatry, 154*, 384–389.

Muehlbach, M. J., & Walsh, J. K. (1995). The effects of caffeine on simulated shift work and subsequent daytime sleep. *Sleep, 18*, 22–29.

National Commission on Sleep Disorders Research. (1993). *Wake up America: A national sleep alert* (Vol. 1). Executive summary and executive report, submitted to the United States Congress and the Secretary U.S. Department of Health and Human Services.

Paradiso, S., Robinson, R G., Andreasen, N.C., et al. (1997). Emotional activation of limbic circuitry in elderly normal subjects in a PET study. *American Journal of Psychiatry, 154*, 384-389.

Partinen, M., & Hublin, C. (2000). Epidemiology of sleep. In M. H. Kryger, T. Roth, & W. C. Dement (Eds.), *Principles and practice of sleep medicine* (3rd ed., pp. 558–579), Philadelphia: W. B. Saunders.

Pivik, R. T. (2000). Psychophysiology of dreams. In M. H. Kryger, T. Roth, & W. C. Dement (Eds.), *Principles and practice of sleep medicine* (3rd ed., pp. 491–501), Philadelphia: W. B. Saunders.

Pollack, C., & Stokes, P. (1997). Circadian rest-activity rhythms in demented and nondemented older community residents and their caregivers. *Journal of the American Geriatric Society*, *45*(4), 446–452.

Randazzo, A. C., Muehlbach, M. J., Schweitzer, P. K., & Walsh, J. K. (1998). Cognitive function following acute sleep restriction in children ages 10–14. *Sleep*, *21*(8), 861–868.

Rechtshaffen, A., & Kales, A. A. (1968). *A manual of standardized terminology, techniques, and scoring system for sleep stages of human subjects*. Bethesda, MD: National Institute of Neurological Diseases and Blindness.

Roehrs, T., & Roth, T. (1994). Chronic insomnias associated with circadian rhythm disorders. In M. H. Kryger, T. Roth, & W. C. Dement (Eds.), *Principles and practice of sleep medicine* (2nd ed., pp. 477–481). Philadelphia: W. B. Saunders.

Rogers, A. E. (1997). Nursing management of sleep disorders: Part I—Assessment. *ANNA Journal*, *24*(6), 666–671.

Valencia-Flores, M., Rebollar, V., Rodriguez, C., et al. (2000). Pulmonary hypertension in obese patients with obstructive sleep apnea syndrome. *Sleep*, *23*(Suppl. 2), A15.

Van Dongen, H. P. A., & Dinges, D. F. (2000). Circadian rhythms in fatigue, alertness, and performance. In M. H. Kryger, T. Roth, & W. C. Dement (Eds.), *Principles and practice of sleep medicine* (3rd ed., pp. 391–399). Philadelphia: W. B. Saunders.

Zadra, J. S., & Montplaisir, J. (2000). Sleep deprivation increases the frequency and complexity of behavioral manifestations in adult sleepwalkers. *Sleep*, *23*(Suppl. 2), A14.

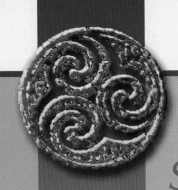

Sexual Disorders

Ronna E. Krozy

SEXUAL DEVELOPMENT
Infancy Through Childhood
Childhood Through Adolescence
Young Adulthood
Adulthood
Later Adulthood
Old Age
The Dying Person

HUMAN SEXUAL RESPONSE
Sexual Desire
Sexual Arousal
Orgasm
Resolution

SEXUAL DISORDERS
Orgasmic Disorders
    Female Orgasmic Disorder

Nursing Management:
Human Response to Disorder
    Biologic Domain

Psychological Domain
Social Domain
Premature Ejaculation
Male Orgasmic Disorder
Sexual Arousal Disorders
    Male Erectile Disorder
    Etiology

Nursing Management:
Human Response to Disorder
    Biologic Domain
    Psychological Domain
    Social Domain
    Female Sexual Arousal Disorder

OTHER SEXUAL DISORDERS
Sexual Desire Disorders
    Hypoactive Sexual
        Desire Disorder
    Sexual Aversion Disorder
Sexual Pain Disorders
    Dyspareunia

Vaginismus
Priapism
Sexual Disorder Caused by
    General Medical Condition
Substance-Induced
    Sexual Dysfunction
Paraphilias
    Exhibitionism
    Fetishism
    Frotteurism
    Pedophilia
    Sexual Masochism
    Sexual Sadism
    Transvestic Fetishism
    Voyeurism
    Paraphilia Not
        Otherwise Specified
Sexual Disorders Not
    Otherwise Specified

**GENDER IDENTITY
DISORDERS**

**LEARNING
OBJECTIVES**

After studying this chapter, you will be able to:

➤ Describe the psychophysiology of the human sexual response cycle.

➤ Distinguish types and etiologies of common sexual dysfunctions and disorders.

➤ Analyze biologic, psychological, and social theories that serve as a basis for caring for people with sexual disorders, paraphilias, and gender identity disorders.

➤ Identify human responses to sexual dysfunctions.

➤ Develop a nursing care plan based on a biopsychosocial assessment of a patient with a sexual disorder.

➤ Identify nursing intervention strategies common to treating those with sexual disorders.

➤ Identify appropriate resources for referring a patient with a sexual dysfunction.

CHAPTER 27

KEY TERMS

advocacy
biosexual identity
dyspareunia
erectile dysfunction
excitement
exhibitionism
fetishism
frotteurism
gender identity
heterosexuality
homosexuality
human sexual
  response cycle
orgasm
orgasmic disorders
paraphilias
plateau
premature ejaculation

primary sexual
  dysfunction
resolution
secondary sexual
  dysfunction
sensate focus
sex role identity
sex therapy
sexual addiction
sexual aversion
  disorder
sexual desire
sexual dysfunction
sexual orientation/
  preference
transvestic fetishism
vaginismus
voyeurism

KEY CONCEPTS

human sexual response
sexuality

Sexuality is a life force that encompasses all that is male or female and all that is human. It refers to the combination of biologic, psychological, social, and experiential factors that mold an individual's sexual development and behavior. Sexuality is also associated with attractiveness, sensuality, pleasure and pleasuring, intimacy, trust, communication, love and affection, affirmation of one's masculinity and femininity, and reverence for life. Sexuality has a large influence on how we view ourselves and one's self-concept and consequently on how we relate to others.

KEY CONCEPT **Sexuality.** Sexuality is a life force that encompasses all that is male or female and all that is human.

The way we feel about ourselves and the way society feels about us is intrinsically tied to our sexuality and thus our self-concept and body image. It is influenced by a person's emotional and physiologic status, beliefs and values, and morals and laws of society. Robinault (1978), an early researcher into the sexual issues of the disabled, noted that personhood is the threshold of sexuality. Yet, society often views sexual rights as belonging only to those who are young and attractive or capable of reproducing, while holding negative sexual attitudes about people who may be "different," such as the physically or mentally challenged, disfigured, obese, aged, institutionalized, or terminally ill. Implicit and explicit messages that a characteristic (such as being aged, mentally ill, or having a disability) has removed all possibility for sexual response often lower the individual's sense of self and sexual functioning. It is important that health professionals, and nurses in particular, erase these stereotypes and recognize that sexual functioning and adaptation have more to do with sexual knowledge, attitudes, experience, and psychological status than with the condition itself. In this way, each individual may be helped to develop his or her fullest sexual capacity. Barriers to sexual fulfillment can arise from medical problems, such as neurologic, musculoskeletal, cardiovascular, respiratory, renal, hepatic, and cognitive impairments; from pain, weakness, and fatigue; and from sequelae of surgical procedures and drugs. More often, sexual problems are a result of the interplay of multiple causes that can include intrapsychic, interpersonal, and sociocultural factors.

Nurses must also be prepared to confront common sexual problems in their practice, such as the pandemic of AIDS (Research Box 27.1); the epidemic of human papillomavirus and other sexually transmitted diseases (STDs) in young women; inadequate sexual knowledge; sexual violence, harassment, and abuse; unplanned pregnancies; and abortion.

As a holistic science, enveloping the total person, nursing's goal is defined as fostering an optimal level of healthy functioning. This role includes promoting sexual health and preventing sexual dysfunction. Nurses are in a unique position to help those with physical or emotional challenges to maximize their sexual capacity through the nursing process. This

includes carrying out a sexual assessment, establishing a nursing diagnosis, and intervening, in the form of sex education, counseling, or referral for sex therapy, as well as assuming the protective role of advocate. Many nurses, however, continue to have difficulty addressing a patient's sexuality, taking a sexual history, or offering sexual advice. This chapter will enhance the nurse's knowledge about sexuality, sexual function, and sexual dysfunction; provide guidelines for identifying actual or potential risks to patients' sexuality; and offer suggestions for intervening with skill and comfort.

SEXUAL DEVELOPMENT

From the moment of conception, each one of us passes through various stages of growth and development, accomplishing specific tasks that are aimed at maturity and self-actualization. All of us are sexual beings, whether or not we are sexually active. Sex is what we are, not what we do—the sum total of all of our biologic and experiential influences. Sexual maturation or psychosexual development is concerned with four phases: biosexual identity, gender identity, sex role identity, and sexual orientation and preference.

Understanding sexual disorders requires a knowledge of the development of normal human sexuality

---

RESEARCH BOX 27.1

Nurse-Expressed Attitudes Toward People Living With AIDS

The purpose of this descriptive correlational research study was (1) to examine baccalaureate nursing students' attitudes toward people living with AIDS (PLWAs) according to how the individuals contracted the disease, and (2) to identify variables associated with the students' attitudes.

The nonrandom sample population consisted of 256 baccalaureate nursing students from five universities, ranging in experience from sophomore to RN-BS level. Results showed that nursing students held more positive attitudes toward PLWAs who contracted the AIDS virus through transfusion or maternal transmission and held less positive, even stigmatizing, attitudes toward those who contracted the disease through drug taking or sexual activity. There was no significant relationship between students' attitudes toward PLWAs and student demographic variables, including age, religion, ethnicity, ideology, work experience, experience with a PLWA, or source of information about AIDS. A more recent study by Olson and Hanchett (1997) supports the hypothesis that empathy expressed by a nurse

and perceived by the patient significantly decreases the patient's distress.

Utilization in the Clinical Setting: These findings suggest that nursing students are more empathic toward those viewed as blameless for their disease and more stigmatizing toward those perceived as actively causing their illness. The study supports the need for nursing education to address the attitudinal component of nursing care and to prepare humanistic care providers to demonstrate nonjudgmental acceptance of people with diverse backgrounds. Patient comfort and self-acceptance or acceptance of diagnosis are greatly affected by caretaker attitudes. Therefore, this study demonstrates that nurses in clinical settings must recognize their feelings, whether positive or negative, about certain types of patients or behaviors; examine the basis for their attitudes and beliefs; be aware of the impact of their feelings on patient outcomes; and provide care that enhances patient self-esteem and sense of genuine acceptance.

West, A. M., Leasure, R., Allen, P., & LaGrow, P. (1996). Attitudes of baccalaureate nursing students toward persons with acquired immunodeficiency syndrome according to mode of human immunodeficiency virus transmission. *Journal of Professional Nursing, 12,* 225–232.

and its terminology. **Biosexual identity** concerns the anatomic and physiologic state of being male or female and results from genetic and hormonal influences. **Gender identity** is the internal sense of one's self as male or female. It is established by 18 months to 3 years of age, after which it is believed to be fixed for life (Strickland, 1995). According to social learning theory, gender identity results from a rearing process whereby the child internalizes the message of being a boy or girl. Socializing agents in the environment, together with social expectations, enforce and reinforce the acquisition of gender identity. Psychodynamic theory suggests that gender identity results from role modeling, identifying with a same-sex parent or other individual. Cognitive theory posits gender identity as arising from the child's intellectual capacity to construct categories of boy and girl in the mind, applying this system of thought to the self, and differentiating the behavior of the sexes. Biologic theory ties gender identity to sexual dimorphism, which begins in utero and which not only contributes to the anatomic development of the child but also is believed to influence chemically the child's self-concept as male or female.

Sex role identity (or gender role) is the outward expression of one's gender. Sex role identity refers to the behaviors, feelings, and attitudes that are determined to be appropriate for males, females, or both. Labels used to describe sex role identity include *masculine* or *feminine*; *traditional* or *conforming*; and *gender-neutral* (also called *cross-roled* or *androgynous*). Gender-neutral terms apply to nonconforming or nontraditional roles, such as female truck drivers or male homemakers. Gender roles are learned by the individual and are influenced by one's religion, parents, peers, schools, social messages, and other socializing agents.

Sexual orientation/preference refers to an individual's feelings of sexual attraction and erotic potential. Both male and female homosexual orientation are thought to occur prepubescently. **Heterosexuality** refers to the sexual arousal or sexual activity involving individuals of the opposite sex. **Homosexuality** may be defined as the erotic arousal of an individual by another person of the same gender or sexual relations between individuals of the same gender. A person who is either heterosexual or homosexual may also practice celibacy.

Infancy Through Childhood

Sexual development starts biologically at conception with the combination of the mother's X chromosome and the father's X or Y chromosome, creating, respectively, a female (XX) or male (XY) embryo. Rudimentary sex organs remain undifferentiated until the seventh week of development. Chromosomes and hormones influence gonadal development. In the female fetus, there is no production of androgen; in the male, androgen promotes the growth of male genitalia and the suppression of female genital growth.

A small number of children survive the chromosomal anomalies that affect sexual appearance, behavior, or function in later life. Two common examples are Klinefelter's syndrome, which usually occurs in males, causing dysfunctional gonads, sterility, and some developmental disability; and Turner's syndrome in females, causing short stature, primary amenorrhea, and other somatic problems. Hormonal aberrations in the developing male or female fetus can give rise to sex ambiguity. Gender dysphoria (a persistent aversion toward some or all of the physical characteristics or social roles that connote one's own biologic sex) may also have a hormonal or genetic basis.

At birth, gender assignment of a healthy infant begins a series of adult interactions that steer the child's development. The colors used to dress the baby, the baseball and bat or baby doll brought to the infant, the gentle rocking or "rough-housing" by a parent, are each reinforcers of future expected masculine or feminine behavior. In modern times, some of these differences are melting away in favor of fostering more androgynous characteristics.

Sexual discovery begins with early genital exploration and touching. Male fetuses have also been observed to develop erections in utero. Genital stimulation usually begins as soon as the child develops coordination. The impaired child will equally self-stimulate, although there may be a lack of coordinated touching replaced with rocking or rubbing thighs.

Between 1 and 3 years of age, children observe body differences, demonstrate interest in bathroom habits and urination, and handle their genitals for pleasure and comfort. Between ages 3 and 5, children comment on the differences in male and female sexual organs. Their curiosity leads them to want to look at and touch adult bodies and breasts. Mutual genital exploration or urination may be seen at this time along with questions about where babies come from. Beyond 5 years of age, boys will often ask the function of their testicles, and associations are made between male and female genitals.

Because human sexual behavior is not biologically impelled by a reproductive period, as in the animal world, but by sexual desire, the human must first learn to separate sexual desire from reproductive desire and then learn how to control it (Robinault, 1978). This requires teaching children about sexual body function and emotions while instilling cultural and religious tenets. Children are frequently thought of as nonsexual, and parents may try to keep them innocent or ignore or punish a child's natural sexual curiosity, thus sending confused messages to the child regarding sexuality. Parents who are threatened by their child's natural sexual curiosity and respond with hostility, punishment, or inducement of fear may permanently alter their child's sexual development.

From preadolescence to adolescence, children develop sexual feelings, a level of sexual interest, and sexual body changes. Issues pertaining to menstruation, nocturnal emissions, masturbation, sexual activity, and sex education normally arise. Parents and health professionals must recognize that these are normal growth steps and address them with positive, healthy attitudes.

Childhood Through Adolescence

As biologic maturation or puberty occur, boys and girls develop primary and secondary sex characteristics, a high level of sexual responsiveness, and the capacity for reproduction. Many youngsters begin to be sexually active in the middle grades, even as early as seventh grade.

Sex may be engaged in because of peer pressure, which seems to work most in the person with weak self-esteem and a questionable future, or because friends or social groups condone sex. Having sex when one is uncomfortable can cause guilt and anxiety. The need to be convinced of being in love, pretending that one is not planning to be sexually active, wanting to feel loved, and fear of rejection all precipitate risk-taking behavior.

To understand teen sexual behavior as it exists today requires broadening our definition of sex to include oral sex, mutual masturbation, and anal intercourse. Ample research addresses teen intercourse, pregnancy, and STDs. However, controlled studies of noncoital practices are nonexistent because of lack of funding, parental unwillingness to have their children questioned, and taboos surrounding these practices. More importantly, teens have adopted the cultural norm of defining sex as vaginal intercourse, and many teens and college students are practicing oral or anal sex, equating these practices with abstinence, virginity, and protection from STDs (Bogart et al., 2000; Remez, 2000). Unfortunately, various STDs are transmissible through noncoital sex, and emotional issues arise from these practices. Until health professionals have a consensus on what constitutes sex, how teens define sex, and who is practicing what, they will not be effective in reducing the physical or emotional risks in this population.

Although lack of knowledge still contributes to unwanted pregnancies and STDs, issues of motivation and attitudes have greater impact. For this reason, sex education programs are focusing on helping teens, particularly young women, to assert their rights to practice abstinence (refuse to have sex) or to make wise decisions about safer sexual practices, such as consistent and correct use of all forms of contraceptives with any sexual encounter (American Pediatrics Association, 1999).

Special attention should be given to chronically ill or disabled adolescents to educate them. Chronically ill adolescents have an only slightly later mean age of beginning intercourse (Nelson, 1995). Health professionals should therefore include sexuality and contraceptive information when working with chronically ill adolescents because pregnancy may be a far greater risk for girls with serious illnesses, such as diabetes or lupus erythematosus.

Adolescents with chronic illness and disability may experience a disruption in their sexual development with eventual sexual dysfunction. Reduced testosterone levels associated with hyperthyroidism may cause erectile or ejaculatory dysfunction; cerebral palsy may precipitate vaginismus and masturbatory dysfunction; and sickle cell anemia may cause priapism and gonadal atrophy. Growth failure and delayed pubescence can also exaggerate the difference in appearance that disabled adolescents have from their peers. They may have difficulty in becoming independent and separating from their parents, possess poor self-concept and body image, or have inadequate socializing skills. They may experience loneliness or feel excluded or not accepted. Loneliness is correlated with such characteristics as low self-esteem, shyness, self-consciousness, lower affiliative tendencies, and external locus of control. It not only is painful for the person but also is a form of stigma that may precipitate withdrawal, illness, or depression as well as suicide or sexually indiscrete behavior. Lack of knowledge and noncompliant, aggressive, or acting-out behavior may also be seen.

Young Adulthood

During young adulthood, young adults must choose careers, decide whether to marry or remain single, whether to engage in sex with one partner or many, whether to practice birth control or get information, and whether or not they want to have children. Tasks of this stage involve attaining sexual maturity and developing a close intimate bond with another individual. Intimacy is both physical and psychological, and engagement in frequent sexual activity is common at this stage, creating great risk for STDs.

Young adults may still lack adequate knowledge about sexuality. College students frequently have questions about ways to deal with an aggressive partner, contraceptive methods, body image, sexual trends, causes and treatments of sexual problems, homosexuality, when and whether a sexual relationship is morally appropriate before marriage, and STDs.

Adulthood

After achieving the tasks of early adulthood—establishing independence, sexual adjustment, and an intimate relationship—the next stage usually involves marriage and parenting. However, adult sexual expression may differ greatly in accordance with culture, emotional readiness, choice, situation, or opportunity, including cohabitation of heterosexual or homosexual partners, celibacy, casual sex, or sex outside of marriage.

The ability to achieve and give sexual satisfaction, to perform adequately, and to communicate about one's needs are considered desired outcomes. Sexual issues arising during adulthood often evolve around family planning and deciding whether to have children (and if so, when and how many), methods of contraception, or a changing sexual relationship during pregnancy. Once children are in the household, the time, place, and energy for sexual activity may be problematic. For most married young adults, sexual pleasure becomes balanced with other life processes, but many couples experience sexual frustration and dissatisfaction and may need marital, family, or sexuality counseling.

Adults with developmental disabilities face more complex sexual issues. The effects of developmental disability differ in learning capacity, emotional stability, and social skills, although institutionalization may have a more negative effect on sexual behavior than the disability. The needs, capabilities, and goals of mild to moderately developmentally disabled people can be the same as those of the "normal population," although there may be weaker sexual impulses among the severely disabled. They can have feelings of love, affection, and passion, but lack of opportunity or instruction can cause misdirected sex drives, leading to increased homosexuality or masturbation.

Developmentally disabled adults are entitled to experience friendship and love, to achieve sexual potential, and to make decisions about life, including marriage and the right to have children. They can benefit from the companionship and stability of marriage, although childrearing may be stressful and require a number of support services.

Later Adulthood

Middle age is most often characterized as a time of transition, when people begin to confront the aging process and mortality and reassess their life, goals, and future expectations. All body systems undergo growth, development, and eventual decline. Although changes in physical appearance and the sexual system begin about the third decade of life, it is during the fourth to fifth decade of life that these changes become more obvious, and a number of chronic illnesses, such as hypertension or arthritis, may also begin. As a result of decreased endocrine production, gradual changes to body tissues occur over a 15- to 20-year span. Most of the physical symptoms arise from vasomotor instability, which can include morning fatigue, vague pains, hot flashes, dizziness, chills, sweating, nervousness, cry-

ing spells, decreased sexual potency, and palpitations. Although these symptoms often characterize female menopause, they have been reported to occur in a small percentage of men.

Menopause results from the gradual cessation of menstruation and ovulation, which ends reproductive capacity. This usually occurs between the ages of 45 and 55 years, with an average age of 51 years. Estrogen deficiency affects the sexual system by causing a gradual thinning of the vaginal mucosa, decreasing elasticity of muscles and orgasmic force, and increasing breast involution (sagging of breast tissue). Vaginal lubrication decreases, often requiring the use of a water-soluble lubricant or saliva. Although most women experience little or no change in sexual function, both decreased and increased sexual activity and interest have been reported.

Male sexual changes are a result of decreasing testosterone production. The amount and viability of sperm decrease, erections become less firm, and more direct sexual stimulation is needed. The testicles begin to decrease in elasticity and size, ejaculation time increases, and the force of ejaculation decreases. Prostatic enlargement begins in about 20% of men during middle age, which can cause urinary frequency and nocturia.

Although many people adapt to this transition from youth to older adulthood, some have difficulty coping with the aging process and losing their youth. Because our society emphasizes and values youth and beauty, aging is difficult for some to accept. If they experience added stress or frustration from a disappointing marriage, illness, or failure to achieve goals, they may experience midlife crises in which they try to recapture or retain feelings of youthfulness by using cosmetics and plastic surgery, seeking younger mates, and engaging in flirtatious or other adolescent behaviors; some may even become depressed and withdrawn. The man may perceive he is losing his masculinity through loss of sexual power, whereas the woman perceives her loss of attractiveness and desirability to be the cause.

Old Age

Sexual activity among senior adults can continue throughout life and does under favorable conditions. Numerous studies have indicated that elderly people can continue functioning even into their 80s and 90s. Although the frequency and types of sexual encounters may decline, the quality need not change. For some individuals, there may even be an increase in frequency and interest.

Sexual continuity depends to a great extent on good physical health and the availability of an interested and interesting partner (Masters & Johnson, 1966). Comfort (1974) postulated a disuse phenomenon, suggesting that continuous sexual activity is required (through masturbation or with a partner) if sexual function is to be retained. Other determinants for sexual continuity are positive self-image, self-esteem, positive adaptation and preparedness for aging, and factual information. The enjoyment and importance of sex in the earlier years often determine the role of sex in later years.

The gradual changes in cellular structure and in female function brought about by the aging process similarly affect the sexual system. Over time, the gonadal hormones, testosterone and estrogen, are decreased, resulting in genital tissue change and, in females, infertility. This does not cause inevitable loss of desire unless the circulating blood level of testosterone is severely low.

After menopause, the female hormone, estrogen, decreases. The ovarian, uterine, and vaginal tissues gradually atrophy, and lubrication is decreased. Breast tissue also atrophies and causes sagging. Thinning vaginal walls, owing to a flattening of uterine rugae, and decreased lubrication may cause **dyspareunia** (pain during intercourse). An increase in time is required to lubricate the vulvovaginal areas and to strengthen clitoral response, but orgasmic capacity and breast response remain fairly constant in appropriately stimulated women.

In men, sexual decline, often termed *climacteric*, starts later than in women. The production of testosterone lowers. The testicles decrease in size and lie in a lower position as a result of decrease in the elastic tissue of the scrotal sacs. Spermatogenesis decreases, although viable sperm, capable of impregnation, continue to be produced. Seminal fluid is less voluminous and viscous, and ejaculatory force is decreased. Erection is less firm, requiring more time and more direct stimulation, and ejaculatory demand is decreased. The older man, however, is capable of sustaining erection much longer with decreased ejaculatory demand, potentially benefiting the older woman, who requires increased time to reach orgasm. Coupled with the woman's increased sexual enjoyment in the later years, sexual activity is often perceived as more satisfactory than previously experienced.

Thus, in the healthy adult, sexual function, although modified by the aging process, should remain satisfying despite a differently timed sequence. Frequent sexual activity, whether by coitus or masturbation, usually preserves sexual potency. Female masturbation preserves lubrication capacity, but lack of intercourse may hasten vaginal shrinkage with dyspareunia should coitus be attempted. Masturbation, considered a harmless release of sexual tension and an alternative to intercourse, is practiced by both sexes, but some older adults may feel it is sinful or juvenile.

The Dying Person

Death is often viewed as the last stage of growth and development. Although most people are fortunate to live into their 70s and beyond, death may occur at any place along life's continuum. As a total part of the individual's personhood, sexuality remains a human force throughout life.

Patients who have a terminal illness or who are dying do not necessarily lose their desire to remain sexually active. Sexual dysfunction can result from the physical and emotional impact of the disease process. Many dying patients continue to have sexual feelings, a need for closeness with another person, and the desire to be touched, hugged, and talked to. Health professionals, as well as the patient and family, may be surprised or embarrassed by the continuing sexual interest, believing that sex should not be important or that it might hasten dying. The patient may inadvertently be rejected because the partner is afraid of causing harm, fears contracting illness, or is beginning the process of anticipatory grieving. There may be taboos of touching the person. Self-imposed abstinence may result from the patient's religious preoccupation and attempts to purify the self, as well as from self-repugnance.

Nurses who work with dying patients should encourage the patient and family to discuss sexual issues and needs. It is important to emphasize that intimacy may be expressed in many ways but that continued sexual activity need not be eliminated. It may be hypothesized that patients who experience satisfactory orgasm may benefit from the neurochemically induced release of tension and feeling of well-being.

HUMAN SEXUAL RESPONSE

The dynamics of human sexual response are still not fully understood, although most theories suggest that sexual behavior, including sexual arousal, is learned (O'Donohue & Plaud, 1994).

KEY CONCEPT   Human   Sexual   Response. The **human sexual response** cycle consists of four phases: desire, excitement, orgasm, and resolution.

In the healthy adult, sexual expression is mediated through interrelated body circuits or neurobiologic mechanisms (Schiavi & Segraves, 1995). Sex drive is integrated through the central nervous system and is believed to be located in the limbic system of the forebrain. Emotion is thought to be located in the hypothalamus. The autonomic nervous system governs extragenital changes, causing such reactions as increased respiration and heart rate. The parasympathetic nervous system is believed to largely control arousal, and the sympathetic nervous system, orgastic discharge. The exact mechanism is unknown; however, hormonal interaction with neurotransmitters in the brain is thought to promote sexual expression. Although body systems and structures are normally intact and function together, sexual response is often possible despite various impairments.

Sexual stimulation brings about a total-body response with dramatic changes seen in the genitals and breasts. In 1966, Masters and Johnson described the **human sexual response cycle** as consisting of four phases: **excitement, plateau, orgasm,** and **resolution.** Table 27-1 summarizes the physiologic changes related to each phase of human sexual response. In addition, for most men, immediately after orgasm and before resolution, there is a refractory period when no response is possible.

Following Masters and Johnson's work, Kaplan (1979) proposed a three-phase model of sexual response—desire, excitement, and orgasm—and identified low-desire states as a frequent cause of sexual dysfunction. Today, the sexual response cycle is conceptualized as consisting of four phases: desire, arousal, orgasm, and resolution. However, current researchers in women's sexuality consider these models "phallocentric" and not reflecting women's actual experience.

There are several key dynamics of women's sexual response that may differ significantly from those of the man. Many women do not appear to have a strong innate sexual drive, and sexual motivation may be stimulated by nonsexual interpersonal factors, such as a desire for physical connection rather than simply sexual release. Arousal and desire appear to be interchangeable and inseparable from one another, with one reinforcing the other. Subjective feelings of interest may follow the sensation of arousal, and sexual satisfaction may be felt without orgasm.

Sexual Desire

Sexual desire may be described as the ability, interest, or willingness to receive, or a motivational state to seek, sexual stimulation. Sexual desire (or sex drive) is believed to be mediated by neurotransmitters that are found in the limbic system of the brain and have inhibitory and excitatory function. Kaplan (1979) posited that sex drive is physiologically connected to both pleasure and pain centers and that nerve pathways connect the central sex centers and spinal reflex centers controlling genital response. Thus, pain (psychological or physiologic) can inhibit sexual desire and affect sexual function. Current research supports the theory that that both anger and anxiety result in lowered levels of self-reported desire (Beck, 1995). Sex hormones, particularly androgen, influence desire in both genders, but less is known about hormonal influence in women. That the higher centers of the brain apparently mediate the lower

reflex response centers supports the relationship between cognitive and affective states and sexual function.

Sexual Arousal

Excitement or arousal refers to an arousal state of mounting sexual tension characterized by vasoconstriction and myotonia. In the male, erection is a neurologic and hemodynamic event. In the unimpaired male, intact pathways between the brain and the sex organs and within the sacral arc permit stimuli to reach the nerves in the penis. Psychogenic and tactile stimulation promote the release of chemicals, which dilate penile arteries. A rapid inflow of arterial blood to the corpora cavernosa causes stiffening and elongation of the penis. Smooth muscle tissues in the walls of the penile arteries and lacunar spaces relax. This creates a high degree of pressure against the penile veins, almost occluding the venous drainage (Morgentaler, 1999).

The neurologic control of erection involves both central and peripheral nervous systems, with primary mediation by the parasympathetic branch of the autonomic nervous system. The cerebral cortex processes various sexual stimuli that are transmitted to the sacral spinal cord. The sacral parasympathetic nerves (nervi erigentes) provide the major motor supply to the penis, whereas sensation is transmitted through the pudendal sensory nerves. The thoracolumbar sympathetic nervous system is thought to produce engorgement of the corpus spongiosum. A strong relationship between plasma testosterone and sexual function has been shown in the animal world, although it is less clear in humans. Although some castrated males have demonstrated no change in erectile capacity, most researchers have observed loss of libido with androgen deficiency (Krane, 1986).

Female arousal is also a neurologic and hemodynamic event, and the genitosexual innervation in females appears to be analogous to that in males. For example, the parasympathetic nervous system brings about vaginal lubrication (a transudate of fluid from the vaginal mucosa), pelvic congestion, and clitoral swelling, as well as enlargement of breasts and labia, expansion of the vaginal barrel, tenting of the cervix and uterine body, flattening of the labia majora, retraction of the clitoris, and nipple erection.

Androgen promotes libido in both genders by activating the cerebral sex centers. Women who have received testosterone as a medical treatment have reported higher arousal states than previously experienced, whereas those with depleted sources of androgen due to drugs or surgery lose their libido. The role of estrogens and progesterone in governing sexual arousal remains somewhat inconclusive. Some women report increased libido during the outset of the menstrual cycle when the estrogen level is high; others report

TABLE 27.1 Physiologic Changes During Phases of Sexual Response

	Excitement	Plateau	Orgasm	Resolution
Male and Female				
General response	Vasocongestion and myotonia. Increased respiration, heart rate, blood pressure. Skin mottling on many women, some men.	Peaking of excitement phase. Increased muscle tension; involuntary pelvic thrusting; increased skin flush.	Release of sexual tension; loss of voluntary muscle control; ejaculatory inevitability in male. Peak heart rate 110–180; blood pressure 30–100 systolic, 20–50 diastolic > normal.	General feeling of well-being. Muscular tension dissipates. Gradual return to normal of skin color, heart rate, etc.
Breasts	*Female:* Nipples erect, areolae tumesce, breasts engorge. *Male:* partial to complete nipple erection.	Continuation of responses in both genders.	Unchanged.	Return to normal size, more rapid in females than males.
Male				
Penis	Erection results from vasocongestion of corpora cavernosa; distention of glans.	Corpus spongiosum engorges; penile bulb enlarges two to three times; coronal ridge of glans distends.	Ischiocavernosa and bulbospongiosa muscles contract at 0.8-s intervals; ejaculation of semen through urethra.	Penis detumesces rapidly as blood leaves corpora; complete detumescence may take up to 30 min.
Scrotum, vas deferens, prostate, seminal vesicles	Engorgement of walls of scrotal sac; scrotum elevates from contraction of cremaster muscles and shortening of vas deferens.	Engorgement of scrotum and testes continues; testes elevate against perineum before ejaculation; may emit clear pre-ejaculate fluid from Cowper's gland that can contain sperm.	No change in scrotum. Vas deferens, seminal vesicles, and prostate contract at emission phase, producing sense of inevitability of ejaculation, followed by rapid occurrence of orgasm.	Rapid detumescence in most men.
Female				
Clitoris	Engorgement of vestibular bulbs, corpus cavernosa, and corpus spongiosum. Shaft widens and may elongate.	Shaft and glans retract against pubic bone.	Retraction continues.	Tumescence may continue 5–10 min after orgasm; then retracts to normal within 5–10 min.
Labia	Vasocongestion, more pronounced in women who have had children.	Labia majora continue to swell with slight separation; in nullipara may flatten against perineum; color may range from pink to red, darker in multipara.	Labia majora remain unchanged; labia minora may contract.	If orgasmic, return to normal size in 1–2 min for nullipara and 10–15 min multipara.

(continued)

TABLE 27.1	Physiologic Changes During Phases of Sexual Response (Continued)			
	Excitement	**Plateau**	**Orgasm**	**Resolution**
Vagina	Lubrication or transudate produced from vaginal walls. Congestion in lower third of vagina with ballooning of inner two thirds. Color changes to purple-red.	Slowing of lubrication. Lower third of vagina highly engorged, decreases lumen, width and length of vagina increases; called orgasmic platform. Color deepens.	Contractions of circumvaginal muscles at 0.8-s intervals. Color unchanged.	Orgasmic platform decreases rapidly with gradual return of color.
Uterus	Engorgement of uterus and broad ligaments. Moves up and back from pelvic floor.	Engorgement continues; elevation complete.	Uterine contractions occur; may be unfelt or cause discomfort in pregnancy or postmenopause.	Decrease in vasocongestion within 10 min nullipara; 10–20 min multipara; 20–60 min if not orgasmic. Uterus returns to normal position in 5–10 min.

no cyclic fluctuations. When estrogen levels are low, however, replacement therapy has resulted in improved vaginal lubrication and integrity of tissue in the breast and vaginal mucosa.

Nongenital changes in both genders include increased heart rate, blood pressure, respiration, and myotonia.

Orgasm

Orgasm, formerly termed *climax*, is largely controlled by cerebral function and is characterized by clonic reflex muscular contractions. The orgasmic response in men often differs from that in women. There are two stages to male orgasm. Emission is a reflex mediated by the sympathetic nervous system that is located in the lateral horn of the thoracolumbar spinal cord (T-11 to L-2). Rhythmic contraction of the smooth muscle in the seminal vesicles, vas deferens, and prostate transports semen to the prostatic urethra, giving rise to the sensation that ejaculation is inevitable. Ejaculation, mediated by somatic nerves exiting from the sacral spinal cord (S-2 to S-4), results from pelvic muscle contractions at 0.8-second intervals and seminal expulsion. Simultaneously, sympathetic innervation arising from the thoracolumbar fibers contracts the bladder sphincter so that semen does not back up into the bladder. This neurologic schema accounts for the altered response, called *retrograde ejaculation*, in men with spinal cord injury or multiple sclerosis. Generally, the man experiences one orgasm after ejaculatory demand (or inevitability) and requires a period of time before erection and orgasm are again possible.

In women, three patterns of orgasmic response have been reported. The first is similar to that in men. The second pattern is described as a rippling effect of multiorgasms at the plateau level; the third shows mounting excitement levels, bypassing the plateau, to orgasm and resolution (Masters & Johnson, 1966). Orgasm may occur through clitoral stimulation, intercourse, breast stimulation, or combined stimuli and occasionally through mental stimulation alone. It is characterized by 0.8-second contractions of the uterus, pubococcygeal muscles, and anal sphincter and is perceived as a diffuse, pleasurable body sensation. Researchers have reported seeing an area on the anterior wall of the uterus along the urethra, called the *Grafenberg* (or *G*) *spot*, that swells with manual stimulation and secretes a similar fluid as the male prostate. They consider this an analogous gland that suggests female ejaculation (Ladas et al., 1981).

Resolution

Resolution is the gradual return of the organs and body systems to the unaroused state. Muscle tension and vasocongestion subside. Breathing and heart rate gradually return to normal rates. Usually, the person feels a sense of relaxation, relief of tension, and satisfaction. Some women may be capable of additional orgasms if properly stimulated; a small number of men also possess this capacity, but most experience a refractory period immediately after orgasm and before resolution when no response is possible.

Lieblum (2000) noted that both men and women can experience the physiologic changes associated with the sexual response cycle without feeling pleasure or satisfaction. Thus, there is a need to include the subjective outcome of satisfaction as an additional phase of the human response cycle.

SEXUAL DISORDERS

A sexual problem becomes a sexual disorder when there is a disturbance in the sexual response cycle or pain associated with intercourse. Problematic sexual behaviors are classified as **sexual dysfunctions** (or disorders), paraphilias, and gender identity disorders (American Psychiatric Association [APA], 2000). Sexual disorders are characterized by alterations in sexual desire and response and by emotional and interpersonal distress. These disorders are classified according to orgasmic disorders, sexual arousal disorders, sexual desire disorders, sexual pain disorders, and sexual dysfunctions due to a general medical condition. The paraphilias are characterized by recurrent, intense sexual urges, fantasies, or behaviors involving unusual objects, activities, or situations. These urges cause significant distress to the individual or impair social or occupational functioning. The paraphilias include exhibitionism, fetishism, voyeurism, pedophilia, sexual masochism and sadism, transvestic fetishism, frotteurism, and paraphilia not otherwise specified. Gender identity disorders constitute a category of dysfunctions that is used only when there is a persistent cross-gender identification with accompanying discomfort about one's assigned sex (APA, 2000).

Sexual disorders may occur during the desire, arousal/excitement, or orgasm/release phase of sexual response. Each phase of the human sexual response cycle may be impaired by physical, emotional, or environmental factors. **Primary sexual dysfunction** occurs when the appropriate sexual response was never experienced, and **secondary sexual dysfunction** occurs with a decline or cessation of previously experienced appropriate response. This chapter highlights two of the more common sexual disorders: female orgasmic disorder and male erectile disorder.

Orgasmic Disorders

Female Orgasmic Disorder

Female orgasmic disorder, formerly called *inhibited female orgasm*, is a dysfunction characterized by the inability of a woman to experience orgasm. Female orgasmic dysfunction may be lifelong or primary (lack of orgasm despite circumstance or stimulation), acquired or secondary (loss of former orgasmic capacity), and generalized or situational (orgasm occurs during special circumstances only). **Orgasmic disorder** may appear as inability to reach orgasm by any means, either alone or with a partner, or achieving orgasm only during masturbation or partner stimulation, but not during intercourse (Table 27-2).

Women with orgasmic dysfunction often desire, enjoy, and initiate sexual activity. Most obtain both the excitement and plateau stages of the sexual response cycle, but they do not progress to orgasm. Physiologically, it may be difficult for a woman to feel stimulation in the sensitive vaginal areas that trigger orgasm during actual intercourse. It has been questioned whether this response constitutes an actual dysfunction if a woman can reach orgasm in other ways. However, if the condition causes distress, it should be treated as a disorder.

Epidemiology. Female orgasmic disorder is considered the most common female sexual difficulty presented to practitioners, with a frequency rate estimated to be 25% (APA, 2000). The variability in prevalence rates may reflect differences in assessment procedures (ie, interview versus community survey), sample (ie, United States versus other countries), type of disorder (ie, lifelong versus acquired, global versus situational), and changes in prevalence and incidence over time.

Etiologic Factors

Biologic Theories. The causes of orgasmic dysfunction are both physiologic and psychogenic. There are a large number of potential biologic precipitants of orgasmic dysfunction. In general, any local genital or pelvic pathology, trauma, or surgery that causes pain on intercourse can produce impaired response to sexual stimulation. Any disorder that damages the spinal cord and thus interferes with the transmission of "sexual" stimuli may also impair ability to reach orgasm. Many endocrine disorders, as well as any condition that reduces the amount of androgen supplied to the female, may impair orgasm. Systemic diseases often decrease orgasmic response and interfere with sexual response because of the pain and general debility they cause. Central nervous system depressants (eg, alcohol, barbiturates, narcotics), psychiatric disorders, infections, inflammatory disorders, and pregnancy have all been associated with female orgasmic disorder. Many medications also affect the sexual response cycle (Table 27-3).

Psychological Theories. Orgasmic dysfunction is maintained by a cluster of emotions and cognitions. The general emotional states that seem to mediate inhibition of orgasm are (1) sexual anxiety and guilt, (2) anger or hostility toward one's partner, (3) indifference toward one's partner, (4) depression, or (5) excessive and intrusive thoughts. Misinformation or ignorance is an immediate correlate of orgasmic dysfunction that may produce any of these orgasm-inhibiting states.

Sexual dysfunction arises from immediate and specific or remote psychological causes, which create intrapsychic conflict leading to anxiety and blockage of erotic feeling toward lovemaking. The need to feel val-

TABLE 27.2	Key Diagnostic Characteristics for Female Orgasmic Disorder 302.73	
Diagnostic Criteria		**Target Symptoms and Associated Findings**

• Persistent or recurrent delay in or absence of orgasm following normal sexual excitement phase (based on less than that reasonable for the person's age, sexual experience, and adequacy of sexual stimulation received)
• Marked distress or interpersonal difficulty resulting from disturbance
• Not better accounted for by another Axis I disorder
• Not exclusively a direct physiologic effect of a substance or medical condition
  Lifelong type: present since onset of sexual functioning
  Acquired type: develops after a period of normal functioning
  Generalized type: not limited to certain types of stimulation, situations, or partners
  Situational type: limited to certain types of stimulation, situations, or partners
  Due to psychological factors: psychological factors play major role in onset, severity, exacerbation, or maintenance of the sexual dysfunction
  Due to combined factors: psychological factors play a role in onset, severity, exacerbation, or maintenance of sexual dysfunction and a general medical condition or substance use is also contributory but not sufficient enough to account for the sexual dysfunction
		• Possible body image or self-esteem disturbance
		• Possible interference with relationship satisfaction

ued and loved may place unrealistic performance demands on a partner, thus promoting sexual failure. Another barrier is failing to engage in sexually stimulating behavior, a factor often complicated by inability to communicate. It is necessary to determine whether marital discord predates the onset of a sexual dysfunction or has occurred as a result of the problem. Hostility can lead to withholding pleasure deliberately through sexual sabotage—creating tension before lovemaking, suggesting sex at an inopportune time, making oneself deliberately unattractive, or producing deliberate frustrations (Kaplan, 1979).

Fear of losing personal control over body functions, particularly those that permit satisfying, unconflicted sexual expression, often precipitates anxiety. Performance failure or worry that one will not satisfy one's partner may promote deliberate blockage of erotic stimuli. Depression is a common response to failed attempts at satisfying sexual activity and a common cause of low sexual energy.

Social Theories. Cultural expectations play an important role in the sexual experience. Religious prohibitions and cultural taboos often contribute to a woman's view of her sexuality. If a woman believes that sexual relationships are sinful or "a woman's duty," she is not as likely to explore her own sexual potential.

Risk Factors. If a woman has been sexually abused as a child, she may not be able to engage in an intimate relationship. In psychiatric patients, a history of sexual abuse may affect the presentation of symptoms or response to treatment (Mitchell et al., 1996). For example, these patients often have difficulty trusting others and may be reluctant to describe their symptoms or engage in a therapeutic relationship. It is also hypothesized that 1 of every 3 women will be raped in her lifetime. Many will suffer "silent rape syndrome," the aftermath of unreported rape, and may experience chronic depression, relationship problems, and sexual dysfunction (see Chap. 37).

Interdisciplinary Treatment. The overall goal of treatment of the woman with a primary orgasmic disorder is to improve her sexual functioning by focusing on the underlying reason for her inability to experience an orgasm. A variety of biologic factors, such as endocrine, neurologic, and metabolic illnesses, medications, such as antidepressants, antihypertensives, and alcohol can impair orgasm. Once identified, these factors can be modified or altered by teaching adaptive techniques or use of alternative drug therapies. If complicated interpersonal factors exist or the woman needs to learn specific techniques (such as erotic fantasy), she will be referred to a therapist trained and certified in sex therapy. These specialists have been trained to use a variety of interventions aimed at reducing anxiety, improving communication between partners regarding

TABLE 27.3 Effect of Medications on Sexual Functioning

Generic (Trade)	Affects Desire	Affects Arousal	Affects Orgasm
acetazolamide (Diamox)	X		
alprazolam (Xanax)	X		X
amitriptyline (Elavil)	X	X	X
amoxapine (Asendin)	X	X	X
bendroflumethiazide (Naturetin)	X	X	
chlordiazepoxide (Librium)	X		X
chlorpromazine (Thorazine)	X	X	X
chlorprothixene (Taractan)			X
chlorthalidone (Hygroton)	X	X	
cimetidine (Tagamet)	X	X	
clofibrate (Atromid S)	X	X	
clomipramine (Anafranil)	X	X	X
clonidine (Catapres)	X	X	
clorazepate (Tranxene)	X		
desipramine (Norpramin)	X	X	X
diazepam (Valium)	X		
dichlorphenamide (Daranide)	X		
disulfiram (Antabuse)		X	
doxepin (Sinequan)	X	X	X
fenfluramine (Pondimin)	X		
fluoxetine (Prozac)		X	X
guanethidine (Ismelin)	X	X	X
haloperidol (Haldol)	X	X	X
hydrochlorothiazide (Diuril)	X	X	
imipramine (Tofranil)	X	X	X
lithium (Eskalith, Lithonate)	X	X	
lorazepam (Atavan)	X		X
maprotiline (Ludiomil)	X	X	X
mesoridazine (Serentil)			X
nortriptyline (Aventyl, Pamelor)	X	X	X
paroxetine (Paxil)			X
perphenazine (Trilafon)			X
phenelzine (Nardil)	X	X	X
phenobarbital (Solfoton)	X		
pimozide (Orap)		X	
primedone (Mysoline)	X		X
propranolol (Inderal)	X	X	
protriptyline (Vivactil)	X	X	X
reserpine (Serpasil)	X	X	
sertraline (Zoloft)			X
spironolactone (Aldactone)	X	X	
thiabendazole (Mintezol)		X	
thiothixene (Navane)	X	X	X
tranylcypromine (Parnate)		X	X
trazodone (Desyrel)		X	X
trifluoperazine (Stelazine)			X

sexual preferences, and possibly teaching women to engage in sex play that corresponds with the techniques they use for masturbation (Table 27-4). Sex therapy for primary orgasmic dysfunction involves teaching the woman to produce orgasm through masturbation. The therapist should discuss any negative attitudes the woman may have about this behavior, affirm the patient's right to enjoy her sexuality, and re-assure her of the appropriateness of this method. If manual stimulation is terminated because of tension or anxiety, use of a vibrator can be advised to provide the highest level of stimulation. Teaching Kegel exercises, which strengthen the pubococcygeal muscle, has been used as a self-exploratory aspect of therapy and often results in increased sexual pleasure during intercourse.

TABLE 27.4 Interventions for Common Sexual Dysfunctions

Sexual Dysfunction	Intervention	Goal
Hypoactive sexual desire	Medical examination Facilitative communication Psychotherapy Education	Rule out hormonal imbalance Awareness and resolution of personal, sexual, and relationship issues
Sexual aversion	Psychotherapy Education Therapeutic controlled exposure to real or simulated sexual situation	Promote insight into inner conflicts Extinguish fear of aversive stimulus under safe conditions
Erectile dysfunction	Medical examination Organic etiology: penile implant, vascular surgery, intracavernosal pharmacotherapy, vacuum pump, drugs Sensate focus Counseling or psychotherapy Education Marital or couples therapy	Rule out penile hemodynamic, neurological, hormonal, or other organic causes Treat, control, or reverse physiologic cause Decrease pressure to perform Eliminate spectatoring Relearn new response Awareness and resolution of personal, sexual, and relationship issues
Premature ejaculation	Sensate focus Squeeze technique: includes progressive exercises from partner masturbation to controlled intromission and thrusting Counseling or psychotherapy Marital or couples therapy Education	Decrease pressure to perform Increase awareness of ejaculatory inevitability Learn new ejaculatory control responses Awareness and resolution of personal, sexual, and relationship issues Knowledge of arousal-orgasm mechanism
Female orgasmic dysfunction	Medical examination Sensate focus: progressive exercises from nongenital to genital stimulation and intercourse Masturbation Vibrator Assertiveness training Facilitative communication Counseling or psychotherapy Marital or couples therapy Education	Rule out organic etiology Decrease pressure to perform Increase awareness of pleasurable sensations Eliminate spectatoring Increase partner awareness of sites and methods of pleasuring Teach self-pleasuring, reaching orgasm Teach entitlement to and approach to request pleasurable sexual stimuli Increase awareness of personal, sexual, and relationship issues Knowledge of anatomy and physiology of human sexual response
Male orgasmic dysfunction	Medical examination Sensate focus Desensitization Manual or oral stimulation Vibrator Counseling or psychotherapy Education	Rule out organic etiology Decrease pressure to perform Increase awareness of pleasurable sensations Eliminate spectatoring Decrease anxiety or fear Increase pleasurable sensations Uncover deeper feelings, such as fear or hostility, blocking intravaginal orgasm Increase awareness and resolution of sexual and relationship issues Teach mechanism of sexual response

(continued)

	TABLE 27.4 Interventions for Common Sexual Dysfunctions (Continued)	
Sexual Dysfunction	**Intervention**	**Goal**
Vaginismus	Counseling or psychotherapy	Uncover deeper feelings, etiology of problem
	Dyadic counseling with men and women co-therapists	Promote feeling of safety and trust in woman
		Increase awareness and resolution of sexual and relationship issues
	Relaxation exercises	Promote relaxation of pubococcygeal muscle
	Insertion of graduated sizes of vaginal dilators, progressing to finger and penis	Promote tolerance of vaginal containment
	Assertiveness training	Teach communication skills
Dyspareunia	Medical examination	Rule out organic etiology
	Organic etiology: hormone replacement, localized infections or inflammation, etc.	Treat, control, or reverse physiologic cause
	In women, artificial lubricant, oral stimulation	Teach need for and promote increased lubrication to decrease susceptibility to abrasion
	Education	Teach relationship of sexual response and changes related to age, illness, or emotions
	Assertiveness training	Teach communication skills
	Sensate focus	Decrease performance anxiety; promote relaxation
	Counseling or psychotherapy	Promote self-knowledge; uncover sexual or relationship issues

In treating secondary orgasmic dysfunction, sex therapy using sensate focus and sexual stimulation exercises has been successful (McCabe & Delaney, 1992). The therapist must use open, factual, and sensitive instruction and be alert to any anxiety that either partner may be experiencing. **Sensate focus** is a method for partners to learn what each finds arousing and to learn to communicate those preferences. It begins with nongenital contact and gradually includes genital touch and sexual intercourse. The man caresses the woman as she desires during foreplay, usually through noncoital stimulation. After several sessions, she is then instructed to insert the erect penis, concentrate on the vaginal sensations elicited, and then begin thrusting. A method using dismounting and reinsertion, or interspersing clitoral stimulation with thrusting, has been successful.

NURSING MANAGEMENT: HUMAN RESPONSE TO DISORDER

Comprehensive information is essential to recognize, conceptualize, and manage a sexual problem correctly. The nurse will most likely be seeing the patient for another problem (psychiatric problem, acute or chronic physical health problem) and will discover the sexual problem. Even though most of the treatment is delivered by a mental health specialist, such as a sex thera-

pist, the generalist psychiatric–mental health nurse has a responsibility to assess the patient's sexual health carefully, determine the presence of any problems, and initiate interventions within his or her scope of practice—counseling, sex education, problem-solving, or referral. In addressing a patient's sexuality, the nurse completes a sexual history, establishes a nursing diagnosis and develops outcomes, plans and implements appropriate interventions, and then evaluates outcomes. The purpose of a sexual assessment is to gather historical and physical data to assess the impact of an illness on sexuality or identify actual or potential threats to sexual health. Through sexual assessment and the identification of a nursing diagnosis, patients may discuss sexual concerns, receive factual information, and obtain appropriate assistance.

Attention should be paid to special populations at high risk for sexual problems. People who are developmentally disabled may need help in developing satisfying sexual relationships. Psychiatric disorders often interfere with the physical and psychosocial aspect of sexuality. People who are institutionalized may have little opportunity for sexual partners.

Gays and lesbians can suffer from social stigma, confusion, and guilt that seriously affect self-esteem and overall mental health. People with same-sex orientation may be reluctant to discuss any sexual problems because of the social stigma associated with their lifestyle. Elderly people may also be reluctant to discuss any sexual problems. These populations need reassurance that nurses are knowledgeable about the topic of sexual dysfunction and are able to provide help in the area of sexual health.

Some misconceptions and myths exist regarding patients' sexuality and reluctance to talk about it. It is a myth that older adults are disinterested in sex or unwilling to talk about it. Experience shows that a warm, encouraging, and permissive atmosphere appears to have a freeing-up effect on older people and that many elderly individuals not only discuss their sexuality willingly but also are open to new information (Krozy, 1987). Some may mistakenly believe that many disabled people are incapable of sexual activity and that sex talk will unnecessarily frustrate them. This is not true.

Generally, a sexual history includes the patient's perception of real or potential problems, past sexual expression or preexisting sexual problems, history of presenting problems (lifelong or secondary) and situational factors (global versus situational), type and quality of relationship, level of knowledge, and coexisting drug therapy or illness. The depth and context of a sexual history depend on the patient's life status and condition. Often, the nurse must first address sexuality before patients realize they can broach the subject. It is possible that neglecting to address sexuality may precipitate anxiety or negative behavior. Verbal and nonverbal cues signal a patient's readiness for altered sexuality information. It is the nurse's role to be aware of such cues, promote readiness behavior, and demonstrate support for the patient's sexual needs.

Nurses must be knowledgeable and feel comfortable regarding their own sexuality to assess their patients' sexuality. Nurses can increase their knowledge fairly easily given the availability of literature, workshops, and sex education courses. One study of oncology nurses suggested that positive sexual attitudes do foster more sexuality-related nursing interventions (Wilson & Dibble, 1993). Sexual comfort may be fostered through such techniques as desensitization (repeated exposure to dissonant material), role play, and values clarification. Characteristics of the nurse with sexual self-comfort include accepting oneself as a sexual being, being able to discuss any aspect of sexuality with people of any age, and possessing factual information (Krozy, 1978). Changing nurses' misconceptions and attitudes will have a positive effect on removing barriers to sexual assessment and will promote competence in addressing sexuality.

Give the patient permission to discuss sexuality by raising the topic or indicating that sexuality will be part of the health history. Acknowledge that some people find it difficult to discuss intimate issues. Explain that your rationale for asking questions is to uncover problems and provide assistance. Privacy must be guaranteed so that others will not overhear intimate information. When a patient is in the home setting, it may be difficult to find a quiet place or to ask a partner to leave. This may be facilitated during the contract-setting period by indicating that occasionally you will want to speak with each individual privately.

Questions should require a descriptive answer, which allows patients to share their experiences, beliefs, and attitudes. Because sexual information is personal (eg, sexual fantasies, fidelity, masturbation), it should be collected in individual sessions, especially when assessing couples (Risen, 1995). Proceed from the least to the more sensitive questions and be prepared for unexpected answers or unsophisticated street language. Remember that appearing shocked might impede further communication. Respond with honesty and sensitivity, admitting when you might not have the answer.

Emphasize normality by starting questions with "many people feel" or ". . . are concerned about . . ." or "practice . . . ." If a patient is surprised by sexual questions, explain that you are seeking factual information rather than making assumptions.

Learn to tolerate silence and respect a patient's refusal to answer but indicate your willingness to approach the subject at a later time. Avoid judging the person by your own beliefs and practice. Sometimes, it is important to clarify terms and use slang if necessary. Assess only those areas that are pertinent for the patient at this time. Several sessions may be necessary to complete the interview.

Observation and listening are especially important in taking a sexual history. Because sex is often a forbidden subject, patients frequently provide cues or clues to sexual difficulties. A skilled nurse can learn a great deal from an individual's body language. Inappropriate sexual behavior may arise because of multiple psychosocial etiologies, such as the need to validate one's masculinity or femininity, hostility, need for attention, desire to punish another person, loneliness, social isolation, or organic brain disease and confusion. The nurse must identify the underlying causes of this behavior before attempting to intervene.

The Sexual Assessment Guide provides important content area for a sexual assessment (Text Box 27-1). Other assessment data from the general history, including demographic information, may affect the findings from the patient's sexual history. It is the nurse's responsibility to identify and include this information as necessary.

Biologic Domain

Assessment. The nursing assessment of the woman who is experiencing orgasmic difficulties considers her current sexual functioning, age, physical health, and the

TEXT BOX 27.1

Sexual Assessment Guide

Sexual Development and Reproduction

How did you learn about sex and how were your questions answered?

What did you learn from your family, school, religion?

How did you feel about being a male or female? Problem?

Beliefs about body; satisfaction with looks/function?

Diet, drugs, anorexia/bulimia, steroids, fitness/exercise regimen?

Menstruation or menopause experience? Issues? Questions?

Contraceptive practices? Pregnancies? Problems? Questions?

Infertility problems, treatments, outcomes?

Health Conditions and Practices

Females

Do you practice breast self-examination? Vaginal self-examination?

How often have you had a pelvic examination? Pap smear?

Males

Do you practice testicular self-examination?

Females and Males

Health promotion activities? What type? Frequency?

Have you had any discharge, itching, swelling, genital surgery?

Any STDs? Frequency? Treatment? Outcomes?

Medical conditions? Injuries? Medications, prescribed and nonprescribed?

Amount, type; frequency of alcohol, tobacco, other drugs?

Psychiatric conditions? Appearance, mood, state.

Social and Sexual Activity

How would you describe your social life? Often feel lonely? What do you do about these feelings?

Have you ever been sexually active? Currently sexually active?

How would you describe your current sexual activity? Satisfactory/unsatisfactory? What would you change?

Is it a problem for you being sexually active? How so? Or if not sexually active, how have you dealt with this?

At this time, how important is having a sexual relationship?

How have you dealt with your sexual needs since changing your status (ie, becoming single/unattached/divorced)?

Do you ever feel guilty or anxious about anything pertaining to your sexual lifestyle/behavior?

What types of sexual practices do you engage in? Penile–vaginal intercourse? Oral–genital sex? Anal sex?

Are you aware of sexual practices that may put you at risk? What do you do to protect yourself?

Have you had a past sexual trauma? Treatment or counseling received?

Sexual Function

Do you feel that you have a sexual problem? For how long? Did you always have this problem? What happens?

Are you interested in having sex? All the time? Some of the time? Never?

Does the thought of sex make you fearful or anxious? Do you avoid it?

Do you ever have difficulty becoming sexually aroused?

Males

Do you ever have difficulty achieving or maintaining an erection?

Have you noticed any change in the rigidity, size, or circumference of your penis? Other changes?

Do you feel you ejaculate too quickly? Too slowly? Unable to ejaculate in the vagina? Other?

Females

Do you have difficulty becoming lubricated?

Do you tighten up before intercourse so that penile insertion is impossible?

Problems reaching orgasm? How often? Under what circumstance?

Females and Males

Do you ever experience pain? On intromission? Thrusting? Orgasm? What happens?

Do you have sexual or other problems with your partner? What are they?

Do you feel your partner has problems? What are they?

Can you communicate your sexual concerns or preference?

Orientation

Have you had/are you in a sexual relationship with someone of your own gender?

Do you consider yourself to be exclusively heterosexual? Bisexual? Exclusively gay/lesbian? Are others aware of your sexual orientation?

How has your sexual orientation affected your life?

General

Do you have any questions about sexuality or sexual function?

Do you want to speak with someone who specializes in sexual problems? Marital issues? Other?

Cues/Clues

Sexual humor, ribald remarks, obscene gestures

Self-deprecation

Genital exposure, public masturbation

Inappropriate touching of care provider or other person

Questions pertaining to sexual relationship of care provider

Statements or questions beginning with "I have a friend who . . . "

Nervousness related to sexual topic

presence of any medical or psychiatric problems. The biologic aspect of the assessment will consider sexual functioning (sexual response cycle) as well as factors that contribute to sexual functioning (eg, rest, nutrition, personal hygiene). The use of alcohol and substances can negatively affect an individual's sexual functioning. A careful medication history is important when assessing sexual functioning because so many medications have a negative effect on sexual performance (see Chap. 10).

An important assessment area is determining how comfortable the person is with her own sexuality and her own body. Is the inability to have an orgasm recent? Has she ever experienced orgasms? Under what conditions? Does she masturbate, and is orgasm reached? Nonverbal communication is just as important as verbal communication when discussing sexual functioning. A disgusted look on a patient's face when discussing masturbation is a clear indication that she is not comfortable with self-stimulation.

Interventions. The planning process for nursing intervention requires mutual collaboration from assessment to evaluation, sharing the purpose of assessment, and establishing priorities. Intervention is based on the patient's needs, nursing diagnosis, problem severity, and nurse's competence (Fig. 27-1). The assessment data usually lead to a nursing diagnosis of either Ineffective Sexuality Patterns or Sexual Dysfunction. Ineffective

Sexuality Patterns is used as the nursing diagnosis if the person is at risk for or has already experienced a change in sexual functioning. Sexual Dysfunction refers to problematic sexual function that the individual perceives as unsatisfying, unrewarding, or inadequate and for which nursing can intervene. Sexual Dysfunction can be used as a nursing diagnosis when patient characteristics include problems with sexual relationships, value conflicts, frequent need to confirm desirability, sexual dissatisfaction, and change of interest in self and others. This diagnosis is also used by physicians and therapists to describe a disruption in any of the phases of the human sexual response cycle.

Physical health and fitness enhance sexuality. Getting adequate rest, maintaining optimal nutrition, and exercising regularly promote sexual health. Nurses should be aware of the processes, techniques, and adaptive devices that can improve the sexual function of patients, particularly those who report impaired sexual response. For example, patients can be taught the benefits of using imagery and fantasy in lovemaking, increasing foreplay, being flexible in timing sexual interactions, improving hygiene, using adaptive positions for intercourse, or using a vibrator. Explaining the dynamics of sexual response and facilitating sexual communication between partners are also important nursing actions.

Adults with chronic illness and those who have become disabled after marriage experience other psycho-

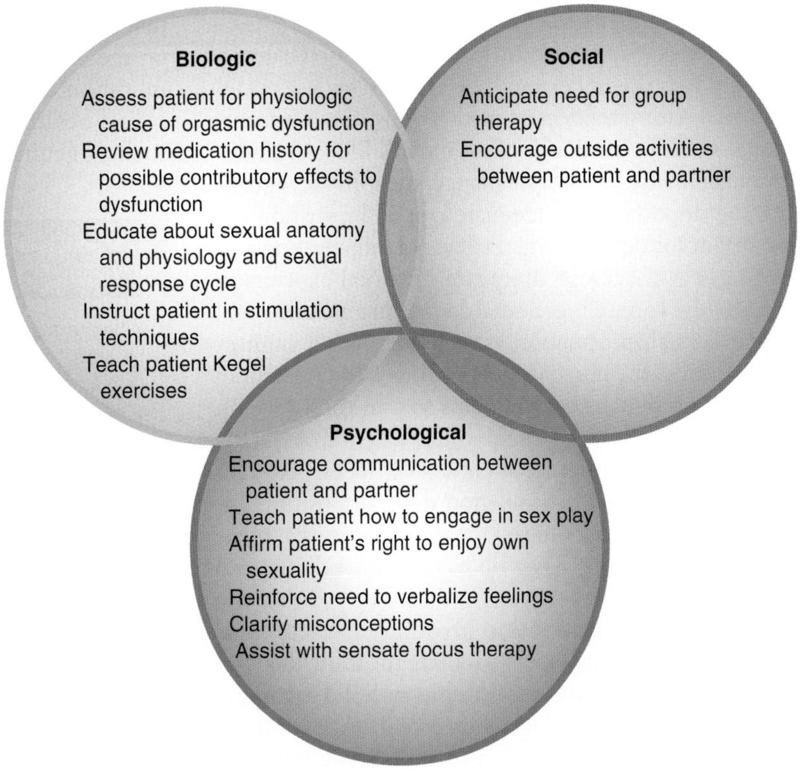

FIGURE 27.1 Biopsychosocial interventions for patients with female orgasmic disorder.

sexual stressors due to problems with sensation, movement, body structure, fertility, energy, or negative self-image or by affecting the partner's motivation. Disabled women may require assistance with menstrual hygiene. Pregnancy, though usually possible, can pose risks that include hypertension, decubitus ulcers, premature labor, or inability to perceive labor. Contraception may also be more difficult when the birth control pill is contraindicated, as in the woman with a spinal cord injury, or when the individual is unable to manipulate a diaphragm or a condom, as might occur with cerebral palsy. A patient's impairment often requires altering standard positioning for pelvic or rectal examinations.

Nurses should be aware that most individuals who report difficulties with sexual response often benefit from factual information and helpful suggestions and are not in need of sex therapy. However, when longstanding, highly complex problems have been assessed, it is better to refer the individual or couple to a formally trained, certified sex therapist.

Psychological Domain

Assessment. The psychological assessment focuses on the woman's self-concept and body image. A poor self-concept can prevent a woman from engaging in sexual relationships. Mood states, such as chronic depression and grief, also seriously affect the woman's ability to have an orgasm. The amount of stress and its relationship to the ability to relax and focus on her own sexuality are important assessment data. Very important are the quality of her relationship and her partner's ability to meet her sexual needs.

The woman's sexual knowledge should also be determined. Does she understand the sexual response cycle? Knowledge of the effect of medications, the hormonal changes that occur during the woman's life cycle (adolescence, menstruation, pregnancy, menopause, aging), and the importance of adequate rest and nutrition are important for determining the level of intervention.

Interventions. Any alteration in sexual expression may require counseling. Sexual counseling includes providing factual information as well as offering suggestions. Ideally, the nurse will help patients to understand the basis of their sexual problems so that they develop problem-solving skills. Patients often benefit from learning how to communicate their sexual needs better in such areas as type of stimulation desired, positioning, and amount of time required for maximum sexual pleasure. The nurse may also wish to recommend resource materials.

Interpersonal relationship problems are often the basis for orgasmic problems. Helping the individual examine the quality of the relationship with the partner is the first step in psychological interventions. Communication skills training to improve dialogue between partners is effective in treating secondary orgasmic dysfunction (McCabe & Delaney, 1992). This teaches partners to listen, verbalize, reflect feelings, manage conflict, and use assertive behavior. However, much less success was seen with secondary orgasmic dysfunction resulting from marital disharmony. This suggests the need to combine various interventions with marital therapy (see Psychoeducation Checklist: Female Orgasmic Disorder).

Sex education is the process of teaching factual information and helping individuals to develop healthy sexual behaviors and attitudes. Sex education as a single treatment mode has not been effective, although teaching about anatomy and physiology, sexual behaviors and response, and clarification of misconceptions remain an important intervention. The provision of sex education represents conscious cultivation of sexual potential by assisting individuals to understand, adjust, and enjoy their sexuality according to their desire and opportunities. However, a number of groups, such as elderly people and those with identifiable physical or mental disability, have been viewed as sexually oppressed and have not been the recipients of such education. For the nurse working with chronically ill individuals, sex education might include sexual anatomy and physiology, sexual response, hygiene, risk factors, the effect of various illnesses and drugs on sexual function, and methods to minimize negative effects. Parents with developmentally disabled children often benefit from anticipatory guidance.

The role of the nurse who works with young adults may be one of assisting in the transition from reliance on the family for health care and health advice to promoting independent health decisions, teaching about sexual health, and explaining unfamiliar procedures, such as genital examinations or Papanicolauo's (Pap)

PSYCHOEDUCATION CHECKLIST
Female Orgasmic Disorder

When caring for the patient with female orgasmic disorder, be sure to include the following topics in your teaching plan for the patient and partner:

• Possible etiologic factors
• Anxiety reduction techniques
• Communication skills
• Sexual preferences
• Sexual play
• Sensate focus
• Kegel exercises
• Erotic fantasy
• Group therapy
• Sex therapy

smears. Young women often prefer same-gender health professionals to perform genital examinations and may be more at ease with the gynecologic nurse practitioner.

Developmentally disabled adults are capable of learning about sex through the use of models and repetitious language. Nurses have the opportunity to teach acceptable standards of behavior and to protect this population from sexual exploitation or abuse and report incidents if they become aware. **Advocacy** includes preventing involuntary sterilization. Some states require that the patient be represented by a court-appointed lawyer who argues against sterilization. Parents and medical staff are not involved, especially when parents may be the ones who desire the sterilization.

Although most patients may be helped with competent sexual counseling, some patients with sexual dysfunctions will require sex therapy. **Sex therapy** blends education and counseling along with psychotherapy and specific sexual exercises. In referring a patient to a sex therapist, the nurse must ascertain that the therapist is certified by the American Association of Sex Educators, Counselors and Therapists (AASECT). Generally, the skill required to practice sex therapy surpasses the expertise of the nurse, although nurses have become sex therapists through advanced education and supervised clinical experience.

Elderly patients with emotional or functional sexual problems should be given treatment, be it hormonal replacement therapy or counseling. Sex therapy is appropriate at any age because sexual dysfunction, even when long-standing, can be reversed (Masters & Johnson, 1970).

Poor physical health and lack of a partner are often common barriers to sexual continuity for older adults. Other barriers include lack of privacy or institutionalization, where elderly may be overmedicated to prevent sexual "acting out." Sensory and sexual deprivation may lead to sexual regression or the unconscious sexualization of eating, urination, and defecation.

Demographically, elderly women outlive men, are often less ill than men, are younger at widowhood than men, and statistically outnumber men. Additionally, the need for a socially approved, legal partner; reticence to seek extramarital partners; proscriptions against dating or marrying a younger man; and difficulty taking the initiative in sexual activity present greater sexual barriers for women. Women may consciously suppress their sexual interest to cope with the loss of a partner or the partner's sexual ability.

Lack of knowledge about the impacts of aging or health conditions on sexuality, the normality of continued sexual desire and interest, and the alternatives for sexual gratification may inhibit sexual activity. This may be detrimental because maintaining sexual activity and interest are positive forms of exercise for the mind and body and deterrents to suicide. Patients may also require that their sexual rights, choices, and personal dignity be protected by an advocate.

Patients may need assistance with problem solving and assertiveness. When an individual has a condition that might be passed on to offspring or that impairs the individual's ability to parent, decisions about reproduction, such as whether to have a child or an abortion, may be especially difficult. The nurse must be able to explore options with the patient, help the patient make choices without undue personal or outside influence, and support the patient's decision. Sexual advocacy can also involve the facilitation of privacy and space for conjugal visits for the individual who is institutionalized as well as challenging policies that separate married couples or prevent sexual contact between consenting adults through medication or other methods (Krozy, 1984).

Social Domain

Assessment. The social dimension is important in the area of sexuality. Is the patient's gender identity (sense of being male or female) the same as her sex role identity (outward expression of her gender)? Living within a heterosexual relationship when the gender and sex role identities are not the same could seriously affect the patient's ability to experience sexual satisfaction. Some women reach adult life, have a male partner, and have children, but never experience orgasm until they have a female partner. For these women, successful treatment of their orgasmic disorder may mean a complete change in lifestyle.

Cultural and family values play an important role in understanding a patient's response to orgasmic dysfunction. Lifestyle disruptions, a birth of a child, a move to another city, or a change in financial or social status may coincide with sexual dysfunction.

Interventions. Women with orgasmic dysfunction can benefit from a support group that includes women with similar problems. Group modalities, such as psychoeducation groups, are useful in helping patients decrease their embarrassment and uneasiness about sexual topics and increase their knowledge. Partner support is critical and should be encouraged throughout treatment.

Evaluation and Treatment Outcomes. Outcomes related to sexual functioning cannot be developed without the patient because they are too personal. Examples of specific behavioral outcome statements include the following:

- Correctly describes sexual anatomy and physiology
- Correctly identifies relationship between drug therapy and sexual dysfunction
- Verbalizes satisfaction with alternate mode of sexual expression

- Seeks further information by requesting written material
- States positive change in sexual relationship with partner
- Correctly explains proper use of contraceptive
- Reports improved body image with breast prosthesis (or reconstructive surgery)

Evaluation of nursing interventions for patients with altered sexual expression or sexual dysfunction is an important aspect of the nursing process. Because the patient and nurse collaborate throughout the nursing process, the patient outcomes are based on the patient's expectations. Outcomes range from learning about anatomy and physiology to improving body image to enhance sexuality.

Nursing Care Plan 27-1 demonstrates the nursing process in a patient with multiple sclerosis who has developed altered sexual expression and sexual dysfunction.

Premature Ejaculation

Premature ejaculation is a male orgasmic disorder defined as (1) the inability to control ejaculation before, during, or shortly after intromission; and (2) ejaculation before the individual desires it. Diagnostic characteristics are listed in Table 27-5. Premature ejaculation may be recurrent or persistent and is either primary, lifelong, or secondarily acquired. It may occur only in certain situations or may be generalized, occurring in almost all situations regardless of partner, location, or present life situation. Premature ejaculation is not diagnosed in a man whose difficulty is caused by drug or alcohol abuse. In those cases, a substance abuse diagnosis is made, with the sexual disorder generally resolving once the substance abuse is treated. Psychological causes are implicated in most cases.

A marked degree of distress about the prematurity of the ejaculation needs to be present to diagnose the disorder. An occasional episode of premature ejaculation is not considered dysfunctional. The age of the male, the contentment within his relationship, current life stressors, preexisting medical conditions, medication use, past sexual experience, and recent sexual activity are all areas to be carefully assessed when trying to determine whether dysfunction is actually present.

Epidemiology. Premature ejaculation has been viewed as the most common male sexual dysfunction, affecting up to 40% of adult men at some point in their lifetime. Unlike erectile dysfunction, which has been studied formally and for which most sexual therapy is sought, information on premature ejaculation has arisen primarily through self-report. It is estimated that about 27% of men seeking treatment report premature ejaculation as a problem. Many cases are unreported. Even when it

is not defined as a problem by the man, it still affects partner satisfaction.

Etiology. Current theories about the etiology of premature ejaculation point to an interaction of psychogenic and organic factors. Although premature ejaculation may arise from a purely organic cause, performance anxiety and fear of negative outcomes may be additional triggers. Interestingly, when tested in self-stimulation studies, eliminating these factors to a great degree, premature ejaculators still reached orgasm in half the time as nonpremature ejaculators. This may be a result of heightened sympathetic dominance early in the sexual response cycle (Rowland & Burnett, 2000).

Premature ejaculation frequently begins in the teen years when sexual activity is beginning and delaying orgasm has not been learned. It may occur after a period of abstinence or, on occasion, an older man will lose the learned ability to delay the ejaculation and seek treatment. Neurobiologic impairment of ejaculatory reflex, both in premature and retarded ejaculation, has also been reported.

Nursing Management. The problem of premature ejaculation will come to the attention of the nurse during a thorough health history that includes specific sexual data. It is unlikely that the nurse will be seeing the patient primarily for sexual dysfunction. Through a careful assessment, the generalist psychiatric–mental health nurse can determine whether the problem is causing distress to the individual. If so, the nurse can explore with the patient the possibility of further assessment and treatment. Patients need assurance that many men have similar problems and that treatment is possible (see Psychoeducation Checklist: Premature Ejaculation).

In addition to counseling, sensate focus is used to treat premature ejaculation. This involves "paradoxical intent," whereby the couple is asked not to engage in intercourse or any other sexual activity until directed to do so. Prohibiting the activities that cause frustration decreases performance anxiety. Both partners are taught to give and receive pleasure in a nondemanding way while learning what each finds desirable.

After several days of sensate focus, patients shift to using the "squeeze technique," pressing the frenulum of the penis and the area on the opposite side, just above and below the coronal ridge. This is done with manual stimulation and then with withdrawal after vaginal insertion. Pressure applied to the base of the penis after some control has been achieved may also prolong ejaculation while the penis is contained in the vagina.

With premature ejaculation, the purpose of these exercises is to increase the man's awareness of the sensations occurring before ejaculation, enhance voluntary control, and lengthen the plateau or pre-ejaculatory

(text continues on page 710)

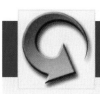

NURSING CARE PLAN 27.1
A Patient With Multiple Sclerosis and Sexual Dysfunction

AD is a 35-year-old woman, happily married for 11 years, and the mother of two children. She attended college, earning a master's degree in education. She has been employed as a sixth grade teacher but is currently not working.

AD was diagnosed with multiple sclerosis 3 years ago. She is being seen for a periodic check-up by the nurse practitioner. Some of Ms. Davidson's present symptoms include transitory visual blurring, weakness of the lower extremities, and mood swings. She also has had problems with urinary leakage and occasional bowel incontinence. She admits, with some obvious discomfort, that she is experiencing sexual difficulty and that her sexual activity is far less frequent than before her illness. Although AD claims her husband has remained attentive and affectionate, she feels she is no longer attractive nor able to fulfill her functions as a wife. She says she wouldn't blame her husband if he found someone else.

Physical examination has demonstrated decreased sensation and reflexes in lower extremities, decreased hand grasp, slight delayed blink response and nystagmus, clear speech pattern, nondistended bladder, normal bowel sounds, BP 124/76, P 76, R 24. Patient wears absorbent pad for urinary incontinence with slight odor of urine. Is weepy, wrings hands, and eyes are downcast when discussing marital relationship. Husband accompanied patient to appointment, holding her hand in waiting room. Offered to be present during examination or answer questions if desired.

SETTING: OUTPATIENT CLINIC

Baseline Assessment: AD is a 35-year-old, happily married woman diagnosed with multiple sclerosis 3 years ago. Present symptoms: visual blurring, weakness of extremities, mood swings, urinary leakage, occasional bowel incontinence. Experiencing decreased sexual enjoyment, low self-esteem, low body image. Has had difficulty experiencing orgasm for 2 years. Has difficulty communicating needs.

Associated Psychiatric Diagnosis	*Medications*
Axis I: Female orgasmic disorder Rule Out: Major depressive episode Axis II: None Axis III: Multiple sclerosis Axis IV: Primary support group (discord with husband) Axis V: GAF = Current 70 　　　　　　　Potential 85	Interferon-β (Betaseron) 8 mIU (0.25 mg) subcutaneously every other day Oxybutynin (Ditropan) 5 mg tid

NURSING DIAGNOSIS 1: INEFFECTIVE SEXUALITY PATTERNS

Defining Characteristics	*Related Factors*
Feels unattractive, can't fulfill roles, would understand husband finding another woman. "How would you feel if you had an 'accident' right before you were supposed to make love?" States husband has remained attentive, considerate, but believes it's because he feels pity. States she has moods, ". . . really feeling sorry for myself. I suppose . . . I'm depressed . . . frustrated . . . MS affects you that way."	States she often feels tired and weak. Has some difficulty with mobility, requires assistance with bathing in tub and fastening back buttons and hooks. Frequently has urinary incontinence and occasional loss of bowel control. States she is usually unable to hold urine and sometimes bowels. Satisfactory sexual relationship before onset of illness, although had difficulty verbalizing sexual needs. Altered self-esteem Chronic illness

OUTCOMES

Initial	*Long-Term*
1. Patient and partner will identify three barriers and three enhancers to effective communication regarding their sexual needs and problems.	2. Patient will adapt to limitations and regain positive body image. 3. Patient and partner will experience comfortable and satisfactory sexual expression.

(continued)

NURSING CARE PLAN 27.1 (Continued)

INTERVENTIONS

Interventions	Rationale	Evaluation
Deficient Knowledge Educate patient and family; provide written materials; encourage questions.	Patients and families need factual information on the trajectory, treatment, and impact of multiple sclerosis.	Patient and partner correctly explain emotional aspects and pathophysiology of multiple sclerosis.
Communication Demonstrate empathy for the patient's difficulty in communicating sexual needs.	Talking about sex makes some people embarrassed.	Patient and partner correctly identify factors that promote or impede their communication.
Explain common reasons for experiencing difficulty when discussing sexual issues.	Individuals may not know how to phrase what they mean. They may be afraid of insulting their partner or have religious or cultural taboo.	Couple increase comfort in discussing sexual needs.
Emphasize the importance of being able to tell each other what is personally satisfying.	Clear communication is more successful than "telepathy."	Patient able to identify need for more time and foreplay.
Help patients establish effective communication patterns by using role play or teaching assertive communication skills, ie, beginning statements with "I really like it when you. . . ."	Becoming assertive often requires changing male/aggressive and female/passive learned behavior patterns. Use of a fictional situation that can be role played and analyzed is an instructive nonthreatening model for learning new behaviors.	Patient and partner report more open communication, which allows more sharing of true feelings and fears.
Encourage the establishment of a consistent, mutually agreeable, relaxed time to talk.	Communication is easier when it is planned and viewed as a value.	Patient and partner report that communication is improved by allotting one-half hour for "together time" each evening.
Encourage use of support or self-help groups.	Communication can be enhanced through sharing thoughts, feelings, and experiences with others.	Has contacted Multiple Sclerosis Society.
Describe sexual concerns commonly identified by partners.	Partner may feel guilt about sexual desire when mate is ill; fear of harming, increasing discomfort, or overburdening mate; difficulty when mate assumes caretaking and lover role, often helped by use of a home health aide.	Couple beginning to address issues; express difficulty in adapting to the current and inevitable changes of the disease; express fear of complete loss of function in all aspects of function, not just sexuality.
Disturbed Body Image/ Altered Self Concept related to illness and change in function.	Common sequelae of chronic illness.	Patient able to express thoughts and feelings about the effects of the disease.
Help patient confront reality but identify positive aspects of personality.	Allows patient to focus on health function and inner being.	Sees self as good mother, teacher, wife.
Encourage patient to maintain good hygiene, dress attractively, use grooming aids such as perfume, treat self to manicure.	Optimizing appearance is a mood enhancer.	States she is having friend take her to hairdresser every other week, bought new outfit through catalog.
Fatigue/Weakness Identify optimal time for sexual interaction.	Decreases stress; increases relaxation.	Reports using time when children are with grandparents for intimacy.
Do not eat or drink before activity.	Decreases expenditure of energy and potential for incontinence.	Able to cite correct rationale for food/fluid limitations.
Teach use of side-lying or rear entry position during intercourse.	Decreases energy expenditure of patient.	Reports ability to use these positions.
Use pillows to support weakened extremities.	Assists positioning when there is muscle weakness.	Reports increased satisfaction in sexual activity when pillows used for positioning.

NURSING CARE PLAN 27.1 (Continued)

INTERVENTIONS

Interventions	Rationale	Evaluation
Inform patient of effect of medications being taken.	Some drugs cause impaired sexual response and fatigue.	Not applicable at this time.
Impaired Mobility Teach active or passive range-of-motion exercises.	Helps to prevent contractures.	Has been evaluated by physical therapist; reports range-of-motion exercises done twice daily.
Consider use of a waterbed. Teach possibility and treatment of contractures or adductor spasms.	Assists with movement. Antispasmodics may be needed and are effective when taken 10–15 min before sexual activity.	Not applicable at this time.
Bladder Incontinence For urinary leakage teach to empty bladder in accordance with prescribed bladder training program. Discuss decreasing fluids a few hours before sexual activity, having padding or towels on hand. Before sexual activity, void on cue or via intermittent catheterization. If indwelling catheter, may advise temporary removal or moving clamp and taping catheter to one side.	To maximize urinary function, bladder training should be initiated as early as possible. These techniques decrease urinary leakage or incontinence; protect bed linens if accident occurs. Permits patient with urinary retention or indwelling catheter to have coitus.	Reports following bladder training program. Patient empties bladder and decreases fluid before attempting sexual intercourse; pads bed. If indwelling catheter, tapes catheter over abdomen.
Bowel Incontinence Establish a regular bowel program. Cover bed linens with towels.	Helps decrease occurrence of accidental bowel elimination; may require use of suppository or enema. Helps prepare for accidents.	Reports following a regulated bowel training program.

NURSING DIAGNOSIS 2: SEXUAL DYSFUNCTION

Defining Characteristics	Related Factors
Verbalizes difficulty with vaginal lubrication occasional discomfort and decreased genital sensations; "weird feelings," during orgasm; frequent inability to achieve orgasm; some loss of desire.	Disease process; knowledge deficit; difficulty verbalizing sexual needs.

OUTCOMES

Initial	Long-Term
1. Patient and partner will cite at least five effects of multiple sclerosis on sexual function and at least five adaptive methods to promote satisfactory sexual expression.	2. Patient and partner will use methods that minimize the psychological and organic effects of multiple sclerosis on sexual function. 3. Patient and partner will experience comfortable and satisfactory sexual expression.

INTERVENTIONS

Interventions	Rationale	Evaluation
Deficient Knowledge Teach sexual effects of multiple sclerosis.	Disease precipitates numerous biopsychosocial effects.	Patient and partner correctly explain emotional aspects and pathophysiology of disease and its relationship to sexual dysfunction.

(continued)

NURSING CARE PLAN 27.1 (Continued)

INTERVENTIONS

Interventions	Rationale	Evaluation
Suggest sexuality handbook from local chapter of Multiple Sclerosis Society and resources for self-help, counseling, and respite.	Resources include: MS Toll-Free Information 1-800-FIGHT-MS (1-800-344-4687)	Sexual information requested from the Multiple Sclerosis Society.
Identify local resources, ie, individual service providers, Planned Parenthood, hospital departments of sexual health care, national organizations offering professional and nonprofessional sexual information.	Sex Information and Educational Council of the United States (SIECUS) 130 W. 42nd St. Suite 350 New York, NY 10036	
Dyspareunia		
	Multiple sclerosis can cause unusual sensations, but this effect is often transitory.	Able to cite rationale for sensations, but finds them distressing.
Rule out or treat infection.	Infectious processes can cause painful intercourse.	No infection noted on examination.
Decreased Lubrication		
Substitute natural lubrication with water-based lubricant such as K-Y jelly; benefits of oral sex and lubricating effect of saliva.	Vaginal dryness is a result of disease as well as stress.	Dyspareunia lessened with K-Y jelly.
Teach need for relaxation.	Sexual function is greatly affected by stress.	Report more relaxation during intimacy when children at grandparents' home.
Teach partner to increase foreplay and stimulation.	When sensations decreased, longer and more direct stimulation is required.	
Secondary Orgasmic Dysfunction		
Encourage discussion of concerns.	Often fear rejection or abandonment.	Reports communication has improved.
Suggest individual or couples counseling if difficulties cannot be resolved.	If partner planning to leave, refer patient/family for social and other necessary support services.	Not applicable at this time.
Assess mental status.	Depression may result from organic or psychological factors; may also require medication.	Demonstrates appropriate level of grieving; may need counseling at later time.
Teach experimenting with new erotic areas, techniques, ie, fantasy, visual aids.	Enhances excitement and orgasmic stages of sexual response.	Have not begun yet.
If sex therapy desired or necessary, refer to AASECT-certified sex therapist only.	Important to access qualified counselor.	Not desired at this time.

phase of the response cycle. When some control has been demonstrated, the couple proceed first to penile insertion with the woman on top with no thrusting to gradual and then full thrusting. Couples are taught to practice the squeeze technique periodically after therapy.

Pharmacologic treatment to delay ejaculation is being studied, with clomipramine and paroxetine showing promising results in controlled studies (Schiavi & Segraves, 1995; McMahon & Touma, 1999). Other techniques include topical anesthetics applied to the head of the penis to decrease sensation, and distraction (ie, focusing on negative or nonstimulating thoughts); the latter has had limited success but is often viewed as depersonalizing.

Male Orgasmic Disorder

Male orgasmic disorder, formerly called *ejaculatory incompetence* and later *inhibited male orgasm*, is the inability to ejaculate into the vagina (Masters & Johnson, 1970).

TABLE 27.5 Key Diagnostic Characteristics for Premature Ejaculation 302.75

Diagnostic Criteria	Target Symptoms and Associated Findings

• Persistent or recurrent ejaculation with minimal sexual stimulation before, on, or shortly after penetration and before the person wishes it.
• Not better accounted for by another Axis I disorder
• Not exclusively a direct physiologic effect of a substance or medical condition
   Lifelong type: present since onset of sexual functioning
   Acquired type: develops after a period of normal functioning
   Generalized type: not limited to certain types of stimulation, situations, or partners
   Situational type: limited to certain types of stimulation, situations, or partners
   Due to psychological factors: psychological factors play major role in onset, severity, exacerbation, or maintenance of the sexual dysfunction
   Due to combined factors: psychological factors play a role in onset, severity, exacerbation, or maintenance of sexual dysfunction and a general medical condition or substance use is also contributory but not sufficient enough to account for the sexual dysfunction
	• Association with sexual anxiety, fear of failure, concerns about sexual performance, fear of embarrassment
	• Disruption of existing marital or sexual relationships or fear of initiating new relationships

The APA's (2000) *Diagnostic and Statistical Manual of Mental Disorders*, 4th edition, Text revision (*DSM-IV-TR*) defines it as the persistent or recurrent delay in achieving orgasm following normal excitement. Diagnostic characteristics are given in Table 27-6. This dysfunction may result from congenital genitourinary anomalies, drugs, or other impairments of the sympathetic nervous system, such as spinal cord injury (Althof & Seftel, 1995). Often, it is viewed as a psychological reaction to negative attitudes about sex, interpersonal problems, or fear of consequences, such as impregnating one's partner. Sensitive dyadic counseling is required, particularly when a woman wishes to conceive.

PSYCHOEDUCATION CHECKLIST
Premature Ejaculation

When caring for the patient with premature ejaculation, be sure to include the following topics in your teaching plan for the patient and partner:

• Possible etiologic factors
• Pharmacologic agents, if indicated, including drug, dosage, action, frequency, and possible adverse effects
• Measures to decrease anxiety performance
• Communication skills
• Sexual counseling
• Sensate focus
• Sex therapy

Separate or combined interventions include vibratory and electrical stimulation; sensate focus, which gradually teaches the man to transfer the sensation of ejaculatory demand from manual stimulation to intravaginal ejaculation; and psychotherapy.

Sexual Arousal Disorders

Male Erectile Disorder

The diagnosis of male erectile disorder was formerly referred to as *impotence*, a term now considered pejorative. **Erectile dysfunction** refers to the inability of a man to achieve or maintain an erection sufficient for completion of the sexual activity. Although most men experience an occasional lack of erection, intervention is required when there is consistent (more than a year) erectile inefficiency during masturbation, intercourse, or on awakening.

Epidemiology. Estimates of the number of American men experiencing erectile dysfunction range from 10 to 20 million, accounting for the most common complaint for which sex therapy is sought (Feldman et al., 1994). This prevalence is believed to be the basis for the establishment of Impotence Anonymous for patients and I-ANON for partners. Public discussion of this problem has emerged because, until recently, psychological causes were blamed for most erectile dysfunction; it is now believed that 60% or more of the cases have an organic basis. Erectile dysfunction may occur at any age,

TABLE 27.6   Summary of Key Diagnostic Characteristics of Sexual Disorders

Disorder	Diagnostic Characteristics
Other Sexual Disorders	• Marked distress or interpersonal difficulty • Not better accounted for by another Axis I disorder • Not a direct physiologic effect of a substance or general medical condition
Premature ejaculation 302.75	• As listed above for other sexual disorders • Persistent or recurrent onset of orgasm and ejaculation with minimal stimulation; occurring before, on, or shortly after penetration before the person wishes

Hypoactive sexual desire disorder
302.71
	• As listed above for other sexual disorders
	• Deficiency or absence of sexual fantasies or desire for sexual activity
	    Global low sexual desire encompassing all forms of sexual expression or situational low sexual desire
	    Lack of initiating sexual activity or reluctantly engages in it when initiated by partner

Female sexual arousal disorder 302.72	• As listed above for other sexual disorders • Persistent or recurrent inability to attain or maintain adequate lubrication or swelling response associated with sexual excitement until completion of sexual activity Lack of pelvic vasocongestion, vaginal lubrication and expansion, and external genitalia swelling

Sexual aversion disorder
302.79
	• As listed above for other sexual disorders
	• Aversion to or active avoidance of genital sexual contact with a sexual partner
	    Anxiety, fear, or disgust when confronted with sexual opportunity
	    Isolated to a particular aspect of sexual experience or generalized revulsion to all sexual stimulation

Male orgasmic disorder 302.74	• As listed above for other sexual disorders • Persistent or recurrent delay in or absence of orgasm after normal sexual excitement phase Inability to reach orgasm during intercourse, but able to ejaculate with manual or oral stimulation
Sexual Pain Disorders	• Marked distress or interpersonal difficulty • Not caused by vaginismus or lack of lubrication • Not better accounted for by another Axis I disorder • Not a direct physiologic effect of a substance or general medical condition
Dyspareunia 302.76	• As listed above for sexual pain disorders • Genital pain associated with sexual intercourse In both males and females before, during, or after coitus
Vaginismus 306.51	• As listed above for sexual pain disorders • Recurrent or persistent involuntary contraction of the perineal muscles with vaginal penetration Involving the outer one third of the vagina
Paraphilias	• Recurrent intense sexually arousing fantasies, sexual urges, or behaviors Over a period of at least 6 months • Significant distress or impairment in social, occupational, or other important areas of functioning
Exhibitionism 302.4	• Behaviors described above involving exposure of genitals to unsuspecting strangers
Fetishism 302.81	• Behaviors described above involving the use of nonliving objects • Objects not limited to female clothing used in cross-dressing or devices used for tactile genital stimulation
Frotteurism 302.89	• Behaviors described above involving touching or rubbing against a nonconsenting person
Pedophilia 302.2	• Behaviors described above involving sexual activity with prepubescent child or children (13 y and younger) • Perpetrator at least 16 y old and at least 5 y older than child
Sexual masochism 302.83	• Behaviors described above involving real acts of being humiliated, beaten bound, or made to suffer

(continued)

TABLE 27.6 **Summary of Key Diagnostic Characteristics of Sexual Disorders** (Continued)

Disorder	Diagnostic Characteristics
Sexual sadism 302.84	• Behaviors described above involving real acts causing a victim psychological or physical suffering that sexually excites other person
Transvestic fetishism 302.3	• Behaviors described above involving acts of cross-dressing
Voyeurism 302.82	• Behaviors described above involving acts of observing an unsuspecting person who is naked, in process of undressing, or engaging in sexual activity
Paraphilia not otherwise specified 302.9	• Behaviors described above involving obscene phone calls, corpses, focusing on a body part, animals, fires, enemas, or urine
Gender Identity Disorders	• Strong and persistent cross-gender identification Desire to be or insistence that one is of the opposite sex • Persistent discomfort about one's assigned sex or sense of appropriateness in that role • Not a concurrent physical intersex condition • Significant distress or impairment in social, occupational, or other important area of functioning
Sexual disorder not otherwise specified 302.9	• Marked feelings of inadequacy about sexual performance or other traits related to self-imposed standards of gender • Distress about a pattern of repeated sexual relationships Experiencing of others as things to be used • Persistent and marked distress about sexual orientation

although the incidence increases with aging. Men with diabetes, cardiovascular disease, or chronic renal failure also have a higher incidence of erectile dysfunction. Erectile disorders may be subdivided into several types according to the length of time for development, the frequency of occurrence, the type of sexual experience, and the cause of the disorder. A distinction is usually made between biologic and psychogenic cause.

Etiology

Biologic Theories. Although it may be classified as primary (never having occurred) or secondary, this dysfunction may be better categorized according to type: failure to initiate (lack of or faulty innervation), failure to fill (inability of the blood to fill the corpora or for the corpora to expand), and inability to store (related to rapid leakage of blood from the veins) (Goldstein & Rothstein, 1990). Common biologic causes of erectile dysfunction include genital trauma, vascular insufficiency, renal disease, hormonal deficiencies, Parkinson's disease, diabetes, multiple sclerosis, surgical procedures, antihypertensive and antidepressant drugs, and heavy cigarette smoking. It is also more common with the aging process. In psychiatric patients, many of the medications affect sexual functioning.

Psychological Theories. Erectile dysfunction may also have a psychological basis. Numerous psychosocial etiologies have been identified. Fear of failure, relationship stress, poor body image, fear of rejection, partner hostility, guilt, cultural taboos, religious pro-

scriptions, lack of knowledge, and negative attitudes are some of the identified etiologic factors. Not surprisingly, one may observe psychological sequelae to biologically based erectile failure, validating the multifactorial basis often identified and the imperative need to pursue a thorough investigation of causes before instituting a treatment regime.

NURSING MANAGEMENT: HUMAN RESPONSE TO DISORDER

Erectile dysfunction may be related to numerous physical causes—hypertension, diabetes, alcohol dependency or abuse, and obesity. Medications are also implicated in erectile disorder. Treatment of erectile dysfunction requires both a thorough health history and physical examination to seek an organic cause and a psychological evaluation. Erectile dysfunction is often diagnosed by dynamic infusion cavernosometry and cavernosography. This four-part examination consists of (1) creating a drug-induced erection by injection of phentolamine and papaverine and recording the penile blood pressure, (2) infusing saline into the corpora to test storage ability, (3) testing penile arterial blood pressure with ultrasound, and (4) visualizing the storage mechanism of the erect penis by radiography (Goldstein & Rothstein, 1990).

Biologic Domain

Assessment. Most men are not comfortable discussing sexuality and sexual problems. The assessment should be conducted in an atmosphere of trust and understanding. In many cultures, male self-esteem is related to the ability to perform sexually. When a man has problems with maintaining an erection, it is embarrassing and demeaning to him. Sensitivity to the patient's feelings should be reflected throughout the assessment (see Therapeutic Dialogue: Mr. J).

The nursing diagnoses usually generated from the assessment data are similar to those of the female orgasmic disorder—Ineffective Sexuality Patterns or Sexual Dysfunction.

Interventions. Promotion of positive health practices that focus on adequate nutrition, rest, and exercise is important in promoting erectile functioning. Weight loss may improve overall health and enhance the strength of the erection. Regular exercise is also related to sexual health. Helping the patient develop a new lifestyle is important in promoting sexual functioning. Reducing alcohol consumption can also improve sexual performance.

When erection is determined to be permanently impaired, several options may be considered to facilitate intercourse. An external penile prosthesis can be placed over the flaccid penis; some find this not esthetically pleasing. A pumping device that creates a vacuum can be used for blood entrapment, followed by placement of a rubber band at the base of the penis. Surgical techniques for improving vascular sufficiency are also showing promising results.

Surgical implant of a penile prosthesis into each of the corpora has been a popular alternative. Several types exist. Mechanical or nonhydraulic implants may be a pair of semirigid rods that are bent up or down or activated by a switch that shortens a cable and pulls the device into a rigid position. Hydraulic prostheses use pumped fluid to expand hollow cylinders in the corpora. Multicomponent prostheses require implantation of two penile cylinders, a fluid reservoir implanted within the abdomen, a pump in the scrotum, and connective tubing. This system requires extensive surgery. The potential for complications is lessened with use of a two-piece or one-piece prosthesis. The one-piece or self-contained inflatable prosthesis uses a pump implanted on each side of the coronal ridge that transfers fluid from an outer to an inner cylinder; bending the penis releases a valve and detumescence occurs (Goldstein & Rothstein, 1990).

Pharmacologic Interventions. Sildenafil citrate (Viagra) has become the treatment of choice for erectile dysfunction. Sildenafil enhances the effect of nitric oxide, which is released in the corpus cavernosum during sexual stimulation. This medication is rapidly absorbed, with maximum observed plasma concentrations reached within 30 to 120 minutes of oral dosing in the fasted state. Seldenafil is contraindicated in individuals who are using organic nitrates (Pfizer, 2000).

Before the introduction of sildenafil, intracavernosal pharmacotherapy was the treatment of choice for erec-

---

THERAPEUTIC DIALOGUE   Mr. J

Ineffective Approach

Nurse: Mr. J, are you currently sexually active?
Patient: I'm married. Of course, I am.
Nurse: How would you describe your sexual activity?
Patient: OK.
Nurse: What do you mean, OK?
Patient: Just OK. (Getting irritated)
Nurse: Is there a problem?
Patient: Look, I just don't want to talk about it.

Effective Approach

Nurse: Mr. J, are you currently sexually active?
Patient: I'm married. Of course I am.
Nurse: Well, . . . sometimes it can be difficult to maintain a sexual relationship with the same partner over many years.
Patient: Yeah, you got that right.
Nurse: (Silence)
Patient: I wish I were younger. Then, sex was really good.
Nurse: Oh, has it changed?
Patient: Well, yeah.
Nurse: (Silence)
Patient: I just wish I could satisfy my wife.
Nurse: Is there a specific problem, such as becoming aroused, maintaining an erection, having an ejaculation?

Patient: Yes, I can't keep my erection. It's so frustrating.
Nurse: Are you able to become excited?
Patient: That part's OK. I just wish I could keep an erection long enough to satisfy my wife.
Nurse: Have you talked to her about it?
Patient: Yeah, she wants me to go to that clinic.
Nurse: The male sexuality clinic?
Patient: That's the one. Do you know anything about it?
Nurse: Yes, the staff are all well qualified. I would be happy to make a referral for you.

Critical Thinking Challenge

• Compare the course of the first dialogue with the second one. What did the second nurse do differently to elicit information about the patient's erectile dysfunction?

• What is problematic about the first dialogue?

• The nurse in the second dialogue did not continue to ask questions. Instead, this nurse chose to discuss the general topic of sexual relationships within marriage and then made a referral. Debate whether or not the nurse should have pursued more details about the sexual dysfunction.

tile dysfunction. Papaverine hydrochloride, a vascular smooth muscle relaxant, and phentolamine mesylate, a short-acting smooth muscle relaxant and α-blocker are directly injected into the corpus cavernosum by the patient or partner. This increases arterial flow of blood into the corpora and decreases venous outflow. Neurogenic rather than vascular erectile dysfunction appears to respond better. Complications can include excessive bleeding, scarring and priapism, and potential liver involvement. Counseling, strict monitoring, and specific teaching are required (Payton & Goldstein, 1986). Prostaglandin E$_1$, a cardiovascular smooth muscle relaxant, is also used because of its efficiency and lessened incidence of liver damage and priapism compared with papaverine (Robinson, 1994).

Another treatment is the use of alprostadil (prostaglandin) in microsuppository form inserted into the urethra using a special applicator. The system called MUSE causes a rapid absorption of the medication through the urethral mucosa into the corpus spongiosum. It is particularly useful for men unable to inject themselves.

Yohimbine, an α-adrenergic receptor blocking agent and alkaloid plant derivative, has been used as an aphrodisiac to treat erectile dysfunction with some success. Bromocriptine has had similar success but has not been tested in a wide-scale controlled study (Schiavi & Segraves, 1995).

Psychological Domain

Interventions. Education is important for the patient with erectile disorder. Teaching the patient about positive health practices and treatment options (ie, mechanical devices, medications, surgical procedures) is usually needed (see Psychoeducation Checklist: Male Erectile Disorder). The patient's concern about his partner's satisfaction needs to be explored. Many times,

---

PSYCHOEDUCATION CHECKLIST
Male Erectile Disorder

When caring for the patient with male erectile disorder, be sure to include the following topics in your teaching plan for the patient and partner:

- Possible etiologic factors
- Psychopharmacologic agents (such as intracavernosal therapy or yohimbine), including drug, action, frequency, administration technique, and possible adverse reactions
- Alternative methods of sexual expression
- Prosthesis use
- Sexual education and counseling
- Communication skills
- Sex therapy

---

men believe that partner satisfaction is related only to penile penetration and the ability to sustain an erection. Encouraging the patient to talk with his partner about her (or his) sexual needs and other aspects of their sexual experience (physical closeness, kissing, hugging, mutual exploration of their bodies) helps him broaden his understanding of the sexual experience.

Social Domain

Interventions. Men with erectile dysfunction can benefit from supportive men's groups that address sexual issues. Patients should be encouraged to include their partner in lifestyle changes that are being made.

Evaluation and Treatment Outcomes. The major outcome is improved sexual functioning. Acceptance of change of physical status is an outcome that is difficult to obtain. Improvement in sexual satisfaction may include increasing the ability for erectile functioning. If erectile dysfunction is permanent, exploration of other avenues of sexual expression may indicate a successful outcome. In this disorder, partner satisfaction is usually of prime concern. Improved communication with his partner may also be a positive outcome.

Female Sexual Arousal Disorder

Female sexual arousal disorder is a persistent or recurrent inability to attain or maintain an adequate lubrication-swelling response until completion of sexual activity (APA, 2000). A woman may be considered to have sexual arousal disorder if she does not experience a subjective sense of sexual excitement or pleasure related to the physiologic changes associated with sexual arousal and if this causes marked personal or interpersonal distress.

The female sexual arousal disorder may be the least studied of the sexual disorders but more common than we believe, necessitating more accurate assessment and research. Its actual prevalence is unknown because objective measurement of arousal is more difficult for women than for men (Everaerd & Laan, 1994), desire and orgasmic disorders often overlap, and some women may be unaware of having a disorder because of lack of knowledge about their normal anatomy and sexual responses.

A female sexual arousal disorder may occur at any age and is either lifelong or acquired. Although there are usually no visible signs of a sexual arousal disorder, it may cause relationship difficulties and personal stress along with avoidance of sexual activity and impaired communication.

Although not well researched, sexual arousal disorders may be caused by psychological factors, such as anxiety, guilt, and history of sexual abuse, as well as by biophysiologic factors. Changes in androgen levels during the menstrual cycle have been shown to affect arousal. During ovulation, arousal has been found lower than during other times of the menstrual phase, although the basis for this may be related to fear of pregnancy (Silber, 1994). During pregnancy, stimulation in the presence of natural genital vasocongestion may produce less sexual change than it would in a nonpregnant woman, resulting in perceived decreased sexual arousal. Aging also affects sexual arousal because vasocongestion develops more slowly in older women, there is decreased vaginal lubrication after menopause, and lower estrogen levels at this life stage may affect sexual arousal.

Female sexual arousal disorder is hypothesized to result from a negative feedback loop between faulty cognitive and physiologic components (eg, mislabeling bodily cues) (Palace & Gorzalka, 1992). Intervention should aim to modify the negative cognitions and enhance the physiologic response, although there is still question about the interactive mechanisms that mediate arousal.

OTHER SEXUAL DISORDERS

Sexual Desire Disorders

Hypoactive Sexual Desire Disorder

Hypoactive sexual desire disorder has been called *inhibited sexual desire, low libido, sexual anesthesia, general sexual dysfunction,* and *frigidity* (pejoratively applied to women). It refers to a recurrent deficiency or absence of sexual fantasies and desire for sexual activity. It may be primary or secondary and may include all forms of sexual expression or be specific to a partner or activity. Individuals with this disorder report that they are uninterested in sex, do not or cannot get "turned on," and require no sexual gratification. There may be active avoidance of potential sexual relationships.

The population prevalence rate for hypoactive sexual desire is about 20%, with a female-to-male ratio of 2 : 1 (Rosen & Lieblum, 1995). The age of onset for individuals with lifelong forms of hypoactive desire disorder is puberty. Often, the disorder develops in adulthood, after a period of adequate sexual interest, in association with psychological distress, stressful life events (eg, childbirth), or relationship difficulties. It may be continuous or episodic, the latter suggesting problems with intimacy and commitment.

Hypoactive sexual desire can result from depression, stress, aging, endocrine disease, drugs that disrupt the balance of serotonin, dopamine, and hormones as well as illnesses or surgical procedures, making sexual activity unpleasant or uncomfortable. Kaplan (1979) further identifies anxiety, fear, and anger as having the most effect on lowering desire for sexual stimulation.

The disorder may be the primary dysfunction or may be the consequence of emotional distress induced by disturbance in excitement or orgasm. Individuals with hypoactive sexual desire disorder may have diffi-

culties developing stable sexual relationships and may have marital dissatisfaction and disruption. A total lack of interest is likely to have its roots in childhood experiences. Schreiner-Engel and Schiavi (1986) note that there may be a correlation between hypoactive sexual desire and lifelong affective disorder.

Therapy for nonorganic hypoactive sexual desire (as well as hypersexuality) aims at helping the patient to gain insight into the problem and permit erotic impulses to emerge in a naturally appropriate fashion. Depending on etiologic factors, treatment approaches may include individual and couples therapy, sex therapy techniques, clinical hypnosis, cognitive-behavioral therapy, guided fantasy exercises, and sexual assertiveness training. Use of drugs and hormones, however, has not shown much success (Rosen & Lieblum, 1995).

Sexual Aversion Disorder

Sexual aversion disorder is characterized by a phobic reaction to real or anticipated sexual activity and occurs far more frequently in women than men. **Sexual aversion disorder** is defined as a persistent or recurrent extreme discomfort with or avoidance of most or all genital contact with a partner. Manifestations may include nausea, diarrhea, profuse perspiration, and palpitations. It frequently results from a traumatic past sexual experience as well as intrapsychic conflicts about intimacy, sexual guilt, relationship problems, and severely negative parental attitudes about sex. Faith and Schare (1993) found that in both men and women, sexual avoidance was strongly correlated with cognitively fixating on negative body characteristics. Sexual aversion is a significant source of emotional distress and may seriously restrict the individual's ability to form intimate relationships.

Sexual Pain Disorders

Dyspareunia

Dyspareunia is a sexual pain disorder characterized by genital pain in men or women, associated with sexual intercourse. It may occur during intromission or thrusting as well as before or after coitus. In women, it is often a result of interpersonal or emotional factors such as sexual dissatisfaction or poor technique leading to inadequate relaxation and lubrication. Biologic etiologies include intact or biperforate hymen, postmenopausal atrophic changes, trauma, malignancy, intestinal disease, or other pelvic disorders. In men, painful intercourse may result from an irretractable foreskin, localized infection or irritation of the genitourinary tract, intestinal disease or constipation, or trauma. Although rare, male dyspareunia may arise from ejaculatory anxiety, which results in painful, involuntary genital muscle spasm. Resolution consists of identifying and treating organic causes or counseling the patient and partner about techniques such as use of water-soluble lubricants or oral sex to increase readiness.

Vaginismus

Vaginismus is characterized by a psychologically induced spastic, involuntary constriction of the perineal and outer vaginal muscles, fostered by imagined, anticipated, or actual attempts at vaginal penetration. Vaginismus may be an acquired or life-long conditioned response to past episodes of organically caused painful intercourse, negative conditioning, fear of pregnancy, homosexual orientation, or rape. Women in treatment for vaginismus often have a normal sexual drive and have masturbated and experienced orgasm through means other than intercourse (Hawton & Katalan, 1990). Treatment includes a thorough health history and sexologic examination, conjoint sex therapy with a male and female therapist, and instructing the patient to self-insert graduated plastic dilators to reprogram response, as well as teaching normal anatomy and physiology and Kegel exercises.

Priapism

Priapism is a rare condition of prolonged and painful erection, usually without sexual desire, and often the result of a neurologic or vascular impairment. It is not considered a sexual disorder. Patients must be taught that priapism that results from intracavernosal pharmacotherapy (ie, pharmacologic treatment by penile injection for erectile dysfunction) constitutes a medical emergency necessitating pharmacologic reversal. Damage to tissues from ischemia may occur in as little as 4 hours (Sidi, 1988). Treatment often consists of repeatedly withdrawing corporal blood and irrigating the cavernous bodies with a saline–phenylephrine hydrochloride mixture until detumescence occurs; in rare instances, surgical shunting may be necessary.

Sexual Disorder Caused by General Medical Condition

Sexual dysfunction can result from physical illness or physical problems and can be temporary or permanent. Numerous conditions directly impede sexual response by interfering with endocrine levels, blood circulation, respiration, nerve transmission, or mobility, or by creating fatigue or genital or generalized pain. Surgical procedures and drugs may equally affect the body. Ill health can be one of the greatest detriments to sexual expression, not only because it prioritizes energy used toward recuperation, but also because it often lowers an individual's sense of personal worth and attractiveness, prerequisites to seeing oneself as a lover or sexual part-

ner. Physical conditions that commonly affect sexual response are listed in Text Box 27-2.

Substance-Induced Sexual Dysfunction

Substance-induced sexual dysfunction may involve impaired desire, arousal, orgasm, or painful intercourse. It may resemble a primary sexual dysfunction; however, the problem is completely explained by direct physiologic effects of a substance—drug of abuse, medication, or toxic exposure (APA, 2000). The aim of treatment is to eliminate the substance affecting sexual dysfunction. In the case of a necessary medication, interventions that enhance sexual functioning despite the presence of the medication should be considered. Alternative forms of the problematic medication may be available.

Paraphilias

Paraphilias are a group of psychosexual disorders that include sexual behaviors most people would define as unusual, deviant, or perverse (APA, 2000). Characteristics of the paraphilias include recurrent, intense sexual

TEXT BOX 27.2

Medical Conditions and Substances Affecting Sexual Function

- Cardiovascular conditions and vascular conditions
- Endocrine conditions, particularly diabetes mellitus, which causes gradual impotence in 50% of men and orgasmic dysfunction in one third of women
- Cancer or cancer treatments, such as radiation
- Surgery, particularly hysterectomy, mastectomy, prostatectomy, bowel surgery
- Arthritis and neuromuscular disorders
- Spinal cord injury
- Head injury
- Cerebrovascular accident (stroke)
- Organic brain syndrome (senile dementia, Alzheimer's disease)
- Cerebral palsy
- Asthma, emphysema, and chronic obstructive pulmonary disease
- Chronic renal failure
- Obesity
- Localized genital conditions, such as Sjögren's syndrome, balanitis, vulvar ulcers, psoriasis
- Prescription medications (antihypertensive drugs, anticholinergic drugs, some antidepressants)
- Chronic use of most recreational drugs
- Chronic alcohol abuse

urges, fantasies, or behaviors involving unusual objects, activities, or situations that cause emotional distress or impairment in social, occupational, or other areas of functioning. Paraphilic acts often involve a preference for nonhuman objects for sexual arousal or repetitive sexual activity causing real or simulated suffering to consenting or nonconsenting partners.

Another term that has appeared in the literature is **sexual addiction,** defined by Schneider (1988) as out-of-control sexual behaviors that are somewhat tolerated by society (eg, compulsive masturbation, promiscuity, and excess time or money spent on pornography and prostitution), unacceptable (eg, voyeurism, exhibitionism, and obscene calls), and major crimes (eg, rape and incest). Schneider found that sexual addiction responds best to group therapy. Sexaholics Anonymous, fashioned after Alcoholics Anonymous, was formed in California to promote sexual sobriety and restore self-esteem and healthier relationships. Four models of sexual behavior can be defined that defy easy classification (Travin, 1995). These are termed *compulsive sexual behaviors* and may be a symptom of obsessive-compulsive disorder, affect disorder, sexual addiction, or sexual impulse disorder. Nonparaphilic compulsive sexual behaviors may be normative behaviors carried to the extreme.

Paraphilias are rarely diagnosed, although the large commercial market in paraphiliac pornography and paraphernalia suggests a much higher prevalence than that which is presented. One half of the individuals with paraphilias seen clinically are married (APA, 2000). Diagnosis is complicated across cultures because acceptability of sexual practices varies across cultures, except for sexual masochism, for which the gender ratio is 20 men for each woman (APA, 2000). Treatment of paraphilias is rarely sought by the individual; rather, it is a result of the psychosocial or criminal ramifications.

Certain behaviors and fantasies associated with paraphilias are said to begin in childhood and become more elaborate and better defined during adolescence and early adulthood. The disorders are often found to be chronic and lifelong, with the fantasies and behavior diminishing with old age. The following are those classified by *DSM-IV-TR.*

Exhibitionism

Exhibitionism involves exposing one's genitals to strangers, with occasional masturbation. There may be an awareness of the desire to shock the individual or the fantasy that the individual will become sexually aroused on observation of the exposure.

Fetishism

Use of an object for sexual arousal is called **fetishism.** Sexual excitement results when items such as women's undergarments, foot apparel, or other objects are held, rubbed, or smelled. The individual usually masturbates with the item, or it is worn by a partner during sexual activity. Absence of the fetishistic item may result in male erectile dysfunction. Fetishism usually begins in adolescence and continues throughout life.

Frotteurism

Frotteurism is characterized by sexually arousing urges, fantasies, and behaviors resulting from touching or rubbing one's genitals against the breasts, genitals, or thighs of a nonconsenting person. This paraphilia usually begins in early adolescence or young adulthood and diminishes with age.

Pedophilia

Pedophilia involves sexual activity with a child usually 13 years of age or younger by an individual at least 16 years of age or 5 years older than the child. There is often a preference for gender and age range. Pedophilic acts include fondling, oral sex, and anal or vaginal intercourse with the penis, fingers, or objects, with varying amounts of force. Reasons for pedophilic acts are cognitively distorted and include educating the child, providing pleasure, or perceiving the child as sexually provocative.

Sexual abuse is said to occur in at least 156,000 children yearly, with about 15% of all girls and 7% of boys molested by 18 years of age. Child molestation occurs in all economic, social, and cultural groups. Perpetrators, or pedophiles, tend to arise from four groups. Those younger than 18 years of age use the child to experiment with sex; those 35 to 45 years of age often involve their children or friends' children; those older than 55 years of age, who may have central nervous system disease, are responding to stress or may have lost their partner; and the chronic pedophile has a lifelong sexual attraction to children. Although male perpetrators constitute the majority of offenders, various studies report that between 13% and 40% of victims of incest and abuse in day care centers identify women as the abusers (Abel & Rouleau, 1995).

Sexual Masochism

The focus of sexual masochism involves the real act of being humiliated, beaten, bound, or made to suffer. Self-induced masochistic acts include use of electric shock, pin sticking, restraints, and mutilation; partner-induced acts may include bondage, whipping, being urinated or defecated on, and being forced to crawl, bark, or wear diapers. One dangerous form of sexual masochism that may be practiced alone or with a partner is "hypoxyphilia." Oxygen deprivation by means of a noose, plastic bag, chest compression, or drug effect is used during sexual activity to heighten orgasmic sensation. However, deaths have occurred as a result of these techniques.

Sexual Sadism

The focus of sexual sadism involves the real act of experiencing sexual excitement from causing physical or psychological suffering of another individual. Not uncommonly, the individual with sadistic behavior interacts with a masochistic partner. Sadistic behavior includes various forms of physical punishment, use of restraints, rape, burning, stabbing, strangulation, torture, and murder. This is usually a chronic paraphilia that begins as early sexual fantasies and increases in severity over time. When practiced with a nonconsenting partner, it is likely to be repeated until the perpetrator is arrested.

Transvestic Fetishism

Transvestic fetishism applies generally to the heterosexual man who cross-dresses for the purpose of sexual excitement. The fantasies, sexual urges, or behaviors associated with the cross-dressing are recurrent and cause clinically significant distress or impairment in social, occupational, or other important areas of functioning.

Voyeurism

Voyeurism involves "peeping," for the purpose of sexual excitement, at unsuspecting people who are nude, undressing, or engaged in sexual activity.

Paraphilia Not Otherwise Specified

The *DSM-IV-TR* reserves this category for paraphilias not meeting criteria for specific categories. Examples include sexual fantasies, urges, and activities involving animals (zoophilia), corpses (necrophilia), feces (coprophilia), urine (urophilia), body parts (partialism), and obscene telephone calls (telephone scatalogia).

Sexual Disorders Not Otherwise Specified

An example in this *DSM-IV-TR* category is a sexual disorder characterized by distress related to a pattern of repeated sexual relationships and successive lovers who are perceived and used as sexual objects. This may be similar to hypersexuality, formerly called *satyriasis* or *nymphomania*, that Kaplan (1979) defined as a psychological need for continued sexual stimulation.

GENDER IDENTITY DISORDERS

Gender identity disorders are characterized by a strong and persistent identification with the opposite sex and the desire or perception that one is of that gender.

There must also be evidence of persistent discomfort about one's assigned sex or a sense of inappropriateness in the gender role of that sex.

In child clinical samples, there are about 5 boys for each girl referred with this disorder; in adult clinical samples, the ratio is 2 to 3 men for each woman. No recent epidemiologic studies provide data on the prevalence of gender identity disorder (APA, 2000). As a result of extensive population studies in the United States and abroad, Diamond (1993) suggested that about 5% to 6% of men and 2% to 3% of women constitute the gay population, a figure somewhat less than the 10% usually cited. According to Mattison and McWhirter (1995), acceptance of one's identity as gay or lesbian and presenting oneself to the world as such ("coming out") are considered vital to psychological, social, spiritual, and even physical health.

However, positive self-identification can be difficult given the existence of homophobia, prejudice, and stigma. The individual may initially feel self-hatred, with fear of rejection from family and friends. Some marry and have children as a way to suppress their inner knowledge, hide their true orientation, or try to maintain the "normal order" as dictated by society. These individuals, however, are not experiencing gender identity disorder; rather, they are responding to the negative attitudes still promulgated in many sectors of society.

Mattison and McWhirter (1995) report that a well-integrated sexual orientation is highly resistant to change and that attempts to change sexual orientation are not successful. Further, the APA is considering viewing such attempts as malpractice because of the devastating effects on the homosexual individual.

Summary of Key Points

➤ Sexuality is a basic dimension of every individual's personality, undergoing periods of growth and development and influenced by biologic and psychosocial factors.

➤ People can maintain their sexuality throughout their lives. It is a myth that elderly people are not sexually active.

➤ The sexual response cycle consists of four phases: desire, excitement, orgasm, and resolution. Sexual disorders are characterized by changes in sexual desire and sexual response that cause emotional and interpersonal distress.

➤ Female orgasmic disorder is one of the most common disorders affecting women; erectile dysfunction and premature ejaculation are the most common disorders affecting men.

➤ A sexual history is a key part of the nursing assessment. A nurse should be comfortable with his or her own sexuality to collect meaningful assessment data.

➤ Nursing interventions for people experiencing sexual dysfunction include (but are not limited to) counseling, education, and referral to sex therapists.

➤ Various medications negatively affect the sexual response cycle. Education about medication side effects and sexual experiences is important in maintaining health.

➤ Paraphilias are rarely diagnosed, but the prevalence may be higher than usually presented.

➤ Gender identity disorders occur when the individual is uncomfortable with assigned sex or gender role.

Critical Thinking Challenges

1. Compare the physiologic changes of the male and female during the phases of sexual response.

2. A 36-year-old woman was recently diagnosed with depression and treated with a selective serotonin reuptake inhibitor (antidepressant). Her depression is improving, but she has not been interested in sexual relations with her husband. Her lack of sexual interest is beginning to cause problems in her marriage. What could account for the changes in sexual interest? Develop a brief care plan for this patient.

3. Differentiate the sexual disorders of desire, arousal, and orgasm and relate their symptoms to the phases of sexual response.

4. A 52-year-old married man who is being successfully treated with lithium carbonate for his bipolar disorder was recently diagnosed with diabetes mellitus. He was told that his diabetes could be controlled by weight loss and diet. His major worry is that the diabetes and lithium are causing his impotence. He casually mentions that he is considering stopping the lithium. What issues should the nurse explore with the patient? What actions could the patient begin that would improve his sexual health?

5. During a nursing assessment, a young adult woman reveals that she is a lesbian and that she is currently living with her partner. She has not yet told her parents about her sexual orientation and is experiencing some anxiety about sharing this part of her life with her family. Her partner is supportive and encourages the young woman to take her time in telling her family members. Is this patient experiencing symptoms of a gender identity disorder? Explain.

6. A man is having considerable distress about his wife's inability to enjoy sexual relations after the birth of their third child. He has never been unfaithful to his wife but is frustrated with their current relationship. He is considering having an affair with one of his coworkers. What would be the best approach for this patient? Is referral to a sex therapist appropriate?

WEB LINKS

www.priory.com/sex This Sexual Disorders website includes extracts from *Psychiatry in General Practice*, with information on classification, treatment, self-assessment, and referral.

www.med.nyu.edu This site of the New York University School of Medicine provides online sexual disorders screening for men.

www.dr-bob.org This site has psychopharmacology tips from the University of Chicago.

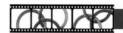

MOVIES

The Birdcage: 1996. In this remake of the 1978 French comedy, *La Cage aux Folles*, Robin Williams stars as Armand Goldman, a gay cabaret owner who lives in Miami's South Beach with his partner Albert, the club's star performer. Armand and Albert must try to disguise their gay relationship when the inlaws of Armand's son, Val, come for dinner.

Viewing Points: Would anyone in the film meet any criteria for having a mental disorder, including a gender identity disorder? Observe your feelings about Armand and Albert's lifestyle.

REFERENCES

Abel, G. G., & Rouleau, J. L. (1995). Sexual abuses. *Psychiatric Clinics of North America, 18*(1), 139–153.

Althof, S. E., & Seftel, A. D. (1995). The evaluation and management of erectile dysfunction. *Psychiatric Clinics of North America, 18*(1), 171–192.

American Pediatrics Association. (1999). Contraception and adolescents. *Pediatrics, 104,* 1161–1166.

American Psychiatric Association. (2000). *Diagnostic and statistical manual of mental disorders* (4th edition, Text revision). Washington, DC: Author.

Beck, J. G. (1995). Hypoactive sexual desire disorder: An overview. *Journal of Consulting and Clinical Psychology, 63*(6), 919–927.

Bogart, L. M., Cecil, H., Wagstaff, D. A., et al. (2000). Is it 'sex'?: College students' interpretations of sexual behavior terminology. *Journal of Sex Research, 37,* 108–116.

Comfort, A. (1974). Sexuality in old age. *Journal of the American Geriatrics Society, 22,* 440–442.

Diamond, M. (1993). Homosexuality and bisexuality. *Archives of Sexual Behavior, 22,* 291–310.

Everaerd, W., & Laan, E. (1994). Cognitive aspects of sexual functioning and dysfunctioning. *Sexual and Marital Therapy, 9,* 225–230.

Faith, M. S., & Schare, M. L. (1993). The role of body image in sexually avoidant behavior. *Archives of Sexual Behavior, 22,* 345–356.

Feldman, H. A., Goldstein, I., & Hatzichristou, D. G. (1994). Impotence and its medical and psychosocial correlates:

Results of the Massachusetts male aging study. *Journal of Urology, 151*(54), 54–61.

Goldstein, I., & Rothstein, L. (1990). *The potent male.* Los Angeles: The Body Press.

Gregoire, A. (1999). Assessing and managing male sexual problems. *British Medical Journal, 318,* 315(1); **http://web1.infotrac.galegroup,** Article A53984541.

Hawton, K., & Katalan, J. (1990). Sex therapy for vaginismus: Characteristics of couples and treatment outcome. *Sexual and Marital Therapy, 5*(1), 31–48.

Kaplan, H. S. (1979). *Disorders of sexual desire and other concepts and techniques in sex therapy.* New York: Simon & Schuster.

Krane, R. J. (1986). Sexual function and dysfunction. In M. F. Campbell (Ed.), *Campbell's urology* (5th ed.) (pp. 700–735). Philadelphia: W. B. Saunders.

Krozy, R. (1978). Becoming comfortable with sexual assessment. *American Journal of Nursing, 78,* 1036–1038.

Krozy, R. E. (1984). Assessment: Sexuality and nursing care. In L. P. Higgins & J. W. Hawkins (Eds.), *Human sexuality across the life span: Implications for nursing practice* (pp. 109–149). Monterey, CA: Wadsworth.

Krozy, R. E. L. (1987). A human sexuality program for older adults: Effect on sexual knowledge and attitudes, attendance factors and outcomes. *Dissertation Abstracts International, 48,* 1123A.

Ladas, A. K., Whipple, B., & Perry, J. D. (1981). *The G spot and other recent discoveries about human sexuality.* New York: Dell Publishing.

Lieblum, S. R. (2000). Redefining female sexual response. *Contemporary OB/GYN, 45,* 120–126.

Masters, W. H., & Johnson, V. E. (1970). *Human sexual inadequacy.* Boston: Little, Brown.

Masters, W. H., & Johnson, V. E. (1966). *Human sexual response.* Boston: Little, Brown.

Mattison, A. M., & McWhirter, D. P. (1995). Lesbians, gay men, and their families. *Psychiatric Clinics of North America, 18*(1), 123–137.

McCabe, M. P., & Delaney, S. M. (1992). An evaluation of therapeutic programs for the treatment of secondary inorgasmia in women. *Archives of Sexual Behavior, 21,* 69–89.

McMahon, C. G., & Touma, K. (1999). Treatment of premature ejaculation with paroxetine hydrochloride. *International Journal of Impotence Research, 11,* 241–246.

Mitchell, D., Grindel, C. G., & Laurenzano, C. (1996). Sexual abuse assessment on admission by nursing staff in general hospital psychiatric settings. *Psychiatric Services, 4,* 159–164.

Morgentaler, A. (1999). Male impotence. *Lancet, 354,* 1713–1718.

Nelson, M. R. (1995). Sexuality in childhood disability. *Physical Medicine and Rehabilitation: State of the Art Review, 9,* 451–462.

Olson, J., & Hanchett, E. (1997). Nurse-expressed empathy, patient outcomes, and development of a middle-range theory. *Image—The Journal of Nursing Scholarship, 29,* 71–76.

Palace, E. M., & Gorzalka, B. B. (1992). Differential patterns of arousal in sexually functional and dysfunctional women: Physiological and subjective components of sexual response. *Archives of Sexual Behavior, 21,* 135–159.

Payton, T. R., & Goldstein, I. (1986). Intracavernosal pharmacotherapy. *Journal of Urological Nursing, 5,* 611–616.

Pfizer. (2000). *Viagra.* Prescribing Information. New York: Pfizer Labs.

Remez, L. (2000). Oral sex among adolescents: Is it sex or is it abstinence? *Family Planning Perspectives, 32,* 298–304.

Risen, C. B. (1995). A guide to taking a sexual history. *Psychiatric Clinics of North America, 18,* 39–53.

Robinault, I. P. (1978). *Sex, society, and the disabled: A developmental inquiry into roles, reactions, and responsibilities.* Hagerstown, MD: Harper & Row.

Robinson, P. (1994). An observational study of prostaglandin E-1: Comparing trial and maintenance dose. *Urologic Nursing, 14*(3), 76–78.

Rosen, R., & Lieblum, S. (1995). Hypoactive sexual desire. *Psychiatric Clinics of North America, 18*(1), 107–121.

Rowland, D. L., & Burnett, A. L. (2000). Pharmacotherapy in the treatment of male sexual dysfunction. *Journal of Sex Research, 37,* 226–236.

Schiavi, R. C., & Segraves, R. T. (1995). The biology of sexual function. *Psychiatric Clinics of North America, 18*(1), 7–22.

Schneider, J. P. (1988). Effective group therapy for sex addicts. *Medical Aspects of Human Sexuality, 22*(7), 42.

Schreiner-Engel, P., & Schiavi, R. C. (1986). Lifetime psychopathology in individuals with low sexual desire. *Journal of Nervous and Mental Disease, 174,* 646–651.

Sidi, A. A. (1988). Vasoactive intracavernous pharmacotherapy. *Urologic Clinics of North America, 15,* 95–101.

Silber, M. (1994). Menstrual cycle and work schedule: Effects on women's sexuality. *Archives of Sexual Behavior, 23,* 397–404.

Strickland, B. (1995). Research on sexual orientation and human development. *Developmental Psychology, 31*(10), 137–140.

Travin, S. (1995). Compulsive sexual behaviors. *Psychiatric Clinics of North America, 18*(1), 155–169.

Wilson, P., & Dibble, S. (1993). Rehabilitation nurses' knowledge of and attitude toward sexuality. *Rehabilitation Nursing Research, 2*(2), 69–74.

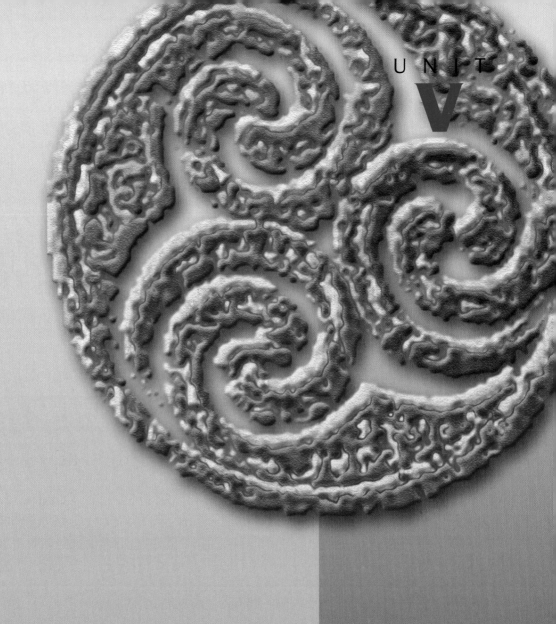

Care of Special Populations

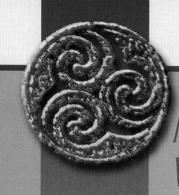

Mental Health Promotion With Children and Adolescents

Catherine Gray Deering and Lawrence Scahill

CHILDHOOD AND ADOLESCENT MENTAL HEALTH

COMMON CHILDHOOD PROBLEMS
Death and Grieving
Preschool-Aged Children

School-Aged Children
Adolescents
Separation and Divorce
Sibling Relationships
Physical Illness
Adolescent Risk-Taking Behaviors

RISK FACTORS FOR CHILDHOOD PSYCHOPATHOLOGY
Poverty and Homelessness
Child Abuse and Neglect
Out-of-Home Placement
Children of Alcoholics

INTERVENTION APPROACHES

LEARNING OBJECTIVES

After reading this chapter, the student will be able to:

➤ Identify protective factors in the mental health promotion of children and adolescents.
➤ Identify risk factors for the development of psychopathology in childhood and adolescence.
➤ Analyze the role of the nurse in mental health promotion with children and families.

attachment
bibliotherapy
child abuse and neglect
developmental delay
early intervention
  programs
family preservation
fetal alcohol syndrome

formal operations
normalization
protective factor
psychoeducational
  programs
risk factor
social skills training

*C*hildren are not miniature adults. They respond to the stresses of life in different ways according to their developmental levels. This chapter examines the importance of childhood and adolescent mental health, discusses the effects of common childhood stressors, identifies stressors that create risk for psychopathology, and provides guidelines for mental health promotion and risk reduction. Nurses are in a key position to identify and intervene with children and adolescents at risk for psychopathology by virtue of their close contact with families in health care settings and their roles as educators. Knowing the difference between normal child development and psychopathology is crucial in helping parents to view their children's behavior realistically and to respond appropriately.

CHILDHOOD AND ADOLESCENT MENTAL HEALTH

Supportive social networks and positive childhood and adolescent experiences maximize the mental health of children and adolescents. Children are more likely to be mentally healthy if they have (1) normal physical and psychosocial development, (2) an easy temperament, and (3) secure **attachment** at an early age. These three areas are considered in the mental health assessment of children (see Chap. 11). **Developmental delays** not only slow the child's progress but also can interfere with the development of positive self-esteem. Children with an easy temperament can adapt to change without intense emotional reactions. A secure attachment helps the child test the world without fear of rejection.

COMMON CHILDHOOD PROBLEMS

Death and Grieving

Loss is an inevitable part of life. All children experience significant losses, the most common being death of a grandparent, parental divorce, death of a pet, and loss of friends through moving or changing schools. Learning to mourn losses can lead to a renewed appreciation of the precious value of life and close relationships. Vast research shows that both children and adults who experience major losses are at risk for the development of psychopathology, particularly if the natural grieving process is impeded. The grieving process differs somewhat for children than for adults (Table 28-1). Children tend to grieve in stages. They begin without understanding the full effects of the loss and experience some numbness or dulling of emotional

TABLE 28.1 Grieving in Childhood, Adolescence, and Adulthood		
Children	**Adolescents**	**Adults**
• View death as reversible: do not understand that death is permanent until about age 7 years	• Understand that death is permanent but may flirt with death (eg. reckless driving, unprotected sex) due to omnipotent feelings	• Understand that death is permanent: may struggle with spiritual beliefs about death
• Experiment with ideas about death by killing bugs, staging funerals, acting out death in play	• May be fascinated by death, enjoy morbid books and movies, listen to rock music about death and suicide	• May try not to think about death, depending on cultural background
• Mourn through activities (eg, mock funerals, playing with things owned by the loved one); may not cry	• Mourn by talking about the loss, crying, and reflecting on it, sometimes becoming dramatic (eg, over-identifying with the lost person, developing poetic or romantic ideas about death)	• Mourn through talking about the loss, crying, reviewing memories, and thinking privately about it
• May not discuss the loss openly, but express grief through regression, somatic complaints, behavior problems, or withdrawal	• Often withdraw when mourning or seek comfort through peer groups; may feel parents do not understand their feelings	• Usually discuss loss openly, depending on level of support available, may feel there is a "time limit" on how long it is socially acceptable to grieve
• Need repeated explanations to fully understand the loss; it may be helpful to read children's books that explain death	• Need permission to grieve openly because they may believe they should act strong or take care of the adults involved; need acceptance of their sometimes extreme reactions	• Need friends, family, and other supportive people to listen and allow them to mourn for however long it takes; need opportunities to review their feelings and memories

pain. This stage progresses to a greater acceptance of the reality of the loss, which leads to more intense psychological pain. Finally, they undergo a reorganization of identity to incorporate the loved person, which may involve engaging in new activities and interests (Van Epps et al., 1997).

Children respond differently to loss according to their developmental level. As early as age 3 years, children have some understanding of the concept of death. For example, the death of a goldfish provides an opportunity for the small child to grasp the idea that the fish will never swim again. Not until about age 7 years, however, can most children understand the permanence of death. Before this age, they may verbalize that someone has "died" but in the next sentence ask when the dead person will be "coming back." Even adolescents sometimes flirt with death by driving dangerously or engaging in other risky behaviors, as if they believe they are immune to death. If the concept of death is difficult for adults to grasp, they should be particularly sensitive to the child's struggle to understand and cope with it. Most children closely watch their parents' response to grief and loss and use fantasy to fill the gaps in their understanding. Many times, family members take turns grieving, with children sensing that their parents are so overwhelmed by their own emotional pain that they cannot bear the children's grief, and parents taking turns being strong for each other.

Preschool-Aged Children

The preschool-aged child may react more to the parents' distress about a death than to the death itself. Because young children depend totally on their parents, they may be frightened when they see their parents upset. Anything the parent can do to alleviate the child's anxiety, such as reassuring him or her that the parent will be okay and continuing the child's normal routine (eg, normal bedtimes, snacks, play times) will help the child to feel secure. Because preschool-aged children have limited ability to verbalize their feelings, they may need to express them through fantasy play and activities such as mock funerals. Books that explain death, such as *Charlotte's Web* by E. B. White, may also be helpful. Parents should take care not to use euphemisms that could fuel misconceptions of death, such as "He went to sleep," "She went on a long journey," or "Jesus took him." Young children may interpret these messages literally and fear going to sleep (because they might die) or focus their natural, grief-related anger on the irrational idea that the person deliberately has not returned. The best approach is to explain honestly that the person has died and is not coming back, elicit the child's understanding and questions about what has happened, and then repeat this process continually as the child gradually begins to grasp the reality of the situation. The decision of whether to take a small child to a funeral may be particularly complex. Figure 28-1 enumerates some factors to consider.

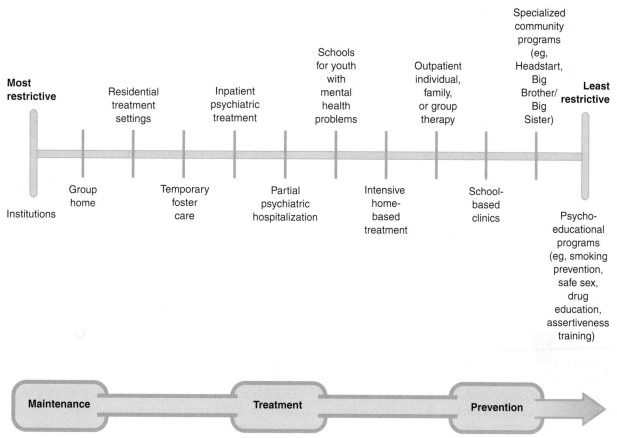

FIGURE 28.1 The continuum of mental health care for children and adolescents.

School-Aged Children

School-aged children better understand the permanence of death, but they may be unable to express their feelings about it in the same way that adults do. Children in this age group may express their grief through somatic complaints, regression, behavior problems, withdrawal, and even hostility toward parents. They may feel that others expect them to cry and react with immediate emotional intensity to the death; when they do not react this way, they feel guilty.

Adolescents

Adolescents who are in Piaget's stage of formal operations can better understand death as an abstract concept. **Formal operations** is the period of cognitive development characterized by the ability to use abstract reasoning to conceptualize and solve problems. Because adolescents tend to be idealistic and to think in extremes, they may even have poetic or romantic notions about death. Many teenagers become fascinated with morbid rock music, movies, and books. Although they may be able to express their thoughts and feelings about death more clearly than younger children, they are often reluctant to do so for fear of being viewed as childish.

Some adolescents assume a parental role in the family after a death, denying their own needs. School settings may be particularly helpful in providing group and individual support for grieving adolescents, particularly as a preventive intervention (Van Epps et al., 1997).

Separation and Divorce

Nearly half of all marriages in the United States end in divorce. Many more couples separate without ever filing for divorce. Parental separation and divorce create changes in the family structure, usually resulting in a substantial reduction in the contact that children have with one of their parents. The child's response to divorce is similar to the response to death. In some ways, divorce may be harder for the child to understand because the noncustodial parent is gone but still alive, and the parents have made a conscious choice to separate. Research shows that children of divorce are at increased risk for emotional, behavior, and academic problems (Hetherington et al., 1998). The response to the loss that divorce imposes, however, varies depending on the child's temperament, the parents' interventions, and the level of stress, change, and conflict surrounding the divorce.

The first 2 or 3 years after the marital breakup tend to be the most difficult. Typical childhood reactions include confusion, guilt, depression, regression, somatic symptoms, acting-out behaviors (eg, stealing, disobedience), fantasies that the parents will reunite, fear of losing the custodial parent, and alignment with one parent against the other. After an initial period of adjustment, children usually accept the reality of the situation and begin coping adaptively. Most divorced parents eventually remarry to new partners, which often imposes another period of coping difficulties for the children. Children with stepparents and stepsiblings are at renewed risk for the development of emotional and behavior problems as they struggle to cope with the establishment of these relationships (Hetherington et al., 1998).

Protective factors against the development of emotional problems in children of divorce and remarriage include a structured home and school environment with reasonable and consistent limit setting and a warm, supportive relationship with stepparents (Hetherington et al., 1998). Helpful interventions for children of divorce include education regarding children's reactions; promotion of regular and predictable visitation; reduction of conflict between the parents through counseling, mediation, and clear visitation policies; continuance of usual routines and limit setting; and family counseling to facilitate adjustment after remarriage (Table 28-2). Some evidence has shown that it is not the divorce itself but rather the continuing conflict between the parents that is most damaging to the child. Parents manage the divorce better if they can remember that children naturally idealize and identify with both parents and need to view both of them positively. Therefore, it is helpful for parents to reinforce each other's good qualities and focus on evidence of their former partner's love and respect for the child.

Sibling Relationships

Until recently, the role of siblings in a child's development was underemphasized. A growing body of research shows that sibling relationships significantly affect personality development. Moreover, research shows that positive sibling relationships can be protective factors against the development of psychopathology, particularly in troubled families in which the parents are emotionally unavailable (Jenkins, 1992). Thus, nurses should emphasize that whatever parents can do to minimize sibling rivalry and maximize cooperative behavior among their children will benefit their children's social and emotional development throughout life.

Sibling rivalry begins with the birth of the second child. Often, this child's birth is traumatic for the first child who, up until then, was the sole focus of the parents' attention. The older sibling usually reacts with

anger and may reveal not-so-subtle fantasies of getting rid of the new sibling (eg, "I had a dream that the new baby died."). Parents should recognize that these reactions are natural and allow the child to express feelings, both positive and negative, about the baby while reassuring the child that he or she has a very special place in the family. Allowing the older child opportunities to care for the baby and reinforcing any nurturing or affectionate behavior will help to establish a positive bond.

Some degree of sibling rivalry is natural and inevitable, even into adulthood. Intense rivalry and conflict between siblings, however, has been correlated with the development of behavior problems in children (Dunn, 1992). One factor that can exacerbate this problem is differential treatment of children. Some studies have shown that less affection and more control given toward older than younger siblings predicts the development of internalizing (eg, depression, anxiety) and externalizing (eg, oppositional and conduct disorder) behavior problems in the older children (Dunn et al., 1990). Although it is natural and appropriate for parents to use different methods to manage children with different personalities, parents must be sensitive to their children's perceptions of their behavior and emphasize each child's strengths. Helping each child to develop a separate identity based on unique talents and interests can minimize rivalry and perceptions of favoritism.

Children with emotionally disturbed siblings are at increased risk for the development of psychopathology. For example, the risk for depression in siblings of a depressed youth is 20%, as compared to 5% in the general population. The correlations for juvenile delinquency among siblings are between 0.38 for brothers and 0.50 for sisters (Slomkowski et al., 2001). Logically, some heightened risk can be attributed to genetics alone, but other factors in the family environment may combine to increase this underlying vulnerability. Nurses working with emotionally disturbed children should be alert to the development of behavior problems among siblings and include them in any family interventions (Rowe, 1992).

Physical Illness

Many children suffer from a major physical illness or injury at some point during development. About 13% of children in the United States suffer from a chronic medical condition. The experience of hospitalization and intrusive medical procedures is at least acutely traumatic for most children. The likelihood of more lasting psychological problems that result from physical illness depends on the child's developmental level and previous coping mechanisms, the family's level of functioning before and after the illness, and the nature and severity of the illness. As with any major stressor,

TABLE 28.2	Play Therapy With a 4-Year-Old Child Whose Parents Are Divorcing	

Patient Statement	Nurse Response	Analysis and Rationale
(Child smashes two cars together and makes loud, crashing sound.)	That's a loud crash. They really hit hard.	Child may be experiencing anger and frustration nonverbally through play. Nurse attempts to establish rapport with child by relating at child's level, using age-appropriate vocabulary.
Crrrash!	I know a kid who gets so mad sometimes that he feels like smashing something.	Child is engrossed in fantasy play, typical of preschoolers. Children often use toys as symbols of human figures (animism). Nurse uses indirect method of eliciting child's feelings because preschoolers often do not express feelings directly. Reference to another child's anger helps to normalize this child's feelings.
Yeah!	Sounds like you feel that way sometimes, too.	Child is beginning to relate to nurse and sense her empathy. Nurse reflects the child's feelings to facilitate further communication.
Yeah, especially when my mom and dad fight.	It's hard to listen to parents fighting. Sometimes It's scary. You wonder what's going to happen.	Child is experiencing frustration and helplessness related to family conflict. Nurse expresses empathy and attempts to articulate child's feelings because preschool children have a limited ability to identify and label feelings.
My mom and dad are getting a divorce.	That's too bad. What's going to happen when they get the divorce?	Child has basic awareness of the reality of parents' divorce, but may not understand this concept. Nurse expresses empathy and attempts to assess the child's level of understanding of the divorce.
Dad's not going to live in our house.	Oh, I guess you'll miss having him there all the time. It would be so nice if you all could live together, but I guess that's not going to happen.	Preschool child focuses on the effects the divorce will have on him (egocentrism). Child seems to have a clear understanding of the consequences of the divorce. Nurse articulates the child's perspective and reinforces the reality of the divorce to avoid fueling denial and reconciliation fantasies that the child may have.
(Silently moves cars across the floor.)	What do you think is the reason your parents decided to get a divorce?	Child expresses sadness nonverbally. Nurse further attempts to assess the child's understanding of the circumstances surrounding the divorce.
Because I did it.	What do you mean—you did it?	Child provides clue that he may be feeling responsible. Nurse uses clarification to fully assess child's understanding.
I made them mad. When I left my bike in the driveway and Dad ran over it.	How? So you think that's why they're getting the divorce?	Child uses egocentric thinking typical of a preschooler to draw conclusion that his actions caused the divorce. Nurse continues to clarify the child's thinking. The goal is to elicit the child's perceptions so that the nurse can correct any misperceptions.
Yeah, they had a big fight that night	They may have been upset about the bike, but I don't think that's why they're getting a divorce.	The nurse goes on to explain why parents get divorced and to provide opportunities for the child to ask questions.
Why?	Because parents get divorced when they're upset at *each other*—when they can't get along—not when they're upset with their children.	

the perception of the event (ie, meaning of the illness) will influence the family's ability to cope.

Common childhood reactions to physical illness include regression (eg, loss of previous developmental gains in toilet training, social maturity, autonomous behavior), sleep and feeding difficulties, behavior problems (negativism, withdrawal), somatic complaints that represent masked attempts at emotional expression (eg, headaches, stomach aches), and depression. Infants and preschool-aged children are particularly vulnerable to separation anxiety during illness and may regress to earlier levels of anxiety about strangers, becoming fearful of health care providers. Young children often have magical thinking about the illness, and their tendency to process information in concrete terms often leads to misperceptions about the nature of the illness and treatment procedures (eg, dye = die; stretcher = stretch her) (Boggs, 1999). Adolescents may be concerned about body image and maintaining their sense of independence and control.

Nurses must remember that parents are the primary resource to the child and the experts who know the child's needs and reactions. Thus, nurses must maintain a collaborative approach in working with parents of physically ill children. If the child is a sick infant, nurses should take care to allow the normal attachment process between parents and the infant to unfold, despite the intervention of health care professionals who may be tempted to assume many parenting functions. Parents who come to view their children as physically and emotionally fragile will feel disempowered in decision making and limit setting and may develop helpless or overprotective styles of dealing with their children.

Many parents react with guilt to their child's illness or injury, especially if the illness is genetically based or partially the result of their own behavior (eg, drug or alcohol abuse during pregnancy). Parents may project their guilt onto each other or health care professionals, lashing out in anger and blame. Nurses should view this behavior as a natural part of the grieving process and help parents to move forward in caring for their children and regaining competence. Teaching parents how to care for their children's medical problems and reinforcing their successes in doing so will help.

Chronic physical illness in childhood has been linked with the development of various emotional and behavior problems. Although only about 33% of chronically ill children develop psychological difficulties, they are about 250% more likely to develop psychiatric problems than physically healthy children. Conditions that affect the central nervous system (CNS) (eg, infections, metabolic diseases, CNS malformations, brain and spinal cord trauma) are particularly likely to result in psychiatric difficulties (Wasserman, 1990). Nurses who understand pathophysiologic processes are in a unique position to assess the interaction between biologic and psychological factors that contribute to mental health problems in chronically ill children (eg, lethargy from high blood sugar or respiratory problems; mood swings from steroid use). Inactivity and lack of sensory stimulation from hospitalization or bed rest may contribute to neurologic deficits and development delays. The major challenge for a chronically ill child is to remain active despite the limitations of the illness and to become fully integrated into school and social activities. Children who view themselves as different or defective will suffer from low self-esteem and be more vulnerable to depression, anxiety, and behavior problems.

Adolescent Risk-Taking Behaviors

Adolescence is a time of growing independence and, consequently, experimentation. Emotional extremes prevail. To adolescents, the world seems great one day and terrible the next; people are either for them or against them. Adolescents are struggling to consolidate their abilities to control their impulses and react to the many "crises" that may seem trivial to adults but are very important to teens. Biologic changes (eg, onset of puberty, height and weight changes, hormone changes), psychological changes (increased ability for abstract thinking), and social changes (dating, driving, increased autonomy from parents) are all significant. The primary developmental task of identity formation leads teenagers to test different roles and struggle to find a peer group that fits their unfolding self-image.

During this process, many adolescents experiment with risk-taking behaviors, such as smoking, using alcohol and drugs, having unprotected sex, engaging in truancy or delinquent behaviors, and running away from home. Although most youths eventually become more responsible, some develop harmful behavior patterns and addictions that endanger their mental and physical health. Adolescents who have already developed psychiatric problems are particularly vulnerable to engaging in risky behaviors because they have limited coping skills, may attempt to self-medicate their symptoms, and may feel increased pressure to fit in with other teens. Moreover, research shows that risky behaviors tend to be interrelated (Eggert et al., 1994).

Several approaches to mental health promotion with adolescents are recommended. First, intervening at the peer group level through education programs, alternative recreation activities, and peer counseling is most successful (Research Box 28-1). Adolescents are skeptical of authority figures and tend to listen most to one another. Nurses working with teenagers should use a discussion approach that encourages questioning and argument, as opposed to talking down to or "talking at" teenagers. Second, research has shown that training in values clarification, problem solving, social skills, and assertiveness helps give adolescents the skills to cope with situations in which they are pressured by their peers (Kazdin, 1993). Social psychological research shows that if just one person can find the strength to express an unpopular viewpoint in a group and decline to participate in a destructive activity, others will quickly follow. It takes enormous courage, as well as concrete knowledge and practice with assertiveness, to speak up in these situations. A third type of intervention is a program that uses team efforts by teachers, parents, community leaders, and teen role models. These programs help at-risk youth by building self-esteem, setting positive examples, and working to involve the youth in community activities. Approaches that have not proved effective include mere education and information about danger-

RESEARCH BOX 28.1

*Effectiveness of a
Psychoeducational Group*

This study investigated the effectiveness of a 10-session psychoeducational group intervention for adolescents at risk for depression and acting out behaviors. The researchers tested the intervention with 40 high school students who scored in the moderate range for depression and difficulties coping. Teams of advanced practice nurses and school nurses or guidance counselors conducted the program in the high school setting. A training manual for the program was used to prepare all group leaders to intervene consistently, with a specific agenda for each group session. The program combined education, group support, and cognitive-behavioral strategies for solving typical teenage problems such as dealing with peer pressure, family conflict, and decisions about risky behaviors. At the end of the program, the adolescents reported reduced depressive symptoms and improved coping behaviors on several questionnaires. Additionally, they commented that the group intervention was a positive, enjoyable experience.

Implications for Nursing Practice. This study demonstrated the usefulness of psychoeducational approaches for the prevention of mental health problems in adolescents. It represents one step in a line of research that these nurses have done, who have previously investigated sources of stress and coping difficulties for teens and who have a major federal grant that is funding their continued research on preventive interventions. The researchers hypothesize that learning general coping skills will help adolescents choose alternatives to substance abuse, pregnancy, violence, and risky lifestyles. Exploring these issues in a group context is particularly useful during the peer-oriented years of adolescence. Although the long-term effectiveness of this program is yet to be determined, the intervention holds promise as a well-designed, detailed approach that could be adapted in various clinical and community settings.

Puskar, K. R., Lamb, J., & Tusaie-Mumford, K. (1997). Teaching kids to cope: A preventive mental health nursing strategy for adolescents. *Journal of Child and Adolescent Psychiatric Nursing, 10*, 18–28.

ous activities without behavior training and programs that provide inadequate training and support for the professionals implementing them.

RISK FACTORS FOR CHILDHOOD PSYCHOPATHOLOGY

Poverty and Homelessness

An estimated 19.2% of children in the United States live below the poverty line (U.S. Bureau of the Census, 1999), and a disproportionate number of children from minority groups live in poverty. The effects of poverty on child development and family functioning are numerous and pervasive. Lack of proper nutrition and access to prenatal and mother–infant care place children from poor families at risk for the development of both physical and mental health problems. Children from poor rural areas often lack access to educational and other resources. Urban children living in ghetto areas are vulnerable to violent crime, crowded living conditions, and drug-infested neighborhoods. Although crime, drug abuse, gang activity, and teenage pregnancy are seen in adolescents from all socioeconomic backgrounds, children living in poverty may be more vulnerable to these problems because they may view their options as limited. Thus, they may have an increased need to maintain a tough image and struggle more for a sense of control over their environment. The obstacles inherent in overcoming the effects of poverty can seem insurmountable to young people and are difficult to imagine for those professionals raised in middle-class families.

A major focus of nursing preventive intervention with poor families involves simply forming an alliance that conveys respect and willingness to work as an advocate to help them gain access to resources. In terms of Maslow's need hierarchy, families living in poverty may be more focused on survival needs (eg, food, shelter) than self-actualization needs (eg, insight-oriented psychotherapy for themselves or their children). Unless the nurse can work as a partner with the family and address the issues most pressing for the family with an active, problem-solving approach, other types of intervention may be impossible. At the same time, it is inappropriate to assume that poor families will be resistant to or unable to benefit from psychotherapy or other mental health interventions.

An estimated 1.5 million children and adolescents in the United States are homeless. Homelessness in children and teens may result from no shelter for the entire family, running away, or being thrown out of their homes. Chapter 32 reviews in detail mental health issues related to homelessness, but some mention of the specific effects of homelessness on youth deserves mention here. Research reveals an increased risk for physical health problems (eg, nutrition deficiencies, infections, chronic illnesses), mental health problems (particularly developmental delays in language, fine or gross motor coordination, and social development; depression; anxiety; disruptive behavior disorders), and educational underachievement in homeless youth (Menke, 1998; Rafferty & Shinn, 1991). The living conditions of many shelters place children at risk for lead poisoning and communicable diseases and make the regular sleep, feeding, play, and bathing patterns important for normal development nearly impossible. Nurses working with homeless families need to be aware of the effects of this lifestyle on children because they have a limited ability to speak for themselves and because their needs are often ignored.

Studies show that the demands of parenting often overwhelm parents in homeless shelters. The unstable nature of their living conditions limits the ability of these parents to nurture their children (Gorzka, 1999).

Runaway youth typically have experienced extreme levels of stressful life events even before they have run away, with most fleeing temporary living arrangements (eg, foster homes, friends, relatives) (Warren et al., 1997). Thus, their runaway experience serves only to compound an already chronic history of trauma and disruption. The key is to prevent the conditions that preceded the runaway behavior.

Child Abuse and Neglect

Victimization within the family system is covered elsewhere in this text (see Chap. 37). Early recognition and reduction of risk factors are the keys to the prevention of **child abuse and neglect** (Research Box 28-2). This section briefly reviews the risk factors, signs and symptoms, effects on development, and methods for prevention of child abuse and neglect.

Risk factors for child abuse and neglect include high levels of family stress, drug or alcohol abuse, a stepparent or parental boyfriend or girlfriend who is unstable or unloving toward the child, and lack of social support for the parents (Fennel & Fishel, 1998). Additionally, young children (particularly those younger than age 3 years) and children with a history of prematurity, medical problems, and severe emotional problems are at high risk because they place great demands on the parents. Abuse has a well-known intergenerational pattern, such that children who are abused and neglected are more likely to repeat this behavior when they become parents (Helfer et al., 1997).

Table 28-3 lists signs of physical, emotional, and sexual abuse in children. Nurses should be aware that they are legally mandated to report any reasonable suspicion of abuse and neglect to the appropriate authorities in their given state. Mandated reporting laws are designed to allow the state to investigate the possibility of abuse, provide protection to children, and link families with the support and services that they need to reduce the risk for further abuse. Nurses are immune from liability for reporting suspected abuse, but they may be held legally accountable for not reporting it. The decision to report abuse sometimes poses an ethical dilemma for nurses as they try to balance the need to maintain the family's trust against the need to protect the child (Lewin, 1994). This decision is further complicated by the knowledge that, if temporary out-of-home placement is necessary, the quality of the placement may not be optimum, and the child and family may suffer in the process of the separation. Experts recommend that nurses report abuse in the presence of the parents, preferably with the parent initi-

RESEARCH BOX 28.2

Screening Tool for Abuse Potential

This work involves the development of a tool for assessing levels of risk for child abuse and neglect in families of children aged 3 years and younger. The nurses who developed the tool did a comprehensive review of the literature on risk factors for child maltreatment and combined these data with ideas from other screening and research tools. The result was a 19-question interview protocol that can be administered in 5 minutes or less. The researchers' goal was to provide a tool that could be used efficiently in primary care settings, because other available tools are more cumbersome and impractical. They piloted the instrument in a primary care clinic, and the nurses who administered it reported that it was concise and easy to use. The tool includes an interview screening protocol with carefully worded questions designed to avoid accusatory attitudes and a scoring guide that indicates the need for referral to community resources.

Implications for Nursing Practice. The nurses who developed this tool assert that assessment of risk for abuse and neglect should be a standard of practice in child health care programs. Screening for possible risk for maltreatment allows nurses to identify families who are most in need of tracking and preventive intervention. Doing so maximizes the efficient use of resources by both families and health care providers. Assessment tools must be brief and designed with specific, helpful questions that can be adapted by both experienced and novice professionals. Because primary care providers may be a family's only formal source of support in the early years of childrearing, this is a key setting for assessment. The development of this tool is a useful contribution to nursing practice, and it provides the potential to intervene with families early enough to make a difference.

Murry, S. K., Baker, A. W., & Lewin, L. (2000). Screening families with young children for child maltreatment potential. *Pediatric Nursing, 26,* 47–54.

ating the phone call, and that the professional should explain the reporting as necessary to provide safety for the child and to obtain services for the family, which is obviously under stress (McNair, 1992). If the parents cannot be present when the report is made, the nurse should, at minimum, notify the family that he or she has made the report and explain why to minimize damaging the professional relationship. A major protective factor against psychopathology stemming from abuse and neglect is the establishment of a supportive relationship with at least one adult, who can provide empathy, consistency, and a possibly corrective experience (eg, a fos-

TABLE 28.3 Signs of Possible Child Abuse

Sexual Abuse	Physical Abuse
• Bruises or bleeding in genitals or rectum • Sexually transmitted disease (eg. HIV, gonorrhea, syphilis, herpes genitalis) • Vaginal or penile discharge • Sore throats • Enuresis or encopresis • Foreign bodies in the vagina or rectum • Pregnancy, especially in a young adolescent • Difficulty in walking or sitting • Sexual acting out with siblings or peers • Sophisticated knowledge of sexual activities • Preoccupation with sexual ideas • Somatic complaints, especially abdominal pain and constipation • Sleep difficulties • Hyperalertness to environment • Withdrawal • Excessive daydreaming or seeming preoccupied • Regressed behavior	• Bruises or lacerations, especially in clusters on back, buttocks, thighs, or large areas of torso* • Fractures inconsistent with the child's history • Old and new injuries at the same time • Unwilling to change clothes in front of others: wears heavy clothes in warm weather • Identifiable marks from belt buckles, electrical cords, or handprints • Cigarette burns • Rope burns on arms, legs, face, neck, or torso from being bound and gagged • Adult-size bite marks • Bald spots interspersed with normal hair • Shrinking at the touch of an adult • Fear of adults, especially parents • Apprehensive when other children cry • Scanning the environment, staying very still, failing to cry when hurt • Aggression or withdrawal • Indiscriminant seeking of affection • Defensive reactions when questioned about injuries • History of being taken to many different clinics and emergency rooms for different injuries

Note: Because many injuries do not represent child abuse, a careful history must be taken.

---

ter parent or other family member) for the child (for review, see Houck & King, 1993).

Prevention of child abuse and neglect takes place through any intervention that supports the parents with physical, financial, mental health, and medical resources that will reduce stress within the family system. Early intervention and family support programs (see later) are considered the cornerstone of preventive efforts. Nurses working with abused children should resist the temptation to view the child as the only victim. Remembering that most abusive parents were abused themselves as children and, therefore, may have limited coping mechanisms or access to positive parental role models will help the nurse maintain empathy toward the parents. Once intervention by state agencies has established the child's safety, a family systems approach that provides support to the whole family unit will be most effective.

Out-of-Home Placement

The tendency to blame parents and view out-of-home placement as a refuge for children has sharply declined in recent years. This change in attitudes has resulted from public awareness of the deficiencies in the foster care system, greater support for parents' rights, and increased knowledge of the biologic basis for many of the disorders of parents and children that lead to out-of-

home placement. **Family preservation** means efforts made by professionals to preserve the family unit by preventing the removal of children from their homes through parental support and education and work to facilitate a secure attachment between the child and parent.

Children now are being removed from their homes only as a last resort. The U.S. Congress recently passed a bill commonly known as the Family Preservation and Support Services Act. This Act establishes and expands services to help children return to their birth families, when appropriate, or at least to facilitate permanent placement with a relative, in an adoptive home, or in some other planned living arrangement (Stanley, 1994). Family support services are designed to assist families with access to resources and education regarding child-rearing, to monitor and facilitate the development of the bond between child and caretaker, and to increase the caretaker's confidence in his or her abilities. Pothier and Kools (1994), nursing experts in foster care reform, recommend that for those children who must be placed out of the home temporarily, review boards should closely monitor their progress and develop plans for permanent living arrangements within 2 years of placement. They also point to the needs for mandatory training programs for foster parents, increased support and consultation for foster homes of children with severe physical and behavior problems, better data systems to track the child's assessment and treatment throughout placement changes, increased access to physical and mental health care, and increased funding for preventive services designed to maintain the family structure.

Despite recent trends toward family preservation, an increasing number of children are being placed in foster homes, group homes, or residential treatment centers annually, often for months to years. Factors leading to the increased number of children in out-of-home placement include increased willingness of the public and professionals to report child abuse and neglect, the epidemic proportions of substance abuse and cases of AIDS, and the increasing number of families living in poverty, which may lead to abuse, neglect, and homelessness (Pothier & Kools, 1994). About 50% of children in out-of-home placement are adolescents, but numbers of infants and young children are growing, particularly those with serious physical and emotional problems, who pose particular challenges for placement (Pothier & Kools, 1994). Infants who are abandoned by drug-abusing parents and HIV-positive children whose parents are sick or deceased need permanent out-of-home placements, which are often difficult to find.

The process of adjustment to an out-of-home placement can be viewed through the conceptual framework of Bowlby's stages of coping with parental separation. According to Bowlby (1960), the child initially responds to separation from parents with protest (crying, kicking, screaming, pleading, and attempting to elicit the parent's return). The child then moves to a state of despair (listlessness, apathy, and withdrawal, which lead to some acceptance of caretaking by others, but a reluctance to reattach fully). Finally, the child experiences detachment if the child and new parent cannot manage to form an emotional bond. Because children often experience multiple placements, the potential for a disrupted attachment may be great by the time the child faces the prospect of a permanent family. After repeatedly undergoing the process of separation and mourning, the child learns that rejection is inevitable and may automatically maintain distance from a new caretaker.

Typical coping styles seen in children exposed to multiple placements include detachment, diffuse rage, chronic depression, antisocial behavior, low self-esteem, and chronic dependency or exaggerated demands for nurturing and support (Steinhauer, 1983). It takes a very committed and resilient parent to continue caring for a child who does not reinforce attempts at caretaking and who exhibits these kinds of significant emotional and behavior problems.

Children of Alcoholics

An estimated 28 million children in the United States grow up in families in which one or both parents are alcoholics. Alcoholism is a biologically based disease that is highly resistant to treatment and characterized by frequent relapses. The codependency movement, which emphasizes the effects of addiction on family members, and groups such as Adult Children of Alcoholics (ACOA) and Al-Anon have brought increasing attention to the effects of parental alcoholism on child development. Any review of this topic must examine the role of both biologic-genetic mechanisms and environmental mechanisms in creating increased risk for psychological problems among children of alcoholics.

Biologic factors affecting children of alcoholics include **fetal alcohol syndrome**, nutritional deficits stemming from neglect, and neuropsychiatric dysfunction related to overstimulation or understimulation (Kaemingk & Paquette, 1999). Genetic factors are at least partly responsible for the well-documented increased risk for substance abuse among children of alcoholics. Recent studies are beginning to establish a link between a family history of anxiety disorders and alcoholism, with genetically transmitted anxiety disorders possibly acting as a precursor to alcohol abuse (Haack, 1990). The precise mechanism of family transmission of alcoholism remains complex and unknown. Fitzgerald and colleagues (1994) cite recent studies suggesting that children of alcoholics may inherit a predisposition to a nonspecific form of biologic dysregulation that may be expressed phenotypically either as alcoholism or some other psychiatric disorder (eg, hyperactivity, conduct disorder, depression), depending on the individual's developmental history.

Children of alcoholics are at high risk for the development of both substance abuse and behavior disorders. Moreover, some evidence has shown that other factors related to alcoholism, such as family stress, violence, divorce, dysfunction, and other concurrent parental psychiatric disorders (eg, depression, anxiety), are as important as the alcoholism itself in increasing this risk (Fitzgerald et al., 1994). The experience of growing up in an alcoholic family is marked by unpredictability, fear, and helplessness because of the cyclic nature of addictive patterns. The literature on children of alcoholics has described several typical roles that children assume, including the "hero" (overly responsible children who may ignore their own needs to take care of parents and other children), "scapegoat" (problem children who divert attention away from the alcoholic parent), "mascot" (family clowns who relieve tension and mask feelings through joking), and "lost child" (children who suffer in silence but may exhibit difficulties at school or in later life). These roles, combined with the enabling behaviors of other family members who attempt to cover up and minimize the effects of the addiction, may become so rigid and effective in masking the problem that children of alcoholics may not come to the attention of mental health professionals until *after* the parent stops drinking and the family roles are disrupted. Even among children who do not develop significant psychopathology, the experience of growing up in an alcoholic family can lead to a poor self-concept when children feel responsible for their parents' behavior, become isolated, and learn to mistrust their own perceptions because the family denies the reality of the addiction.

INTERVENTION APPROACHES

Mental health promotion with children, adolescents, and their families encompasses the full range of preventive efforts discussed in Chapter 3. The overall philosophy of nursing is to advocate for the least restrictive type of intervention possible. This means focusing on interventions that allow maximal autonomy for the child and family, that keep the family unit intact, if possible, and that provide the appropriate level of care to meet the child and family's needs. A continuum of modalities of care is available to children and families (Fig. 28-2).

Professional nursing emphasizes an interdisciplinary approach in which the nurse acts as coordinator, case manager, and advocate to establish linkages with physicians and nurse practitioners, teachers, speech and language specialists, social workers, and other professionals to develop and implement a comprehensive biopsychosocial plan of intervention. Foremost in the nurse's philosophy should be the view of parents as partners. In the past, parents were viewed as the culprits in the creation of child mental health problems and were treated as patients themselves. Recent insights into the biologic and genetic origins of psychiatric disorders have contributed to a refreshing

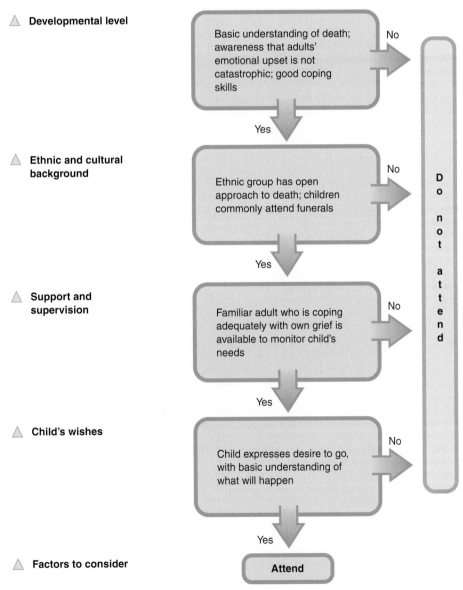

Figure 28.2 Decision tree: should a child attend a funeral?

shift away from blame and pathologizing of parents to a more collaborative approach (Text Box 28-1).

Psychoeducational programs are a particularly effective form of mental health intervention. These programs are designed to teach parents and children basic coping skills for dealing with various stressors. Among other techniques, they use the process of **normalization** to provide families with information about normal child development and expected reactions to various stressors so that they will feel less isolated, know what to expect, and put their reactions into perspective. For example, if families learn that anger is a natural part of grieving, they will be less likely to view it as abnormal and more likely to accept and cope with it constructively. Parallel curricula can be established, with concurrent psychoeducational groups for adults and children. Most foster care agencies now provide a program of education and training for prospective foster parents to help them know what to expect and how to help the child adjust to the placement.

Social skills training is one psychoeducational approach that has been useful with youth who have low self-esteem, aggressive behavior, or a high risk for substance abuse (Forman, 1993). Social skills training involves instruction, feedback, support, and practice with learning behaviors that help children to interact more effectively with peers and adults. When combined with assertiveness training, social skills training can be particularly helpful in providing children with coping skills to resist engaging in addictive or antisocial behaviors and to prevent social withdrawal under stress. Social skills training may be particularly helpful for children who are bullies or rejected by their peers (Fopma-Loy, 2000).

Bibliotherapy involves the use of books and other reading materials to help individuals cope with various life stressors. It is a particularly potent form of intervention because it empowers families to learn and develop coping mechanisms on their own. A wide variety of books are available to help children understand issues such as death, divorce, chronic illness, stepfamilies,

TEXT BOX 28.1

Case Study: A Family Approach to Mental Health Promotion

A teacher refers John, an 8-year-old boy, to the community mental health center because of disruptive behavior. John's grandmother, Doris, brings John to the center. Doris is the custodial parent of John and his 6-year-old sister Lisa. She reports that her daughter Marsha abandoned the children after becoming addicted to cocaine 5 years ago. Since that time, John has had periodic behavior problems, such as lying, stealing, and fighting with other children. Lisa has been depressed and withdrawn, with a tendency to cling to her grandmother. Despite these problems, the children have been functioning reasonably well at school until recently. Doris reports that she has developed a good relationship with the children and provides them with emotional support and limit-setting.

Recently, Marsha returned to live with Doris after completing her third drug treatment program followed by placement in a halfway house for 6 months. She has been drug free for almost 1 year, and she wants to resume parenting of her children. The children are expressing excitement about their mother's return, but they are having some difficulty relating to her. Lisa constantly climbs into her mother's lap and demands attention. John ignores his mother and does not respond to her attempts at discipline. Doris reports that she has had difficulty trusting that Marsha will stay clean and sober, and she still considers herself the children's real mother. She is angry with Marsha for abandoning the children and stealing money from her when she was drug addicted, but she does not say anything to Marsha because she is afraid to upset her.

The nurse at the community mental health center sees several problems that need intervention in this case:

- Family role conflict between Marsha and Doris regarding parenting responsibilities
- Potential for John to develop a disruptive behavior disorder (eg, oppositional defiant disorder, conduct disorder)

- Potential for Lisa to develop an affective disorder (eg, anxiety, depression)
- Potential for Marsha to have a drug addiction relapse because of the stress of attempting to assume the parenting role with two needy, young children and their understandably resentful and mistrusting grandmother

The nurse's approach will be to intervene with the family system as a whole. She will meet periodically with Marsha and Doris to give them an opportunity to express their feelings about their relationship and to divide parenting responsibilities. During these sessions, the nurse will need to assist Marsha with her reintegration into the family unit as the primary caretaker and decision maker for her children. At the same time, the nurse must support the grandmother's relationship with the children because she is the primary attachment figure, based on her consistent, supportive contact with the children over the past few years. A major goal will be to help Marsha and Doris work together in disciplining and parenting the children so that their messages will be consistent and they can maintain a united front. Marsha will be referred to a psychoeducational group on parenting skills, and she and Doris will be given reading materials regarding positive ways to discipline their children. The nurse will also meet with John and Lisa together to help them express their feelings about the changes in the family system and to provide support for their sibling relationship. After obtaining the necessary consent forms to release information, the nurse will maintain close contact with the teacher who referred John to the clinic, in order to facilitate the teacher's efforts to set limits and provide support for John. Marsha will continue attending regular meetings of Cocaine Anonymous and Alcoholics Anonymous, and Doris will be referred to Al Anon for support and assistance in dealing with her anger, mistrust, and fears about Marsha relapsing.

adoption, and birth of a sibling. In addition, many mental health organizations and public health agencies have pamphlets designed to educate parents about various physical and psychological problems. Besides providing concrete information and advice, these reading materials help to reduce anxiety by pointing out common reactions to the various stressors so that families do not feel alone.

Support groups are available for just about every kind of stressor that a family can experience, including substance abuse, death, divorce, and coping with a chronic illness. Both parents and children in groups can experience Yalom's (1985) healing effects of group therapy, including group cohesiveness, universality (awareness of the normalcy and commonality of one's reactions), catharsis, hope, and altruism (being able to help others).

Finally, **early intervention programs** are perhaps the most important form of primary prevention available to children and families. In 1989, U.S. Public Law 99-457 was extended to mandate that infants and toddlers who were diagnosed with physical or mental health problems that created a risk for developmental delays should have access to early intervention programs. This law gave individual states the flexibility to provide services to other young children assumed to be at risk. It increased family support programs to provide regular home visits and offer support, education, and concrete services to families. The assumptions underlying family support programs are that parents are the most consistent and important figures in children's lives; families should be afforded the opportunity to define their own needs and priorities; and emotional support, information, and education will increase parents' abilities to respond effectively to their children (Roberts et al., 1991).

Although nurses have been historically underutilized in school-based mental health efforts, schools are good locations for other early intervention programs because they are physically near the families that they serve and are less intimidating than mental health centers. One such model program is the PIVOT program for adolescent mothers developed by the Department of Mental Health Nursing at Oregon Health Sciences University. This program provides mental health services to teenage mothers and their children in an alternative high school setting. The adolescents involved in this program reportedly have significant histories of abuse and neglect, depression, and conduct disorder, and their children often show evidence of developmental delays (Kendall & Peterson, 1996). By intervening in the school setting, the nurses who have developed this program have been able to have a small but significant effect on two generations of children at risk. Early intervention programs with high-risk families have helped to reduce child abuse and neglect and may be the key to preventing the placement of children outside the home (Fennel & Fishel, 1998).

In conclusion, undertaking interventions to promote the mental health of children and adolescents is time and effort well spent. Many adult mental health problems can be prevented, coped with more effectively, or at least reduced in their scope and severity through focused intervention with children and families. Children lack the power and voice to fight for their own needs, making them one of the most vulnerable groups in society. By virtue of their close interaction with families, nurses are in a key position to identify the mental health needs of children and intervene, particularly in times of crisis. The feeling that comes from making a difference can be fulfilling and long-lasting.

Summary of Key Points

- Nurses working with children and adolescents are in a key position to identify risk and protective factors for psychopathology and to intervene to reduce risk.
- Nurses who are aware of normal developmental processes can educate parents about their children's behaviors, help them better understand their children's reactions to stress, and decide when intervention may be warranted.
- If the process of normal biologic maturation in childhood is disrupted through trauma or neglect, developmental delays and disorders can occur, some of which may have irreversible effects.
- From early infancy, children exhibit different kinds of temperaments that are at least partially biologically determined.
- Studies of attachment show that the quality of the emotional bond between the child and parental figure is an important determinant of the success of later relationships.
- Research shows that children who experience major losses, such as death or divorce, are at risk for the development of psychopathology.
- Sibling relationships have significant effects on personality development. Positive sibling relationships can be protective factors against the development of psychopathology.
- Medical problems in childhood and adolescence may cause psychological problems when illness leads to regression or lack of full participation in family, school, and social activities.
- Striving for identity and independence may lead adolescents to participate in high-risk activities (eg, drug use, unprotected sex, smoking, delinquent behaviors) that may lead to mental health problems.
- Poverty, homelessness, abuse, neglect, and parental alcoholism all create conditions that undermine a

child's ability to make normal developmental gains and contribute to vulnerability for various emotional and behavioral problems.

➤ Children who experience disrupted attachments because of out-of-home placements may have difficulty forming close relationships with their new parents and trusting others.

➤ Family support services and early intervention programs are designed to prevent removal of the child from the family as a result of abuse or neglect and to maintain a strong, nurturing family system.

➤ Psychoeducational approaches such as training opportunities, group experiences, and bibliotherapy provide children and families with the information and skills to foster their own mental health.

➤ The nurse's role in primary, secondary, and tertiary mental health promotion is to act as an advocate, partner, and educator who empowers families to identify and meet their own needs.

Critical Thinking Challenges

1. Analyze a case of a family that is grieving a loss and compare the parents' and children's reactions. Include an evaluation of how each child's reactions differ, depending on his or her developmental level.

2. Watch a movie or read a book that provides a child's view of death, divorce, or some other loss and consider how adults may be insensitive to the child's reactions.

3. Examine your own developmental history and pinpoint periods when stressful life events might have increased risk for emotional problems for you or other family members. What protective factors in your own personality and coping skills and in the environment around you helped you to maintain your good mental health?

4. What aspects of life are more stressful for children than for adults (ie, how is it different to experience life as a child)?

5. Examine how your own social and cultural background may either facilitate or create barriers to your ability to interact with families from other ethnic groups or those who are poor or homeless.

6. Allow yourself to reflect on how your own judgmental attitudes might interfere with your ability to communicate effectively with families who have abused or neglected their children.

7. Why is the process of normalization of feelings such a powerful intervention with children and families? What kinds of mental health issues, developmental processes, or both would benefit from teaching related to normal reactions? How can nurses incorporate this kind of intervention into their practice roles?

8. How can nurses expand their roles to have maximal effects on primary, secondary, and tertiary mental health intervention with children and families?

 WEB LINKS

www.nncc.org/Child.dev.page.html   This site gives detailed accounts of expected developmental milestones from birth through adulthood and provides links to numerous articles on topics of child development and parenting.

www.aacap.org/publications/factsfam/index.htm The American Academy of Child and Adolescent Psychiatry website provides an exhaustive list of links to short articles on many mental health issues and is geared toward families and consumers.

www.indiana.edu/~eric'rec/ieo/bibs/bibl-pre.html This site includes guidelines for bibliotherapy with children and links to books geared toward various issues in child development.

www.ispn.org/html/acapn.html   This is the website of the Association of Child and Adolescent Psychiatric Nurses. This nursing organization is dedicated to support, networking, advocacy, and education of mental health of children and families.

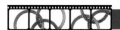 **MOVIES**

My Girl: 1991. This story lovingly portrays a young girl coping with her mother's death. It provides a thoughtful general analysis of death since the family runs a funeral parlor.
Viewing Points: How is the depiction of the child's grieving process in this film typical of childhood mourning? What aspects of it appear to be uniquely influenced by her family and the circumstances? How could the adults in the film have been more sensitive to the child's fears and anxieties about death?

To Kill a Mockingbird: 1962. The narrator of this beautiful film is a young girl growing up in the South before the Civil Rights Movement. The story illustrates several important factors that can influence a child's development, including single-parent families, cultural factors, the effects of abuse and alcoholism, and the child's attempt to reconcile good and evil forces in the world.
Viewing Points: How effective is this single-parent family in coping with life stresses and developmental changes? What aspects of the family's functioning appear particularly strong? Compare Scout and Jem's upbringing to that of the young woman from the family with alcoholism. In what ways does this

young girl appear to be at risk for the development of mental health problems?

The Breakfast Club: 1985. This funny, poignant portrayal of adolescence is told through the eyes of several teens from different backgrounds brought together when they are assigned to detention. It illustrates the heightened sense of drama that typifies adolescence, identity concerns, and peer relationship struggles.

Viewing Points: Which of these adolescents do you consider to be most at risk for the development of mental health problems? State the reasons for your argument. What are some factors that appear to be contributing to the risk-taking and acting-out behaviors among these adolescents?

The Color Purple: 1985. This film illustrates the effects of emotional and sexual abuse on the self-esteem of a girl growing up in the rural south. More importantly, it illustrates the healing effect of love and the indomitable strength of the human spirit.

Viewing Points: How does the experience of growing up with abuse appear to have affected the development of the young girl in this movie? What are some of the positive and maladaptive coping mechanisms that the young girl uses to cope with the family dysfunction?

What's Eating Gilbert Grape?: 1997. Johnny Depp, as Gilbert plays a frustrated young man who struggles to be free from emotional stagnation, his sleepy Iowa town, and his 500-pound recluse mother. This story is about the dynamics of a complex family and revolves around the relationship of Gilbert's mentally handicapped brother played by Leonardo De Caprio.

Significance: Family interaction revolves around food and the impact of the mother's obesity on the rest of the family.

Viewing Points: Observe the interaction of the family during meal times. How has the mother's disability impacted the family? How would you provide nursing care to this very complex family?

REFERENCES

Boggs, K. U. (1999). Communicating with children. In E. Arnold & K. U. Boggs (Eds.), *Interpersonal relationships: Professional skills for nurses* (3rd ed.). Philadelphia: W. B. Saunders.

Bowlby, J. (1960). Grief and mourning in infancy and early childhood. *Psychoanalytic Study of the Child, 15,* 9–52.

Dunn, J. (1992). Sisters and brothers: Current issues in developmental research. In F. Boer & J. Dunn (Eds.), *Children's sibling relationships: Developmental and clinical issues.* Hillsdale, NJ: Erlbaum.

Dunn, J., Stocker, C., & Plomin, R. (1990). Nonshared experiences within the family: Correlates of behavioral problems in middle childhood. *Development and Psychopathology, 2,* 113–126.

Eggert, L. L., Thompson, E. A., Herting, J. R., & Nicholas, L. J. (1994). Prevention research program: Reconnecting at-risk youth. *Issues in Mental Health Nursing, 15,* 107–135.

Fennel, D. C., & Fishel, A. H. (1998). Parent education: An evaluation of STEP on abusive parents' perceptions and abuse potential. *Journal of Child and Adolescent Psychiatric Nursing, 11*(3), 107–120.

Fitzgerald, H. E., Davies, W. H., Zucker, R. A., & Klinger, M. (1994). Developmental systems theory and substance abuse: A conceptual and methodological framework for analyzing patterns of variation in families. In L. L'Abate (Ed.), *Handbook of developmental family psychology and psychopathology* (pp. 350–372) York: Wiley.

Fopma-Loy, J. (2000). Peer rejection and neglect of latency-age children: Pathways and a group psychotherapy model. *Journal of Child and Adolescent Psychiatric Nursing, 13,* 29–38.

Forman, S. G. (1993). *Coping skills interventions for children and adolescents.* San Francisco: Jossey-Bass.

Gorzka, P. (1999). Homeless parents' perceptions of parenting stress. *Journal of Child and Adolescent Psychiatric Nursing, 12,* 7–16.

Haack, M. R. (1990). Collaborative investigation of adult children of alcoholics with anxiety. *Archives of Psychiatric Nursing, 4,* 62–66.

Helfer, M. E., Kemper, S., Kongman, R. D. (1997). *The battered child.* Chicago, IL: University of Chicago Press.

Hetherington, E. M., Bridges, M., & Insabella, G. M. (1998). What matters? What does not? Five perspectives on the association between marital transitions and children's adjustment. *American Psychologist, 53*(2), 167–184.

Houck, G. M., & King, M. C. (1993). Cognitive functioning and behavioral and emotional adjustment in maltreated children. *Journal of Child and Adolescent Psychiatric and Mental Health Nursing, 6,* 5–17.

Jenkins, J. (1992). Sibling relationships in disharmonious homes: Potential difficulties and protective effects. In F. Boer & J. Dunn (Eds.), *Children's sibling relationships: Developmental and clinical issues.* Hillsdale, NJ: Erlbaum.

Kaemingk, K., & Paquette, A. (1999). Effects of prenatal alcohol exposure on neuropsychological functioning. *Developmental Neuropsychology, 15,* 111–140.

Kazdin, A. E. (1993). Adolescent mental health: Prevention and treatment programs. *American Psychologist, 48,* 127–141.

Kendall, J., & Peterson, G. (1996). A school-based mental health clinic for adolescent mothers. *Journal of Child and Adolescent Psychiatric Nursing, 9,* 7–17.

Lewin, L. (1994). Child abuse: Ethical and legal concerns for the nurse. *Journal of Psychosocial Nursing and Mental Health Services, 32,* 15–18.

McNair, R. (1992). Ethical dilemmas of child abuse reporting: Implications for mental health counselors. *Journal of Mental Health Counseling, 14,* 127–136.

Menke, E. M. (1998). The mental health of homeless school-age children. *Journal of Child and Adolescent Psychiatric Nursing, 11,* 87–98.

Murry, S. K., Baker, A. W., & Lewin, L. (2000). Screening families with young children for child maltreatment potential. *Pediatric Nursing, 26,* 47–54.

Pothier, P. C., & Kools, S. (1994). Position paper on foster care reform. *Journal of Child and Adolescent Psychiatric Nursing, 7,* 41–43.

Puskar, K. R., Lamb, J., & Tusaie-Mumford, K. (1997). Teaching kids to cope: A preventive mental health nursing strategy for adolescents. *Journal of Child and Adolescent Psychiatric Nursing, 10,* 18–28.

Rafferty, Y., & Shinn, M. (1991). The impact of homelessness on children. *American Psychologist, 46,* 1170–1179.

Rowe, J. (1992). In support of sibling inclusion: A literature review. *Journal of Child and Adolescent Psychiatric Nursing, 5,* 27–33.

Slomkowski, C., Rende, R., Conger, K. J., et al. (2001). Sisters, brothers, and delinquency: Evaluating social influence during early and middle adolescence. *Child Development, 72*(1), 271–283.

Stanley, S. (1994). Family preservation support services. *Journal of Child and Adolescent Psychiatric Nursing, 7,* 32.

Steinhauer, P. D. (1983). Issues of attachment and separation: Foster care and adoption. In P. D. Steinhauer & Q. Rae-Grant (Eds.), *Psychological problems of the child in the family* (pp. 69–99). New York: Basic Books.

U.S. Bureau of the Census. (1999). Poverty in the United States, 1998. *Current population reports,* Series P-60, No. 181. Washington, DC: Government Printing Office.

Van Epps, J., Opie, N. D., & Goodwin, T. (1997). Themes in the bereavement experience of inner city adolescents. *Journal of Child and Adolescent Psychiatric Nursing, 10,* 25–36.

Warren, J. K., Gary, F. A., & Moorhead, M. S. (1997). Runaway youths in a southern community: Four critical areas of inquiry. *Journal of Child and Adolescent Psychiatric Nursing, 10*(2), 26–35.

Wasserman, A. L. (1990). Principles of psychiatric care of children and adolescents with medical illnesses. In B. A. Garfinkel, G. A. Carlson, & E. B. Weller (Eds.), *Psychiatric disorders in children and adolescents* (pp. 486–502). Philadelphia: W. B. Saunders.

Yalom, I. D. (1985). *The theory and practice of group psychotherapy* (2nd ed.). New York: Basic Books.

Care of Children and Adolescents With Psychiatric Disorders

Lawrence Scahill, Vanya Hamrin,
and Catherine Gray Deering

LEARNING OBJECTIVES

After studying this chapter, you will be able to:

➤ Identify the disorders usually first diagnosed in infancy, childhood, or adolescence, according to the *DSM-IV-TR*.

➤ Differentiate between mental retardation and pervasive developmental disorders.

➤ Identify the biopsychosocial dimensions of the developmental disorders of childhood.

➤ Discuss the nursing management of children with pervasive developmental disorders.

➤ Compare the disruptive behavior disorders: attention deficit hyperactivity disorder, oppositional defiant disorder, and conduct disorder.

➤ Relate the assessment data of children with attention deficit hyperactivity disorder to the development of nursing diagnoses, interventions, and evaluation of outcomes.

➤ Identify the steps involved in fundamental behavior modification interventions, such as "time out," for children.

➤ Discuss the epidemiology, etiology, psychopharmacologic interventions, and nursing management of children with disorders of mood and anxiety.

➤ Discuss the epidemiology, etiology, psychopharmacologic interventions, and nursing management of children with tic disorders.

➤ Discuss behavioral intervention strategies for the treatment of encopresis.

KEY TERMS

autism
communication
  disorders
dyslexia
encopresis
enuresis
externalizing disorders

internalizing disorders
learning disorder
mental retardation
phonologic processing
school phobia
stereotypic behavior

KEY CONCEPTS

attention
developmental delay
hyperactivity
impulsiveness
tics

The understanding of child psychiatric disorders has bene-fited from advances in several related fields, including developmental biology, neuroanatomy, psychopharmacology, genetics, and epidemiology. Before the introduction of the third edition of the American Psychiatric Association's (APA's) Diagnostic and Statistical Manual of Mental Disorders (DSM-III) in 1980, clinicians based their diagnostic decisions on subjective impressions rather than on clearly defined diagnostic criteria. Because the clinician's theoretic orientation directly influenced these subjective impressions, psychiatric diagnoses were notoriously unreliable.

The aims of any diagnostic system are (1) to foster communication between clinicians, (2) to provide insight concerning etiology, and (3) to predict long-term outcomes. A reliable method for making psychiatric diagnoses, therefore, is necessary for ongoing research efforts concerning the etiology and outcome of childhood disorders. Because they are categorical in nature without clear categorical boundaries, current psychiatric diagnoses for children and adolescents provide only limited explanations of a condition's etiology or outcomes. The clear diagnostic criteria and the multiaxial system introduced by DSM-III, however, facilitate communication among clinicians. This chapter uses the current DSM-IV-TR criteria (APA, 2000) in defining childhood disorders. The DSM-IV-TR contains 10 categories of disorders, as listed in Table 29-1. Despite their limitations, the DSM-III and DSM-IV-TR represent major steps forward in defining psychiatric disorders of childhood.

Child psychopathology can be classified according to several broad categories: developmental disorders, disruptive behavior disorders, mood and anxiety disorders, tic disorders, and psychotic disorders. The prevalence of child psychiatric disorders varies across these categories. For example, child schizophrenia is rare, whereas the disruptive behavior disorder, attention deficit hyperactivity disorder (ADHD), is relatively frequent. In cited estimates of prevalence for psychiatric disorders of childhood, the numbers usually include adolescents; however, it should be noted that some of these disorders vary with age. For example, depression is more common in adolescents than in younger children. Gender ratio may also vary with some disorders according to age. For example, depression is probably more common in boys in all children younger than 12 years of age but is more common in girls during adolescence.

This work was supported in part by the following USPHS grants: Children's Clinical Research Center Grant MO1-RR06022; Program Project Grant PO1-MH49351 from the National Institute of Mental Health; Program Project Grant HD-03008 from the National Institute of Child Health and Human Development and Research Units on Pediatric Psychopharmacology; contract NO1-MH-70009 from the National Institute of Mental Health; and a grant from the Tourette Syndrome Association.

The Center for Mental Health Services estimates that 5% to 9% of all 9- to 17-year-olds have serious emotional disturbances with extreme functional impairments, and another 4% to 6% have serious emotional disturbances with some functional impairment (Friedman et al., 1996). These percentages translate into an estimated 8 million American children younger than age 18 years with a psychiatric disorder. Of these, only a small percentage is in active treatment. This discrepancy appears to be the result of limited access to treatment facilities, either because of financial constraints or because specialized mental health services for children are simply unavailable (Institute of Medicine, 1989; Satcher, 2001). Psychiatric problems are less easily diagnosed in children than they are in adults. One factor contributing to this difference is that sometimes the symptoms of disorders are indistinguishable from the turbulence of normal growth and development. For example, a 4-year-old who has an invisible imaginary friend is normal; however, an adolescent with an invisible friend might be experiencing a hallucination. The certainty of current estimates for the frequency of the various psychiatric disorders is also inconsistent, partly because of changing definitions of these disorders.

This chapter presents an overview of the childhood disorders that the generalist psychiatric–mental health nurse may encounter and discusses the nursing care of children with these problems. Because it is beyond the scope of this text to present all child psychiatric disorders, this chapter focuses on developmental, disruptive behavior, mood and anxiety, and tic disorders. It highlights in detail ADHD. It also briefly describes childhood schizophrenia and elimination disorders.

DEVELOPMENTAL DISORDERS OF CHILDHOOD

Under the primary influences of genes and environment, development may be said to proceed along several pathways such as attention, cognition, language, affect, and social and moral behavior. The developmental disorders of childhood include several conditions that are etiologically unrelated; however, their common feature is a significant delay in one or more lines of development. Some of these developmental pathways and developmental delays are closely interwoven. For example, a language delay can interfere with a child's social development and contribute to behavior problems (Cohen et al., 1998). The *DSM-IV-TR* classifies developmental disorders in several categories, including mental retardation, pervasive developmental disorders, and specific developmental disorders. It places mental retardation on Axis II and records pervasive developmental disorders and specific developmental disorders on Axis I. This is a change from the *DSM-III*, which could be a source of confusion when reading child psychiatric literature or past medical records.

TABLE 29.1 Disorders Usually First Diagnosed in Infancy, Childhood, or Adolescence

Disorder	Characteristics
Mental Retardation	
Mild	Significantly below-average intellectual functioning (IQ about 70
Moderate	or below) with onset before age 18 years and concurrent im-
Severe	pairments in adaptive functioning
Profound	
Severity unspecified	
Learning Disorders	
Reading disorder	Academic functioning substantially below that expected given
Mathematics disorder	the person's chronologic age, measured intelligence, and
Disorder of written expression	age-appropriate education
Learning disorders not otherwise specified	
Motor Skills Disorders	
Developmental coordination disorder	Motor coordination substantially below that expected given the
	person's chronologic age and measured intelligence
Communication Disorders	
Expressive language disorder	Significant delay or deviance in speech or language
Mixed receptive–expressive language disorder	
Phonologic disorder	
Stuttering	
Communication disorder not otherwise specified	
Pervasive Developmental Disorders	
Autistic disorder	Severe deficits in multiple areas of development; these include
Asperger's disorder	impairment in reciprocal social interaction, impairment in
Pervasive developmental disorder not otherwise specified	communication, and the presence of stereotyped behavior, restricted interests, and activities
Rett's disorder	
Childhood disintegrative disorder	
Attention-Deficit and Disruptive Behavior Disorders	
Predominantly inattentive type	Prominent symptoms of inattention and/or hyperactivity–
Predominantly hyperactive–impulsive type	impulsivity
Combined type	
Conduct disorder	A pattern of behavior that violates the basic rights of others or major age-appropriate societal norms or rules
Oppositional defiant disorder	A pattern of negativistic, hostile, and defiant behavior
Feeding and Eating Disorders of Infancy or Early Childhood	
Pica	Persistent disturbances in feeding and eating
Rumination disorder	
Feeding disorder of infancy or early childhood	
Tic Disorders	
Tourette's disorder	Vocal or motor tics
Chronic motor or vocal tic disorder	
Transient tic disorder	
Tic disorder not otherwise specified	
Elimination Disorders	
Encopresis	Repeated passage of feces into inappropriate places
Enuresis	Repeated voiding of urine into inappropriate places

(continued)

TABLE 29.1 Disorders Usually First Diagnosed in Infancy, Childhood, or Adolescence (Continued)	
Disorder	**Characteristics**
Other Disorders of Infancy, Childhood, or Adolescence	
Separation anxiety disorder	Developmentally inappropriate and excessive anxiety concerning separation from home or those to whom the child is attached
Selective mutism	A consistent failure to speak in specific social situations despite speaking in other situations
Reactive attachment disorder of infancy or early childhood	Markedly disturbed and developmentally inappropriate social relatedness that occurs in most contexts and is associated with grossly pathogenic care
Stereotypic movement disorder	Repetitive, seemingly driven, and nonfunctional motor behavior that markedly interferes with normal activities and at times may result in bodily injury

Data from American Psychiatric Association. (2000). *Diagnostic and statistical manual of mental disorders* (4th ed., Text revision) (pp. 39–41). Washington, DC: Author.

MENTAL RETARDATION

Mental retardation is defined by significantly below-average intelligence accompanied by impaired adaptive functioning (Table 29-2). Mental retardation can be difficult to diagnose because of its overlapping symptomatology with other disorders. The diagnosis is made through clinical assessment of behavioral features, historical accounts from parents and teachers, and performance on standardized tests (Elder, 1996), such as the Stanford-Binet or the Wechsler Intelligence Scales for Children. Because intelligence tests have been standardized to a mean of 100 with a standard deviation of 15 points, the usual threshold for mental retardation is an intelligence quotient (IQ) of 70 or less (ie, two standard deviations below the population mean). The emphasis is not only on intelligence but also on adaptive behavior and developmental delays. Impaired adaptive functioning is primarily a clinical judgment based on the child's capacity to manage age-appropriate tasks of daily living. Standardized assessments, however, such as the Vineland Adaptive Behavior Scales (Sparrow et al., 1984), are available to assist with determination of the child's capabilities.

Because the diagnosis of mental retardation includes deficits in adaptive functioning, the classification of an individual as mentally retarded is not necessarily lifelong. Some children may be diagnosed at school age as mentally retarded, but the diagnosis is no longer appropriate in adulthood because their social skills and occupational functioning have improved.

> Mental retardation is below average intelligence accompanied by impaired adaptive functioning.

Epidemiology and Etiology

No large prevalence study for mental retardation comparable with the Epidemiological Catchment Area (ECA) program for mental disorders has been conducted within the general population. Using the intelligence threshold of an IQ below 70 (or two standard deviations below the population mean), the prevalence of mental retardation has been estimated at 2%, with a range from 1% to 2.5%. Nearly 90% of those who are mentally retarded are in the mildly retarded range. Although there is consensus that the rate of mental illness is quite high in the mentally retarded population, variation in reported frequency of comorbid conditions is wide, ranging from 15% to 35% (Hardan & Sahl, 1997). Estimates are that psychosis occurs in 5% to 12% of individuals who are mentally retarded. Some children display symptoms of pervasive development disorders (discussed later), such as poor eye contact, extreme difficulty in managing transitions, and repetitive behavior.

Mental retardation has no single cause. Recent evidence indicates that a significant number of cases of mental retardation result from specific genetic abnormalities, such as fragile X syndrome, trisomy 21 (Down's syndrome), and phenylketonuria. Many other cases appear to result from multifactorial causes, in which several genes combine with environmental factors (eg, perinatal exposures) to produce the handicap.

| **TABLE 29.2** | **Key Diagnostic Characteristics of Mental Retardation**
317 Mild mental retardation
318.0 Moderate retardation
318.1 Severe mental retardation
318.2 Profound mental retardation
319 Mental retardation, severity unspecified |

Diagnostic Criteria and Target Symptoms	Associated Findings
• Significantly subaverage general intellectual functioning 　Mild: IQ level 55 to 69 　Moderate: IQ level 40 to 54 　Severe: IQ level 25 to 39 　Profound: IQ level below 25 　Severity unspecified: strong presumption, but IQ 　　testing cannot be completed. • Impairments in adaptive functioning in at least two 　areas: 　Communication 　Self-care 　Social/interpersonal skills 　Ability to use of community resources 　Capacity for self-direction 　Functional academic skills 　Work 　Leisure • Onset before age 18 years	*Behavioral (none specifically unique to mental retardation):* • Possible passiveness and dependency • Possible hyperactivity and impulsivity • Possible aggressiveness and self-injurious behavior *Physical examination:* • Features of clinical syndrome (such as Down's syndrome 　or fragile X) • Increased likelihood of neurologic, neuromuscular, 　visual, auditory, and cardiovascular conditions with 　increasing severity of retardation

Nursing Management

The assessment of a child who is mentally retarded focuses on current physical abilities, intellectual status, and social functioning. A developmental history is a useful way to gather information about past and current capacities (Text Box 29-1). The nurse compares these data with normal growth and development. Developmentally delayed children who have not had a psychological evaluation should be considered for referral. These children also require evaluation for other comorbid psychiatric disorders, which may be a challenge because of the child's cognitive limitations. Discussions about feelings and behavior may be too complex for these children.

The nurse also assesses the child's support systems (family, school, rehabilitative, and psychiatric) to ensure that the child's special needs have been identified and are being addressed. For example, a previous evaluation may have recommended occupational therapy to improve the child's motor coordination. The family, however, may lack transportation to the recommended center for these services, requiring identification of an acceptable alternative that is closer to home. Institutionalized people who are mentally retarded may also have a psychiatric disorder and may require carefully

TEXT BOX 29.1

Salient Points of Developmental History for Disorders in Childhood and Adolescence

• Maternal age and health status during pregnancy

• Exposure to medication, alcohol, or other substances during pregnancy

• Course of pregnancy, labor, and delivery

• Infant's health at birth

• Eating, sleeping, and growth in first year

• Health status in first year

• Interest in others in first 2 years

• Motor development

• Mastery of bowel and bladder control

• Speech and language development

• Activity level

• Response to separation (eg, school entry)

• Regulation of mood and anxiety

• Medical history in early childhood

• Social development

• Interests

constructed behavioral care plans and administration of psychotropic medications (Hurley, 1996).

The complexity of the child and family's response to mental retardation and other comorbid conditions will determine the nursing diagnoses, planning, and implementation of nursing interventions. Some nursing diagnoses that may be appropriate include Ineffective Coping, Delayed Growth and Development, and Interrupted Family Processes. The overall goals are an optimal level of functioning for the family and eventual independent functioning within a normal social environment for the child. For most children with mental retardation, achieving independence in adulthood will be delayed, but not impossible. Nursing interventions include promoting coping skills (interventions directed at building strengths, adapting to change, and maintaining or achieving a higher level of functioning), patient education, and parent education (McCloskey & Bulechek, 1996).

Continuum of Care

Children and families may require varying levels of interventions at different times throughout the life cycle. When a child is young, the family will require special academic support and, for some, residential services. The need for psychiatric intervention will vary according to severity of retardation, family functioning, and the existence of other disorders. Feelings of grief and loss in family members (especially parents) related to having a child with a disability may need special attention. Family therapy may be beneficial to help the family cope with the stresses of raising a child with special needs.

PERVASIVE DEVELOPMENTAL DISORDERS

A developmental delay means that the child's development is outside the norm, including delayed socialization, communication, peculiar mannerisms, and idiosyncratic interests. Pervasive developmental disorders (PDDs) are a group of syndromes marked by severe developmental delays in several areas. In this group of disorders, the developmental delays cannot be attributed to mental retardation. Children with PDDs may or may not be mentally retarded, but they commonly show an uneven pattern of intellectual strengths and weaknesses. Children with PDDs may show a lifelong pattern of being rigid in style, intolerant of change, and prone to behavioral outbursts in response to environmental demands or changes in routine.

> **KEY CONCEPT** **Developmental Delay. Developmental delay** means that the child's development is outside the norm, including delayed socialization, communication, peculiar mannerisms, and idiosyncratic interests.

> Pervasive developmental disorders are a group of syndromes marked by severe developmental delays in several areas that cannot be attributed to mental retardation.

Types

The *DSM-IV-TR* includes several categories of PDDs, but it is beyond the scope of this chapter to review all of them (Koenig & Scahill, in press). This section will focus on autistic disorder and Asperger's disorder.

Autistic Disorder

Autistic disorder, or **autism,** is defined as marked impairment of development in social interaction and communication with a restrictive repertoire of activity and interest. Autism has been a subject of considerable interest and research effort since its original description more than 50 years ago, when Leo Kanner (1894 to 1981) described the profound isolation of these children as well as their extreme desire for sameness. Two features distinguish autism from other PDDs: early age of onset (before age 30 months) and severe disturbance in social relatedness. These children appear aloof and indifferent to others and often seem to prefer inanimate objects.

The impairment in communication is severe and affects both verbal and nonverbal communication (APA, 2000). Autistic children manifest delayed and deviant language development as evidenced by *echolalia* (repetition of words or phrases spoken by others) and a tendency to be extremely concrete in interpretation of language. Pronoun reversals and abnormal intonation are also common. Other common features of autism categorized as **stereotypic behavior** include repetitive rocking, hand flapping, and an extraordinary insistence on sameness. The child may also engage in self-injurious behavior, such as hitting, head banging, or biting. Some interests may evolve into unusual fascination with specific objects, such as fans, air conditioners, or a particular topic, such as Civil War generals.

> Autistic disorder is marked impairment of development in social interaction and communication with a restrictive repertoire of activity and interest.

Epidemiology and Etiology. As currently defined, autism affects between 2 and 20 people per 10,000 in the general population (Chakrabarti & Fombonne, 2001). It occurs in boys more often than girls, with the ratio ranging from 2:1 to 5:1. When girls are affected, however, they tend to be more severely impaired and have poorer outcomes (Cohen & Volkmar, 1997). About half of children with autism are mentally retarded, and about 25% have seizure disorders.

Since Kanner's description, numerous theories have been offered concerning the cause of autism, including perinatal insult and impaired parent–child interactions (Kanner, 1943). It was fashionable in the 1950s and 1960s to believe that the "indifference" of professional parents was a contributing cause of autism. This explanation is no longer seriously considered and almost certainly reflected an **ascertainment bias** (a bias that occurs when the method of identifying cases creates a sample that differs from the population it purports to represent) because professional families were more likely to use the services of major medical centers. It also represents a failure to recognize that the child's disability may have contributed to disturbed parent–child interactions rather than the effect.

Low IQ and autism recur at a higher than expected rate in the siblings of children with autism, and monozygotic twins are more likely to be **concordant** (mutually affected) than dizygotic twins, suggesting that genetic factors play a role in the disorder. Other proposed causes include perinatal complications, such as exposure to infectious agents or medications during gestation, prematurity, and gestational bleeding. The presence of minor physical anomalies in these children has led to a hypothesis of a first-trimester insult, but controlled studies fail to support a prominent role for perinatal complications in autism (Bolton et al., 1997). Biochemical studies have shown increased platelet serotonin levels, excessive dopaminergic activity, and alteration of endogenous opioids (Anderson & Hoshino, 1997) (Fig. 29-1). Despite the substantial body of evidence pointing to a neurobiologic basis, the specific cause remains unknown and may result from multiple factors.

Psychopharmacologic Interventions. No medication has proved effective at changing the core social and linguistic deficits of autism. Numerous psychiatric med-

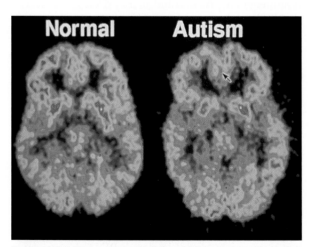

FIGURE 29.1 The patient with autism (*right*) may have decreased metabolic rates in the cingulate gyrus and other associated areas; however, wide heterogeneity in brain metabolic patterns is seen in patients with autism. (Courtesy of Monte S. Buchsbaum, MD, The Mount Sinai Medical Center and School of Medicine, New York, NY.)

ications, however, have been used to treat the associated developmental deficits and behavioral difficulties (see McDougle et al., 2000 for a detailed review). Medications can reduce the frequency and intensity of behavioral disturbances, including hyperactivity, agitation, mood instability, aggression, self-injury, and stereotypic behavior. Haloperidol has demonstrated efficacy in reducing hyperactivity, stereotypic behavior, and emotional lability (Anderson et al., 1989). Despite these reported benefits, haloperidol is associated with a range of side effects. Findings from a recent review of 224 children with autism treated with haloperidol showed that 12.5% had either tardive dyskinesia (n = 5) or withdrawal dyskinesias (n = 23) (Campbell et al., 1997). Given these findings, drug holidays every 6 to 12 months are often recommended to observe the child's continued need for medication. Some children may also show rebound effect (worsening of behavior) for up to 8 weeks after stopping medication (Dulcan et al., 1995). The less potent antipsychotics, such as chlorpromazine, tend to cause excessive sedation without clinical improvement. Clinical reports of the efficacy of the newer atypical antipsychotics for the treatment of autism have shown promising results (reviewed in McDougle et al., 2000). The atypical antipsychotic medications have not been studied in controlled trials in autism; thus, it would be premature to endorse their use. A multisite placebo-controlled study of risperidone is currently underway, which should provide definitive information about the efficacy of risperidone in treating autism (Arnold et al., 2000).

Methylphenidate (Ritalin) may reduce target symptoms of inattention, impulsivity, and overactivity in some higher functioning children and adolescents. Stimulants, however, may increase internal preoccupations, social withdrawal, and stereotypic behavior (Aman, 1996). Several controlled studies of the opioid antagonist naltrexone have found modest improvements in activity level reported, but this was not supported in a recent study. The selective serotonin reuptake inhibitors (SSRIs) may be helpful in managing the compulsive behavior, withdrawal, and irritability but they have not been well studied in children with PDD (McDougle et al., 2000). Lithium has been reported to reduce manifestations of mood disturbances in individuals with autism. Finally, there is an open study showing buspirone may reduce agitation and explosive outbursts in some individuals (Buitelaar et al., 1998).

Continuum of Care

Autism is a chronic disorder usually requiring long-term care at various levels of intensity. Treatment consists of designing academic, interpersonal, and social experiences that support the child's development. In early school-age, the child may be able to live at home and attend a special school for children with autism that uses behavioral modification. Other outpatient services may include family counseling and home care. As the child gets older, living at home may become more difficult because of physical size, disruptive behavior, and the need for a highly structured environment. Thus, in some cases, residential placement may be the best alternative.

Asperger's Disorder

Although Asperger's disorder was also described about 50 years ago, it was not included in *DSM-III* or *DSM-III-R*. It has been incorporated into *DSM-IV-TR* and is defined as severe and sustained impairment in social interaction and restricted, repetitive patterns of behavior, interests, and activities (APA, 2000). This disorder is less strongly associated with mental retardation, as is autism, and the linguistic handicap is typically less severe (Cohen & Volkmar, 1997). These children have profound social deficits, however, marked by inappropriate initiation of social interactions, inability to respond to usual social cues, and a tendency to be concrete in their interpretation of language. Many children with Asperger's disorder display stereotypic behaviors, such as rocking and hand flapping, and these children tend to be inflexible in the performance of their daily living tasks. Signs of developmental delay may not be apparent until preschool or school age when social deficits become evident (Text Box 29-2). The differences in intelligence, language development, and age of clear onset suggest that Asperger's is distinguishable from autism. It may not be differentiated from autism, however, in the literature (Cohen & Volkmar, 1997).

> Asperger's disorder is defined by severe and sustained impairment in social interaction and restricted, repetitive patterns of behavior, interests, and activities not associated with mental retardation. Linguistic handicaps are typically less severe than in autism.

Epidemiology and Etiology. The prevalence of this disorder is difficult to determine because of shifts in its definition and lack of population data on the newly established diagnostic criteria. The current estimate is in the range of 1 to 3 per 1,000. Asperger's disorder appears to be more common in boys. Although no genetic marker has been identified, the disorder often runs in families, with high recurrence in fathers (Cohen & Volkmar, 1997; Volkmar et al., 2000).

Psychopharmacologic Interventions. Psychopharmacologic management is targeted to specific manifestations, such as compulsive behavior, or comorbid conditions, such as depression. Although no medication studies have been conducted on a sample of children carefully diagnosed with Asperger's, approaches to the

TEXT BOX 29.2

Clinical Vignette: Frank (Asperger's Disorder)

A pediatrician refers Frank, age 5 years and 6 months, for an evaluation because of Frank's unusual preoccupation with ceiling fans and lawn sprinklers. According to his mother, Frank became interested in ceiling fans at age 3 years when he began drawing them, tearing pictures of them out of magazines, and engaging others in discussions about them. In the months before the evaluation, Frank also became fascinated by lawn sprinklers. These preoccupations so dominated Frank's interactions with others that he was practically incapable of discussing any other topics. He remained on the periphery of his kindergarten class and had few friends, though he tried.

Frank was the product of a full-term uncomplicated pregnancy, labor, and delivery to his then 25-year-old mother. It was her first pregnancy, and both parents eagerly anticipated Frank's birth. As an infant, Frank was healthy but seemed to cry a lot and was difficult to comfort, causing his mother to feel inadequate and depleted. His motor development was also delayed, and at age 3 years, nonfamily members had difficulty understanding his speech. His articulation, however, was within normal limits at the time of consultation. Frank received regular pediatric care and had no history of serious illness or injury. There was no family history of mental retardation or psychiatric illness; results of genetic testing for chromosomal abnormality were negative.

In addition to his unusual preoccupations, Frank resisted any change in his routine, was easily frustrated, and was prone to temper tantrums. His parents sharply disagreed about the nature of and appropriate response to his problems. This conflict appears to have contributed to their separation and divorce.

treatment of depression and anxiety disorders would be the same as those used in typically developing young children.

Continuum of Care. Asperger's disorder has been recognized only recently. As with autism, the family needs help in supporting the child's development and symptomatic management.

NURSING MANAGEMENT: HUMAN RESPONSE TO DISORDER

Biologic Domain

Assessment

The assessment of children with PDDs is a complex endeavor (Koenig & Scahill, in press). Biologic assessment should include a review of physical health and neurologic status, giving particular attention to coordination, childhood illnesses, injuries, and hospitalizations. The nurse should assess sleep, appetite, and activity patterns because they may be disturbed in these children. Lack of adequate sleep can increase irritability. Comorbid seizure disorders are common in autism, and depression is often seen concurrently with Asperger's. Thus, the nurse should consider these conditions in the assessment.

Youngsters with additional psychiatric disorders or seizures may be receiving multiple medications and require the care of several clinicians. Therefore, the assessment should include a careful review of current medications and treating clinicians.

Nursing Diagnosis and Outcomes: Biologic Domain

Assessment data generate a variety of potential nursing diagnoses. Self-Care Deficits, Impaired Verbal Communication, Disturbed Sensory Perceptions, Delayed Growth and Development, and Disturbed Sleep Pattern are common diagnoses in the biologic domain for children with PDD. Outcomes need to be individualized to the child, family, and social environment.

Interventions for the Biologic Domain

In teaching self-care skills, the nurse needs to consider the child's current adaptive skills and language limitations. Developing a list of activities for the child to post on his or her bedroom may be effective for some children. Drawings or symbols may be useful for nonverbal children. Physical safety is an important concern for children who are cognitively delayed and may have impaired judgment.

As noted earlier, children with PDD may be treated with multiple medications in novel combinations. In some cases, these unusual combinations are the result of careful management. In other cases, the combinations are the result of clinical mismanagement, perhaps because of poor coordination among treating prescribers. Consequently, the nurse should carefully review the target symptoms for each drug treatment with the parents. This review includes possible drug interactions that are especially important for this clinical population.

Psychological Domain

Assessment

Critical elements to evaluate include intellectual ability, linguistic competence, and adaptive functioning. Direct behavioral observation is critical to evaluate the child's ability to relate to others, to select age-appropriate activities, and to watch for stereotypic behaviors. Children with PDD often need specific behavioral interventions to reduce the frequency of inappropriate or aggressive behavior. These interventions follow from a careful evaluation of the circumstances that precede or accompany the behavior and the usual consequences of the behavior (Coucouvanis, 1997). For example, a child may exhibit angry outbursts in response to routine transitions. If the tantrum is dramatic, the consequence may be that the transition does not take place. By structuring the environment and using visual cues to signal the end of one activity and the start of another, it may be possible to reduce the number and intensity of responses to transitions (Coucouvanis, 1997).

Nursing Diagnosis and Outcomes: Psychological Domain

Assessment data generate a variety of potential nursing diagnoses. Anxiety and Disturbed Thought Processes are common diagnoses in the psychological domain for children with PDD. Because of the long-term nature of these disorders, outcomes may change over time.

Interventions for the Psychological Domain

Managing the repetitive behaviors of these children will depend on the specific behavior and its effects on others or the environment. If the behavior, such as rocking, has no negative effects, ignoring it may be the best approach. If the behavior, such as head banging, is unacceptable, redirecting the child and using positive reinforcement are recommended. In some cases, especially in severely delayed children, these strategies may not work, and environmental alterations and perhaps protective headgear are needed.

Social Domain

Assessment

The nursing assessment is an ongoing process in which attention is given to establishing a positive relationship with the child and the family. These children exhibit various behavioral problems and have varying degrees of adaptive deficits. Therefore, the assessment should include a review of the child's capacity for self-care and maladaptive behaviors (Coucouvanis, 1997). Self-injury and aggression are sometimes present, and children may need to be protected from hurting themselves and others. Inquiry should also include the presence of perseverative behaviors and preoccupation with restricted interests. These odd behaviors may not necessarily cause a problem, but they may interfere with the child's relationships.

Another important domain to consider in the nursing assessment is the effects of the child's developmental delays on the family. The PDDs invariably affect family interaction, and responding to the child's needs may adversely affect family functioning. For example, sleep disruption in family members who manage these children may increase family stress.

Nursing Diagnosis and Outcomes: Social Domain

Assessment data generate a variety of potential nursing diagnoses. Social Isolation is a common social diagnosis in children with PDD. The family may be grieving the loss of the normal child they had expected and are trying to cope with the multitude of problems inherent in raising a child with a disability. Because of the long-term nature of these disorders, the aims of treatment may change over time. Throughout childhood, however, the focus should be on the development of age-appropriate social skills.

Interventions for the Social Domain

Planning interventions for youngsters with severe developmental problems considers the child, family, and community supports such as schools, rehabilitation centers, or group homes. First and foremost, the various clinicians involved in the child's treatment should collaborate with the family toward the same general goals. As the number of clinicians and educators involved increases, the chance of fragmentation in treatment planning also increases. The nurse can serve as a case coordinator.

Interventions for social isolation should fit the child's cognitive, linguistic, and developmental levels. Interventions fostering nonverbal social interactions may be more useful than those based on speech. For higher functioning children, activities such as getting the mail, passing out snacks, or taking turns in the context of simple games can engage the child in social activities without requiring the use of their limited language skills. Structuring social interactions so that the child has to share a task with another, such as carrying a load of books, may help to boost confidence in relating to others.

When children with PDD are hospitalized, milieu management—a consistent, structured environment with predictable routines for activities, mealtimes, and bedtimes—is necessary for successful treatment. Changes in routine may provoke disorganization in the child with PDD, leading to emotional disequilibrium and explosive behavior. The safety of the inpatient unit offers an opportunity to try behavioral strategies, such as rewards for managing transitions. Health care professionals can pass on successful strategies to parents or primary caretakers. Because children with PDD have difficulty relating to others, they should spend most of their time within the therapeutic environment of the unit. These children can learn social and linguistic skills, such as taking turns in conversation and warning the listener before changing the subject in the context of milieu. If a child requires isolation for control of aggressive or assaultive behavior, a brief "time out" followed by prompt reentry into unit activities is optimum.

Autism and related disorders are chronic conditions that call for extraordinary patience and determination. Unfortunately, lack of integration of medical, psychiatric, social, and educational services can add to the family's burden. Parents may manifest denial, grief, guilt, and anger at various points as they adjust to their child's disability. The nurse can offer parents the opportunity to express their frustrations and disappointments and can be alert for indications that parents are in need of additional assistance such as parent support groups or respite care.

Residential care may be necessary in some cases. After making the decision to place a child into a residential facility, family members may experience guilt, loss, and a sense of failure concerning their inability to manage the child at home. Family interventions include support, education, counseling, and referral to self-help groups. Whenever possible, the nurse provides education to help parents determine appropriate expectations for their child with PDD and to meet the child's special needs. The following are examples of potentially useful nursing interventions focusing on the family:

- Interpreting the treatment plan for parents and child
- Modeling appropriate behavior modification techniques
- Including the parents as cotherapists for the implementation of the care plan
- Assisting the family in identifying and resolving their sense of loss related to the diagnosis
- Coordinating support systems for parents, siblings, and family members
- Maintaining interdisciplinary collaboration

Evaluation and Treatment Outcomes

Evaluation of patient and family outcomes is an ongoing process. Short-term outcomes might consist of discrete behavioral improvements, such as reducing self-injurious behavior by 50%. The long-term goal is for the patient to achieve the highest level of functioning. The prognosis depends on the severity of the impairments, the interventions available, and the cognitive ability of the child. The use of standardized rating scales before and after treatment can improve the precision of outcome measurement (Arnold et al., 2000).

SPECIFIC DEVELOPMENTAL DISORDERS

In contrast to mental retardation and PDD, specific developmental disorders are characterized by a narrower range of deficits. These more discrete delays can occur in various developmental domains. Some children, however, have more than one specific developmental disorder, and some of these disorders may have a common etiology (Beitchman & Young, 1997).

Types

Specific developmental disorders are generally classified as learning, communication, and motor skills disorders. This section focuses primarily on learning and communication disorders.

Learning Disorder

The precise definition of **learning disorder** (also called *learning disability*) varies depending on the source and state statute. In general, however, learning disorder is defined as a discrepancy between actual achievement and expected achievement based on the person's age and intellectual ability. Learning disorders are typically classified as verbal (reading and spelling) or nonverbal (mathematics). This distinction between verbal and nonverbal learning disorders comes from the presumed differences in the nature and etiology (see later). Recent evidence supports the validity of these presumptions (Beitchman & Young, 1997).

> Generally, learning disorder is defined as a discrepancy between actual achievement and expected achievement based on the person's age and intellectual ability.

Reading disability, also called **dyslexia,** has been recognized for more than 50 years. It is defined as a significantly lower score for mental age on standardized tests in reading that is not the result of low intelligence or inadequate schooling. This relatively common problem affects about 5% of school-aged children, with some studies reporting higher prevalence. In clinical samples, dyslexia affects boys more often than girls; however, a large community-based sample of children with reading disorders found no gender difference. This discrepancy suggests that the observed difference in clinic samples may be related to biases in seeking treatment rather than a true gender difference (Shaywitz et al., 1990).

Although it is clear that no single cause will provide a sufficient explanation for reading disability, the underlying problem appears to be a deficit in **phonologic processing,** which involves the discrimination and interpretation of speech sounds. A disturbance in the development of the left hemisphere is believed to cause this deficit. Both genetic and environmental factors have been implicated in the etiology of reading disability. Data from family studies show that reading disability is familial and that shared environmental factors alone cannot explain the high rate of recurrence in affected families. Additional evidence from twin studies indicates that specific weaknesses in phonologic processing are more likely to be observed in monozygotic twins compared with dizygotic twins (Willcutt et al., 2000).

Less is known about the prevalence of nonverbal learning disorder (mathematics disorder), with estimates ranging from 0.1 to 1.0% and no apparent difference between boys and girls. Mathematics disorder (which is manifested by significant delay in learning mathematics) appears to be a right-hemisphere disorder. Right-hemisphere dysfunction and math problems have been shown in fragile X syndrome and Turner's syndrome, both of which are genetic syndromes. Other reports from clinical populations have shown that acquired problems, such as early onset seizure disorders, can produce right hemisphere dysfunction and mathematic disability.

Communication Disorders

Communication disorders involve speech or language impairments. *Speech* refers to the motor aspects of speaking; *language* consists of higher-order aspects of formulating and comprehending verbal communication. A large community survey of 5-year-olds in Canada found a combined prevalence of 19% for speech and language disorders (Beitchman et al., 1986a), suggesting they are fairly common in school-aged children. Although evidence suggests that many communication deficits appearing at this age do resolve, speech and language disorders are also associated with psychiatric disability (Tomblin et al., 2000; Toppelberg & Shapiro, 2000). As with reading disability, there are undoubtedly multiple causes of speech or language handicap.

A delay in speech or language development can adversely affect the child's socialization and education. For example, peers may rebuff or tease a child with an articulation defect or stutter, contributing to withdrawal and a negative self-image. The resulting isolation could limit opportunities to negotiate rules, take turns, and learn cooperation. These same tasks could also be difficult for children with language delay. Moreover, language appears to play a role in the regulation of behavior and impulses. Not surprisingly, impaired language appears to be a risk factor for ADHD (Fletcher et al., 1999; Toppelberg and Shapiro, 2000). Children with language delays may also be at greater risk for reading disability, which may share the same underlying phonologic defect (Tomblin et al., 2000; Willcutt et al., 2000).

NURSING MANAGEMENT: HUMAN RESPONSE TO DISORDER

Nursing assessment of children with a known specific developmental disorder includes (1) evidence of interference in daily life, (2) determination of the youngster's ability (and limitations) to communicate during the interview, (3) assessment of the child's perception about his or her disability, (4) observation for impaired learning and communication, and (5) past and current interventions for the learning or communication deficit, with data gathered through direct interview of the child and significant others such as parents. Several nursing diagnoses can be generated from these data, such as Impaired Verbal Communication, Low Self-Esteem, and Social Isolation. For the child with learning disabilities, nurses can focus on building self-esteem and helping the family connect with guidance and educational resources that support the child's development into adulthood. For the child with communication disorders, the interventions focus on fostering social and communication skills and making referrals for specific speech or language therapy. Modeling appropriate communication in spontaneous situations with the child can be a useful intervention for some children. The following is an overview of nursing interventions for the child with specific developmental difficulties:

- Introduce strategies for increasing communication skills (eg, initiating conversation, taking turns in conversation, facing the listener).
- Identify and develop specific intervention strategies for problems secondary to learning communication disorders, such as low self-esteem (Tomblin et al., 2000).
- Provide parental support for coping with the disorder.
- Maintain interdisciplinary medical, dental, speech therapy, and educational collaboration.
- Refer to learning or speech specialist for evaluation and assistance (Toppelberg & Shapiro, 2000).

Continuum of Care

Children with learning disabilities obviously require careful psychoeducational and cognitive testing to identify their strengths and deficits. School or clinical psychologists usually perform this type of specialized testing. When a learning disability has been identified, the Education for the Handicapped Act (PL 94-142) mandates that public school systems provide remedial services in the least restrictive educational setting. Families occasionally need help in advocating for these services.

The same is true for children with communication disorders, although the services requested may be different. Speech pathologists conduct the diagnostic assessment of speech and language disorder. Nurses may be involved with formal screening for communication disorders (Tomblin et al., 2000). Services such as speech therapy (directed at the motor aspects of speaking) or social skills groups (directed at the social and interpersonal aspects of language) are often available in school districts and can be obtained if a speech or lan-

guage disorder has been identified. For some children with communication disorders, the services offered by the school may be insufficient. In such cases, the nurse can help the family locate a facility that can provide these needed services.

DISRUPTIVE BEHAVIOR DISORDERS

The disruptive behavior disorders, which include ADHD, oppositional defiant disorder, and conduct disorder, are a group of syndromes marked by significant problems of conduct. Because these disorders are characterized by "acting-out" behaviors, they are sometimes referred to as **externalizing disorders.** In contrast, disorders of mood (eg, anxiety, depression) are classified as **internalizing disorders** because the symptoms tend to be within the child.

The disruptive behavior disorders are more common in boys and are associated with lower socioeconomic status, urban living (Scahill et al., 1999b; Szatmari et al., 1989b), learning disabilities (Fletcher et al., 1999; Tomblin et al., 2000), and language delay (Toppelberg & Shapiro, 2000). These disorders are relatively common in school-aged children and frequently are part of the presenting complaint in child psychiatric treatment settings.

ATTENTION DEFICIT HYPERACTIVITY DISORDER

ADHD is a common disorder in school-aged children. It is almost certainly a heterogeneous disorder with multiple etiologies. The relatively high frequency of ADHD and associated behavior problems virtually guarantees that nurses will meet these children in all pediatric treatment settings.

Clinical Course and Diagnostic Criteria

Parents and teachers describe children with ADHD as restless, always on the go, highly distractible, unable to wait their turn, heedless, and frequently disruptive. Indeed, it is often disruptive behavior that brings these children into treatment. The historical debate concerning the nature of ADHD is reflected in the labels used to describe it: organic brain syndrome, hyperkinetic impulse disorder, minimal brain dysfunction, hyperkinetic reaction of childhood, hyperkinesis, attention deficit disorder, and most recently, in *DSM-IV-TR*, attention deficit hyperactivity disorder. This long list of terms also implies the various theories regarding the cause and the presumed site of the primary defect. The *DSM-IV-TR* represents yet another formulation of ADHD by defining ADHD as predominantly hyperactive type, predominantly inattentive type, or combined type (Table 29-3).

TABLE 29.3 Key Diagnostic Characteristics of Attention Deficit Hyperactivity Disorder
314.10: Attention deficit hyperactivity disorder, combined type
314.00: Attention deficit hyperactivity disorder, predominantly inattentive type
314.01: Attention deficit hyperactivity disorder, predominantly hyperactive–impulsive type
314.9: Attention deficit hyperactivity disorder, not otherwise specified

Diagnostic Criteria and Target Symptoms	Associated Findings

• Symptoms of inattention (at least six):
  Lacks close attention to details; makes careless mistakes in activities
  Has difficulty sustaining attention
  Appears to not listen when spoken to directly
  Has difficulty following through on instructions; fails to finish work or activities
  Has difficulty organizing tasks and activities
  Has difficulty with tasks requiring sustained mental effort; commonly avoids, dislikes, or is reluctant to engage in them
  Loses items necessary for tasks
  Is easily distracted by outside stimuli
  Is often forgetful in daily activities
• Symptoms of hyperactivity-impulsivity (at least six):
  Hyperactivity
    Fidgets or squirms
    Gets up when expectation is to remain seated
    Excessively runs about or climbs inappropriately
    Has difficulty with quiet leisure activities
    Often appears "on the go" or "driven by a motor"
    Talks excessively
  Impulsivity
    Blurts out answers before question completion
    Has difficulty awaiting turn
    Is interruptive or intrusive of others
• Symptoms are maladaptive and inconsistent with developmental level, persisting for at least 6 months
• Some symptoms present before age 7 years
• Evidence of significant impairment in social, academic, or occupational functioning
• Not exclusive during other psychiatric disorder; not better accounted for by another mental disorder
	• Low frustration tolerance
	• Temper outbursts
	• Bossiness, stubbornness
	• Excessive and frequent insistence for requests to be met
	• Mood lability
	• Demoralization
	• Dysphoria
	• Rejection by peers
	• Low self-regard
	• Resentment and antagonism within family
	• Reduced vocational achievement

Despite the historical shifts in terminology and the various proposals regarding the etiology of ADHD, the accumulated consensus over the past several decades is that three core symptoms define the disorder: inattention, impulsiveness, and hyperactivity.

Attention deficit hyperactivity disorder is a persistent pattern of inattention, hyperactivity, and impulsiveness that is pervasive and inappropriate for developmental level (APA, 2000).

Attention is a complex mental process that involves the ability to concentrate on one activity to the exclusion of others as well as the ability to sustain focus over time. Children with ADHD are easily distracted and lack persistence in the performance of age-appropriate tasks, reflecting an inability to filter out stimuli, sustain attention, or both. The inability to screen out stimuli leaves the child unable to identify salient stimuli. The child may then treat all incoming stimuli with equal regard and respond to multiple incoming stimuli. Alternatively, it has been argued that the distractibility seen in ADHD is the result of stimulus-seeking behavior. Given the heterogeneity of ADHD, either of these models may be true for subgroups of affected children.

KEY CONCEPT   **Attention. Attention** is a complex process that involves the ability to concentrate on one activity to the exclusion of others as well as the ability to sustain that focus over time.

Impulsiveness is the tendency to act on urges, notions, or desires without adequately considering the consequences. Both clinical observation and laboratory studies support the conclusion that children with ADHD are prone to impulsive, risk-taking behavior (Barkley, 1998). A fundamental question that some have raised is that impulsiveness may not be truly separate from distractibility or hyperactivity. Alternatively, some have argued that children with ADHD have an impaired capacity to learn through reinforcement, which predisposes them to impulsive behavior. Indirect support for this view comes from studies showing that animals with lesions of the frontal lobe are less able to make use of reinforcement without additional external structure and greater rewards (Barkley, 1998). In behavioral terms, children with ADHD often fail to consider the consequences of their actions, exercise poor judgment, and tend to have more than usual lumps, bumps, and bruises because of their risk-taking behavior. They often require a high degree of structure and supervision.

KEY CONCEPT   **Impulsiveness. Impulsiveness** is the tendency to act on urges, notions, or desires without adequately considering the consequences.

Hyperactivity is excessive motor activity as evidenced by restlessness, inability to remain seated, and high levels of physical motion and verbal output. Although hyperactivity is a characteristic often associated with ADHD, controversy is long-standing about whether attention deficit can occur without overactivity. The decision by *DSM-IV-TR* to define ADHD as predominately hyperactive, predominately inattentive, or combined offers a compromise in the debate over attention deficit disorder with or without hyperactivity. Even those who argue in favor of attention deficit disorder without hyperactivity acknowledge that it is probably much less common than attention deficit disorder with hyperactivity.

In many cases, it is the hyperactivity that prompts the search for treatment. Parents typically report that the child's hyperactivity was manifest early in life and evident in most situations. The child's overactivity may be more noticeable in the classroom, however, because it is poorly tolerated there (Barkley, 1998).

KEY CONCEPT   **Hyperactivity. Hyperactivity** is excessive motor activity, as evidenced by restlessness, inability to remain seated, and high levels of physical motion and verbal output.

Epidemiology and Risk Factors

Although prevalence estimates vary depending on the diagnostic criteria used, the sources of data, and the sampling procedure, ADHD is a common psychiatric disorder of childhood. The current estimate in school-aged children is about 6%, with a range of 2% to 14%. Boys are affected three to eight times more often than are girls (for a review, see Scahill & Schwab-Stone, 2000). Longitudinal studies that followed groups of children with ADHD into adulthood have shown that 30% to 40% continued to have problems with impulsiveness and inattention, although hyperactivity seemed to be slightly less evident (Mannuzza et al., 1998). Young adults with a history of ADHD were more likely to have multiple arrests and arrests for more serious offenses than the control group. Another study of teenagers has shown similar findings (Fischer et al., 1993). Clearly, then, a substantial minority of children do not "grow out of" ADHD. These findings bolster the connection between ADHD and antisocial behavior (see Chap. 22).

Etiologic Factors

Despite more than a half century of investigation, the etiology of ADHD remains unclear (Barkley, 1998). Numerous environmental exposures, including perinatal insult, head injury, psychosocial disadvantage, lead poisoning, and diet (eg, food allergies or sensitivity to food additives), have been proposed as potential causes. Although these hypotheses may explain some cases, none of these exposures alone is likely to account for a significant portion of children with ADHD (Barkley, 1998). The claim that food additives or allergies cause ADHD has very limited empiric data to support it (Scahill & DeGraft-Johnson, 1997).

Biologic Factors

Although the etiology of ADHD is uncertain, persuasive evidence from several lines of research has shown that the frontal lobe and functional connections with specific subcortical structures are dysregulated in patients with ADHD. For example, a structural magnetic resonance imaging (MRI) study in 57 boys with ADHD compared with 55 controls showed reduced volumes of the right dorsolateral frontal region and in selected regions of the basal ganglia (Castellanos et al., 1996). Using single-photon emission computed tomography (SPECT) to measure brain activity, Lou and colleagues (1990) found reduced blood flow in these same subcortical regions (caudate and putamen) compared with controls. Additional evidence linking ADHD to dysfunction of the frontal lobe comes from a positron emission tomography (PET) scan study of adults who had a personal history of ADHD and were parents of children with ADHD. This study found hypoperfusion (decreased metabolic activity) in the frontal lobe of the adults with a history of ADHD compared with the control group (Zametkin et al., 1990). These investigators used similar techniques to evaluate frontal lobe functioning in a group of adolescents with ADHD. Although the findings were in the same direction, the difference between normal controls and the adolescents with ADHD was not statistically significant (Zametkin et al., 1993). More recently, Vaidya and colleagues (1998) showed differences in frontal-subcortical function during an attentional task. The difference between normal subjects and subjects with ADHD was reduced when the subjects with ADHD received methylphenidate.

Genetic factors have also been implicated in the etiology of ADHD and clearly play a fundamental role for at least a subgroup of children. Several twin studies have shown that, although identical twins are not fully concordant for ADHD, they are far more likely to be mutually affected than dizygotic twins (Goodman & Stevenson, 1989a, 1989b). A more recent twin study examined the concordance of ADHD symptoms in a large community sample of monozygotic and dizygotic twins across a wide range of symptoms, from none to severe (Levy et al., 1999). In that study, the monozygotic twins not only showed higher concordance for ADHD than the dizygotic twins but also showed greater similarity across the full range of symptoms. By contrast, the dizygotic twins showed much greater variability in their expression of ADHD symptoms. These findings suggest that ADHD can be viewed as one or more heritable traits (eg, attention and impulsiveness) on a continuum form mild to severe. Family genetic studies also support a prominent role for genetics in the etiology of ADHD. In the largest family study to date, Biederman and colleagues (1992) showed that ADHD is more likely to affect biologic relatives of children with ADHD than biologic relatives of pediatric controls.

Psychological and Social Factors

Although genetic endowment clearly plays a fundamental role in the etiology of ADHD, environmental factors are also important. Psychosocial influences (family stress and marital discord) are associated with ADHD, but the direction of causality is difficult to determine (DuPaul & Stoner, 1994; Scahill et al., 1999b; Szatmari et al., 1989b). Other psychosocial correlates that have been observed in large community samples (Scahill et al., 1999b; Szatmari et al., 1989b) and community samples (Biederman et al., 1995) are poverty, overcrowded living conditions, and family dysfunction.

NURSING MANAGEMENT: HUMAN RESPONSE TO DISORDER

Biologic Domain

Assessment

The nursing assessment may be initiated either before or after the diagnosis of ADHD is made. In the school setting, the nurse may suspect ADHD and collect similar assessment data as the nurse in a psychiatric facility. In the school setting, the primary focus of the assessment is the impact of ADHD on classroom behavior and school performance. In the hospital, the nurse tries to determine the contribution of ADHD to the acute psychiatric problem. In both cases, the nurse collects assessment data through direct interview and observation of the child. Because children with ADHD may have difficulty sitting through long sessions, interviews are typically brief. Parents and teachers are extremely important sources for assessment data. To this end, the nurse can make use of several standardized instruments (Text Box 29-3).

TEXT BOX 29.3

Standardized Instruments for Parent and Teachers for the Diagnosis of Attention Deficit Hyperactivity Disorder (ADHD)*

The Conners Parent Questionnaire is a 48-item scale that a parent completes about his or her child. Each item is a statement that the parent rates on a 4-point scale from 0 (not at all) to 3 (very much). The Conners Teacher Questionnaire is a 28-item questionnaire that the child's teacher completes according to the same 4-point scale as the Parent Questionnaire. Both questionnaires have been standardized by age and gender for a mean of 50 and a standard deviation of 10 (Conners, 1989; Goyette et al., 1978).

The ADHD Rating Scale is a recently developed measure that asks parents or teachers to respond directly to 18 items in the *DSM-IV-TR* criteria (see Barkley, 1998, for a description of this scale). A similar scale called the SNAP-IV is available on-line for free at www.adhd.com.

The Child Behavior Checklist (CBCL) is a 118-item questionnaire that a parent completes. In addition to the 118 questions about specific behaviors and psychiatric symptoms, the CBCL also includes questions concerning the child's competence in social and academic spheres as well as age-appropriate activities. Normative data are available allowing the conversion of raw scores to standard scores for age and gender. There is also a teacher version of this scale.

---

*Note that the diagnosis of ADHD is not made on the basis of questionnaires alone. Data from these rating scales augment the information gathered through interview and observation. These questionnaires can be especially useful before and after initiating a treatment plan to measure change.

As with other psychiatric disorders with onset in childhood, the nursing assessment of children with ADHD begins with identification and exploration of the presenting problem. This typically entails a review of the child's developmental course, the onset and pattern of the current symptoms, factors that have worsened or improved the child's problems, and prior treatment or self-initiated efforts to remedy the situation. The association of ADHD and communication disorders suggests a need for careful consideration of language development and current linguistic functioning. Medical history is also essential, consisting of perinatal course, childhood illnesses, hospitalizations, injuries, seizures, tics, physical growth, general health status, and timing of the child's last physical examination.

Behavior of these children is characteristically very active and can easily be observed. They cannot sit still. They fidget. Even in sleep, they may be more active than normal children. Thus, a careful assessment of eating, sleeping, and activity patterns is essential. Assessing daily food intake, typical diet, and frequency of eating will help identify any nutrition problems. Caffeinated products can contribute to hyperactivity. Sleep is often disturbed for children with ADHD and consequently the family. A detailed sleep assessment can provide points for interventions and help the interpretation of drug effects.

Nursing Diagnoses and Outcomes: Biologic Domain

Depending on the severity of the responses, family situation, and school environment, several nursing diagnoses could be generated from the assessment data. In the biologic domain, possible diagnoses include Self-Care Deficit, Risk for Imbalanced Nutrition, Risk for Injury, and Disturbed Sleep Pattern. The outcomes should be individualized to the child.

Interventions for the Biologic Domain

Planning of nursing interventions must be done within the context of the family, treatment setting, and school environment. With the parents, clinical team members, and school personnel, the nurse participates in designing a plan of care that fits the child's and family's needs. Medication can help the hyperactivity, impulsiveness, and inattention. Therefore, teaching the parent, child, and school personnel about the importance of the medication in ADHD and the potential side effects is a place to begin. Explaining to the child that the medication improves concentration and the ability to sit still can help strengthen patient motivation.

Several medications may be used in the treatment of ADHD, though the stimulants are by far the most common (Table 29-4). Commonly used stimulants include methylphenidate, D-amphetamine, and D, L-amphetamine. Although each of these medications has demonstrated efficacy in controlled studies, methylphenidate has received considerably more research effort and is typically the first medication tried in the treatment of ADHD (Barkley, 1998; MTA Group, 1999). Another psychostimulant, pemoline, has fallen out of use because of concerns about liver toxicity. It should be noted that the stimulants are not effective in all cases; hence, alternatives to the stimulants may be prescribed for children who do not respond to the stimulants or develop tics when taking them (Scahill et al., 2001a).

Methylphenidate is short-acting medication that peaks in about 90 minutes to 2 hours and has a total duration of action of about 4 hours. Hence, parents or teachers often describe a return of overactivity and distractibility as the first dose of medication wears off. This "rebound effect" can often be managed by moving the second dose of the day slightly closer to the first dose. Similar phenomena may be observed with the amphetamines, though the rebound typically occurs later because the duration of action is slightly longer than methylphenidate (see Drug Profile: Methylphenidate).

A national survey estimated that just less than 5% of elementary school children have been prescribed medication for inattention and hyperactivity. Of these, more than 90% were prescribed methylphenidate

TABLE 29.4	Stimulant Medications Used in the Treatment of Attention Deficit Hyperactivity Disorder	
Medication	**Total Daily Dosage**	**Common Side Effects**
Methylphenidate	10–60 mg in two or three divided doses	Loss of appetite, insomnia, rebound activation, increase in tics or compulsive behavior, psychotic reaction
D-Amphetamine	5–40 mg in two divided doses	Similar to methylphenidate
D, L-Amphetamine	5–40 mg in two divided doses	Similar to methylphenidate

---

DRUG PROFILE: Methylphenidate
(Central Nervous System Stimulant)
Trade Name: Ritalin and Various Generic Formulations

Receptor affinity: The mechanisms through which methylphenidate exerts its effects are not completely clear. At low doses, such as those used in the treatment of children and adolescents with ADHD, it provides mild cortical stimulation similar to that of amphetamines. This stimulation results from methylphenidate's ability to block the reuptake of dopamine and norepinephrine in the synaptic cleft. Main sites appear to be the cerebral cortex, striatum, and pons.

Indications: Treatment of narcolepsy, attention deficit disorders, and hyperkinetic syndrome; unlabeled uses for treatment of depression in elderly patients and patients with cancer or stroke.

Routes and dosage: Available in 5- or 10-mg immediate release tablets and 20-mg sustained-release tablets (Ritalin-SR). Newer long-acting preparations, such as Concerta and Metadate, are also available.

Adult dosage: Must be individualized; range from 10 to 60 mg/d, orally in divided doses bid to tid, preferably 15 to 30 min before meals. If insomnia is a problem, drug should be administered before 6 PM.

Child dosage: Initially, 5 mg orally before breakfast and lunch, with gradual increases of 5 to 10 mg weekly. Usually given on a tid schedule, with the last dose being roughly half that of the first and second dose. Daily dosage of >60 mg not recommended. Discontinue after 1 month if no improvement.

Peak effect: 1 h; *half-life:* 3–4 h for the immediate-release preparations.

Select adverse reactions: Nervousness, insomnia, dizziness, headache, dyskinesias (including tics), toxic psychosis, anorexia, nausea, abdominal pain, increased or decreased pulse and blood pressure, tachycardia, angina, dysrhythmias, palpitations, tolerance, psychological dependence.

Warning: The drug is discontinued periodically to assess the patient's condition. Contraindications include marked anxiety, tension and agitation, glaucoma, severe depression, and obsessive-compulsive disorder. Use cautiously in patients with a personal or family history of tic disorders, seizure disorders, hypertension, drug dependence, alcoholism, or emotional instability.

Specific patient/family education:

- Do not chew or crush sustained-release tablets—they must be swallowed whole.

- Take the drug exactly as prescribed; if insomnia is a problem, time and dose may need adjustment. The drug is rarely taken after 5 PM.

- Avoid alcohol and OTC products, including decongestants, cold remedies, and cough syrups—these could accentuate side effects of the stimulant.

- Keep appointments for follow-up, including laboratory tests and evaluations for monitoring the child's growth.

- Note that the prescriber may discontinue the drug periodically to confirm effectiveness of therapy.

(Safer et al., 1996). This figure represents a gradual increase over the first half of the 1990s. Nonetheless, claims that methylphenidate is overprescribed are probably not justified (Jensen et al., 1999).

Psychological Domain

Assessment

Hyperactivity, impulsivity, and inattention are typically pervasive problems that are evident both at school and at home. Discipline is frequently an issue because parents may have difficulty controlling their child's behavior, which at times can become destructive.

Nursing Diagnoses and Outcomes: Psychological Domain

Assessment of the psychological domain may generate several diagnoses. Possibilities include Anxiety and Defensive Coping. The outcomes should be individualized to the child.

Interventions for the Psychological Domain

As a complement to medication, behavioral programs based on rewards for positive behavior, such as waiting turns and following directions, can foster new social skills. Interventions may also include specific cognitive behavioral techniques in which the child learns to "stop, look, and listen" before doing. These approaches have been refined, and several useful treatment manuals are now available (Barkley, 1998). In general, these manuals emphasize problem solving and development of prosocial behavior. Interactions with children can be guided by the following:

- Set clear limits with clear consequences. Use few words and simplify instructions.
- Establish and maintain a predictable environment with clear rules and regular routines for eating, sleeping, and playing.
- Promote attention by maintaining a calm environment with few stimuli. These children cannot filter extraneous stimuli and react to all stimuli equally.
- Establish eye contact before giving directions; ask child to repeat what was heard.
- Encourage the child to do homework in a quiet place, outside of a traffic pattern.
- Assist the child to work on one assignment at a time (reward with a break after each completion).

Social Domain

Assessment

Dysfunctional interactions can develop within the family. Reviewing the problem behaviors and the situations in which they occur is a way to identify negative interaction patterns. These children are often behind in their work at school because of poor organization, off-task behavior, and impulsive responses. They exhaust their parents, aggravate teachers, and annoy siblings with their intrusive and disruptive behavior. Because ADHD often occurs in the context of psychosocial adversity, it is important to review the family situation, including parenting style, stability of household membership, consistency of rules and routines, and life events such as divorce, moves, deaths, and job loss. Identification of these factors can be useful in shaping a care plan that builds on potential strengths and mitigates the effects of environmental factors that may perpetuate the child's disruptive behavior. Data regarding school performance, behavior at home, and comorbid psychiatric disorders are essential for developing school interventions, behavior plans, and establishing the baseline severity for medication.

Nursing Diagnoses and Outcomes: Social Domain

Depending on the severity of the responses, family situation, and school environment, several nursing diagnoses could be generated from the assessment data. Impaired Social Interaction, Ineffective Role Performance, and Compromised Family Coping are typical diagnoses in the social domain. The outcomes should be individualized to the child. Short-term outcomes, such as decreasing the number of classroom ejections within a 2-week period, may be useful for one child. Minimizing the frequency and amplitude of angry outbursts at home may be relevant to the next child.

Interventions for the Social Domain

Family treatment is nearly always a component of cognitive behavioral treatment approaches with the child. This may involve parent training that focuses on principles of behavior management, such as appropriate limit setting and reward systems, as well as revising expectations about the child's behavior.

School programming often involves increasing structure in the child's school day to offset the child's tendency to act without forethought and to be easily distracted by extraneous stimuli. Specific remediation is required for the child with comorbid deficits in learning or language. Some children may require small, self-contained classrooms.

Evaluation and Treatment Outcomes

Sometimes, children do not notice any effects following medication, but people in their environment do. Often, within 1 to 2 weeks of initiating therapy, children with ADHD become more attentive, less impulsive, and less active. Parents and teachers are often the first to notice improvement. Useful tools for tracking changes in behavior are the Parent and Teacher Conners Questionnaires or the ADHD Rating Scale (Conners, 1989). Over time, academic achievement may also improve (Fig. 29-2).

Continuum of Care

The treatment of ADHD may be multimodal (includes several types of interventions), encompassing four main areas: individual treatment for the child, family treatment, school accommodations, and medication. Rarely is a child hospitalized for ADHD only. Treatment is carried out in the community mental health clinic, school, home, and primary care clinic. See Nursing Care Plan 29-1.

OPPOSITIONAL DEFIANT DISORDER AND CONDUCT DISORDER

Oppositional defiant disorder is characterized by a persistent pattern of disobedience, argumentativeness, angry outbursts, low tolerance for frustration, and tendency to blame others for misfortunes, large and small. These children have trouble making friends and often find themselves in conflict with adults. This disorder is distinguishable from conduct disorder, which is characterized by more serious violations of social norms, including aggressive behavior, destruction of property, and cruelty to animals. Youngsters with conduct disorder often lie to achieve short-term ends, may be truant from school, may run away from home, and may engage in petty larceny or even mugging (Text Box 29-4).

> Oppositional defiant disorder is characterized by a persistent pattern of disobedience, argumentativeness, angry outbursts, low tolerance for frustration, and tendency to blame others for misfortunes, large and small.

> Conduct disorder is characterized by serious violations of social norms, including aggressive behavior, destruction of property, and cruelty to animals.

The prevalence of conduct disorder is greater in boys and ranges from 6% to 16%, compared with a range of 2% to 9% in girls. Conduct disorder is one of the most frequently diagnosed disorders in children in mental health facilities. Individuals with conduct disorder are at

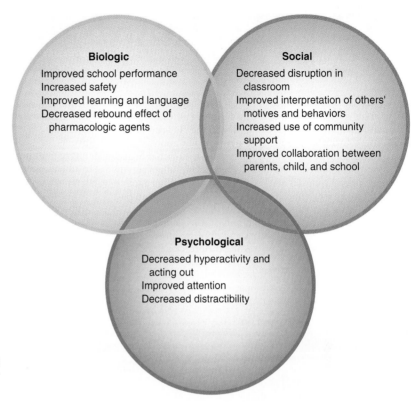

Biologic
Improved school performance
Increased safety
Improved learning and language
Decreased rebound effect of
    pharmacologic agents

Social
Decreased disruption in
    classroom
Improved interpretation of others'
    motives and behaviors
Increased use of community
    support
Improved collaboration between
    parents, child, and school

Psychological
Decreased hyperactivity and
    acting out
Improved attention
Decreased distractibility

FIGURE 29.2 Biopsychosocial outcomes for patients with attention deficit hyperactivity disorder.

greater risk for developing mood or anxiety disorders and substance-related disorders (APA, 2000). Other common comorbid conditions that may precede conduct disorder include specific developmental delays such as learning disabilities and language delay, ADHD, and oppositional defiant disorder. Several recent reports from large community surveys, family studies, and studies of clinical samples confirm the high comorbidity among these disorders (Barkley, 1998; Beitchman et al., 1986b; Biederman et al., 1992; Lahey et al., 1992; Scahill et al., 1999b; Szatmari et al., 1989b).

Children with ADHD, a learning disability, or a language deficit may frequently encounter failure and acquire a bitter and hostile attitude. Appropriate treatment focused on the ADHD or the specific developmental delay may foster more positive interactions and promote success at school. Success in these areas may lead to more positive behavior in some cases.

The etiology of oppositional defiant disorder and conduct disorder is complex. More attention has been paid to conduct disorder, probably because it is the more serious of the two. Models used to understand antisocial personality disorder (see Chap. 22) and aggressiveness (see Chap. 36) are useful in examining these childhood disorders, which appear to have both genetic and environmental components. For example, the risk for conduct disorder is increased in the offspring of individuals with conduct disorder. Physical abuse by fathers, however, whether biologic or adoptive, also increases the risk for conduct disorder (Blackson et al., 1999).

NURSING MANAGEMENT: HUMAN RESPONSE TO DISORDER

Biologic Domain

Assessment

The nurse gathers data from multiple sources and domains, including biologic, psychological (mood, behavioral, cognitions), and social. These adolescents are at high risk for physical injury as a result of fighting and impulsive behavior. Sexual promiscuity is common, resulting in an increased frequency of pregnancy and sexually transmitted diseases.

Another important aspect of assessment of adolescents presenting with defiance or aggressive behavior is to rule out comorbid conditions that may partially explain or complicate their lack of behavioral control. These conditions include ADHD, learning disabilities, chemical dependency, depression, bipolar illness, or generalized anxiety. Young people who are chronically depressed may be irritable and easily frustrated. Given the tendency of adolescents to act out their frustration, chronic depression may exacerbate their behavior.

(text continues on page 764)

NURSING CARE PLAN 29.1
A Patient With Attention Deficit Hyperactivity Disorder

Jamie, age 6 years, comes to the primary health care clinic with his mother Lillian because of motor restlessness, distractibility, and disruptive behavior in the classroom. According to Lillian, Jamie had a reasonably good year in kindergarten, but early in the first grade, the teacher began to report disruptive behavior. On reflection, Lillian recalls that kindergarten was a half-day program with more activity. By contrast, Jamie is expected to sit in his seat and pay attention for longer periods in first grade.

Jamie's medical history is unremarkable. Lillian's pregnancy with Jamie was her first and unplanned. Although there were no complications during the pregnancy, the period was marked by significant marital discord, culminating in divorce before Jamie's first birthday. Jamie was born by cesarean section after a long, unproductive labor. He was healthy at birth and grew normally, with no develop-

mental delays. Despite genuine interest in other children, his intrusive style and inability to wait his turn has resulted in frequent conflicts with them. The family history is positive for substance abuse in his father. In addition, Lillian reports that her ex-husband was disruptive in school, had trouble concentrating, and was highly impulsive, problems that have continued into adulthood.

During the three evaluation sessions, Jamie is active but cooperative. His speech is fluent and normal in tone and tempo, but somewhat loud. His discourse is coherent, but at times he makes rather abrupt changes in conversation without warning his listeners. Psychological testing done at the school revealed average to above-average intelligence. Parent and teacher questionnaires concurred that Jamie was overactive, impulsive, inattentive, and quarrelsome, but not defiant.

SETTING: PSYCHIATRIC HOME CARE AGENCY

Baseline Assessment: Jamie is a 6-year-old boy with prominent hyperactivity and disruptive behavior living with Lillian, his single mother. These problems interfere with his interpersonal relationships and academic progress. Lillian is discouraged and feels unable to manage Jamie's behavior.

Associated Psychiatric Diagnosis	*Medications*
Axis I: Attention deficit hyperactivity disorder Axis II: None Axis III: None Axis IV: Problems with primary support (mother is exhausted) Educational problems (failing in school) Economic problems (mother in entry-level job with no health insurance) Axis V: GAF = 52	Methylphenidate 5 mg at breakfast to start, gradually increasing to 5 mg at 8 AM, 5 mg between 11 AM and 12 noon, and 5 mg between 3 PM and 4 PM. Raise or lower dose slightly depending on response.

NURSING DIAGNOSIS 1: IMPAIRED SOCIAL INTERACTION

Defining Characteristics	*Related Factors*
Cannot establish and maintain developmentally appropriate social relationships Has interpersonal difficulties at school Fails to complete tasks Is not well accepted by peers Is easily distracted Interrupts others Cannot wait his turn in games Speaks out of turn in the classroom	Impulsive behavior Overactive Inattentive Risk-taking behavior (tried to climb out the window to get away from Lillian) Failure to recognize effects of his behavior

OUTCOMES

Initial	*Discharge*
1. Decrease hyperactivity and disruptive behavior. 2. Improve attention and decrease distractibility. 3. Decrease frequency of acting without forethought.	4. Improve capacity to identify alternative responses in conflicts with peers. 5. Improve capacity to interpret behavior of age-mates.

NURSING CARE PLAN 29.1 (Continued)

INTERVENTIONS

Intervention	Rationale	Ongoing Assessment
Educate mother and teach about ADHD and use of stimulant medication.	Better understanding helps to ensure adherence; also parents and teachers often miscast children with ADHD as "troublemakers."	Determine extent to which parent or teacher "blames" Jamie for his problems.
Monitor adherence to medication schedule.	Uneven compliance may contribute to failed trial of medication.	Administer parent and teacher questionnaires; inquire about behavior across entire day.
Ensure that medication is both effective and well tolerated.	Stimulants can affect appetite and sleep and can cause "behavioral rebound" (Barkley, 1998).	Administer parent and teacher questionnaires; check height and weight; ask about sleep and appetite.

EVALUATION

Outcomes	Revised Outcomes	Interventions
Jamie shows decreased hyperactivity and less disruption in the classroom.	Improve ability to identify disruptive classroom behavior.	Initiate point system to reward appropriate behavior.
Jamie shows improved attention and decreased distractibility.	Improve school performance.	Move to front of classroom as an aid to attention.
Mother and teacher attest to Jamie's decreased impulsive behavior.	Increase Jamie's capacity to recognize effects of his behavior on others.	Encourage participation in structured activities.
Jamie identifies alternative responses such as walking away until it is his turn.	Increase frequency of acting on these alternative approaches.	Inquire about social skills group at school, if needed.
Jamie improves interpretation of motives and behaviors of others.	Improve acceptance by peers.	Encourage participation in community activities.

NURSING DIAGNOSIS 2: INEFFECTIVE COPING (LILLIAN)

Defining Characteristics	Related Factors
Verbalizes discouragement and inability to handle situation with Jamie	Chronicity of ADHD Childrearing problems

OUTCOMES

Initial	Discharge
1. Verbalize frustration at trying to raise a child with ADHD alone. 2. Identify positive methods of interacting and disciplining Jamie that will support the parent–child relationship as well as meet Jamie's development needs.	3. Identify coping patterns that decrease the sense of frustration and increase parental competence. 4. Initiate a collaborative relationship with schoolteacher. 5. Identify sources of support in the community and begin to access these resources.

INTERVENTIONS

Intervention	Rationale	Ongoing Assessment
Assess mother's discouragement and feelings about parenting, identifying specific problem areas.	Helping the mother verbalize her feelings and identify problem areas helps in formulating problem-solving strategies.	Assess the severity of the problems with which she is living.
Refer mother to Community Mental Health Center for free parenting class.	Parent training based on clear limits and rewards can be effective for decreasing impulsive and disruptive behavior.	Monitor mother's level of confidence and perceived change in Jamie's behavior.

(continued)

NURSING CARE PLAN 29.1 (Continued)

INTERVENTIONS

Intervention	Rationale	Ongoing Assessment
Refer mother to self-help organization.	Parent groups such as Children and Adults With Attention Deficit Disorder (CHAAD) can be sources of support and information.	Determine whether contact was made and whether it was helpful.
Make contact with school to enhance collaboration with mother.	To assess effectiveness of medication and other interventions, need feedback from teachers.	Determine whether mother has been able to contact teacher.

EVALUATION

Outcomes	Revised Outcomes	Interventions
After two sessions, Lillian expresses her frustrations, but she has begun to identify different ways of relating to Jamie and his developmental needs.	None	None
Through attending the parenting class and joining a support group, Lillian begins to change her coping patterns, decrease her frustrations, and increase parental competence.	Complete parenting class; attend at least two support group meetings each month.	If necessary, refer for additional parent counseling.
Lillian initiates a collaborative relationship with Jamie's teacher.	Lillian and teacher mutually develop and implement behavior plans for home and school.	Have mother observe in the classroom; have mother visit highly structured classroom.

Conduct problems can also elevate the risk for depression because young people who regularly elicit negative attention from parents and teachers and are constantly at odds with their environment may become despondent.

Nursing Diagnoses and Outcomes: Biologic Domain

Typical nursing diagnoses in the biologic domain that are generated from the assessment are Risk for Other-Directed Violence, Risk for Self-Directed Violence, and Impaired Verbal Communication. Even though the outcomes are individualized for each patient, some outcomes for these patients are as follows:

- Maintenance of physical safety in the milieu (or other treatment setting)
- Decreased frequency of verbal and physical aggressive episodes

Interventions for the Biologic Domain

Children with oppositional defiant disorder or conduct disorder who also have specific developmental disorders should be placed in appropriate programs for remediation. If a diagnosis of ADHD or depression emerges from the evaluation, appropriate pharmaco-

therapy should be considered (see previous discussion of ADHD and discussion below regarding depression).

Several medications have been used to treat extremely aggressive behavior, including antipsychotics, such as haloperidol and thioridazine; the anticonvulsant carbamazepine; the α-blocking agent propranolol; and the antimanic medication lithium carbonate. Each of these medications has shown some support for its use in children and adolescents, but the evidence appears the strongest for haloperidol (Werry & Aman, 1998).

Psychological Domain

Assessment

Adolescents with conduct problems are usually brought or coerced into the mental health system by family, school, or the court system because of fighting, truancy, speeding tickets, car accidents, petty crimes, substance abuse, or suicide attempts. These young people may be hostile, sarcastic, defensive, and provocative. At the same time, they may appear calm, outgoing, and engaging. Inconsistencies, distortions, and misrepresentations of the truth are common when interviewing these children, so obtaining a clear history may be difficult. Therefore, instead of asking if an event or behavior occurred, it may be better to ask when it occurred. A structured interview

TEXT BOX 29.4

Clinical Vignette: Leon (Conduct Disorder)

Leon, a 14-year-old Hispanic boy, was admitted to the child psychiatric inpatient service from the emergency department after a fight with his mother. His mother reported that she and Leon had argued earlier in the evening and that he stormed out of the house screaming and vowing he would never return. Several hours later, Leon came back, yelling and demanding entry into the apartment. Leon's father was working. While his mother was getting up to open the door, Leon continued to yell and scream, waking the neighbors. This led to further arguing between Leon and his mother. Before long, the police were called, and Leon was taken to the emergency department.

The admission interview revealed that Leon had run away on several occasions and had even stayed away overnight. Although he strongly denied drug use, he had gotten drunk on several occasions. He had also been in several fights, the latest of which resulted in an expulsion from school. Three months before admission, he was caught trying to steal a cassette tape from a music store. More recently, he boasted that he and his friends had snatched a purse at an outdoor concert and had broken into a car to steal its contents. Leon's school performance had been declining; he was truant on several occasions and will probably have to repeat ninth grade.

Leon was born in Puerto Rico and is the oldest of three children. His family moved to the mainland shortly after his birth, and the primary language at home is Spanish. His father is employed as a janitor and speaks very little English. His mother works as a secretary and has achieved fairly good command of English. He has received no treatment except for consultation with the school social worker.

such as the Diagnostic Schedule for Children (DISC) or self-reports such as the Youth Self-Report (Achenbach, 1991) can aid the assessment. These adolescents are adept at changing the subject and diverting discussions away from sensitive issues. They often use denial, projection, and externalization of anger as defense mechanisms when asked for self-disclosure. The assessment, which may take several sessions, should be conducted in a nonjudgmental fashion.

Nursing Diagnoses and Outcomes: Psychological Domain

In the psychological domain, a typical nursing diagnosis generated from the assessment data is Ineffective Coping. Even though the outcomes are individualized for each patient, outcomes for these patients include the following:

- Increased personal responsibility for behavior
- Increased use of problem-solving skills as evidenced by decreased interpersonal conflicts
- Decreased rule violations and conflicts with authority figures

Interventions for the Psychological Domain

In planning interventions for patients with oppositional defiant disorder or conduct disorder, the nurse must target problem behaviors. Therapeutic progress may be slow, at least partly because these patients often lack trust in authority figures. The nurse should communicate behavioral expectations clearly and enforce them consistently. Consequences of appropriate and inappropriate actions should also be clear. Specific approaches for improving social and problem-solving skills are fundamental features for school-aged children and adolescents.

Insofar as children and adolescents with conduct problems fail to recognize the adverse effects of their verbal and nonverbal behavior, their deficit can be formulated as an interpersonal problem. Social skills training teaches adolescents with these behavior disorders to recognize the ways in which their actions affect others. Training involves techniques such as role playing, modeling by the therapist, and giving positive reinforcement to improve interpersonal relationships and enhance social outcomes.

In contrast to social skills training, which proposes that problems of conduct are the result of poor interpersonal skills, problem-solving therapy conceptualizes conduct problems as the result of deficiencies in cognitive processes. These processes include assessment of situations, interpretation of events, and expectations of others that are congruent with behavior. As reviewed by Kazdin (1997), these children often misinterpret the intentions of others and may perceive hostility with little or no cause. Problem-solving skills training teaches these children to generate alternative solutions to social situations, to sharpen thinking concerning the consequences of those choices, and to evaluate responses after interpersonal conflicts.

Social Domain

Assessment

High levels of marital conflict, parental substance abuse, and parental antisocial behavior often mark family history.

Nursing Diagnoses and Outcomes: Social Domain

In the social domain, nursing diagnoses generated from the assessment include Compromised Family Coping and Impaired Social Interaction. Even though the outcomes are individualized for each patient, some outcomes for these patients are as follows:

- Increased use of problem-solving skills as evidenced by decreased interpersonal conflicts
- Decreased rule violations and conflicts with authority figures

Interventions for the Social Domain

 Parent education for preschool- and school-aged children with disruptive behavior problems appear to be most effective. Parent training begins with educating parents about disruptive behavior disorders, focusing particularly on impulsiveness, impaired judgment, and self-control. Children with long-standing problems in these areas often elicit punitive responses and negative attributions about their behavior from their parents. Ironically, because these parental responses focus on the child's failure, they may contribute to the child's behavior problems. An important second step is to clarify parental expectations and interpretation of the child's behavior. Parent management training may be offered to a group of parents or to individuals (Barkley, 1997; Webster-Stratton & Hammond, 1997).

The aims of parent education are to provide parents with new ways of understanding their child's behavior and to promote improved interactions between parent and child. The most commonly presented techniques include the importance of positive reinforcement (praise and tangible rewards) for adaptive behavior, clear limits for unacceptable behavior, and use of mild punishment, such as time out (Text Box 29-5).

TEXT BOX 29.5

Time Out

Time Out Procedure

- *Labeling behavior:* Identify the behavior that the child is expected to perform or cease. The aim of this statement is to make clear what is required of the child. It typically takes the form of a simple declarative sentence: "Threatening is not acceptable."

- *Warning:* In this step, the child is informed that if he or she does not perform the expected behavior or stop the unacceptable behavior, he or she will be given a "time out." "This is a warning: if you continue threatening to hit people, you'll have a time out."

- *Time out:* If the child does not heed the warning, he or she is told to take a time out in simple straightforward terms: "take a time out."

- *Duration:* The usual duration for a time out is 5 minutes for children 5 years of age or older.

- *Location:* The child sits in a designated time-out chair without toys and without talking. The chair should be located away from general activity but within view. A kitchen timer can be used to mark the time, but the clock does not start until the child is sitting quietly in the designated spot.

- *Follow-up:* The child is asked to recount why he or she was given the time out. The explanation need not be detailed, and no further discussion of the matter is required. Indeed, long discourse about the child's behavior is not helpful and should be avoided.

Family therapy is directed at assisting the family with altering maladaptive patterns of interaction or improving adjustment to stressors, such as changes in membership or losses. Multisystemic family therapy, which considers the child in the context of multiple family and community systems, has shown promise in the treatment of adolescents with conduct disorder (Henggeler et al., 1999).

Evaluation and Treatment Outcomes

The nurse can review treatment goals and objectives to assess the child's progress with respect to verbal and physical aggression, socially appropriate resolution of conflicts, compliance with rules and expectations, and better management of frustration. As is true for the initial assessment, evaluation of treatment outcomes relies on input from parents, teachers, and other team members.

Continuum of Care

Children and adolescents with disorders of conduct may be involved in many different agencies in the community, such as child welfare services, school authorities, and the legal system. Mental health services are requested when a child or adolescent's behavior is out of control or a comorbid disorder is suspected. Helping the youngster and the family negotiate their way through this maze of services may be an essential part of the treatment plan.

DISORDERS OF MOOD AND ANXIETY

ANXIETY DISORDERS

Anxiety is a universal human emotion. Indeed, it may well be that common anxiety-provoking stimuli have biologically protective value. For example, a fear of snakes and the dark may have contributed to the survival of early humans through vigilance and avoidance behavior. Some degree of worry and specific fears is considered normal over the course of childhood (eg, anxiety about strangers in the 1-year-old). When the level of anxiety is excessive and hinders daily functioning, however, the diagnosis of an anxiety disorder may be appropriate. This section focuses on separation anxiety, a disorder diagnosed in childhood, and obsessive-compulsive disorder (OCD), which is an adult disorder that occurs in both adults and children (see Chap. 21).

SEPARATION ANXIETY DISORDER

Some have suggested that separation anxiety disorder is the childhood equivalent of panic disorder in adults. Although many children experience some discomfort on separation from their mothers or major attachment figures, children with separation anxiety disorder suffer great distress when faced with ordinary separations, such as going to school. In most cases, the mother is the focus of the child's concern, but this may not be so, especially if the mother is not the primary caretaker. The child may exhibit extraordinary reluctance or even refusal to separate from the primary caretaker. When asked, most children with separation anxiety disorder will express worry about harm or permanent loss of their major attachment figure. Other children may express worry about their own safety.

For a diagnosis of separation anxiety disorder, *DSM-IV-TR* specifies excessive anxiety on separation from home or major attachment figure before 18 years of age as evidenced by such features as acute distress, frequent nightmares about separation, and reluctance or refusal to separate. This excessive anxiety must be present for at least 1 month and cause clinically significant impairment in social or academic functioning (Table 29-5).

A common manifestation of anxiety is **school phobia,** in which the child refuses to attend school, preferring to stay at home with the primary attachment figure. It should be noted, however, that school phobia is a common presenting complaint in child psychiatric clinics and may be part of separation anxiety disorder, general anxiety disorder, social phobia, OCD, depression, or conduct disorder. In rare cases, school phobia can be a side effect of haloperidol. The term school phobia was coined to distinguish it from truancy—whether it is a phobia in the usual sense is a matter of some debate. When another disorder such as depression is identified, it becomes the focus of treatment. In some cases, the school phobia may resolve when the primary disorder is successfully treated.

> Separation anxiety disorder is excessive anxiety on separation from home or major attachment figure before age 18 years. It is evidenced by such features as acute distress, frequent nightmares about separation, and reluctance or refusal to separate. It lasts for at least 1 month and causes clinically significant impairment in social or academic functioning.

Epidemiology and Etiology

The prevalence of separation anxiety disorder is estimated at 4% of school-aged children. Thus, separation anxiety disorder is relatively common in children. Anxiety disorders run in families, and it appears that both environmental and genetic factors affect the risk for separation anxiety disorder. For example, it may emerge after a move, change to a new school, or death of a family member or pet. By contrast, recent evidence suggests that traits such as shyness and behavioral inhibition (reluctance in new situations) are inherited (Schwartz et al., 1999). Furthermore, not only are children with an enduring "inhibited" temperament at

TABLE 29.5 **Key Diagnostic Characteristics of Separation Anxiety Disorder 309.21**

Diagnostic Criteria and Target Symptoms	Associated Findings

• Inappropriate and excessive anxiety about being away from home or primary attachment figure
    Excessive distress when separation occurs or is anticipated
    Persistent, excessive worry about losing or having harm come to attachment figures
    Persistent and excessive worry about an event that might cause separation from attachment figure
    Persistent reluctance or refusal to go to school or somewhere else because of separation anxiety
    Reluctance to be alone without attachment figures at home or without significant adults in other settings
    Persistent reluctance or refusal to go to sleep without being near attachment figure or sleep away from home
    Repeated nightmares about being separated
    Repeated complaints of physical symptoms when separated or when separation from attachment figures is anticipated
• Duration of at least 4 weeks
• Onset before age 18 years (for early-onset type, onset before age 6 years)
• Not exclusively occurring during course of other psychotic disorder; not better accounted for by panic disorder with agoraphobia
	• Social withdrawal, apathy, sadness
	• Difficulty concentrating
	• Fears of other situations, such as animals, monsters, accidents, and plane travel
	• Concerns about death and dying
	• School refusal and subsequent academic difficulties
	• Anger or lashing out with prospect of separation
	• Unusual perceptual experiences when alone
	• Demanding and needing constant attention and reassurance
	• Somatic complaints
	• Possible depressed mood
	• Other recurring worries that do not involve attachment figure

greater risk for anxiety disorders themselves, but their immediate family members are also at greater risk for anxiety disorders compared with a psychiatric control group (Rosenbaum et al., 1991). Others have argued in favor of environmental determinants of separation anxiety, contending that anxious parents communicate to the child that the world is inhospitable and menacing to keep the child near. Recent data suggest that the long-term outcome of childhood disorders is generally favorable (Last et al., 1996).

Psychopharmacologic Interventions

The tricyclic antidepressant medication imipramine has been used as an adjunct to behavioral treatment or as a primary therapy for several years (Velosa & Riddle, 2000). In a controlled study, however, imipramine was no better than a placebo in managing separation anxiety (Klein et al., 1992). In addition, some children display drowsiness and irritability when taking imipramine. Other side effects may include tachycardia, dry mouth, constipation, urinary retention, and dizziness. As a class of medications, the tricyclics can alter cardiac conduction; hence, baseline and follow-up electrocardiograms are recommended (Scahill et al., 2000a). A recent multicenter study showed that the specific serotonin inhibitor, fluvoxamine, is effective for reducing separation anxiety (RUPP Anxiety Group, 2001).

Nursing Management

School phobia is often what prompts the family to seek consultation for the child. The onset of school refusal may be gradual or acute. Because school phobia can be a behavioral manifestation of several different child psychiatric disorders, it requires careful assessment. Issues to consider are whether the parents are aware that the child is avoiding school; what efforts the family has used to return the child to school; the presence of significant subjective distress in the child with anticipation of going to school; and whether the school refusal occurs in the context of other behavioral, social, or emotional problems. The nurse should also review the purpose and dose of current medications.

The child's developmental history and response to new situations and prior separations provide essential background information for understanding the child's current separation anxiety. The assessment should also include a review of recent life events and the methods the family has used to promote the child's return to school. Finally, the family history with respect to anxiety, panic attacks, or phobias is also informative.

Most clinicians agree that the child should return to school as soon as possible because resistance to attending school invariably mounts the longer the child remains absent. Several therapeutic approaches are used in the treatment of separation anxiety disorder, including individual psychotherapy, behavioral treatment, and pharmacotherapy. Although individual psychotherapy is commonly used to treat separation anxiety disorder, data to support this approach are sparse. By contrast, evidence suggests that behavioral techniques can be effective in reducing separation anxiety. These techniques include flooding (rapid and forcible return to school) and desensitization in which the child is gradually returned to school (Bernstein et al., 1996). To be successful, these techniques require close collaboration with the family and the school. Treatment of school phobia itself may involve medication, such as the antidepressant medication fluvoxamine.

OBSESSIVE-COMPULSIVE DISORDER

OCD is now recognized as far more common than previously supposed. It may have onset in childhood and is characterized by intrusive thoughts that are difficult to dislodge (obsessions) and ritualized behaviors that the child feels driven to perform (compulsions). Historically, OCD was regarded as a neurosis, and the primary symptoms were viewed as the expression of unresolved sexual and aggressive impulses. Recent evidence from family genetic studies, pharmacologic trials, and neuroimaging studies has dramatically shifted the conceptualization of OCD (Fitzgerald et al., 1999) (see Chap. 21). The notion that OCD is the manifestation of internal conflict concerning sexual and aggressive impulses is giving way to a more biologic model (Insel, 1992).

> Obsessive-compulsive disorder is characterized by intrusive thoughts that are difficult to dislodge (obsessions) and ritualized behaviors that the child feels driven to perform (compulsions).

Epidemiology and Etiology

Until recently, OCD was considered uncommon in adults and even more rare in children. Recent findings from the multicenter ECA study provided an estimate of 2% to 3% in the general population for adults. In addition, many of these adults reported that their symptoms began in childhood (Karno et al., 1988). A large community sample of high school students found a prevalence of about 2% (Flament et al., 1988). Thus, OCD is far more prevalent than previously supposed and can be expressed in childhood (Riddle et al., 1990).

Family genetic studies indicate that OCD recurs with a greater than expected frequency in the families of patients with OCD or Tourette's disorder, suggesting an inherited vulnerability in some cases (Lenane et al., 1990; Pauls & Alsobrook, 2000). OCD has also been associated with other movement disorders, such as Sydenham's chorea (Swedo et al., 1998). This observation has led to speculation that autoimmune mechanisms may underlie some cases of OCD (Swedo & Kiessling, 1994). Regardless of etiology, most researchers now conceptualize OCD as a disorder of the basal ganglia (Fitzgerald et al., 1999; Insel, 1992). Results from neuroimaging studies, which have shown functional abnormalities in the brain circuits connecting the frontal cortex and basal ganglia structures such as the caudate nucleus, strongly support this view (see Fitzgerald et al., 1999 and Insel, 1992 for a review). OCD is frequently accompanied by anxiety disorders in some cases or tic disorders in others.

Psychopharmacologic Interventions

Double-blind trials with clomipramine, fluoxetine, fluvoxamine, and sertraline have demonstrated the effectiveness of these agents in reducing symptoms of OCD in children and adolescents (DeVeaugh-Geiss et al., 1992; March et al., 1998; Riddle et al., 1992, 2001; Scahill et al., 1997a). Although the precise mechanism for their positive effects on OCD is not completely clear, these agents block the reuptake of serotonin in the brain. This property appears to be essential to the therapeutic effects of these agents because other antidepressants that do not block the reuptake of serotonin are not effective in treating OCD (Leonard et al., 1989; Goodman et al., 1990).

Nursing Management

Recurrent worries and ritualistic behavior can occur normally in children at particular stages of development. The first step in the assessment of OCD in children is to distinguish between normal childhood rituals and worries on one hand and pathologic rituals and obsessional thoughts on the other (King & Scahill, 1999). Obsessional thoughts are recurrent, nagging, and bothersome. Although children may describe obsessions as occurring "out of the blue," external events may trigger obsessions. For example, a child may fear contamination whenever he or she is in contact with a certain person or object. Likewise, compulsions waste time, cause distress, and interfere with daily living (Text Box 29-6).

Several measures are now available to assist in the assessment of OCD in children. The Leyton Survey is a 20-item self-report version of an earlier instrument. This shorter version has been used in both epidemiologic studies and clinical trials; high scores appear to be predictive of a clinical diagnosis of OCD (Flament et al., 1988). The Children's Yale-Brown Obsessive Compulsive Scale (CY-BOCS) is a semistructured interview

TEXT BOX 29.6

Clinical Vignette: Kimberly (Obsessive-Compulsive Disorder)

Kimberly, an 11-year-old fifth grader, comes for evaluation because her mother and teacher have become increasingly concerned about her repetitive behaviors. In retrospect, Kim's mother recalls first noticing repetitive rituals about 2 years before, but she did not become alarmed about these behaviors until recently when they began to interfere with daily living. At the time of referral, Kim exhibits complicated jumping rituals that involve a specific number of jumps and a particular manner of jumping. She also turns light switches off and on and performs complex movements, such as blinking in patterns and thrusting her arms back and forth a certain number of times. Her mother also reports Kim's near-constant request for reassurance about her own safety. In recent months, her incessant demands for reassurance have been more frequent and elaborate. For example, Kim's mother has to answer three times that everything is all right and then say, "I swear to it."

At the evaluation, Kim expresses fears that some ill fate, such as catastrophic illness or injury, will befall her. This fear is triggered by contact with any individual who seems sick, chance exposures to foul smells or dirt, or minor scrapes or bumps. Once the fear is triggered, she becomes increasingly anxious and consumed with the fear that she will develop an illness and die. Sometimes, her fears are specific, such as cancer or AIDS. Other times, her fears are more ambiguous, as evidenced by statements such as, "something bad will happen" if she doesn't complete the ritual. Kim acknowledges that the ritual is probably not related to the feared event, but she is reluctant to take a chance. If the ritual does not reduce her anxiety, she seeks reassurance from her mother.

Kim's medical history was negative for serious illness or injury. She was born after an uncomplicated pregnancy, labor, and delivery and achieved developmental milestones at appropriate times. Indeed, her mother could recall no unusual problems in the first few years of life except that Kim was typically anxious in new situations. Kim's mother reports a prior history of panic attacks, but the family history is otherwise negative for anxiety disorders, including obsessive-compulsive disorder.

designed to measure the severity of OCD once the diagnosis has been made. The CY-BOCS is a revision of the original adult instrument (Goodman et al., 1989a, 1989b), and preliminary evidence suggests that it is a reliable and valid measure of OCD severity in children (Scahill et al., 1997b).

The severity of the child's and family's response to OCD will determine the appropriate nursing diagnoses. When the obsessions and compulsions emerge, these children or adolescents are in distress because of the disturbing and relentless nature of the symptoms. Parents may be pulled into the child's rituals (Riddle et al., 1990; Scahill et al., 1996). Ineffective Coping, Compromised

Family Coping, and Ineffective Role Performance are likely nursing diagnoses. Treatment goals focus on reducing the obsessions and compulsions and their effects on the child's development.

Behavior modification techniques have demonstrated benefit in reducing the primary symptoms of OCD in adults. Behavior therapy, however, has not been well studied in children and adolescents (March et al., 1994; Scahill et al., 1996). The techniques that have been consistently effective in the treatment of OCD are exposure and response prevention (Piacentini, 1999). Exposure consists of gradual confrontation with events or situations that trigger obsessions and cause the urge to ritualize. According to the theory behind behavior therapy, repeated exposure works because the patient learns that the immediate anxiety will subside even if he or she does not complete the ritual. Response prevention complements exposure and consists of instructing the patient to delay execution of the ritual. When exposure and response prevention are combined, the patient is confronted with a triggering stimulus such as dirt (exposure) but agrees not to do the hand washing for a brief period (response prevention) and tracks the anxiety level during the exercise. Successful cognitive behavioral treatment of children with OCD includes parents, both to include them in the treatment plan and to reduce parental involvement in the ritualized behavior. For example, the child may demand that the parent participate in a washing and checking ritual (Piacentini, 1999; Scahill et al., 1996).

MOOD DISORDERS: MAJOR DEPRESSIVE DISORDER

The *DSM-IV-TR* includes several mood disorders, among them major depressive disorder, dysthymic disorder, bipolar I and bipolar II disorders, and cyclothymic disorder. Although these disorders occur in children and adolescents, they are less common in prepubertal children. These disorders are reviewed in detail in Chapter 20. Hence, this section is confined to a brief discussion of major depressive disorder in children and adolescents.

Depression is characterized by profound sadness, loss of interest in usual activities, loss of appetite with weight loss, sleep disturbance, loss of energy, feeling worthless or guilty, and recurrent thoughts of death or suicide. To meet *DSM-IV* criteria, these symptoms must be present on a daily basis and persist for at least 2 weeks (see Chap. 20).

Epidemiology

The prevalence of depression in children and adolescents is estimated at 1% to 5%, with adolescents being at the high end of this range and school-aged children at the low end. Boys appear to be at higher risk for depression until adolescence, when depression becomes more common in girls.

Nursing Management

The clinical picture of a child with depression may be similar to that of adults, but children may not spontaneously express feelings of sadness and worthlessness. Thus, clinical experience is helpful when trying to elicit the symptoms of depression from young children. Reports from parents are important sources of information about changes in sleep patterns, appetite, activity level and interests, and emotional stability. Also, quantitative measures, such as the Children's Depression Rating Scale (Poznanski et al., 1984) and the Children's Depression Inventory (Kazdin, 1989), can assist in the assessment of childhood depression (for a review of clinical ratings, see Scahill & Ort, 1995).

Nursing diagnoses for children or adolescents who are depressed are similar to those for adults. Included are Ineffective Coping, Chronic Low Self-Esteem, Disturbed Thought Processes, Self-Care Deficit, Imbalanced Nutrition, and Disturbed Sleep Pattern. Treatment goals include improving the depressed mood and restoring sleep, appetite, and self-care.

Interventions for responses to major depressive disorder in children and adolescents are also similar to those for adults. The psychiatric nurse develops a therapeutic relationship with the child and provides parent education and support. These children may act out their feelings rather than discuss them. Thus, behavior problems may accompany depression. Developing sensitivity to the influence of environmental events on the child is important for the nurse, parents, and teachers (Text Box 29-7). These children are likely to be treated with an antidepressant medication and may also be in psychotherapy with a mental health specialist. Unfortunately, outcome data concerning the superiority of any psychotherapeutic method are scarce. In addition, there are surprisingly few studies supporting the use of antidepressant medications in children (Emslie et al., 1997; Ambrosini et al., 1999). Much more research is needed to confirm the best methods of treating children with major depression.

TIC DISORDERS AND TOURETTE'S DISORDER

Tics are sudden, rapid, repetitive, and stereotyped motor movements or vocalizations. Motor tics are usually quick, jerky movements of the eyes, face, neck, and shoulders, although they may involve other muscle groups as well. Occasionally, tics involve slower, more purposeful, or dystonic movements. Phonic tics typically

Text Box 29.7

Decision Tree: Behavior and Social Events

Mrs. S has just returned with her son Jared to the child psychiatric inpatient services following an overnight pass. She reports that the visit did not go well due to Jared's anger and defiance. She remarked that this behavior was distressingly similar to his behavior before the hospitalization. She expressed additional concern because of the upcoming discharge from the hospital. After saying goodbye to Jared, she pulled the nurse aside and stated that she had decided to file for divorce.

Mrs. S indicated that she had not told her husband or the family therapist. When asked whether Jared knew about her decision, Mrs. S suddenly realized that he may have overheard her discussing the matter with her sister on the telephone during this home visit.

How should the nurse approach this situation?

Choice	Possible Outcomes
Discuss her hypothesis about Jared's behavior and his uncertainty	Mother can see relationship between Jared's behavior and her plan for divorce
	Mother ignores the nurse
	Mother is interested, but does not see the connection
Ignore the statement	Child and family did not learn about the connection between Jared's behavior and the events at home
Encourage mother to sort out her problems	The focus is then on mother's problems

Analysis
The best response is focusing on the possible relationship between Jared's recent behavioral deterioration and his uncertainty of his family's future. If the nurse ignores the statement or focuses on the mother's interpretation of Jared's behavior, the mother is less likely to appreciate the connection between pending divorce and Jared's behavior. The nurse should also emphasize the importance of discussing the matter in family therapy.

---

include repetitive throat clearing, grunting, or other noises but may also include more complex sounds, such as words, parts of words, and, in a minority of patients, obscenities. Transient tics by definition do not endure over time and appear to be fairly common in school-aged children.

 KEY CONCEPT **Tics.** **Tics** are sudden, rapid, repetitive, stereotyped motor movements or vocalizations.

Tic disorder is a general term encompassing several syndromes that are chiefly characterized by motor tics, phonic tics, or both. The *DSM-IV-TR* includes four tic disorders: Tourette's syndrome or disorder, chronic motor or vocal tic disorder, transient tic disorder, and tic disorder not otherwise specified. This section focuses on the most severe tic disorder, Tourette's disorder. Tourette's disorder is defined by the presence of multiple motor and phonic tics for at least 1 year (Table 29-6).

TABLE 29.6   Key Diagnostic Characteristics of Tourette's Syndrome 307.23

Diagnostic Criteria and Target Symptoms	Associated Findings

• Multiple motor tics and one or more vocal tics
  Sudden rapid recurrent, nonrhythmic, stereotyped motor movements or vocalizations
  Motor tics typically involving the head and other parts of body
  Vocal tics typically involving throat clearing, grunting, and occasionally words or parts of words
• Tics occurring many times a day, present for at least 1 year
  Appear simultaneously or at different periods during the illness
  No tic-free period of more than 3 consecutive months
• Onset before age 18 years
• Not a direct physiologic effect of a substance or general medical condition
	• Obsessions and compulsions
	• Hyperactivity, distractibility, and impulsivity
	• Social discomfort, shame, self-consciousness, and depressed mood
	• Impaired social, academic, and occupational functioning
	• Possible interference with daily activities if tics are severe

Because no diagnostic tests are used for this disorder, the diagnosis is based on the type and duration of tics present (Leckman & Cohen, 1999). The typical age of onset for tics is about 7 years, and motor tics generally precede phonic tics. Parents often describe the seeming replacement of one tic with another. In addition to this changing repertoire of motor and phonic tics, Tourette's disorder exhibits a waxing and waning course. The child can suppress the tics for brief periods. Thus, it is not uncommon to hear from parents that their child has more frequent tics at home than at school. Older children and adults may describe an urge or a physical sensation before having a tic. The general trend is for tic symptoms to decline by early adulthood (Leckman et al., 1998).

Tourette's disorder is defined by multiple motor and phonic tics for at least 1 year.

Epidemiology and Etiology

The prevalence of Tourette's disorder is estimated to be between 1 and 3 per 1,000 in school-aged children, with boys being affected three to six times more often than girls (Scahill et al., 2000b). The precise nature of the underlying pathophysiology is unclear, but the basal ganglia and functionally related cortical areas are presumed to play a central role (Leckman et al., 1992; Leckman & Cohen, 1999). The observation in the 1970s that the potent dopamine blocker, haloperidol, could reduce tics sparked interest in the biologic mechanisms, with particular focus on central dopaminergic systems.

Although the etiology of Tourette's disorder is unknown, several lines of evidence point to failed inhibition of specific brain circuits at the level of the basal ganglia (Leckman et al., 1992). The basal ganglia, which consist of the caudate, putamen, and globus pallidus, are located at the base of the cortex and play an important role in planning and executing movement. This functional role is accomplished by means of parallel circuits that connect the basal ganglia to the cortex and the thalamus. To date, no specific lesions in the basal ganglia have been found in Tourette's disorder. Nonetheless, findings from neuroimaging studies are consistent with the possibility that there may be some abnormality of the basal ganglia (Peterson et al., 1993, 1998a, 1998b; Singer et al., 1993).

In the 1980s, data from family-genetic studies began to emerge, indicating that Tourette's disorder is inherited as a single autosomal dominant gene. More recent studies, however, suggest that the inheritance may involve more than a single gene (Tourette Syndrome Association, 1999). The range of expression is presumed to be variable and includes Tourette's disorder, chronic motor or chronic vocal tics, and OCD as well. Twin studies have shown that monozygotic twins are far more likely to be concordant for Tourette's disorder than

dizygotic twins, further supporting the genetic hypotheses. Even when monozygotic twins are concordant, however, the twins may not be equally affected. Thus, although substantial evidence supports a genetic etiology, environmental factors affect the expression of the gene (for a more complete review, see Walkup et al., 1996).

Several neurochemical systems have been implicated in the etiology of Tourette's disorder, including dopamine systems, noradrenaline, endogenous opioids, and serotonin. The consistent observation that boys are more likely to be affected than girls has also led to speculation about the potential role of androgens in the pathophysiology of tic disorders. Treatment strategies based on this theory, however, appear to be ineffective (Peterson et al., 1998b). It is possible that newer neuroimaging techniques, genetic investigations, and pharmacologic studies will elucidate the complex interaction of these various neurochemical systems as well as the anatomic site of interest.

Psychopharmacologic Interventions

Two classes of drugs are commonly used in the treatment of tics: antipsychotics and α-adrenergic receptor agonists. The most commonly used antipsychotics include haloperidol and pimozide. These agents are not in the phenothiazine group, and both are potent dopamine blockers. Low doses are often sufficient to reduce the frequency and intensity of tics. Attempts to eradicate all tics by increasing the dosages of these antipsychotics almost certainly results in diminishing therapeutic returns and additional side effects. The most frequently encountered side effects include drowsiness, dulled thinking, muscle stiffness, akathisia, increased appetite and weight gain, and acute dystonic reactions. Long-term use carries a small risk for tardive dyskinesia. Recently, the atypical antipsychotics ziprasidone and risperidone have been evaluated for the treatment of tics in children and adolescents (Sallee et al., 2000; Scahill et al., 2001b). Ziprasidone was superior to placebo in the study by Sallee and colleagues (2000). Risperidone was also superior to placebo (Scahill et al., 2001).

The α_2-adrenergic receptor agonist clonidine has been used in the treatment of Tourette's disorder for more than 20 years. Guanfacine is a newer α_2-adrenergic receptor agonist that has only recently been studied in children with Tourette's disorder. Both drugs were originally developed as antihypertensive agents, but their regulatory action on the brain's norepinephrine system led researchers to try these medications in patients with Tourette's disorder. Results from double-blind, placebo-controlled studies indicate that both clonidine and guanfacine are effective in reducing tics (Leckman et al., 1991; Scahill et al., 2001a). The level of improvement in tic symptoms, however, is generally less than that observed with the antipsychotics. In the study by Scahill and colleagues (2001a), guanfacine was also effective in reducing symptoms of ADHD. (For further discussion of pharmacotherapy in Tourette's disorder, see Scahill et al., 1999a.)

Nursing Management

Nursing assessment of a child with tics includes a review of the onset, course, and current level of the symptoms. The goals of the assessment are to identify the frequency, intensity, complexity, and interference of the tics and their effects on functioning; determine the child's highest adaptive functioning; identify the child's areas of strength and weakness in general and in school; and identify social supports for the child and family (Leckman & Cohen, 1999). Another important aspect of the assessment is to determine the effects of the tic symptoms on the child and family. Some children and families adjust well; however, others are embarrassed or devastated and tend to withdraw socially. About half of school-aged children with Tourette's disorder have ADHD, and a substantial percentage have symptoms of OCD (Leckman & Cohen, 1999). Therefore, in addition to inquiring about tics, the nurse should assess the child's overall development, activity level, and capacity to concentrate and persist with a single task, as well as the presence of repetitive habits and recurring worries. Nursing diagnoses could include Ineffective Coping, Impaired Social Interaction, Anxiety, and Compromised Family Coping.

Children with Tourette's disorder typically have normal intelligence, although clinical samples may show a higher frequency of learning problems. These learning problems may include subtle problems of organization and planning or more severe problems with reading (Pennington, 1991; Schultz et al., 1998). Handwriting is another common problem for these youngsters, including both speed and legibility. The use of a computer can obviate difficulties with handwriting in some cases.

The approach to planning nursing interventions depends on the primary source of impairment: tics themselves, OCD symptoms, or the triad of hyperactivity, inattention, and poor impulse control. The nurse can provide counseling and education for the patient, education for the parents, and consultation for the school. Most children and their families need some education about Tourette's disorder. Individual psychotherapy with a mental health specialist (such as a psychologist or an advanced practice nurse) may be indicated for some children and adolescents with Tourette's disorder to deal with maladaptive responses to the chronic condition.

Before evaluation and diagnosis of Tourette's disorder, most families struggle with various explanations for the child's tics. Because tics fluctuate in severity over time and may be more prominent in some settings than in others, family members may have difficulty understanding their involuntary nature. Some parents may be convinced that the tics are deliberate and done to secure attention; others may judge that the tics are "nervous habits" indicative of underlying trouble. Such views require reconciliation with the currently accepted view that tics are involuntary. Some parents may conclude that the child is incapable of controlling any behavior because of Tourette's disorder. They may subsequently feel uncertain about setting limits. In these families, delineating the boundaries of Tourette's disorder can be helpful (Leckman & Cohen, 1999).

On learning that this disorder is probably genetic, some parents may harbor guilt for having passed it on to their child. The nurse can assist such families by listening to these concerns and providing information about the natural history of Tourette's disorder—it is not a progressive condition, tics often diminish in adulthood, and it need not restrict what the child can achieve in life.

Teachers, guidance counselors, and school nurses may need current information about Tourette's disorder and related problems. Discussions with school personnel often include issues such as how to deal with tic behaviors that are disruptive in the classroom, how to manage teasing from other children, and how to handle medication side effects. A careful discussion of the boundaries of Tourette's disorder and tic symptomatology usually can resolve these matters. Teachers who understand the involuntary nature of tics can often generate creative solutions, such as excusing the child for errands. This maneuver allows the child to step out of the classroom briefly to release a bout of tics, thereby reducing stress. In some situations, a brief presentation about Tourette's disorder to the class will reduce teasing and help both teachers and classmates tolerate the tic symptoms (Leckman & Cohen, 1999) (see Therapeutic Dialogue: Response to Tic Symptoms and Disruptive Behavior).

Before initiating these interventions, it is essential to identify the child's needs and to pursue these strategies in collaboration with the family and other clinical team members. The Education for the Handicapped Act (Public Law 94-142) ensures that children with conditions such as Tourette's disorder are eligible for special education services even if they do meet full criteria for learning disability. Thus, if evidence shows that Tourette's disorder is hindering academic progress, parents can demand special education services for their child. Nurses can help families negotiate with the school to obtain appropriate services.

THERAPEUTIC DIALOGUE	Response to Tic Symptoms and Disruptive Behavior

Ineffective Approach

Teacher: I see the tics. He jerks his head, makes faces, and flicks his hands.

Nurse: What do you do about them?

Teacher: What can I do? If he isn't disrupting the class, I leave him alone. Even when he is throwing spitballs.

Nurse: Spitballs! He shouldn't be allowed to throw spitballs.

Teacher: Oh, I thought that was a part of his problem.

Nurse: Well, throwing spitballs has nothing to do with tics.

Effective Approach

Teacher: I see the tics. He jerks his head, makes faces, and flicks his hands.

Nurse: He cannot help the tics that you are seeing. Tic disorders can exhibit a wide range of severity, from mild to severe and from simple to complex. Some complex tics may be difficult to distinguish from habits or rituals.

Teacher: What about things like throwing spitballs? When he does things like that, I try to ignore that behavior.

Nurse: You are very sensitive to him. (Validation) However, the spitball is not a tic behavior.

Teacher: What should I do?

Nurse: How do you usually handle that type of behavior? (A modification of reflection)

Teacher: I'd ask him to stop and sometimes go into the hall.

Nurse: Disruptive behavior that is voluntary in a student with a tic disorder should be handled as you would handle any other child.

Critical Thinking Challenge

• Compare the responses of the nurse in these scenarios. What made the difference in the teacher's responsiveness to the nurse?

CHILDHOOD SCHIZOPHRENIA

Childhood (early-onset) schizophrenia is diagnosed by the same criteria as those used in adults (see Chap. 18). The difficulty in diagnosing children with a psychiatric disorder has led to years of debate and controversy regarding whether childhood schizophrenia differs from the adult type or is merely an early manifestation of the same disorder. For many years, it was believed that autism represented the childhood form of schizophrenia. In recent years, however, autism and childhood schizophrenia have been differentiated (Cohen & Volkmar, 1997). As currently defined, childhood schizophrenia is rare, with an estimated 2 cases per 100,000 in the population. Diagnosis of childhood schizophrenia is even less common in children younger than age 5 years (King, 1994). By way of comparison, the adult disorder, which usually has its onset in middle to late adolescence, has a prevalence of 2 to 10 cases per 1,000. Childhood schizophrenia is usually characterized by poorer premorbid functioning than later-onset schizophrenia. Common premorbid difficulties include social, cognitive, linguistic, attentional, motor, and perceptual delays (King, 1994). Early-onset schizophrenia shows a higher concordance in monozygotic twin pairs than that reported for adult-onset schizophrenia. In addition, although the frequency of schizophrenia in parents of those with childhood-onset schizophrenia is no different from that observed in the parents of those with adult-onset schizophrenia, the frequency of the disease in the siblings is higher in the early-onset type (King, 1994). Taken together, these findings suggest that early-onset schizophrenia is a more severe form of the disorder.

Nursing care for these children follows a similar approach to that used in treatment of PDDs. Antipsychotic medication will be prescribed for symptoms (Kumra, 2000). Increasingly, clinicians are using the newer atypical neuroleptics, such as risperidone, olanzapine, and quetiapine (Kumra, 2000). These medications have both dopamine-blocking and serotonin-blocking properties. This combined effect is presumed to decrease the risk for neurologic side effects associated with the traditional neuroleptics (see Chaps. 8 and 18 for more detailed description of the atypical neuroleptics). Development of an individualized care plan for children with schizophrenia begins with a nursing assessment to identify functional problems specific to the child. Similarly, the recognition that childhood schizophrenia is a chronic and severe condition should guide the identification of outcomes. Goals should be realistic, and the nurse should pay special attention to the child's support systems. Parent education about the disorder, medications, and long-term management (including use of community resources) are essential parts of the treatment plan. Long-term management also requires monitoring of chronic neuroleptic therapy. Although the newer, atypical neuroleptic medications appear to have a lower risk for neurologic effects, other side effects such as weight gain also warrant careful monitoring (Martin et al., 2000).

ELIMINATION DISORDERS

ENURESIS

Enuresis is the involuntary excretion of urine after the age at which the child should have attained bladder control. Enuresis is usually means bedwetting, although repeated urination on clothing during waking hours can occur (diurnal enuresis). For nocturnal enuresis, the *DSM-IV-TR* specifies that bedwetting occurs at least twice per week for a duration of 3 months and that the child is at least age 5 years. Even without treatment, 50% of these children can achieve dryness by age 10 years.

Enuresis is the involuntary excretion of urine after the age at which the child should have attained bladder control.

Epidemiology and Etiology

The prevalence of nocturnal enuresis varies with age and gender, being most common in young boys. For example, an estimated 6.7% of 5-year-old boys, 3% of boys aged 9 to 11 years, and 1% of 14-year-old boys have nocturnal enuresis. The frequency in girls is about half that of boys in each age group. The etiology of enuresis is unknown, with probably no single cause. Most children with nocturnal enuresis are urologically normal. Some evidence has shown that at least some children with nocturnal enuresis secrete decreased amounts of antidiuretic hormone during sleep, which may play a role in enuresis (Reiner, 1995).

Nursing Management

The nursing assessment should include the child's developmental history, the onset and course of enuresis, prior treatment, presence of emotional problems, and medical history. The nurse should also explore the family's home environment, family attitudes about the child's enuresis, and the family's medical history. Routine laboratory tests such as urinalysis and a urine culture are used to determine the presence of infection. The nurse should obtain baseline data regarding toileting habits, including daytime incontinence, urinary frequency, and constipation. He or she should refer children with persistent daytime enuresis for consultation with a urologist (Reiner, 1995).

In many cases, limiting fluid intake in the evening is sufficient to decrease the frequency of bedwetting. If conservative methods fail, both drug and behavioral treatment have been beneficial for nocturnal enuresis. Imipramine has shown efficacy in the treatment of enuresis (Gittleman-Klein, 1980). The nasal spray preparation of desmopressin (DDAVP) has also shown promise in the treatment of enuresis, but beneficial effects may not endure over time (Hamano et al., 2000). DDAVP is a synthetic antidiuretic hormone that actually inhibits the production of urine. A recent review suggests that DDAVP helps about 25% of children who use it, with minimal risk for adverse effects (Harari & Moulden, 2000).

The most effective nonpharmacologic treatment is the use of a pad and buzzer. In this form of behavioral treatment, the bed is equipped with a pad that sets off a buzzer if the child wets. The buzzer then wakes up the child, thereby reminding the child to void. Bedwetting can often be extinguished with this method in a relatively brief period.

ENCOPRESIS

Encopresis is defined as soiling clothing with feces or depositing feces in inappropriate places. Additional diagnostic criteria include that the child is older than age 4 years, that the soiling occurs at least once per month, and that the soiling is not the result of a medical disorder such as aganglionic megacolon (Hirschsprung's disease). The most common form of encopresis is fecal impaction accompanied by leakage around the hardened mass of stool. Because of the loss of muscle tone in the lower bowel, the child loses the usual urge to defecate and may not feel the leakage. Surprisingly, the child may not detect the smell of the stool because the olfactory apparatus becomes accustomed to the odor. If left untreated, this problem generally resolves independently by middle adolescence.

Encopresis is defined as soiling clothing with or depositing feces in inappropriate places.

Epidemiology and Etiology

As with enuresis, encopresis is more common in boys, and the frequency of the condition declines with age. The current estimate of prevalence is 1.5% of school-aged children, with boys three to four times more likely to have encopresis than girls (Zuckerman, 1995).

The reasons for withholding stool and starting the cycle of fecal impaction are unclear but are usually not the result of physical causes. As noted previously, however, once the fecal impaction occurs, there is a loss of tone in the bowel and leakage.

Nursing Management

The assessment includes a detailed interview with the child and parent regarding the pattern of the encopresis. A calm, matter-of-fact approach can help to reduce the child's embarrassment. A physical examination is also necessary; hence, collaboration with the child's primary care provider or consulting pediatric specialist is essential. For the most part, children with encopresis do not have severe emotional or behavioral disturbances, but the nurse should inquire about other

(*text continues on page 778*)

TABLE 29.7   Summary of Diagnostic Characteristics

Disorder	Diagnostic Characteristics

Pervasive Developmental Disorders Not Otherwise Specified	• Impairment of reciprocal social interaction
	    Marked impairment in use of nonverbal behaviors
	    Failure to develop appropriate peer relationships
	    Absence of spontaneously seeking to share enjoyment, interest, or achievements (eg, pointing out things of interest)
	    Lack of social or emotional reciprocity (oblivious to others, not noticing another's distress)
	• Repetitive and stereotypic behavior patterns and activities
	    Preoccupation with pattern that is abnormal in intensity or focus
	    Inflexible adherence to nonfunctional routines or rituals
	    Stereotypic, repetitive motor mannerisms
	    Persistent preoccupation with idiosyncratic interests (eg, train schedules, air conditioners)

Autism	• As listed above for pervasive developmental disorders
	• Severe impairment in communication
	    Delay or total lack of spoken language
	    Impaired ability to initiate or sustain a conversation
	    Use of stereotypic, repetitive, or idiosyncratic language
	    Lack of varied, spontaneous make-believe or social imitative play
	• Abnormal social interaction, use of language for social communication, or symbolic or imaginative play before age 3 years
	• Not better accounted for by another psychiatric disorder

Asperger's disorder	• As listed above for pervasive developmental disorders • Clinically significant impairment in social, occupational, or other areas of functioning • No general delay in language • Less likely to have delay in cognitive development or age-appropriate self-help skills or adaptive behavior • Not better accounted for by another pervasive developmental disorder or schizophrenia
Learning Disorders	• Discrepancy between academic achievement and intellectual ability
Reading disorders	• Reading achievement substantially below that expected for age, intelligence, and education
Mathematics disorders	• Mathematic ability substantially below that expected for age, intelligence, and education
Disorders of written expression	• Writing skills substantially below that expected for age, intelligence, and education
Communication Disorders	• Interference with academic or occupational achievement or social communication

Expressive language disorder	• Deficits not explained by retardation or deprivation
	• Impairment of expressive language development
	    Limited amount of speech
	    Limited range of vocabulary
	    Vocabulary errors
	    Sentence structure problems
	    Unusual word order
	    Slow rate of language development
	    Difficulty in communication, both verbally and with sign language
	• As listed above for communication disorders
	• Deficits cannot be explained by pervasive developmental disorder

Mixed receptive-expressive language disorder	• Impairment of receptive and expressive language development
	    Markedly limited vocabulary
	    Errors in tense
	    Difficulty recalling words or appropriate-length sentences
	    General difficulty expressing ideas
	    Difficulty understanding words, sentences, or types of words or statements
	    Multiple disabilities such as inability to understand basic vocabulary or simple sentences; deficits in sound discrimination, storage, recall, and sequencing
	• As listed above for communication disorders
	• Deficits not explained by pervasive developmental disorder

(continued)

TABLE 29.7 Summary of Diagnostic Characteristics (Continued)

Disorder	Diagnostic Characteristics

Phonologic disorder	• Failure to use appropriate developmentally expected speech sounds
	    Errors in sound production
	    Substitution of one sound for another
	    Omission of sounds
	• As listed above for communication disorders

Stuttering	• Disturbed fluency and timing patterns of speech
	    Repetition of sounds and syllables
	    Prolongation of sound
	    Interjections
	    Broken words
	    Filled or unfilled pauses in speech
	    Substitutions of words to avoid problematic sounds
	    Production of words with an excess of physical tension
	    Repetitions of monosyllabic whole word
	• As listed above for communication disorders

Disruptive Behavior Disorders	• Significant impairment in social, academic, or occupational functioning • Not accounted for by antisocial personality disorder if over age 18 years

Conduct disorder	• Repetitive and persistent behavior that violates the rights of others or major age-appropriate societal norms
	    Aggression to people and animals
	    Destruction of property
	    Deceitfulness or theft
	    Serious violations of rule
	• As listed above for disruptive behavior disorders

Oppositional defiant disorder	• Negativistic, hostile behavior pattern
	    Loss of temper
	    Frequently argumentative
	    Active defiance or refusal to comply with adult requests or rules
	    Deliberate annoyance of others
	    Blaming of others for own mistakes or misbehavior
	    Anger and resentment
	    Spitefulness and vindictiveness
	• As listed above for disruptive behavior disorders
	• Not exclusive during course of psychotic or mood disorder

Anxiety Disorders Obsessive-compulsive disorders	See Chap. 22.
Mood Disorders Major depressive disorder	See Chap. 20.
Tic Disorders	• Single or multiple tics • Onset before age 18 years • Not a direct physiologic effect of substance or general medical condition • Not better accounted for by criteria for Tourette's disorder
Chronic motor or vocal tic disorder 307.22	• Motor or vocal tics • Occurring many times per day nearly every day or intermittently throughout more than 1 year: never a tic-free period greater than 3 months • As listed above for tic disorders
Transient tic disorder 307.21	• Motor or vocal tics • Occurring many times during the day for at least 4 weeks: not longer than 12 consecutive months • As listed above for tic disorders • Not better accounted for also by chronic motor or vocal tic disorder

(continued)

TABLE 29.7	Summary of Diagnostic Characteristics (Continued)
Disorder	**Diagnostic Characteristics**
Childhood Schizophrenia **Elimination Disorders**	See Chap. 19.
Enuresis 307.6	• Repeated voiding into bed or clothes (involuntary or intentional) • Occurring twice a week for at least 3 consecutive months or significant impairment in social, academic, or other area of functioning • At least 5 years of age or developmental equivalent • Not a physiologic effect of a substance or general medical condition
Encopresis 307.7 without constipation and overflow incontinence 787.6 with constipation and over- flow incontinence	• Repeated passage of feces into inappropriate places, such as clothing or floor • Occurring at least once a month for at least 3 months • At least 4 years of age or developmental equivalent • Not the physiologic effect of a substance or general medical condition except involving constipation

psychiatric disorders. The diagnosis of encopresis is presumed given a history of intermittent constipation and soiling. Collaboration with primary care consultants is often helpful to rule out rare medical conditions, such as Hirschsprung's disease. Primary care practitioners can also provide advice concerning the method of evacuating the lower bowel and evaluating the success of that effort (Zuckerman, 1995).

Effective intervention begins with educating the parents and the child about normal bowel function and the self-perpetuating cycle of fecal impaction and leakage of stool around the hardened mass of feces. The short-term goal of this educational effort is to decrease the anger and recrimination that often complicate the picture in these families. Because encopresis often results in a loss of bowel tone over time, it may help to motivate children by emphasizing the need to strengthen their muscles. In many cases, cleaning out the bowel is necessary before initiating behavioral treatment. The bowel catharsis is usually followed by mineral oil, which is often continued during the bowel retraining program. A high-fiber diet is often recommended. The behavioral treatment program involves daily sitting on the toilet after each meal for a predetermined period (eg, 10 minutes). The child and parents can measure the time with an ordinary kitchen timer, and the parents can encourage the child to read or look at picture books while sitting. They can give the child rewards in the form of stars, stickers, or points for complying with the retraining program and add bonuses for successful defecation. The family can tally stickers or points on a calendar, and the child can "cash in" collected points for small prizes (see Issenman et al., 1999 and Papenfus, 1998 for more details on managing encopresis).

All the disorders discussed in this chapter are summarized in Table 29-7.

Summary of Key Points

➤ Improved methods of assessing for and defining psychiatric disorders have enhanced appreciation for the frequency of psychiatric disorders in children and adolescents.

➤ An estimated 8 million children and adolescents have a psychiatric disorder in the United States (12% of individuals younger than age 18 years).

➤ The developmental disorders include mental retardation, pervasive developmental disorders (PDDs), and specific developmental disorders. Mental retardation often complicates PDDs. Assessment findings should guide nursing management. Specific developmental disorders include communication disorders and learning disorders. These disorders are fairly common in the general population, but they are more frequent in children with other primary psychiatric disorders.

➤ Child psychiatric disorders can be divided into externalizing and internalizing disorders. Externalizing disorders include the disruptive behavior disorders: attention deficit hyperactivity disorder (ADHD), oppositional defiant disorder, and conduct disorder. Internalizing disorders include depression and anxiety disorders.

➤ ADHD is defined by the presence of inattention, impulsiveness, and, in most cases, hyperactivity. As currently defined, ADHD is the most common disorder of childhood. This heterogeneous disorder affects boys more often than girls.

➤ Effective treatment of ADHD often involves multiple approaches, including medication, parent training, and child behavioral treatment.

➤ Primary features of oppositional defiant disorder include persistent disobedience, argumentativeness, and tantrums.

➤ Conduct disorder is characterized by lying, truancy, stealing, and fighting.

➤ Assessment of children with disruptive behavior problems involves securing data from multiple sources, including the child, parents, and school personnel.

➤ Standardized rating instruments can assist data collection from multiple informants.

➤ Separation anxiety and obsessive-compulsive disorder (OCD) are relatively frequent anxiety disorders in school-aged children.

➤ Treatment of separation anxiety and OCD may include medication, behavioral therapy, or a combination of these treatments.

➤ Major depression in children is believed to be similar to major depression in adults.

➤ The efficacy of antidepressant medications is less well established in children and adolescents compared with adults.

➤ Tourette's disorder is a tic disorder characterized by motor and phonic tics. Common comorbid conditions include ADHD and OCD.

➤ Childhood schizophrenia is a rare disorder in children.

➤ Elimination disorders include encopresis and enuresis. Behavioral therapy approaches are the most effective treatment for these disorders. Medication may also be used.

Critical Thinking Challenges

1. Discuss the distinguishing features of ADHD and conduct disorder.
2. What brain region is believed to play a fundamental role in the pathophysiology of Tourette's disorder?
3. Discuss the differences and similarities between mental retardation, pervasive developmental disorders, and learning disability.
4. Analyze how genetic and environmental factors may interact in the etiology of child psychiatric disorders.
5. Learning disabilities and communication disorders are more frequent in children with psychiatric disorders when compared with the general population. How might a learning disability or a communication disorder further complicate a psychiatric illness in a school-aged child?
6. Compare and contrast nursing approaches for a child with ADHD with those used for a child with autistic disorder. How are they different? How are they similar?
7. Discuss the significance of the Education for the Handicapped Act. What are some of the implications for nurses working with children with a psychiatric disorder and their families?

8. How would you answer this question from a parent: "What causes ADHD—is it my fault?"

 WEB LINKS

www.chadd.org This site of the Children and Adults With Attention-Deficit/Hyperactivity Disorder (CHADD) organization provides information and resources on ADHD.

www.adhd.mentalhelp.net The Mental Health Disorders and Treatment website provides information about ADHD.

www.wpi.edu/~trek/aspergers.html This website describes Asperger's disorder.

www.autism-society.org The Autism Society of America advances the understanding of autism.

www.autism.org The website of the Center for Study of Autism contains information and resources about autism and related disorders.

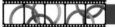 **MOVIES**

Rain Man: 1988. This classic film stars Dustin Hoffman as Raymond Babbit, a man who has autism (savant). Tom Cruise plays his brother Charlie, a self-centered hustler who believes that he has been cheated out of his inheritance. Discovering Raymond in an institution, Charlie abducts Raymond in a last ditch effort to get his fair share of the family estate. The story evolves around the relationship that develops as the brothers drive cross-country.

Dustin Hoffman brilliantly portrays the behaviors and symptoms of high functioning autism, such as the monotone speech, insistence on sameness, and repetitive behavior.

Viewing Points: Identify and describe Raymond's ritualistic behaviors. Identify the behaviors that depict extreme autistic isolation. Observe Raymond's language patterns and any distinct abnormalities. What happens when Raymond's rituals are interrupted?

REFERENCES

Achenbach, T. (1991). *Manual for the child behavior checklist and behavior profile.* Burlington, VT: University of Vermont.

Aman, M. G. (1996). Stimulant drugs in developmental disabilities revisited. *Journal of Developmental and Physical Disabilities, 8,* 347–365.

Ambrosini, P. J., Wagner, K. D., Biederman, J., et al. (1999). Multicenter open-label Sertraline study in adolescent outpatients with major depression. *Journal of the American Academy of Child and Adolescent Psychiatry, 38*(5), 556–572.

American Psychiatric Association. (2000). *Diagnostic and statistical manual of mental disorders* (4th ed., Text revision). Washington, DC: Author.

Anderson, G. M., & Hoshino, Y. (1997). Neurochemical studies of autism. In D. J. Cohen & F. R. Volkmar (Eds.), *Handbook of autism and pervasive developmental disorders* (2nd ed.) (pp. 325–343). New York: Wiley.

Anderson, L. T., Campbell, M., Adams, P., et al. (1989). The effects of haloperidol on discrimination learning and behavioral symptoms in autistic children. *Journal of Autism and Developmental Disorders, 19,* 227–239.

Arnold, L. E., Aman, M. G., Martin, A., et al. (2000). Assessment in multisite randomized clinical trials (RCTs) of patients with autistic disorder. *Journal of Autism Development, 30,* 99–111.

Barkley, R. A. (1998). *Attention deficit hyperactivity disorder: A handbook for diagnosis and treatment.* New York: Guilford Press.

Barkley, R. A. (1997). *Defiant children: A clinician's manual for parent training.* New York: Guilford Press.

Beitchman, J. H., & Young, A. R. (1997). Learning disorders with a special emphasis on reading disorders: A review of the past 10 years [Review]. *Journal of the American Academy of Child and Adolescent Psychiatry, 36*(8), 1020–1032.

Beitchman, J. H., Nair, R., Clegg, M., & Patel, P. G. (1986a). Prevalence of speech and language disorders in 5-year-old kindergarten children in the Ottawa-Carleton Region. *Journal of Speech and Hearing Disorders, 51,* 98–110.

Beitchman, J. H., Nair, R., Clegg, M., et al. (1986b). Prevalence of psychiatric disorders in children with speech and language disorders. *Journal of the American Academy of Child and Adolescent Psychiatry, 25,* 528–535.

Bernstein, G. A., Borchardt, C. M., & Perwien, A. R. (1996). Anxiety disorders in children and adolescents: A review of the past 10 years. *Journal of the American Academy of Child and Adolescent Psychiatry, 35,* 1110–1119.

Biederman, J., Faraone, S. V., Keenan, K., et al. (1992). Further evidence for family-genetic risk factors attention deficit disorder. *Archives of General Psychiatry, 49,* 728–738.

Biederman, J., Milberger, S., Faraone, S. V., et al. (1995). Family-environment risk factors for attention-deficit hyperactivity disorder. *Archives of General Psychiatry, 52,* 464–470.

Blackson, T. C., Butler, T., Belsky, J., et al. (1999). Individual traits and family contexts predict sons' externalizing behavior and preliminary relative risk ratios for conduct disorder and substance use disorder outcomes. *Drug and Alcohol Dependence, 56*(2), 115–131.

Bolton, P. F., Murphy, M., Macdonald, H., et al. (1997). Obstetric complications in autism: Consequences or causes of the condition? *Journal of the American Academy of Child and Adolescent Psychiatry, 36*(2), 272–281.

Buitelaar, J. K., van der Gaag, R. J., & van der Hoeven, J. (1998). Buspirone in the management of anxiety and irritability in children with pervasive disorders: Results of an open-label study. *Journal of Clinical Psychiatry, 59*(2), 56–59.

Campbell, M., Armenteros, J. L., Malone, R. P. et al. (1997). Neuroleptic-related dyskinesias in autistic children: A prospective, longitudinal study. *Journal of the American*

Academy of Child and Adolescent Psychiatric Nursing, 36, 835–843.

Castellanos, F. X., Giedd, J. N., Marsh, W. L., et al. (1996). Quantitative brain magnetic resonance imaging in attention-deficit hyperactivity disorder. *Archives of General Psychiatry, 53*(7), 607–616.

Chakrabarti, S., & Fombonne, E. (2001). Pervasive developmental disorders in preschool children. *Journal of the American Medical Association, 285*(24), 3093–3142.

Cohen, D. J., & Volkmar, F. R. (1997). *Handbook of autism and pervasive developmental disorders* (2nd ed.). New York: Wiley.

Cohen, D. J., & Volkmar, F. R. (1997). *Handbook of autism and pervasive developmental disorders* (2nd ed.). New York, Wiley.

Cohen, N. J., Barwick, M. A., Horodezky, N. B., et al. (1998). Language, achievement, and cognitive processing in psychiatrically disturbed children with previously identified and unsuspected language impairments. *Journal of Child Psychology and Psychiatry and Allied Disciplines, 39*(6), 865–877.

Conners, C. K. (1989). *Conners' rating scales manual.* North Tonawanda, NY: Multi-Health Systems.

Coucouvanis, J. (1997). Behavioral intervention for children with autism. *Journal of Child and Adolescent Psychiatric Nursing, 10,* 37–44.

DeVeaugh-Geiss, J., Moroz, G., Biederman, J., et al. (1992). Clomipramine hydrochloride in childhood and adolescent obsessive-compulsive disorder: A multicenter trial. *Journal of American Academy of Child and Adolescent Psychiatry, 31,* 45–49.

Dulcan, M., Bregman, J., Weller, E., & Weller, R. (1995). Treatment of childhood and adolescent disorders. In A. Schatzberg & C. Nemeroff (Eds.), *The American Psychiatric Press textbook of psychopharmacology.* Washington, DC: American Psychiatric Press.

DuPaul, G., & Stoner, G. (1994). *ADHD in the schools: Assessment and intervention strategies.* New York: Guilford Press.

Elder, J. (1996). Behavioral treatment of children with autism, mental retardation, and related disabilities: Ethics and efficacy. *Journal of Child and Adolescent Psychiatric Nursing, 9*(3), 28–36.

Emslie, G. J., Rush, A. J., Weinberg, W. A., et al. (1997). A double-blind, randomized, placebo-controlled trial of fluoxetine in children and adolescents with depression. *Archives of General Psychiatry, 54,* 1031–1037.

Feldman, H. M., Kolmen, B. K., & Gonzaga, A. M. (1999). Naltrexone and communication skills in young children with autism. *Journal of the American Academy of Child and Adolescent Psychiatry, 38*(5), 587–593.

Fischer, M., Barkley, R. A., Fletcher, K. E., & Smallish, L. (1993). The stability of dimensions of behavior in ADHD and normal children over an 8-year followup. *Journal of Abnormal Child Psychology, 21*(3), 315–337.

Fitzgerald, K. D., MacMaster, F. P., Paulson L. D., & Rosenberg, D. R. (1999). Neurobiology of childhood obsessive-compulsive disorder. *Child and Adolescent Psychiatric Clinics of North America, 8*(3), 533–575.

Flament, M. F., Whitaker, A., Rapoport, J. L., et al. (1988). Obsessive compulsive disorder in adolescence. *Journal of* the *American Academy of Child and Adolescent Psychiatry, 27,* 764–771.

Fletcher, J. M., Shaywitz, S. E., & Shaywitz, B. A. (1999). Comorbidity of learning and attention disorders: Separate but equal. *Pediatric Clinics of North America, 46*(5), 885–897.

Friedman, R. M., Katz-Leavy, J. W., Manderscheid, R. W., & Sondheimer, D. L. (1996). Prevalence of serious emotional disturbance in children and adolescents. In R. Manderscheid & M. Sonnenschein (Eds.), *Mental health, United States, 1996* (DHHS Publication no. SMA 96-3098, pp. 71–89). Washington, DC: U.S. Government Printing Office.

Gittleman-Klein, R. (1980). Diagnosis and drug treatment of childhood disorders. In D. F. Klein, R. Gittleman-Klein, F. Quitkin, & A. Rifkin (Eds.), *Diagnosis and drug treatment of psychiatric disorders: Adults and children* (pp. 576–775). Baltimore: Williams & Wilkins.

Goodman, R., & Stevenson, J. (1989a). A twin study of hyperactivity I: An examination of hyperactivity scores and categories from Rutter teacher and parent questionnaires. *Journal of Child Psychology and Psychiatry, 30,* 671–689.

Goodman, R., & Stevenson, J. (1989b). A twin study of hyperactivity II: The aetiological role of genes, family relationships and perinatal adversity. *Journal of Child Psychology and Psychiatry, 30,* 691–709.

Goodman, W. K., Price, L. H., Delgado, P. L., et al. (1990). Specificity of serotonin reuptake inhibitors in the treatment of obsessive compulsive disorder. *Archives of General Psychiatry, 47,* 577–585.

Goodman, W. K., Price, L. H., Rasmussen, S. A., et al. (1989a). The Yale-Brown Obsessive Compulsive Scale: Development, use and reliability. *Archives of General Psychiatry, 46,* 1006–1011.

Goodman, W. K., Price, L. H., Rasmussen, S. A., et al. (1989b). The Yale-Brown Obsessive Compulsive Scale: Validity. *Archives of General Psychiatry, 46,* 10.

Goyette, C. H., Conners, C. K., & Ulrich, R. F. (1978). Normative data on revised Conners' Parent and Teacher Rating Scales. *Journal of Abnormal Child Psychology, 6*(2), 221–236.

Hamano, S., Yamanishi, T., Igarashi, T., et al. (2000). Functional bladder capacity as predictor of response to desmopressin and retention control training in monosymptomatic nocturnal enuresis. *European Urology, 37*(6), 718–722.

Harari, M. D., & Moulden, A. (2000). Nocturnal enuresis: What is happening? *Journal of Pediatrics and Child Health, 36*(1), 78–81.

Hardan, A., & Sahl, R. (1997). Psychopathology in children and adolescents with developmental disorders. *Research in Developmental Disabilities, 18*(5), 369–382.

Henggeler, S. W., et al. (1999). Home-based multisystemic therapy as an alternative to the hospitalization of youths in psychiatric crisis: Clinical outcomes. *Journal of the American Academy of Child & Adolescent Psychiatry, 38*(11), 1331–1339.

Henggeler, S. W., Melton G. B., & Smith, L. A. (1992). Family preservation using multisystemic therapy: An effective alternative to incarcerating serious juvenile offenders. *Journal of Consulting and Clinical Psychology, 60,* 953–961.

Hurley, A. (1996). Identifying psychiatric disorders in persons with mental retardation: A model illustrated by depression in Down syndrome. *Journal of Rehabilitation, 62*(1), 27–33.

Insel, T. R. (1992). Toward a neuroanatomy of obsessive-compulsive disorder. *Archives of General Psychiatry, 49,* 739–744.

Institute of Medicine. (1989). *Research on children and adolescents with mental, behavioral, and developmental disorders* (Division of Mental Health and Behavioral Medicine). Washington, DC: National Academy Press.

Issenman, R. M., Filmer, R. B., & Gorski, P. A. (1999). A review of bowel and bladder control development in children: How gastrointestinal and urologic conditions relate to problems in toilet training. *Pediatrics, 103*(6 Pt 2), 1346–1352.

Jensen, P. S., Bhatara, V. S., Vitiello, B., et al. (1999). Psychoactive medication prescribing practices for U.S. children: Gaps between research and clinical practice. *Journal of the American Academy of Child and Adolescent Psychiatry, 38,* 557–565.

Kanner, L. (1943). Autistic disturbances of affective contact. *Nervous Child, 2,* 217–250.

Karno, M., Golding, J. M., Sorenson, S. B., & Burnam, M. A. (1988). The epidemiology of obsessive compulsive disorder in five US communities. *Archives of General Psychiatry, 45,* 1094–1099.

Kazdin, A. E. (1997). Practitioner review: Psychosocial treatments for conduct disorder in children. *Journal of Child Psychology and Psychiatry, 38*(2), 161–178.

Kazdin, A. E. (1989). Identifying depression in children: A comparison of alternative selection criteria. *Journal of Abnormal Child Psychology, 17*(4), 437–454.

King, R. A. (1994). Childhood-onset schizophrenia. *Child and Adolescent Clinics of North America, 3*(1), 1–13.

King, R. A., & Scahill, L. (1999). The assessment and coordination of treatment of children and adolescents with OCD. *Child and Adolescent Psychiatric Clinics of North America, 8*(3), 577–597.

Klein, R. G., Koplewicz, H. S., & Kanner, A. (1992). Imipramine treatment of children with separation anxiety. *Journal of the American Academy of Child and Adolescent Psychiatry, 31,* 21–28.

Koenig, K., & Scahill, L. (In press). Assessment of children with pervasive developmental disorders.

Kumra, S. (2000). The diagnosis and treatment of children and adolescents with schizophrenia: "My mind is playing tricks on me." *Child and Adolescent Psychiatric Clinics of North America, 9*(1), 183–199.

Lahey, B. B., Loeber, R., Quay, H. C., et al. (1992). Oppositional defiant and conduct disorders: Issues to be resolved for *DSM-IV. Journal of the American Academy of Child and Adolescent Psychiatry, 31,* 539–546.

Last, C. G., Perrin, S., Hersen, M., & Kazdin, A. E. (1996). A prospective study of childhood anxiety disorders. *Journal of the American Academy of Child and Adolescent Psychiatry, 35*(11), 1502–1510.

Leckman, J. F., Zhang, H., Vitale, A., et al. (1998). Course of tic severity in Tourette syndrome: The first two decades. *Pediatrics, 102,* 14–19.

Leckman, J. F., Hardin, M. T., Riddle, M. A., et al. (1991). Clonidine treatment of Gilles de la Tourette's syndrome. *Archives of General Psychiatry, 48,* 324–328.

Leckman, J. F., & Cohen, D. J. (1999). *Tourette's syndrome. Tics, obsessions, compulsions: Developmental psychopathology and clinical care.* New York: John Wiley & Sons.

Leckman, J. F., Pauls, D. L., Peterson, B. S., et al. (1992). Pathogenesis of Tourette's syndrome: Clues from the clinical phenotype. In T. N. Chase, A. J. Friedhoff, & D. J. Cohen (Eds.), *Advances in neurology* (58) (pp. 15–24). New York: Raven Press.

Lenane, M. C., Swedo, S. E., Leonard, H. L., et al. (1990). Psychiatric disorders in first degree relatives of children and adolescents with obsessive compulsive disorder. *Journal of the American Academy of Child and Adolescent Psychiatry, 29,* 407–412.

Leonard, H. L., Swedo, S. E., Rapoport, J. L., et al. (1989). Treatment of obsessive-compulsive disorder with clomipramine and desipramine in children and adolescents. *Archives of General Psychiatry, 46,* 1088–1092.

Levy, F., Hay, D. A., McStephen, M. et al. (1999). Attention-deficit hyperactivity disorder: A category or a continuum? Genetic analysis of a large-scale twin study. *Journal of the American Academy of Child and Adolescent Psychiatry, 36,* 737–744.

Lou, H. C., Henriksen, L., & Bruhn, P. (1990). Focal cerebral dysfunction in developmental learning disabilities. *Lancet, 335,* 8–11.

Mannuzza, S., Klein, R. G., Bessler, A., et al (1998). Adult psychiatric status of hyperactive boys grown up. *American Journal of Psychiatry, 155*(4), 493–498.

March, J. S., Biederman, J., Wolkow, R., et al. (1998). Sertraline in children and adolescents with obsessive-compulsive disorder: A multi-center randomized controlled trial. *Journal of the American Medical Association, 280,* 1752–1755.

March, J. S., Mulle, K., & Herbel, B. (1994). Behavioral psychotherapy for children and adolescents with obsessive-compulsive disorder: An open trial of a new protocol-driven treatment package. *Journal of the American Academy of Child and Adolescent Psychiatry, 33,* 333–341.

Martin, A., Landau, J., Leebens, P., et al. (2000). Risperidone-associated weight gain in children and adolescents: A retrospective chart review. *Journal of Child and Adolescent Psychopharmacology, 10,* 259–268.

McCloskey, J., & Bulechek, G. (1996). *Nursing Interventions Classification* (NIC). St. Louis: Mosby.

McDougle, C. J., Scahill, L., McCracken, J., et al. (2000). Research units on Pediatric Psychopharmacology (RUPP). Autism Network: Background and rationale for the initial controlled study of risperidone. *Child Psychiatric Clinics of North America, 9*(1), 201–224.

MTA Cooperative Group. (1999). A 14-month randomized clinical trial of treatment strategies for attention-deficit/hyperactivity disorder. *Archives of General Psychiatry, 56,* 1073–1086.

Papenfus, H. A. (1998). Encopresis in the school-aged child. *Journal of School Nursing, 14*(1), 26–31.

Pennington, B. F. (1991). *Diagnosing learning disorders, a neuropsychological framework.* New York: Guilford.

Peterson, B. S., Leckman, J. F., Tucker, D., et al. (1998a). Preliminary findings of antistreptococcal antibody titers and basal ganglia volumes in tic, obsessive-compulsive, and attention deficit/hyperactivity disorders. *Archives of General Psychiatry, 57*(4), 364–372.

Peterson, B. S., Riddle, M. A., Cohen, D. J., et al. (1993). Reduced basal ganglia volumes in Tourette's syndrome, using 3-dimensional reconstruction techniques from MRIs. *Neurology, 43,* 941–949.

Peterson, B. S., Zhang, H., Anderson, G. M., & Leckman, J. F. (1998b). A double-blind, placebo-controlled, crossover trial of an antiandrogen in the treatment of Tourette's syndrome. *Journal of Clinical Psychopharmacology, 18*(4), 324–331.

Piacentini, J. (1999). Cognitive behavioral therapy of childhood OCD. *Child and Adolescent Psychiatric Clinics of North America, 8*(3), 599–616.

Poznanski, E. O., Grossman, J. A., Buchsbaum, Y., et al. (1984). Preliminary studies of the reliability and validity of the Children's Depression Rating Scale. *Journal of the American Academy of Child Psychiatry, 23*(2), 191–197.

Reiner, W. G. (1995). Enuresis in child psychiatric practice. *Child and Adolescent Psychiatric Clinics of North America, 4,* 453–460.

The Research Unit on Pediatric Psychopharmacology Anxiety Study Group. (2001). Fluvoxamine for the treatment of anxiety disorders in children and adolescents. *New England Journal of Medicine, 344*(17), 1279–1285.

Riddle, M. A., Reeve, E. A., Yaryura-Tobias, J. A., et al. (2001). Fluvoxamine for children and adolescents with obsessive-compulsive disorder: A controlled multicenter trial. *Journal of American Academy of Child and Adolescent Psychiatry, 40*(2), 222–229.

Riddle, M. A., Scahill, L., King, R. A., et al. (1990). Obsessive compulsive disorder in children and adolescents: Phenomenology and family history. *Journal of the American Academy of Child and Adolescent Psychiatry, 29*(5), 766–772.

Riddle, M. A., Scahill, L., King, R. A., et al. (1992). Double-blind, crossover trial of fluoxetine and placebo in children and adolescents with obsessive compulsive disorder. *Journal of the American Academy of Child and Adolescent Psychiatry, 31,* 1062–1069.

Rosenbaum, J. F., Biederman, J., Hirshfeld, D. R., et al. (1991). Further evidence of an association between behavioral inhibition and anxiety disorders: Results from a family study of children from a non-clinical sample. *Journal of Psychiatry Research, 25,* 49–65.

Safer, D. J., Zito, J. M., & Fine, E. M. (1996). Increased methylphenidate usage for attention deficit disorder in the 1990s. *Pediatrics, 87*(6), 1084–1088.

Sallee, F. R., Kurlan, R., Goetz, C. G., et al. (2000). Ziprasidone treatment of children and adolescents with Tourette's syndrome: A pilot study. *Journal of the American Academy of Child and Adolescent Psychiatry, 39*(3), 292–299.

Satcher, D. (2001). *Report of the Surgeon General's Conference on Children's Mental Health*. National Institute of Mental Health. Bethesda, MD.

Scahill, L., Chappell, P. B., Kim, Y. S., et al. (2001). A placebo-controlled study of guanfacine in the treatment of children with tic disorders and attention deficit hyperactivity disorder. *American Journal of Psychiatry, 158*(7), 1067–1074.

Scahill, L., Chappell, P. B., Kim, Y. S., et al. (2001a). A placebo-controlled study of guanfacine in the treatment of attention deficit hyperactivity disorder and tic disorders. *American Journal of Psychiatry, 158*(7), 1064–1074.

Scahill, L., Chappell, P. B., King, R. A., & Leckman, J. F. (2000a). Pharmacologic treatment of tic disorders. *Child and Adolescent Psychiatric Clinics of North America, 9*(1), 99–117.

Scahill, L., & DeGraft-Johnson, A. (1997). Food allergies, asthma, and attention deficit hyperactivity disorder. *Journal of Child and Adolescent Psychiatric Nursing, 10*, 36–40.

Scahill, L., Leckman, J. F., Katsovich, L., & Peterson, B. S. (2001b). *A controlled study of risperidone in children and adults with Tourette syndrome*. Presented at the American Psychiatric Association Meeting, May 2001, New Orleans, LA.

Scahill, L., & Ort, S. I. (1995). Clinical ratings in child psychiatric nursing. *Journal of Child and Adolescent Psychiatric Nursing, 8*, 33–41.

Scahill, L., Riddle, M. A., King, R. A., et al. (1997a). Fluoxetine has no marked effect on tic symptoms in patients with Tourette's syndrome: A double-blind placebo-controlled study. *Journal of Child and Adolescent Psychopharmacology, 7*(2), 75–85.

Scahill, L., Riddle, M. A., McSwiggan-Hardin, M., et al. (1997b). Children's Yale-Brown Obsessive Compulsive Scale: Reliability and validity. *Journal of the American Academy of Child and Adolescent Psychiatry, 36*, 844–852.

Scahill, L., & Schwab-Stone, M. (2000). Epidemiology of attention deficit hyperactivity disorder in school-age children. *Child and Adolescent Psychiatric Clinics of North America, 9*(3), 541–555.

Scahill, L., Schwab-Stone, M., Merikangas, K. R., et al. (1999). Psychosocial and clinical correlates of ADHD in a community sample of school-age children. *Journal of the American Academy of Child and Adolescent Psychology, 38*(8), 976–984.

Scahill, L., Tanner, C., & Dure, L. (2000b) Epidemiology of tic disorders and Tourette syndrome: Toward a common definition. *Advances in Neurology, 85*, 261–272.

Scahill, L., Vitulano, L. A., Brenner, E., et al. (1996). Behavioral therapy for children and adolescents with obsessive-compulsive disorder: A pilot study. *Journal of Child and Adolescent Psychopharmacology, 6*, 191–202.

Schultz, R. T., Carter, A. S., Gladstone, M., et al. (1998). Visual-motor integration functioning in children with Tourette syndrome. *Neuropsychology, 12*(1), 134–145.

Schwartz, C. E., Snidman, N., & Kagan, J. (1999). Adolescent social anxiety as an outcome of inhibited temperament in childhood. *Journal of the American Academy of Child and Adolescent Psychiatry, 38*(8), 1008–1015.

Shaywitz, S. E., Shaywitz, B. A., Fletcher, J. M., & Escobar, M. D. (1990). Prevalence of reading disability in boys and girls: Results of the Connecticut longitudinal study. *Journal of the American Medical Association, 264*, 998–1002.

Singer, H., Reiss, A., Brown, J., et al. (1993). Volumetric MRI changes in basal ganglia of children with Tourette's syndrome. *Neurology, 43*, 950–956.

Sparrow, S. S., Balla, D. A., & Cicchetti, D. V. (1984). *Vineland Adaptive Behavior Scales*. Circle Pines, MN: American Guidance Clinic.

Swedo, S. E., Leonard, H. L., Garvey, M., et al. (1998). Pediatric autoimmune neuropsychiatric disorders associated with streptococcal infections: clinical description of the first 50 cases. *American Journal of Psychiatry, 155*(2), 2164–2271.

Szatmari, P., Boyle, M., & Offord, D. R. (1989a). ADHD and conduct disorder: Degree of diagnostic overlap and differences among correlates. *Journal of the American Academy of Child and Adolescent Psychiatry, 28*, 865–872.

Szatmari, P., Offord, D. R., & Boyle, M. H. (1989b). Ontario Child Health Study: Prevalence of attention deficit disorder with hyperactivity. *Journal of Child Psychology and Psychiatry, 30*, 219–230.

Tomblin, J. B., Zhang, X., Buckwalter, P., & Catts, H. (2000). The association of reading disability, behavioral disorders, and language impairment among second-grade children. *Journal of Child Psychology and Psychiatry and Allied Disciplines, 41*(4), 473–482.

Toppelberg, C. O., & Shapiro, T. (2000). 10-year update review: Language disorders. *Journal of the American Academy of Child and Adolescent Psychiatry, 39*(2), 143–152.

Tourette Syndrome Association International Consortium for Genetics. (1999). A complete genome screen in sib pairs affected by Gilles de la Tourette syndrome. *American Journal of Human Genetics, 65*(5), 1428–1436.

Vaidya, C. J., Austin, G., Kirkorian, G., et al. (1998). Selective effects of methylphenidate in attention deficit disorder: A functional magnetic resonance study. *Proceedings National Academy of Sciences, 95*, 14494–14499.

Velosa, J. F., & Riddle, M. A. (2000). Psychopharmacologic treatment of anxiety disorders in children and adolescents. *Child and Adolescent Psychiatric Clinics of North America, 9*(1), 119–133.

Volkmar, F. R., Klin, A., Schultz, R. T., Rubin, E., & Bronen, R. (2000). Asperger's disorder. *American Journal of Psychiatry, 157*(2), 262–267.

Walkup, J. T., LaBuda, M. C., Singer H. S., et al. (1996). Family study and segregation analysis of Tourette syndrome: Evidence of a mixed model of inheritance. *American Journal of Human Genetics, 59*, 684–693.

Webster-Stratton, C., & Hammond, M. (1997). Treating children with early-onset conduct problems: A comparison of child and parent training interventions. *Journal of Consulting and Clinical Psychology, 65*(1), 93–109.

Werry, J. S., & Aman, M. G. (1998). Practitioner's guide to psychoactive drugs for children and adolescents. New York: Plenum Press.

Willcutt, E. G., Pennington, B. F., & DeFries, J. C. (2000). Twin study of the etiology of comorbidity between reading disability and attention-deficit/hyperactivity disorder. *American Journal of Medical Genetics, 96*(3), 293–301.

Zametkin, A. J., Liebenauer, L. L., Fitzgerald, G. A., et al. (1993). Brain metabolism in teenagers with attention-deficit hyperactivity disorder. *Archives of General Psychiatry, 50,* 333–340.

Zametkin, A. J., Nordahl, T. E., Gross, M., et al. (1990). Cerebral glucose metabolism in adults with hyperactivity of childhood onset. *New England Journal of Medicine, 323*(20), 1361–1366.

Zuckerman, B. (1995). Encopresis. In S. Parker & B. Zuckerman (Eds.), *Behavioral and developmental pediatrics* (pp. 126–132). Boston: Little, Brown.

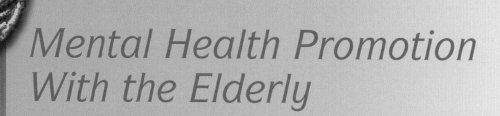

Mental Health Promotion With the Elderly

Bonnie J. Wakefield, Linda A. Gerdner, and Toni Tripp-Reimer

ELDER SPHERE
Late Life Transitions
  Normative Biologic Involution
  Late Life Illness and Comorbidity
  Cognitive Transcendence
    Transitions
  Social Role Transitions
  Social Support Transitions

Health
  Functional Status
  Health Behaviors
  Well-Being
ENVIRONMENT SPHERE
Social Dimension
Cultural Dimension
Physical Dimension

Residential Care
  Assisted Living
Spiritual Dimension
NURSING SPHERE
Nursing Diagnoses
Nursing Interventions
Nursing-Sensitive
  Patient Outcomes

LEARNING OBJECTIVES

After studying this chapter, you will be able to:

➤ Describe a conceptual model for guiding the nursing care of older adults.
➤ Discuss five late life transitions and their effects on elders.
➤ Define three elements of health in elders.
➤ Discuss the effects of environmental factors on elders.
➤ Discuss factors that contribute to nervous system plasticity.
➤ Identify factors that may affect memory in older adults.
➤ Discuss the implications of changes in reaction time in older adults for the assessment process.
➤ Identify five effects of aging related to pharmacokinetics and nursing implications associated with each.
➤ Identify three risks associated with polypharmacy.
➤ List risk factors for poverty and suicide in elders.
➤ Describe the features and benefits of residential care settings.
➤ Discuss nursing interventions that are especially effective with elderly patients.

adverse drug reactions   self-care
functional status   transition
half-life

*E*lderly people are at somewhat greater risk than younger age groups for the development or recurrence of mental health problems. Both functional and organic disorders increase with age, and the social conditions under which many elders live can exacerbate stress and emotional problems. About 15% to 25% of people older than 65 years of age are purported to suffer from mental illness or emotional distress that affects their quality of life; this percentage increases with institutionalization. Yet, despite the high prevalence of psychiatric disorders and mental health problems in later life, elderly people remain vastly underserved by the current mental health system. All too often, geropsychiatric disorders are misdiagnosed, mistreated, or simply overlooked. The consequences are high comorbidity, increased health care costs, needless suffering, and diminished ability of affected elders to live life to the fullest (Buckwalter, 1992). Yet, nurses must recognize that elderly patients benefit from the same psychotherapeutic interventions used with younger individuals.

Gerontology, *the study of human aging, is a broad field that crosses several disciplines. Within each discipline, multiple theories have evolved to both inform and shape gerontologic research. Because each field views human aging through its own disciplinary lens, each employs different constructs, foci, and methods. As a result, there is a large mass of disparate perspectives. Although these theories are not necessarily contradictory, they do not form a cohesive unit. No unified theory of aging has yet been established, and even the desirability of such a formulation is debated (Achenbaum & Bengtson, 1994; Marshall, 1994). In part, the lack of a unified theory stems from the multiple competing*

theoretic orientations within each discipline. Table 30-1 provides a summary of many of the major discrete gerontologic theories.

The limited development of theory and theory-based research in gerontologic nursing has been consistently noted (Bahr, 1992; Basson, 1967; Brimmer, 1979; Kayser-Jones, 1981; Knowles, 1983; Martinson, 1985; Murphy & Freston, 1991; Reed, 1989, 1991; Wolanin, 1983). When theory-based research has been conducted, however, it generally has employed one of the models shown in Table 30-1. The focus of gerontologic nursing differs depending on the theoretic perspective employed. Practitioners may select various discrete theories depending on the particular clinical situation, the nature of the patient, the health issue, the environmental context, and the therapeutic goal. An integrative approach could assist gerontologic nurses to provide more comprehensive and contextually relevant care. Conceptually delineating the scope of gerontologic nursing is a first step in understanding the nature of gerontologic phenomena and the ways in which nursing promotes health and facilitates transitions for older adults.

This chapter describes a holistic framework from which to view nursing care for elderly individuals. This framework is based on the Iowa conceptual model of gerontological Nursing presented in Figure 30-1 (Glick & Tripp-Reimer, 1996). Each section summarizes and highlights important issues relative to mental health promotion in elderly people. In this model, gerontologic nursing encompasses three spheres: elder, environment, and nursing. The elder sphere emphasizes the centrality of developmental and health processes in late life.

(text continues on page 791)

TABLE 30.1   Major Theoretic Perspectives in Gerontology

Discipline	Theory	Key Elements	Proponents
Philosophy	Dialectic gerontology	Acknowledges contradictory features of aging and locates those contradictions within a developmental or historical framework	Wershow (1981)
	Hermeneutic gerontology	Emphasizes understanding over explanation of sciences as well as for aging individuals	Prado (1983)
	Critical gerontology	Focuses on emancipation from domination	Moody (1988)
Sociology-anthropology Sociocultural	Age grading	Cultural system of group organization based on structural (not chronologic) age	Bernardi (1985)
	Subculture	The aged form their own subculture in American society.	Rose (1964)
	Exchange	Rational economic model; elders have less power because they control fewer resources and make fewer exchanges.	Dowd (1975)
	Modernization	Status of aged is inversely related to level of societal industrialization.	Cowgill & Holmes (1972)
	Status: reciprocity	Elder status is related to control over knowledge, economic resources, prior achievements.	Press & McCool (1972)
	Double jeopardy hypothesis	Minority group elders face discrimination related to ethnicity and age.	Jackson (1980)
	Social networks	Networks of elders decrease with role loss.	Sokolovsky (1986)
	Social support: formal and informal	As age increases, reliance on formal support systems increases, and reliance on informal systems decreases.	Cantor & Little (1985)
Social psychology	Activity theory	Importance of active role participation for positive adjustment	Havighurst & Albrecht (1953); Havighurst et al. (1963)
	Disengagement	Mutual withdrawal between elder and society	Cumming & Henry (1961)
	Social competence/ breakdown	Breakdowns in social competence occur with crises (losses) of aging; social reconstruction syndrome can reverse downward spiral.	Kuypers & Bengtson (1973)
	Person-environment fit	Physical, cognitive, social model; competent individuals tolerate more change.	Lawton & Nahemow (1973)
		Optimal fit model: congruence between individual and environment.	Kahana (1982)
		Four-factor model: individual and environmental characteristics; mediators and behavior change	Parr (1980)
		Field fit (field theory): interaction between individual and psychological environment	Schaie (1962)
	Life course	Aging as a lifelong process; biopsychosocial integration; social change (history) affects cohort; new patterns of aging can cause social change	Clausen (1972); Riley (1979); Hagestad & Neugarten (1985)

TABLE 30.1 Major Theoretic Perspectives in Gerontology (Continued)			
Discipline	**Theory**	**Key Elements**	**Proponents**
	Age stratification	Unique movement and experience of social cohorts (cohort flow)	Riley (1971); Foner (1974)
Psychology			
Personality development	Analytic	Aging: time of reflection and introversion	Jung (1933, 1960)
	Neo-freudian social theorists	Aging issue: ego integrity versus ego despair	Erikson (1963)
		Ego differentiation versus work role preoccupation; body and ego	Peck (1968)
		Dialectic operations: fifth period of cognitive development	Riegel (1973)
	Life-span transitions	Developmental tasks: adjustment to changes in health, work, social roles, physical living arrangements	Havighurst (1972)
		Developmental tasks: physical adjustments, new roles, life acceptance, death view	Newman & Newman (1984)
		Changes in cognitive and functional ability result in increased attention to aging and mortality	Levinson (1978)
	Moral reasoning	Life crises product of moral dilemmas that result in patterning or moral decisions	Kohlberg (1973)
	Continuity	Pattern of personality traits (established early) become more pronounced in response to stresses.	Neugarten (1973); McCrae & Costa (1982); Schaie & Parham (1976); Atchley (1989)
	Script	Elders order the script in the scenes of their lives to maintain sense of continuity.	Carlson (1981)
Personality dimensions	Traits	Sense of coherence	Sagy & Antonovsky (1990)
		Stability versus change	Bengston et al. (1985); McCrae & Costa (1982)
		Locus of control	Rodin (1986)
		Rigidity versus flexibility	Riley & Foner (1968); Butler (1974)
	Types	Four personality types (integrated, armored defended, passive dependent, unintegrated) related to satisfaction	Neugarten et al. (1968)
		Five subtypes (mature, rocking chair, armored, angry, self-haters)	Reichard et al. (1962)
Cognitive psychology	Generalized slowing hypothesis	Age deficits distributed throughout information processing system; not localized in particular stages	Salthouse (1985)
	Schema–neural network theory	Cognition occurs on neural network rather than staged succession of information processing	
	Crystallized versus fluid intelligence	Crystallized (accumulation) intelligence remains stable or increases; flexible (novel) intelligence declines.	Horn (1982)

(continued)

TABLE 30.1   Major Theoretic Perspectives in Gerontology (Continued)

Discipline	Theory	Key Elements	Proponents
	Information loss model	Task complexity retards process times; slowing results from information loss.	Hale et al. (1987)
	Single-peak creativity model	Creativity peaks in early 30s or 40s, followed by gradual decline.	Lehman (1953)
	Divergent thinking decline	Attributed to CNS slowing, decreased motivation, and cohort effect	Kogan (1987)
	Levels of processing model	Depth of processing is dependent on meaning to elder; elders encode less deeply.	Craik (1977)
	Processing deficit model		Eysenck (1974)
	Signal detection theory	Separate indicators for ability to detect, discriminate, and remember target events versus predispositional biases	Botwinick (1973)
	Terminal drop	Decline in cognitive functioning immediately before death	Kleemeier (1962)
	Expert schema theory	Expert's domain-specific knowledge and performance remain stable	Perlmutter (1988)
	Compensatory skill acquisition	Expert's increased skills compensate for decreased speed	Charness (1985)
Biology System level	Neuroendocrine	Homeostatic mechanisms decline; pathologic stress responses increase	Shock (1979); Timiras et al. (1984)
	Immunologic	Decreased immune efficacy and accuracy result in increased infections and autoimmune processes.	Zatz & Goldstein (1985)
Cellular	Wear and tear (rate of living)	Internal (basal metabolic rate) and external (temperature, altitude) affect life span.	Sacher (1980)
	Free radical accumulation	Oxidants (free radicals) directly damage cell membrane and cytoplasm.	Harman (1956)
	Lipofuscin (age pigment) accumulation	Increasing lipofuscin deposits in aging cells result in decreased mitochondria, cytoplasm, and endoplasmic reticulum.	Sohal (1981)
	Cross-linking	Protein (collagen) molecules form bonds over time, resulting in decreased elasticity and function.	Verzar (1963)
Molecular and genetic	Codon fidelity	Inability to decode mRNA triple codons (basepairs) impairs accuracy of mRNA message.	Agris et al. (1985)
	Somatic mutation	Radiation exposure increases mutations, resulting in fewer functional genes.	Sziland (1959); Curtis & Miller (1971)
	Error (catastrophe)	Increased RNA errors result in accumulation of protein abnormalities.	Orgel (1963) Medvedev (1972)
	Hayflick limit (genetic clock)	Finite number of cell divisions programmed in DNA (species specific)	Hayflick (1965)
	Dysdifferentiation	Accumulation of molecular damage impairs gene activity.	Cutler (1975)
	Antagonistic pleiotropy	Delayed expression of deleterious genes	Williams (1957) Medawar (1957)

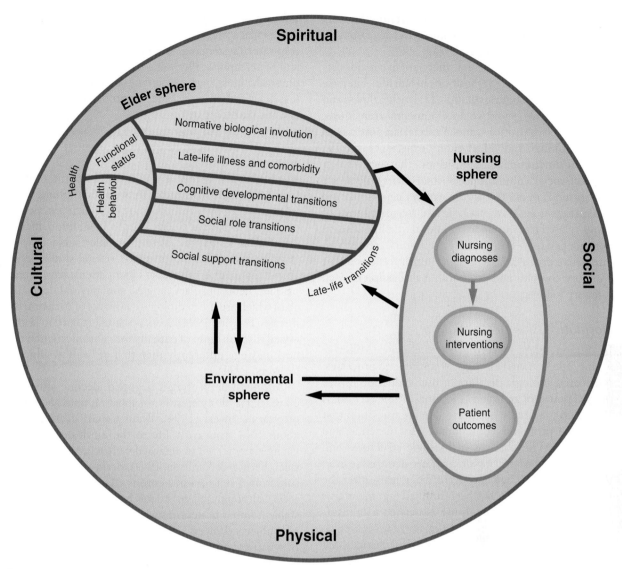

Figure 30.1 Iowa conceptual model of gerontologic nursing.

Developmental and health processes occur in a physical, social, cultural, and spiritual context, that is, environment, which constitutes a second sphere. Nursing, the third sphere, emphasizes interventions based on accurate diagnosis of responses to personal, environmental, or person–environment phenomena toward the outcome (goal) of optimal health.

The focus on developmental processes is grounded in the belief that the life course is an interpretation of biopsychosocial phenomena. In this model, late life events reflect life transitions that evoke responses affecting the level of health, which is experienced as well-being and is composed of the elements of functional status, health behavior, and life satisfaction. The gerontologic phenomena of concern to nursing incorporate the nature of late life transitions, the responses to these events, the environmental context, and the consequent functional health and well-being of older adults. Nursing interventions assist older adults in identifying and integrating

effects of late life transitions and support the developmental responses toward higher levels of well-being. These assistive actions are directed toward the individual as well as the surrounding microenvironmental and macroenvironmental systems that affect the health of adults in later life. Each portion of the model is described in subsequent sections.

ELDER SPHERE

Late Life Transitions

Many events that represent temporary or relatively permanent transitions from one pattern of being to another characterize the course of life. A **transition** is "a passage from one life phase, condition or state to another" (Meleis & Trangenstein, 1994, p. 256). Aging may be viewed as both positive and negative. Late life transitions can be viewed as positive avenues for personal growth and ultimately as advancing development and health (Jones & Meleis, 1993).

As depicted in Figure 30-1, there are five major categories of aging-related transitions in late life. They are (1) normative biologic involution, (2) late life illness and comorbidity, (3) cognitive developmental transitions, (4) social role transitions, and (5) social support transitions. Although individual elders experience specific personal environmental transitions, the surrounding physical, social, cultural, and spiritual environments are the "ground" or context within which the personal and social transitions take place. These five categories of aging-related transitions are neither mutually exclusive nor independent. Rather, they are mutual, reciprocal, interactive processes resulting in health responses that are more complex and profound. A discussion of each category follows.

Normative Biologic Involution

Involution refers to retrogressive change (Miller & Keane, 1983) in vital biologic structures and processes. Normative biologic involution, the "reduction in size or vital power of an organ" (Thomas, 1989, p. 939), is a universal, naturally occurring late life transition that may have profound consequences for function and well-being. The changes in biologic structures and processes can occur in a particular organ or tissue or in the whole body. They may occur from disuse after the function of the organ has been fulfilled (eg, the uterus or thymus gland) or from disuse associated with insufficient exercise or movement (eg, in neuromusculoskeletal systems). Distinguishing physical changes that occur with biologic aging, however, from those that occur because of decreased physical activity, level of motivation, influence of societal expectations, or cumulative effects of disease is difficult (Fiatarone & Evans, 1993; Kane, 1993; Spirduso & MacRae).

Aging-related biologic involution encompasses major changes in all organ systems, thus altering functional capacity in all dimensions (Pendergast et al., 1993). Many older adults, however, can integrate profound decrements in physical capacity without affecting the ability to function under normal conditions (Arking, 1991). What is actually compromised is functional reserve, that is, the degree of plasticity that one sees in younger adults. A discussion of the important neurobiologic changes follows.

Neurologic system changes that occur with aging include central and peripheral neuronal cell loss; slowed transmission of nervous impulses; slowed reaction time; diminished proprioception, balance, and postural control; poor thermoregulation; and altered sleep patterns. The effects of changes in the nervous system are con-

founded by changes in other systems, such as the cardiovascular system (eg, decreased arterial elasticity) and respiratory system (eg, diminished response to hypoxia and hypercapnia). Physiologic changes occurring with physical illness may precipitate altered mental status (eg, delirium) or exacerbate symptoms of existing psychiatric illness (eg, depression).

The brain, like most other body organs, undergoes changes with aging. These changes occur at a variable rate across individuals and are affected by genetic and environmental factors as well as by systemic disease outside the nervous system. In fact, determining what is "normal" aging is complicated by the high prevalence of chronic disease in elderly people. In addition, markers of disease may be present in older subjects who show no symptoms. For instance, several studies have shown that cognitively intact older patients have senile plaques, neurofibrillary tangles, and amyloid deposits, all of which are the pathologic hallmarks of Alzheimer's disease (Powers, 1994). Also, researchers have hypothesized that the brain of patients with chronic mental illness may age differently than that of healthy subjects (Powers, 1994).

Although brain weight begins to decline after age 30 years, visible atrophy is not apparent until about age 60 years (Powers, 1994). Brain weight decreases by about 10% from early life to the ninth decade; this change is reflected in enlarged ventricles and widened sulci (Barclay & Wolfson, 1993). Brain atrophy may result from a net loss of neurons (Barclay & Wolfson, 1993), although recent studies have shown a relatively stable number of neurons when comparing young and old subjects (Powers, 1994). Reduction in the number of synapses with aging is variable (Powers, 1994).

Although in the past it was believed that cerebral blood flow and the metabolic rate of oxygen release decreased with aging, this finding may have been related to conditions such as Alzheimer's disease rather than to aging alone (Barclay & Wolfson, 1993).

Even though people are born with all the neurons that they will have throughout life, the nervous system has a considerable degree of plasticity. This plasticity enables it to sustain structural losses without necessarily losing function (Drachman & Barclay, 1993). Mechanisms that contribute to this plasticity include a large reserve of redundant neurons; the ability of neurons to form new connections or to substitute for damaged neurons; the ability to increase presynaptic synthesis of neurotransmitters and to increase the postsynaptic sensitivity to signals from impaired systems; and secondary hypertrophy of remaining elements of partially denervated structures (eg, hypertrophy of innervated muscle fibers in a partially denervated muscle) (Drachman & Barclay, 1993). These mechanisms allow normal function despite losses over the decades, although remaining neurons become increasingly important to maintain function.

The effects of aging on the transmitter system have been measured. Levels of chemical transmitters may be reduced at the presynaptic level; postsynaptic reception and changes in signal transduction have been found (Powers, 1994).

Whether age-related changes result from physiologic consequences of aging or unrecognized disease is still uncertain.

All five senses decline with age. This factor is important when assessing psychiatrically ill elderly patients because diminished senses may affect attention and perception, potentially affecting interpretation of standard mental status examinations. Structural changes in the eye include rigidity of the iris, accumulation of yellow substance in the lens, and diminished lens elasticity. These changes result in decreased pupil size, alteration in color perception, presbyopia, impaired adaptation to darkness, and significant vision impairment in the presence of glare (Ferri & Fretwell, 1992). Auditory changes are noticeable as early as age 40 years; age of onset, however, varies according to lifestyle (eg, previous exposure to occupational noise). There is a loss of cochlear neurons, resulting in hearing loss (Ferri & Fretwell, 1992). Evidence suggests that IQ need not necessarily decline with age, but hearing loss may affect performance on intelligence tests (Sands & Meredith, 1989). Several other factors beyond loss of hearing, however, can influence age-related differences in performance on intelligence tests. Research on taste, touch, and smell is sparse, but a uniform dulling of these senses occurs with aging. Again, the rate of decline is highly variable among individuals. Suggestions for communicating with frail elderly people are listed in Text Box 30-1.

Late Life Illness and Comorbidity

Late life is also characterized by prevalence of disease, illness, and comorbidity (multiple chronicities). Although the frequency of acute conditions declines with advancing age, estimates are that about 90% of older adults have chronic medical conditions (Young & Olson, 1991) that can adversely affect function. The major chronic conditions experienced by older adults are ischemic heart disease, hypertension, vision impairment, hearing impairment, musculoskeletal impairment, and diabetes (Van Nostrand et al., 1993). Disease states often reduce physiologic capacity and consequently increase functional dependency. Further, during acute episodes of illness, many elders lose functional ability because they have limited reserves or cannot mobilize reserves to regain their premorbid performance levels (Margitic et al., 1993; Sager et al., 1996; Svanborg, 1993).

Primary and secondary mental health problems compromise function and quality of life. For example,

TEXT BOX 30.1

Communicating With Elderly People

- Focus the person's attention on the exchange of communication; the older adult may need extra time to begin to process information.
- Face the elder when speaking to him or her.
- Minimize distractions in the room, including other people, objects in your hands, noise, and other activities.
- Reduce glare from room lighting by dimming too-bright lights. Conversely, avoid sitting in shadows.
- Speak slowly and clearly. Elders may depend on lip-reading, so ensure that the individual can see you. Speak loudly, but don't shout.
- Use short, simple sentences and be prepared to repeat or revise what you have said.
- Limit the number of topics discussed at one time to prevent information overload.
- Ask one question at a time to minimize confusion. Allow plenty of time for the elder to answer and express ideas.
- Frequently summarize the important points of the conversation to improve understanding and comprehension.
- Avoid the urge to finish sentences.
- If the communication exchange is going poorly, postpone it for another time.

Adapted from (1998). Tips for communicating with frail, elderly patients. *American Nurse, 30*(6).

an elder's interpretation of an impairment may generate mental health responses that limit cognitive, affective, or physical capacities. The net effect is reduced physical and social activity. For example, one group of inactive, socially isolated older adults living at home was found to be more "tired," to give lower perceived health ratings, and to visit physicians and use sedatives more often than elders who were not experiencing social isolation (Svanborg, 1993). Thus, the psychological representation of and response to actual or potential disability, as well as the social context in which it occurs, are important determinants of actual function (Schultz & Williamson, 1993).

Because of the higher number of chronic illnesses in elderly people, those older than are 65 years purchase 30% of all prescription drugs and 40% of all over-the-counter drugs (Cohen, 2000; Salom & Davis, 1995). The aging process affects pharmacokinetics (primarily the mechanisms of drug absorption, distribution, metabolism, and excretion) and the strength and number of protein-binding sites. These changes place the elderly person at increased risk for adverse drug reactions. In fact, patients between ages 60 and 70 years are twice as likely to experience adverse drug reactions as patients aged 30 to 40 years.

Adverse drug reactions are fundamentally different from drug allergies. **Adverse drug reactions** are undesired, dose-dependent pharmacologic responses to drugs and a leading cause of morbidity and mortality (Cohen, 2000). It is important to note that when adverse drug reactions occur, they may develop gradually over time and may be difficult to recognize (LeSage, 1991). Therefore, recommendations are for the physician to conduct an individual assessment for the establishment of low loading and maintenance doses that minimize adverse drug reactions (Cohen, 2000).

As individuals age, changes occur in the splanchnic circulation and gastrointestinal tract that may alter absorption of medications (Douglas & Rush, 1988). The following factors may also influence rate of absorption (Meyers, 1989):

- Type of capsule or coating on the pill (ie, enteric)
- Amount, fat content, or both of food in the stomach
- Emotional state
- Body position (positioning on right side increases gastric emptying)
- Interaction with other medications

Body composition and blood flow are important factors in the distribution of medications (Larson & Hoot Martin, 1999). As a person ages, the following changes occur related to the proportion of body fat, lean body weight, and total body water (Meyers, 1989):

- Body fat increases 18% to 36% in men.
- Body fat increases 33% to 48% in women.
- Total body water decreases 10% to 15%.
- Muscle mass decreases.

These changes affect the relationship between the medication's concentration and solubility in the body (Larson & Hoot Martin, 1999). As a result, fat-soluble drugs, such as tricyclic antidepressants and certain benzodiazepines, become sequestered in fatty tissue rather than remaining in the circulating plasma. These factors increase the drug's **half-life** (the time required to decrease the amount of drug in the body by 50%), thereby increasing the risk for accumulation and drug toxicity (Douglas & Rush, 1988).

Most drugs are metabolized or biotransformed in the liver. This process is defined as the enzymatic alteration of the drug structure. Cardiovascular and hepatic changes that may occur in elderly people affect drug metabolism.

Blood flow in the liver tends to decrease with advancing age, with estimated reduction as much as 40% to 50% by age 65 years. Decreased cardiac output is the major factor slowing blood flow through the liver. Reduction of blood flow decreases the liver's opportunity to metabolize medications. Consequently, medication may remain in the blood longer, increasing the risk for toxicity.

Metabolism in the liver cell has two phases. Phase I typically decreases with age and consists of oxidation, hydrolysis, or reduction. Examples of drugs that are transformed by phase I include tricyclic antidepressants, phenothiazines, and some benzodiazepines. In contrast, phase II involves the process of conjugation, which the aging process does not affect.

Even without disease, a predictable decline in glomerular filtration and tubular secretion occurs with aging. Renal blood flow decreases by as much as 10% every decade after age 40 years. Renal clearance is estimated to decrease by as much as 35% between ages 20 and 90 years. These changes result in decreased renal excretion, which is of particular concern because the kidneys excrete most drugs (Douglas & Rush, 1988). Lithium carbonate is one example of a water-soluble drug that the kidneys excrete unchanged. Impaired renal function in individuals taking this drug could lead to toxicity (Meyers, 1989).

The number of protein-binding sites and the strength of protein–drug binding tend to decrease with age (Smith et al., 1993). The result is fewer binding sites for protein-bound drugs. Most psychotropics have high binding affinity to protein (Table 30-2). The loss of protein binding sites can potentially result in the following:

- Increased "free" concentration of a drug in the body tissues, intensifying the effect of the drug
- Increased amount of drug available for excretion through the liver or kidneys
- Increased risk for drug-binding and drug interactions

TABLE 30.2   Psychotropic Medications With a High Binding Affinity to Plasma Proteins

Drug	Percentage Bound to Protein Plasma
Amitriptyline	96
Diazepam	99
Imipramine	92
Lorazepam	93
Nortriptyline	95
Oxazepam	88
Trazodone	90

Polypharmacy is the concurrent use of multiple medications by a single patient (Larsen & Hoot Martin, 1999). Polypharmacy increases the potential for adverse drug reactions, interactions, and poor compliance (Garne & Barr, 1984, pp. 9–10; LeSage, 1991; Walker et al., 1999).

Polypharmacy is often associated with chronic illness and long-term drug therapy (LeSage, 1991). Eighty percent of people older than age 65 years have at least one chronic condition, and 50% have more than one chronic condition (Swonger & Burbank, 1995). In this age of medical specialization, treatment by more than one physician is not uncommon. Serious problems result, however, when coordination of the care delivery and treatment regimen specific to prescribed medications is lacking (Larsen & Hoot Martin, 1999; LeSage, 1991). These problems are compounded when the patient uses over-the-counter drugs, herbal remedies, and home or folk remedies without considering their potential interaction with prescribed drugs (LeSage, 1991). Nurses can follow the principles delineated in Text Box 30-2 to improve drug therapy in the elderly population.

As previously mentioned, enhancing health self-care capability is a major area for nursing intervention. Education of elderly patients and their families is crucial to ensuring compliance and minimizing untoward effects of medications. Basic principles regarding neurobiologic changes in normal aging (as previously dis-

cussed) should be applied when designing teaching strategies. The nurse must consider the elder's pace of learning as well as visual and hearing deficits. Education should include the reason for administering the drug and important side effects of the drug. The nurse should provide instructional aids, large-print labeling, and devices such as medication calendars that encourage compliance. The nurse should inform patients of the option to waive the requirements for childproof containers if they have trouble opening them (LeSage, 1991; Smith et al., 1993).

Cognitive Transcendence Transitions

In nursing, although health has been linked to developmental issues throughout the life span (Reed, 1989, 1991), late life adult developmental phenomena have not been well defined (Kogan, 1990; Stevenson, 1977). Jung (1933), Erikson (1963), and Peck (1968) conducted pioneering work in psychology, describing issues in ego development in late life. Although Erikson identified "integrity versus despair" as a developmental task specific to late adulthood, Peck contended that Erikson's stage applied generally to post–middle-age development and was not specific to late life. Jung, however, pioneered the notion of ego transcendence as a late life phenomenon.

Developmental psychologists expanded on the classic notions of ego development and identified several

TEXT BOX 30.2

Drug Therapy Interventions

- Minimize the number of drugs that the patient uses, keeping only those drugs that are essential. One third of the residents in one long-term care facility received 8 to 16 drugs daily (Lamy, 1984).

- Always consider alternatives among different drug classifications or dosage forms that are more suitable for elderly patients (Garne & Barr, 1984; Smith et al., 1993).

- Implement preventive measures to reduce the need for certain medications. Such prevention includes health promotion through proper nutrition, exercise, and stress reduction (LeSage, 1991).

- Most age-dependent pharmacokinetic changes lead to potential accumulation of the drug. Therefore, physicians usually start both the loading and maintenance doses at low levels (Cohen, 2000; Garne & Barr, 1984).

- Exercise caution when administering medication with a long half-life or in an older adult with impaired renal or liver function. Under these conditions, the physician may extend the time between doses (Miller, 1998).

- Be knowledgeable of each drug's properties, including such factors as half-life, excretion, and adverse effects. For example, venlafaxine HCl (Effexor), a structurally novel antidepressant that inhibits the reuptake of sero-

tonin and norepinephrine, requires regular monitoring of the patient's blood pressure.

- Assess the patient's clinical history for physical problems that may affect excretion of medications.

- Monitor laboratory values (eg, creatinine clearance) and urinary output in patients receiving medications eliminated by the kidneys.

- Monitor plasma albumin levels in patients receiving drugs that have high binding affinity to protein.

- Regularly monitor the patient's reaction to all medications to ensure a therapeutic response.

- Look for potential drug interactions that may complicate therapy. Antacids lower gastric acidity and may decrease the rate at which other medications are dissolved and absorbed. Phenothiazines, tricyclics, and benzodiazepines interact with antacids, resulting in decreased absorption. Anticholinergics, phenothiazines, and tricyclic antidepressants may delay the absorption of many other drugs but increase the total absorption of digoxin (Smith et al., 1993).

- Instruct patients to consult with their physicians or pharmacists before taking any over-the-counter medications.

tasks specific to development beyond 70 years of age (Havighurst, 1972; Newman & Newman, 1984). They identified major developmental tasks as adjustments to changes in physical status, roles, work, living arrangements, and mortality. The ego theorists, however, emphasized acceptance of existence that transcends the mortal body.

The developmental perspective on aging as posited by theories of gerotranscendence and self-transcendence offer a positive view of aging. Rather than emphasizing decrements in physical capacity for function, developmental theory provides for continued growth in dimensions such as spirituality, generativity, and inner strength in the context of aging-related transitions in late life (Ebersole & Hess, 1994). The phenomenon of gerotranscendence may also explain aging-related differences in coping with changes in health status and residence (Meeks et al., 1989).

Social Role Transitions

Several major aging-related social role transitions potentially alter personal and social identity (George, 1990). Evidence also supports the possibility of profound gender differences in aging-related role experiences (Theriault, 1994). Major transitions discussed here are retirement and changes in family roles, including widowhood. Both retirement and widowhood place elders at risk for poverty in late life. Finally, changes in sexuality are discussed.

Retirement. The transition during retirement from a paid work role to a potentially less structured and purposeful pattern of living can lead to alterations in self-concept. Retirement is frequently characterized as a stressful life event that may bring psychological, social, and economic uncertainty (Midanik et al., 1995). Even though potentially stressful, the average age of retirement has decreased from 1955 to 1960 (about age 66 years) to 1985 to 1990 (about age 63 years) (Gendell & Seigel, 1996).

Retirement affects social roles, income, use of health services, and participation in leisure activities. As with many of the changes associated with aging in the current cohort of elderly individuals, gender plays an important role in adjustment to retirement. Ozawa and Lum (1998) analyzed a sample of participants (4,447 women and 4,062 men) from the New Beneficiary Survey administered by the Social Security Administration. Analyzed data included income status and changes in income status over 10 years (1982 to 1992). Income status was defined as a person's income level considering the number of household members. The study found that the percentage of women who became widowed over the 10-year period was higher than that of men, and that the net effect of spouse loss on postretirement income

was different for men and women. Never-married women, however, fared relatively well economically in old age, because of human capital variables (ie, education, occupation, and labor force attachment). Although the effect of marital status on financial status after retirement is still strong, the effect of marital status is expected to weaken in future cohorts of elderly women. Future studies of retirement will need to adapt new paradigms (Mein et al., 1998).

Use of formal health services is also variable after retirement. Again, using the New Beneficiary Survey, Ozawa and Tseng (1999) selected 2,983 participants who reported at least three physical limitations and analyzed their use of three types of services during the 10 years after retirement: out-of-home services, in-home services, and transportation. Out-of-home services included services at senior citizen centers, adult day care services, and congregate meals. In-home services included visiting nurses, home health service, homemaker services, home-delivered meals, and telephone services. Use of out-of-home services was strongly related to age, marital status, and education. In general, younger, nonmarried (divorced or widowed), and more educated respondents were more likely to use out-of-home services. There was no relationship between use of out-of-home services and health status or income. Conversely, older, nonmarried respondents with a greater number of health impairments were more likely to use in-home services; income did not affect use of services. More health impairments and nonwhite race were positively associated with use of transportation. Number of children was unrelated to use of formal services. Therefore, nonmarried elderly people were more likely to use formal services after retirement, most likely because they lack the informal support of a spouse.

Health conditions may also prevent participation in leisure activities after retirement. Holmes and Dorfman (2000) investigated the relationship of two sets of health conditions and activities after retirement. They categorized the health conditions as life-threatening (eg, heart disease, cancer, diabetes) and non–life-threatening (eg, arthritis and fractures). They defined four activity domains, including informal social activities (eg, talking on the phone), formal social activities (eg, attendance at religious services, meetings of organizations, and volunteer activities), active leisure (eg, participation in active sports, walking, gardening), and home maintenance activities (eg, housework, yard work). As expected, the number of health conditions reduced time spent in the defined activities. The most commonly affected activities were active leisure pursuits, such as walking, gardening, active sports, and home maintenance activities. Among life-threatening conditions, lung disease showed the most persistent negative effects on activities in retirement, with diabetes the second most restrictive. Heart disease and cancer showed few negative effects, indicating that individuals with those conditions had learned to adapt to their illness to allow continued participation. More prevalent, non–life threatening conditions showed fewer effects on activities in retirement. Increased age was associated with decreased participation. Conversely, higher education levels were associated with increased participation in both formal and informal activities.

Loss of Spouse. A second group of aging-related role transitions is changes in family roles. Events such as retirement, death of a spouse, or death of one's own parents bring about these changes (Hagestad, 1990). Loss of one's spouse, particularly when the relationship has been long and satisfying, constitutes a major life event for the elderly person. Most often, loss of a spouse occurs through death because, after age 65 years, divorce occurs only at the rate of 0.9% in women and 1.7% in men (U.S. Bureau of the Census, 1991). For the most part, researchers and social services have ignored divorce in late life. Because it is relatively rare and few empirical data support interventions, the nurse must assess the individual person to determine his or her reaction to this role loss. Reaction to divorce may be similar to the grieving process a person experiences after the death of a spouse; however, the social and cultural norms are different.

Evidence regarding the role of gender reactions to and during bereavement is conflicting. In a study of 150 community-dwelling elderly people, Barer (1994) found interesting differences in reactions to loss of a spouse. Although the men in the study were more physically and economically advantaged, women had more extensive social networks, including closer ties with and more help from children. More women lose their spouses; however, they tend to be widowed at a younger age than men and therefore have more time to adjust and develop substitute social relationships to replace the spouse. Conversely, men tend to lose their wives at an older age, have fewer social networks to replace the spouse, and express feelings of loneliness and abandonment. Because of differences in longevity, men and women usually experience life events at different ages. Women are more likely to expect to become widowed than men and may therefore prepare early on for this adjustment (Barer, 1994).

More recently, Benedict and Zhang (1999) also found gender differences in reactions to loss through death. In this study, 391 individuals who had lost a spouse, parent, child, other relative, or friend were asked to recall their experiences at the time of the loss. Significantly more women than men recalled being highly emotional at the time of the loss, and the recovery period after the loss was longer for women. More men than women, however, wished that they could have changed past relationships with their families. One possible explanation for the findings in this study is that a significantly higher percentage of women (38.5%) than men (15.1%) had lost a spouse, whereas men more often reported the loss of a parent (52.4% for men versus 39.8% for women). When responses to spousal death only were studied, other investigators (Quigley & Schatz, 1999) found no differences between men and women.

Regardless of gender differences, survivors are at higher risk for depression and face financial issues after the death of a loved one. Health care professionals should work closely with grieving survivors to help them understand that their lives will be displaced for some time. Support sessions on the grief process and financial and employment planning could become a standard part of care (Wyatt et al., 1999).

Poverty. Because retirement and widowhood are common events in late life, elders can be at higher risk for poverty than other age groups. Two groups of poor elderly include those who have lived in poverty all their lives and those who become impoverished in late life. Poverty may result from inadequate retirement income, illness and medical bills, discrimination against women in pension plans, and financial exploitation of older individuals. Health care costs are probably the largest contributor to economic insecurity in elderly people. A profile of a typical impoverished older adult is a nonwhite (African American or Hispanic), rural dwelling individual who lives alone and has one or more chronic illnesses (Matteson et al., 1997). Poverty has significant effects on the elderly population, including higher mortality rates, poorer health, lower health-related quality of life, lower likelihood of participating in health screening programs, and higher likelihood of using the emergency department for acute illness (Matteson et al., 1997).

Sexuality. As in younger people, sexuality in older individuals involves a complex interplay of physical, psychological, social, and moral dimensions. Unfortunately, the major surveys of sexual practices have included few, if any, elderly individuals (Bortz et al., 1999). Misinformation and attitudinal barriers continue to plague the study of sexuality in the aging individual. Several generalizations have emerged from the existing literature: (1) older persons can retain interest in sex; (2) frequency of sexual activity is reported to be less than desired; and (3) increasing problems with sexual performance are associated with increasing age in both men and women (Bortz et al., 1999).

Several physical changes with aging affect sexual functioning. For women, these changes include decreasing estrogen levels, alterations in the structural integrity of the vagina (eg, decreased blood flow, decreased flexibility, diminished lubrication, and diminished response during orgasm), and decreased breast engorgement during arousal (Wright, 2001). For men, changes include a decline in testosterone production, increased time to achieve erection, less firm erections, decreased urgency for ejaculation, decreased sperm production, and a longer refractory period (ie, the amount of time before the man can achieve another erection) (Wright, 2001). Problems with sexual performance in aging men are centered around physical changes, that is, erectile dysfunction. In contrast, sexual performance in aging women involves social opportunity (Bortz et al., 1999). Despite physical changes, interest in and enjoyment of sexual activities can continue until one's death.

For older women, sexual response continues as in younger women, but with less intensity. As with other physical changes with age, differentiating normal age-related changes from sexual dysfunction can be challenging, particularly in elderly people, in whom a higher rate of chronic illness and use of medications complicate accurate diagnosis. Even with chronic illness, many older women describe themselves as interested in and satisfied with a variety of sexual activities (Johnson, 1998). Although being older is negatively correlated with sexual interest in women, sexual attitudes and knowledge were also important predictors of interest, participation, and satisfaction with sexual activity (Johnson, 1998).

In men, both the reported frequency and desired frequency for coitus declines as age increases (Bortz et al., 1999). Men are more likely to be sexually active, but less satisfied with their level of sexual activity compared with women (Matthias et al., 1997). As with women, partner availability and willingness influence the frequency of sexual activity, and the availability and willingness of partners declines with increasing age. Age alone, however, does not account for sexual function and satisfaction in aging men. The receptivity of the partner and medical illness are important predictors of sexual activity in older men (Bortz et al., 1999). For both men and women, a strong predictor of sexual satisfaction is positive mental health (Matthias et al., 1997).

Several factors contribute to whether a person engages in sex in later life: age, health, desire to remain sexually active, access to a partner, and a conducive environment (Levy, 1994; Matthias et al., 1997). Age and health have been discussed previously. Desire to remain sexually active is affected by self-perception as an attractive, sexual being; attitudes, beliefs and values about sexual behavior; and the effects of poor health and use of medications. Access to a partner may be prevented through death of a spouse or divorce, and subsequently, adult children's attitudes about widowed or divorced parents becoming sexually involved (Travis, 1987). Access to a conducive environment may be hindered if the parent resides with an adult child or is a nursing home resident. Although nursing home residents may remain interested in maintaining sexual relationships, the attitudes of the staff and physicians constitute an additional barrier for this population beyond those noted previously (Bauer,

1999). Health care professionals are often uncomfortable discussing sexuality with patients and may erroneously believe that older adults are not interested, or worse yet, should not be interested in sex. Suggested interventions to remove barriers for nursing home residents include improving privacy (eg, "do not disturb" signs), educating staff about sexuality in the elderly, allowing conjugal or home visits, encouraging forms of sexual expression other than intercourse (eg, hugging, kissing), assessing medications that may affect sexual function, and providing counseling about sexuality to interested residents (Richardson & Lazur, 1995). Finally, as with younger adults, older people, particularly those with risk factors for HIV, should be counseled about safe-sex practices and the use of condoms (Gordon & Thompson, 1995).

Social Support Transitions

Social support and interest in its relationship to health emerged in the 1970s, at a time when social isolation and low levels of social integration were associated with negative health consequences (Hogue, 1985; Norbeck, 1988). Most research in social support conceptualizes social support as a buffer to stress, which, in turn, advances health. Other investigators hypothesize that social support directly affects stress and health (Norbeck, 1988). More recently, researchers have proposed the negative effects of social support (or its "burden") (Krause & Jay, 1991).

Isreal and Antonucci (1987) examined the relationship between social network characteristics and psychological well-being in a sample of men and women aged 50 to 95 years. They found that most of the network characteristics were not significantly related to psychological well-being. The qualitative dimensions of affective support and reciprocal affective support, however, were strongly associated with psychological well-being. In a later study, Connidis and McMullin (1993) confirmed the importance of the qualitative aspect of social support. They found that having children enhanced the well-being of older adults only if the parents viewed their relationship as being "close." These investigators concluded that having a small network or fewer social contacts is not necessarily detrimental to well-being in older adults. Older adults may compensate for loss of family by expanding friendship networks, and employment may become an important source of establishing a network in late life.

Suicide. A lack of social support has been linked to the rate of suicide in the elderly. After falls and motor vehicle collisions, suicide is the third leading cause of death from injury among people older than age 65 years. Age-specific rates for suicide are consistently higher among the elderly than any other age group. Of people aged 65 years or older, men account for 81% of suicides. Rates are the highest for divorced or widowed men (Lehmann

& Rabins, 1999). Risk factors for suicide in elderly people include being white, male, widowed or divorced, retired or unemployed, living alone in an urban area, in poor health (including poor mental health), or lonely, and having a history of poor interpersonal relationships (Matteson et al., 1997). Older people make fewer attempts per successful suicide; firearms are the most common method of suicide by both men and women older than age 65 years (Lehmann & Rabins, 1999).

Health

A second major construct in the model of the elder sphere is health. In this model, health is viewed as being in process and as an outcome of developmental responses to late life transitions. That is, health as an outcome is not simply a state of being; rather, it is a process of becoming in the context of late life transitions. In this context, definitions of health for older adults focus on objective functional status (Wells, 1993), health behaviors, and subjective qualitative indicators such as well-being (Burgener & Chiverton, 1992) and life satisfaction (George, 1990).

Functional Status

Physical Function. **Functional status** is defined as the extent to which a person has the ability to carry out independently personal care, home management, and social functions in everyday life in a way that has meaning and purpose. It is frequently measured by assessing an individual's ability to perform basic and instrumental activities of daily living (ADLs). Tasks concerning fundamental daily activities, such as personal care or basic mobility, are classified as "basic" activities of daily living (BADLs). More complex tasks associated with independent community living, such as home management or shopping, are considered "instrumental" activities of daily living (IADLs) (Guccione & Jette, 1988). Many intrinsic and extrinsic factors influence functional status. Intrinsic factors include biologic and behavioral characteristics, whereas extrinsic factors include the amount and type of health care provided as well as supportive physical and social environments (Kane, 1993; Schulz & Williamson, 1993).

Estimates of the prevalence of functional dependency vary across surveys. In general, however, studies have shown that difficulty in performing ADLs increases with advancing age and that rates of dependency are significantly higher for women than for men, particularly for women who live alone (Guralnik & Simonsick, 1993; Van Nostrand et al., 1993).

Cognitive Function. Cognitive function greatly influences physical functional. Because of physical and physiologic changes in the brain in aging, cognitive function is assumed to decline. Although many aspects of cognition remain stable over time, several diseases associated with alterations in cognition are more prevalent in the elderly, including depression, dementia, and delirium.

Normal aging does not impair consciousness. Alertness is required for attention, but the alert patient may not necessarily be able to attend. Attention has two aspects: sustained attention (vigilance) and selective attention (ability to extract relevant from irrelevant information). Numerous studies indicate that elderly people perform well on tests of both sustained and selective attention. Earlier findings of poor performance on tests of selective attention have been attributed to lack of control for perceptual difficulties (eg, vision and hearing deficits) (Albert, 1994).

Intelligence and personality are stable across the life span in the absence of disease. Although intelligence is stable, learning abilities of older people may be more selective, requiring motivation ("how important is this information?"), meaningful content ("why do I need to know this?"), and familiarity with the idea or content. Although age causes no differences in the ability to process knowledge to learn a skill, younger people are more likely to employ strategies to learn tasks (Swanson & Lee, 1992). Level of education needs to be considered in evaluating responses on mental status examinations because it may represent (serve as a proxy measure for) socioeconomic status and occupation, both of which are correlated with performance on mental status examinations (Launer et al., 1993; Frisoni et al., 1993).

Reaction time slows (Salthouse, 1993), which may affect how quickly the elder responds to questions. Hurrying elders to answer questions may interfere with their ability to provide the correct answer. This has been labeled the *speed–accuracy shift*, by which the elderly person focuses more on accuracy than on speed in responding (Hertzog et al., 1993). Caution tends to increase, whereas risk-taking behavior tends to decrease; older adults are more likely to make errors of omission (leave the answer out) than errors of commission (make a guess) (Cerella, 1990).

Other than overall intelligence, age-related memory alterations have been more widely studied than any other aspect of cognition. Primary memory, or short-term memory, is the ability to retain a small amount of information over a brief period. Secondary memory, or long-term memory, is a memory store containing an unlimited amount of information over an indefinite period. Although some assert that primary memory shows few, if any, losses with aging (Albert, 1994), others believe age-related differences in performance on short-term memory tasks are striking (Morris & McManus, 1991; Verhaeghen et al., 1993). Age decrements are greater when subjects are asked to recall information than when they are asked to recognize stimuli to which they were previously exposed (memory versus recognition) (Albert,

1994). Memory problems in later life are believed to result from problems encoding, or "getting" the information in the first place. This problem may be related to sensory problems, not paying attention, or a general failure to link the "to be remembered" information to existing knowledge through association or to strengthen the memory through repetition. It is important, however, not to confuse decline with deficit. Although a decline in memory ability may be frustrating for the older individual, it does not necessarily hamper his or her ability to function daily. Threats to memory include medications, depression (impairs concentration and attention), poor nutrition, infection, heart and lung disease (lack of oxygen), thyroid problems (can cause symptoms of depression or confusion that mimic memory loss), alcohol use, and sensory loss (interferes with perception).

Memory loss is not a normal part of aging. To remember events, humans must first attend to information and process it. Older people may well dismiss information that is not important to them (remember motivation, meaningfulness, familiarity).

Changes in cognition are most likely accounted for by structural and functional changes in the brain. Structural and functional alterations are probably highly specific, since aspects of cognitive decline are very specific (eg, secondary memory) and many abilities are preserved. Moreover, external factors may modify the development or expression of age-related changes in cognition, including activity levels, socioeconomic status, education, and personality (Albert, 1994; Hultsch et al., 1993; Inouye et al., 1993).

Health Behaviors

Health behaviors, or health **self-care,** include all actions that a person performs to promote his or her own health, prevent disease, limit illness, and restore health (Levin & Idler, 1984; Dean, 1992). This broad definition emphasizes the individual rather than the professional sphere. As a result, health activities, including use of professional health care and adherence to therapeutic regimens, are viewed as options under the control of the elder rather than professional dictums.

Researchers have focused considerable attention on the health self-care of elders (Cox, 1986; Hickey et al., 1986; Jirovec & Kasno, 1990; Kart & Dunkle, 1989; Lenihan, 1988; Vickery et al., 1988). Most research has been concerned with the use of traditional professional health services. This body of literature consistently shows that older adults are the largest single group of consumers of formal or professional health services. Health utilization, however, is disproportionately spread over this group: a relatively small proportion of elders use a relatively large proportion of both inpatient and outpatient services (Kraus, 1990).

Elders engage in various activities to promote their own health and to maintain a sense of well-being. The scope of these self-determined behaviors and their efficacy, however, have not been fully explored (Sokolovsky & Vesperi, 1991; Tripp-Reimer & Cohen, 1987). Rather, professional standards are generally applied to assess elders' level of activity in predetermined categories of health promotion and illness prevention activities (Brown & McCreedy, 1986; Duffy, 1993; Rakowski et al., 1992; Walker et al., 1988). Current programs to promote healthy lifestyles for elders include the Healthy Lifestyles for Seniors Program (Santa Monica) and the New Mexico Health Promotion With Elders Project (New Mexico). These programs generally include components of exercise, nutrition, health screening, and health habits (Alford & Futrell, 1992). The degree to which they build on the established practices and beliefs of elders, however, has not yet been assessed.

Well-Being

Health and well-being are terms that are frequently used in tandem to denote a goal or standard for preventive and therapeutic intervention. Health is associated with absence of diagnosed disease, whereas well-being represents qualitative, subjective judgments about quality of life. A primary goal in gerontology is finding ways to enhance the quality of life of older adults. Quality of life is a global construct, however, that encompasses a broad range of personal, environmental, and social variables. Moreover, no definition of quality of life is universally accepted. The most frequent measures of quality of life are life satisfaction, morale, and happiness, three constructs that are highly correlated (George, 1990). These quality of life indicators, however, may not be measurable in segments of older adult populations. Three problems have been identified in applying quality of life indicators to elderly adults with dementia. First, many of the variables used as indicators of quality of life require subjective evaluations by the individual, which may or may not be feasible with cognitive impairment. Second, the broad domains of quality of life are not relevant for older adults who have little or no control over where they live. Finally, a network of family and friends may not exist, and even if family and friends are present, people with cognitive impairments may be unable to relate to them (Burgener & Chiverton, 1992).

In contrast to quality of life, the concept of well-being offers an alternative qualitative health standard. Well-being may convey a global meaning as in Webster's definition, which describes it as "a state of being happy, healthy or prosperous" (*Webster's Ninth New Collegiate Dictionary,* p. 1339). Similarly, Isreal and Antonucci (1987) defined well-being as the "extent to which positive feelings outweigh negative feelings" (p. 465), whereas George (1990, p. 190) viewed it as "an individual's perceptions of overall life quality." Burgener and Chiverton (1992), on the other hand, conceptualized well-being as having two major components: affect and life satisfaction. Affect may be positive (eg, happy) or negative (eg, depressed), and it is an indicator of the emotional component of well-being. Life satisfaction is a cognitive-judgmental aspect that requires a subjective evaluation by the respondent.

ENVIRONMENTAL SPHERE

The effects of the environment on health have been identified as a major concern throughout nursing's history (Williams, 1988). Early studies of environment examined it as a source of stress and disease. Several reviews have shown that nursing theory and research on environmental issues focused more on the immediate physical environment than on larger societal influences embedded in social, political, and economic structures (Chopoorian, 1986; Kleffel, 1991; Stevens, 1989). Although it is impossible to distinguish precise dimensional boundaries, the environmental sphere of the conceptual model (see Fig. 30-1) specifies four dimensions: social, cultural, physical, and spiritual.

Social Dimension

According to Chopoorian (1986), environment bridges personal and societal dimensions. She proposed three major components: (1) sociopolitical structures, (2) human social relations, and (3) everyday life. In this schema, everyday life is defined as personal habits and routine activities.

Chopoorian (1986) believed that individuals interpret from everyday experience. Moreover, she argued that, in the United States, social structures such as government, private industry, health care, and educational institutions operate within highly stratified, hierarchic power systems. In turn, the power systems filter downward to microsocial systems, such as the family and work groups, in a way that actually reproduces organizational life in everyday life. Of particular concern to the well-being of elders is the fact that the power relations that characterize these organizational systems generate ideologies such as ageism, sexism, and classism, all of which limit alternatives open to individuals and populations. This view is consistent with the notion that policy decisions actually shape life trajectories (Hagestad, 1990) and that the sociopolitical and economic environment is often the origin of patients' most serious problems (Kleffel, 1991). Inducing sociopolitical change to equalize the distribution of power and resources at all levels of social exchange, as well as to change ideologies that characterize elders as socioeconomic liabilities, requires the concerted efforts of elders themselves as well as professional and social groups concerned with enhancing late life development and well-being.

Cultural Dimension

The cultural (values, beliefs, and patterns of behavior) dimension of elder–environment interaction is based in ethnic affiliation (race, national origin, religion, language) and is closely related to social structures and processes in its influence on the experience of aging (Jackson et al., 1990; Keith, 1990; Tripp-Reimer et al., 1995). Keith (1990) noted that the influence of cultural values and traditional behaviors on older adults' experiences is mediated by an exchange between the traditions and changing social contexts as experienced by new generations, and also by the elders' attempts to blend traditional resources with social change. Thus, identifying cultural affiliation provides a context from which nurses may anticipate individual differences in values, religions, family structures, lines of authority, and other life patterns (Tripp-Reimer et al., 1995). Understanding and accepting individual differences that arise from cultural variation enhances the ability to facilitate late life development in a culturally sensitive manner. This in turn preserves the personhood of individual elders, that is, it "accords a complete and normal identity" (Keith, 1990, p. 100).

Tripp-Reimer and colleagues (1995) identified several reasons for considering the cultural dimension in gerontologic nursing. First, cultural factors largely determine the definition and status of elders. Second, an elder's beliefs, values, and behaviors are established through a history of enculturation, through which individual pattern and meaning are derived. Thus, although cultural heritage is a significant context for planning care, it does not predict behavior at an individual level. For example, ethnic elders do not experience the same patterns of eligibility, access, and use of health care services as their younger counterparts.

Physical Dimension

The model of person-environment fit has provided a theoretic basis for examining the effects of personal (physical) environment on function and well-being in late life (Parmelee & Lawton, 1990). One of the major issues in addressing living space for late life is housing and the proximity of "home" to social resources such as church, community centers, shopping, health care, and related social services. Although most elders live in their own homes (Czaja et al., 1993), housing options that reduce or eliminate many of the functional demands of home management have been designed and continue to be studied and developed. As in other late life social transitions, however, relocating to smaller and more protective housing may be welcomed by some and fiercely resisted by others.

For every person currently in institutional care, an estimated four others who require some form of long-term care are in the community. How and by whom will they be provided care?

Approaches to this looming problem include the following:

- Reducing the need for home care by improving the health of older people
- Finding and paying for home care when disability and frailty preclude continued independence
- Ensuring better integration across the total continuum of care and coordination of different care providers who subscribe to a biopsychosocial view of health care that includes both medical and social components

In keeping with this last point, more emphasis should be placed on community care options, services that provide both sustenance and growth. Examples of supportive services necessary to foster independent community living include information and referral services, transportation and nutrition services, legal and protective services, comprehensive senior centers, homemaker and handyman services, matching of older with younger individuals to share housing, and use of the supports available through churches, community groups, or mental health and other community agencies (ie, area agencies on aging) to maintain elderly individuals in the community for as long as possible. The availability and accessibility of these services vary greatly, and eligibility requirements may exist. Also, some mentally ill older patients may be resistant to accepting services. If resistance to service use is widespread, the problem must be addressed and innovative delivery mechanisms developed and tested.

Most nursing homes violate all the elements traditionally associated with culturally and socially relevant definitions of "home," in that residents have little control over with whom they live, who comes and goes in their personal space, and other aspects of the environment such as furnishings and appointments (Wilson, 1994). Not surprisingly, perceived quality of life and life satisfaction decrease as elders transition from independent living to more dependent levels of care (eg, assisted living to nursing home care) (Crist, 1999; Schroeder et al., 1998).

Residential Care

Various residential care models are in part a response to the medical model emphasis in most long-term care facilities, and the need to develop alternatives to nursing home care. Residential care models include a spectrum of state-licensed residential living environments such as foster care homes, family homes, personal care homes, residential care facilities, and assisted living arrangements. The latter care option, which links housing and

services, is described in more detail later to illustrate some of the key features of one of the fastest growing types of residential care approaches (Alzheimer's Association, 1994; Gramann, 1999; Hawes, 1999).

Although residential care settings vary in size from small private homes for up to four residents to large congregate care facilities that may care for more than 100 residents, all offer assistance and care to their residents and share with them the responsibilities for activities of daily living. Ideally, the care provided is flexible, resident and family oriented, and intended to optimize individual dignity, functioning, health, and well-being. The physical environment and design features of the facility should support the functioning of the impaired older adult and accommodate behaviors and diminished abilities (Alzheimer's Association, 1994; Hawes, 1999).

There is a lack of federal guidelines to standardize residential care. Rather, state regulations usually specify and define factors such as environmental adaptations, assessment procedures, care planning and services, and minimum staffing ratios, which are generally quite low. Some states require new facilities to undergo an extensive process for licensure, or obtain a Certificate of Need before plans are approved. Definitions of required levels of nursing care vary markedly in regulations from state to state. A number of residential settings have been developed to care for special populations, such as people with varying levels of cognitive impairment. Many facilities offer a range of care options along a continuum of care that anticipate and adjust to the changing needs of residents (Alzheimer's Association, 1994; Melia, 2000; Tinsley, 1998).

Consumers should question residential providers about all aspects of services in order to determine whether the older adult's needs and abilities match the care provided in that facility, including staff training and staffing patterns, medication supervision, approaches to behavior management, activities provided, services available (eg, care management, family support, counseling, day care), safety and security issues, provision of personal care with attention to dignity and privacy, health and nutrition concerns, and full disclosure of costs and funding and payment issues (Alzheimer's Association, 1994).

Assisted Living

The assisted living concept is one alternative model of supportive housing that is growing at a phenomenal rate because of consumer preferences, costs associated with traditional long-term care, and changes in the attitudes of health care professionals (Hawes, 1999; Wilson, 1994). The state of Oregon has been a leader in developing standards of care and licensure conditions and in evaluating resident outcomes associated with assisted living projects. In Oregon's model program, residents (including Medicaid recipients) are entitled to a private apartment, shared only by choice, that includes a kitchen, bath with roll-in shower, locking doors, and temperature control capability. The overall shelter costs in assisted living are not substantially higher than in nursing facilities (Wilson, 1994). In addition, routine nursing services and case management for ancillary services are provided.

Perhaps the most important feature of these assisted living facilities is not the environment or even the services provided; rather, it is the orientation toward the elderly resident that is paramount. That orientation is one that empowers the frail older adult by sharing responsibilities for care and activities of daily living, enhancing their choices and managing risks (Gramann, 1999; Wilson, 1994). The need for alternative long-term care strategies for this population is expected to continue, with the growing number of older adults in need of supportive services.

The desire for elders to remain in their own homes is often met with family and societal judgments of being emotional, sentimental, and irrational. Similarly, the subjective value of home is often weighed against objective measures of housing quality, such as size and structural conditions, and adequacy of utilities, such as plumbing and heating. Parmelee and Lawton (1990) describe the tension between the need for autonomy and the need for security when designing physical environments for older adults. Autonomy refers to a state in which elders feel or are capable of managing daily life and pursuing goals using their own resources. Autonomy implies a freedom of choice and action—the regulation of one's own life and life space. Central to the idea of facilitating autonomy is the issue of control and individual differences in the desire for control. Security, on the other hand, refers to the dependability of physical, social, and interpersonal resources for managing daily life. It addresses physical safety as well as psychological comfort (ie, peace of mind) (Parmelee & Lawton, 1990). Balancing autonomy and security extends beyond the immediate living space to the neighborhood, where developing a sense of community contributes to physical safety and emotional security.

Spiritual Dimension

Despite the fact that spirituality has been addressed for centuries and from a wide variety of perspectives, scientists have been reluctant to approach this topic directly. Levin (1994, p. xvi), for example, described the "collective amnesia" of scientists regarding the significance of spiritual issues and religion for health and aging. The spiritual dimension, however, is a key element in elders' lived experience.

Spirituality emerges as humans address the eternal mythic questions of life: the purpose and meaning of life, truth, love, desire, evil, suffering, and death. It may be viewed as the *life principle* that pervades and integrates a person's entire being. Moberg (1974, p. 259) defined spiritual as pertaining "to the inner resources of people, their ultimate concern around which all other values are focused, their central philosophy in life (whether designated as religious or non-religious) which guides their conduct, and all the supernatural and non-material dimensions of human nature."

In the Western, classical sense, spirituality includes the transcendent (or that which exists apart from the material world—beyond basic human knowledge). More recently, however, the idea of spirituality incorporates the humanistic perspective, which may exclude ideas of transcendence. Humanistic (Third Force) psychologists such as Carl Rogers and Rollo May have their roots in the existential (phenomenologic) movement in European philosophy. They propose that insight into our own mortality forms the impetus to shift from the ordinary state of human existence to a higher state: from an ontic to an ontologic mode. The ontic mode is characterized by forgetfulness of being, treating self and other as object ("inauthentic"). On the other hand, the ontologic mode is characterized by mindfulness of being, treating self and other as subject ("authentic") (Yallom, 1980; Tiryakian, 1968). The humanists suggest that the main purpose of life is to find meaning, and that this can be accomplished through creations (or accomplishments), experiences in the world, and attitude toward suffering (Frankl, 1963). Here, spirituality is the mystery in striving to be in unity with others.

In nursing, spirituality is recognized as a basic quality, inherent in all humans. The spiritual perspective has been identified as having three critical attributes: (1) connectedness (with other humans, nature, universal forces, or God); (2) beliefs in powers or forces beyond the self, and a faith that affirms life; and (3) a creative energy. Further, the spiritual perspective provides a path for the quest for the meaning of life, organizes and guides human values and motivations, and results in self-transcendence (Haase et al., 1992; Reed, 1992).

Whereas spirituality is "internal" and individual based, it may be aided or guided in its development through religion. Religion is a component of the environment external to the person and provides "options" for engaging the sacred. Religion is a universal social institution, which generally is composed of three major elements: (1) a set of organized beliefs about the nature of the nonmaterial (supernatural) world, often but not always including concepts of a god or deities; (2) myths or sacred stories about the history and actions of the supernatural powers, beings, or forces; and (3) rituals involving symbolic acts or objects that mediate between the human and the suprahuman spheres (Campbell, 1986; Moore, 1992).

NURSING SPHERE

The nursing sphere in the conceptual model (see Fig. 30-1) incorporates three nursing knowledge domains: diagnoses, interventions, and outcomes (Iowa Intervention Project, 1992). Diagnoses and outcomes represent patient phenomena, whereas the intervention domain represents nursing therapeutics that are carried out to achieve health outcomes (Iowa Intervention Project, 2000).

Nursing Diagnoses

Nursing diagnoses are clinical judgments about individual, family, or community responses to actual or potential health problems and life processes (North American Nursing Diagnosis Association, 2001). In the context of late life transitions, diagnoses consider the timing of the transition and at what point the elder is in the transition process. Diagnoses also reflect emotional, attitudinal, and functional responses to the challenges posed by developmental, situational, or health–illness transitions. As described earlier, change introduces uncertainty and is stressful; thus, readiness for the transition is another major focus for diagnosis. The nurse can assess this variable by exploring the meanings that a particular life change has for the elder. Similarly, diagnosis involves identifying what knowledge and skills the elder requires to develop a new identity and manage changing roles and physical capacities (Schumacher & Meleis, 1994). Ebersole and Hess (1994) suggest that late life transitions require very different adaptive capacities than earlier stages of the life course. In late life, existential issues such as experiencing losses, redefining meanings in existence, and living in the present become the standard, replacing the performance and future orientation that characterize earlier adulthood.

In addition to individual responses, assessment and diagnosis include the physical, social, cultural, and spiritual environmental resources for, and barriers to, achieving optimal health behavior, functional status, and well-being. As previously shown, environmental phenomena are critical to enhancing developmental and functional capacities in late life.

The extent to which the current North American Nursing Diagnosis Association taxonomy represents the phenomena of aging-related late life transitions and the environments in which they occur will need to be examined. Work is underway to identify relevant diagnoses in the current taxonomy and to develop diagnoses that are needed.

Nursing Interventions

Nursing interventions focus on assisting elders to achieve health outcomes when experiencing aging-related tran-

sitions. Meleis and Trangenstein (1994) argued that the process of facilitating transitions to enhance a sense of well-being gives nursing a unique perspective. Interventions target personal and environmental resources and barriers to achieving health outcomes. Although it is not feasible to include a detailed description of all relevant interventions in this chapter, interventions identified as "core" to geriatric nursing are listed in Text Box 30-3 (Iowa Intervention Project, 1996). Several areas for intervention, however, are included here for purposes of illustration.

TEXT BOX 30.3

Core Nursing Interventions Defined by the National Gerontological Nursing Association

Abuse Protection: Elder

Active Listening

Activity Therapy

Behavior Management

Bowel Incontinence Care

Bowel Training

Caregiver Support

Communication Enhancement: Hearing Deficit

Constipation/Impaction Management

Coping Enhancement

Delirium Management

Dementia Management

Dying Care

Emotional Support

Environmental Management: Comfort

Exercise Promotion

Exercise Therapy: Ambulation

Fluid/Electrolyte Management

Foot Care

Grief Work Facilitation

Medication Administration

Nutrition Management

Patient Rights Protection

Positioning

Pressure Management

Reminiscence Therapy

Respite Care

Self-Care Assistance

Urinary Habit Training

Urinary Incontinence Care

From: Iowa Intervention Project. (1996). *Core interventions by specialty.* Iowa City, IA: Nursing Classifications Center.

One area for intervention is assisting the elder to prepare for the transition by providing information about internal developmental processes, sources of social support, and opportunities for personal growth and role supplementation (Schumacher & Meleis, 1994). According to Ebersole and Hess (1994), individuals are usually ill prepared for major life transitions. Similarly, elders do not perceive planning for changes, such as retirement, as being a health concern (Bevil et al., 1993). As researchers learn more about late life transition experiences, health care professionals will be better equipped to facilitate elders, families, and communities in their development.

Another major focus of intervention is lifestyle. As with all life stages, health promotion and primary and secondary prevention have become national and local strategies for improving health (U.S. Department of Health and Human Services, 1990). Lifestyle interventions such as exercise promotion and nutrition counseling are particularly important in late life because a tendency to slow down and become more sedentary usually accompanies aging. Moreover, lack of exercise was shown to be as predictive of functional decline as several medical conditions and variables such as visual impairment (Mor et al., 1989). For example, muscle function appears to be the most important aging-related physical change in that it interferes with ADL function as well as endurance. Studies have shown that resistance exercise that targets specific muscle groups used in functional tasks (eg, lifting, grasping, locomotion) can improve muscle strength (Hughes et al., 1994). Similarly, such exercise can help maintain or improve joint flexibility even with musculoskeletal disease. Hughes and associates (1994) suggested that because of its high prevalence among older adults, musculoskeletal disease is often ignored when, in fact, any joint impairment should be considered a risk factor for functional dependence. This suggestion has implications for interventions of health screening, risk appraisal, and risk reduction.

A third major area for intervention is the facilitation of role supplementation and role enhancement. Adelmann (1994) found that elders who occupied multiple roles experienced higher levels of psychological well-being than elders with fewer roles. Ebersole and Hess (1994) also suggest that nurses can assist elders to develop ways to enhance the exchange process through reciprocal activities and interpersonal reliance. Similarly, engaging elders in life review (eg, reminiscence therapy) can facilitate developmental processes such as gerotranscendence.

A fourth area of nursing intervention is management of the environment. Although safety is a priority, interventions directed toward the environment go beyond physical safety to include use of sociopolitical processes to bring about change in constraining social processes and structures. Facilitating the use of social structures and processes can be done through individual efforts, such as assisting elders to perceive and describe their own environments in a way that helps them recognize constraints on their health and freedom to participate (Kleffel, 1991). It can also be done through sociopolitical processes (Kleffel, 1991; Stevens, 1989). Although nursing has a tradition of managing the immediate physical environment to reduce its negative effects on function and well-being, Kleffel (1991) suggested that nurses' lack of awareness about the effects of the social, economic, and political environment on function and well-being has contributed to the peripheral role of nursing in influencing change in these systems.

Enhancing health self-care capability is another major area for nursing intervention. Many chronic symptoms and illnesses require major self-care efforts to maintain health and to obtain optimal benefit from treatment and rehabilitation (Kart & Engler, 1994). One mechanism for enhancing health self-care is patient education that is designed in accordance with elder characteristics and the requisite knowledge (Dellasega et al., 1994). Patient education focusing on self-monitoring for early detection of disease is also an important dimension of health self-care. For example, instruction in breast cancer self-examination has been shown to be effective in increasing the frequency, proficiency, and perceived skill in conducting breast self-examination (Lierman et al., 1994).

Nursing-Sensitive Patient Outcomes

The third component of the nursing sphere in the conceptual model is the development and evaluation of desired health outcomes. As shown in the elder sphere of the model, health outcomes in late life include functional status, health behavior, and well-being. A nursing-sensitive patient outcome refers to a variable client (or patient) state, condition, or perception largely influenced by and sensitive to nursing intervention (Iowa Outcomes Project, 2000). Late life transitions are complex processes that have many contexts. Similarly, treatment is multidimensional and often interdisciplinary. Consequently, health outcomes are difficult to classify because they are influenced by multiple inputs, including the patient.

In general, the desired effect of interventions is successful elder management of late life transitions and meaningful living. Indicators of successful management include, but are not limited to, emotional well-being, mastery of new skills and roles, meaningful relationships, functional ability, and personal transformation. As previously noted, transitions occur over time; thus, outcomes occur throughout the process and are not universally associated with a defined end point (Meleis & Trangenstein, 1994). Again, work is underway to develop observable outcome indicators that can be used to examine the effects of nursing intervention in practice and research.

Summary of Key Points

➤ The five major categories of aging-related transitions are (1) normative biologic involution, (2) late life illness and comorbidity, (3) cognitive developmental transitions, (4) social role transitions, and (5) social support transitions.

➤ Major changes in social roles with aging include retirement, widowhood, and changes in residence.

➤ The brain changes with aging; these changes include a decline in weight and reduction in synapses.

➤ The nervous system has a considerable degree of plasticity and can sustain some structural losses without losing function.

➤ All five special senses (sight, hearing, touch, taste, and smell) decline with age.

➤ Intelligence and personality are stable over the life span; however, reaction time slows with age.

➤ Threats to memory in the elderly include medications, depression, poor nutrition, infection, heart and lung disease, thyroid problems, alcohol use, and sensory loss.

➤ People between 60 and 70 years of age are twice as likely to experience an adverse drug reaction than those 30 to 40 years of age.

➤ Elderly people are at higher risk for poverty and suicide.

➤ Although older adults experience many physical changes, they can and have the desire to remain sexually active.

➤ Aging affects pharmacokinetics, including drug absorption, distribution, metabolism, and excretion; it also affects the strength and number of protein-binding sites.

➤ Residential care environments ideally emphasize family-oriented care that optimizes existing functional capacities.

➤ Assisted living is a supportive housing environment that provides routine nursing services and case management within a philosophy of patient empowerment.

➤ The risk for adverse drug reactions increases with the number of drugs that the elderly person is receiving.

Critical Thinking Challenges

1. What factors contribute to nervous system plasticity in older adults?

2. What five factors may affect the absorption of medications in elderly people?

3. How do changes in the proportion of body fat, lean body weight, and total body water in elderly people affect the distribution of fat-soluble medications?

4. What classifications of drugs does the liver metabolize?

5. How does aging affect renal function?

6. What information must the nurse determine before the safe administration of medication in elderly people?

7. What nursing interventions and care environments have been useful in treating older patients with mental health problems?

 WEB LINKS

www.aarp.org American Association of Retired Persons. This useful website provides information and resources related to the elderly.

www.nasmhpd.org/consurdiv.htm National Association of Consumer/Survivor Mental Health Administrators (NAC/SMHA) Older Persons Division. This site provides mental health service regulations.

www.elderweb.com Elder Web Newsletter. This site is a consumer's newsletter for older adults.

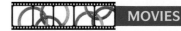 **MOVIES**

Driving Miss Daisy: 1989. This delightful film stars Jessica Tandy as Daisy Werthan, a cantankerous old woman. Morgan Freeman plays Hoke Colburn, Daisy's chauffeur. This beautiful story examines a relationship between two people who have more in common than just getting old. *Driving Miss Daisy* challenges some of the myths about getting old.

Viewing Points: Identify the normal behaviors in the growth and development of the elderly. Observe the verbal and nonverbal communication of Daisy and Hoke. How do they support each other?

REFERENCES

Achenbaum, W. A., & Bengtson, V. L. (1994). Re-engaging the disengagement theory of aging: On the history and assessment of theory in gerontology. *Gerontologist, 34,* 756–763.

Adelmann, P. K. (1994). Multiple roles and psychological well-being in a national sample of older adults. *Journals of Gerontology: Social Sciences, 49*(6), S277–S285.

Agris, P. F., Boak, A., Basler, J. W., et al. (1985). Analysis of cellular senescence through detection and assessment of

RNAs and proteins important to gene expression: Transfer RNAs and autoimmune antigens. *Advances in Experimental Medicine & Biology, 190*, 509–539.

Albert, M. S. (1994). Cognition and aging. In W. R. Hazzard, E. L. Bierman, J. P. Blass, et al. (Eds.), *Principles of geriatric medicine and gerontology* (3rd ed., pp. 1013–1019). New York: McGraw-Hill.

Alford, D., & Futrell, M. (1992). Wellness and health promotion of the elderly. *Nursing Outlook, 40*, 221–226.

Alzheimer's Association. (1994). *Residential settings: An examination of Alzheimer issues*. Chicago: Author.

Arking, R. (1991). Modifying the aging process. In R. F. Young & E. A. Olson (Eds.), *Health, illness and disability in later life* (pp. 11-24). Newbury Park, CA: Sage.

Atchley, R. C. (1989). A continuity theory of normal aging. *Gerontologist, 29*, 183–190.

Bahr, Sr., R. T. (1992). Personhood: A theory for gerontological nursing. *Holistic Nursing Practice, 7*(1), 1–6.

Barclay, L., & Wolfson, L. (1993). Normal aging: Pathophysiologic and clinical changes. In L. Barclay (Ed.), *Clinical geriatric neurology* (pp. 13–20). Philadelphia: Lea & Febiger.

Barer, B. M. (1994). Men and women aging differently. *International Journal of Aging and Human Development, 38*(1), 29–40.

Basson, P. (1967). The gerontological nursing literature. *Nursing Research, 16*(3), 267–272.

Bauer, M. (1999). Their only privacy is between their sheets: Privacy and the sexuality of elderly nursing home residents. *Journal of Gerontological Nursing, 25*(8), 37–41.

Benedict, A., & Zhang, X. (1999). Reactions to loss among men and women: A comparison. *Activities, Adaptation & Aging, 24*(1), 29–38.

Bengtson, V. L., Reedy, M., & Gordon, C. (1985). Aging and self-conceptions: Personality processes and social contexts. In J. Birren & K. Schaie (Eds.), *Handbook of psychology of aging* (pp. 544–593). New York: Van Nostrand Reinhold.

Bernardi, B. (1985). *Age class systems: Social institutions and polities based on age*. London: Cambridge.

Bevil, C. A., O'Connor, P. C., & Mattoon, P. M. (1993). Leisure activity, life satisfaction and perceived health status in older adults. *Gerontology & Geriatrics Education, 14*(2), 3–17.

Bortz, W. M., Wallace, D. H., & Wiley, D. (1999). Sexual function in 1,202 aging males: Differentiating aspects. *Journals of Gerontology: Medical Sciences, 54A*, M237–241.

Botwinick, J. (1973). *Aging and behavior*. New York: Springer.

Brimmer, P. F. (1979). Past, present and future in gerontological nursing research. *Journal of Gerontological Nursing, 5*(6), 27–34.

Brown, J., & McCreedy, M. (1986). The hale elderly: Health behavior and its correlates. *Research in Nursing & Health, 9*, 317–329.

Buckwalter, K. C. (1992). *Geriatric mental health nursing: Current and future challenges*. Thorofare, NJ: Slack.

Burgener, S. C., & Chiverton, P. (1992). Conceptualizing psychological well-being in cognitively-impaired older persons. *Image—The Journal of Nursing Scholarship, 24*(2), 209–213.

Butler, R. N. (1974). Successful aging. *Mental Health, 58*(3), 7–12.

Campbell, J. (1986). *The inner reaches of outer space: Metaphor as myth and religion*. Toronto: St. James Press.

Cantor, M., & Little, V. (1985). Aging and social care. In R. Binstock & E. Shanas (Eds.), *Handbook of aging and the social sciences* (pp. 745–781). New York: Van Nostrand Reinhold.

Carlson, R. (1981). Studies in script theory: Adult analogs of a childhood nuclear scene. *Journal of Personality and Social Psychology, 40*, 501–510.

Cerella, J. (1990). Aging and information-processing rate. In J. E. Birren & K. W. Schaie (Eds.), *Handbook of the psychology of aging* (3rd ed., pp. 201–221). San Diego: Academic Press.

Charness, R. (1985). Aging and problem solving performance. In R. Charness (Ed.), *Aging and human performance* (pp. 225–260). New York: Wiley.

Chopoorian, T. J. (1986). Reconceptualizing the environment. In P. Moccia (Ed.), *New approaches to theory development*. New York: NLN Press.

Clausen, J. A. (1972). The life course of individuals. In M. W. Riley, M. Johnson, & A. Foner (Eds.), *Aging and society. III. A sociology of age stratification* (pp. 457–515). New York: Russell Sage.

Cohen, J. S. (2000). Avoiding adverse reactions: Effective lower-dose drug therapies for older patients. *Geriatrics, 55*(2), 54–64.

Connidis, I. A., & McMullin, J. A. (1993). To have or have not: Parent status and the subjective well-being of older men and women. *Gerontologist, 33*(5), 630–636.

Cowgill, D. O., & Holmes, L. D. (Eds.). (1972). *Aging and modernization*. New York: Appleton-Century-Crofts.

Cox, C. (1986). The interaction model of client health behavior: Application to the study of community based elders. *Advances in Nursing Science, 9*, 40–57.

Craik, F. I. (1977). Age differences in human memory. In J. E. Birren & K. Schaie (Eds.), *Handbook of the psychology of aging* (pp. 384-420). New York: Van Nostrand Reinhold.

Crist, P. A. (1999). Does quality of life vary with different types of housing among older persons? A pilot study. *Physical and Occupational Therapy in Geriatrics, 16*(3/4), 101–116.

Cummings, J. L., & Coffey, C. E. (1994). Neurobiological basis of behavior. In C. E. Coffey & J. L. Cummings (Eds.), *Textbook of geriatric neuropsychiatry* (pp. 71–96). Washington, DC: American Psychiatric Press.

Curtis, H. J., & Miller, K. (1971). Chromosome aberrations in liver cells of guinea pigs. *Journals of Gerontology, 26*, 292–293.

Cutler, R. G. (1975). Evolution of human longevity and the genetic complexity governing aging rate. *Proceedings of the National Academy of Sciences (USA), 72*, 4664–4668.

Czaja, S. J., Weber, R. A., & Nair, S. N. (1993). A human factors analysis of ADL activities: A capability-demand approach. *Journals of Gerontology, 48* (Special Issue), 44–48.

Dean, K. (1992). Health related behavior: Concepts and methods. In M. G. Ory, R. P. Abeles, & P. D. Lipman

(Eds.), *Aging, health, and behavior* (pp. 27–56). Newbury Park, CA: Sage.

Dellasega, C., Clark, D., McCreary, D., et al. (1994). Nursing process: Teaching elderly clients. *Journal of Gerontological Nursing, 20*(1), 31–38.

Douglas, K. C., & Rush, D. R. (1988). Aging changes and drug-related illness in the elderly. *Geriatric Medicine Today, 7*(4), 61–71.

Dowd, J. J. (1975). Aging as exchange: A preface to theory. *Journals of Gerontology, 30*, 584–594.

Drachman, D. A., & Barclay, L. (1993). Overview of geriatric neurology. In L. Barclay (Ed.), *Clinical geriatric neurology* (pp. 3–8). Philadelphia: Lea & Febiger.

Duffy, M. E. (1993). Determinants of health-promotion lifestyles in older people. *Image—The Journal of Nursing Scholarship, 25*, 23–28.

Ebersole, P., & Hess, P. (1994). *Toward healthy aging* (4th ed.). St. Louis: Mosby–Year Book.

Erikson, E. H. (1963). *Childhood and society.* New York: Norton.

Eysenck, M. W. (1974). Age differences in incidental learning. *Developmental Psychology, 10*, 936–941.

Ferri, F. F., & Fretwell, M. D. (1992). *Practical guide to the care of the geriatric patient.* St. Louis: Mosby–Year Book.

Fiatarone, M. A., & Evans, W. J. (1993). The etiology and reversibility of muscle dysfunction in the aged. *Journals of Gerontology, 48* (Special Issue), 77–83.

Foner, A. (1974). Age stratification and age conflict in political life. *American Sociological Review, 39*, 1081–1104.

Frankl, V. (1963). *Man's search for meaning: An introduction to logotherapy.* New York: Pocket Books.

Frisoni, G. B., Rozzini, R., Bianchetti, A., & Trabucchi, M. (1993). Principal lifetime occupation and MMSE score in elderly persons. *Journals of Gerontology, 48*(6), S310–S314.

Garne, H. W. R., & Barr, W. H. (1984). *Geriatric pharmacokinetics.* Richmond, VA: Virginia Commonwealth University.

Gendell, M., & Siegel, J. S. (1996). Trends in retirement age in the United States, 1955–1993, by sex and race. *Journals of Gerontology: Social Sciences, 51B*, S132–139.

George, L. (1990). Social structure, social processes and social-psychological states. In R. H. Binstock & L. K. George (Eds.), *Handbook of aging and the social sciences* (3rd ed., pp. 186–204). San Diego: Academic Press.

Glick, O., & Tripp-Reimer, T. (1996). Iowa conceptual model for gerontological nursing. In E. A. Swanson & T. Tripp-Reimer (Eds.), *Advances in gerontological nursing* (Vol. 1, pp. 11–55). New York: Springer.

Gordon, S. M., & Thompson, S. (1995). The changing epidemiology of human immunodeficiency virus infection in older persons. *Journal of the American Geriatrics Society, 43*, 7–9.

Gramann, D. (1999). New frontiers in integrated care. *Caring, 18*(4), 14–17.

Guccione, A. A., & Jette, M. A. (1988). Assessing limitations in physical function in patients with arthritis. *Arthritis Care & Research, 1*(3), 170–176.

Guralnik, J., & Simonsick, E. (1993). Physical disability in older Americans. *Journals of Gerontology, 48* (Special Issue), 84–88.

Haase, J. E., Britt, T., Coward, D. O., et al. (1992). Simultaneous concept analysis of spiritual perspective, hope, acceptance and self-transcendence. *Image—The Journal of Nursing Scholarship, 24*, 141–147.

Hagestad, G. O. (1990). Social perspectives on the life course. In R. H. Binstock & L. K. George (Eds.), *Handbook of aging and social science* (3rd ed., pp. 151–168). San Diego: Academic Press.

Hagestad, G. O., & Neugarten, B. L. (1985). Age and the life course. In R. Binstock & E. Shanas (Eds.), *Handbook of aging and the social sciences* (pp. 35–61). New York: Van Nostrand Reinhold.

Hale, S., Myerson, J., & Wagstaff, D. (1987). General slowing of nonverbal information processing: Evidence for a power law. *Journals of Gerontology, 42*, 131–136.

Harman, D. (1956). Aging: A theory based on free radical and radiation chemistry. *Journals of Gerontology, 11*, 298–300.

Havighurst, R. J. (1972). *Developmental tasks and education.* New York: McKay.

Havighurst, R. J., & Albrecht, R. (1953). *Older people.* New York: Longmares, Green.

Havighurst, R. J., Neugarten, B. L., & Tobin, S. S. (1963). Disengagement, personality and life satisfaction in the later years. In P. Hansen (Ed.), *Age with a future* (pp. 419–425). Copenhagen: Munksgaard.

Hawes, C. (1999). A key piece of the integration puzzle: Managing the chronic care needs of the frail elderly in residential care settings. *Generations, 23*(2), 51–55.

Hayflick, L. (1965). The limited in vitro lifetime of human diploid cell strains. *Experimental Cell Research, 57*, 614–636.

Hertzog, C., Vernon, M. C., & Rympa, B. (1993). Age differences in mental rotation task performance: The influence of speed/accuracy tradeoffs. *Journals of Gerontology, 48*(3), P150–P156.

Hickey, T., Dean, K., & Holstein, B. E. (1986). Emerging trends in gerontology and geriatrics. *Social Science and Medicine, 23*, 1363–1369.

Hogue, C. C. (1985). Social support. In J. E. Hall & B. R. Weaver (Eds.), *Distributive nursing practice: A systems approach to community health* (2nd ed., pp. 58–81). Philadelphia: Lippincott.

Holmes, J. S., & Dorfman, L. T. (2000). The effects of specific health conditions on activities in retirement. *Activities, Adaptation & Aging, 25*(1), 47–65.

Horn, J. L. (1982). The theory of fluid and crystallized intelligence in relation to concepts of cognitive psychology and aging in adulthood. In F. M. Craik & S. Trehub (Eds.), *Aging and cognitive processes* (pp. 237–278). New York: Plenum.

Hughes, S. L., Dunlop, D., Edelman, P., et al. (1994). Impact of joint impairment on longitudinal disability in elderly persons. *Journals of Gerontology: Social Sciences, 49*(6), S291–S300.

Hultsch, D. F., Hammer, M., & Small, B. J. (1993). Age differences in cognitive performance in later life: Relationships to self-reported health and activity life style. *Journals of Gerontology, 48*(1), P1–P11.

Inouye, S. K., Albert, M. S., Mohs, R., et al. (1993). Cognitive performance in a high-functioning community-dwelling elderly population. *Journals of Gerontology, 48*(4), M146–M151.

Iowa Intervention Project. (1992). Need and significance. In J. M. McCloskey & G. M. Bulechek (Eds.), *Nursing interventions classification (NIC)* (pp. 3–16). St. Louis: Mosby.

Iowa Intervention Project. (1996). *Core interventions by specialty.* Iowa City, IA: Nursing Classification Center.

Iowa Intervention Project. (2000). J. M. McCloskey & G. M. Bulechek (Eds.), *Nursing interventions classifications (NIC)* (3rd ed.). St. Louis: Mosby.

Iowa Outcomes Project. (2000). M. Johnson, M. Maas, & S. Moohead, (Eds.), *Nursing outcomes classification (NOC)* (2nd ed.) St. Louis: Mosby.

Isreal, B. A., & Antonucci, T. C. (1987). Social network characteristics and psychological well-being: A replication and extension. *Health Education Quarterly, 14*(4), 461–481.

Jackson, J. J. (1980). *Minorities and aging.* Belmont, CA: Wadsworth.

Jackson, J. S., Antonucci, T. C., & Gibson, R. C. (1990). Social support and health. In J. Birren & K. W. Schaie (Eds.), *Handbook of psychology of aging* (3rd ed., pp. 103–123). San Diego: Academic Press.

Jirovec, M., & Kasno, J. (1990). Self-care agency as a function of patient-environment factors among nursing home residents. *Research in Nursing & Health, 13*, 303–309.

Johnson, B. K. (1998). A correlational framework for understanding sexuality in women age 50 and older. *Health Care for Women International, 19*, 553–564.

Jones, P. S., & Meleis, A. I. (1993). Health is empowerment. *Advances in Nursing Services, 15*(3), 1–14.

Jung, C. G. (1933). *Modern man in search of a soul.* New York: Harcourt, Brace.

Jung, C. G. (1960). The stages of life. In: *Collected works (8): Structure and dynamics of the psyche.* New York: Pantheon.

Kahana, E. A. (1982). A congruence model of person-environment interaction. In M. P. Lawton, P. G. Windley, & T. O. Byerts (Eds.), *Aging and the environment: Theoretical approaches* (pp. 97–121). New York: Springer.

Kane, R. L. (1993). The implications of assessment. *Journals of Gerontology, 48* (Special Issue), 27–31.

Kart, C. S., & Engler, C. A. (1994). Predisposition to self-health care: Who does what for themselves and why? *Journals of Gerontology: Social Science, 49*(6), S301–S308.

Kart, C., & Dunkle, R. (1989). Assessing capacity for self-care among the aged. *Journal of Aging and Health, 1*, 430–450.

Kayser-Jones, J. S. (1981). Gerontological nursing research revisited. *Journal of Gerontological Nursing, 7*, 217–223.

Keith, J. (1990). Age in social and cultural context: Anthropological perspectives. In R. H. Binstock & L. George (Eds.), *Handbook of aging and the social sciences* (pp. 91–111). San Diego: Academic Press.

Kleemeier, R. W. (1962). Intellectual changes in the senium. *Proceedings of the American Statistical Association, 1*, 181–190.

Kleffel, D. (1991). Rethinking the environment as a domain of nursing knowledge. *Advances in Nursing Science, 14*(1), 40–51.

Knowles, L. (1983). Gerontological nursing '82. *International Journal of Nursing Studies, 20*(1), 45–54.

Kogan, N. (1987). Creativity. In G. L. Maddox (Ed.), *Encyclopedia of aging* (pp. 153–155). New York: Springer.

Kogan, N. (1990). Personality and aging. In J. Birren & K. W. Schaie (Eds.), *Handbook of the psychology of aging* (3rd ed., pp. 330–346). San Diego: Academic Press.

Kohlberg, L. (1973). Continuities in childhood and adult moral development revisited. In P. Boltes & K. W. Schaie (Eds.), *Life span developmental psychology: Personality and socialization* (pp. 179–204). New York: Academic Press.

Kraus, N. (1990). Illness behavior in late life. In R. H. Binstock & K. J. George (Eds.), *Handbook of aging and the social sciences* (pp. 227–244). New York: Academic Press.

Kraus, N., & Jay, G. (1991). Stress, social support, and negative interaction in later life. *Research on Aging, 13*, 333–363.

Kuypers, J. A., & Bengtson, V. L. (1973). Social breakdown and competence: A model of normal aging. *Human Development, 16*, 181–201.

Larson, P., & Hoot Martin, J. (1999). Polypharmacy and elderly patients. *AORN Journal, 69*(3), 619, 621–622, 625, 627–628.

Launer, L. J., Dinkgreve, M., Jonker, C., et al. (1993). Are age and education independent correlates of the mini-mental state exam performance of community-dwelling elderly? *Journals of Gerontology, 48*(6), P271–P277.

Lawton, M. P., & Nahemow, L. (1973). Ecology and the aging process. In C. Eisdorfer & M. P. Lawton (Eds.), *Psychology of adult development and aging* (pp. 619–674). Washington, DC: American Psychological Association.

Lehman, H. C. (1953). *Age and achievement.* Princeton, NJ: Princeton University Press.

Lehmann, S. W., & Rabins, P. V. (1999). Clinical geropsychiatry. In J. J. Gallo, J. Busby-Whitehead, P. V. Rabins, et al. (Eds.), *Reichel's care of the elderly: Clinical aspects of aging* (5th ed., pp. 179–189). Philadelphia: Lippincott Williams & Wilkins.

Lenihan, A. A. (1988). Identification of self-care behaviors in the elderly. *Journal of Professional Nursing, 4*, 285–288.

LeSage, J. (1991). Polypharmacy in geriatric patients. *Nursing Clinics of North America, 26*(2), 273–289.

Levin, J. S. (1994). *Religion in aging and health.* Newbury Park, CA: Sage.

Levin, L., & Idler, E. (1984). Self-care in health. *Annual Review of Public Health, 4*, 181–201.

Levinson, D. J. (1978). *The seasons of a man's life.* New York: Knopf.

Levy, J. A. (1994). Sexuality and aging. In W. R. Hazzard, E. L. Bierman, J. P. Blass, et al. (Eds.), *Principles of geriatric medicine and gerontology* (3rd. ed.). New York: McGraw-Hill.

Lierman, L. M., Young, H. M., Powell-Cope, G., et al. (1994). Effects of education and support on breast self-examination in older women. *Nursing Research, 43*(3), 158–163.

Margitic, S. E., Inouye, S. K., Thomas, J. L., et al. (1993). Hospital outcomes project for the elderly (HOPE): Rationale and design for a prospective pooled analysis. *Journal of the American Geriatrics Society, 41*, 258–267.

Marshall, V. W. (1994). Sociology, psychology, and the theoretical legacy of the Kansas City Studies. *Gerontologist, 34*, 768–774.

Martinson, I. (1985). Gerontology comes of age. *Journal of Gerontological Nursing, 10*(7), 8–17.

Matteson, M. A., Bearon, L. B., & McConnell, E. S. (1997). Psychosocial problems associated with aging. In M. A. Matteson, E. S. McConnell, & A. D. Linton (Eds.), *Gerontological nursing: Concepts and practice* (2nd ed., pp. 603–659). Philadelphia: W. B. Saunders.

Matthias, R. E., Lubben, J. E., Atchison, K. A., & Schweitzer, S. O. (1997). Sexual activity and satisfaction among very old adults: Results from a community-dwelling Medicare population survey. *Gerontologist, 37*, 6–14.

McCrae, R. R., & Costa, P. T. (1982). Self-concept and the stability of personality: Cross-sectional comparisons of self-reports and ratings. *Journal of Personality and Social Psychology, 43*, 1282–1292.

Medawar, P. B. (1957). *The uniqueness of the individual.* London: Methuen.

Medvedev, Z. A. (1972). Repetition of molecular-genetic information as a possible factor in evolutionary changes of life-span. *Experimental Gerontology, 7*, 227–234.

Meeks, S., Carstensen, L. L., Tamsky, B., et al. (1989). Age differences in coping: Does less mean worse. *International Journal of Aging and Human Development, 28*(2), 127–140.

Mein, G., Higgs, P., Ferrie, J., & Stansfeld, S. A. (1998). Paradigms of retirement: The importance of health and ageing in the Whitehall II Study. *Social Science & Medicine, 47*, 535–545.

Meleis, A., & Trangenstein, P. (1994). Facilitating transitions: Redefinition of the nursing mission. *Nursing Outlook, 42*, 255–259.

Melia, M. (2000). Regulation: The state of the states. *Nursing Homes, 49*(5), 67–68.

Midanik, L., Soghikan, K., Ransom, L., & Tekawa, I. (1995). The effect of retirement on mental health and health behaviors: The Kaiser Permanente retirement study. *Journals of Gerontology: Social Sciences, 50B*(1), 559–561.

Miller, C. A. (1998). Frail elders: Handle with care when using medications. *Geriatric Nursing, 19*(4), 239–240.

Moberg, D. O. (1974). Spiritual well-being in late life. In J. F. Gubrium (Ed.), *Late life communities and environmental policy.* Springfield, IL: C. Thomas.

Moody, H. R. (1988). Toward a critical gerontology: The contribution of the humanities to theories of aging. In J. E. Birren & V. L. Bengtson (Eds.), *Emergent theories of aging* (pp. 19–40). New York: Springer.

Moore, T. (1992). *Care of the soul: A guide for cultivating depth and sacredness in everyday life.* New York: Harper Collins.

Mor, V., Murphy, J., Masterson-Allen, S., et al. (1989). Risk of functional decline among well elderly. *Journal of Clinical Epidemiology, 42*(9), 895–904.

Morris, J. C., & McManus, D. Q. (1991). The neurology of aging: Normal versus pathologic change. *Geriatrics, 46*(8), 47–54.

Murphy, E., & Freston, M. S. (1991). An analysis of theory-research linkages in published gerontological nursing studies 1983–1989. *Advances in Nursing Science, 13*(4), 1–13.

Neugarten, B. L. (1973). Personality changes in late life: A developmental perspective. In C. Eisdorfer & M. P. Lawton (Eds.), *The psychology of adult development and aging* (pp. 311–338). Washington, DC: American Psychological Association.

Neugarten, B. L., Havighurst, R. J., & Tobin, S. S. (1968). Personality and patterns of aging. In B. L. Neugarten (Ed.), *Middle age and aging* (pp. 173–180). Chicago: University of Chicago Press.

Newman, B. M., & Newman, P. R. (1984). *Development through life: A psychosocial approach.* Homewood, IL: Dorsey.

Norbeck, J. (1988). Social support. *Annual Review of Nursing Research, 6*, 85–109.

North American Nursing Diagnosis Association (NANDA). (2001). *Nursing diagnoses: Definitions and classification.* Philadelphia: Author.

Orgel, L. E. (1963). The maintenance of the accuracy of protein synthesis and its relevance to aging. *Proceedings of the National Academy of Sciences (USA), 49*, 517–521.

Ozawa, M. N., & Lum, Y. (1998). Marital status and change in income status 10 years after retirement. *Social Work Research, 22*(2), 116–128.

Ozawa, M. N., & Tseng, H. (1999). Utilization of formal services during the 10 years after retirement. *Journal of Gerontological Social Work, 31*, 3–20.

Parmelee, P., & Lawton, M. (1990). The design of special environments for the aged. In J. Birren & K. W. Schaie (Eds.), *Handbook of the psychology of aging* (pp. 465–488). San Diego: Academic Press.

Parr, J. (1980). The interaction of persons and living environments. In L. W. Poon (Ed.), *Aging in the 1980s* (pp. 393–406). Washington, DC: American Psychological Association.

Peck, R. C. (1968). Psychological developments in the second half of life. In B. Neugarten (Ed.), *Middle age and aging* (pp. 88–92). Chicago: University of Chicago Press.

Pendergast, D. R., Fisher, N. M., & Calkins, E. (1993). Cardiovascular, neuromuscular, and metabolic alterations with age leading to frailty. *Journals of Gerontology, 48* (Special Issue), 61–67.

Perlmutter, M. (1988). Cognitive potential through life. In J. E. Birren & V. L. Bengtson (Eds.), *Emergent theories of aging* (pp. 247–268). New York: Springer.

Powers, R. E. (1994). Neurobiology of aging. In C. E. Coffey & J. L. Cummings (Eds.), *Textbook of geriatric neuropsychiatry* (pp. 35–69). Washington, DC: American Psychiatric Press.

Prado, C. G. (1983). Aging and narrative. *International Journal of Applied Philosophy, 1*, 1–14.

Press, I., & McKool, M. (1972). Social structure and status of the aged: Toward some valid cross-cultural generalizations. *Aging and Human Development, 3*, 279–306.

Quigley, D. G., & Schatz, M. S. (1999). Men and women and their responses in spousal bereavement. *Hospice Journal, 14*(2), 65–78.

Rakowski, W., Rice, C., & McHorney, C. (1992). Information seeking about health among older adults. *Behavior, Health and Aging, 2*, 181–198.

Reed, P. (1989). Mental health of older adults. *Western Journal of Nursing Research, 11*(2), 143–163.

Reed, P. G. (1992). An emerging paradigm for the investigation of spirituality in nursing. *Research in Nursing & Health, 15,* 349–357.

Reed, P. G. (1991). Toward a nursing theory of self-transcendence: Deductive reformulation using developmental theories. *Advances in Nursing Science, 13*(4), 64–77.

Reichard, S., Levson, F., & Peterson, P. G. (1962). *Aging and personality.* New York: Wiley.

Reigel, K. F. (1973). Dialectical operations: The final period of cognitive development. *Human Development, 16,* 346–370.

Richardson, J. P., & Lazur, A. (1995). Sexuality in the nursing home patient. *American Family Physician, 51*(1), 121–124.

Riley, M. W. (1971). Social gerontology and the age stratification of society. *Gerontologist, 11,* 79–87.

Riley, M. W. (1979). Life-course perspectives. In M. W. Riley (Ed.), *Aging from birth to death: Interdisciplinary perspectives* (pp. 3–13). Washington, DC: Westview.

Riley, M. W. & Foner, A. (Eds.). (1968). *Aging and Society.* New York: Russell Sage.

Rodin, J. (1986). Aging and health: Effects of the sense of control. *Science, 233,* 1271–1276.

Rose, A. M. (1964). A current theoretical issue in social gerontology. *Gerontologist, 4,* 46–50.

Sacher, G. A. (1980). Theory in gerontology. *Annual Review of Gerontology and Geriatrics, 1,* 3–24.

Sager, M. A., Rudberg, M. A., Jalaluddin, M., et al. (1996). Hospital admission risk profile (HARP): Identifying older patients at risk for functional decline following acute medical illness and hospitalization. *Journal of the American Geriatrics Society, 44,* 251–257.

Sagy, S., & Antonovsky, A. (1990). Explaining life satisfaction in later life: The sense of coherence model and activity theory. *Behavior, Health and Aging, 1*(1), 11–25.

Salom, I. L., & Davis, K. (1995). Prescribing for older patients: How to avoid toxic drug reactions. *Geriatrics, 50*(10), 37–43.

Salthouse, T. A. (1985). *A theory of cognitive aging.* Amsterdam: North-Holland.

Salthouse, T. A. (1993). Attentional blocks are not responsible for age-related slowing. *Journals of Gerontology, 48*(6), P263–P270.

Sands, L. P., & Meredith, W. (1989). Effects of sensory and motor functioning on adult intellectual performance. *Journals of Gerontology, 44*(2), P56–P58.

Schaie, K. W. (1962). A field-theory approach to age changes in cognitive behavior. *Vita Humana, 5,* 129–141.

Schaie, K. W., & Parham, I. (1976). Stability of adult personality traits: Fact or fable? *Journal of Personality and Social Psychology, 34,* 146–158.

Schroeder, J. M., Nau, K. L., Osness, W. H., & Potteiger, J. A. (1998). A comparison of life satisfaction, functional ability, physical characteristics, and activity level among older adults in various living settings. *Journal of Aging and Physical Activity, 6,* 340–349.

Schulz, R., & Williamson, G. M. (1993). Psychosocial and behavioral dimensions of physical frailty. *Journals of Gerontology, 48* (Special Issue), 39–43.

Schumacher, K. D., & Meleis, A. (1994). Transitions: A central concept in nursing. *Image—The Journal of Nursing Scholarship, 26*(2), 119–127.

Shock, N. W. (1979). Systems physiology and aging. *Federal Proceedings, 38,* 161–169.

Smith, M., Buckwalter, K. C., & Mitchell, S. (1993). *Geriatric mental health training series.* New York: Springer.

Sohal, R. S. (1981). *Age pigments.* Amsterdam: Elsevier.

Sokolovsky, J. (1986). Network methodologies in the study of aging. In C. L. Fry, & J. Keith (Eds.), *New methods for old age research* (pp. 231–262). South Hadley, MA: Bergin & Garvey.

Sokolovsky, J., & Vesperi, M. D. (1991). The cultural context of well-being in old age. In *Generations, 15*(1), 21–24.

Spirduso, W., & MacRae, P. G. (1990). Motor performance and aging. In J. Birren & K. W. Schaie (Eds.), *Handbook of the psychology of aging* (3rd ed., pp. 184–200). San Diego: Academic Press.

Stevens, P. (1989). A critical reconceptualization of environment in nursing: Implications for methodology. *Advances in Nursing Science, 11*(4), 56–68.

Stevenson, J. S. (1977). *Issues and crises during middlescence.* New York: Appleton-Century-Crofts.

Svanborg, A. (1993). A medical-social intervention in a 70-year old Swedish population: Is it possible to postpone functional decline in aging? *Journals of Gerontology, 48* (Special Issue), 84–88.

Swanson, L. R., & Lee, T. D. (1992). Effects of aging and schedules of knowledge of results on motor learning. *Journals of Gerontology, 47*(6), P406–P411.

Swonger, A., & Burbank, P. (1995). *Drug therapy and the elderly.* Boston: Jones & Bartlett.

Sziland, L. (1959). On the nature of the aging process. *Proceedings of the National Academy of Sciences (USA), 45,* 30–45.

Theriault, J. (1994). Retirement as a psychosocial transition: Process of adaption to change. *International Journal of Aging and Human Development, 38*(2), 153–170.

Timiras, P. S., Hudson, D. B., & Segall, P. E. (1984). Lifetime brain serotonin: Regional effects of age and precursor availability. *Neurobiology of Aging, 5*(3), 235–242.

Tinsley, R. K. (1998). 1998 ALFA survey highlights. *Nursing Homes, 47*(8), 58–59.

Tiryakian, E. A. (1968). The existential self and the person. In C. Gordon & K. J. Gergen (Eds.), *The self in social interaction* (pp. 75-86). New York: Wiley.

Travis, S. S. (1987). Older adults sexuality and remarriage. *Journal of Gerontological Nursing, 13*(6), 8–14.

Tripp-Reimer, T., & Cohen, M. (1987). Using phenomenology in health promotion research. In M. J. Duffy & N. J. Pender (Eds.), *Conceptual issues in health promotion research* (pp. 121–127). Indianapolis: Sigma Theta Tau.

Tripp-Reimer, T., Johnson, R., & Rios, H. (1995). Cultural dimensions in gerontological nursing. In M. Stanley & P. Gauntlett Beare (Eds.), *Gerontological nursing.* Philadelphia: F. A. Davis.

U.S. Bureau of the Census. (1993). *Statistical abstract of the United States* (113th ed.). Washington, DC: Author.

U.S. Department of Health and Human Services. (1990). *Healthy People 2000: National health promotion and disease prevention objectives*. PHS 91-50213. Washington, DC: Author.

Van Nostrand, J., Furner, S., & Suzman, R. (Eds.). (1993). Health data on older Americans: United States, 1992. *National Center for Vital Statistics, Vital Health Statistics, 3*, 27.

Venes, D., & Thomas, C. L. (Eds.). (2001). *Taber's cyclopedic medical dictionary* (19th ed.). Philadelphia: F. A. Davis.

Verhaeghen, P., Marcoen, A., & Goossens, L. (1993). Facts and fiction about memory aging: A quantitative integration of research findings. *Journals of Gerontology, 48*(4), P157–P171.

Verzar, F. (1963). *Lectures on experimental gerontology*. Springfield, IL: CC Thomas.

Vickery, D., Golaszewski, T., Wright, E., & Kalmer, H. (1988). Effect of self-care interventions on the use of medical service within a Medicare population. *Medical Care, 26*, 580–588.

Walker, M. K., Foreman, M. D., & the NICHE Faculty. (1999). Medication safety: A protocol for nursing action. *Geriatric Nursing, 20*(1), 34–39.

Walker, S., Volken, K., Sechrist, K., & Pender, N. (1988). Health promoting life styles of older adults. *Advances in Nursing Science, 11*(1), 76–90.

Wells, T. (1993). Setting the agenda for gerontological nursing education. In C. Heine (Ed.), *Determining the future of gerontological nursing education*. New York: NLN Press.

Webster's ninth new collegiate dictionary (1990). Springfield, MA: Merriam-Webster, Inc.

Wershow, H. J. (1981). *Controversial issues in gerontology*. New York: Springer.

Williams, G. C. (1957). Pleiotropy, natural selection, and the evolution of senescence. *Evolution, 11*, 398–411.

Williams, M. A. (1988). The physical environment and patient care. *Annual Review of Nursing Research, 6*, 61–83.

Wilson, K. B. (1994). Assisted living: Model program may signify the future. *Long Term Care Quality Letter, 6*(15), 1–4.

Wolanin, M. O. (1983). Clinical geriatric nursing research. *Annual Review of Nursing Research, 1*, 77–99.

Wright, L. (2001). Sexuality-reproductive pattern: Normal changes with aging. In M. L. Maas, K. C. Buckwalter, M. D. Hardy, et al. (Eds.), *Nursing care of older adults: Diagnoses, outcomes, and interventions* (pp. 729–732). St. Louis: Mosby.

Wyatt, G. K., Friedman, L., Given, C. W., & Given, B. A. (1999). A profile of bereaved caregivers following provision of terminal care. *Journal of Palliative Care, 15*(1), 13–25.

Yallom, I. D. (1980). *Existential psychotherapy*. New York: Basic Books.

Young, R. F., & Olson, E. A. (1991). Overview of health and disease in later life. In R. F. Young, & E. A. Olson (Eds.), *Health, illness and disability in later life* (pp. 1–7). Newbury Park, CA: Sage.

Zatz, M. M., & Goldstein, A. L. (1985). Thymosins, lymphokines, and the immunology of aging. *Gerontology, 31*, 263–277.

Delirium, Dementias, and Other Related Disorders

Mary Ann Boyd, Linda Garand, Linda A. Gerdner, Bonnie J. Wakefield, and Kathleen C. Buckwalter

After studying this chapter, you will be able to:

➤ Distinguish the clinical characteristics, onset, and course of delirium and Alzheimer's disease.

➤ Analyze the prevailing biologic, psychological, and social theories that relate to delirium and Alzheimer's disease in elderly people.

➤ Integrate biopsychosocial theories into the analysis of human responses to delirium and dementia, with emphasis on the concepts of impaired cognition and memory.

➤ Discuss various etiologies for cognitive impairment in other patients (other than those with delirium and dementia).

➤ Interpret the impact of culture and education on mental status testing.

➤ Formulate nursing diagnoses based on a biopsychosocial assessment of patients with impaired cognitive function.

➤ Identify expected outcomes for patients with impaired cognition and their evaluation.

➤ Discuss nursing interventions used for patients with impaired cognition.

KEY TERMS

acetylcholine (ACh)
acetylcholinesterase (AChE)
acetylcholinesterase inhibitors (AChEI)
agnosia
aphasia
apraxia
butyrylcholinesterase (BuChE)
bradykinesia
catastrophic reactions
cortical dementia
disinhibition
disturbance of executive functioning
hyperkinetic delirium
hypokinetic delirium
hypersexuality
hypervocalization
illusions
neuritic plaques
neurofibrillary tangles
subcortical dementia

KEY CONCEPTS

cognition
delirium
dementia
memory

*C*ognition and memory are important in many psychiatric disorders, but in this chapter, they are the key concepts. Cognition was defined in Chapter 10 as the ability to think and know. Now the definition is further refined to be understood as a relatively high level of intellectual processing in which perceptions and information are acquired, used, or manipulated. Cognition involves both how reality is perceived and how those perceptions are understood in relation to internal representations of reality previously acquired. In the broadest sense, cognition denotes how the brain processes information. Cognition includes a number of specific functions, such as the acquisition and use of language, the ability to be oriented in time and space, and the ability to learn and solve problems. It includes judgment, reasoning, attention, comprehension, concept formation, planning, and the use of symbols, such as mathematics or writing.

Memory, a facet of cognition, refers to the ability to recall or reproduce what has been learned or experienced. It is more than simple storage and retrieval; it is a complex cognitive mental function that includes most areas of the brain, especially the hippocampus, which is believed to be essential to the transfer of some memories from short-term to long-term storage. Defects of memory are an essential feature of many cognitive disorders, particularly dementia.

KEY CONCEPT Cognition. **Cognition** is based on a system of interrelated abilities, such as perception, reasoning, judgment, intuition, and memory, that allow one to be aware of oneself and one's surroundings. Impairments in these abilities can result in a failure of the afflicted person to recognize that he or she is ill and in need of treatment.

KEY CONCEPT Memory. **Memory** is a facet of cognition concerned with retaining and recalling past experiences, whether they occurred in the physical environment or internally as cognitive events.

The disorders discussed in this chapter, delirium, dementia, and other cognitive disorders, are characterized by deficits in cognition or memory that represent a clearcut deterioration from a previous level of functioning. Delirium is a disorder of acute cognitive impairment and can be caused by a medical condition (eg, infection) or substance abuse, or it may have multiple etiologies. Dementia is characterized by chronic cognitive impairments and is differentiated by underlying cause, not by symptom patterns, which are often similar. Some dementias are irreversible and progressive, such as Alzheimer's type, but not all dementias are irreversible. For example, some organic compounds and chemicals, such as lead, aluminum, manganese, and toluene (one of the toxins in glue and paint), may produce symptoms of dementia (Table 31-1). Once evaluated and treated, the

TABLE 31.1	Examples of Organic Compounds and Chemicals That May Produce Dementia	
Organic Compound or Chemical	**Related Symptoms**
Arsenic	Headache Drowsiness Confusion
Mercury	Tremors Extrapyramidal signs Upper and lower extremity ataxia Depression Confusion
Lead	Abdominal cramps Anemia Peripheral neuropathy Encephalopathy (rare)
Manganese	Extrapyramidal symptoms Delirium
Aluminum	Myoclonus Speech disorders Seizure disorders Cognitive impairment
Toluene (methyl benzene)	Profound cognitive impairment Tremor Ataxia Loss of vision and hearing

symptoms of dementia resolve in many of these disorders, such as endocrine disorders.

KEY CONCEPT Delirium. **Delirium** is a disorder of acute cognitive impairment and is caused by a medical condition (eg, infection), substance abuse, or multiple etiologies.

KEY CONCEPT Dementia. **Dementia** is characterized by chronic cognitive impairments and is differentiated by underlying cause, not by symptom patterns, which are often similar.

Dementia can be further classified as cortical or subcortical to denote the location of the underlying pathology. **Cortical dementia** results from a disease process that globally afflicts the cortex. **Subcortical dementia** is caused by dysfunction or deterioration of deep gray- or white-matter structures inside the brain and brain stem. Symptoms of subcortical dementia may be more localized and tend to disrupt arousal, attention, and motivation, but they can produce a variety of clinical behavioral manifestations. In this chapter, a type of cortical dementia, Alzheimer's, is highlighted because it the most prevalent form of dementia.

DELIRIUM

Clinical Course of Disorder

Delirium is a disturbance in consciousness and a change in cognition that develops over a short period of time. It is usually reversible if the underlying cause is identified and treated quickly. It is a serious disorder and should be always treated as an emergency.

These individuals are brought to the emergency room in a state of confusion and disorientation that developed over a few hours or days. If delirium is not treated in a timely manner, irreversible neurologic damage can occur. About 25% of patients do not survive.

Diagnostic Criteria

Impairment of consciousness is the key diagnostic criterion. The patient becomes less aware of his or her environment and loses the ability to focus, sustain, and shift attention. There are usually other associated cognitive changes that include problems in memory, orientation, and language. The patient may not know where he or she is, may not recognize familiar objects, or may not be able to carry on a conversation. Another important diagnostic indicator is that the problem developed over a short period of time (compared with dementia, which develops gradually) (American Psychiatric Association [APA], 2000). Table 31-2 presents the diagnostic criteria of delirium owing to a general medical condition. Delirium is different than dementia, but the presenting symptoms are often similar. Table 31-3 lists the differences between delirium and dementia.

Delirium in Special Populations

Children

Delirium can occur in children and may be related to medications (anticholinergics) or fever. Children seem to be especially susceptible to this disorder, probably because of their immature brain. However, it may be hard to diagnose and may be mistaken for uncooperative behavior.

Elderly People

Although delirium may occur in any age group, it is most common among the elderly. In this age group, delirium is often mistaken as dementia, which in turn leads to inappropriate treatment.

Epidemiology and Risk Factors

Statistics concerning prevalence are based primarily on elderly individuals in acute care settings. Estimated prevalence rates range from 10% to 30% of patients. In nursing homes, the prevalence is much higher, approaching 60% of those older than the age of 75 years.

TABLE 31.2 Key Diagnostic Characteristics for Delirium Caused by a General Medical Condition 293.0

Diagnostic Criteria	Associated Findings

• Disturbance of consciousness
   Reduced clarity of awareness
   Decreased ability to focus, sustain, or shift attention
• Developing over a short period of time—usually hours to days; fluctuating during the course of the day
• Cognitive changes
   Memory deficit, disorientation, language disturbance
   Development of perceptual disturbance not better accounted for by a pre-existing, established, or evolving dementia
• History physical examination, or laboratory tests indicating change as a direct cause of physiologic effects of medical condition
	Associated Behavioral Findings
	• Attention wandering
	• Perseveration
	• Easily distracted
	• Recent memory changes
	• Dysnomia, dysgraphia
	• Speech is rambling, irrelevant, incoherent
	• Misinterpretations, illusions, and hallucinations
	
	Associated Physical Findings
	• Daytime sleepiness
	• Nighttime agitation
	• Difficulty falling asleep
	• Restlessness, hyperactivity, or sluggishness and lethargy
	• Anxiety, fear, irritability, anger, euphoria, and apathy
	• Rapid unpredictable shifts from one emotional state to another

Etiologies • Substance intoxication delirium • Substance withdrawal delirium • Multiple etiologies (due to more than one medical condition, substance effect, or medication side effect) • Not otherwise specified	***Associated Laboratory Findings*** • Abnormal electroencephalogram

TABLE 31.3 Differentiating Delirium From Dementia

Dimensions	Delirium	Dementia
Onset	Sudden	Insidious
24-h course	Fluctuating	Stable
Consciousness	Reduced	Clear
Attention	Globally disoriented	Usually normal
Cognition	Globally disoriented	Globally impaired
Hallucinations	Visual auditory	May be present
Orientation	Usually impaired	Often impaired
Psychomotor activity	Increased, reduced, or shifts	Often normal
Speech	Often incoherent, slow or rapid	Often normal
Involuntary movement	Often asterixis or coarse tremor	Often absent
Physical illness or drug toxicity	One or both	Often absent

Adapted from Lipowski, Z. J. (1990). *Delirium: Acute confusional states* (p. 192). New York: Oxford University Press.

Delirium occurs in up to 30% of hospitalized cancer patients and in 30% to 40% of those hospitalized with AIDS. Near death, 80% of patients experience delirium (APA, 2000).

Because of greater longevity, the prevalence of delirium is higher for women than for men. However, one study identified male gender as a risk factor (Schor et al., 1992). No investigations of delirium have suggested familial trends.

Delirium is particularly common in elderly, postsurgical patients. One study showed 41% (51 of 126) of elderly patients studied who were admitted to the hospital for hip fractures experienced delirium during the hospitalization, and in 20 of the patients, delirium persisted at discharge (Marcantonio et al., 2000). Patients experiencing mental confusion are also more likely to be victims of falls and fractures. Text Box 31-1 lists proposed risk factors for delirium. See Text Box 31-2 for a clinical vignette of a patient who experienced delirium after trying an over-the-counter (OTC) sleeping medication.

Etiology

The etiology of delirium is complex and usually multifaceted. A lack of generally accepted theories of causation has resulted in considerable variability in the research. Thus, integrating the research and applying it to practice has been difficult. To date, studies have focused almost exclusively on biologic causes of delirium, with psychosocial factors viewed as contributing or facilitating. Because environmental and psychosocial factors have been studied only in small, uncontrolled studies, conclusions cannot yet be drawn about these factors. For this reason, the following discussion of etiology covers biologic theories of causation.

The most commonly identified causes of delirium, in order of frequency, are as follows:

- Medications
- Infections (particularly urinary tract and upper respiratory)
- Fluid and electrolyte imbalance; metabolic disturbances

The probability of developing the syndrome is increased if certain predisposing factors, such as advanced age, brain damage, or dementia, are also present. Sensory overload or underload, immobilization, sleep deprivation, and psychosocial stress also contribute to the development of delirium.

Because delirium has multiple causes, a wide variety of brain alterations may also be responsible for its development. The major theories of causation are as follows:

TEXT BOX 31.1

Risk Factors for Delirium

- Advanced age
- Pre-existing dementia
- Functional dependence
- Pre-existing illness
- Bone fracture
- Infection
- Medications (both number and type)
- Changes in vital signs (including hypotension and hyper- or hypothermia)
- Electrolyte or metabolic imbalance
- Admission to a long-term care institution
- Postcardiotomy
- AIDS
- Pain

- A general reduction in cerebral functioning, which can result from a decrease in the supply, uptake, or use of substances for brain metabolic activity
- Damage of enzyme systems, the blood–brain barrier, or cell membranes
- Reduced brain metabolism resulting in decreased acetylcholine synthesis
- Imbalance of neurotransmitters, such as acetylcholine, norepinephrine, and dopamine
- Raised plasma cortisol level in response to acute stress, which affects attention and information processing
- Involvement of the white matter, especially in the thalamocortical projections (Tune, 2000).

Interdisciplinary Treatment and Priority Care Issues

Although delirium may be recognized and diagnosed in any health care setting, appropriate intervention requires that the patient be admitted to an acute care setting for rigorous assessment and rapid treatment. The priority in care is identification of the underlying cause of the delirium. Interdisciplinary management of delirium includes two primary aspects: (1) elimination or correction of the underlying cause, and (2) symptomatic and supportive measures (eg, adequate rest, comfort promotion, maintenance of fluid and electrolyte balance, and protection from injury) (House, 2000).

When developing a treatment plan for a patient in whom delirium is suspected, close attention must be paid to correction of any organic or disease-related factors. Initially, life-threatening illnesses, such as cerebral hypoxia, hypertensive encephalopathy, intracranial hemorrhage, meningitis, severe electrolyte and metabolic imbalances, hypoglycemia, and intoxication, must be ruled out or corrected. If possible, all suspected medications should be stopped and vital signs monitored at least every 2 hours. Because many patients with delirium are seriously ill, good nursing care is vital. The plan of care requires close observation of the patient with particular regard to changes in vital signs, behavior, and mental status. Patients are followed until the delirium clears or until discharge. If the delirium still exists at discharge, it is critical that referrals for postdischarge follow-up assessment and care be implemented.

NURSING MANAGEMENT: HUMAN RESPONSE TO DISORDER

By definition, a biologic insult must be present for delirium to occur, but psychological and environmental factors are often involved. Because delirium develops quickly over a matter of hours or days and has been associated with increased mortality, nurses should be particularly vigilant in assessing individuals who are at increased risk for this syndrome. If the patient is a child, the assessment process presented in Chapter 11 should be used. If the patient is an elderly person, the assessment in Chapter 12 should serve as a guide. Special efforts should be made to include family members in the nursing process.

Biologic Domain

Biologic Assessment

The onset of symptoms is typically signaled by a rapid or acute change in behavior. To assess the onset of symptoms, the nurse will need to know what is normal for the individual; caregivers, family members, or significant others should be interviewed because they can often provide valuable information. Family members may be the only resource for accurate information.

Past and Present Health Status. Past history should include a description of the onset, duration, range, and intensity of associated symptoms. The presence of chronic physical illness, dementia, depression, or other psychiatric illnesses should be identified. Sorting out historic information may be particularly problematic when delirium is accompanied by an acute illness, recent surgery, or infection.

Physical Examination and Review of Systems. If the patient is cooperative, a physical examination will be conducted in the emergency room. Vital signs are crucial. A review of systems must be conducted in each patient suspected of having delirium or other organic mental disorders. Laboratory data, including a complete blood count, glucose, blood urea nitrogen, creatinine, electrolytes, liver function, and oxygen saturation, as well as fluid balance, signs of constipation, or a recent history of diarrhea, should be assessed in an attempt to discover an underlying cause.

Physical Functions. Functional assessment includes physical functional status (activities of daily living), use of sensory aids (glasses and hearing aids), usual activity level and any recent changes, and pain assessment. Because sleep is often disturbed in patients with delirium, sleep patterns must be assessed, including what is typical for the individual and recent changes. Often, the sleep–wake cycle of the patient with delirium becomes reversed, with the individual attempting to sleep during the day and to be awake at night. Not only are sleep disturbances a symptom of delirium, but also sleep deprivation may add to confusion. Restoration of a normal sleep cycle is extremely important.

Pharmacologic Assessment. A substance abuse history (including alcohol intake and smoking history) should be obtained (see Chaps. 11 and 12). In addition, information regarding the use of medications must be obtained, with particular attention given to new medications or changes in dose of current medications. Table 31-4 lists some of the drugs that can cause delirium. Special attention should be given to combinations of these medications because delirium is often the result of the use of multiple medications, especially those with anticholinergic side effects.

Information regarding OTC medications should be included in this assessment. OTC medications are often thought of as harmless, but a number of these, such as cold medications, taken in sufficient quantities may produce confusion, especially in elderly patients.

Findings from the medication assessment are integrated with findings of the physical assessment, including such things as fluid and electrolyte balance, lack of adequate pain management, or serum drug levels, if available. For example, chronic pain may lead an individual to use more medication for pain relief than has been intended. Careful monitoring of the effectiveness of pain medications may lead to the use of a different medication that is more effective with less potential for misuse. Because many classes of medica-

tions have been associated with delirium, the focus is on changes in the type and number of medications and how medications relate to other findings in the history and physical assessment.

Nursing Diagnoses Related to Biologic Domain

The nursing diagnoses typically generated from assessment data are Acute Confusion, Disturbed Thought Processes, or Disturbed Sensory Perception (visual or auditory) (North American Nursing Diagnosis Association [NANDA], 2001). However, an astute nurse will also use nursing diagnoses based on other indicators, such as Hyperthermia, Acute Pain, Risk for Infection, and Disturbed Sleep Pattern.

Biologic Interventions

Important interventions for a patient experiencing acute confusional state include providing a safe and therapeutic environment, maintaining fluid and electrolyte balance and adequate nutrition, and preventing aspiration and decubitus ulcers, which are often complications (Text Box 31-3). Other interventions relate to a particular nursing diagnosis focused on individual symptoms and underlying causes, for example, for patients with Altered Sleep Patterns, the intervention Sleep Enhancement is appropriate (McCloskey & Bulechek, 1996). For more information, see Chapter 26.

Safety Interventions. Behaviors exhibited by the delirious patient, such as hallucinations, delusions or illusions, and aggression or agitation (restlessness or excitability), may pose safety problems. The patient must be protected from physical harm by using low beds, guard rails, and careful supervision. The intervention Surveillance: Safety or Fall Prevention may be implemented (McCloskey & Bulechek, 1996). See Text Box 31-4.

Pharmacologic Interventions. The goal of psychopharmacologic management is treatment of the behaviors associated with delirium, such as symptoms of agitation, inattention, sleep disorder, and psychosis, so that the patient can be more comfortable. The decision to use medications should be based on the presence of these specific symptoms. Dosages are usually kept very low, especially with elderly patients. There is no consensus on the use of psychopharmacologic agents to control the symptoms of delirium, and limited studies have been conducted. Consideration of the use of these medications is usually related to the appearance of agitation, combativeness, or hallucinations. However, the choice of medication should be made with consideration of the likelihood of side effects (particularly anticholinergic effects, hypotension, and respiratory suppression) and the potential for making the delirium worse. For most

TABLE 31.4 Examples of Drugs That Can Cause Delirium

Class	Specific Drugs	Class	Specific Drugs
Anticholinergic Teldrin)	antihistamines chlorpheniramine (Ornade and antiparkinsonian drugs (eg, benztropine [Cogentin], biperiden [Akineton], or trihexyphenidyl) atropine belladona alkaloids diphenhydramine (Benadryl) phenothiazines promethazine (Phenergan) scopolamine tricyclic antidepressants	Cardiac	β-blockers propranolol (Inderal) clonidine (Catapres) digitalis (Digoxin and Lanoxin) lidocaine (Xylocaine) methyldopa (Aldomet) quinidine procainamide (Pronestyl)
Anticonvulsant	phenobarbital phenytoin (Dilantin) sodium valproate (Depakene)	Sedative-hypnotic	barbiturates benzodiazepines
		Sympathomimetic	amphetamines phenylephrine phenylpropanolamine
Antiinflammatory	corticosteroids ibuprofen (Motrin and Advil) indomethacin (Indocin) naproxen (Naprosyn)	Over-the-counter	Compoz Excedrin P.M. Sleep-Eze Sominex
Antiparkinsonian	amantadine (Symmetrel) carbidopa (Sinemet) levodopa (Larodopa)	Miscellaneous	acyclovir (antiviral) aminophylline amphotericin (antifungal) bromides cephalexin (Keflex) chlorpropamide (Diabinese) cimetidine (Tagamet) disulfiram (Antabuse) lithium metronidazole (Flagyl) theophylline timolol ophthalmic
Antituberculous	isoniazid rifampin		
Analgesic	opiates salicylates synthetic narcotics		

Adapted from Wise, M. G., & Gray, K. F. (1994). Delirium, dementia, and amnestic disorders. In R. E. Hales, S. C. Yudofsky, & J. A. Talbott (Eds.), *Textbook of psychiatry* (2nd ed., p. 320). Washington, DC: American Psychiatric Press.

delirious patients, short-term use of an antipsychotic, such as risperidone (Risperdal), is the medication of choice. The use of antipsychotics in elderly patients is discussed in greater detail later in the chapter.

Benzodiazepines have also been tried, especially when the delirium is related to alcohol withdrawal. However, in some patients, these medications may produce further impairment of cognition because of the sedation, and, in some cases, a paradoxic agitation may develop. Using these medications alone is not recommended for the treatment of delirium, but in conjunction with antipsychotics such as risperidone, low doses of medications such as lorazepam have been useful (Drugs & Therapy Perspectives, 1997).

Administration and Monitoring of Medications. Patients experiencing delirium may resist taking medication because of their confusion. If medication is given, ideally it should be oral.

Side-Effect Monitoring and Management. Monitoring action and side effects is especially important because the cause of the delirium may not be known and the patient may inadvertently be affected by the medication. Patients should be monitored for the presence of sedation, hypotension, or extrapyramidal symptoms. Although mental status often fluctuates during delirium, it may also be influenced by these medications, and any changes or worsening of mental status after administration of the medication should be reported to the prescriber immediately. Some side effects may also be confused with the symptoms of delirium. For example, akathisia (see Chap. 8) may appear to be agitation or restlessness. The patient's physical condition and concurrent medications may also influence the bioavailability, metabolism, and elimination of these medications. Adequate hydration and nutrition must be maintained. When using antipsychotic medications, closely monitor the patient for symptoms of neuroleptic malignant syndrome (see Chap. 18). The appearance of these symptoms may be missed because many may be confused with those related to delirium.

Finally, the use of antipsychotics or other medications for treating symptoms related to delirium should

TEXT BOX 31.3

Interventions: Providing a Safe and Therapeutic Environment for the Delirious Patient

- Identify etiologic factors causing delirium.
- Initiate therapies to reduce or eliminate factors causing the delirium.
- Monitor neurologic status on an ongoing basis.
- Provide unconditional positive regard.
- Verbally acknowledge the patient's fears and feelings.
- Provide optimistic but realistic assurance.
- Allow the patient to maintain rituals that limit anxiety.
- Provide patient with information about what is happening and what can be expected to occur in the future.
- Avoid demands for abstract thinking if patient can only think in concrete terms.
- Limit need for decision making if frustrating or confusing to patient.
- Administer medications PRN for anxiety or agitation.
- Encourage visitation by significant others as appropriate.
- Recognize and accept the patient's perceptions or interpretation of reality (hallucinations or delusions).
- State your perceptions in a calm, reassuring, and non-argumentative manner.
- Respond to the theme or feeling tone, rather than the content, of the hallucination or delusion.
- When possible, remove stimuli that create misperception in a particular patient (eg, pictures on the wall, television).
- Maintain a well-lit environment that reduces sharp contrasts and shadows.
- Assist with needs related to nutrition, elimination, hydration, and personal hygiene.
- Maintain a hazard-free environment.

- Place identification bracelet on patient.
- Provide appropriate level of supervision or surveillance to monitor patient and to allow for therapeutic actions as needed.
- Use physical restraints as needed.
- Avoid frustrating patient by quizzing with orientation questions that cannot be answered.
- Inform patient of person, place, and time as needed.
- Provide a consistent physical environment and daily routine.
- Provide caregivers who are familiar to the patient.
- Use environmental cues (eg, signs, pictures, clocks, calendars, color coding of environment) to stimulate memory, reorient, and promote appropriate behavior.
- Provide a low-stimulation environment for the patient in whom disorientation is increased by overstimulation.
- Encourage use of aids that increase sensory input (eg, eyeglasses, hearing aids, dentures).
- Approach patient slowly and from the front.
- Address patient by name when initiating interaction.
- Reorient patient to the health care provider with each contact.
- Communicate with simple, direct descriptive statements.
- Prepare patient for upcoming changes in usual routine and environment prior to occurrence.
- Provide new information slowly and in small doses, with frequent rest periods.
- Focus interpersonal interactions on what is familiar and meaningful to the patient.

Adapted from Iowa Intervention Project. (1995). J. C. McCloskey & G. M. Bulechek (Eds.), *Nursing interventions classification (NIC)* (2nd ed.). St. Louis: Mosby–Year Book.

---

be discontinued as soon as possible. These medications should not be stopped abruptly, but rather should be withdrawn gradually over several days or weeks.

Drug–Drug Interactions. The etiology of delirium is often a drug–drug interaction. OTC sleeping, cold, or allergy medication may be the cause. If medication is the underlying cause, it is important to identify accurately which medications are involved before administering any other drugs. A consultation from a clinical pharmacist may also be helpful.

Teaching Points. One of the most important objectives is to help the patient and family identify the underlying cause of the delirium in order to prevent future occurrences. If the delirium is not resolved before discharge, family members will need to know how to manage the patient at home.

Psychological Domain

Psychological Assessment

Psychological assessment of the individual with delirium focuses on cognitive changes revealed through the mental status examination as well as resulting behavioral manifestations. Changes in mental status must be monitored frequently for early detection of delirium, especially in elderly patients. In addition, other factors, such as stressors and environmental change, may contribute to the symptoms.

Mental Status. Rapid onset of global cognitive impairment that affects multiple aspects of intellectual functioning is the hallmark of delirium. Mental status evaluation reveals a number of changes:

TEXT BOX 31.4

Fall Prevention

Definition

Instituting special precautions with patient at risk for injury from falling.

Activities

Identify cognitive or physical deficits of the patient that may increase potential of falling in a particular environment.

Identify characteristics of environment that may increase potential for falls (eg, slippery floors and open stairways).

Monitor gait, balance, and fatigue level with ambulation.

Assist unsteady individual with ambulation.

Provide assistive devices (eg, cane and walker) to steady gait.

Maintain assistive devices in good working order.

Lock wheels of wheelchair, bed, or gurney during transfer of patient.

Place articles within easy reach of the patient.

Instruct patient to call for assistance with movement, as appropriate.

Teach patient how to fall to minimize injury.

Post signs to remind patient to call for help when getting out of bed, as appropriate.

Use proper technique to transfer patient to and from wheelchair, bed, toilet, and so on.

Provide elevated toilet seat for easy transfer.

Provide chairs of proper height, with backrests and armrests for easy transfer.

Provide bed mattress with firm edges for easy transfer.

Use physical restraints to limit potentially unsafe movement, as appropriate.

Use side rails of appropriate length and height to prevent falls from bed, as needed.

Place a mechanical bed in lowest position.

Provide a sleeping surface close to the floor, as needed.

Provide seating on beanbag chair to limit mobility, as appropriate.

Place a foam wedge in seat of chair to prevent patient from arising, as appropriate.

Use partially filled water mattress on bed to limit mobility, as appropriate.

Provide the dependent patient with a means of summoning help (eg, bell or call light) when caregiver is not present.

Answer call light immediately.

Assist with toileting at frequent, scheduled intervals.

Use a bed alarm to alert caretaker that individual is getting out of bed, as appropriate.

Mark doorway thresholds and edges of steps, as needed.

Remove low-lying furniture (eg, footstools and tables) that present a tripping hazard.

Avoid clutter on floor surface.

Provide adequate lighting for increased visibility.

Provide nightlight at bedside.

Provide visible handrails and grab bars.

Place gates in open doorways leading to stairways.

Provide nonslip, nontrip floor surfaces.

Provide a nonslip surface in bathtub or shower.

Provide sturdy, nonslip step stools to facilitate easy reaches.

Provide storage areas that are within easy reach.

Provide heavy furniture that will not tip if used for support.

Orient patient to physical "setup" of room.

Avoid unnecessary rearrangement of physical environment.

Ensure that patient wears shoes that fit properly, fasten securely, and have nonskid soles.

Instruct patient to wear prescription glasses, as appropriate, when out of bed.

Educate family members about risk factors that contribute to falls and how they can decrease these risks.

Instruct family on importance of handrails for stairs, bathrooms, and walkways.

Assist family in identifying hazards in the home and modifying them.

Instruct patient to avoid ice and other slippery outdoor surfaces.

Institute a routine physical exercise program that includes walking.

Post signs to alert staff that patient is at high risk for falls.

Collaborate with other health care team members to minimize side effects of medications that contribute to falling (eg, orthostatic hypotension and unsteady gait).

McCloskey, J., & Bulechek, G. (1996). *Nursing interventions classification (NIC).* St. Louis: Mosby.

- Fluctuations in level of consciousness with reduced awareness of the environment
- Difficulty focusing and sustaining or shifting attention
- Severely impaired memory, especially immediate and recent memory

Patients may be disorientated to time and place, but rarely to person. Environmental perceptions are often altered. The patient may believe shadows are actually a person in their room. Thought content is often illogical, and speech may be incoherent or inappropriate to the context. Each of these variations in mental status will tend to fluctuate over the course of the day. During the same day, an individual with delirium may appear confused and uncooperative, whereas later, that person may be more lucid and able to follow instructions. Nurses must continually assess the cognitive status of the individual throughout the day so that their approach to the interventions may be modified accordingly.

Several rating scales are available for use in assessing the cognitive and behavioral fluctuations of delirium (Text Box 31-5). The Mini-Mental State Examination (MMSE) quantifies the severity of cognitive impairment, but it does not differentiate delirium from other forms of cognitive decline. When interpreting the MMSE, scores of 20 to 30 indicate mild delirium, 10 to 20 moderate delirium, and 0 to 10 severe delirium (Ross et al., 1991). Calculations, orientation (especially to time), and recall are most affected in delirium, whereas naming and registration are relatively preserved. Other scales, such as the Confusion Assessment Method (Inouye et al., 1990), incorporate the criteria for diagnosing delirium from the *Diagnostic and Statistical Manual of Mental Disorders* (APA, 2000) and

are more sensitive for detecting delirium. Finally, the Confusion Rating Scale (CRS) (Williams et al., 1988) was developed specifically for nurses to rate behavioral change in delirium across shifts. The CRS showed a 78% agreement with measures of mental status and may provide an effective method for nurses to standardize assessments of the fluctuating behavioral impact of delirium across a group of nurses. This relatively simple scale is provided in Text Box 31-6.

Behavior. Delirious patients exhibit a wide range of behaviors, complicating the process of making a diagnosis and planning interventions. At times, the individual may be restless or agitated, and at other times lethargic and slow to respond. Delirium can be categorized into three types. Patients with **hyperkinetic delirium** exhibit behaviors most commonly recognized as delirium, that is, psychomotor hyperactivity, marked excitability, and a tendency toward hallucinations. Patients with **hypokinetic delirium** may be lethargic, somnolent, and apa-

---

TEXT BOX 31.5

Rating Scales for Use With Delirium

The Confusion Assessment Method (CAM)
Inouye, S. K., van Dyck, C. H., Alessi, C. A., et al. (1990). Clarifying confusion: The confusion assessment method. *Annals of Internal Medicine, 113,* 941–948.

Confusion Rating Scale (CRS)
Williams, M. A., Ward, S. E., & Campbell, E. B. (1988). Confusion: Testing versus observation. *Journal of Gerontological Nursing, 14*(1), 25–30.

Delirium Symptom Interview
Levkoff, S., Liptzin, B., Cleary, P., et al. (1991). Review of research instruments and techniques used to detect delirium. *International Psychogeriatrics, 3,* 253–271.

Delirium Rating Scale (DRS)
Trzepacz, P. T., Baker, R. W., & Greenhouse, J. (1988). A symptom rating scale for delirium. *Psychiatry Research, 23,* 89–97.

High Sensitivity Cognitive Screen (HSCS)
Faust, D., & Fogel, B. S. (1989). The development and initial validation of a sensitive bedside cognitive screening test. *Journal of Nervous and Mental Disease, 177,* 25–31.

NEECHAM Confusion Scale
Neelon, V. J., Champagne, M. T., McConnell, E., et al. (1992). Use of the NEECHAM confusion scale to assess acute confusional states of hospitalized older patients. In S. G. Funk, E. M. Tornquist, M. T. Champagne, & R. A. Wiese (Eds.), *Key aspects of elder care.* New York: Springer.

TEXT BOX 31.6

Confusion Rating Scale

1. Disorientation to place, time, or recognition of persons as assessed by spontaneous remarks of the patient or by informal questioning by the caregiver	0	1	2
2. Communication unrelated or inappropriate to the situation or unusual for the person, such as shouting, nonsensical or garbled conversation, or lack of communication when deviating from the person's usual pattern	0	1	2
3. Behaviors inappropriate to the situation such as pulling at tubes or attempting to get out of bed when contraindicated	0	1	2
4. The presence of illusions or hallucinations	0	1	2

0 = not present at any time during an 8-h period (shift)

1 = present at some time during the shift in a mild form   Total___

2 = present at some time during the shift in a marked form

Scores range from 0 = no impairment to 8 = severe impairment

Adapted and used with permission from Williams, M. A., Ward, S. E., & Campbell, E. B. (1988). Confusion: Testing versus observation. *Journal of Gerontological Nursing, 14*(1), 25–30.

thetic and exhibit reduced psychomotor activity; this is the "quiet" patient for whom the diagnosis of delirium is often missed. The third, a mixed variant, involves behavior that fluctuates between the hyperactive and hypoactive states.

Nursing Diagnoses Related to Psychological Domain

The nursing diagnosis Acute Confusion is also associated with impaired cognitive functioning. Even though the underlying cause of confusion is physiologic, nursing care should focus on the psychological domain as well as the physical. Other typical nursing diagnoses related to the psychological domain include Disturbed Thought Process, Ineffective Coping, and Disturbed Personal Identity.

Psychological Interventions

Staff should have frequent interaction with patients and support them if they are confused or hallucinating. Patients should be encouraged to express their fears and discomforts that result from frightening or disconcerting psychotic experiences. Adequate lighting, easy-to-read calendars and clocks, a reasonable noise level, and frequent verbal orientation may lessen this frightening experience. If the patient wears eyeglasses or uses a hearing aid, these devices should be used. Including familiar personal possessions in the environment may also help. Interventions that may be useful for these individuals will be discussed in detail later in the chapter (see the section on Dementia).

Social Domain

Social Assessment

Discussion should be initiated with the family to determine whether the patient's behaviors are new. An assessment of living arrangements may provide information about sensory stimulation or social isolation. Cultural and educational background must be considered when the patient's mental capacity is evaluated. Individuals from certain ethnic backgrounds may not be familiar with the information used in tests of general knowledge (eg, names of presidents, geographic knowledge), memory (eg, date of birth in cultures that do not routinely celebrate birthdays), and orientation (eg, sense of placement and location may be conceptualized differently in some cultures) (APA, 2000). Some cultural practices may involve the use of some substances, such as elixirs, containing chemicals that may exacerbate the symptoms of delirium. Assessment should address these practices.

Family support for the individual and their understanding of the disorder must be assessed. The behaviors exhibited by the person experiencing delirium may be frightening or at least confusing for family members. Some family members may actually increase the agitation of the individual. Assessment of family interactions and their ability to understand the symptoms of delirium is important. If available, their calm and reassuring presence can be helpful to the individual.

Nursing Diagnoses Related to Social Domain

Several nursing diagnoses associated with the social domain can be generated. Interrupted Family Processes, Ineffective Protection, Ineffective Role Performance, and Risk for Injury are the most typical. Risk for Injury is a high-priority diagnosis because these individuals are more likely to fall or injure themselves during a confused state.

Social Interventions

The environment needs to be a safe one that protects the patient from injury. A predictable, orienting environment will help to re-establish order to the patient's life. That is, provide a calendar, clocks, and other items that help orient the patient to time, place, and person. If the patient is agitated, de-escalation techniques should be used. Physical restraint should be avoided and reserved for very rare circumstances. It is important to explain the patient's behavior to family members in terms of the diagnosis of delirium. During a delirious episode, the presence of close family members can be helpful. Families can work with staff in reorienting the patient and providing a supportive environment. Families will need to understand that important decisions requiring the patient's input should be delayed if at all possible until the patient has recovered. Although patients may be able to participate in decision making, they may not remember the decision later; therefore, it is important to have several witnesses present.

Evaluation and Treatment Outcomes

The primary goal of treatment is prevention or resolution of the delirious episode with return to previous cognitive status. Outcome measures include (1) correction of the underlying physiologic alteration, (2) resolution of confusion, (3) family member verbalization of understanding of confusion, and (4) prevention of injury. Resolution of confusion is the primary goal; however, the nurse makes important contributions to all four of these outcomes. The end result of delirium is either full recovery, incomplete recovery, incomplete recovery with some residual cognitive impairment, or a downward course leading to death.

Continuum of Care

The nurse may encounter delirious patients in a number of treatment settings (eg, home, nursing home, ambulatory care, day treatment, outpatient setting, hospital). Commonly, patients are admitted to an acute care setting for rapid evaluation and treatment of the underlying etiology. An abrupt change in cognitive status can also occur while the patient is hospitalized for another reason. Delirium often persists beyond discharge from the hospital. Discharge planning should routinely include family education and referrals to community health care providers. If the patient will be returning to a residential long-term care setting, communication with facility staff about the patient's hospital stay and treatment regimen is crucial. For more information on caring for patients with delirium, see Psychoeducation Checklist: Delirium.

DEMENTIA OF THE ALZHEIMER'S TYPE

Clinical Course of Disorder

Alzheimer's disease (AD) is a degenerative, progressive neuropsychiatric disorder that results in cognitive impairment, emotional and behavioral changes, physical and functional decline, and ultimately death.

Gradually, the patient's ability to carry out activities of daily living declines, although physical status often remains intact until late in the disease process. A disorder of elderly people, AD has been diagnosed in patients as young as 35 years of age. The person with AD lives an average of 8 years after initial diagnosis and may live as many as 20 years after the onset of symptoms (which appear long before the diagnosis is made).

Two subtypes have been identified: early-onset AD (age 65 years and younger) and late-onset AD (age older than 65 years). Late-onset AD is much more common

---

PSYCHOEDUCATION CHECKLIST
Delirium

When caring for the patient with delirium, be sure to include the caregivers, as appropriate, and address the following topic areas in the teaching plan:

• Psychopharmacologic agents, if used, including drug action, dosage, frequency, and possible adverse effects
• Underlying cause of delirium
• Mental status changes
• Safety measures
• Hydration and nutrition
• Avoidance of restraints
• Decision-making guidelines

---

than early-onset AD, but early-onset AD has a more rapid progression. AD is also routinely conceptualized in terms of three stages: mild, moderate, and severe. Signs and symptoms of AD change as the patient passes from one phase of the illness to another (Fig. 31-1). It is unclear whether all patients with AD pass through a specific sequence of deterioration and whether the staging of a patient at initial assessment has any prognostic implications in terms of speed of decline. Nevertheless, staging is a useful technique for determining the patient's current cognitive status and provides a sound basis for decisions in clinical management.

Diagnostic Criteria

The diagnosis of AD is made on clinical grounds, and verification of Alzheimer's etiology is confirmed at autopsy by the presence of abnormal degenerative structures, neuritic plaques, and neurofibrillary tangles. The essential feature of dementia of the Alzheimer's type is the development of multiple cognitive deficits, especially memory impairment, and at least one of the following cognitive disturbances: **aphasia** (alterations in language ability), **apraxia** (impaired ability to execute motor activities despite intact motor functioning), **agnosia** (failure to recognize or identify objects despite intact sensory function), or a **disturbance of executive functioning** (ability to think abstractly, plan, initiate, sequence, monitor, and stop complex behavior). The cognitive deficits must be sufficiently severe to cause impairment in occupational or social functioning and must represent a decline from a previously higher level of functioning (APA, 2000). These symptoms are common to all presentations of the symptoms of dementia, regardless of the underlying pathology. Table 31-5 provides a list of the essential symptoms of dementia, along with other possible behavioral and psychological changes that may or may not be present. To make a diagnosis of AD, all other known causes of dementia must be excluded (eg, vascular, AIDS, Parkinson's disease).

Epidemiology and Risk Factors

Currently, an estimated 4 million Americans are afflicted with AD, and conservative projections estimate that by the year 2040, the number of cases of AD in the United States may exceed 6 million. About 10% of people older than 65 years of age and up to 47.2% of those older than 85 years of age suffer from AD, which accounts for more than 50% of all dementia. The age of onset of dementia depends on the etiology but is usually late in life, with the highest prevalence after the age of 85 years (Alzheimer's Disease and Related Disorders Association [ADRDA],

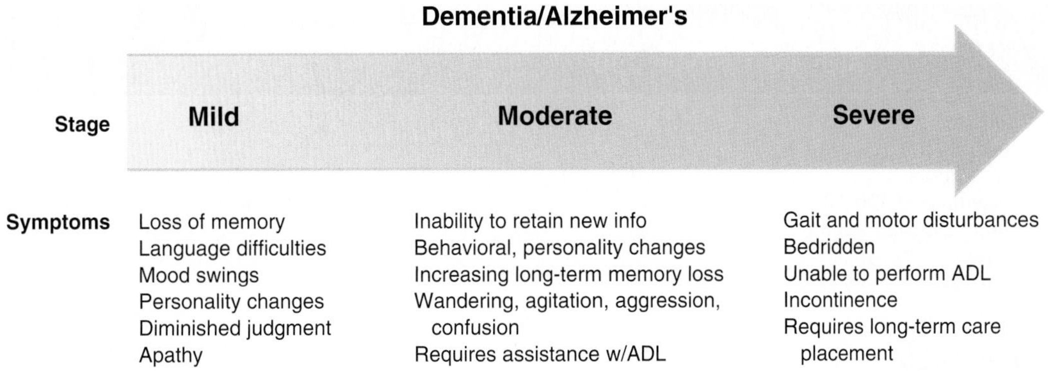

Dementia/Alzheimer's

Stage	Mild	Moderate	Severe

Symptoms	Loss of memory	Inability to retain new info	Gait and motor disturbances
	Language difficulties	Behavioral, personality changes	Bedridden
	Mood swings	Increasing long-term memory loss	Unable to perform ADL
	Personality changes	Wandering, agitation, aggression,	Incontinence
	Diminished judgment	confusion	Requires long-term care
	Apathy	Requires assistance w/ADL	placement

FIGURE 31.1 Alzheimer's disease progression.

2001). AD appears to be present in all groups, but studies are lacking on the incidence and prevalence of AD among each of the major ethnic groups. At present, AD follows heart disease, cancer, and stroke as the fourth leading cause of death among elderly people in the United States. About 70% of all patients with dementia live at home, and about 60% of nursing home residents have a dementing illness (ADRDA, 2001).

To date, only age, a familial tendency for either AD or Down's syndrome, head trauma, and low educational level or illiteracy are identified risk factors for AD. Studies evaluating impaired immunity, viruses, and environmental toxins (eg, aluminum) as potential risk factors have proved inconclusive.

Age is the major risk for Alzheimer's. All studies conducted to date consistently indicate a steep increase in both the prevalence and incidence of AD with age. Alzheimer's type dementia is twice as common in women as in men, but this may be because women tend to live longer than men and the incidence of AD increases with advanced age.

AD can run in families. Compared with the general population, first-degree biologic relatives of individuals with early-onset AD are more likely to develop the disorder. About 10% of AD patients report other affected family members, and about 50% of adults with early-onset AD have a positive family history. However, about 60% of patients with AD do not show any familial aggregation. Patients with Down's syndrome frequently and precociously develop pathologic lesions that cannot be distinguished from AD. So far, studies point toward genetically related risk factors only in familial AD. However, the familial form accounts for only a small proportion of cases of Alzheimer's disease (less than 5%) (Cummings et al., 1998).

The hypothesis that low educational level may increase the risk for Alzheimer's remains controversial. The connection between AD and education is unclear at this time. One theory is that education has a direct biologic effect on the brain, which increases synaptic reserve. The educational effect may also be an indirect association resulting from as yet undetermined socioeconomic or environmental factors (eg, poor diet or exposure to toxins during gestation or early childhood), or it might be an invalid finding because of measurement inadequacies or other technical problems. One recent study suggests that the association of education with AD is related to women, not men (Letenneur et al., 2000).

Prior head injury leading to unconsciousness may represent a significant risk factor for the later development of AD, perhaps accounting for 5% to 10% of the attributable risk (Graves et al., 1990; Mortimer et al., 1991). Further study is needed to ascertain whether this finding is robust or the result of "selective recall" on the part of spouses or relatives of AD patients (Advisory Panel on Alzheimer's Disease [APAD], 1991). Other data suggest that brief periods of brain ischemia caused by coronary stenosis might predispose a person to AD (Aronson et al., 1990).

Etiology

Researchers have not yet identified a definitive cause of AD. It is possible that a combination of mechanisms may be operating or that different mechanisms are responsible for dementia in different people. In general, the brain appears normal in the early phases of AD, but it undergoes widespread atrophy as the disease advances.

Plaques and Tangles

One piece of the puzzle is partially explained by a leading theory that, in Alzheimer's, β-amyloid deposits destroy cholinergic neurons, in a similar manner to cholesterol causing atherosclerosis. It is hypothesized that **neuritic plaques,** extracellular lesions consisting of β-*amyloid protein* and *apolipoprotein A* (apoA) cores, form in the nucleus basalis of Meynert, gradually increase

TABLE 31.5   Key Diagnostic Characteristics for Dementia of the Alzheimer's Type 290

With early onset:
With delirium 290.11
With delusions 290.12
With depressed mood 290.13
Uncomplicated 290.10
With late onset:
With delirium 290.3
With delusions 290.20
With depressed mood 290.21
Uncomplicated 290.0

Diagnostic Criteria	Target Symptoms and Associated Findings

• Development of multiple cognitive deficits
• Involvement of both memory impairment and one or more of the following cognitive disturbances: aphasia, apraxia, agnosia, or disturbance in executive functioning
• Significant impairment in social or occupational functioning resulting from cognitive deficits; significant decline from previous level of functioning
• Cognitive deficits not due to: other CNS conditions causing progressive deficits in memory or cognition; systemic conditions known to cause dementia; substance-induced conditions
• Not occurring exclusively during course of a delirium
• Not better accounted for by another Axis I disorder
    Early onset: age 65 y or less
    Late onset: over age 65 y
	• Memory impairment
	• Cognitive disturbances
	
	Associated Behavioral Findings
	• Spatial disorientation and difficulty with spatial tasks
	• Poor judgment and poor insight
	• Little or no awareness of memory loss or other cognitive abnormalities
	• Unrealistic assessment of abilities; underestimation of risks involved in activities
	• Possible suicidal behaviors (usually in early stages when individual is more capable of carrying out a plan of action)
	• Possible gait disturbances and falls
	• Disinhibited behavior, such as inappropriate jokes, neglect of personal hygiene, undue familiarity with strangers, or disregard for conventional rules of social conduct
	• Delusions, especially ones involving persecution
	• Superimposed delirium
	
	Associated Physical Examination Findings
	• Few motor or sensory signs (in the first year of illness)
	• Myoclonus and gait disorder (later)
	• Seizure possible
	
	Associated Laboratory Findings
	• Brain atrophy (with computed tomography or magnetic resonance imaging)
	• Senile plaques, neurofibrillary tangles, granulovascular degeneration, neuronal loss, astrocytic gliosis, and amyloid angiopathy on microscopic examination

in number, and are abnormally distributed throughout the cholinergic system. The nucleus basalis of Meynert is the major brain center for cholinergic neurons, which have the principal role in mediating memory formation. The more neuritic plaques, the more impairment in cognitive functioning. Alzheimer's may be a problem of too much formation of β-amyloid, or too little removal of it (Stahl, 2000).

Neurofibrillary tangles are fibrous proteins, or *tau proteins*, that are chemically altered and twisted together and spread throughout the brain, interfering with nerve functioning in cholinergic neurons. It is hypothesized that formation of these neurofibrillary tangles is related to the apolipoprotein E4 (apoE$_4$). Apolipoprotein (apoE) is a normal cholesterol-carrying protein produced by a gene on chromosome 19, which has three forms: apoE$_2$, apoE$_3$, and apoE$_4$. It appears that apoE$_3$ protects against abnormal changes in proteins that lead to neurofibrillary tangles, associated with late-onset dementia, but apoE$_4$ appears to leave these proteins unprotected and increases the patient's risk for AD (Stahl, 2000) (Fig. 31-2).

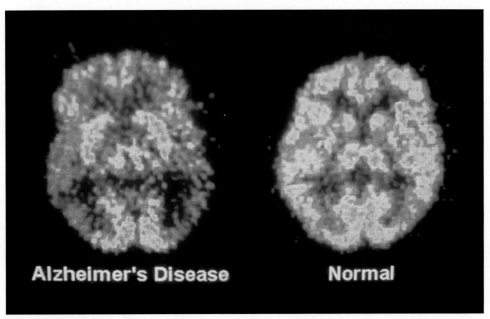

FIGURE 31.2 Metabolic activity in a subject with Alzheimer's disease (*left*) and in a control subject (*right*). (Courtesy of Monte S. Buchsbaum, MD, The Mount Sinai Medical Center and School of Medicine, New York, NY.)

Cholinergic Hypothesis

Acetylcholine (ACh) is an important neurotransmitter associated with cognitive functioning, and disruption of cholinergic mechanisms damages memory in animals and humans (see Chap. 7). In AD, ACh is reduced, but the number of ACh receptors is relatively unchanged. The reduced ACh is related to a decrease in *choline acetyltransferase* (a critical enzyme in the synthesis of ACh), especially in the forebrain. That is, there are fewer enzymes available to synthesize ACh, which leads to a reduction in cholinergic activity. Positron emission tomography scans in Figures 31-3 and 31-4 clearly show changes in brain function.

Genetic Factors

Initially, scientists hoped to find a singular, identifiable genetic basis for AD, but it is now recognized that even in early-onset AD, genetic factors are heterogeneous. Chromosomes 21, 14, and 19 are implicated in the development of AD. Chromosome 21 is associated because amyloid plaques and neurofibrillary tangles accumulate consistently in older people with Down's syndrome (trisomy 21) who develop AD. A locus on chromosome 14 is found in 70% of people with familial AD (Mullan et al., 1992; Schellenberg et al., 1992; Peskind, 1996). The role of chromosome 19 in the production of apoE was previously discussed.

Other Theories

The use of certain medications, such as nonsteroidal antiinflammatory drugs and estrogen replacement ther-

apy, may delay the onset of the disorder (Andersen et al., 1995; McGeer, et al., 1996; and Benson, 1999). Vitamin E and the drug selegiline (deprenyl) appear to delay important milestones in the course of Alzheimer's, including nursing home placement and severe functional impairments, even as the disease progresses (Sano et al., 1997). All of these findings are being pursued in the quest for additional knowledge related to the etiology of Alzheimer's.

Interdisciplinary Treatment

In designing services and interventions, the interdisciplinary team must keep in mind that AD has a progressively deteriorating clinical course, and that the anatomic and neurochemical changes that occur in the brains of its victims are accompanied by impairments in cognition, sensorium, affect (facial expression representing mood), behavior, and psychosocial functioning. The nature and range of services needed by patients and families throughout the full course of the illness can vary dramatically at different stages.

Initial assessment of the patient suspected of having dementia has three main objectives: (1) confirmation of the diagnosis, (2) establishment of baseline levels in a number of functional spheres, and (3) establishment of a therapeutic relationship with the patient and family that will continue through subsequent phases of the disease process. Treatment efforts currently focus on managing the cognitive symptoms, delaying the cognitive decline (eg, memory loss, confusion, and problems with learning, speech, and reasoning), treating the noncognitive

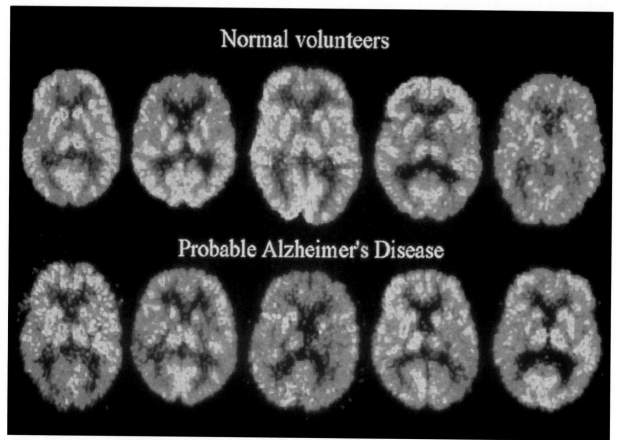

FIGURE 31.3 Series comparison of elderly control subjects (*top row*) and patients with Alzheimer's disease (*bottom row*). Although there are some decreases in metabolism associated with age, in most patients with Alzheimer's disease, there are marked decreases in the temporal lobe, an area important in memory functions. (Courtesy of Monte S. Buchsbaum, MD, The Mount Sinai Medical Center and School of Medicine, New York, NY.)

symptoms (eg, psychosis, mood symptoms, agitation), and supporting the caregivers as a means of improving the quality of life for both patients and their caregivers.

Priority Care Issues

The priority of care will change throughout the course of the disorder. Initially, the priority is delaying cognitive decline and supporting family members. Later, the priority changes to protecting the patient from hurting him or herself because of lack of judgment. Near the end, the physical needs of the patient become the focus of care.

 Family Response to Disorder

Families are the first to be aware of the cognitive problem, often before the patient, who can be unaware of the extent of memory impairment. When finally confirmed, the actual diagnosis can be devastating to the family. Unlike delirium, a diagnosis of AD means long-term care responsibilities, while at the same time losing the essence of a family member day by day. Most families

keep their relative at home as long as possible in order to maintain contact and to avoid costly nursing home placement. The two symptoms that often result in nursing home placement are incontinence that cannot be managed and behavioral problems, such as wandering and aggression.

Especially in dementia, the needs of family members should also be considered. Caring for a family member with dementia takes its toll. Caregivers' health is often compromised and normal family functioning threatened. Caregiver distress is a major health risk for the family, and "caregiver burnout" is a common cause of institutionalization of patients with dementia. One study demonstrated the effectiveness of an AD caregiver support program in delaying nursing home placement of patients with AD. The program included counseling sessions and participation in a support group. The caregivers receiving the support program allowed a greater proportion of patients to remain in their home environment for a longer period of time (an average of 329 days) than the caregivers who did not receive the support (Mittelman et al., 1996).

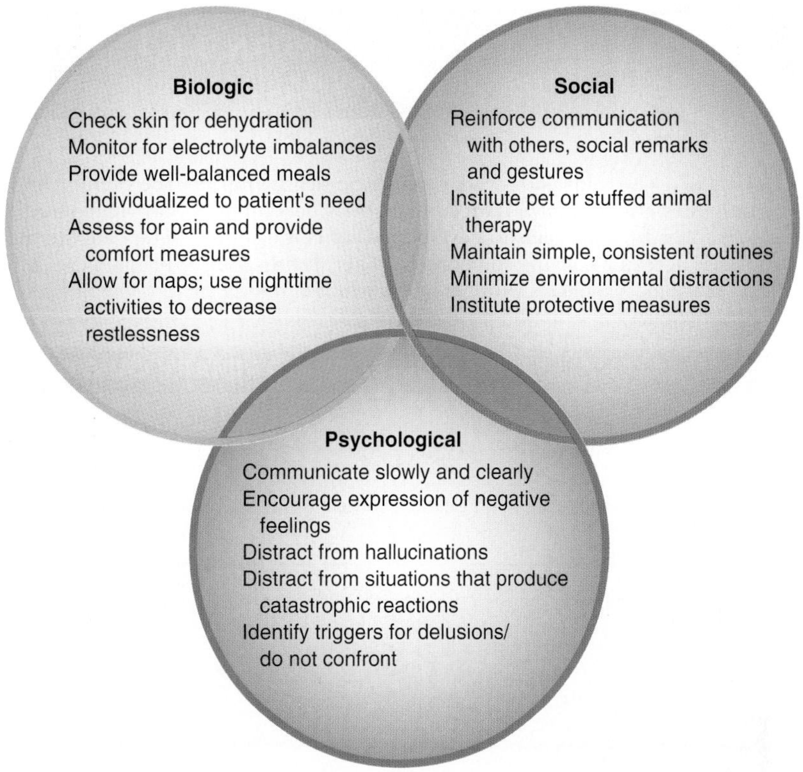

Biologic

Check skin for dehydration
Monitor for electrolyte imbalances
Provide well-balanced meals
    individualized to patient's need
Assess for pain and provide
    comfort measures
Allow for naps; use nighttime
    activities to decrease
    restlessness

Social

Reinforce communication
    with others, social remarks
    and gestures
Institute pet or stuffed animal
    therapy
Maintain simple, consistent routines
Minimize environmental distractions
Institute protective measures

Psychological

Communicate slowly and clearly
Encourage expression of negative
    feelings
Distract from hallucinations
Distract from situations that produce
    catastrophic reactions
Identify triggers for delusions/
    do not confront

FIGURE 31.4 Biopsychosocial interventions for patients with dementia.

NURSING MANAGEMENT: HUMAN RESPONSE TO DISORDER

The development and implementation of appropriate, effective, and safe nursing services for the care and support of patients with dementia and their families is a particular challenge because of the complex nature of the illness (see Nursing Care Plan 31-1). Even though AD is caused by biologic changes, the psychological and social domains are seriously affected by this disorder. The assessment of the patient with AD should follow the geropsychiatric nursing assessment in Chapter 12.

Biologic Domain

Biologic Assessment

Past and Present Health Status. The nursing assessment should include a medical history, current medication profile (prescription and OTC medications or home remedies), substance abuse history (including alcohol intake and smoking history), presence of chronic physical or psychiatric illness, and a description of the onset, duration, range, and intensity of symptoms associated with dementia. The onset of symptoms in dementia is typically gradual, with insidious changes in behavior. To conduct a thorough assessment of the patient with dementia, the nurse needs to know what is typical for the individual; therefore, caregivers, family members, or significant others can be sources of valuable information.

Physical Examination and a Review of Body Systems. A review of body systems must be conducted on each patient suspected of having dementia. Specific biologic assessment parameters for a patient with dementia include vital signs, neurologic status, nutritional status, bladder and bowel function, hygiene (including oral hygiene), skin integrity, rest and activity level, sleep patterns, and fluid and electrolyte balance. The AD patient's neurologic function is usually preserved through the early and middle stages of the disease, although seizures, gait disturbances, and tremors may occur at any time. In the later stages of the disease, neurologic signs, such as flexion contractures and primitive reflexes, are prominent features.

Physical Functions. At first, limitations may primarily involve instrumental activities, such as shopping, preparing meals, and performing other household chores. Later in the disease process, basic physical dysfunctions occur, such as incontinence, ataxia, dysphagia, and contractures (Seltzer et al., 1988). Incontinence can be a major source of stress and a considerable burden to family caregivers. Evaluation of the patient's functional abilities includes bathing, dressing, toileting, feeding, nutritional status, physical mobility, sleep patterns, and pain.

Assessment of physical functions includes activities of daily living, recent changes in functional abilities, use of sensory aids (glasses and hearing aids), activity level, and assessment of pain. Glasses and hearing aids may need to be in place before other assessments can be made.

NURSING CARE PLAN 31.1
Patient With Dementia

LW is a 76-year-old widow who lives independently. Recently, her children have noticed that she is becoming more forgetful and seems to have periods of confusion. She has agreed to having someone help her during the day. Her oldest son lives with her and is with her during the evening and night. LW refuses to see a health care provider but did agree to go in for a routine checkup. Her daughter helped her get dressed and took her to the primary care office.

SETTING: PRIMARY CARE OFFICE

Baseline Assessment: A well-groomed woman is accompanied by her daughter. LW says there is nothing wrong, but daughter disagrees. A review of body systems reveals poor hearing and vision but is otherwise unremarkable. MMSE score is 19. Daughter reports that LW has become very suspicious of neighbors and has changed her locks several times.

Associated Psychiatric Diagnosis	Medications

Axis I: Probable dementia of the Alzheimer's type
Axis II: None
Axis III: History of breast cancer, unilateral mastectomy
   Arthritis
Axis IV: Social problems (suspiciousness)
   GAF = Current 70
        Potential 70
	Galantamine (Reminyl) 4 mg bid, titrate to 8 mg
	   bid over 4 weeks.
	Consider risperidone 0.5–1 mg od, if psychotic
	   symptoms occur.

NURSING DIAGNOSIS 1: IMPAIRED MEMORY

Defining Characteristics	Related Factors
Inability to recall information Inability to recall past events Observed instances of forgetfulness Forgets to perform daily activities—grooming	Neurocognitive changes associated with dementia

OUTCOMES

Initial	Long-Term
Maintain or improve current memory	Delay cognitive decline associated with dementia

INTERVENTIONS

Interventions	Rationale	Ongoing Assessment
Develop memory cues in home. Have clocks and calendars well displayed. Make lists for patients. Teach patient and family about taking an acetylcholinesterase inhibitor. Review expected effects, side effects, and adverse effects. Develop a titration schedule with family to decrease the appearance of side effects.	Maintaining current level of memory involves providing cues that will help patient recall information. Confidence and self-esteem improve when a person looks well-groomed.	Contact family members for patient's ability to use memory cues. Monitor response to suggestions.
Observe patient for visuospatial impairment. If present, sequence habitual activities, such as eating, dressing, bathing, etc.	Visuospatial impairment is one of the symptoms of dementia.	Observe for appropriate dress, bathing, eating, etc.

NURSING CARE PLAN 31.1 (Continued)

EVALUATION

Outcomes	Revised Outcomes	Interventions
LW did have some improvement in memory. Suspiciousness and behavioral symptoms improved.	Continue maintaining memory.	Continue with memory cues and galantamine.

Self-Care. Alterations in the central nervous system (CNS) associated with dementia impair the patient's ability to collect information from the environment, retrieve memories, retain new information, and give meaning to current situations. Therefore, patients with dementia often neglect self-care activities. It is especially important to reevaluate periodically biologic assessment parameters because patients with dementia may neglect activities such as bathing, eating, or skin care.

Sleep–Wake Disturbances. The sleep-wake disturbances that commonly occur in dementia are hypersomnia, insomnia, and reversal of the sleep–wake cycle (see Chap. 26). These disturbances may be partly due to physiologic changes, neurotransmitters, or metabolic changes that occur as a result of a dementia-causing disease or injury, but they are often of environmental or iatrogenic origin. Patients with dementia have frequent daytime napping and nighttime periods of wakefulness, with little rapid eye movement (REM) sleep. Lowered levels of REM sleep are associated with restlessness, irritability, and general sleep impairment (Turner et al., 2000).

Activity and Exercise. One of the earliest symptoms of Alzheimer's is withdrawal from normal activities. The patient may just sit staring at a blank wall.

Nutrition. Eating can become a problem for a patient with dementia. As the disease progresses, patients may lose the ability to feed themselves or recognize what is offered as food. The hyperactive patient requires frequent feedings of a high-protein, high-carbohydrate diet in the form of finger foods (which they can carry while on the go). It may be wise to secure a fanny pack around the patient's waist with an assortment of nutritious finger foods appropriate for the patient who can no longer use eating utensils properly. Most patients with dementia prefer to feed themselves with their fingers rather than have someone feed them.

Some patients with dementia are bulimic or hyperoral (eating or chewing almost everything possible and sometimes with an insatiable appetite). In fact, some patients with advanced dementia put inedible objects into their mouths, presumably because they fail to recognize the objects as nonfood items. Other dementia patients develop anorexia and have no appetite. It is important to monitor patients with altered appetites for hydration and electrolyte imbalances. Maintenance of weight and proper hydration status are signs of effective nursing interventions with a dementia patient.

Pain. Assessment and documentation of any physical discomfort or pain the patient may be experiencing is a part of any geropsychiatric nursing assessment (see Chap. 12). Although AD is not usually thought of as a physically painful disorder, patients often have other comorbid physical diseases that may be painful. In the early stages of AD, the patient can usually respond to verbal questions regarding pain. Later, it is often difficult to assess objectively the comfort level, especially if the patient is noncommunicative. Some patients in the end stage of dementia become hypersensitive to touch.

Pain can be assessed by obtaining vital signs, completing a physical assessment, and using one of the pain assessment scales (see Chap. 12). Sometimes, laboratory tests must be conducted to help identify the source of discomfort. Subtle behavioral changes, such as lethargy, anxiety, or restlessness, or more obvious physical signs, such as pyrexia, tachypnea, or tachycardia, may be the only indications of actual or impending illness. Observing for changes in patterns of nonverbal communication, such as facial expressions, can help the nurse identify indicators of pain. Hypervocalizations (disturbed vocalizations), restlessness, and agitation are other signs that may indicate the presence of pain.

Nursing Diagnoses Related to Biologic Domain

The unique and changing needs of these patients present a challenge for nurses in all settings. A multitude of potential nursing diagnoses focusing on the biologic domain can be identified for this population. A sample of common nursing diagnoses include Imbalanced Nutrition: Less (or More) Than Body Requirements; Feeding Self-Care Deficit; Impaired Swallowing; Bathing/Hygiene Self-Care Deficit; Dressing/Grooming Self-Care Deficit; Toileting Self-Care Deficit; Constipation (or Perceived Constipation); Bowel Incontinence; Impaired Urinary Elimination; Functional Incontinence; Total Incontinence; Deficient Fluid Volume; Risk for

Impaired Skin Integrity; Impaired Physical Mobility; Activity Intolerance; Fatigue; Disturbed Sleep Pattern; Pain; Chronic Pain; Ineffective Health Maintenance; and Impaired Home Maintenance.

Biologic Interventions

The numerous interventions for the biologic domain vary throughout the course of the disorder. Initially, the patient requires simple directions for self-care activities and initiation of psychopharmacologic treatment. At the end of the disorder, total patient care is required.

Self-Care Interventions. Patients should be encouraged to maintain as much self-care as possible. Promotion of self-care supports cognitive functioning and a sense of independence. In the early stages, the nurse should maximize normal perceptual experiences by making sure that the patient and family have appropriate eyeglasses and working hearing aids. If eyeglasses and hearing aids are needed, but not used, patients are more likely to have false perceptual experiences (hallucinations). Monitoring changing levels of self-care is necessary and ongoing throughout the course of the disorder.

Oral hygiene can be a problem and requires excellent basic nursing care. Aging and many medications reduce salivary flow, which can lead to a painfully dry and cracking oral mucosa. Drugs that have *xerostomia* (dry mouth) as a side effect and are commonly prescribed for patients with progressive dementia include antidepressants, antispasmodics, antihypertensives, bronchodilators, and some antipsychotics. If xerostomia is present, hard candy or gum can be used to stimulate salivary flow, or modification of the drug regimen may be necessary. Glycerol mouthwash can provide as much symptomatic relief from xerostomia as artificial saliva.

Nutritional Interventions. Maintenance of nutrition and hydration are essential nursing interventions. The patient's weight, oral intake, and hydration status should be monitored carefully. Dementia patients should eat well-balanced meals that are appropriate to their activity level and eating abilities, with special attention given to electrolyte balance and fluid intake.

When swallowing is a problem for the patient, thick liquids or semisoft foods are more effective than traditionally prepared foods. If a patient is prone to choke or aspirate food, less liquid (pureed) and more semisolid foods should be included in the diet because liquid flows into the pharyngeal cavity quicker than solid food. It may also benefit the patient to consume less milk-based foods because these foods may increase respiratory mucus.

The dining environment should be calm and food presentation appealing. If the patient eats only a small portion of food at one meal, reduce the presentation of food in terms of the amount and number of choices. One-dish meals, such as a casserole, are ideal for the dementia patient. If the patient is stressed or upset, it is better to delay feeding because eating,

chewing, and swallowing difficulties are accentuated (Research Box 31-1).

As dementia progresses, intensive feeding efforts are needed to ensure adequate food and fluid intake. If food intake is low, vitamin and mineral supplements may be indicated. If weight loss cannot be stopped by skillful feeding or dietary adjustments, then enteral or parenteral feedings may be considered. The patient's quality of life is an important issue to consider when the family or other health care proxy must decide whether to use artificial feeding mechanisms. By inserting a feeding tube, the goal of sustaining weight can be met, but patient comfort may be jeopardized, especially if restraints are used to keep the tube in place.

The dementia patient should be presented food that is of proper temperature and easy to chew (soft) and swallow. In the later stages of progressive dementia, some patients hoard food in their mouths without actually swallowing it; others swallow too rapidly or fail to chew their food sufficiently before attempting to swallow. The nurse is cautioned to observe for swallowing difficulties that place the demented patient at risk for aspiration and asphyxiation. Problems in swallowing may be a result of changes in esophageal motility and decreased secretion of saliva.

RESEARCH BOX 31.1

Quality of Mealtime Experience for Nursing Home Residents

One of the most basic nursing actions is nutritional care. Many nursing home residents are malnourished and suffer inadequate intake and weight loss. Consequently, residents are often fed by direct care staff who may find the task of feeding patients routine. The purpose of this study was to determine whether the quality of interaction between staff and patient made a difference in the quality of the mealtime experience and patient's nutritional status. The interaction between caregivers and patients were observed for 12 months. Caregiver behavior was either task-driven and mechanistic or empathic and creative. Those patients whose caregivers were empathic and creative during mealtime had a better experience and nutritional status than those who were fed in a mechanistic manner.

Utilization in Clinical Setting: Common sense says that the more pleasant the meal experience, the more an individual will eat. This study supports that common sense notion. For nurses, this study provides support for a creative approach to feeding patients. Empathy really does make a difference in physical outcomes.

Schell, E. S., & Kayser-Jones, J. (1999). The effect of role-taking ability on caregiver-resident mealtime interaction. *Applied Nursing Research, 12,* 38–44.

Interventions Supporting Bowel and Bladder Function. Urinary or bowel incontinence occurs in many patients with dementia. During middle phases of the disease, incontinence may be caused by the patient's inability to communicate the need to use the toilet; to locate a toilet quickly; to undress appropriately to use the toilet; to recognize the sensation of fullness indicating the need to micturate or defecate; or to apathy with lack of motivation to remain continent. Later in the disease process, incontinence is thought to be related to cortical damage (Alzheimer's Association, 1995).

For the patient who is incontinent because of an inability to locate the toilet, orientation may be helpful. Signs and active training should help to modify disorientation in elderly patients. Displaying pictures or signs on bathroom doors provides visual cues; words should use appropriate terminology.

If the patient is unable to recognize the need to void because of a loss of sensory perception of fullness, increasing fluid intake can help to fill the bladder sufficiently to give a clear message of the need to urinate. Also, getting to know the patient's habits and moods can help the nurse to identify signals that indicate a need to void. The patient can then be assisted to reach the bathroom in time. Placing the patient near the toilet or supplying a commode nearby may help if the patient is incontinent because of an inability to reach the toilet in time. If the patient demonstrates dressing apraxia (cannot undress appropriately), clothing can be modified with easy-to-open fasteners in place of zippers or buttons. Urinating in inappropriate locations can be controlled by carefully assessing the patient's voiding pattern and then taking the patient to the toilet at appropriate intervals. Once brought into the bathroom, many patients void appropriately, although some may need further reminding and gentle assistance. For nocturnal incontinence, other strategies may be effective. Limiting the amount of fluid consumed after the evening meal and taking the patient to the toilet just before going to bed or upon awakening during the night should reduce or eliminate nocturia.

Indwelling urinary catheters are contraindicated in patients with dementia because they are generally not well tolerated and because hand restraints are often used to prevent them from removing the catheter. Additionally, indwelling urinary catheters foster the development of urinary tract infections and may compromise the patient's dignity and comfort. Urinary incontinence can be managed with the use of disposable, adult-sized diapers that must be checked regularly and changed expeditiously when soiled.

Dementia patients often experience constipation, although they may not be able to tell the nurse about changes in bowel activity; therefore, subtle signs such as lethargy, reduced appetite, and abdominal distention need to be assessed frequently. Medications, decreased food and liquid intake, lack of motor activity, and decreased intestinal motility contribute to the development of constipation. Patients should be given a diet high in fiber, including bran or whole grains, vegetables, and fruit. Adequate oral intake (minimum of 1,500 to 2,000 mL/d) helps to prevent constipation. A gentle laxative such as milk of magnesia (1 to 2 tablespoons every other evening) is commonly used to promote bowel elimination. Enemas and harsher chemical cathartics should be avoided because they may increase pain or discomfort. Care must be taken to ensure that the patient does not become dehydrated in the process of treating constipation.

Sleep Interventions. Disturbed sleep cycles are particularly stressful to both family caregivers and nursing staff. Not only is disturbed sleep difficult to manage from a behavioral perspective, but also the patient's overall level of health may suffer because sleep serves a restorative function. Sedative-hypnotics may be prescribed for a short time for restlessness or insomnia but may cause a paradoxic reaction of agitation and insomnia (especially in elderly patients).

Sleep hygiene interventions discussed in Chapter 26 are appropriate for dementia patients, although morning and afternoon naps (or rest periods for patients who do not nap) may be the most effective intervention for a dementia patient with altered diurnal rhythms. Morning naps are likely to produce REM sleep patterns and may help patients who are restless from a loss of REM sleep, whereas afternoon naps produce deep sleep and are suitable for restlessness associated with fatigue. Rest periods (in reclining chairs) in the morning and afternoon may help to eliminate late-day confusion (sundowning) and night awakenings (Hall et al., 1995).

Activity and Exercise Interventions. Activity and exercise are important nursing interventions for patients with dementia. To promote a feeling of success, any activity or exercise plan must be culturally sensitive and adapted to the patient's functional ability and interests. The activity or exercise must be designed to prevent excess stress (both physical and psychological), which means that it must be individualized for each patient with dementia, based on their relative strengths and deficits. If the program of rest, activity, and exercise is truly individualized, the resultant feelings of value and competency will enhance the patient's morale and self-esteem.

Pain and Comfort Management. Nursing care of noncommunicative dementia patients in pain can be challenging because of the difficulty in identifying and monitoring the pain. Consequently, patients with dementia who are experiencing pain are often undertreated (see Chap. 12). There must be several measures by which the efficacy of pharmacologic interventions are determined, such as improvement in restlessness and decreased agitation. Small doses of oral morphine solution appear to reduce discomfort during routine nursing procedures. If used in small doses (5 to 10 mg every 4 to 6 hours), morphine does not cause substantial respiratory depression, vomiting, or tolerance (Volicer, 1988). The main side effect of morphine is constipation.

Relaxation. Approaching patients in a calm, confident, unhurried manner; maintaining a soothing, quiet environment; avoiding unnecessary noise or chatter around patients and lowering vocal tone and rate when addressing them; maintaining eye contact; and using touch judiciously are likely to promote a sense of security conducive to patient relaxation and comfort. Simple relaxation techniques can be used to reduce stress. These exercises should be done with the patient.

Pharmacologic Interventions. Because there is no medication that will cure AD, psychopharmacologic interventions have two goals: (1) restoration or maintenance of cognitive function, and (2) treatment of related psychiatric and behavioral disturbances that cause discomfort for the individual, interfere with treatment, or worsen the individual's cognitive status. Medications for AD must used with caution. Doses must be kept extremely low, and individuals should be monitored closely for the appearance of any side effects or worsening of cognitive status. "Start low and go slow" is the principle guiding the administration of psychopharmacologic agents in elderly patients.

Administration and Monitoring Medications. Often, convincing the patient to take the medication is one of the biggest nursing challenges. Patients may be unwilling, even though they previously agreed to take the drugs. The nurse will need to investigate and hypothesize the reason for the reluctance to take medication. It may be because of difficulty swallowing pills, paranoid ideas, or lack of understanding. The underlying reason for medication refusal will determine the strategy. If the patient has difficulty swallowing, most medications come in concentrate liquid form and can be easily swallowed. Some medication can also be mixed in food. If suspicion or paranoia is the reason, the nurse will need to try to identify the conditions under which the patient feels safe to take the medication, such as for a favorite nurse or relative.

Cholinesterase Inhibitors. **Acetylcholinesterase** (AChE) is the key enzyme that inactivates the neurotransmitter acetylcholine. AChE is found in high concentrations in the brain and is one of two cholinesterase enzymes capable of breaking down ACh. **Butyrylcholinesterase** (BuChE), a nonspecific cholinesterase, is also found in the brain, but especially in the glial cells.

Both AChE and BuChE work in the gastrointestinal tract. If these enzymes are inhibited, the destruction of ACh will be delayed, resulting in an increase in ACh activity. The increase in ACh activity helps maintain cognitive functioning and delay its decline. **Acetylcholinesterase inhibitors** (AChEI) are the mainstay of pharmacologic treatment of dementia because they inhibit AChE, resulting in an enhancement of cholinergic activity. Because these medications have been shown to delay the decline in cognitive functioning, but generally do not improve cognitive function once it has declined, it is important that this medication be started as soon as the diagnosis is made. The primary side effect of these medications is gastrointestinal distress—nausea, vomiting, and diarrhea.

The first AChEI approved by the U.S. Food and Drug Administration for use in the treatment of mild to moderate AD in 1992 was tacrine hydrochloride (Cognex). Although Cognex does increase ACh levels, it inhibits both AChE and BuChE. The side effects are problematic because there is considerable gastrointestinal distress, and liver enzymes are elevated in 50% of patients. Cognex is administered 2 to 3 times throughout the day and has to given between meals for maximum absorption.

In late 1996, the second-generation medications were launched with the approval of donepezil HCl (Aricept), a specific and potent AChEI that has demonstrated modest efficacy in tests of global functioning and cognition (Tariot et al., 1997). Donepezil differs from tacrine in that it does not inhibit BuChE and has a much better side-effect profile. Donepezil can be given twice a day. The second-generation medications are longer acting than tacrine and have greater selectivity and fewer side effects. Two other AChEIs have since been approved: rivastigmine (Exelon) in 2000 and galantamine (Reminyl) in 2001. Rivastigmine inhibits both cholinesterase enzymes, AChE and BuChE. Galantamine is selective to AChE and does not inhibit BuChE. Galantamine is unique in that it acts as modulator to the nicotinic receptor, causing a boost in the release of ACh and other neurotransmitters. See Drug Profile: Galantamine Hydrobromide.

The cholinesterase inhibitors are oral medications usually taken once or twice a day. The most frequent side effects are nausea and diarrhea. If the patient is suspicious or paranoid, the most difficult aspect in administering the drug is convincing the patient to take it. The earlier in the disease process these medications are initiated, the more likely they will delay cognitive decline.

There are no special monitors for these medications. With cholinesterase inhibitors, patients should not be taking any anticholinergic medication.

Antipsychotics. Antipsychotics are often effective in reducing psychosis, agitation, or aggressive behaviors that are frequently present in the moderate to severe

---

DRUG PROFILE: Galantamine Hydrobromide
(Acetylcholinesterase inhibitor)
Trade Name: Reminyl

Receptor affinity: Competitive and reversible inhibitor of acetylcholinesterase (AChE); modulates the acetylcholine nicotinic receptors.
Indications: For mild to moderate dementia in Alzheimer's dementia.
Routes and dosage: Available in 4-mg, 8-mg, 12-mg tablets. Start with low dose 4-mg bid for at least 4 weeks. May increase to 8- to 12-mg bid.
   Dose titration recommended. Dose increases should follow minimum of 4 weeks at prior dose.
   If medication interrupted for several days, patient should be restarted at lowest dose and escalate up.
Half-life (peak effect): Half life is 7 hours; peak effect in 1 hour.
Select adverse reactions: Initially, nausea, vomiting may occur. Tends to decrease over time.

Warning: Can affect the ability to drive or operate machinery. A lower dose may be prescribed if taking antidepressants, paroxetine, quinidine, ketoconazole, or ritonavir. Should not be used in patients with severe liver impairment.
Specific patient/family education:
- Take medication as prescribed, usually twice a day, preferably with meals.
- If gastrointestinal upset occurs, take with meals.
- Do not abruptly discontinue drug (positive effects will be lost).
- Report any signs and symptoms of adverse effects.
- Use caution if driving or performing tasks that require alertness if dizziness, confusion, or lightheadedness occurs.

---

stages of AD. With the introduction of the atypical antipsychotics, the use of conventional antipsychotics, such as haloperidol, in elderly patients immediately declined. Risperidone, quetiapine, and olanzapine have all been studied in elderly patients. Clozaril is not prescribed as a front-line agent because of its side-effect profile.

When using atypical antipsychotics in elderly patients, the dosage should be much lower than in younger adults. These medications can usually be given once a day, except for quetiapine, which has a shorter half-life than the others. It is also important for the nurse to monitor side effects of these medications and recognize that their side effects are different from each other (see Chap. 8).

Antidepressants and Mood Stabilizers. A depressed mood is common in patients with dementia. Depressed dementia patients often respond to psychotherapeutic intervention alone (individual or group therapy) or in combination with pharmacotherapy. Low doses of the selective serotonin reuptake inhibitors and other newer antidepressive agents should be considered.

Antianxiety Medications (Sedative-Hypnotics). Hypnotics and sedatives should be used with caution in elderly patients. If used, these medications should be administered on a short-term basis. For example, during a crisis, the use of an antianxiety medication may be considered. Ideally, the patient should try a nonbenzodiazepine before being prescribed a benzodiazepine. In elderly people, the benzodiazepines can cause a paradoxic reaction.

Other Medication Issues. Additionally, clinical observations indicate that elderly patients with defects in the cholinergic system are more vulnerable to the effects of anticholinergic drugs that can cause confusion and amnesia. Anticholinergic medications should be avoided in patients with AD if at all possible. See Table 31-6 for examples of medications that are commonly prescribed in elderly patients, all of which have been shown to have anticholinergic receptor activity.

Other Somatic Interventions. Restorative therapy is used to enhance the survival and function of neurons that are prone to degeneration in AD. One of the most direct ways to restore neuronal function is the administration of neurotrophins (neuron nourishment). Nerve growth factor is the best characterized neurotrophin and, because of its action on cholinergic cells, is the most relevant to AD. Most of the ACh in the cerebral cortex and hippocampus comes from cholinergic cells located in the ventral forebrain. Cholinergic forebrain neurons degenerate early in the course of AD and are also highly responsive to nerve growth factor (Growdon, 1992).

TABLE 31.6 Medications With Anticholinergic Effects

Commonly prescribed in the elderly
- Cimetidine
- Ranitidine
- Prednisolone
- Theophylline
- Warfarin
- Dipyridamole
- Codeine
- Nifedipine
- Isosorbide
- Digoxin
- Furosemide
- Triamterene and hydrochlorothiazide
- Captopril

Tune, L., Carr, S., Hoag, E., Cooper, T. (1992). Anticholinergic effects of drugs commonly prescribed for the elderly: Potential means for assessing risk of delirium. *Am J Psychiatry, 149,* 1393–1394.

Psychological Domain

Psychological Assessment

Responses to Mental Health Problems. Personality changes almost always accompany dementia and can take the form of either an accentuation or a marked alteration of a patient's previous lifelong character traits. The neural substrates underlying personality change in AD are not understood, but researchers have identified two contrasting patterns. One is marked by apathy, lack of spontaneity, and passivity. The other involves growing irritability, sarcasm, self-preoccupation, and intolerance of and lack of concern for others. Assessment of the psychological domain includes sexuality and spirituality.

Cognitive Status. The mental status should always be assessed and can follow the process suggested in Chapter 12. The MMSE continues to be used, but there are other tools that can be administered. The Cognitive Abilities Screening Instrument was discussed is Chapter 12.

Cognitive disturbance is the clinical hallmark of dementia. Intellectual status of the patient is usually assessed by the traditional, neurologically oriented mental status assessment. If cognitive deterioration occurs rapidly, delirium should be suspected. The pa-tient should be quickly evaluated by a physician because the presence of delirium calls for immediate attention to diagnose and treat the underlying cause (Text Box 31-7).

Memory. The most dramatic and consistent cognitive impairment is in memory. These patients appear mildly forgetful and repetitive in conversation. They misplace objects, miss appointments, and forget what they were just doing. They may loose track of a conversation or television story. Initially, they may complain of memory problems, but rapidly in the course of the illness, insight is lost and they become unaware of what is lost. Sometimes, they may confabulate, making what appears to be an appropriate explanation of why the information or object is missing. Eventually, all aspects of memory are impaired, and even long-term memories are affected. During the interview, short-term memory loss is usually readily evident by the patient's inability to recall three or four words given to him or her at the beginning of the assessment. Often, the earliest symptom of AD is the inability to retain new information.

Language. Language is also progressively impaired. Individuals with AD may initially have agnosia, difficulty finding a word in a sentence or in naming an object.

TEXT BOX 31.7

Rating Scales for Use With Dementia

Mental Status Questionnaires

Mini-Mental State Examination
Folstein, M. F., Folstein, S. E., & McHugh, P. R. (1975). "Mini mental state" a practical method for grading the cognitive state of patients for the clinician. *Journal of Psychiatric Research, 12,* 189–198. See Chap. 10.

Dementia Rating Scale
Mattis, S. (1976). Mental status examination for organic mental syndrome in the elderly patient. In L. Bellak & T. B. Karasu (Eds.), *Geriatric psychiatry: A handbook for psychiatrists and primary care physicians* (pp. 79–121). New York: Grune & Stratton.

Cognitive Abilities Screening Instrument (CASI)
Teng, E. L., Hasegawa, K., Homma, A., et al. (1994). The cognitive abilities screening instrument (CASI): A practical test for cross-cultural epidemiological studies of dementia. *International Psychogeriatrics, 6,* 45–58.

Short Portable Mental Status Questionnaire
Pfeiffer, E. (1975). A short portable mental status questionnaire for the assessment of organic brain deficit in elderly patients. *Journal of the American Geriatrics Society, 23,* 433–441.

Information–Memory–Concentration
Mental Status Questionnaire
Blessed, G., Tomlinson, B. E., & Roth, M. (1968). The association between quantitative measures of dementia and of senile changes in the cerebral grey matter of elderly patients. *British Journal of Psychiatry, 114,* 797–911.

Combination of Cognitive and Functional Assessment

Brief Cognitive Rating Scale
Reisberg, B., Schneck, M. K., & Ferris, S. H. (1983). The brief cognitive rating scale (BCRS): Findings in primary degenerative dementia. *Psychopharmacology Bulletin, 19,* 47–50.

Includes five scales: concentration, recent memory, remote memory, orientation, and functioning and self-care.

Alzheimer's Disease Assessment Scale
Rosen, W. G., Mohs, R. C., & Davis, K. L. (1984). A new rating scale for Alzheimer's disease. *American Journal of Psychiatry, 141,* 1256–1364.

Includes 21 items in the cognitive section and 10 items that are noncognitive, such as mood, appetite, delusions, and pacing.

Ratings Scales for Relatives

Geriatric Evaluation by Relatives Rating Scale Instrument (GERRI)
Schwartz, G. E. (1983). Development and validation of the Geriatric Evaluation by Relatives Rating Instrument (GERRI). *Psychological Reports, 53,* 478–488.

They may be able to talk around it, but the loss is noticeable. Later, fluent aphasia develops, comprehension diminishes, and, finally, they become mute and unresponsive to directions or information.

Visuospatial Impairment. Deficits in visuospatial tasks that require sensory and motor coordination develop early, drawing is abnormal, and ability to write may change. Inaccurate drawings on the MMSE or clock drawings (see Chap. 12) is diagnostic of impairment in this area. Sequencing tasks, such as cooking or other self-care skills, become impaired. The individual becomes unable to complete complex tasks that require calculations, such as balancing the check book.

Executive Functioning. Judgment, reasoning, and the ability to problem solve or make decisions are also impaired later in the disorder, closer to the time of nursing home placement. It is hypothesized that as the disease progresses, the degeneration of neurons is spread diffusely throughout the neocortex.

Psychotic Symptoms. Delusional thought content and hallucinations are common in people with dementia. These psychotic symptoms differ from those of schizophrenia.

Suspiciousness and Delusion and Illusion Formation. During the early and middle stages of dementia, many patients are aware of their cognitive losses and compensate with hyperalertness. In a hyperalert state, one becomes aware of many environmental stimuli that are not readily understood. Suspiciousness is a variant of the hyperalert or hypervigilant state in which stimuli are interpreted as dangerous. **Illusions,** or mistaken perceptions, also occur commonly in dementia patients. For example, a woman with dementia mistakes her husband for her father. He resembles her father in that he is roughly her father's age when he was last alive. If an illusion becomes a false fixed belief, it is a delusion.

As the disease progresses, delusions develop in 34% to 50% of the people with dementia. These characteristic delusions are different from those discussed in the psychotic disorders. Common delusional beliefs include the following:

- Belief that his or her spouse is engaging in marital infidelity
- Belief that other patients or staff are trying to hurt him or her
- Belief that staff or family members are impersonators
- Belief that people are stealing his or her belongings
- Belief that strangers are living in his or her home
- Belief that people on television are real

Hallucinations. Hallucinations frequently occur in dementia and are often visual or tactile in nature (but can also be auditory, gustatory, or olfactory). Unlike in schizophrenia, visual hallucinations (not auditory) are the most common in dementia. A frequent complaint is that children, adults, or strange creatures are entering the house or the patient's room. These hallucinations may not seem unusual to the patient. If possible, the content and form of hallucination should be ascertained because this information may suggest a treatable disorder. For example, auditory hallucinations commanding patients to kill themselves may be caused by a treatable depression, not the dementia. Often, hallucinations in dementia are pleasant, such as children being in the room. These individuals may conduct conversations with nobody in particular. Hallucinations may also be frightening or uncomfortable for patients.

Mood Changes

Depression. Recognition of coexisting (and often treatable) psychiatric disorders in patients with dementia is often ignored. A depressed mood is common and is reported in 40% to 50% of AD cases. A diagnosis of major depression is less frequent, occurring in 10% to 20% of AD patients. A number of people with AD develop one or more depressive episodes with symptoms such as psychomotor retardation, anxiety, feelings of guilt and worthlessness, sadness, frequent crying, insomnia, loss of appetite, weight loss, and suicidal rumination. Depressive symptoms are most prevalent in the early stages of dementia, which may be attributed to the patient's awareness of cognitive changes, memory loss, and functional decline. However, dysphoric symptoms can occur at any stage, even in the most disoriented elderly patients. In more advanced stages of dementia, assessment of depression depends more on changes in behavior than on verbal complaints (Alexopoulos & Abrams, 1991).

Anxiety. Symptoms of anxiety develop in a high proportion of demented and nondemented geriatric patients with major depression (Alexopoulos, 1991). Therefore, it is important to assess a demented patient for depression when signs of anxiety are present. Moderate anxiety is a natural reaction to the fear engendered by gradual deterioration of intellectual function and the realization of impending loss of control over one's life. Failure to complete a task once regarded as simple creates a source of anxiety in the AD patient. As patients with AD become unsure of their surroundings and the expectations of others, they frequently react with fear and distress. It is thought that anxious behavior occurs when the patient is pressed to perform beyond his or her ability.

Catastrophic Reactions. **Catastrophic reactions** are overreactions or extreme anxiety reactions to everyday situations. Catastrophic responses occur when environmental stressors are allowed to continue or increase beyond the patient's threshold of stress tolerance. Behaviors indicative of catastrophic reactions typically include verbal or physical aggression, violence, agitated or anxious behavior, emotional outbursts, noisy behavior, compulsive or repetitive behavior, agitated night awakening, and other behaviors in which the patient is cognitively or socially inaccessible. Factors that contribute to catastrophic responses in patients with progressive cognitive decline include fatigue, change in routine (pace or caregiver), demands beyond the patient's ability, overwhelming sensory stimuli, and physical stressors, such as pain or hunger (Hall, 1988a).

Behavioral Responses

Apathy and Withdrawal. Apathy, the inability or unwillingness to become involved with one's environment, is common in AD, especially during the moderate to later stages. Apathy leads to withdrawal from the environment and a gradual loss of empathy for others. The lack of empathy is very difficult for families and friends to understand. In a study comparing the prevalence of symptoms of those with dementia ($n = 329$) and those with no dementia ($n = 629$), the most prevalent symptom (27.4%) of those with dementia was apathy (no dementia, 3.1%). (Lyketsos et al., 2000).

Restlessness, Agitation, and Aggression. Restlessness, agitation, and aggression are relatively common in moderate to later stages of dementia (Lyketsos et al., 2000). Restlessness should be further evaluated to determine its underlying cause. If the restlessness occurs during medication change or adjustment, side effects should be suspected.

Agitation and aggressive physical contacts are among the most dangerous behavior management problems encountered in any setting. They often result in placement of a family member in a nursing home. Careful evaluation of the antecedents leading up to the behavior enable the nurse to plan nursing care that prevents future occurrences.

Aberrant Motor Behavior. Symptoms such as fidgeting, picking at clothing, wringing hands, loud vocalizations, and wandering may all be signs of such underlying conditions as dehydration, medication reaction, pain, or infection (suggesting delirium). One of the most difficult behaviors for which to determine an underlying cause is **hypervocalization,** the screams, curses, moans, groans, and verbal repetitiveness that are common in the later stages of cognitively impaired elderly patients, often occurring during a hospitalization or nursing home placement. In the assessment of these hypervocalizations, it is important to identify when the behavior is occurring, antecedents of the behavior, and any related events, such as a family member leaving or a change in stimulation.

Disinhibition. One of the most frustrating symptoms of AD is **disinhibition,** acting on thoughts and feelings without exercising appropriate social judgment. In AD, the patient may decide that he or she is more comfortable naked than with clothes. Or the patient may not be able to find his or her clothes and may walk into a room of people without any clothes on. This behavior is extremely disconcerting to family members and can also lead to nursing home placement.

Hypersexuality. A closely related symptom is **hypersexuality,** inappropriate and socially unacceptable sexual behavior. The patient begins talking and behaving in ways that are uncharacteristic of premorbid behavior. This behavior is very difficult for family members and nursing home staff.

Stress and Coping Skills. Patients with dementia seem extremely sensitive to stressful situations and often do not have the coping abilities to deal with the situation. The Behavioral Assessment for Low Stimulus Care Plan (BALSCP) is an instrument used to assess for behavioral manifestations of dementia and to determine whether patients would benefit from a low-stimulus environment and plan of care (Hall, 1988b). Use of the BALSCP to assess the patient's baseline behaviors assists the nurse when evaluating outcomes of specific nursing interventions (Text Box 31-8).

Nursing Diagnoses Related to Psychological Domain

A multitude of potential nursing diagnoses can be identified for the psychological domain of this population. A sample of common nursing diagnoses includes Impaired Memory; Disturbed Thought Processes; Chronic Confusion; Disturbed Sensory Perception; Impaired Environmental Interpretation Syndrome; Risk for Violence: Self-Directed or Directed at Others; Risk for Loneliness; Risk for Caregiver Role Strain; Ineffective Sexuality Patterns; Ineffective Individual Coping; Hopelessness; and Powerlessness (NANDA, 2001).

Psychological Interventions

The therapeutic relationship is the basis for interventions for the patient and family with dementia. Care of the patient entails a long-term relationship needing much support and expert nursing care. Interventions should be delivered within the relationship context (Research Box 31-2).

Interventions for Cognitive Impairment

Validation Therapy. Validation therapy (VT) emerged in the 1970s as a method for communicating with patients with AD. It was developed as a contrast to reality therapy, which attempted to provide a here-and-now, factual focus to the interaction. VT focuses on the emotions and subjective reality of the patients. In VT, the nurse does not try to reorient the patient, but rather respects the individual's sense of reality (Day, 1997). VT is a useful model for nursing care of the patient with dementia.

(text continues on page 843)

TEXT BOX 31.8

Behavioral Assessment for Low Stimulus Care Plan

Directions: This form will assist nursing staff in evaluating patients for potential cognitive decline or need for a low-stimulus environment. The following behaviors are associated with progressive dementing illness and are indicative of general cognitive decline.

Check off the following behaviors that you have observed in your patient or have been reported by staff or family members. Award 1 point for each reported behavior and 2 additional points for behaviors you directly observe. Place the total sum obtained on each symptom cluster where indicated. If the patient accumulates 2 points in the "Progressively Lowered Stress Threshold" category or 6 more points in either the cognitive, conative, or affective categories, the patient should be considered for dementia evaluation, and a lowered stimulus care plan should be implemented. All positive scores should be recorded in the patient's health care record.

DATE: _____

I. Progressively Lowered Stress Threshold

                                 Cluster Total___

    1. Catastrophic Behaviors . . . . ___
        A. Becomes confused
        B. Becomes agitated
        C. Wakes up confused at night
        D. Has panic attacks
        E. Becomes violent or combative
        F. Sudden psychotic symptoms
        G. "Sundowning behaviors" such as late-day confusion
        H. Fearful behavior
        I. Purposeful wandering to get away from environment
        J. Packs to leave dwelling

    2. Purposeless Behavior . . . . ___
        A. Purposeless wandering, touching everything
        B. Continuous sorting through objects
        C. Daytime sleeping other than nap time
        D. Staring into space
        E. Fantasy behavior such as carrying briefcase, dolls, stuffed animals; or patients stating they are at a place other than where they really are
        F. Purposeless conversation to others or no person in particular

    3. Avoidance of stimuli . . . . ___
        A. Refusal to participate (in activity, care, etc)
        B. Avoidance of potentially misleading stimuli, such as TV, radios, social gatherings

II. Conative (planning) and Functional Losses

                                   Cluster Total___

    1. Starts activity, wanders away . . . . ___
    2. Starts activity, becomes confused (mixed up).. ___
    3. Starts activity, becomes frustrated . . . . ___
    4. Refuses to start activity . . . . ___
    5. Unable to initiate activities but can perform once started . . . . ___
    6. Is confused or loses function if daily routine is changed . . . . ___
    7. Incontinent . . . . ___
    8. Motor apraxia . . . . ___
        A. Gait disturbances
        B. Problems with sitting or standing
        C. Becomes "frozen" when walking
        D. Rigidity
    9. Unable to plan day . . . . ___
   10. Unable to plan events . . . . ___
   11. Any sign of decline in function in . . . . ___
        A. Money management
        B. Legal affairs
        C. Shopping
        D. Transportation
        E. Housecleaning
        F. Home maintenance
        G. Bathing
        H. Choosing clothing or dressing
        I. Cooking

III. Cognitive Losses   Cluster Total___

    1. Loss of Memory . . . . ___
        A. Difficulty remembering recent events
        B. Distorts past events
        C. Difficulty remembering past events
        D. Asks same question repeatedly
        E. Misses appointments

    2. Loss of sense of time . . . . ___
        A. Repeatedly asks what time or day it is
        B. Preoccupied with a coming event as to when it will occur
        C. Dresses or prepares for appointments or events early
        D. Confuses day with night, or time of day
        E. Obvious confusion over time of past events (occurred 1 week or 1 year ago)

    3. Inability to use abstract thought . . . . ___
        A. Inability to calculate checkbook
        B. Inability to respond to reasoning or explanations
        C. Lack of concern for safety
        D. Inability to problem solve

TEXT BOX 31.8 (*Continued*)

4. Inability to make choices or decisions . . . . . ___

   A. Cooks same food for dinner repeatedly

   B. Wears same clothing for days

   C. Asks others what to order when in restaurant

   D. Defers most choices to others

   E. Defers answers to direct questions to others (family members)

5. Poor judgment . . . . ___

   A. Has problems with financial matters

   B. Has legal problems

   C. Has made unusually large or inappropriate purchases

   D. Dresses inappropriately for weather

   E. Drives unsafely, refuses to stop

   F. Refuses to pay bills

   G. Eats spoiled food

   H. Sweeps, rakes leaves, mows grass, or performs similar task for hours and despite completion, inclement weather, or other cues to stop

   I. Unrealistic about limitations and abilities

6. Loss of language ability . . . . ___

   A. Unable to read or comprehend writing

   B. Has word-finding difficulties or substitutes inappropriate word

   C. Does not initiate conversation in social situations

7. Attempts to compensate for losses . . . . ___

   A. Defers judgments, decisions, questions to others

   B. Keeps lists, calendars

   C. Becomes increasingly secretive

   D. Makes statements such as "I think I'm going crazy," "I think I'm losing my mind," "something is wrong with my (head, memory, mind)"

IV. Affective Losses   Cluster Total___

   1. Loss of affect . . . . ___

      A. Loss of "sparkle" (bland facial expression)

      B. Loss of sense of humor

      C. Loss of spontaneity

      D. Loss of personality, increasingly dull affect

      E. Loss of quickness, slow to respond to environment or in social situations

   2. Inability to inhibit . . . . ___

      A. Emotionally labile, quick to anger or cry

      B. Makes spontaneous or inappropriate remarks

      C. Displays disinhibited behavior, such as public undressing, or making socially inappropriate comments

   D. Lack of patience

   E. Negative personality traits intensify or become dominant, person is "more" of who they have always been

   F. Increase in temper over increasingly trivial things

3. Social withdrawal . . . . ___

   A. Withdraws from past social groups

   B. Prefers to stay at home

   C. Leaves or requests to leave social gatherings early

   D. Leaves dinner table early or abruptly

   E. Quits club or social organizations

   F. Avoids large groups, such as day room activities

   G. Intolerant or becomes upset after multiple or high-stimulus activities

4. Self-preoccupation . . . . ___

   A. Apparent selfishness

   B. Apparent lack of concern or ability to understand needs of others, including spouse

   C. Need for immediate gratification (food, activity, toileting)

   D. Withdrawal from family group

   E. Appears to withdraw into self or become seclusive or even reclusive

   F. Develops preoccupation with bodily functions, such as bowels, toileting, pain, food consumption, fear of gaining weight, or constant eating

5. Psychotic manifestations . . . . ___

   A. Paranoia, making accusations

   B. Hallucinations or delusion

   C. Distorted perceptions of environmental stimuli such as thinking TV pictures or situations are real, misinterpreting pictures, or mirror images (illusions)

6. Loss of recognition of people . . . . ___

   A. Friends

   B. Family

   C. Self in mirror

7. Antisocial behavior . . . . ___

   A. Loss of social graces

   B. Family complains of being embarrassed

   C. Inappropriate use of everyday objects, such as stuffing objects into toilet, taking down drapes, or ingesting cleaning fluids

   D. Smearing food or body waste

   E. Yelling or screaming

Hall, G. R. (1988). *Behavioral assessment of low stimulus care plan.* Unpublished manuscript. The University of Iowa Hospitals and Clinics, Department of Nursing, Iowa City, IA. Reprinted by permission.

RESEARCH BOX 31.2

Therapeutic Relationship in the Later Stages of Alzheimer's Disease

This study explored the possibility of developing a therapeutic relationship with individuals in the later stages of Alzheimer's disease. Forty-two nursing home residents with Alzheimer's disease ranging in age from 76 to 103 years (mean age, 87 years), primarily female (83%), with an MMSE ranging from 0 to 18 agreed to participate in the study. Advance practice nurses met with participants three times a week for 16 weeks. Sessions were recorded during weeks 1, 8, and 16. Each nurse entered the relationship with the participant with the expectation and willingness to establish a meaningful relationship. Nurses initiated the conversations but followed participants' lead if they raised a topic of interest or concern. The nurses did not use life review, reality orientation, or validation ap-

proaches during the sessions but tried to make the discussions as meaningful as possible. Narrative analysis was used to identify evidence of the development of a therapeutic relationship. The results indicated that there were evident patterns in the way participants behaved at different stages of the relationship. The results challenge the assumption that therapeutic work with moderate to severely impaired patients is impossible or futile.

Utilization in the Clinical Setting: Nursing care for patients with moderate to severe Alzheimer's disease should include the use of the therapeutic relationship. Through this relationship, nurses likely will be able to recognize depression, anxiety, and pain.

Williams, C., & Tappen, R. (1999). Can we create a therapeutic relationship with nursing home residents in the later stages of Alzheimer's Disease? *Journal of Psychosocial Nursing, 37*(3), 28–35.

Memory Enhancement. Interventions for progressive memory impairment should always be a part of the treatment plan. The sooner patients are placed on AChE inhibitors, the slower the cognitive decline. However, pharmacologic agents are only a small part of the intervention picture. The nursing goal is to maintain memory functioning as long as possible. The nurse should make a concerted effort to reinforce short- and long-term memory. For example, reminding patients what they had for breakfast, which activity was just completed, or who were their visitors a few hours ago will reinforce their short-term memory. For long-term memory, encouraging patients to tell the stories of their earlier years will help bring these memories into focus. In the earlier stages, there is considerable frustration when the patient realizes that he or she has short-term memory loss. In a matter-of-fact manner, the nurse should "fill in the blanks" and then redirect to another activity. Pictures of familiar people, places, and activities are also important tools in memory retrieval. Using scents (perfume, shaving lotions, spices, different foods) to stimulate memory retrieval and asking patients to relate memories are also useful. Formalized reminiscence groups also help patients relive their earlier experiences and support long-term memories.

Orientation Interventions. Attempts should be made to remind patients of the day, time, and location in order to enhance cognitive functioning. However, if the patient begins to argue with the nurse that he or she is really at home or that it is really 1992, *do not* confront the patient with the facts. Any confrontation could easily escalate into an argument. Instead, the nurse should

either redirect the patient or focus on the topic at hand. See Therapeutic Dialogue: The Patient With Dementia of the Alzheimer's Type.

Maintenance of Language Functions. Losing the ability to name an object (agnosia) is very frustrating. For example, the patient may describe a flower in terms of color, size, and fragrance but never be able to name it as a flower. When this happens, the nurse should immediately say the name of the item. This reinforces cognitive functioning and prevents disruption in the interaction. Referral to speech therapists may also be useful if the language impairment is a barrier in communication.

Supporting Visuospatial Functioning. The patient with visuospatial impairments loses the ability to sequence automatic behaviors, such as getting dressed or eating with silverware. For example, patients often put their clothes on backward, inside out, or with undergarments over outer garments. Once dressed, they become confused as to how they arrived at their current state. If this happens, the nurse should begin to place clothes for dressing in a sequence so that the patient can move from one article to the next in the correct sequence. This same technique can be used in other situations, such as eating, bathing, and toileting.

Interventions for Psychosis. Patients who are experiencing psychosis usually are prescribed an antipsychotic. Interventions associated with antipsychotic therapy were presented earlier in this chapter.

Managing Suspicions, Illusions, and Delusions. Patients suspiciousness and delusional thinking must be

---

THERAPEUTIC DIALOGUE | **The Patient With Dementia of the Alzheimer's Type**

Lois's daughter has told the home health agency nurse that on several occasions Lois has been found cowering and fearful under the kitchen table, saying she was hiding from voices. The nurse also knows that Lois denies having any difficulty with her memory or her ability to care for herself.

Ineffective Approach

Nurse: I'm here to see you about your health problems.
Patient: I have no problems. Why are you here?
Nurse: I'm here to help you.
Patient: I do not need any help. I think there is a mistake.
Nurse: Oh, there is no mistake. Your name is Ms. W, isn't it?
Patient: Yes, but I don't know who you are or why you are here. I'm very tired, please excuse me.
Nurse: OK. I will return another day.

Effective Approach

Nurse: Hello, my name is Susan Miller. I'm the home health nurse and I will be spending some time with you.
Patient: Oh, alright. Come in. Sit here.
Nurse: Thank you.
Patient: There is nothing wrong with me, you know.
Nurse: Are you wondering why I am here? (open-ended statement)
Patient: I know why you are here. My children think that I cannot take care of myself.
Nurse: Is that true? Can you take care of yourself? (re-statement)
Patient: Of course, I can care for myself. When people get older they slow down. I'm just a little slower now and that upsets my children.

Nurse: You are a little slower? (reflection)
Patient: I sometimes forget things.
Nurse: Such as . . . (open-ended statement)
Patient: Sometimes, I cannot remember a telephone number or a name of a food.
Nurse: Does that cause problems?
Patient: According to my children, it does!
Nurse: What about you? What causes problems for you?
Patient: Sometimes the radio says terrible things to me.
Nurse: That must be frightening. (acceptance)
Patient: It's terrifying. Then, my daughter looks at me as if I am crazy. Am I?
Nurse: It sounds like your mind is playing tricks on you. Let's see if we can figure out how to control the radio. (validation)
Patient: Oh, OK. Will you tell my daughter that I am not crazy?
Nurse: Sure, I would be happy to meet with both you and your daughter if you would like. (acceptance)

Critical Thinking Challenge

• How did the nurse's underlying assumption that the patient would welcome the nurse in the first scenario lead to the nurse's rejection by the patient?

• What communication techniques did the nurse use in the second scenario to open communication and set the stage for the development of a sense of trust?

---

addressed to be certain that they do not endanger themselves or others. Often, delusions are verbalized when patients are placed in a situation they cannot master cognitively. The principle of nonconfrontation is most important in dealing with suspiciousness and delusion formation. No efforts should be made to ease the patient's suspicions directly or to correct delusions. Efforts should be directed at determining the circumstances that trigger suspicion or delusion formation and creating a means of avoiding these situations.

Frequent causes of suspicion are changes in daily routine and the presence of strangers. The common accusations that "Someone has entered my room," or "Someone has changed my room," can be managed by asking, "Do you want to see if anything is missing?" Such accusations usually arise when a patient cannot remember what the room looked like or when the room was rearranged or cleaned.

Dementia patients often hide or misplace their belongings and later complain that the item is missing. It is helpful if the nurse and other caregivers pay attention to the patient's favorite hiding places and communicate this so that objects can be more easily retrieved. An out-

burst of delusional accusations following a social outing or other activity may indicate that the activity was too long, the setting was too stimulating, there was too much activity, or the pace was too fast for the patient. All of these elements can be modified, or it may be necessary to exclude or significantly diminish the delusional patient's participation in overstimulating activities.

Dementia patients have delusions that a spouse, child, or other significant person is an impostor. If this situation occurs, it is important to assert in a matter-of-fact manner that "This is your wife, Barbara" or "I am your daughter, Jenny." More vigorous assertions, such as offering various types of proof, tend to increase puzzlement as to why a person would go so far to impersonate the spouse or child.

When dementia patients experience illusions, the nurse needs to find the source of the illusion and remove it from the environment if possible. For example, if a dementia patient is watching a television program featuring animals and then verbalizes that the animal is in the room, switch the channel and redirect the conversation. Demented patients may no longer recognize the reflection in the mirror as self and become agitated, thinking that a stranger is staring at them. Potentially misleading or disturbing stimuli, such as mirrors or art work, can be easily covered or removed from the environment (Text Box 31-9).

Managing Hallucinations. If at all possible, it is best to use reassurance and distraction with the hallucinating patient. For example, an 89-year-old AD patient would get up each night and walk to the nursing station (she lived in a residential care facility). She would whisper to the nurses, "There's a man in my bed who won't let me sleep. You should patrol this place better!" If the hallucination is not too disturbing for the patient, it can often be dismissed calmly with diversion or distraction. Because this patient does not seem too concerned by the man in her bed, the nurse may gently respond by saying, "I'm sorry you have to put up with so much. Just wait here (or come with me) and I'll make sure your room is ready for you." The nurse should then take the patient back to her room and tuck her in bed (Gwyther, 1985).

Frightening hallucinations and delusions usually require antipsychotic medications to dampen the patient's emotional reactions, but they can also be dealt with by optimizing perceptual cues (cover mirrors or turn off the television) and by encouraging patients to stay physically close to their caregivers. For example, one patient frequently told the visiting nurse that she was being poisoned by deadly bugs. She knew the bugs were real because they crawled up and down her arms and legs while she tried to sleep at night. As a consequence, the patient was not getting adequate sleep. For this patient, antipsychotic medication may help her sleep at night, and she would also likely benefit from reassurance and protection. Patients benefit more if nurses give them a specific intervention to help the hallucination. For example, this patient may benefit from having the home care nurse massage her legs and arms with body lotion when making a visit. The patient could be told that the lotion should help keep the bugs off her at night. The nurse does not have to agree with the patient's hallucination or delusion but should let the patient know that the feelings are justified based on the patient's perception of the threat.

Interventions for Alterations in Mood

Managing Depression. Psychotherapeutic nursing interventions for the depression that often accompanies dementia are similar to interventions for any depression. It is important to spend time alone with patients and to personalize their care as a way of communicating the patient's value (see Therapeutic Dialogue: The Patient With Dementia of the Alzheimer's Type). Encourage expression of negative emotions because it is often helpful for patients to talk honestly to a nonjudgmental person about his or her feelings. Although depressed patients with dementia are likely to be too disorganized to commit suicide, it is wise to remove potentially harmful objects from the environment.

Do not force depressed patients to interact with others or participate in activities, but encourage activity and exercise. One of the psychogenic aspects of depression is a sense of lowered worth related to the patient's actual decreased competence to work and to deal with the problems of daily living. Therefore, it may be helpful to involve the person in a simple repetitive task or project (such as folding linens or setting the table), especially one that involves helping someone else. Assist the patient in meeting self-care needs while encouraging independence when possible.

Managing Anxiety. Cognitively impaired patients are particularly vulnerable to anxiety. As patients with dementia become more unsure of their surroundings or of what is expected of them, they tend to react with fear and distress. They may feel lost, insecure, and left out. Failure to complete a task once regarded as simple creates anxiety and agitation. Often, demented individuals are unable to explain the source of their anxiety, common symptoms of which include fidgeting, picking at clothing, wringing hands, or wandering. The difficulty in developing interventions for the anxious dementia

---

TEXT BOX 31.9

Critical Thinking Dilemma: Dementia of Alzheimer's Type

It is 8 o'clock and you are working as a nurse on an inpatient general medical unit of a large urban hospital. A 72-year-old man is admitted to your unit with symptoms of disorientation to time and place, and he is intermittently exhibiting signs of agitation. He thinks you are his child, and he falls asleep while you ask him questions about his symptoms. When you ask him to sign a consent form and hand him a pen, he looks at you as if he didn't understand your request.

The patient's wife tells you that he has had trouble with his memory for the past 3 or 4 years but that her husband has been "acting strange for the past 4 days." The patient's wife denies any history of substance abuse or head injury, but states that her husband has been recently diagnosed as having dementia of the Alzheimer's type.

The patient's physician gives a verbal order to restrain the patient "as needed" while writing orders for lab work. Given this information:

- What assessment techniques would you use to determine whether this patient has dementia, delirium, or both?

- What nursing diagnosis would be included in the patient's plan of care?

- What nursing interventions would promote comfort and safety for this patient?

- What would be the possible outcomes of physically restraining this patient (eg, would restraints be helpful or harmful for the patient)?

patient is that the symptoms may also be a sign of underlying illnesses, such as depression, pain, infection, or other physical illnesses.

In many cases, lowering the demands or perceived demands placed on the patient will be conducive to promoting comfort. Although maintaining autonomy in any remaining function is a high priority in nursing care of the patient with dementia, it may decrease the patient's anxiety or stress level to have things done for him or her at certain points along the illness continuum. In addition, being sensitive to the pronounced startle reflexes and potential hypersensitivity to touch also helps reduce the stress.

The threshold for stress is progressively lowered in AD and other progressive dementias. A healthy person frequently uses cognitive coping strategies when under stress, whereas the person with dementia can no longer use many of these strategies. Effective nursing interventions include simplifying routines, making routines as consistent and predictable as possible, reducing the number of choices the patient must make, identifying areas in which control can be maintained, and creating an environment in which the patient feels safe. With any of the therapeutic interventions discussed, the nurse is reminded that each patient has relative strengths and weaknesses and that sound nursing judgment must be used in each situation.

Commonly used therapeutic approaches may exacerbate anxiety in a patient with dementia. For example, reality orientation is usually an effective intervention for acutely confused patients. With the dementia patient, reality orientation is contraindicated because it is possible that the patient's disoriented behavior or language has inherent meaning. If the disoriented behavior or language is continuously neglected or corrected by the nurse, the patient's sense of isolation and anxiety may increase.

Another therapeutic intervention that may (or may not) be contraindicated in patients with dementia is providing the patient with information before a difficult or painful procedure. Anticipatory preparation for nonroutine events may produce anxiety because the dementia patient is unable to retain information, use reasoning skills, or make sound judgments. Telling the patient that he or she is scheduled for an upcoming diagnostic test only communicates, on an emotional level, that something distressing is about to happen. A simple explanation immediately before the event may be more therapeutic (Beck & Heacock, 1988).

Managing Catastrophic Reactions. If a dementia patient reacts catastrophically, remain calm, minimize environmental distractions (quiet the environment), get the patient's attention, and softly verbalize what you think he or she is feeling with the assurance that he or she is safe. Give information slowly, clearly, and simply, one step at a time. Let the patient know that you understand the fear (or other possible emotional response, such as anger or anxiety).

As the nurse becomes skilled at identifying antecedents to the patient's catastrophic reactions, it becomes possible to avoid situations that provoke such reactions. Patients with AD respond poorly to change and respond well to structure. Attempts to argue or reason with them only escalate their dysfunctional behavioral responses.

Interventions for Behavior Problems

Managing Apathy and Withdrawal. As the patient withdraws and becomes more apathetic, the nurse is challenged to engage the patient in meaningful activities and interactions. To provide this level of care, the nurse must know the premorbid functioning of the patient. Close contact with family helps give the nurse ideas about meaningful activities.

Managing Restlessness and Wandering. Restlessness and wandering are major concerns for caregivers, especially in the community (home) or long-term care setting. The principal means of dealing with restless patients who wander into other patient's rooms or out the door is to have an adequate number of staff (or caregivers, in the home setting) to provide supervision, as well as electronically controlled exits. Wandering behavior may be interrupted in more cognitively intact patients by distracting them verbally or visually. Patients who are beyond verbal distraction can be distracted by physically joining them on their walk and then interrupting their course of action and gently redirecting them back to the house or facility. Many times, wandering is a result of a patient's inability to find his own room or may represent other agenda-seeking behaviors.

Managing Aberrant Behavior. When patients are picking in the air or wringing hands, simple distraction may work. Hypervocalizations are another story. Direct care staff tend to avoid these patients, which only makes the vocalizations worse. In reality, these vocalizations may have meaning to the patient. The nurse should develop strategies to try to reduce the frequency of vocalizations (Table 31-7).

Managing Agitated Behavior. Agitated behavior is likely to occur when patients are pressed to assist in their own care. A calm, unhurried, and undemanding approach is usually most effective. Attempts at reasoning may only aggravate the situation and increase the patient's resistance to care. If the nurse is unable to determine the source of the patient's anxiety, the patient's restless energy can often be channeled into activities such as walking. Relaxation techniques can be effective for reducing behavioral problems and anxiety in demented patients as well.

Reducing Disinhibition. Anticipation of disinhibiting behavior is the key to nursing interventions for this problem. Disinhibition can take many forms, from undressing in a public setting, to touching someone inappropriately, to making cruel, but factual statements. This behavior can usually be viewed as normal by itself,

TABLE 31.7 Possible Meanings Underlying Challenging Vocal Behaviors of Demented Elders and Related Management Strategies

Possible Underlying Meanings	Related Management Strategies
"I hurt!" (eg, from arthritis, fractures, pressure ulcers, degenerative joint disease, cancer)	• Observe for pain behaviors (eg, posture, facial expressions, and gait in conjunction with vocalizations) • Treat suspected pain judiciously with analgesics and nonpharmacologic measures (eg, repositioning, careful manipulation of patient during transfers and personal care, warm/cold packs, massage, relaxation)
"I'm tired." (eg, sleep disturbances possibly related to altered sleep–wake cycle with day–night reversal, difficulty falling asleep, frequent night awakenings)	• Increase daytime activity and exercise to minimize daytime napping and promote nighttime sleep • Promote normal sleep patterns and biorhythms by strengthening natural environmental cues (eg, provide light exposure during the day, avoid bright, artificial lights at night), provide large calendars and clocks • Establish a bedtime routine • Reduce night awakenings: avoid excess fluids, diuretics, caffeine at bedtime; minimize loud noises, consolidate nighttime care activities (eg, changing, medications, treatments)
"I'm lonely."	• Encourage social interactions between patients and their family, caregivers, and others • Increase time the patient spends in group settings to minimize time in isolation • Provide opportunity to interact with pets
"I need . . . " (eg, food, a drink, a blanket, to use the toilet, to be turned or repositioned)	• Anticipate needs (eg, assist patient to toilet soon after breakfast when the gastrocolic reflex is likely) • Keep patient comfort and safety in mind during care (eg, minimize body exposure to prevent hypothermia)
"I'm stressed." (eg, inability to tolerate sensory overload)	• Promote rest and quiet time • Minimize "white noise" (eg, vacuum cleaner) and background noise (eg, televisions and radios) • Avoid harsh lighting and busy, abstract designs • Limit patient's contacts with other agitated people • Reduce behavioral expectations of patient, minimize choices, promote a stable routine
"I'm bored." (eg, lack of sensory stimulation)	• Maximize hearing and visual abilities (eg, keep external auditory canals free from cerumen plugs, ensure glasses and hearing aids are worn, provide reading material of large print, soften lighting to reduce glare) • Play soft, classical music for auditory stimulation • Offer structured diversions (eg, outdoor activities)
"What are you doing to me?" (eg, personal boundaries are invaded)	• Avoid startling patients by approaching them from the front • Always speak before touching the patient • Inform patients what you plan to do and why *before* you do it • Allow for flexibility in patient care
"I don't feel well." (eg, a urinary or upper respiratory tract infection, metabolic abnormality, fecal impaction)	• Identify etiology through patient history, examination, possible tests (eg, urinalysis, blood work, chest radiograph, neurologic testing) • Treat underlying causes
"I'm frustrated—I have no control." (eg, loss of autonomy)	• When possible, allow patient to make own decisions • Maximize patient involvement during personal care (eg, offer patient a washcloth to assist with bathing) • Treat patients with dignity and respect (eg, dress or change patient in private)
"I'm lost." (eg, memory impairment)	• Maintain familiar routines • Label the patient's room, bathroom, drawers, and possessions with large name signs • Promote a sense of belonging through displays of familiar personal items, such as old family pictures

(continued)

TABLE 31.7 Possible Meanings Underlying Challenging Vocal Behaviors of Demented Elders and Related Management Strategies (Continued)

Possible Underlying Meanings	Related Management Strategies
"I feel strange." (eg, side effects from medications that may include psychotropics, corticosteroids, β-blockers, nonsteroidal antiinflammatories)	• Minimize overall number of medications; consider nondrug interventions when possible • Begin new medications one at a time; start with low doses, titrate slowly. Suspect drug reaction if patient's behavior (eg, vocal) changes • Educate caregivers about patient medications
"I need to be loved!"	• Provide human contact and purposeful touch • Acknowledge or verify patient's feelings • Encourage alternate, nonverbal ways to express feelings, such as through music, painting, or drawing • Stress a sense of purpose in life, acknowledge achievements, reaffirm that the patient is still needed

Clavel, D. S. (1999). Vocalizations among cognitively impaired elders. *Geriatric Nursing, 20,* 90–93.

but abnormal within its social context. With keen behavioral assessment of the patient, the nurse should be able to anticipate the likely socially inappropriate behavior and redirect the patient or change the context of the situation. If the patient starts undressing in the dining room, offering a robe and gently escorting him or her to another part of the room might be all that is needed. If a patient is trying to fondle a staff member or another patient, having the staff member leave the immediate area or redirecting the patient may alleviate the situation.

Social Domain

Social Assessment

Dementia interferes with a person's ability to interact socially as much as it disrupts intellectual functioning. The social domain assessment should include those areas explained in Chapter 12, including functional status, social systems, spiritual assessment, legal status, and quality of life (see Chap. 12). The Global Assessment of Functioning scale presented in Chapter 4 can be used also.

The patient's whole social network is affected by dementia, and the primary caregiver of a person with dementia (usually the spouse or daughter in a community setting) is often considered a co-patient. It is important to assess the family caregiver's ability to use supportive mechanisms to maintain his or her own integrity throughout the disease process.

The extent of the primary caregiver's personal, informal, and formal support systems must also be assessed, as well as personal resources, skills, and stressors. The assessment of the social domain provides objective data on the patient's social circumstances and impressions of the patient's family structure, sociocultural beliefs, attitudes toward health and disease, myths about dementia, patterns of communication, and degree of psychopathology (such as potential for abuse). If the patient still resides in the community, a home visit will prove useful because it gives the nurse information about the patient in the natural environment. From this assessment, the nurse can identify the situational and psychosocial stressors that affect the family and patient and can begin to develop interventions to strengthen coping strategies, including the ability to seek help from appropriate community resources.

Nursing Diagnoses Related to Social Domain

Typical nursing diagnosis for the social domain are Deficient Diversional Activity; Impaired Social Interaction; Social Isolation; Risk for Loneliness; Caregiver Role Strain; Ineffective Coping; Hopelessness; and Powerlessness (NANDA, 2001). Outcomes are determined according to nursing diagnoses.

Social Interventions

Safety Interventions. One of the primary concerns of the nurse should be patient safety. In the early stages of the illness, safety may not seem to be a prime issue because the individual is cognitively intact. Early behaviors suggesting dementia, however, are often related to safety, such as the patient getting lost while driving or going the wrong way on the highway. Patients may be prevented from driving even though they can continue to live at home. Safety continues to be an issue in the home when patients engage in unsupervised cooking, cleaning, or household tasks. Day care centers provide a structured yet safe environment for these individuals. Family members should be encouraged to assess continually the abilities of members to live at home safely.

During hospitalizations or nursing home care, the safety issues are different. There are more people with the patient, which presents more opportunity for wandering into unsafe areas. Most geropsychiatric units are locked and in a dementia unit, and there is often an electronic alarm system to alert staff of patients attempting to leave the secured floor. Staff and visitors need to be constantly on the lookout for situations that could jeopardize the safety of the patients.

Environmental Interventions. The need for stimulation can also be an antecedent to catastrophic reactions. The need for stimulation varies from individual to individual and can change, depending on many factors, including cognitive intactness, alertness, emotional state, and physical state. The amount of stimulation received also influences each patient's behavior. Lack of stimulation or intense stimulation may cause emotional distress and aggression. Generally speaking, the more severe the dementia, the less stimulation can be integrated. The nurse should attempt to determine each patient's optimal level of stimulation at various times of the day. For example, it may be that stimulating environments can be tolerated early in the morning, but not in the afternoon when the patient is fatigued.

Socialization Activities. Overlearned social skills are rarely lost in patients with AD. It is not unusual for the patient with dementia to respond appropriately to a handshake or smile well into the disease process. Even those patients who are no longer able to communicate coherently will carry on long discussions with people who are willing to listen and respond (to language that does not make sense). There is a strong risk for social isolation in patients with dementia because of communication difficulties. Reinforcing social remarks and gestures, such as eye contact, smiling, greetings, and farewells, can promote a sense of competency and self-esteem. Pet therapy and "stuffed animal" therapy can also enhance social interaction in cognitively impaired individuals. A study conducted by Francis and Baly (1986) evaluated the therapeutic effect of stuffed plush animals as "pets" for nursing home residents. The introduction of personal plush animals made a significant positive difference in the patient's social interaction. They also had a positive effect on depressive symptoms. Finally, it is important to remember that patients with dementia do not lose their ability to laugh and play, and the psychosocial benefits of humor are well known.

The nurse who engages a dementia patient in an activity is encouraged to (1) avoid confronting the patient with the disability; (2) allow the level of autonomy best tolerated by the patient; (3) simplify activities and directions to the point that they can be mastered (eg, avoid directions such as "use right or left arm" because it may be frustrating for the patient to distinguish one from the other); (4) provide adequate structure or directions; and (5) do not expect instructions to be carried out correctly. It is important to monitor the length of time, crowding, and noise level when the patient participates in a group activity because all of these factors may increase the patient's stress level (Gwyther, 1985).

Activities that elicit pleasant memories from an earlier time in the patient's life (reminiscence) may produce a soothing effect. Eliciting pleasant memories may be enhanced by gentle stimulation of the patient's senses, for example, viewing and discussing photo albums, looking at personal memorabilia, providing a favorite food item, playing a musical instrument, or listening to music the person preferred in younger years. Studies have shown that music can reduce agitated behavior in patients with dementia.

It may be useful to incorporate movement or dance along with a singing exercise. If the patient with dementia resists structured exercise, it may be because of a fear of falling or injury, or of demonstrating to others that his or her health is failing. Demented patients often forget how to move or how to coordinate their movements in relation to objects. Therefore, exercise should be light and enjoyable. Encourage the patient to take rest periods at intervals throughout the activity in an effort to minimize stress.

Home Visits. The goal of in-home and community-based long-term care services is to maintain patients in a self-determining environment that provides the most home-like atmosphere possible, allows maximum personal choice for care recipients and caregiver, and encourages optimal family caregiving involvement without overwhelming the resources of the family network. All services for patients with dementia and their families must be provided within a context of continuity of care, a concept that mandates access to a variety of health and supportive services over an unpredictable and changing clinical course.

The effectiveness of nursing home visits was recently demonstrated. In a randomized study, elderly residents with psychiatric disorders living in six public housing sites in Baltimore were identified by building staff. Residents in three of the buildings were assigned to receive nursing interventions by visiting nurses, whereas the residents in the other three did not. The interventions included patient counseling and education, liaisons with the patient's social worker, preparation of patient medication with monitoring of adherence and side effects, facilitation of care and support for patient physical health problems, discussion with home health care providers about medication, and monitoring of patient vital signs. Each patient was seen an average of five times. At the end of 26 months, patients receiving the interventions were significantly less depressed and had fewer psychiatric symptoms than those who did not receive the intervention (Rabins et al., 2000).

Community Actions. Nurses working with dementia patients are especially knowledgeable about all aspects of the illness and care. These nurses are often involved in local organizations, such as the Alzheimer's Association. Even though consumer driven, issues of care and safety and reimbursement of services often require professional expertise and influence.

⮕ Family Interventions

Caregivers are faced with extreme pressures. Caregivers are either spouses of the person with Alzheimer's Disease or children, usually a daughter, who also have other responsibilities, such as children and a job. The caregiver often feels isolated, frustrated, and trapped. The potential for patient abuse is significant, especially if agitated and aggressive behaviors are present in the relative. The use of home health nurses has been investigated relative to their impact on the burden and depression of elderly caregivers. The caregivers who used the home health services were significantly less burdened and less depressed than those who did not use these services (Mignor, 2000).

It is important that the nurse recognize the need of the caregivers for support and relief from the 24-hour responsibility. Determining availability of family members or friends to assist with personal care of the patient should be included in the assessment. Caregivers should be encouraged to attend support groups and carve out personal time. Educational and training programs may help in understanding the complex nature of the disorder. Community resources, such as day care centers, home health agencies, and other community services, can be important aspect of nursing care for the patient with dementia.

Evaluation and Treatment Outcomes

The objectives of nursing interventions are to help the patient with dementia remain as independent as possible and to function at the highest cognitive, physical, emotional, spiritual, and social levels. The maximum level of functional ability can be promoted when nursing care is related to and based on the remaining abilities of the patient. Patients who are diagnosed with AD or other types of dementia have a wide and varying range of functional abilities. As cognitive decline progresses, there is a tendency for caregivers to perform more and more tasks for the patient. It is essential to assess for strengths and to assist in the maintenance of existing skills. Adaptive and appropriate behaviors continue to some degree in people with dementia, even in the presence of increasing

cognitive decline. It is important for nursing interventions to focus on more than the maintenance of optimal physical functional ability; interventions also must focus on meeting psychological, social, and spiritual needs of the patient with dementia.

Nurses can maintain quality of life if they protect a patient's overall well-being by balancing physical, mental, social, and spiritual health. Figure 31-4 illustrates the truly biopsychosocial aspects of the treatment of individuals with dementia by summarizing potential outcomes of nursing care.

Continuum of Care

Community Care

It is estimated that more than 7 of 10 people with Alzheimer's disease live at home. Almost 75% of home care is provided by family and friends. The remainder is paid care, costing an average of $12,500 per year, most of which is covered by families (ADRDA, 2001). Use of community-based services (eg, home health aides, home-delivered meals, adult day care, respite care, caregiver support groups) often extends the amount of time an individual with AD or a related disorder can safely remain in the home. However, the progressive impairment associated with dementia often culminates with placement in a long-term care facility. The nurse working in a physician's office or ambulatory setting may provide ongoing information about management and problem solving. The public health nurse may provide intermittent assessment and ongoing case management. Nurses working in programs designed specifically for patients with dementia, such as adult day care, also practice the role of educator. The nurse who is simply a neighbor or family member is often asked to advise about management of the person with dementia.

The complex and interrelated problems often observed in patients with neuropsychiatric disorders will increasingly demand the attention of nurses in all health care settings. Cooperation between health care providers of different disciplines and in various settings is needed to meet the highly individualized needs of patients with neuropsychiatric deficits.

Inpatient-Focused Care

Comprehensive admission assessment, followed by the development of an individualized (and constantly updated) care plan that involves the patient, significant others, and a variety of health care professionals, is the foundation of an effective and efficient postdischarge plan. Attention to all aspects of this process is necessary to ensure that the goal of continuity of care is achieved. The hospital-based nurse may initiate family education and counseling as part of discharge planning. For more information on caring for the patient with dementia, see Psychoeducation Checklist: Dementia.

Nursing Home Care

As the dementia deteriorates, most patients are placed in a nursing home for care. Nursing care in a nursing home is usually delivered by nurses' aides, who need support and direction during their care. Interestingly, people with dementia require complex nursing care, but the skill level of people caring for these individuals is often minimal. Education and support of the direct caregiver is the focus of most nursing homes.

OTHER DEMENTIAS

Dementia symptoms may occur as a result of a number of disorders and underlying etiologies. The subsequent sections provide a brief description of some of the dementias listed in the *Diagnostic and Statistical Manual of Mental Disorders* (APA, 2000). In each case, the classic symptoms of dementia (eg, memory impairment with a number of other cognitive deficits) must be present. Nursing interventions for all dementias are similar to those described for individuals with AD.

Vascular Dementia

Vascular dementia (also known as *multiinfarct dementia*) is seen in about 20% of patients with dementia, most commonly people between the ages of 60 and 75 years. Slightly more men than women are affected. Vascular dementia results when a series of small strokes damage or destroy brain tissue. These are commonly referred to as "ministrokes" or transient ischemic attacks (TIAs), and several TIAs may occur before the affected individ-

ual becomes aware of the symptoms of vascular dementia. Most often, a blood clot or plaques (fatty deposits) block the vessels that supply blood to the brain, causing a stroke. However, a stroke can also occur when a blood vessel bursts in the brain.

There are several primary causes of strokes, including high blood cholesterol, diabetes, heart disease, and high blood pressure. Of these, high blood pressure is the greatest risk factor for vascular dementia. It is essential that anyone who demonstrates symptoms of dementia or who has a history of stroke should have a complete physical examination that includes neurologic and neuropsychological evaluation, diet and medication history, review of recent stressors, and an array of laboratory tests. Damage to the brain in vascular dementia is usually apparent using computed tomography scans or magnetic resonance imaging. At autopsy, multifocal lesions may be found, rather than the more generalized cortical atrophy characteristic of AD.

The behavior changes that result from vascular dementia are similar to those found in AD, such as memory loss, depression, emotional lability or emotional incontinence (including inappropriate laughing or crying), wandering or getting lost in familiar places, bladder or bowel incontinence, difficulty following instructions, gait changes such as small shuffling steps, and problems handling daily activities such as money management. However, these symptoms usually begin more suddenly rather than developing slowly over time, as is the case in AD. Often, the neurologic symptoms associated with a TIA are minimal and may last only a few days, including slight weakness in an extremity, dizziness, or slurred speech. Thus, the clinical progression is often described as intermittent and fluctuating, or of step-like deterioration, with the patient's cognitive and functional status improving or plateauing for a period of time, followed by a rapid decline in function after another series of small strokes. The Hachinski Ischemia Score in Text Box 31-10 may be helpful in differentiating vascular dementia from AD and in summarizing the symptoms more closely related to vascular dementia.

Treatment is aimed at reducing the primary risk factors for vascular dementia, including hypertension, diabetes, and further strokes. Interventions are implemented to reduce the tendency of the blood to clot and of platelets to aggregate, using medications and lifestyle changes such as diet, exercise, and smoking cessation to control hypertension, high cholesterol, heart disease, and diabetes. Increasingly, doctors are recommending drugs such as aspirin to help prevent clots from forming in the small blood vessels. Occasionally, surgical procedures such as carotid endarterectomy may be needed to remove blockages in the carotid artery. Studies of the efficacy of this procedure in vascular dementia are underway.

Text Box 31.10

Hachinski Ischemia Score

Abrupt onset	2
Stepwise progression	1
Fluctuating course	2
Nocturnal confusion	1
Relative preservation of personality	1
Depression	1
Somatic complaints	1
Emotional incontinence	1
History of hypertension	1
History of stroke	2
Evidence of associated atherosclerosis	1
Focal neurologic symptoms	2
Focal neurologic signs	2
Alzheimer's disease if scores total	4 or less
Vascular dementias if scores total	7 or more

Hachinski, V. C. (1983). Differential diagnosis of Alzheimer's dementia: Multi-infarct dementia. In B. Reisberg (Ed.), *Alzheimer's disease* (pp. 188–192). New York: Free Press/Macmillan.

Dementia Caused by Other General Medical Conditions

People of any age, race, or gender are at risk for dementia caused by a medical condition known to cause cerebral pathology. Elderly people are particularly vulnerable to the development of dementia owing to general medical conditions because so many older people are affected by one or more chronic medical illnesses. Strong relationships have been described between chronic medical illness and the development of dementia. Of the conditions that cause dementia, about 10% are completely treatable, and about 25% to 30% cease to progress as long as treatment is initiated before irreversible brain damage has occurred. Finally, about 50% to 60% of patients with dementia have a disorder for which no specific medical treatment is available.

Dementia Caused by AIDS

Dementia associated with AIDS has been called AIDS dementia complex (ADC). ADC has been observed in nearly two thirds of all AIDS patients, whereas neuropathologic findings occur in more than 90% of patients with AIDS (Navia et al., 1986). AIDS is caused by HIV-1, which infects and destroys T lymphocytes as well as the CNS. HIV-1 directly invades the CNS and allows opportunistic infections of the CNS and other organ systems. It is likely that AIDS will become an important cause of dementia over the next several decades (Weiner et al., 1991).

Dementia Caused by Head Trauma

When head trauma occurs in the context of a single injury, the resulting dementia is usually not progressive, but repeated head injury (eg, from the sport of boxing) may lead to a progressive dementia. When the nurse observes progressive decline in intellectual functioning after a single incident of head trauma, the possibility of another superimposed process must be considered. Head injury associated with a prolonged loss of consciousness (days to months) may be followed by delirium or dementia or a profound alteration in personality.

The degree and type of cognitive impairment or behavioral disturbances demonstrated by a person with head trauma depend on the location and extent of the brain injury (as with other forms of dementia). Repeated head injuries, such as those sustained by young, healthy boxers, may lead to dementia pugi listica, or "punch-drunk syndrome." Although the exact mechanism of this disorder is unknown, it appears likely that early damage to neurons and their connections becomes clinically manifest later, when the combination of normal neuronal cell loss and prior damage summate to reach a threshold of impaired cognitive function.

Dementia Caused by Parkinson's Disease

Parkinson's disease is a neurologic syndrome of unknown etiology, which manifests as a disorder of movement, with a slow and progressive course. Clinical manifestations of Parkinson's disease are **bradykinesia** (the slowing of body movements), rigidity, resting tremor, and postural changes. The person's gait is unstable, which results in frequent falls. Parkinson's disease may appear at any time after a person reaches 30 years of age, but the median age of onset is about 70 years of age. A subcortical dementia can be diagnosed in about 20% to 60% of patients with Parkinson's disease (APA, 2000). Although investigators do not know why, there is considerable pathologic overlap between Parkinson's disease and AD. Joachim and associates (1988) reported that 18% of the AD patients they examined had sufficient neuronal loss and Lewy bodies in the substantia nigra to warrant a diagnosis of Parkinson's disease. Medical treatment of Parkinson's disease is typically with anticholinergics and dopamine agonists. It is important for nurses to know that in patients with dementia caused by Parkinson's disease, anticholinergic medications are contraindicated because they are likely to increase the patient's level of confusion (Cummings, 1991).

Dementia Caused by Huntington's Disease

Huntington's disease is a progressive, genetically transmitted autosomal dominant disorder characterized by choreiform movements and mental abnormalities. The onset is usually between the ages of 30 and 50 years, but onset occurs before 5 years of age in the juvenile form or as late as 85 years of age in the late-onset form. The disease affects men and women equally. A person with Huntington's disease usually lives for 15 to 20 years after diagnosis (APA, 2000). The dementia syndrome of Huntington's disease is characterized by insidious changes in behavior and personality. Typically, the dementia is frontal, which means that the person demonstrates prominent behavioral problems and disruption of attention.

Dementia Caused by Pick's Disease

Pick's disease is a rare form of dementia that is clinically similar to AD. The etiology of Pick's disease is unknown. Pick's disease particularly affects the frontal and temporal lobes of the brain (APA, 2000). The disorder usually manifests in individuals between ages 50 and 60 years, although it can occur among older individuals. Pick's disease is not readily distinguishable from AD until autopsy (APA, 2000), when the distinctive intraneuronal Pick's bodies can be identified microscopically.

Dementia Caused by Creutzfeldt-Jakob Disease

Creutzfeldt-Jakob disease is a rare, rapidly fatal brain disorder. Many of the symptoms seen in Creutzfeldt-Jakob disease are similar to those found in AD and other dementias. However, changes in the brain tissue are different in Creutzfeldt-Jakob disease and are best differentiated by surgical biopsy or on autopsy. Scientists speculate that Creutzfeldt-Jakob disease is caused by a "slow" and "unconventional" virus because it has a relatively long incubation period (3 years or more) before symptoms begin to appear. The precise mechanism by which the virus affects the brain is unknown (APA, 2000).

At present, there is no effective treatment for the disease, and nothing has been found to slow progression of the illness, although antiviral drug studies are ongoing. Because of its rapid clinical course, an important nursing role is assisting family members to understand and come to terms with the illness and to make decisions related to treatment setting and life-sustaining treatments. Creutzfeldt-Jakob disease progresses much more rapidly than most dementias, and death usually occurs within 1 year after onset, although some evidence suggests that extensive changes in the brain may be present before symptoms appear.

Only about 3,000 cases of Creutzfeldt-Jakob disease have been reported in the past 70 years, resulting in an annual incidence of about 1 per 1 million population. The disease strikes both men and women, most commonly between the ages of 50 and 75 years. Interestingly, there appears to be a genetic component to Creutzfeldt-Jakob disease (Bertoni et al., 1992). Inhabitants of certain rural areas of the world, such as Slovakia and Chile, and Libyan-born Jews living in Israel have a much higher incidence of the disease. In the United States, about 15% of people with Creutzfeldt-Jakob disease have a positive family history of early-onset dementia (APA, 2000).

Person-to-person transmission of Creutzfeldt-Jakob disease is rare (but possible), and it can be transmitted from people to animals and between animals. Evidence indicates that the virus can be introduced into the nervous system of healthy patients during medical procedures, such as corneal transplantation, implantation of contaminated electrodes in the brain, and injection of contaminated growth hormones (a few health care workers exposed to the virus, probably through blood and spinal fluids, have developed the disease). Because of the transmissible nature of Creutzfeldt-Jakob disease, and because the virus is not easily destroyed, strict criteria for the handling of infected tissues and other contaminated materials have been developed.

Substance-Induced Persisting Dementia

If dementia results from the persisting effects of a substance (eg, drugs of abuse, a medication, or exposure to toxins), then substance-induced persisting dementia is diagnosed. Other causes of dementia (eg, dementia owing to a general medical condition) must always be considered, even in a person with a dependence on or exposure to a substance. For example, head injuries often result from substance use and may be the underlying cause of the dementia syndrome (APA, 2000).

Drugs of abuse are the most common toxins in young adults, and prescription drugs are the most common toxins in elderly people. In older patients, dementia results from use of long-acting benzodiazepines, barbiturates, meprobamate (Equanil), and a host of other drugs, depending on their dose and the length of time they have been used. Drugs such as flurazepam (Dalmane), with a half-life of more than 120 hours, accumulate rapidly in a person's body. Other drugs accumulate more slowly or require relatively high doses for toxicity to develop. A toxic etiology should be suspected in every patient with a probable diagnosis of dementia. The nurse should inquire about exposure to drugs and toxins (exposure to toxins at work sites, medication use, and recreational drug use) for each patient with dementia, and any substances known to be potentially injurious to the nervous system should be withdrawn if at all possible.

Most of the dementias in this category are related to chronic alcohol abuse. Understanding the cognitive deficits associated with chronic alcohol consumption is complicated. Alcoholic dementia is directly related to the toxic effects of alcohol, although the vitamin deficiencies associated with alcoholism (thiamine and niacin) are also known to be etiologically related to dementia. Alcoholics also have a high incidence of systemic illnesses that can affect cognition (eg, cirrhosis, cardiomyopathy), and they are susceptible to repeated head injuries, which carry cognitive consequences of their own.

Much of our knowledge about cognitive deficits in alcoholics comes from the study of patients with Korsakoff's syndrome, which is a profound deficit in the ability to form new memories and is associated with a variable deficit in recall of old memories despite a clear sensorium. Further careful examination reveals a flattening of drives, unconcern about incapacity, and profound apathy. Nonetheless, Korsakoff's syndrome does not qualify as a dementia; rather, it would be considered an amnestic syndrome (or restricted deficit of memory). In alcohol-induced dementia, the cognitive deficits span a wider range of functioning than with Korsakoff's syndrome (see Chap. 25).

Chemicals and organic compounds that impair functioning of the CNS usually have their primary effects on other body systems: the gastrointestinal, renal, hepatic, blood-forming, and peripheral nervous systems. For example, metal poisonings generally produce gastrointestinal symptoms and peripheral neuropathy. Cognitive changes with poisoning tend to be more characteristic of delirium than dementia, with altered levels of consciousness a prominent feature. See Table 31-1 for a list of some of the organic compounds or chemicals that can cause symptoms of dementia; related distinguishing symptoms are also included.

Many adolescents and indigent adults engage in the act of "huffing" because the cost of purchasing spray paint, hair spray, glue, and other aerosol products is relatively inexpensive (compared with illicit street drugs). The nurse is reminded to evaluate people who abuse drugs for signs of cognitive impairment because neural and cognitive symptoms tend to appear before permanent brain damage occurs. It is also important to realize that the patient's cognitive status may not immediately improve after discontinuation of the offending agent. The effects of drugs taken over a long period may be long lasting, and improvement may follow discontinuation only slowly. In dementia associated with chronic alcoholism, for example, cognition may improve only after many months of abstinence.

AMNESTIC DISORDER

Amnestic disorder is characterized by an impairment in memory that is caused either by the direct physiologic effects of a general medical condition or by the persisting effects of a substance (eg, a drug of abuse, a medication, or exposure to a toxin) (APA, 2000). More specifically, amnestic disorder is diagnosed when there is severe memory impairment without other significant cognitive impairments (eg, aphasia, apraxia, agnosia, or disturbances in executive functioning) or impaired consciousness, which would indicate a diagnosis of either delirium or dementia.

The amnestic disorders share a common symptom, memory impairment, but are differentiated by etiology. Amnestic disorders often occur as the result of pathologic processes. Traumatic brain injury, cerebrovascular events, or specific types of neurotoxic exposure (eg, carbon monoxide poisoning) may lead to an acute onset of an amnestic disorder. Other conditions, such as prolonged substance abuse, chronic neurotoxic exposure, or sustained nutritional deficiency (eg, thiamine deficiency) create a more insidious onset. The age of the patient and course of amnestic disorder may vary, depending on the pathologic process causing the disorder.

Amnestic disorder is characterized by an impaired ability to learn new information or an inability to recall previously learned information (short-term recall) or past events (long-term recall), with preservation of immediate recall (immediate-recall deficits are commonly associated with dementia) (APA, 2000). Although short-term and long-term memory are impaired in most patients who have a form of organic brain disease, the occurrence of memory impairment as a relatively circumscribed deficit is rare. Short-term or recent memory is usually more severely impaired than remote memory with an amnestic disorder, and no deficit may be observed when the patient is asked to recall events or dates that have been overlearned. Most patients with deficits in short-term recall are disoriented to place and time; therefore, disorientation is a common sign of amnestic disorder. In some forms of amnestic disorder, however, the patient may remember information from the very remote past better than more recent events (eg, the patient may have a vivid memory of a hospital stay that occurred many years ago, but may have no idea that he or she is currently in the hospital) (APA, 2000).

Amnestic disorders are often preceded by an evolving and variable clinical picture, which includes confusion and disorientation, occasionally with attentional deficits that suggest a delirium (eg, amnestic disorder caused by thiamine deficiency). Confabulation (filling gaps in memory with imaginary events) may be noted during the early stages of amnestic disorder but usually disappears with time. For this reason, it may be important for the nurse to obtain corroborating information from family members or other informants when gathering historical information on the patient. Most patients with a severe amnestic disorder lack insight into their memory deficits and may adamantly deny the presence of memory impairment despite evidence to the contrary. This lack of insight may lead to accusations against others or, in some instances, to agitation. Some individuals may acknowledge that they have memory problems but appear unconcerned. Apathy, lack of initiative, emotional blandness, or other changes in personality are not uncommon with amnestic disorder.

Summary of Key Points

➤ Neuropsychiatric disorders, such as delirium and dementia, are characterized clinically by significant deficits in cognition or memory that represent a clearcut change from a previous level of functioning. In some disorders, the loss of cognitive function is progressive, such as in Alzheimer's disease.

➤ Two major syndromes of cognitive impairment in elderly people are delirium and chronic cognitive impairments, such as dementia. It is important to recognize the differences because the interventions and expected outcomes for the two syndromes are different.

➤ Delirium is characterized by a disturbance in consciousness and a change in cognition that develops over a short period of time. It requires rapid detection and treatment because in 25% of cases, it is a sign of impending death.

➤ Usually, delirium is caused by a combination of precipitating factors. The most commonly identified causes are medications, infections (particularly urinary tract and upper respiratory tract infections), fluid and electrolyte imbalance, and metabolic disturbances such as electrolyte imbalance or poor nutrition. Other important predisposing factors include advanced age, brain damage, pre-existing dementia, and biopsychosocial stressors.

➤ The primary goal of treatment of delirium is prevention or resolution of the acute confusional episode with return to previous cognitive status and interventions focusing on (1) elimination or correction of the underlying cause and (2) symptomatic and safety and supportive measures.

➤ Dementia is characterized by the gradual onset of decline in cognitive function, especially memory, usually accompanied by changes in behavior and personality. There are numerous causes of the symptoms of dementia, some of which are reversible, such as hypoxia, carbon monoxide poisoning, and vitamin deficiencies.

➤ Alzheimer's disease is an example of a progressive, degenerative dementia. Treatment efforts currently focus on reduction of cognitive symptoms (eg, memory loss, confusion, and problems with learning, speech, and reasoning) in attempts to improve the quality of life for both patients and their caregivers.

➤ No one cause of dementia or Alzheimer's disease has been discovered. A genetic link has been established for Alzheimer's type dementia in about 50% of patients, and current research has implicated three chromosomes (21, 14, and 19). Research efforts continue to pinpoint a singular identifiable genetic basis while focusing on other implicated etiologies, including neurochemical (ie, decreased acetylcholine believed to play a major role in memory impairment), neuropathologic (ie, degeneration of glutamatergic nerve terminals, head injury causing damage to the blood–brain barrier, defects in the immune system), and even some environmental factors (ie, aluminum and other heavy metals).

➤ Some of the psychosocial stressors known to precipitate delirium and contribute to worsening dementia include sensory overload or underload, immobilization, sleep deprivation, fatigue, pain or hunger, change in routine (pace or caregiver), or demands beyond patient's ability. Nursing interventions should include reducing the impact of these stressors on patients and educating their families or caregivers.

➤ Educating families and caregivers about what to expect, progressive cognitive decline and behavior changes, environment safety, and community resources for patients with dementia is essential to ensuring proper care.

➤ Symptoms of dementia may occur as a result of a number of disorders, including vascular and amnestic disorders, head trauma, AIDS, and substance abuse and as a symptom of Parkinson's. Huntington's, Pick's, and Creutzfeldt-Jakob diseases.

Critical Thinking Challenges

1. What factors should the nurse consider in differentiating Alzheimer's disease from vascular dementia?
2. Compare the defining characteristics and related risk factors of acute confusion with those for the NANDA diagnoses of Altered Thought Processes and Sensory/Perceptual Alterations.
3. What are the differences and similarities between the recommended nursing interventions for delirium and dementia? What is the theoretic base for these similarities and differences?
4. Describe three ways in which medical disease can disrupt brain functioning, and relate these mechanisms to the neuropsychiatric disorders presented in this chapter.
5. Suggest reasons that elderly people are particularly vulnerable to the development of neuropsychiatric disorders.
6. In what ways can culture and education influence mental status test scores?

7. The physical environment is particularly important to the patient with dementia. Every effort should be made to modify the physical environment to compensate for the cognitive and functional impairment associated with AD and related disorders, including safety measures and the avoidance of misleading stimuli. Visualize your last experience in a health care setting (hospital, nursing home, day care program, or home care setting). Identify environmental factors that could be misleading or stress producing to a person with impaired cognition (dementia), and identify ways to modify this environment to alleviate some of the stressors or misleading stimuli.

 WEB LINKS

www.alz.org   This Alzheimer's Association website provides information, resources, and consumer and caregiver support.

www.ninds.nih.gov/health_and_medical/disorders/ alzheimersdisease_doc.htm   The National Institute of Neurological Disorders and Stroke website provides useful information about Alzheimer's disease.

www.pdsg.org.uk   This website of the Pick's Disease Support Group provides information on Pick's disease, Lewy bodies, and other dementias.

www.alzheimer.ca/english/misc/redirect.htm   This site of the Alzheimer's Association of Canada provide information and resources related to the disease.

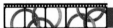 **MOVIES**

The Madness of King George: 1995. This is a true story of King George III, the British monarch credited with losing the American colonies, who developed a mental illness. King George did not have dementia but did have bouts of delirium and psychosis. Today, it is widely believed that the king suffered from porphyria, a rare genetic disorder that interferes with the body's chemical balance. The symptoms include rashes, abdominal pain, and reddish blue urine, all of which George suffered. Untreated, it can affect the nervous system and lead to delirium and psychosis. If King George were alive today, he would be treated with drugs and advised to avoid too much sunlight. *Viewing Points:* Identify the symptoms of psychosis and mood disturbances. How does this film depict the understanding of mental illness? What does the use of the term "madness" in the title imply? If you cared for King George today, what medications would he be given for his psychosis and mood disturbances?

REFERENCES

Advisory Panel on Alzheimer's Disease. (1991). *Second report of the Advisory Panel on Alzheimer's Disease* (DHHS Publication No. ADM 91-1791). Washington, DC: U.S. Government Printing Office.

Alexopoulos, G. S. (1991). Anxiety and depression in the elderly. In C. Salzman & B. D. Lebowitz (Eds.), *Anxiety in the elderly.* New York: Springer.

Alexopoulos, G. S., & Abrams, R. C. (1991). Depression in Alzheimer's disease. *Psychiatric Clinics of North America, 14,* 327–340.

Alzheimer's Disease and Related Disorders Association (2001). *General statistics and demographics.* Chicago: Author.

American Psychiatric Association. (2000). *Diagnostic and statistical manual of mental disorders* (4th ed., Text revision). Washington, DC: Author.

Anderson, K., Launer, L. J., Oh, A. Hoea, A. W., & Breteler, M. M., & Hofman, A. (1995). Do nonsteroidal anti-inflammatory drugs decrease the risk for Alzheimer's disease? The Rotterdam Study. *Neurology, 45*(8), 1141–1145.

Aronson, M., Ooi, W. L., Morgenstern, H., et al. (1990). Women, myocardial infarction and dementia in the very old. *Neurology, 40,* 1102–1106.

Beck, C., & Heacock, P. (1988). Nursing interventions for patients with Alzheimer's disease. *Nursing Clinics of North America, 23*(1), 95–124.

Benson, S. (1999). Hormone replacement therapy and Alzheimer's disease: an update on the issues. *Health Care Women International, 20*(6), 619–638.

Bertoni, J. M., Brown, P., Goldfarb, L. G., et al. (1992). Familial Creutzfeldt-Jakob disease (codon 200 mutation) with supranuclear palsy. *Journal of the American Medical Association, 268,* 2413–2415.

Cummings, J. L., Vinters, H. V., Cole, G. M., & Khachaturian, Z. S. (1998). Alzheimer's disease: Etiologies, pathophysiology, cognitive reserve, and treatment opportunities. *Neurology, 51,* S2–S17.

Cummings, J. L. (1991). Behavioral complications of drug treatment of Parkinson's disease. *Journal of the American Geriatrics Society, 39,* 708–716.

Day, C. (1997). Validation therapy: A review of the literature. *Journal of Gerontological Nursing, 23*(4), 19–34.

Drugs & Therapy Perspectives. (1997). Drug-induced delirium: Diagnosis, management, and prevention. *10*(3), 5–9. Adis International Limited.

Graves, A. B., White, E., Koepsell, T. D., et al. (1990). The association between head trauma and Alzheimer's disease. *American Journal of Epidemiology, 131,* 491.

Growdon, J. H. (1992). Treatment for Alzheimer's disease? *New England Journal of Medicine, 327*(18), 1306–1309.

Gwyther, L. P. (1985). *Care of Alzheimer's patients: A manual for nursing home staff.* Chicago: Alzheimer's Disease and Related Disorders Association; and Washington, DC: American Health Care Association.

Hall, G. R. (1988a). Care of the patient with Alzheimer's disease living at home. *Nursing Clinics of North America, 23*(1), 31–46.

Hall, G. R. (1988b). *Development of an assessment instrument: Behavioral assessment for alterations in thought process due to cognitive loss.* Unpublished manuscript, The University of Iowa Hospitals and Clinics, Department of Nursing, Iowa City, Iowa.

Hall, G. R., Buckwalter, K. C., Stolley, J. M., et al. (1995). Standardized care plan: Managing Alzheimer's patient at home. *Journal of Gerontological Nursing, 21*(1), 41–42.

Inouye, S. K., van Dyke, C. H., Alessi, C. A., et al. (1990). Clarifying confusion: The confusion assessment method. A new method for detection of delirium. *Annals of Internal Medicine, 113,* 941–948.

Joachim, C. L., & Kelkoe, D. J. (1992). The seminal role of b-amyloid in the pathogenesis of Alzheimer's disease. *Alzheimer's Disease and Associated Disorders, 6,* 7–34.

Letenneur, L., Launer, L. J., Andersen, K., et al. (2000). Education and the risk for Alzheimer's disease: Sex makes a difference. EURODEM pooled analyses. EURODEM Incidence Research Group. *American Journal of Epidemiology, 151*(11), 1064–1071.

Lyketsos, C. G., Steinberg, M., Tschanz, J. T., Norton, M. C., Steffan, D. C. & Breither, J. C. (2000). Mental and behavioral disturbances in dementia: Findings from the Cache County Study on memory in aging. *American Journal of Psychiatry, 157,* 707–714.

Marcantonio, E. R., Flacker, J. M., Michaels, M., & Resnick, N. M. (2000). Delirium is independently associated with poor functional recovery after hip fracture. *Journal of the American Geriatrics Society, 48*(6), 618–624.

McCloskey, J. C., & Bulechek, G. M. (1996). *Nursing interventions classification (NIC).* St. Louis: Mosby.

McGeer, P., Schulzer, M., & McGeer, E. G. (1996). Arthritis and anti-inflammatory agents as possible protective factors for Alzheimer's disease: A review of 17 epidemiologic studies. *Neurology, 48*(5), 1473–1474.

Mignor, D. (2000). Effectiveness of use of home health nurses to decrease burden and depression of elderly caregivers. *Journal of Psychosocial Nursing & Mental Health Services, 38*(7), 34–41.

Mittelman, M. S., Ferris, S. H., Shulman, E., et al. (1996). A family intervention to delay nursing home placement of patients with Alzheimer's disease: A randomized controlled trial. *Journal of the American Medical Association, 276,* 1725–1731.

Mortimer, J. A., Van Duijn, C. M., Chandra, V., et al. (1991). Head trauma as a risk factor for Alzheimer's disease: A collaborative re-analysis of case-control studies. *International Journal of Epidemiology, 20,* S28–S35.

Mullan, M., Houlden, H., Windelspecht, M., et al. (1992). A locus for familial early-onset Alzheimer's disease in the long arm of chromosome 14, proximal to the alpha 1-anichymotrypsin gene. *Nature Genetics, 2*(4), 340–342.

Navia, B. A., Jordan, B. D., & Price, R. N. (1986). The AIDS dementia complex. I. Clinical features. *Annals of Neurology, 19,* 517–524.

Peskind, E. (1996). Neurobiology of Alzheimer's disease. *Journal of Clinical Psychiatry, 57*(Suppl. 14), 5–8.

Rabins, P. V., Black, B. S., Roca, R., et al. (2000). Effectiveness of a nurse-based outreach program for identifying and treating psychiatric illness in the elderly. *Journal of the American Medical Association, 283,* 2802–2809.

Ross, C. A., Peyser, C. E., Shapiro, I., & Folstein, M. F. (1991). Delirium: Phenomenologic and etiologic subtypes. *International Psychogeriatrics, 3,* 135–147.

Sano, M., Ernesto, C., Thomas, R. G., et al. (1997). A controlled trial of selegiline, alpha-tocopherol, or both as treatment for Alzheimer's disease. The Alzheimer's Disease Cooperative Study. *New England Journal of Medicine, 336,* 1216–1222.

Schellenberg, G. D., Boehnke, M., Wijsman, E. M., et al. (1992). Genetic association and linkage analysis of the apolipoprotein CII locus and familial Alzheimer's disease. *Annals of Neurology, 31*(2), 223–227.

Schor, J., Levkoff, S., Lipsitz, L., et al. (1992). Risk factors for delirium in hospitalized elderly. *Journal of the American Medical Association, 267,* 827–831.

Seltzer, B., Larkin, J. P., & Fabiszewski, K. J. (1988). Management of the outpatient with Alzheimer's disease: An interdisciplinary team approach. In L. Volicer, K. J. Fabiszewski, Y. L. Rheaume, & K. E. Lasch (Eds.), *Clinical management of Alzheimer's disease* (pp. 13–28). Rockville, MD: Aspen.

Stahl, S. M. (2000). *Essential psychopharmacology: Neuroscientific basis and practical applications* (2nd ed.). New York: Cambridge University Press.

Tariot, P., Schneider, L., & Porsteinsson, A. (1997). Treating Alzheimer's disease: Pharmacologic options now and in the near future. *Postgraduate Medicine, 101*(6), 73–76, 81, 84.

Tune, L. (2000). Delirium. In C. E. Coffey, and J. L. Cummings (Eds.). The American psychiatric press textbook of geriatric neuropsychiatry (2nd ed.) (pp. 441–462). Washington, DC: American Psychiatric Press.

Turner, R. S., D'Amato, C. J., Chervin, R. D., & Blaivas, M. (2000). The pathology of REM sleep behavior disorder with comorbid LEWY body dementia. *Neurology, 55*(11), 1730–1732.

Volicer, L. (1988). Drugs used in the treatment of Alzheimer's disease. In L. Volicer, K. J. Fabiszewski, Y. L. Rheaume, & K. E. Lasch (Eds.), *Clinical management of Alzheimer's disease* (pp. 196–199). Rockville, MD: Aspen.

Weiner, M. F., Tintner, R. J., & Goodkin, K. (1991). Differential diagnosis. In M. R. Weiner (Ed.), *The dementias: Diagnosis and management.* Washington, DC: American Psychiatric Press.

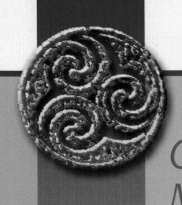

Care of the Homeless Mentally Ill

Ruth Beckmann Murray and Marjorie Baier

LEARNING OBJECTIVES

After studying this chapter, you will be able to:

➤ Define the meaning of homelessness to the person and family.

➤ Describe risk factors for becoming homeless.

➤ Identify risk factors for developing mental illness or chemical dependency among people who are homeless.

➤ Differentiate characteristics of various populations who are homeless.

➤ Discuss personal and societal attitudes and beliefs about homelessness.

➤ Describe assessment of people who are homeless and mentally ill.

➤ Formulate some nursing diagnoses relevant to the homeless population.

➤ Examine ways in which access to health care is limited for people who are homeless and mentally ill.

➤ Summarize interventions for people who are homeless and have psychiatric disorders.

➤ Discuss discharge planning needs of people who are homeless and have psychiatric disorders.

➤ List major community resources to which nurses can refer members of the homeless population.

➤ Discuss trends that target improvement of services to people who are homeless and experiencing psychiatric disorders.

case management
continuum of care
day treatment
deinstitutionalization

homeless
homelessness
safe havens
transitional housing

*T*he Stewart B. McKinney Homeless Assistance Act of 1987 defined a **homeless** person as "one who lacks a fixed permanent nighttime residence or whose nighttime residence is a temporary shelter, welfare hotel, transitional housing for the mentally ill, or any public or private place not designated as sleeping accommodations for human beings" (Interagency Council on the Homeless, 1994, p. 22). Homeless individuals and families can be categorized as those (1) encountering a natural disaster, home fire, some situational crisis or unexpected overwhelming life situation; (2) experiencing severe and persistent mental illness or substance abuse problems; or (3) experiencing comorbidity or dual diagnosis—a combination of mental illness and substance abuse. Text Box 32-1 lists characteristics of people who are homeless and mentally ill.

The Stewart B. McKinney Homeless Assistance Act of 1987 (Public Law 100-77) reflected concern in the United States about people who are homeless. This legislation provided the first comprehensive federal funding program targeted specifically to address the health, education, and welfare needs of the homeless population. It allocated money for (1) non-traditional crises and community services for chronically mentally ill people, (2) alcohol and drug detoxification and treatment programs, (3) psychosocial rehabilitation, (4) families with children at risk for emotional disturbance because of homelessness, (5) long-term case management, (6) supportive housing, (7) training of service providers, and (8) research (Interagency Council on the Homeless, 1994). Subsequent revisions to the McKinney Act incorporated an approach called **continuum of care**, which recognizes that, to be effective, a homeless system must provide three distinct components: an emergency shelter, transitional or rehabilitative services for those who need them, and permanent housing or supportive living arrangements. The continuum of care provides a framework for local and state planners to apply for funding from the Department of Housing and Urban Development (HUD) to address in a comprehensive fashion the needs of all people who are homeless. Because of the gap in services for people who are homeless and mentally ill, amendments were made to the McKinney Act in 1992 that included a provision for the creation of **safe havens**, which are a form of supportive housing that serves hard-to-reach people with severe mental illness (Center for Mental Health Services, 1997). The Shelter Plus Care Program, also a continuum of care program, allows for various housing choices and a range of supportive services funded by other sources (U.S. Department of Housing and Urban Development, 1998).

This chapter explores issues relevant to homeless individuals who are also experiencing mental health problems. It presents nursing care measures for such individuals and also ways to improve services for the homeless population.

HOMELESSNESS

Homelessness is a word that evokes images and feelings in everyone. It means to be without a consistent dwelling place, so meeting basic needs is difficult. It means carrying all one's possessions in a car, suitcase, or bag, or storing necessities in a bus station locker or

TEXT BOX 32.1

Characteristics of People Who Are Mentally Ill and Homeless

Although generalizing about this heterogeneous population is difficult, people with serious mental illnesses who are homeless share several important characteristics:

- They are homeless for longer periods than others who are homeless, living on the streets, in parks, or in subway stops.
- At least half of homeless people with serious mental illnesses also have a concurrent substance use disorder.
- They are generally in poorer physical health than other homeless people.
- Most are eligible for, but relatively few receive, any form of income maintenance, including Social Security income (SSI) or public assistance.
- Minorities, especially people of color, are overrepresented.
- Most are willing to accept help (including mental health or substance abuse treatment), but, at least initially, they are more likely to want assistance in meeting basic survival needs such as food, clothing, and housing.

From National Resource Center on Homelessness and Mental Illness. (2000). *Annotated bibliography: Population characteristics of homeless persons.* Available online at **http://www.prainc.com/nrc/bibliographies/populati_char.shtml.**

under the bed of a night shelter. It means no chest for treasured objects, no closet for next season's clothing, no pantry with goodies to eat, no place to entertain friends or have solitude. Boydell and colleagues (2000) found that if the person is homeless long enough, he or she experiences a sense of depersonalization and fragmented identity, loss of self-worth and self-efficacy, and a stigma of being "nothing," "a bum," "lazy," "stupid," and like an object. Some people automatically associate mental illness, violence, and alcohol or drug addiction with homelessness (Murray, 1993, 1996). The person who is homeless for the first time is more likely to describe himself or herself in positive terms than the person who has been homeless for a long time. Most homeless people, however, describe themselves as resourceful, independent, proud, and a survivor (Boydell et al., 2000).

Biographies and research have presented descriptions of the tragedy and nightmare of being homeless (Humphreys, 2000; Menke & Wagner, 1997; Murray, 1996; Torrey, 1988; Wright, 1989). The person who is homeless is often engaged in a hunting-and-gathering, subsistence strategy or culture: scavenging or hunting for shelter, food, clothing, and cans to recycle, and lacking consistent ways to meet basic needs. This lifestyle and the grinding poverty leave little energy for change

or re-entrance into the mainstream of life. Panhandling, hustling, odd jobs, and selling plasma or aluminum cans are sources of income unless the person receives Social Security or veterans or pension benefits. The person becomes victim to the immediate circumstance—hunger, cold, or assault. People who are homeless make choices and pursue various strategies at different times to meet subsistence needs and overcome fear, loss of freedom, resignation, loneliness, and depression (Koegel et al., 1990; Murray, 1996). There is no one to call for help who knows the person and his or her history and who really cares. The longer the person is homeless, the more likely the person is to suffer mental illness or engage in substance use (Koegel et al., 1990; Murray, 1996).

The healthiest survivors have been those who seek support from other homeless people. Women with children who are homeless have described the need to keep going for the sake of and to avoid losing the children. These women described the importance of spiritual beliefs in developing inner resources, reducing distress, and enhancing the connection to self and to powers beyond the self (Humphreys, 2000; Menke & Wagner, 1997).

Historical Perspectives

The phenomenon of many mentally ill street people began in the mid-1900s. A public outcry followed a photographic essay in 1946 by *Life* magazine about deplorable conditions in state hospitals for the mentally ill. The introduction of chlorpromazine (Thorazine) from France to the United States in 1954 provided a simple means of reducing symptoms of psychosis. In 1958, President Dwight D. Eisenhower established the Joint Commission on Mental Illness and Health. By January 1963, this commission had developed a nationwide plan for treating the mentally ill within their communities (Jones, 1983). President John F. Kennedy proposed this plan to Congress, and the "bold new approach to mental illness" resulted in federal legislation, the Mental Retardation Facilities and Community Mental Health Centers Construction Act of 1963. The Act was the impetus to provide a complete array of neighborhood-located mental health services and to fund staffing. Furthermore, soon after the assassination of President Kennedy, the Civil Rights Movement gained momentum. Advocates for the chronically mentally ill claimed the right to the "least restrictive environment." Unfortunately, the vision for day and night care, halfway houses, group homes, home-visiting mental health teams, 24-hour crisis services, vocational and social programs, and sheltered workshops—all coordinated and implemented by a multidisciplinary treatment team—never fully materialized. Contributing factors included lack of federal or state funding, inadequate numbers of prepared professionals, and communities unprepared or unwilling to participate in the movement (Jones, 1983).

The **deinstitutionalization** of the population with mental illness was a major turning point in mental health care. In 1973, the National Institute of Mental Health defined deinstitutionalization of state mental hospitals as (1) prevention of inappropriate mental hospital admissions through the provision of community alternatives for treatment, (2) release to the community of all institutionalized patients who have been given adequate preparation for such a change, and (3) establishment and maintenance of community support systems for noninstitutional people receiving community mental health services (Jones, 1983). Because of deinstitutionalization, in the late 1960s and 1970s, the census of state hospitals declined from thousands to hundreds. In Philadelphia alone, the census was reduced from 6,000 to 800. Cities were ill-prepared to handle the masses; discharged patients and their families were given little or no preparation (Jones, 1983). The stigma against the mentally ill became greater as cities faced real consequent social and financial problems. Furthermore, homeless, severely persistently mentally ill people experienced fear, suspicion, caution, and disorganized thinking, which interfered with using available services and promoted a homeless lifestyle (Taylor, 1996).

The increase in homelessness among people with mental illness cannot be attributed solely to deinstitutionalization (Interagency Council on the Homeless, 1994). Most individuals who are currently homeless have experienced homelessness much more recently than the deinstitutionalization movement of the 1960s and 1970s. The diversion of admissions from state hospitals to inadequate community-based mental health services and affordable housing results in homelessness for people with severe mental illness. Nevertheless, a return to institutional care is not the solution to this problem. The real need is for accessible integrated systems of care that link housing and mental health services (Interagency Council on the Homeless, 1994). These systems of care and services will be discussed later.

Risk Factors

People prefer to have a home and to be part of a family or social group. People do not choose or purposefully maintain homelessness and living on the streets (Walker, 1998). Homelessness has no single cause; many factors typically combine, over time, to cause the person or family to lose permanent housing. Homelessness is often the result of a trajectory marked by eviction for not paying rent, disturbing behavior, and multiple moves; doubling up with relatives and friends in overcrowded conditions until they can tolerate no more; living in a car or van or

running away from a violent home or being abandoned; and then seeking shelter (Rosenheck et al., 1999). The series of events that results in having no home is the culmination of individual and environmental factors, including factors in the mental health system, society, and family or community (Text Box 32-2).

Homeless Populations

The homeless population includes people of all ages, economic levels, racial and cultural backgrounds, and geographic areas. Homeless people are the new poor who are chronically ill, jobless, or elderly and have lost all financial resources. Or, homeless people may have lived in poverty for years and no longer have a home site. Among the homeless, educational level varies greatly from less than an eighth-grade education to doctoral degrees.

Incidence

Estimates of homeless people have varied from 300,000, according to the 1990 census, to several million. An estimated 7 million Americans were believed to have experienced homelessness at least once in the latter half of the 1980s (Ratnesar, 1999). As many as 12 million Americans may have been homeless at some time in their lives. In a 1994 survey of 1,500 people in the 20 largest cities in the United States, 15% had been homeless at some time; 3.6% had been homeless in the past 5 years; and 6.5% had slept in a car, tent, or box. During the average 280 days of homelessness, 42% had been assaulted or robbed, and 61% had been hungry (Link et al., 1995). The United States Conference of Mayors, in its annual survey of hunger and homelessness in 30 cities, found demand for emergency shelter had increased 500% between 1985 and 1998 (Ratnesar, 1999). The National Coalition for the Homeless (1998) estimated in 1996 that 800,000 people were homeless in the United States on any one night. The San Francisco Coalition for the Homeless estimated 16,000 homeless people nightly in 1998, twice that of the late 1980s (Ratnesar, 1999). Reasons for homelessness, in a recent study of 373 homeless young adults (mostly men) in 24 community-based sites, were as follows: (1) alcohol or drug abuse, 48.2%; (2) no financial resources, 32.5%; (3) no job, 30.7%; and (4) psychiatric problems, 10.3% (O'Toole et al., 1997).

Diverse Groups in the Homeless Population

Homelessness occurs in many groups of people. People with severe mental illness are at much higher risk for homelessness than others. Symptoms of mental illness, such as impulsivity, hypersexuality, and poor judgment, may be related to risky sexual behaviors as

TEXT BOX 32.2

Risk Factors for Homelessness Among People With Serious Mental Illness

Individual Risk Factors

- The nature of mental illness, including unpredictable behavior, inability to manage everyday affairs, and inability to communicate needs, which results in conflicts with family, employers, landlords, and neighbors (Bussuk et al., 1997; Davis & Kutler, 1998; Lezak & Edgar, 1996)

- Concurrent mental illness and substance abuse disorders in youth and adults, with behaviors that place them at high risk for eviction, arrest and incarceration in jails, or repeated admissions and short stays in mental hospitals (Bussak et al., 1997; Caton et al., 2000; Greene et al., 1997; Lezak & Edgar, 1996)

- Coexisting HIV or AIDS with severe persistent mental illness, chemical dependency, or both (Goldfinger et al., 1998; Talbott & Lamb, 1987)

- Coexisting demographic and societal factors of poverty; single-parent family (usually female headed); dependent child; child in foster home; racial or ethnic minority; veteran status; single men and women; ex-offender released from jail or prison (Burt, 1992; Bussuk et al., 1997; Caton et al., 2000; Greene et al., 1997; Herman et al., 1997; Rosenheck et al., 1999; Talbott & Lamb, 1987)

- Coexisting physical illness or developmental disability (Rosenheck et al., 1999)

- Exposure to traumatic events repeatedly, resulting in posttraumatic stress disorder and deficits in independent living skills (Davis & Kutter, 1998; Herman et al., 1997)

- Exposure to victimization (physical and sexual abuse), especially if a family member was the perpetrator (Bussuk et al., 1997; Herman et al., 1997; Koegel et al., 1995; Lezak & Edgar, 1996; Talbott & Lamb, 1987)

- Inability to cope with or manage the requirements of community or group living home (Lezak & Edgar, 1996)

- Lack of high school education or equivalence (Bussuk et al., 1997; Caton et al., 2000)

Environmental Risk Factors

Mental Health System Factors (Lezak & Edgar, 1996; Talbott & Lamb, 1987)

- Inadequate discharge planning with a lack of appropriate housing, treatment, and support services

- Lack of funding for community-based services

- Lack of integrated community-based treatment and support services for individual and group therapy, medication monitoring, and case management

- Lack of community-based crisis alternatives for housing, health care, and respite care for families, with risk for rehospitalization and loss of residence

- Lack of attention to consumer preferences for autonomy, privacy, and integrated regular housing

Societal Structural Factors

- Lack of affordable housing; affluent economic times have caused housing prices to soar out of reach, to reduce construction of low-cost housing, and to create a tight rental market (Burt, 1992; Lezak & Edgar, 1996; Ratnesar, 1999; Talbott & Lamb, 1987)

- Insufficient disability benefits; Social Security income recipients are below the federal poverty level (Lezak & Edgar, 1996; Ratnesar, 1999)

- Lack of coordination between mental health and substance abuse systems (Lezak & Edgar, 1996; Talbott & Lamb, 1987)

- Waiting lists to receive a subsidy that requires the person to pay only 30% of income for rent and utilities (Burt, 1992; Ratnesar, 1999)

- Lack of job opportunities for disabled people (Burt, 1992)

Family and Community Factors (Lezak & Edgar, 1996)

- Stigma and discrimination; resistance to community housing for the mentally ill is widespread.

- Poor family relationships; willingness to help the ill person is exhausted as relatives cope with frightening or disturbing behavior and receive insufficient help from the community or medical profession.

- Parents using drugs in the home with children (Bussuk et al., 1997; Caton et al., 2000; Herman et al., 1997)

---

well. Sexual risk-taking behaviors and drug use practices, such as sharing needles, contribute to the higher rate of HIV infection. Poverty also contributes to unsafe sexual behaviors through the limited availability of condoms, sharing of bedrooms, and lack of planning about sexual contacts. Furthermore, there may be a relationship between use of crack cocaine or other drugs and alcohol and unprotected sexual encounters.

Family homelessness, whether because of poverty, unexpected job loss, or natural disaster, such as fire or flood, has an especially adverse effect on children. According to Rosenheck et al. (1999), homeless children

are generally young children. These children have high rates of both acute and chronic health problems, and they are more likely than children who are not homeless to be hospitalized, have delayed immunizations, and have elevated lead blood levels. In addition, they are at risk for developmental delays and emotional and behavioral difficulties. School attendance is disrupted frequently, and they are vulnerable to violence, either as victims or witnesses. The child who is homeless is more likely to experience homelessness in adulthood (Bussuk et al., 1997; Caton et al., 2000; Herman et al., 1997; Koegel et al., 1995).

Living in shelters is stressful for families for several reasons. To begin with, many shelters exclude men and adolescent boys older than age 12 years (Rosenheck et al., 1999); thus, family members are separated. Overcrowding results in lack of privacy and a sense of loss of personal control. A history of abuse and assault is common for a mother who is homeless (Davis & Kutter, 1998; Rosenheck, et al., 1999). Stressors of poverty and reduced social support compound the trauma of these experiences. Homeless mothers have high lifetime rates of major depressive disorder, posttraumatic stress disorder, and substance use disorders. In addition, they have high rates of attempted suicide (Davis & Kutter, 1998; Rosenheck et al., 1999). Homeless women who have a social network, some cash assistance such as Social Security or welfare, or a housing subsidy are more likely to become and remain housed (Bussuk et al., 1997).

Adolescents can become homeless because of strained family relationships, family dissolution, and instability or residential placements (Greene et al., 1997; Koegel et al., 1995; Rosenheck et al., 1999). As a result of being homeless, young people may resort to drug trafficking and prostitution to support themselves. They are at risk for health and mental health problems, including substance abuse, HIV or AIDS, pregnancy, and suicidal behaviors. Because of their high rates of exposure to violence, they are more likely to develop posttraumatic stress disorder and depression. To compound their problems, they are less likely to use shelters, owing to lack of available shelters that will accept them and to their own distrust and fear of providers.

A greater percentage of people who are homeless have been arrested or incarcerated in the past than the general population (Rosenheck et al., 1999). When people who are poor and have substance abuse problems are incarcerated, they are cut off from their communities and are less likely to be able to re-establish themselves after their release from jail or prison. They are at greater risk for homelessness. Other people with criminal records may have turned to crime after they became homeless in order to support themselves. Another group of people with mental illness who have arrest records are those who have been inappropriately jailed because of inadequacies of the mental health treatment system.

Several other groups are at risk for homelessness or may experience homelessness at some point. New immigrants come to a specific location with the intention of setting up permanent residence. Economic problems or conflicts with the sponsoring family may jeopardize housing. Refugees are poor; they are involuntarily living outside the habitual country of nationality because of persecution related to race, religion, nationality, social group membership, or political opinion. Mental health problems arise because of torture experiences, losses suf-fered in the country of origin, and culture shock and scapegoating upon their arrival in the United States and thereafter. Posttraumatic stress is to be expected; physical health problems are often complex (Andrews & Boyle, 1999; DeSantis, 1997). Migrant workers and their families lack residential stability as they move from one geographic region to another for 6 to 9 months a year for the purpose of agricultural production and harvest. These laborers and their families may be U.S. citizens or foreign born. They are poor and typically lack adequate living quarters and health care. A number of physical health problems, as well as depression, are commonly seen in the adults and the children. After farm labor is completed, families members may be homeless until they are able to return to their place of origin or to a relative's home (DeSantis, 1997; Sandhaus, 1998).

Societal Attitudes and Beliefs

Whenever people are described as part of a group, the individual may not be represented accurately in the description or may be misunderstood by others outside of the group. As a result, unrealistic ideas or beliefs may develop about both the group as a whole and individuals within the group or population. Text Box 32-3 presents common myths and the related facts about homeless people who are mentally ill.

NURSING MANAGEMENT OF INDIVIDUALS AND FAMILIES WHO ARE HOMELESS

Assessment

A holistic perspective is essential for assessing any person or family unit who is homeless because people and the phenomenon of homelessness are complex and multifaceted. The nurse must avoid looking at homeless people as problems with deficiencies. Rather, the nurse should look at the unique individual and the person's or family's transactions with the environment and their interdependence.

The approach to the person or family must be gentle and compassionate; the fast-paced, time-focused approach of the traditional health care system is unlikely to gather the needed information to intervene. In fact, the person may leave the setting rather than be subjected to more depersonalization. The nurse must use the principles of a therapeutic relationship and therapeutic communication described in Chapter 9 to establish rapport and trust.

Biologic Assessment

The assessment must begin at the point of the person's need; often, it is a physical need or health problem (Text

TEXT BOX 32.3

Myths and Facts About People Who Are Homeless and Have Psychiatric Disorders

Myth: Homeless people are all alike.

Fact: Homeless people come from all walks of life. Those with and without psychiatric illness share some characteristics. Being homeless is a leveling experience in that it is a sufficiently handicapping condition in itself to cause altered adaptation. Those with chronic substance abuse may have more difficulty in meeting basic needs than those who are chronically mentally ill.

Myth: Most homeless people are lazy, passive, and do not want to work.

Fact: Homeless people who loiter may be actively trying to survive by avoiding extreme weather, seeking monetary or other assistance, or trying to feel a part of mainstream society. Most desire work, even when physical or mental disabilities interfere.

Myth: Homeless people prefer being alone.

Fact: Peer relations with trusted people are preferred and essential to survival and meeting needs.

Myth: Homeless people are stupid and do not know how to manage life.

Fact: People who are homeless must be creative to secure resources and constantly change life ways to survive. Ability to think clearly, however, is threatened under stress and in hostile environments.

Myth: Homeless people refuse to stay in a shelter because they are ill.

Fact: Homeless people, including the mentally ill, do not use shelters for the following reasons: (1) lack of shelter beds in an accessible area, (2) difficulty in reaching the shelter, (3) overcrowded or unpleasant conditions in specific shelters, (4) restrictions on length of stay or criteria for admission, and (5) availability of alternative options (Murray, 1996).

Myth: Street dwellers are unwilling to accept services.

Fact: Most homeless people recognize the need for help; however, survival needs take priority over need for mental health treatment. Nontraditional approaches may be necessary to work with the mentally ill person who is homeless.

Myth: Most homeless people require acute, inpatient psychiatric care.

Fact: About 5% to 7% of adult mentally ill homeless people need inpatient care.

Myth: Most homeless people, especially the mentally ill, are dangerous.

Fact: High visibility of this population lends itself to frequent reporting of minor crimes, such as loitering, panhandling, public misconduct, minor shoplifting, or efforts to protect self from dangerous others, which can result in a fight.

Data from Cohen & Thompson, 1992; Downing & Cobb, 1990; *Exploring Myths*, 1990; Koegel et al., 1990; Smith et al., 1992, 1993: Torrey, 1988; Wright, 1989.

Box 32-4). Because of past experiences with the health care system or providers or because of mental illness or substance use, the person may not allow a thorough physical examination or may refuse to answer questions about history at the first visit. The nurse should realize that many homeless people consider themselves well as long as they can get to the desired place. It may appear adaptive to the individual to not admit illness. The nurse must be aware of the many health problems that may be present (Text Box 32-5). The homeless child or adolescent may suffer any of those listed as well as diseases that are specific to the age group. If the woman is pregnant, the nurse should recognize indications that she is at high risk for maternal or fetal complications.

Psychological Assessment

Behavior that looks like a mental illness may in reality be an expression of normal emotional or social needs. The homeless person may manifest the need to feel safe, secure, and respected and to be treated as a unique and valued person with overt distancing or aggressive behavior. The nurse should ask how long the person has been homeless and in what context (shelter, street, relatives); such variables can considerably affect behavior, feelings, and psychological function.

People who experience homelessness have their own way of being in the world, as described by Taylor (1996). They feel (1) heightened awareness of being labeled, on display, and judged or stigmatized by outer appearance; (2) that little or nothing is owned and that authorities expect certain behavior; (3) anxiety about having to be at a certain place at preset times to meet daily needs; (4) a sense of community or belonging by being part of a group that goes through rituals of waking, eating, lining up, and sharing facilities, space, and resources; and (5) a sense of humor, amusement, aloofness, and light-hearted optimism about ability to cope with a complicated lifestyle and to be hurt as little as possible.

Just as the physical examination may be incomplete, so may the mental status examination have to be done in part or over several visits. See Text Box 32-6 related to psychological assessment.

TEXT BOX 32.4

Biologic Assessment

- Use unobtrusive observation as a part of physical assessment. Some conditions will be immediately obvious. Other conditions may become apparent during the interview.

- Examine—look, touch, palpate, auscultate—the person to the extent he or she allows. The person may resist anything more than a superficial conversation and observation. The nurse may need to perform initial palpation of the abdomen or auscultation of the lung through several layers of clothes. If the patient perceives the health care provider as too intrusive, the patient may leave the setting even though desperate for care.

- Listen carefully to what the patient does *not* say, and pay attention to nonverbal as well as verbal expressions. Avoid unnecessary directness and probing. Give the person time to answer questions. The blood test or urine screen may have to wait; a patient and nonintrusive manner may ensure that the person returns the next day, or soon thereafter, for needed tests or screening.

- Determine whether the person has been prescribed medications in the past. Often, the homeless person is not taking medications, even if they are prescribed and essential. The person may have difficulty keeping pills dry and easily retrievable. A daily insulin injection, for example, may not seem practical.

TEXT BOX 32.5

Physical Health Problems Experienced by People Who Are Homeless, Including Those With Psychiatric Illness

- Injuries, fractures, epistaxis, or edema from trauma, falls, burns, assault, gunshot wounds
- Influenza, colds, bronchitis, asthma, shortness of breath
- Hypothermia, hyperthermia
- Arthritis, musculoskeletal disorders, headaches, fatigue
- Diabetes mellitus
- Hypertension
- Cardiovascular and peripheral vascular diseases
- Malnutrition
- Pulmonary tuberculosis
- Infestations, such as lice or scabies
- Dermatitis, sunburn or frostbite, bruises
- Sexually transmitted diseases
- Hypothyroidism or hyperthyroidism
- Kidney or liver disease
- Cancer
- Epilepsy
- Impaired vision, glaucoma, cataracts
- Impaired hearing
- Dental caries, periodontal disease

Symptoms of schizophrenia may be difficult to differentiate from emotional responses to the stressors of a homeless lifestyle. Required hypervigilance may augment suspicion or paranoid beliefs. The need for constant awareness of possibilities for meeting basic needs can augment self-preoccupation. Blunted affect, lack of communication, loose associations, ambivalence, isolation, and uncertainty may be the result of life on the streets and in various places. Such symptoms or behaviors may be part of the dynamics of the homeless experience and use of healthy coping mechanism and creative survival techniques, rather than pathology.

Substance abuse must be ruled out because the incidence is increased among homeless people, including the mentally ill. Because homeless people, especially those with psychiatric disorders, are often victims of crime and violence, the incidence of posttraumatic stress disorder may be higher than in the general population. Homeless women are especially in danger of being assaulted, abused, and raped (Taylor, 1996).

When the child or adolescent is homeless, the nurse should ask about the educational history, if the youth is enrolled in school, and perceived progress. Homeless children often have difficulty; the school district may

TEXT BOX 32.6

Psychological Assessment

- Observe for behavior that indicates hallucination and try to validate.

- Listen for delusions or denial over time; try to sense what purpose these may serve to the person.

- Observe and listen for what the person defines as a problem and potential solution and what he or she considers to be a strength or coping strategy; validate and reinforce when applicable.

- View the person and his or her situation from the individual's perspective; be a patient, nonthreatening listener. Such an approach encourages the person to return regularly; the nurse can then observe the patterns of behavior.

- Determine the extent of stability or integration of the person's sense of self, cognitive appraisals, and overt behavior. Lack of sense of integration or stability is an indicator of continued monitoring and therapy.

change every time the parent changes shelters. The nurse must determine whether the child has behavioral or emotional problems and if he or she needs special education services. Zima and colleagues (1997) found that 45% of 169 children in 18 emergency family shelters in Los Angeles met the criteria for special education. Only 22% had received any testing or placement.

Homelessness places parents and children at risk for mental health problems; maternal depression may affect the mother–child relationship and create child behavior problems. The nurse should realize that homeless mothers and children also have great resilience. Smith and associates (1993) found that less than 50% of homeless women had a current psychiatric illness. Conrad (1998) found that homeless mothers were not necessarily depressed, nor did they have inadequate coping skills. Many homeless women are competent and resilient; they made the decision to free themselves of a noxious relationship. Further, acute maternal depression was not associated with child behavior problems in 70% of the mother–child dyads who were studied.

Social and Family Assessment

Cultural value differences exist between homeless people and the dominant American culture, to which most providers of health care subscribe. Thus, providers and the homeless person who needs health care may experience cultural conflict in their (1) norms of health and illness, (2) basic value systems and priorities, and (3) perceptions about health care (Downing & Cobb, 1990). Health care providers expect the person, including homeless mentally ill or chemically dependent patients, to problem solve, become more independent, and be future oriented. These values affect assessment, treatment, and interactions with the person and can interfere with the nursing process and patient response to the health care system (Downing & Cobb, 1990). The nurse must consider how the homeless ill patient perceives his or her everyday life and vary the assessment and therapy approach accordingly.

Homelessness is an expression of and response to certain family, societal, or environmental conditions as well as to individual factors. See Text Box 32-7 for factors in the social and family assessment.

Spiritual Assessment

The nurse should listen for expressions that convey a spiritual faith, a connection to a transcendent being, or a belief system that helps the person endure. Questions about the spiritual dimension may convey an invitation to talk about an aspect of life that is often ignored but that may be very important to the person. Listening to values, beliefs, and preferred practices will help determine relevant therapy approaches.

TEXT BOX 32.7

Social and Family Assessment

- Ask about support systems, people who could be helpful, and what services have been or could be used.
- Determine whether the person is isolated from the family, and if so, if it is by personal choice rather than by family choice.
- Respect that the person who feels isolated may avoid talking about the biologic family.
- Explore if the patient views a homeless peer, local pastor, counselor, or another health care provider as "family" or as the support system.
- Convey genuine interest in the person and convey that others may also care. Questions may be the catalyst to re-establishing family ties.

Nursing Diagnoses

The North American Nursing Diagnosis Association (NANDA, 2001) describes several nursing diagnoses that are relevant to the person who is homeless and who is also mentally ill or substance abusing. One NANDA nursing diagnosis that could be considered for people who are homeless is Impaired Home Maintenance. The definition of this nursing diagnosis is "inability to independently maintain a safe growth-promoting immediate environment." Other potential nursing diagnoses include Imbalanced Nutrition, Risk for Injury, Risk for Loneliness, Social Isolation, Ineffective Role Performance, Hopelessness, Posttrauma Syndrome, Relocation Stress Syndrome, Chronic Low Self-Esteem, Chronic Sorrow, Disturbed Thought Processes, and Disturbed Sensory Perception (NANDA, 2001).

Nursing Interventions

Interventions are to be directed at the social system as well as the individual or family level. Interventions should take advantage of community resources as well as the inner resources and support systems of the individual or family.

Cost and lack of insurance are the biggest barriers to health and hospital care of the homeless. Another barrier is the inability of this population to carry out treatment recommendations; survival is the first priority (Gelber et al., 1997; Murray, 1996). Compliance with medication and treatment regimens are difficult because successful treatment requires collaboration, monitoring, time for medication and other measures to be effective, and a secure place to keep medication (Taylor, 1996). Mentally ill people who are homeless often cannot routinely get prescriptions filled. Medicine may be stolen. It is necessary for the person or family unit to have a place to keep medications that can be reached at the necessary times and to have access to primary care services for regular check-ups, assessment for adverse drug responses, and necessary blood monitoring.

People who have been homeless for several years have greater difficulty readjusting to restabilization and need more time for healing, depending on illness severity, comorbidity, and available support system (Taylor, 1996). Homeless people, including those with psychiatric disorders, become creative at surviving on the streets. The nurse must explore resources with the individual or family. See Text Box 32-8 for appropriate interventions.

Depending on the person's expression, the nurse may explore ways to meet spiritual needs. In one study, respondents listed the following as ways to meet spiritual needs (Murray, 1993): (1) pray and put trust in God, (2) hope that things will get better, (3) obtain strength from religious beliefs and say these beliefs to self daily, (4) seek a religious worker and attend religious services, (5) talk about the meaning of the life situation with

someone who is understanding and cares, and (6) read devotional material, such as the Bible or Koran.

Discharge Planning

A crucial time for intervention occurs at discharge from inpatient or medical treatment. At this time, the nurse can assist in the patient's transition from institutional to community living by providing practical and emotional support (Kuno et al., 2000). According to Kuno and associates (2000), having community outpatient mental health treatment is not sufficient to prevent homelessness for high-risk people with mental illness. People with mental illness who have been homeless need assistance in using available resources, such as medical, psychiatric, substance abuse, emergency department treatment, and other outpatient psychiatric services (Kuno et al., 2000). Adequate discharge planning includes linkages with intensive case management services.

In preparation for discharge, the nurse should make arrangements for transfer to transitional housing, if available. He or she should provide the person with phone numbers and directions for emergency shelters, lunch sites, day treatment programs, mental health hotlines, crisis lines (abuse, suicide), appropriate self-help or support groups, and relevant toll-free numbers. Referral can be to the Community Support Programs, funded in many cities by the National Institute of Mental Health, to provide flexible programs that enable the person to receive living skills training and other services to promote independent living (Levine & Rog, 1990). Predischarge planning involves options, such as alternatives if the first suggested shelter is closed upon arrival. Whatever information is given should be legible; concise; able to fit in a pocket, purse, shoe, or boot; and as portable as possible. Bulky brochures or three-ring binders are impractical. The nurse must never assume the person's literacy level; the person may not admit inability to read. If the person is illiterate, time must be spent with helping him or her memorize essential information.

TRENDS FOR IMPROVING SERVICES

Diverse services and integrated systems are essential to address all aspects of life situations of people who are homeless and experiencing psychiatric disorders. Essential components include (1) Safe Havens or stable shelters or residences; (2) accessible outreach; (3) integrated case management; (4) accessible and affordable housing options; (5) treatment and rehabilitation services; (6) general health care services; (7) rehabilitation, vocational training, and assistance with employment; (8) income support; and (9) legal protection (Leshner, 1992). The agencies that provide these services must develop a physical and emotional atmosphere that conveys

---

TEXT BOX 32.8

Interventions With Homeless People

- Provide a list with addresses and phone numbers of shelters and luncheon sites that provide food; discourage rooting through dumpsters and panhandling.

- Provide a list of facilities that are safe, including shelters that provide clothing, a safe place to sleep, and opportunity for basic hygiene and laundry.

- Give information on city ordinances that forbid sleeping on park benches, in building doorways, on sidewalk grates, at bus or train stations, in vacant buildings, or in viaducts.

- Explore sources of income, such as gathering and selling aluminum cans or engaging in temporary day labor. Discourage selling pints of blood or plasma.

- Assist the person directly or by referral to pursue obtaining entitlements, such as Social Security, veterans, or other benefits.

- Explore how to stay safe. Even in a night shelter, the homeless person may not be safe from assault. It is difficult for the homeless person to know who is trustworthy to accompany; carrying a bag or case is usually considered a marker for being robbed on the streets.

- Explore how to secure privacy, which is difficult to achieve, and how to cope with loneliness, which can be overwhelming.

- Give a list of names, addresses, and telephone numbers of agencies that offer services and socialization, such as the local Mental Health Agency or the local chapter of National Alliance for the Mentally Ill.

- Give information about meetings of Alcoholics Anonymous, Narcotics Anonymous, or Cocaine Anonymous if the person is using substances.

a sense of caring and community (Levine & Rog, 1990; Murray & Baier, 1993). The trend is to develop a "one-stop caring center" so that the person or family does not have to travel to numerous separately located agencies to get needs met. Instead, many community agencies are located at one site, much like a shopping mall.

Emergency Services

Some agencies provide a street outreach or mobile outreach program. As part of this program, a van travels the streets nightly to areas where homeless people will be found outdoors. Food, warm coffee, hygiene kits, and a blanket are the first steps in building trust with staff. The homeless person may accept an offer to be driven to a local shelter for the night. Follow-up the next day by van or bicycle provides a way to recontact the individual and invite him or her to the agency programs or take him or her to other social service or health care services. Luncheon sites for the homeless are a basic step in emergency services (Cunnane et al., 1995). Some agencies have a health clinic on site for treatment of minor problems.

Emergency shelters typically provide refuge at night along with an evening meal and morning coffee. Shelters for homeless women and children usually allow them to remain during daytime hours as well. The child leaves the shelter for school; the mother may attend educational classes, counseling, day treatment, rehabilitation, or employment programs. Text Box 32-9 provides ways to improve shelters further.

TEXT BOX 32.9

How Emergency Shelters Could Improve Services

- Extend hours to allow admission earlier in the afternoon and the opportunity to remain past 6 AM or 7 AM.

- Permit late entry to night shelters for those who had held a temporary day job and could not arrive before 6 PM or 7 PM because of work hours and bus transportation schedules.

- Maintain cleanliness and control bugs and vermin.

- Have adequate helpful staff and use effective security inside and outside the shelter.

- Provide a place to store belongings.

- Provide transportation from various points in the city to the night shelter or to needed health care services.

- Have policy that permits stay beyond 14 to 28 days, especially if the person is actively participating in recovery or employment programs.

Data from Murray, R. (1996). Needs and resources: The lived experience of homeless men. *Journal of Psychosocial Nursing, 34* (5), 18–24.

Housing Services

Transitional housing may consist of a halfway house, short-stay residence or group home, or a room at a hotel designated for homeless people (Text Box 32-10). Some agencies have a transitional home and stabilization center where the atmosphere and staff are a model for residents, who work on specific goals and a treatment plan. Sharing housekeeping tasks, obtaining psychiatric stabilization, and attending residence group meetings, social skills and budgeting classes, day treatment programs, and vocational training are steps to independent housing and employment. A holistic program reduces readmission to the hospital and re-entry to street dwelling (Baier et al., 1996; Carr et al., 1998; Murray & Baier, 1993; Murray et al., 1995) (Research Box 32-1).

The HUD continuum of care approach to homelessness includes both the Safe Havens and Shelter Plus Care programs mentioned at the beginning of this chapter. In addition to serving hard-to-reach people

TEXT BOX 32.10

Example of Transitional Housing Services

One agency provides a program for severely and persistently mentally ill women, many of whom are older. They sleep at the night shelter and attend the day treatment program, receiving meals, hygiene and laundry services, clothing, social interaction, long-term case management and counseling, and health services. Those who become stabilized and express aspirations are encouraged to attend GED or community college classes, pursue employment, and move into independent housing. Others live at the site for many years—safe, psychiatrically stable, and content (Cunnane et al., 1995).

Some social service agencies implement a housing program to assist homeless people within a specific geographic area with emergency monetary assistance for rent or utilities bills. Case management, relevant budgeting and education classes, and assistance with employment are included in the program. Case managers work with landlords on issues of tenant rights and occupancy standards and try to prevent tenant–landlord conflicts. Such a program is particularly useful for people at risk for becoming homeless because of changes in the economy, public housing, or welfare policies. As a result, the clients, usually female-headed families with children, become emotionally stabilized and self-sufficient, avoiding welfare, remaining housed, maintaining employment, and keeping the children in school.

Such housing programs are preventative as well as therapeutic in nature, especially when they follow clients for 1 to 2 years, as needed. The cycle of homelessness is broken. One study found that homeless women and those who had subsistence needs met were more likely to acquire and maintain housing than were men or those who had a substance abuse disorder or mental illness (Pollio et al., 1997).

RESEARCH BOX 32.1

Comparison of Completers and Noncompleters in a Transitional Residential Program for Homeless Mentally Ill

The purpose of this study was to evaluate the effectiveness of a transitional residential program for homeless severely, persistently mentally ill clients and to compare differences in client outcomes related to completion of program goals. Effectiveness of the program was measured by whether client became psychiatrically stabilized, found secure housing (apartment, group home, or home of a relative or friend), and began receiving entitlements. Noncompleters were residents who did not follow through on the admission contract or meet these criteria, including those who left against professional advice and those who were asked to leave.

Clinical records of 228 former clients were examined for demographic data, needs on admission, psychiatric diagnosis, participation in activities, length of stay, and type of discharge. The program discharged 48% (110) of the residents according to the admission contract. Mean length of stay for program completers was 143 days; length of stay varied for noncompleters. Participation in at least two activities while in residence was significantly related to program completion. Subjects who completed the program were more likely to obtain permanent hous-ing than noncompleters. Type of discharge or length of stay did not vary significantly by gender or Axis I psychiatric diagnosis, including chemical dependence.

Implications for Nursing: Findings of this study demonstrate the empowerment-oriented approach with homeless mentally ill people. This approach encourages the person to identify needs, determine goals, set terms about the helping process mutually with the therapy staff, and participate in program planning, thus maximizing the patient's control over the helping process and promoting self-determination and autonomy. Psychiatric nurses can be advocates for or leaders in the implementation of this kind of community-based program (Murray & Baier 1993). Although the focus of such programs must remain on achievement of program outcomes, patients who do not successfully complete a program also receive some level of assistance, to the extent to which they can accept services at the time.

Baier, M., Murray, R., North, C., et al. (1996). Comparison of completers and noncompleters in a transitional residential program for homeless mentally ill. *Issues in Mental Health*, *17*, 337–352.

with severe mental illness who are on the streets and have been unwilling or unable to participate in traditional supportive services, a Safe Haven meets the following criteria: (1) provides 24-hour residence for an unspecified duration, (2) provides private or semiprivate accommodations, and (3) has overnight occupancy limited to 25 persons (U.S. Department of Housing and Urban Development, 2000). "Safe Havens provide more than shelter. They close the gap in housing and services available for those homeless individuals who, perhaps because of their illness, have refused help or have been denied or removed from other homeless programs" (Center for Mental Health Services, 1997, p. 3). Shelter Plus Care provides housing and supportive services on a long-term basis for homeless people with disabilities, primarily those with serious mental illness, chronic problems with alcohol or drugs, or AIDS or related diseases (U.S. Department of Housing and Urban Development, 1998).

Case Management

Case management involves systematic assessment, planning, goal setting, counseling and other interventions, coordination of services, referral as necessary, and monitoring of the person's or family's needs and progress. It enhances self-care capability and quality of care along the continuum of care, decreases fragmentation, provides for cost containment, and reduces unnecessary duplication of services or hospitalization. The case manager is the gatekeeper and facilitator who may at first network with services on the person's or family's behalf and then encourage dealing directly with other service providers to obtain bus passes and transportation, children's services and supplies, medical or obstetric care, or housing. The nurse is the ideal team member to be the case manager because of knowledge about both psychiatric and physical diseases and the ability to develop therapeutic relationships and stay connected with the homeless person or family and with the health care system.

Rehabilitation and Education

Day Treatment Programs

Day treatment provides a bridge between institutional and community care for severely mentally ill and substance-abusing people. Because people who are staying in a transitional residence at night are at a critical point for other interventions, their participation in structured day treatment programs can provide emotional and practical support and strengthen ties to community services and potentially to family and friends (Susser et al., 1997). A day treatment program can provide a mailing address for people who are homeless, legal assistance, and help with finding employment and independent housing. It can provide case management, assistance with goal setting and problem solving, and psychiatric or medical care. The day treatment program may incorporate adult basic education classes to increase literacy and survival skills, GED classes for those who want a high school diploma, and computer skills to improve employment options (Cunnane et al., 1995). A Living Skills Program typically includes content in nutrition, budgeting, parenting, household and family management, tenant responsibilities and rights, and employment readiness. Such classes are especially useful to women who will no longer be receiving welfare benefits (Cunnane et al., 1995). The person can receive assistance with application for government benefits, if qualified, and obtaining identification, such as a birth certificate, if needed. The informal environment of day treatment programs promotes a feeling of camaraderie, self-confidence, trust in staff, and aspirations to independent living. Such extensive services for a 9-month period were found to be effective in an 18-month follow-up study, in that respondents were no longer homeless, and rehospitalization was prevented (Susser et al., 1997).

Alcohol and Drug Treatment

The structure of some day treatment programs follows the 12-step model of Alcoholic Anonymous for people who abuse substances or have a dual diagnosis. Sobriety is the goal; the person attends daily meetings, receives necessary psychiatric and medical treatment, and participates in all the other activities and services available at the day treatment program. No one is terminated for relapse; the person is referred to more intensive services, including hospitalization, if necessary (Cunnane et al., 1995).

Employment Services

Job placement is most likely when an employment program teaches basic job-seeking skills (ie, resume writing; interview skills; appropriate attire, hygiene, and behavior; and work etiquette) as well as offers actual job training in settings that prepare the person for the real world and real jobs. Case management during employment training can increase self-confidence, teach the person how to cope with the stresses of regular employment and budgeting skills, and link the person with community resources. It can also help to teach the person various skills for job retention and career development. The employment service should periodically follow-up with both the client employee and employer to ensure a successful record and movement to independence (Cunnane et al., 1995).

Integrated Services

Ongoing social support groups, membership in day treatment programs, attendance at meetings of Alcoholics Anonymous, Narcotics Anonymous, or Cocaine Anonymous, or the local National Alliance for the Mentally Ill or Mental Health Association can help the person who was severely mentally ill or substance abusing to remain in the community and live independently or with family. Support groups foster peer socialization and problem solving, enhance self-esteem, and offer many activities, such as art and recreation therapy or legal assistance. An example of a support group is an Alumni Club for the "alumni" of a job-training center. The evening, mental health after-care program is attended by those who have become psychiatrically stabilized, are employed, and are living independently. A club-like setting provides a safe, friendly, substance-free environment for seven evenings each week, year round. Case management, including individualized treatment plans and counseling, continues for 6 months or longer. Alcoholics Anonymous meetings, self-improvement classes, and other educational opportunities are integrated with case management. Socialization, fun, and effective leisure activities result (Text Box 32-11).

TEXT BOX 32.11

Community Resources to Aid the Homeless

- The National Data Resource Center on Homelessness and Mental Illness
  262 Delaware Avenue
  Delmar, NY 12054
  800-444-7415
  www.prainc.com/nrc
- VA Homeless Assistance Information
  Department of Veterans Affairs (111C)
  810 Vermont Avenue, NW
  Washington, DC 20420
  800-827-1000
  www.va.gov/health/homeless/AssistProg.htm
- National Alliance for the Mentally Ill
  200 North Glebe Road
  Suite 1015
  Arlington, VA 22203
  800-950-6264
  www.nami.org
- National Coalition for the Homeless
  1612 K Street, NW
  Suite 1004
  Washington, DC 20006
  202-775-1322
  www.nationalhomeless.org

Advocacy

Nurses can share experiences and research findings with the local chapter or national headquarters of the National Alliance for the Mentally Ill and with state legislators and members of Congress who are involved in developing legislation and policies related to people who are homeless, mentally ill, and substance abusing. Continued contacts are essential to convey the perceptions and needs of this population and to influence allocations for needed programs and services.

Summary of Key Points

➤ Homeless people are a heterogeneous, diverse group, some of whom are mentally ill or abuse substances.

➤ There are many risks for being homeless; people do not want to be homeless.

➤ Nursing assessment must be holistic; the nurse must listen to the person's perceptions and observe carefully.

➤ The mentally ill or substance abusing homeless person may suffer various physical health problems.

➤ Intervention must be oriented to the person's or family's perceived needs, culturally sensitive, and compassionate.

➤ The homeless mentally ill person may avoid traditional health care services.

➤ Nurses must incorporate new trends in providing and improving services.

Critical Thinking Challenges

1. What factors might interfere with a homeless mentally ill person's ability to follow through with the plan of care?

2. How might medication compliance be an issue for a homeless mentally ill person?

3. What might nurses do as a group to bring the issue of treatment of the homeless mentally ill into public view?

4. What communication approaches might be particularly useful and which might be especially threatening to the homeless mentally ill?

 WEB LINKS

www.nationalhomeless.org The National Coalition for the Homeless. This site represents a national advocacy network of homeless persons, activists, service providers, and others committed to ending homelessness through public education, pol-

icy advocacy, grassroots organizing, and technical assistance.

www.earthsystems.org/ways Fifty-four ways to help the homeless. This is Rabbi Kroloff's website.

www.hud.gov/hmless.html United States Housing Authority. This site provides information for homeless individuals.

www.nchv.org National Coalition for Homeless Veterans. This is a website for homeless veterans.

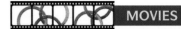 **MOVIES**

The Homeless Home Movie: 1997. This video profiles several different homeless people who struggle with homelessness during 1 year. They range from a pregnant 15-year-old runaway; a couple who live in their car; a Vietnam veteran who lives outside all year; and a man bankrupted after his daughter's long fight with leukemia. This video is available for purchase at faculty and student rates from Media Visions, Inc., 8th Avenue South, South St. Paul, Minnesota 55075.

Viewing Points: Identify the similarities and differences in the lives of those who are homeless. Does your view of homelessness change after seeing this documentary?

REFERENCES

Andrews, M., & Boyle, J. (1999). *Transcultural concepts in nursing care* (2nd ed.). Philadelphia: J. B. Lippincott.

Baier, M., Murray, R., North, C., et al. (1996). Comparison of completers and noncompleters in a transitional residential program for homeless mentally ill. *Issues in Mental Health, 17,* 337–352.

Boydell, K., Goering, P., & Morrell-Bellai, T. (2000). Narratives of identity: Re-presentation of self in people who are homeless. *Qualitative Health Research, 10*(1), 26–38.

Burt, M. R. (1992). *Over the edge: The growth of homelessness in the 1980s* (pp. 1–267). New York: Russell Sage Foundation.

Bussuk, E., Buckner, J., Weinreb, L., et al. (1997). Homelessness in female-headed families: Childhood and adult risk and protective factors. *American Journal of Public Health, 87,* 241–248.

Carr, S., Murray, R., Harrington, Z., & Oge, J. (1998). Discharged residents' satisfaction with transitional housing for the homeless, *Journal of Psychosocial Nursing, 36*(7), 27–33.

Caton, C., Hasin, D., Shrout, P., et al. (2000). Risk factors for homelessness among indigent urban adults with no history of psychotic illness: A case-control study. *American Journal of Public Health, 90,* 258–263.

Center for Mental Health Services and Office of Special Needs Assistance Programs. (1997). *In from the cold: A tool kit for creating safe havens for homeless people on the street*. Washington, DC: U.S. Department of Housing and Urban Development.

Cohen, C., & Thompson, K. (1992). Homeless mentally ill or mentally ill homeless? *American Journal of Psychiatry, 149*(6), 816–823.

Conrad, R. (1998). Maternal depressive symptoms and homeless children's mental health: Risk and resiliency. *Archives of Psychiatric Nursing, 12*(1), 50–58.

Cunnane, E., Wyman, W., Rotermund, A., & Murray, R. (1995). Innovative programming in a community service center. *Community Mental Health Journal, 31*(2), 153–161.

Davis, J., & Kutter, C. (1998). Independent living skills and posttraumatic stress disorder in women who are homeless: Implications for future practice. *American Journal of Occupational Therapy, 52*(1), 39–44.

DeSantis, L. (1997). Building healthy communities with immigrants and refugees. *Journal of Transcultural Nursing, 9*(1), 20–31.

Downing, C., & Cobb, A. (1990). Value orientations of homeless men. *Western Journal of Nursing Research, 12*, 619–628.

Exploring myths about street people. (1990, June). *Access: A publication of the National Resource Center on Homelessness and Mental Illness, 2*(2), 1–3.

Gelber, L., Gallagher, T., Anderson, R., & Koegel, P. (1997). Competing priorities as a barrier to medical care among homeless adults in Los Angeles. *American Journal of Public Health, 87*, 217–220.

Goldfinger, S. M., Susser, E., Roche, B. A., & Berkinan, A. (1998). *HIV, homelessness, and serious mental illness: Implications for policy and practice*. Identifying a population at risk. Available on-line at http://www.prainc.com/nrc/papers/hiv/hiv_toc.shtml.

Greene, J., Enneth, S., & Ringwalt, C. (1997). Substance use among runaway and homeless youth in three national samples. *American Journal of Public Health, 87*, 229–235.

Herman, D., Susser, E., Struening, E., & Link, B. (1997). Adverse childhood experiences: Are they risk factors for adult homelessness? *American Journal of Public Health, 87*, 249–255.

Humphreys, J. (2000). Spirituality and distress in sheltered battered women. *Journal of Nursing Scholarship, 32*, 273–278.

Interagency Council on the Homeless. (1994). *Priority: Home! The federal plan to break the cycle of homelessness*. (HUD Publication No. 1454-CPD). Washington, DC: Author.

Jones, R. (1983). Street people and psychiatry: An introduction. *Hospital and Community Psychiatry, 34*, 807–811.

Kuno, E., Rothbard, A. B., Avery, J., & Culhane, D. (2000). Homelessness among persons with serious mental illness in an enhanced community-based mental health system. *Psychiatric Services, 51*, 1012–1016.

Koegel, P., Burnam, M., & Farr, R. (1990). Subsistence adaptation among homeless adults in the inner city of Los Angeles. *Journal of Social Sciences, 46*(9), 83–107.

Koegel, P., Melamid, E., & Burnam, A. (1995). Childhood risk factors for homelessness among homeless adults. *American Journal of Public Health, 85*, 1642–1649.

Leshner, A. (1992). *Outcasts in Main Street: Report of the Federal Task Force on Homelessness and Severe Mental Illness* (pp. x–xiii). Rockville, MD: Department of Health and Human Services.

Levine, I., & Rog, D. (1990). Mental health services for homeless mentally ill persons. Federal initiatives and current service trends. *American Psychologist, 43*, 963–968.

Lezak, A. D., & Edgar, E. (1996). *Preventing homelessness among people with serious mental illness*. Available on-line at http://www.prainc.com/nrc/papers/prevent/prevent_toc.shtml.

Link, B., Phelan, J., Bresnahan, M., et al. (1995). Lifetime and five-year prevalence of homelessness in the United States: New evidence on an old debate. *American Journal of Orthopsychiatry, 65*, 347–354.

Menke, E., & Wagner, J. (1997). The experience of homeless female-headed families. *Issues in Mental Health Nursing, 18*, 315–330.

Murray, R. (1993). Spiritual care of homeless men. What helps? What hinders? *Journal of Christian Nursing, 10*(2), 30–37, 46.

Murray, R. (1996). Needs and resources: The lived experience of homeless men. *Journal of Psychosocial Nursing, 34*(5), 18–24.

Murray, R., & Baier, M. (1993). Use of therapeutic milieu in a community setting. *Journal of Psychosocial Nursing, 31*(10), 11–16.

Murray, R., Baier, M., North, C., et al. (1995). Components of an effective transitional residential program for homeless mentally ill clients. *Archives of Psychiatric Nursing, 9*, 152–157.

National Coalition for the Homeless. (1998). *NCH Alerts: Legislation and policy*. Washington, DC: Author. Available online at http://www.nationalhomeless.org.

National Resource Center on Homelessness and Mental Illness. (2000). *Annotated bibliography: Population characteristics of homeless persons*. Available online at http://www.prainc.com/nrc/bibliographies/populati_char.shtml.

North American Nursing Diagnosis Association. (2001). *NANDA Nursing Diagnoses: Definitions and classification, 2001–2002*. Philadelphia: Author.

O'Toole, T., Gibbon, J., Hanusa, B., & Fine, M. (1997). Utilization of health care services among subgroups of urban, homeless, and housed poor. *Journal of Health Politics, Policy, and Law, 24*, 91–114.

Pollio, D., North, C., Thompson, S., et al. (1997). Predictors of achieving stable housing in a mentally ill homeless population. *Psychiatric Services, 48*(4), 528–530.

Ratnesar, R. (1999, February 8). Not gone, but forgotten? *Time*, 30–31.

Rosenheck, R., Bassuk, E., & Salomon, A. (1999). Special populations of homeless Americans. In L. B. Fosburg & D. L. Dennis (Eds.), *Practical lessons: The 1998 National Symposium on Homelessness Research*. Available online at http://aspe.hhs.gov/progsys/homeless/symposium/2-Spclpop.htm.

Sandhaus, S. (1998). Migrant health: A harvest of poverty. *American Journal of Nursing, 98*(9), 52–54.

Smith E., North, C., & Spitznagel, E. (1992). A systematic study of mental illness, substance abuse, and treatment in 600 homeless men. *Annals of Clinical Psychiatry, 4*(2), 111–119.

Smith, E., North, C., & Spitznagel, E. (1993). Alcohol, drugs, and psychiatric comorbidity among homeless women: An epidemiologic study. *Journal of Clinical Psychiatry, 54*(3), 82–87.

Susser, E., Valencia, E., Conover, S., et al. (1997). Preventing recurrent homelessness among mentally ill men. A "critical timing" intervention after discharge from a shelter. *American Journal of Public Health, 87,* 256–262.

Talbott, J., & Lamb, H. R. (1987). The homeless mentally ill. *Archives of Psychiatric Nursing, 1,* 379–384.

Taylor, C. (1996, April). Treatment of homeless patients with schizophrenia. *Current approaches to psychoses: Diagnosis and management, 5,* 9–12.

Torrey, E. (1988). *Nowhere to go: The tragic odyssey of the homeless mentally ill.* New York: Harper & Row.

U.S. Department of Housing and Urban Development. (2000). *Continuum of Care and HOPWA Application* (Form HUD040076-CoC). Washington, DC: Author.

U.S. Department of Housing and Urban Development. (1998). *Understanding the shelter plus care program.* Washington, DC: Author.

Walker, C. (1998). Homeless people and mental health: A nursing concern. *American Journal of Nursing, 98*(11), 26–32.

Wright, J. (1989). *Address unknown: The tragedy of homelessness.* Hawthorne, NY: Aldine.

Zima, B., Bussing, R., Forness, S., & Benjamin, B. (1997). Sheltered homeless children: Their eligibility and unmet need for special education evaluations. *American Journal of Public Health, 87,* 236–240.

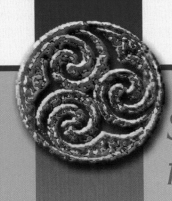

Special Care Concerns for Patients With Dual Disorders

Barbara G. Faltz and Patricia Callahan

RELATIONSHIP OF SUBSTANCE ABUSE TO MENTAL ILLNESS

MANIFESTATIONS OF DUAL DIAGNOSIS

EPIDEMIOLOGY

PSYCHODYNAMIC MODEL OF DUAL DIAGNOSIS

BARRIERS TO TREATMENT
Nature of Substance Abuse
Countertransference
Misunderstandings About and
  Stigmatization of Mental Illness
Health Issues

DISORDER-SPECIFIC ASSESSMENT AND INTERVENTIONS

Psychotic Illnesses
  and Substance Abuse
Anxiety Disorders
  and Substance Abuse
Mood Disorders
  and Substance Abuse
Organic Mental Disorders
  and Substance Abuse
Cognitive Impairment in Early
  Stages of Recovery From
  Substance Abuse
Personality Disorders and
  Substance Abuse

GENERAL TREATMENT ELEMENTS
Setting Priorities When
  Hospitalization Is Necessary
Crisis Stabilization
Engagement

Medication Management
Guidelines for Managing Acute
  Pain in Substance Abusers
Patient Education
Self-Help Groups
Relapse Prevention: Creating a
  New Lifestyle
Continuum of Care
  and Discharge Planning
Case Management
Family Support and Education
Comprehensive Concurrent
  Treatment

PLANNING FOR NURSING CARE

After studying this chapter, you will be able to:

➤ Define the term dual diagnosis.

➤ Discuss the epidemiology of dual diagnosis.

➤ Describe the cycle of relapse.

➤ Describe the effects of alcohol and other drugs on mental illness.

➤ Analyze barriers to the treatment of patients with dual diagnosis.

➤ Discuss four etiologies of dual diagnosis.

➤ Integrate relapse prevention concepts into the care of a patient with dual diagnosis.

We drank for joy and became miserable;
We drank for exhilaration and became depressed;
We drank for friendship and became enemies;
We drank to diminish our problems and saw them
multiply.

Anonymous, from "Positively Negative"

*D**ual diagnosis**, or the coexistence of a substance abuse disorder and a mental health disorder, raises many issues for the psychiatric nurse. Dual diagnosis causes difficulties in making accurate assessments, setting priorities, determining appropriate treatment interventions, and planning the patient's discharge.*

Traditionally, substance abuse and mental health treatment providers have attempted to treat only one aspect of a dual problem. This approach can lead to recurrent relapses into drug or alcohol use or to successive psychiatric hospitalizations. The relapse cycle becomes continuous unless both the mental illness and the substance use disorder are treated.

KEY CONCEPT **Relapse cycle.** In the **relapse cycle**, re-emerging psychiatric symptoms lead to ineffective coping strategies, increased anxiety, substance abuse to avoid painful feelings, adverse consequences, and attempted abstinence, until psychiatric symptoms emerge once more and the cycle repeats itself.

Figure 33-1 shows the relationship between increased psychiatric symptoms and the use of substances as a coping strategy. Without alternative effective coping behaviors, the patient will continue to experience this cycle of relapse and abstinence. The goal of treatment for patients with dual diagnosis is a comprehensive recovery plan for the complex problems presented— one that offers the patient a way out of what can be a downward spiral of debilitation (Fig. 33-1).

This chapter highlights methods of assessing dual diagnoses, explores the psychodynamics of their development, and discusses specific mental illnesses and the adverse effects of concurrent substance abuse. It offers treatment strategies and nursing interventions to address this complex yet common presentation in psychiatric and substance abuse treatment settings. A complete discussion of related substance abuse disorders can be found in Chapter 25.

RELATIONSHIP OF SUBSTANCE ABUSE TO MENTAL ILLNESS

Although it has been prevalent throughout the history of mental illness treatment, the problem of dual diagnosis has been inadvertently magnified by the community mental health reform movement that began in the 1950s. One major facet of this reform was a rational movement toward **deinstitutionalization** of the mentally ill, which

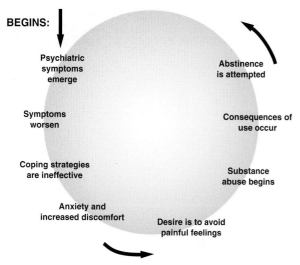

BEGINS:

Psychiatric symptoms emerge

Symptoms worsen

Coping strategies are ineffective

Anxiety and increased discomfort

Abstinence is attempted

Consequences of use occur

Substance abuse begins

Desire is to avoid painful feelings

FIGURE 33.1 Relapse cycle.

resulted in large numbers of homeless mentally ill people living on the streets (Joseph, 1997). Along with homelessness came the increased use of drugs and alcohol and increased incidence of mental illness (Drake & Wallach, 1989).

Chronically mentally ill people are vulnerable to exploitation by others, particularly the more astute and street-wise addicts. It is impossible to make any meaningful distinction between simple recreational use of a substance and actual **substance abuse** with this population because even small amounts of alcohol or other drugs can be damaging to people who have concurrent psychiatric problems. All substances of abuse exert profound effects on mental states, perception, psychomotor function, cognition, and behavior. The specific neurochemical and other biologic mechanisms that evoke these psychological features are discussed in Chapter 25. Table 33-1 lists the psychological effects of abused substances.

The pattern of alcohol and illicit drug use by the mentally ill varies. Some mentally ill people can use alcohol and drugs recreationally, whereas others experience severe problems from the use of these substances. Individuals can become caught in a "revolving door" of repeated hospitalizations because of the distressing symptoms of mental illness that are exacerbated by substance abuse. When the presenting symptoms are stabilized and the patient is released, perhaps with new

TABLE 33.1 Psychological Effects of Substances of Abuse

Substance	Psychological Effects
Alcohol	Organic brain disorders—alcohol amnestic syndrome, dementia Agitation, anxiety disorders, sleep disorders Ataxia, slurred speech Withdrawal symptoms, which may include hallucinations, confusion, illusions, delusions; protracted withdrawal delirium can occur Depression, increased rate of suicide, disinhibition
Cocaine	Anxiety, agitation, hyperactivity, sleep disorders, delusions, paranoia, euphoria, internal sense of interest and excitement Rebound withdrawal symptoms, such as prolonged depression, somnolence, anhedonia
Amphetamines	Similar to cocaine but more prolonged Hyperactivity, agitation, anxiety, increased energy
Hallucinogens and phencyclidine	Hallucinations, delusions, paranoia, confusion Withdrawal can produce severe depression, somnolence Hallucinations, illusions, delusions, perceptual distortions, paranoia, rage, anxiety, agitation, confusion
Marijuana	Acute reactions: panic, anxiety, paranoia, sensory distortions, rare psychotic episodes; patients with schizophrenia use these reactions to distance themselves from painful symptoms and to gain control over symptoms Antimotivational syndrome: apathy, diminished interest in activities and goals, poor job or school performance, memory and cognitive deficits
Opiates	Confusion, somnolence Withdrawal can produce anxiety, irritability, and depression and can trigger suicidal ideation
Sedative-hypnotics	Confusion, slurred speech, ataxia, stupor, sleep disorders, withdrawal delirium, dementia, amnestic disorder, sleep disorders
Volatile solvents	Hallucinations, delusions, hyperactivity, sensory distortions, dementia

Adapted from Segal, B. (1988). *Drugs and behavior.* New York: Gardner Press.

medications or a new discharge plan in place, the patient may fail to follow the therapeutic regimen. The patient may increase use of alcohol or drugs, resulting in an exacerbation of the emotional problem and leading to another episode of hospitalization. This cyclic pattern of mental health or substance abuse decompensation, hospitalization, stabilization, discharge, and decompensation accounts largely for the difficulty in carrying out nursing management with patients who have dual diagnoses.

MANIFESTATIONS OF DUAL DIAGNOSIS

The four possible manifestations of a dual diagnosis and a clinical example describing each follows. For additional information, see Table 33-2.

- *A primary mental illness with subsequent substance abuse.* In this manifestation, a primary mental illness leads to addictive behavior when the patient self-medicates to cope with the symptoms of the illness. It includes abuse resulting from impaired judgment, poor impulse control, impaired social skills, and inappropriate coping strategies.

Sylvia G. was raped when she was 18 years old and held by her assailant for 2 days. She has frequent nightmares, relives the experience almost daily, and is extremely anxious around men whom she does not know. She began drinking heavily after this incident and states that it provides some relief from her anxiety. Drinking also enables her to numb painful feelings. Her alcohol use has had numerous adverse consequences. She was recently fired from her job as a clerk when she was found drinking at her desk. Sylvia has been diagnosed with posttraumatic stress disorder and alcohol dependence.

- *A primary substance abuse disorder with psychopathologic sequelae.* Psychiatric symptoms are consequences of drug or alcohol intoxication, of withdrawal symptoms (such as severe depression after cessation of prolonged cocaine abuse), or of cognitive impairments related to chronic alcohol or drug use.

Ralph D. has been smoking crack cocaine for 3 years. He has lost his job because of absenteeism. His wife has left him, and he is now homeless. He has attempted suicide three times in moments of despair after cocaine binges. He has been unable to stop using crack and continues to be chronically depressed.

- *Dual primary diagnoses.* Psychiatric and substance abuse diagnoses interact to exacerbate each other.

TABLE 33.2 Assessment and Classification of Dual Diagnosis Conditions

Assessment Issue	Primary Mental Illness With Substance Abuse	Substance Abuse With Psychiatric Sequelae	Dual Primary Diagnosis	Common Etiology
Are dual syndromes present?	Yes	Yes	Yes	Yes
Which came first?	Mental illness	Substance abuse	None	None
What is the family history?	Mental illness, if any	Substance abuse, if any	Mental illness, substance abuse, or both	Mental illness, substance abuse, or both, if any
What are the psychosocial factors?	Vulnerable to victimization by peers because of primary mental illness	Often can maintain family and employment during periods of sobriety	Prognosis is less favorable; may often be incarcerated or hospitalized	Common risk factor possible, (eg, homelessness)
What are the treatment and response to treatment?	Treatment for mental illness alleviates both syndromes; discharge plan focuses on mental health maintenance	Treatment for substance abuse alleviates both syndromes; discharge plan focuses on maintenance of sobriety	Treatment for both mental illness and substance abuse required	Treatment for common risk factor alleviates both mental illness and substance abuse

Adapted from Lehman, A. F., Myers, C. P., & Corty, E. (1989). Assessment and classification of patients with psychiatric and substance abuse syndromes. *Hospital and Community Psychiatry, 40*(10), 1019–1024.

Joan K. has a diagnosis of bipolar type II disorder. For many years, she has engaged in heavy drinking, which began in early adolescence. When she is binge drinking, she does not take her medication and experiences manic episodes and deep depressions. She has attempted periods of sobriety but discontinues her medication frequently. She has difficulty controlling impulsive alcohol use.

- *A common etiology.* One common factor causes both disorders. The factor can be (1) genetic; (2) a defect in dopaminergic function that predisposes patients to conditions such as schizophrenia or abuse of dopamine agonists such as amphetamines; or (3) a defect in cholinergic activity that may predispose patients to affective disorders and to substance abuse affecting cholinergic pathways (Lehman et al., 1989).

Frank L. received a diagnosis of attention deficit hyperactivity disorder as a child. His parents, both alcoholics, had a hard time controlling him and would give him alcohol to attempt to "calm him down." Frank continues to have difficulty concentrating, is hyperactive, and has developed numerous medical problems related to his alcohol abuse as an adult.

EPIDEMIOLOGY

The prevalence rates of mental and substance use disorders have been examined in a nationally representative sample of 8,098 individuals in the community. The National Comorbidity Survey (NCS) lifetime prevalence rate of all *DSM-III-R* diagnoses for alcohol, drug, and mental disorders is 48%, with a 12-month rate of 29.5%

(Kessler et al., 1994). The NCS lifetime prevalence for any substance use disorder is 26.6%, for a mental disorder is 21.4%, and for both is 13.7% (Kessler et al., 1994). Miller (1995) reviewed prevalence rate studies of comorbidity in psychiatric and addiction treatment settings (see Table 33-3). Obviously, clinical populations show higher comorbidity rates than in the general population. It is important to note that the overall chance of a comorbid substance use disorder in a patient seeking psychiatric treatment is 1 in 2. Comorbid psychiatric disorders in addiction treatment settings are much lower.

PSYCHODYNAMIC MODEL OF DUAL DIAGNOSIS

Confusion and professional disagreement exist about the etiology of dual diagnosis. Differing views of the etiology affect the proposed treatment strategies. Biologic aspects and theories of mental illness have been integrated into each chapter of the text. Chapter 25 examines several different models of substance abuse etiology. The psychodynamic model is particularly relevant to dual diagnosis. This section examines this model of chemical dependency and dual diagnosis.

Current psychodynamic thought views substance abuse as an attempt by a person to return to homeostasis after experiencing psychological suffering (Brehm & Khantzian, 1997). The person attempts to alleviate or control disturbing feelings such as anxiety, depression, or anger through use of alcohol or drugs. The patient's inability to achieve homeostasis or relief from those feelings without substance abuse is due to "self-regulatory deficiencies" (Brehm & Khantzian, 1997). Table 33-4 describes self-regulatory deficiencies and recommended treatment approaches.

TABLE 33.3 Prevalence of Comorbidity of Mental Health Disorders and Substance Abuse Disorders in U.S. Treatment Settings

Diagnosis	Psychiatry Setting (percentage diagnosed with comorbid substance use disorder by mental illness)	Addiction Setting (percentage of comorbid mental illness by diagnosis)
Depressive disorder	30	5.0
Bipolar disorder	50	0.8
Schizophrenia	50	1.1
Antisocial personality disorder	80	0.6
Anxiety disorder	30	3.0
Phobic disorder	23	6.0

From Miller, N. S. (1995). *Addiction psychiatry: Current diagnosis and treatment* (p. 112). New York: Wiley-Liss.

TABLE 33.4 Self-Regulation Deficiencies That Cause Substance Abuse and Their Treatment

Deficiency	Treatment
Impairment in self-care	Initial stabilization
Vulnerabilities in self	Internalizing self-care functions
Developmental and self-esteem deficiencies	Repairing developmental deficits and enhancing self-esteem
Troubled object relations	Maintaining mature self-object relationships
Deficits in affect tolerance	Modulating affect

From Brehm, N. M., & Khantzian, E. J. (1997). A psychodynamic perspective. In J. H. Lowinson, P. Ruiz, R. B. Millman, & J. G. Langrod (Eds.), *Substance abuse: A comprehensive textbook* (2nd ed., pp. 106–117). Baltimore: Williams & Wilkins. Used with permission.

Ineffective self-regulation leads to the use of substances to achieve emotional homeostasis. Dubey (1997) related that addicts often do not seek a "high" but rather desire to feel "normal" or comfortable in their lives. The purpose of psychotherapy is to help the patient acquire insight into the reasons for the psychological suffering, increase toleration and modulation of painful feelings, learn skills to care for and nurture the self, and adopt a reality that is not based on childhood illusions (Brehm & Khantzian, 1997).

Searches have been numerous for an addictive personality or other personality traits associated with substance abuse. Alcoholism and other drug dependencies have been assumed to be symptomatic of an underlying personality disorder or a disturbance in normal development (Miller & Kurtz, 1994). Examples of the traits proposed for the addictive personality were emotional insecurity, anxiety, unsatisfied dependence needs, narcissism, externalization of blame, and the use of primitive defense mechanisms such as denial (Evans & Sullivan, 1990; Lindstrom, 1992; Miller & Kurtz, 1994).

A person's problematic chemical use may be viewed as a symptom of or a response to family dysfunction. Steinglass (1985) proposed a model of family dysfunction that encourages alcoholism and effectively maintains it because the alcohol abuse serves as a family homeostatic mechanism. He stated that in the areas of home routines and problem solving, a major consequence of the organization of family life around alcoholism is the emphasis on stability rather than long-term family growth and happiness. In this view of the etiology of alcoholism, the dynamics learned as a homeostatic family mechanism are carried into adult relationships.

Models that regard alcohol and drug abuse as symptoms of another primary psychiatric or family dysfunctional problem are problematic. If these models offered

the only explanation for dual diagnosis, the logical treatment would be to seek insight into substance-abusing behavior through psychotherapy. The goal would be to decrease substance abuse as insight emerges. This model of addiction is helpful in viewing the possible etiologies of dual diagnosis, but it is narrowly focused and is only one of many models (see Chap. 25).

Because of the barriers to treatment discussed and differing views on the etiology of addiction, it is essential that a careful and thorough assessment be completed in mental health, chemical dependency, and medical settings. Comprehensive assessment will help ensure that interventions meet patients' needs. Current research trends in dual diagnosis are empiric studies to test the validity of cherished treatment beliefs and efficacy studies of treatment approaches.

BARRIERS TO TREATMENT

High comorbidity rates point to the need for effective dual diagnosis treatment. Patients with dual diagnoses, however, often face barriers to obtaining proper treatment because of specific cultural, economic, and health-related issues. These include the nature of substance abuse, countertransference and the position of substance abusers in society, misunderstandings about and stigmatization of mental illness, and related health issues.

Nature of Substance Abuse

Substance abusers are often unwilling to seek mental health treatment because they may incorrectly attribute disturbing emotions to their drug or alcohol abuse or to withdrawal symptoms. They may view drugs and alcohol as the "cure" rather than the cause of their emotional distress. Conversely, substance-abusing patients may seek mental health treatment for problems associated with the consequences of their abuse but may fail to mention their substance abuse. Also, they may seek medications to alleviate symptoms that are caused by their abuse, such as anxiety, depression, and insomnia, although effective nonpharmacologic interventions are available. Beeder and Millman (1997) pointed out the dilemma facing these patients. The dually diagnosed patient must choose between two equally unsatisfactory options:

1. Take the illicit drug of choice to experience fleeting moments of joy and escape, even though doing so will prompt a decline in overall function and lead to an outcome worsened by the sequelae of increasingly severe psychiatric symptoms.
2. Accept prescribed treatments that might include medications such as neuroleptics or antidepressants, neither of which is intoxicating, even though both promote a better level of functioning and a better treatment outcome.

Countertransference

Mental health professionals in psychiatric treatment programs are often frustrated in their efforts to assist substance-abusing patients. Behavior often associated with addiction, such as denial of a substance abuse diagnosis, manipulative behavior, and noncompliance with health-related protocols, is often regarded as a sign of treatment failure. This type of behavior can provoke hostility from the staff and can make planning for mental health recovery difficult. Drug-abusing patients may have the additional stigma of being regarded as criminals because they commit illegal acts every time they purchase, use, or distribute illicit drugs. Strong public feelings about alcohol-related motor vehicle accidents, negative experiences with family members or friends with drinking problems, and cultural biases against public intoxication can prejudice interactions with patients who are alcohol dependent.

Mental health professionals may have difficulty understanding the compelling nature of drug or alcohol cravings, may not understand differences in drug abuse patterns and behaviors associated with particular drugs of abuse, and may overdiagnose personality disorders in those who take drugs and commit crimes (Beeder & Millman, 1997). Mental health care providers may also be reluctant to endorse the use of 12-step programs, which they may view as nothing more than "prayer meetings," and instead prematurely initiate pharmacotherapy (Beeder & Millman, 1997).

A treatment approach often used in psychodynamic therapies is to seek the underlying cause of the patient's symptoms by uncovering unconscious conflict and thereby producing heightened anxiety (Wallen &

Weiner, 1989). However, if the patient experiences too much anxiety, it may trigger renewed substance abuse. The relapse may then be mistakenly viewed as a failure on the patient's part, not a result of inappropriate treatment.

Misunderstandings About and Stigmatization of Mental Illness

Some substance abuse treatment professionals regard mental illness as outside their area of interest or expertise and may not accept patients with mental health disorders into substance abuse treatment programs. They may lack a general understanding of the nature of mental illness or fear anticipated unpredictable behavior, recurrent substance abuse relapses, and the inability of some dually diagnosed patients to understand or use 12-step programs. Sometimes, patients with cognitive impairment in early recovery are considered lazy, in denial, or unmotivated when what they are actually experiencing is difficulty learning new material (Friedrich & Kuss, 1991). Recovering alcoholics and addicts who are employed in treatment programs may also feel uncomfortable working with mentally ill patients, not only because of a lack of knowledge, but also because of denial of the influence of their own personality or psychopathology on their former drug-taking behaviors (Beeder & Millman, 1997).

Such common symptoms of mental illness as depression, anxiety, and sleep disturbances are often attributed to substance use or withdrawal (Beeder & Millman, 1997). Thus, underlying or concurrent mental health disorders may remain undiagnosed and untreated. Providers may also misunderstand the second step of the Alcoholics Anonymous (AA) program, which states "We came to believe that a power greater than ourselves could restore us to sanity," thinking that mental health-related symptoms will abate if a patient "works the program" (Wallen & Weiner, 1989). In addition, confusion exists about the use of psychoactive medication to treat these common psychiatric symptoms. Chemical dependency programs often require patients to abstain from using any mind-altering drugs, regardless of their purpose, their benefit, or patients' need for them, thereby closing the door needlessly on people who could benefit from these treatment programs.

Health Issues

Numerous health hazards are associated with alcohol and drug abuse (see Chap. 25). Dually diagnosed patients are more likely than others to use emergency departments for primary health care, waiting until they can no longer ignore physical illness. They are more likely to be unclear about the medical plan they need to follow and are more likely to be noncompliant with health care directives. The use of alcohol and illicit substances in addition to medications prescribed for mental illness can lead to drug interactions and the exacerbation of side effects of these medications. Homelessness can increase these patients' medical problems (Joseph, 1997), with inadequate nutrition, poor hygiene, and the adverse effects of exposure to the elements adding to their difficulties. Health care providers often become frustrated with patients' noncompliance and with what they see as difficult behaviors to manage. Their frustration may negatively affect the way they treat dually diagnosed patients. Because of providers' biases against dually diagnosed patients, the nature of these patients' behavior, and confusion about what is the primary and most immediate problem to treat, these patients are often underserved and only partially treated.

DISORDER-SPECIFIC ASSESSMENT AND INTERVENTIONS

Weiss and associates summarized one key challenge in the assessment of dually diagnosed patients when they stated, "Patients with dual diagnoses are not a homogeneous group" (1992, p. 108). Another difficulty is predicting the prognosis for these patients. Stoffelmayr and coworkers (1989) pointed out that the severity of patients' psychological problems and their level of functioning are more important indicators of prognosis than the diagnosis itself. They concluded that, in general, "higher problem severity indicates poorer prognosis" (p. 160). Thorough assessment of mental health and substance use disorders is crucial to making the diagnosis and formulating a treatment plan (Scott et al., 1998).

An important part of assessment is to delineate the relative contribution of each diagnosis to the severity of the current symptoms presented and to prioritize treatment accordingly. Because dually diagnosed patients often make unreliable historians or distort the reality of their mental health problems and the severity of their substance abuse, obtaining objective data is especially important. It is advisable to obtain an objective history of the patient from family, significant others, board and care operators, other health care providers, or anyone familiar with the patient to provide an accurate history. Text Box 33-1 lists basic assessment tools and methods used for dually diagnosed patients. The following concepts are paramount to the discussion of diagnosis and assessment of dual disorders (Ries, 1995):

- Substance use can cause psychiatric symptoms and mimic psychiatric syndromes.

TEXT BOX 33.1

Methods of Assessment of Dual Diagnosis

History and physical examination, laboratory tests (eg, liver function tests, complete blood count) to confirm medical indicators related to substance abuse and also to rule out medical disorders with psychiatric presentations

- Substance abuse history and severity of consequences, and physical symptoms
- Mental status examination and severity of symptoms (eg, suicidal, homicidal, florid psychosis)

Interview with and assessment of family members, to verify or determine: (1) the accuracy of the patient's self-reported substance abuse or mental health history; (2) the patient's history of past mental health problems during periods of abstinence; and, if possible, (3) the sequence of the diagnoses (ie, what symptoms appeared first)

- Interviews with partner, friends, social worker, and other significant people in the patient's life
- Review of court records, medical records, and previous psychiatric and substance abuse treatment
- Urine and blood toxicity screens; use of breath analyzer to test blood alcohol level

Revision of initial assessment by observation of the patient in the clinical setting; full assessment of the underlying psychiatric problem may not be possible until there is a long (up to 6 months) period of total abstinence

- Observation of patient for reappearance of psychiatric symptoms after a period of sobriety
- Assessment of patient's motivation to seek treatment, desire to change behavior, and understanding of diagnoses

- Substance use can initiate or exacerbate a psychiatric disorder.
- Substance use can mask psychiatric symptoms and syndromes.
- Withdrawal from alcohol and other drugs can cause psychiatric symptoms and mimic psychiatric syndromes.
- Psychiatric and substance use disorders can independently coexist.
- Psychiatric behaviors can mimic alcohol and other drug use problems.

Psychotic Illnesses and Substance Abuse

About half of patients with schizophrenia have a concurrent substance use disorder (Bellack & Gearon, 1998). The diagnosis of schizophrenia can be made only if the symptoms as described in the *Diagnostic and Statistical Manual of Mental Disorders*, 4th edition, Text revision

(*DSM-IV-TR*) (American Psychiatric Association [APA], 2000) last at least 6 months. They can only be made accurately without the added complication of substance abuse. The patient with a psychotic disorder may have an altered thought process or delusional thinking and may suffer from auditory hallucinations. He or she may also be cognitively impaired and have poor memory. These patients can have negative symptoms, such as poor motivation and poor hygiene. They often suffer from low self-esteem, have poor social skills, and may have a general sense of not belonging to a community. Their sense of self in relation to the world may be altered. These symptoms can result from intoxication with or withdrawal from substances of abuse (Beeder & Millman, 1997).

Acute and chronic psychotic disorders may be precipitated in predisposed people by the use of cocaine, amphetamines, marijuana, and the hallucinogens as well as during severe withdrawal states (Beeder & Millman, 1997). Whereas all people are vulnerable to the development of psychotic episodes from various drugs at different doses and frequency intervals, one psychotic episode renders a person more susceptible to subsequent episodes (Beeder & Millman, 1997). Rosenthal and Westreich (1999) caution that the default diagnosis for patients presenting with substance use disorders and psychotic symptoms should be that these symptoms are related to substance use until proved otherwise.

Assessing the needs of people with schizophrenia who are also chemically dependent is complicated by the changing interaction among psychotic symptoms, the antipsychotic effects of medications, and the side effects of medications. Management and treatment of the psychotic substance abuser may vary according to the degree of severity of the symptoms. Ries (1995) suggested the following dual focus approach for assessment and treatment:

- Initial focus on severity of presenting symptoms, not on diagnosis of one disorder or another
- Acute crisis intervention and crisis management
- Acute, subacute, and long-term stabilization of the patient
- Ongoing diagnostic efforts
- Multiple-contact longitudinal treatment

The emphatic confrontive approach of addressing a patient's denial of their problems would not benefit this population (see Chap. 25 for further discussion of confrontation). That approach could alienate a patient. A more supportive approach is appropriate. For example, relapses are treated as an expected part of the recovery process. Addressing relapse risk is part of the treatment planning process. Focus is on examining behavior, feelings, and the thinking process that led to the relapse. The nurse must avoid blame and guilt-inducing statements.

Bellack and Gearon (1998) suggest a multifaceted treatment approach for the treatment of the patient with concurrent schizophrenia and substance abuse. Their treatment approach, *behavior treatment for substance abuse in schizophrenia* (BTSAS), consists of four parts:

1. Social skills training to help the patient learn ways to interact in a sober living situation and problem-solving training to review and refine their behaviors
2. Education about the nature of substance abuse, including triggers and cravings
3. **Motivational interviewing**, which helps the patient clarify personal goals and increases commitment to recovery (see Chap. 25)
4. Education regarding relapse prevention techniques

Another important intervention is to integrate the administration of antipsychotic medication into the chemical dependency treatment plan to reduce the chances of relapse. Relapse is frequently secondary to medication noncompliance, especially if patients experience side effects from neuroleptics (Beeder & Millman, 1997).

Anxiety Disorders and Substance Abuse

The *DSM-IV-TR* (APA, 2000) includes acute distress disorder, generalized anxiety disorder, agoraphobia, obsessive-compulsive disorder, panic disorder, post-traumatic stress disorder (PTSD), social phobia, and other specific phobias as some of the anxiety disorders. Nineteen percent of patients with anxiety disorder have a concurrent alcohol problem, and 28% have a drug problem (Scott et al., 1998). PTSD increases the risk for substance abuse relapse and is associated with poorer treatment outcome (Rosenthal & Westreich, 1999). Among patients with substance use disorders, there is a significant likelihood of coexisting anxiety disorder (Ries, 1995).

The symptoms of anxiety may result from an anxiety disorder such as panic attack, or the patient may experience these symptoms secondary to drug or alcohol use as part of a withdrawal syndrome. Symptoms are so subjectively disturbing that they can lead to drug or alcohol abuse as self-medication for the emotional pain and thus require prompt evaluation and treatment. The pharmacologic treatment of anxiety is more difficult because the traditional medications used, the benzodiazepines, are themselves addicting (Sowers & Golden, 1999).

Kushner and colleagues (1990) helped to clarify the relationship between specific anxiety disorders and substance abuse. They found that alcohol problems may be more likely to follow agoraphobia and social phobia from attempts to self-medicate symptoms of anxiety, whereas panic disorder and generalized anxiety disorder may be more likely to follow pathologic alcohol consumption. Confusion about whether alcohol consumption is a cause or an effect of anxiety can be explained by the fact that alcohol use reduces anxiety at first but its abuse increases anxiety over extended periods (Beeder & Millman, 1997).

Patients with anxiety disorders should also pay particular attention to their physical health. Regular, balanced meals, exercise, and sleep are ways to decrease and manage stress levels. Patients should avoid excessive consumption of caffeine and sugars. If the patient has a fear of crowds, he or she may benefit from gradual desensitization techniques. Ries (1995) suggests the following guidelines in treating anxiety and coexisting substance use disorders:

- Treatment can be postponed unless anxiety interferes with substance abuse treatment.
- Anxiety symptoms may resolve with abstinence and substance abuse treatment.
- Affect-liberating therapies should be postponed until the patient is stable.
- Psychotherapy, when required, should be recovery oriented.
- Nonpsychoactive medications are preferred when medication is required.
- Antianxiety treatments such as relaxation techniques can be used with and without medications.
- A healthy diet, aerobic exercise, and avoiding caffeine can reduce anxiety.

Mood Disorders and Substance Abuse

The term *mood disorder* describes various mood disturbances, including major depressive disorder, dysthymic disorder, bipolar I and bipolar II disorders, and cyclothymic disorder (APA, 2000). Thirty-two percent of patients with a mood disorder have a comorbid substance abuse disorder, whereas 56% of patients with a bipolar disorder have a comorbid substance abuse dis-

order (Regier et al., 1990). Substance abuse disorders occur concurrently in 13.4% of patients with any affective disorder (Regier et al., 1990). Substance abuse is more common in bipolar patients than any other Axis I diagnosis. Also, it may contribute to nontreatment compliance and less positive outcomes (Golberg et al., 1999). Mood disorders may be more prevalent among patients using opiates than among other drug users (Ries, 1995). During the first few months of sobriety, symptoms of depression may persist. Initiation of pharmacologic interventions may be delayed until the diagnosis of underlying depression can be made.

Substance abuse is highly correlated with suicide attempts. The incidence of suicide among drug abusers is 20 times that of the general population (Blumenthal, 1988). Seventy percent of teen suicides are associated with substance abuse (Shaffer, 1988). Alcohol abuse is a factor in 25% of all suicides, including those of nonalcoholics (Frances et al., 1987). Depression during withdrawal from alcohol, cocaine, opiates, and amphetamines puts patients at severe risk for suicide. A person's presenting behaviors may not have included depression, but depression may develop as the withdrawal syndrome unfolds. Hyperactivity often appears with stimulant use and at times with alcohol abuse. Patients may be treated for hypomania or bipolar disorder when they are in fact hyperactive. Symptoms usually improve as the person maintains abstinence.

As with anxiety disorders, determining whether mood disorders are the cause or the effect of protracted substance abuse is difficult (Table 33-5). One important assessment is to determine whether drug use relates to mood states. Patients may be attempting to alleviate uncomfortable symptoms such as depression or agitation or to enhance a mood state such as hypomania. Symptoms that persist during periods of abstinence are a clue to the degree that the mood disorder contributes to the presenting symptoms. Whenever possible, the use of medication for mood disorders should be initiated after a period of abstinence (Beeder & Millman, 1997) so that

TABLE 33.5 Drugs That Precipitate or Mimic Mood Disorders

Mood Disorders	During Use (Intoxication)	After Use (Withdrawal)
Depression and dysthymia	Alcohol, benzodiazepines, opioids, barbiturates, cannabis, steroids (chronic use), stimulants (chronic use)	Alcohol, benzodiazepines, opioids, barbiturates, cannabis, steroids (chronic use), stimulants (chronic use)
Mania and cyclothymia	Stimulants, alcohol hallucinogens, inhalants, steroids (chronic and acute use)	Alcohol, benzodiazepines, barbiturates, opiates, steroids (chronic use)

From Ries, R. (1995). *Assessment and treatment of patients with coexisting mental illness and alcohol and other drug abuse* (pp. 29–89). Rockville, MD: U.S. Department of Health and Human Services.

indications are clear as to whether the alcohol or other drug use was not the sole cause of the symptoms.

Patients with bipolar disorders can benefit from chemical dependency treatment if their medications are stabilized and they can tolerate group treatment approaches, focus on and complete simple goals, and follow simple ground rules in a treatment program. Evans and Sullivan (1990) suggested these guidelines for treatment:

- Limit responses in group sessions (eg, to less than 5 minutes total group time).
- Limit the length of responses to simple exercises.
- Work with patients to heal interpersonal relationships that may have become impaired as a result of manic episodes.
- Relate patients' substance abuse and manic episodes to out-of-control behavior for which ongoing treatment (recovery) plans are needed.

For patients who have depression and a substance use disorder, employing interventions centered on examining cognitive distortions (eg, "I'll never get better, no one likes me, alcohol is my only friend") and cognitive therapy techniques can help improve mood. Use of positive self-talk can be helpful for both the depression and the substance use disorders. Working on unresolved grief can be appropriate. Assignments that deal with patients' previous actions, however, can evoke guilt, self-blame, and expressions of low self-esteem, thereby increasing depression (Evans & Sullivan, 1990).

Organic Mental Disorders and Substance Abuse

Current terminology refers to cognitive impairment deficits related to substance abuse as **alcohol-induced persisting amnestic disorder**. **Wernicke's syndrome** is a reversible alcohol-induced amnestic disorder caused by a thiamine-deficient diet. Thiamine is an essential element in the production of fatty acids for synthesis and maintenance of cerebral myelin. Wernicke first called this syndrome "acute superior hemorrhagic polioencephalitis." It is marked by diplopia from palsy of the third or fourth cranial nerves, hyperactivity and delirium from stimulation of cortical brain and thalamic lesions, and coma caused by lesions in cranial nerve nuclei and in the mesencephalon and diencephalon of the brain (Goodwin, 1997). Thiamine treatment can reverse this process if initiated rapidly. All the B vitamins are essential for myelination. Deficiencies can lead to the development of lesions in distal peripheral nerves, causing neuropathies.

A second syndrome, which can occur concurrently with Wernicke's, is **Korsakoff's psychosis**. It is charac-

terized by a loss of recent memory and confabulation (or filling in the blanks in memory by making up facts to cover up this deficit). The patient with this condition is highly suggestible, has poor judgment, and cannot reason critically. Korsakoff's psychosis often follows Wernicke's encephalopathy and is also associated with prior peripheral neuropathy (Goodwin, 1997). It is treated with thiamine and can often be partially reversed.

Patients with alcohol-induced persisting amnestic disorder usually have histories of many years of heavy alcohol abuse, are generally older than age 40 years, can experience sudden onset of symptoms, or may have had symptoms develop over many years (APA, 2000). Impairment can be severe, and once the disorder is established, it can persist indefinitely (APA, 2000). Sedative-hypnotics and anxiolytic agents, as well as anticonvulsants, are also known to cause a persisting amnestic disorder.

Cerebellar degeneration can occur from increased levels of acetaldehyde, a toxic by-product of alcohol metabolism, resulting from years of alcohol abuse. Symptoms are impaired coordination, a broad-based unsteady gait, and fine tremors. Alcohol is directly toxic to the brain, causing atrophy of the frontal cortex and eventually, chronic brain syndrome. Sedative-hypnotic effects of long-term alcohol abuse lead to disturbances in rapid-eye-movement sleep and chronic sleep disorders.

Organic brain disorders resulting from head trauma are more common in substance abusers than in the general population. This discrepancy is largely attributable to motor vehicle accidents, bar fights, physical abuse, and other trauma.

Cognitive Impairment in Early Stages of Recovery From Substance Abuse

Most cognitive impairment in the population of patients seeking alcohol or drug abuse treatment is transitory and resolves within the first month of abstinence. Patients often experience difficulties with abstract reasoning, perceptual-spatial relations, memory, and the ability to learn new concepts (Friedrich & Kus, 1991). In addition to the biologically based etiologies discussed, psychosocial factors can have a negative influence on cognitive ability. Fear of legal or relationship difficulties, depression, grief, and feelings of guilt and shame all may contribute to cognitive impairment (Friedrich & Kus, 1991). Psychological testing and other methods of assessment are necessary to determine whether the patient's cognitive functioning can improve and whether chemical dependency treatment can be used. The nurse must assess the patient's abilities for self-care, independent living, impulse control, control of assaultiveness, direction taking, and development of new responses to new situations and ideas. The nurse must also evaluate changes in mental status over the past 6 months and examine previous treatment outcomes (Evans & Sullivan, 1990).

The basis for intervention in patients with cognitive or memory impairment is clear, direct, simple messages. The following points (Evans & Sullivan, 1990; Friedrich & Kus, 1991) illustrate this approach:

- Use reading material that is relevant to recovery and that can be referred to in short study sessions.
- For patients who have trouble grasping abstract concepts, read first-person accounts of addiction and recovery found in AA and Narcotics Anonymous (NA) literature.
- Concentrate on basic concepts of recovery, such as those in AA slogans, and on patients' need for continuing care after discharge.
- Show films with scenes illustrating relevant family problems or other problems related to abuse. Movies can be more effective than lectures.
- Avoid discussing extraneous issues and avoid theoretic or technical discussions.

Personality Disorders and Substance Abuse

Personality disorders are frequently diagnosed in alcohol and other drug abusers. Regier and associates (1990) noted that 14.3% of people with an alcohol-related disorder and 17.8% of those with a drug-related disorder had a lifetime prevalence rate of antisocial personality disorder. Conversely, people with an antisocial personality disorder had a lifetime prevalence rate of 83.6% for any substance abuse disorder. Those with borderline personality disorder had a 28% rate of substance dependence (Thomas et al., 1999).

Another study suggested a 40% to 50% concurrent diagnosis of antisocial personality disorder and substance dependence. Also, the study reported that 90% of antisocial personality disordered patents who are criminal offenders are substance abusers (Messina et al., 1999). Thomas and colleagues (1999) noted that this population has a higher rate of involuntary hospital admissions, greater resistance to treatment, poor coping skills, poorer interpersonal relationships, and a higher level of impulsivity.

Beeder and Millman (1997) noted that the label *personality disorder* is often incorrectly applied to patients who seek treatment because of legal problems, interpersonal violence, or other difficulties. Chronic drug use can cause personality changes and even psychiatric illness secondary to the actions of the drugs and the behaviors associated with substance abuse. Alcohol and other drug use in patients with personality disorders are often secondary to these disorders. For example, people with antisocial personality disorder may use alcohol and other drugs to enhance their view of the world as fast-paced and dramatic. They may be involved in crime and other sensation-seeking, high-risk behavior that includes polysubstance abuse (Ries, 1995).

Chemical dependency treatment based on tight structure, peer support, and confrontation that addresses the significant destructive behavior on the part of patients with personality disorders appears to be the most useful approach (Beeder & Millman, 1997). Formally structured groups may improve patients' ability to learn new and more appropriate behaviors and to develop new perceptions that may help them in relating to others. Cognitive therapy approaches may help these patients examine the cognitive distortions that contribute to their substance abuse.

GENERAL TREATMENT ELEMENTS

Patients with dual diagnosis enter treatment at various stages of recovery from their disorders. Flexible treatment programs that can meet each patient's different needs are the most effective. Regardless of the patient's degree of recovery or primary diagnosis, some common elements exist in the treatment of dual diagnosis. The following discussion highlights these essential components of treatment.

Setting Priorities When Hospitalization is Necessary

Often, patients with a dual diagnosis can be treated effectively in community mental health settings if their symptoms are stable, they are following their treatment plan, they are compliant with use of psychiatric medications, and they remain alcohol and drug free. Dackis & Gold (1997) specified that patients who meet any of the following criteria should be admitted to the hospital for treatment:

- Serious medical needs, such as the need for detoxification
- An exacerbated medical disorder or an illness that prevents abstinence or outpatient treatment
- Suicidal or homicidal ideation, psychotic disorganization, or other serious psychiatric illnesses
- Failed outpatient treatment
- Addiction severity that prevents any significant period of abstinence
- Serious psychosocial problems such as immediate risk for incarceration, homelessness, or abusive relationships
- Continued abuse of substances during pregnancy

Crisis Stabilization

Setting priorities for patients with a dual diagnosis in a hospital setting is essential. The first priorities are gathering data from a physical examination and nursing assessments, stabilizing psychiatric symptoms, and treating withdrawal symptoms (Beeder & Millman, 1997) (see Chap. 25). After these issues have been addressed, the patient can enter the rehabilitation phase of treatment for both diagnoses. Rehabilitative therapy is appropriate if the patient (1) can participate in a group process, (2) can focus attention on groups or reading material, (3) does not engage in behavior that is detrimental to the group process, (4) can listen to and receive feedback from others, and (5) can benefit from the group process.

Engagement

Engagement entails establishing a treatment relationship, educating the patient about the illnesses, teaching the patient how to maintain stabilization by complying with treatment, and helping the patient overcome denial and other resistances to making a commitment to an ongoing treatment program (Segal, 1988). Substance-abusing patients may experience repeated cycles of detoxification and relapse. Mentally ill patients may have prolonged cycles of "revolving-door" admissions and persistent medication noncompliance before acknowledging the need to engage in continuous treatment (Minkoff, 1989). Each admission is a "window of opportunity." Relapse does not mean that a treatment intervention, the health care provider, or the patient has failed. Readmission and clear, realistic goals can further the patient's engagement in the treatment process. Effective programs emphasize a combination of empathic, long-term relationship building and the use of leverage and possible confrontation by family, other caregivers, or the legal system.

Engaging patients with dual diagnosis in treatment presents two main challenges. The first is developing relationships with people who tend to have difficulties in their relationships and trusting authority figures. The second is patients' lack of motivation and the need to encourage them to enter drug and alcohol treatment programs.

Possible social barriers to patients becoming motivated to seek treatment are homelessness, unemployment, and lack of social support for abstinence. In addition, patients or their therapists may excuse substance abuse because of the patients' psychiatric symptoms. Mental illnesses such as thought disorders, depression, or organic brain disorders may interfere with patients' ability to transcend denial (Osher & Kofoed, 1989). Some patients prefer to regard themselves as victims of circumstance and not as mentally ill or chemically dependent people. They do not seek treatment because they do not view themselves as needing it. These patients do not fully understand their mental illness or the effect of substance abuse on their mood or behavior.

Engagement in treatment is a process that may take many contacts with a patient and requires patience. Patients who struggle with authority and control issues must be convinced that the treatment team members have something to offer and are worth listening to before they will begin to trust them. The engagement process is enhanced if staff can deal with presenting crises concretely (eg, provide help in avoiding legal penalties and obtaining food, housing, entitlements, relief from psychiatric symptoms, vocational opportunities, recreation, and socialization).

The process of engagement is often characterized by approach–avoidance behavior by the patient. Intake and assessment procedures may discourage the patient from engagement or be intolerable if they are protracted and begin with asking the patient numerous pointed personal questions. Adjustments in these procedures may have to be made to tailor treatment to accommodate the needs or reactions of the patient with a dual diagnosis.

Medication Management

One essential feature of dual diagnosis treatment is medication management. Noncompliance with prescribed medications is associated with increased behavior problems after discharge and is a direct cause of relapse and rehospitalization. Impulsive behavior in response to transient exacerbations of psychotic symptoms, depressed mood, or anxiety symptoms may lead to relapse. Disulfiram (Antabuse) is useful to reduce impulsive alcohol use in patients with schizophrenia or with anxiety, affective, or severe personality disorders (Beeder & Millman, 1997). By making alcohol unavailable, disulfiram in effect may reduce the conditioned associations between psychiatric symptoms and drug craving. Furthermore, it may enhance the patient's sense of control (Beeder & Millman, 1997). The use of disulfiram with dually diagnosed patients, however, needs careful evaluation. Patients must be able to refrain from drinking alcohol while taking disulfiram. They must be able to understand the negative consequences that could occur if they were to drink, and they must realize that they cannot give this medication to another person. Disulfiram should not be given to any patient who may deliberately drink after its use as a suicide attempt.

Collaboration between the patient's prescriber and other treatment providers is important to minimize the possible misuse of prescription drugs. Additionally, caution in prescribing medications that can increase the potential of the patient's relapse into abuse of the drug of choice is essential (Zweben & Smith, 1989). The patient in recovery is often reluctant to use potentially mind-altering drugs, and the nurse should explore any concerns (Zweben & Smith, 1989). A cooperative partnership between the health care provider and the patient will help determine which medication is most effective and offers the greatest chance of patient compliance.

The term *abuse* can be applied to the improper use of prescription drugs. Portenoy and Payne (1997) listed the following as clear examples of abuse: (1) prescription forgery; (2) selling of prescription drugs by unauthorized people; (3) acquisition of drugs from nonmedical sources; (4) use of illicit opiates to supplement therapy; (5) unsanctioned drug dose escalation; (6) use of drugs to treat symptoms other than those targeted by the therapy; (7) frequent visits to emergency departments to obtain drugs; (8) contacts with multiple physicians to obtain drug prescriptions; and (9) drug hoarding.

Guidelines for Managing Acute Pain in Substance Abusers

Portenoy and Payne (1997) proposed these guidelines for managing pain related to cancer, AIDS-related neuropathies, or other diseases in chemically dependent patients:

1. Define the pain syndrome and provide treatment for the underlying disorder.
2. Distinguish between the patient who has a remote history of drug abuse, the patient who is receiving methadone maintenance, and the patient who is actively abusing drugs.
3. Apply appropriate pharmacologic principles of opioid use.
   a. Use an appropriate opioid.
   b. Use adequate doses and dosing intervals.
   c. Use an appropriate route.
4. Provide concurrent nonopioid therapies.
5. Recognize specific drug abuse behaviors.
6. Avoid excessive negotiations over specific drugs and doses.
7. Provide early consultation with substance abuse or psychiatric treatment professionals.
8. If the patient is an outpatient, anticipate problems with prescription renewals.

Patient Education

Patient education is an essential element in the treatment of dual diagnosis. Patients with a dual diagnosis often have ego and problem-solving deficits (La Salvia, 1993). Educational group leaders can offer these patients alternative tools for gaining control over their affective state by explaining or demonstrating stress reduction techniques, relaxation techniques, and cognitive therapy tools (La Salvia, 1993). Group sessions can also assist patients in learning interpersonal skills (eg, assertiveness) and problem-solving skills and in relapse prevention planning.

Topics for group sessions should encourage interaction between patients. Sharing their experiences with their peers, patients can enhance these presentations. Topics should be clear, relevant to the group members, and illustrated with charts, handouts, or appropriate films. Each lecture or discussion group should be relatively short and not contain too many new or difficult concepts. Reinforcement and review of previous discussions can be helpful to remind patients of particularly relevant concepts. Text Box 33-2 lists some suitable topics for nurse-led discussion groups. Individual patient education can focus on areas of knowledge deficits and reinforce topics discussed in group settings.

Self-Help Groups

Several self-help groups are appropriate for many patients with a dual diagnosis. The most common groups are **12-step programs**, such as AA and NA (see Chap. 25). Zweben (1987) raised the issue of whether a patient who is taking psychotropic medications may participate in a 12-step program. AA published a landmark report by a group of physicians in AA that addressed this issue. In it, the physicians gave guidelines to members for the sensible use of medications and indicated pitfalls that can occur with psychoactive prescription drug use. The report presented members' stories of abuse and discussed the benefits some members derived from the judicious use of appropriately prescribed medications. The authors concluded: "It becomes clear that just as it is wrong to enable or support any alcoholic to become readdicted to any drug, it's equally wrong to deprive any alcoholic of medication which can alleviate or control other disabling physical and/or emotional problems" (Alcoholic Anonymous World Services, 1984, p. 300). For patients who are concerned that they might not be accepted into AA because of their use of psychiatric medications, this AA literature can be helpful.

The advisability of a patient enrolling in a 12-step program needs to be evaluated on an individual basis. Tailoring AA concepts and work on the 12 steps to the patient's needs can be extremely helpful. Satel and colleagues (1993) discussed ways in which health care providers can help prepare patients for AA. They suggested advising patients about which meetings are likely to have fewer participants and attendees whose background, culture, or emotional difficulties are similar to those of the patient. For example, for Vietnam veterans

TEXT BOX 33.2

Topics for Dual Diagnosis Patient Education Groups

The effects of alcohol and drugs on the body

Alcohol, drugs, and medication—what can go wrong

- What is a healthy lifestyle?
- Triggers for relapse
- What is Alcoholics (or Narcotics) Anonymous?
- What is a sponsor in Alcoholics (or Narcotics) Anonymous?
- What is recovery from mental illness and substance abuse?
- What are tools of recovery?
- The disease of addiction
- The relapse cycle
- How to cope with feelings without using alcohol or other drugs
- Relapse prevention: what works?
- What are cognitive distortions?
- HIV prevention and education

- Leisure time management
- How to manage stress
- Relaxation training
- Assertiveness and recovery
- Common slogans to live by
- Pitfalls in treatment
- The process of recovery
- Creating a relapse prevention plan
- What are my goals? How does the use of alcohol and drugs affect them?

Coping with thoughts about alcohol and drugs

- Problem-solving basics
- Coping with anger
- Negative thinking and how to manage it
- Enhancing social support networks

with PTSD, AA meetings that will meet their needs are often held at Veterans Administration hospitals and outreach centers.

Unrealistic guilt, previous unsatisfactory or negative religion-related incidents or experiences, and fear of crowds or of being self-revealing are examples of patients' emotions and experiences that can interfere with their successful use of 12-step programs. The idea of a "power greater than oneself" can be interpreted as the need for medication and continuing treatment to cope with substance abuse and mental illness. A health care provider familiar with 12-step concepts can often facilitate patients' attempts to use these programs. The numerous advantages of self-help groups make them a potentially powerful support for continued recovery.

Alternative self-help programs similar to 12-step programs are available in some geographic areas. Rational Recovery and Secular Organization for Sobriety are groups that downplay the concept of powerlessness and the spiritual aspects associated with 12-step programs (Satel et al., 1993).

Relapse Prevention: Creating a New Lifestyle

Relapse is the failure to maintain the behaviors needed to remain abstinent (Annis & Davis, 1995). One model of relapse prevention is based on the self-efficacy theory.

It proposes that when a patient enters a situation in which the risk for resuming drinking or drug use is high, his or her expectations of the ability to cope with the situation without substances will predict his or her substance use (Annis & Davis, 1995). If a patient feels confident that he or she can cope with an emotionally charged situation, his or her likelihood of using substances in that situation is lower. See Text Box 33-3 for a list of common situations in which relapse often occurs.

Relapse prevention groups can be valuable sources of support for patients. These groups help patients to (1) analyze which situations are most likely to trigger relapses; (2) examine cognitive, emotional, and behavioral components of high-risk situations; and (3) develop cognitive, behavioral, and effective coping strategies and environmental supports. Role-playing ways out of high-risk situations is a technique that these groups often use (Annis & Davis, 1995; Marlatt & Gordon, 1985). Homework assignments help patients create relapse prevention plans that address new coping strategies for these high-risk situations.

This model uses cognitive-behavioral techniques to help patients plan for stressors that can lead to relapse. The methods highlighted are practical, emphasize and strengthen patients' coping skills, and can be adapted to the needs of individual patients. Relapse prevention plans initiated in treatment are just pieces of paper if they are not implemented after discharge. The follow-

TEXT BOX 33.3

*Categories for Classification
of Relapse Episodes*

I. Intrapersonal and environmental determinants
   A. Coping with negative emotional states
   B. Coping with negative physical and physiologic
      states
   C. Enhancement of positive emotional states
   D. Testing personal control
   E. Giving in to temptations or urges
II. Interpersonal determinants
   A. Coping with interpersonal conflict
   B. Coping with social pressure
   C. Enhancement of positive emotional states

From Marlatt, G. A., & Gordon, J. R. (1985). *Relapse prevention.* New York: Guilford Press. Used with permission.

ing section discusses elements in effective discharge planning for patients with a dual diagnosis.

Continuum of Care and Discharge Planning

Early intervention in crises is important for patients with a dual diagnosis, but equally important is a focus beyond medication management and inpatient treatment episodes. Social interaction skills and coping skills learned in treatment need to be reinforced in community settings to create or enhance a stable living situation and possible vocational opportunities. Active planning and intervention are needed with respect to housing and employment or deterioration may occur, despite gains made during the course of hospitalization.

Establishing a positive social network is regarded as a critical function of any program intended to treat dual diagnosis. Isolation and alienation from prior supports is a problem that most chronic mentally ill substance abusers share. Some patients relate poorly to their families, others are overly dependent on them, and others have difficulty establishing and maintaining social relationships. Some patients' only "families" are peers within the drug subculture who reinforce substance-abusing behavior.

Having opportunities to socialize, access to positive recreational activities, and a supportive peer group are stabilizing influences on patients who may otherwise drop out of treatment altogether. Part of a comprehensive relapse prevention plan is to establish or reinforce the patient's social support network so that he or she can obtain (1) opportunities for substance-free socializing, (2) crisis counseling to prevent readmission to a hospital, and (3) support for sobriety.

Supportive housing is also essential for patients with a dual diagnosis. Supportive housing is especially crucial for patients who are being discharged from the hospital because the risk for relapse is greatest during the first few months after discharge. Halfway houses for substance abusers may de-emphasize medication compliance, and housing designed for the chronically mentally ill may emphasize abstinence enough. Thus, an important part of the multidisciplinary team approach to discharge planning for patients with a dual diagnosis is to help them find the best possible living situation.

Younger patients with severe mental illness may want and expect to find employment. Although some of these patients may be unrealistic about potential professions, they may desire to seek appropriate employment. This desire can be a significant motivator and a useful tool in a treatment program. Referral of patients to halfway houses or residential substance abuse treatment programs that stress vocational skill training can be beneficial. Use of community vocational rehabilitation services and of educational opportunities can be an important part of a discharge plan.

Case Management

Case managers are responsible for conducting outreach activities, linking patients with direct services, monitoring patients' progress through various milieus, educating patients about psychiatric and substance abuse disorders, reiterating treatment recommendations, and coordinating treatment planning across programs (Segal, 1988). Case managers can use four approaches for the delivery of services for patients with a dual diagnosis (Segal, 1988):

Brokerage-generalist. This short-term model seeks to identify the patient's needs and helps gain access to identified resources.

Assertive community treatment. This model involves assertive advocacy, making contact with patients in their homes and natural settings, with the focus on practical problems of daily living.

Strength-based perspective. This model emphasizes providing support for patients to assert direct control over their search for resources and to examine the patients' own strengths in acquiring these resources.

Clinical-rehabilitation. In this model, the clinician provides counseling and is responsible for resource acquisition.

Table 33-6 lists how these models of case management address case management activities for the patient with a dual diagnosis.

TABLE 33.6   Models of Case Management for Patients With Dual Diagnoses

Primary Case Management Activities	Broker-Generalist	Strengths Perspective	Assertive Community Treatment	Clinical Rehabilitation
Engages in outreach and case finding	No	Depends on agency mission and structure	Depends on agency mission and structure	Depends on agency mission and structure
Provides assessment and reassessment	Specific to immediate resource acquisition needs	Strengths based, applicable to any area of need	Broad-based, comprehensive assessment	Broad-based, comprehensive assessment
Assists in goal planning	Brief, related to acquiring resources	Patient driven, teaches specific ways to set and achieve goals	Comprehensive and may include any area of patient's life	Comprehensive and may include any area of patient's life
Makes referrals to needed resources	Patient or case manager may make contact	Patient or case manager may make contact	As needed; resources may be integrated in services	Patient or case manager may make contact
Provides additional services such as therapy, skills teaching	Referral to others for these	Limited; teaches patient to identify strengths and about self-help groups	Provides many services in comprehensive package	Provides services consistent with model
Responds to crisis	Related to resource needs	Related to resource and mental health concerns: active in stabilization and referral	Assertive advocacy on several levels	Assertive advocacy on several levels
Provides direct services related to resource acquisition as part of case management (eg, drop-in center, employment counseling)	Referral to resources that provide direct services	Provides services to prepare patient to gain own resources (eg, role playing, accompanying patient to services)	Provides many direct services as part of comprehensive package	Provides services as part of a rehabilitation services plan; skill teaching

Based on Siegal, H. A. (1998). *Comprehensive case management for substance abuse treatment* (pp. 4–11). Rockville, MD: U.S. Department of Health and Human Services.

Family Support and Education

The families of patients with a dual diagnosis need education and support. The focus of family support groups, such as those under the auspices of the National Alliance for the Mentally Ill, has been both to educate and to help the family cope with a mentally ill relative. Al Anon and Nar Anon take a similar approach to providing peer support to families of substance abusers. These self-help groups aid family members in balancing confrontation of the problem, detachment from forcing a solution to it, and support of the treatment process.

Comprehensive Concurrent Treatment

Several traditional approaches to the treatment of dual disorders are possible:

- Treat the mental illness first.

- Treat the substance use disorder first.
- Treat both conditions concurrently.

Recent literature suggests that a comprehensive concurrent approach is often beneficial after initial stabilization of the presenting problem. Text Box 33-4 presents features of a dual diagnosis outpatient program.

PLANNING FOR NURSING CARE

Numerous challenges face the nurse who provides care to dually diagnosed patients. Comprehensive planning within a multidisciplinary team approach has been highly successful in the management of patients with a dual diagnosis. Community organizations can be valuable sources of support as well. (See Chap. 25 for available community resources.)

TEXT BOX 33.4

Features of a Dual Diagnosis Outpatient Program

Community meeting and goal setting: Patients set small, realistic goals for themselves for the day, which aids them in their ultimate goal of better living in recovery.

Anger management and social communication: Patients learn appropriate ways to express anger and how to socialize with others.

Group therapy: Patients discuss interpersonal issues, get feedback from their peers, and learn problem-solving skills.

Dual recovery anonymous meetings: Patient-run meeting (a modified Alcoholics Anonymous meeting) addresses the specific needs of the patient with dual diagnosis.

Leisure planning: Patients learn skills to enjoy leisure involving clean and sober fun.

Gardening, art therapy, music therapy, swimming: These methods provide alternatives to the use of alcohol and other drugs.

Health education: Patients learn about the effects of drugs and alcohol on the body and about other relevant medical topics.

Medication education: Patients learn about psychiatric medications, their uses, the side effects, and interactions with drugs or alcohol.

Relapse prevention planning: Patients talk about their last relapse; triggers, feelings, and stresses that contributed to the relapse; and the consequences and formulate relapse prevention plans.

Individual counseling: Patients receive individual counseling to develop goals and work on problem-solving techniques.

Psychiatric consultation: Patients are evaluated and followed for medication and other psychiatric interventions.

Note: Patients are *not* discharged from the program if they are intoxicated. They are asked not to come to the program intoxicated, but to return when they are sober to continue work on their recovery.

Summary of Key Points

➤ The incidence of alcohol or drug abuse and one or more comorbid mental health disorders is very high.

➤ A dual diagnosis can consist of a primary mental illness and subsequent substance abuse, a primary substance abuse disorder and psychopathologic sequelae, dual primary diagnoses, or two disorders resulting from a common cause.

➤ In patients with a dual diagnosis, relapse is common if both the substance abuse disorder and the mental health disorder are not addressed concurrently.

➤ Barriers to effective treatment of a dual diagnosis include the nature of substance abuse, countertransference and the position of substance abusers in society, misunderstandings about and the stigmatization of mental illness, and underlying health issues.

➤ Assessment of dual diagnosis often depends on objective data obtained from interviews with family members, reviews of court records, laboratory test results, and physical examination findings.

➤ Alcohol and drug use can cause numerous mental health problems, including organic brain disorders, depression, hallucinations, agitation, confusion, and stupor. These substances interact with common prescription and over-the-counter drugs to cause adverse reactions.

➤ Alcohol and other drugs often exacerbate existing mental health disorders and can lead to noncompliance with prescribed medication regimens and other aspects of treatment.

➤ Elements of treatment for patients with dual diagnosis include possible hospitalization, crisis stabilization, engagement in long-term treatment, medication management, patient education, use of self-help groups, relapse prevention, continuation of care, case management, and family support.

➤ Relapse prevention is crucial in treating dual diagnosis and entails analyzing high-risk situations for relapse; examining the cognitive, emotional, and behavioral components of high-risk situations; and using effective coping strategies and available environmental supports.

Critical Thinking Challenges

1. What criteria would you use to refer an intoxicated and depressed patient in a psychiatric emergency department to the following?
   a. An alcohol detoxification center
   b. An inpatient psychiatric unit
   c. An outpatient alcohol-treatment program
   d. An outpatient community mental health clinic
2. How would you respond to a patient with dual diagnoses who states, "Once my medication is stable, I will be able to drink again."
3. In your opinion, what are the five most important concepts to cover in educating a patient with dual diagnosis?

  WEB LINKS

www.dualdiagnosisfriendly.org Dual Diagnosis Friendly. This website is for those with dual diagnosis.

www.dualdiagnosisresources.com Dual Diagnosis Resources. This site contains program development materials.

www.nmha.org National Mental Health Association Organization. This site provides facts about dual diagnosis.

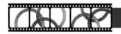 MOVIES

Born on the Fourth of July: 1989. This wrenching, but true, account shows the experiences of Ron Kovic, played by Tom Cruise. Ron was a patriotic teen from a small town who volunteered to serve in Vietnam. During the war, he was shot in the spine, which left him paralyzed from the chest down. He returned home, bitterly alienated from his family, friends, and community. He faced a long and slow rehabilitation process. His depression and abuse of substances only compounded his physical problems. This movie depicts depression and substance abuse coexisting with major physical disabilities.

Viewing Points: How does Ron express his depression? Is he using, abusing, or dependent on alcohol and drugs? How are you feeling throughout this movie? Do your feelings about the character change?

REFERENCES

Alcoholics Anonymous World Services, Inc. (1984). *The A. A. member-medications and other drugs: A report from a group of physicians in A. A.* New York, NY: Author.

American Psychiatric Association. (2000). *Diagnostic and statistical manual of mental disorders* (4th ed., Text revision). Washington, DC: Author.

Annis, H. M., & Davis, C. S. (1995). Relapse prevention. In R. K. Hester & W. R. Miller (Eds.), *Handbook of alcoholism treatment approaches* (2nd ed., pp. 170–181). Boston: Allyn & Bacon.

Beeder, A. B., & Millman, R. B. (1997). Treatment of patients with psychopathology and substance abuse. In J. H. Lowinson, P. Ruiz, R. B. Millman, & J. G. Langrod (Eds.), *Substance abuse: A comprehensive textbook* (3rd ed., pp. 675–690). Baltimore: Williams & Wilkins.

Bellack, A., & Gearon, J. (1998). Substance abuse treatment for people with schizophrenia. *Addictive Behaviors, 23*(6), 749–766.

Blumenthal, S. J. (1988). A guide to risk factors, assessment and treatment of suicidal patients. *Medical Clinics of North America, 72,* 937–971.

Brehm, N. M., & Khantzian, E. J. (1997). A psychodynamic perspective. In J. H. Lowinson, P. Ruiz, R. B. Millman, & J. G. Langrod (Eds.), *Substance abuse: A comprehensive textbook* (3rd ed., pp. 106–117). Baltimore: Williams & Wilkins.

Dackis, C., & Gold, M. S. (1997). Psychiatric hospitals for treatment of dual diagnosis. In J. H. Lowinson, P. Ruiz,

R. B. Millman, & J. G. Langrod (Eds.), *Substance abuse: A comprehensive textbook* (3rd ed., pp. 467–485). Baltimore: Williams & Wilkins.

Drake, R. E., & Wallach, M. A. (1989). Substance abuse among the mentally ill. *Hospital and Community Psychiatry, 40*(10), 1041–1046.

Evans, K., & Sullivan, J. (1990). *Dual diagnosis: Counseling the mentally ill substance abuser.* New York: Guilford Press.

Frances, R., Franklin, J., & Flavin, D. (1987). Suicide and alcoholism. *American Journal of Drug and Alcohol Abuse, 13*(3), 327–341.

Friedrich, R. M., & Kus, R. J. (1991). Cognitive impairments in early sobriety. *Archives of Psychiatric Nursing, 5*(2), 105–112.

Goldberg, J., Garno, J., Leon, A., et al. (1999). A history of substance abuse complicates remission from acute mania in bipolar disorder. *Journal of Clinical Psychiatry, 60*(11), 733–739.

Goodwin, D. W. (1997). Alcohol: Clinical aspects. In J. H. Lowinson, P. Ruiz, R. B. Millman, & J. G. Langrod (Eds.), *Substance abuse: A comprehensive textbook* (3rd ed., pp. 144–151). Baltimore: Williams & Wilkins.

Joseph, H. (1997). Substance abuse and homelessness within the inner cities. In J. H. Lowinson, P. Ruiz, R. B. Millman, & J. G. Langrod (Eds.), *Substance abuse: A comprehensive textbook* (3rd ed., pp. 875–889). Baltimore: Williams & Wilkins.

Kessler, R. C., McGonagle, K. A., & Zhao, S. (1994). Lifetime and 12 months prevalence of *DSM-IIIR* psychiatric disorders in the United States: Results from the National Comorbidity Survey. *Archives of General Psychiatry, 51,* 8–19.

Kushner, M. G., Sher, K. J., & Beitman, M. D. (1990). The relation between alcohol problems and the anxiety disorders. *American Journal of Psychiatry, 147*(6), 685–695.

La Salvia, T. A. (1993). Enhancing addiction treatment through psychoeducational groups. *Journal of Substance Abuse Treatment, 10,* 439–444.

Lehman, A. F., Myers, C. P., & Corty, E. (1989). Assessment and classification of patients with psychiatric and substance abuse syndromes. *Hospital and Community Psychiatry, 40*(10), 1019–1024.

Lindstrom, L. (1992). *Managing alcoholism: Matching clients to treatment.* London: Oxford University Press.

Marlatt, G. A., & Gordon, J. R. (1985). *Relapse prevention.* New York: Guilford Press.

Messina, N., Wish, E., & Nemes, S. (1999). Therapeutic community treatment for substance abusers with antisocial personality disorder. *Journal of Substance Abuse Treatment, 17*(1–2), 121–128.

Miller, N. S. (1995). *Addiction psychiatry: Current diagnosis and treatment* (p. 112). New York: Wiley-Liss.

Miller, W. R., & Kurtz, E. (1994). Models of alcoholism used in treatment: Contrasting AA and other perspectives with which it is confused. *Journal of Studies on Alcoholism, 55*(2), 159–166.

Minkoff, K. (1989). An integrated treatment model for dual diagnosis of psychosis and addiction. *Hospital and Community Psychiatry, 40*(10), 1031–1036.

Osher, F. C., & Kofoed, L. L. (1989). Treatment of patients with psychiatric and psychoactive substance abuse disorders. *Hospital and Community Psychiatry, 40*(10), 1025–1030.

Portenoy, R. K., & Payne, R. (1997). Acute and chronic pain. In J. H. Lowinson, P. Ruiz, R. B. Millman, & J. G. Langrod (Eds.), *Substance abuse: A comprehensive textbook* (3rd ed., pp. 236–246). Baltimore: Williams & Wilkins.

Regier, D. A., Farmer, M. E., Rae, D. S., et al. (1990). Comorbidity of mental disorders with alcohol and other drug abuse: Results from the epidemiologic catchment area (ECA) study. *Journal of the American Medical Association, 264*, 2511–2518.

Ries, R. (1995). *Assessment and treatment of patients with coexisting mental illness and alcohol and other drug abuse* (pp. 29–89). Rockville, MD: U.S. Department of Health and Human Services.

Rosenthal, R. N., & Westreich, L. (1999). Treatment of persons with dual diagnosis of substance use disorders and other psychological problems. In *Addictions: A comprehensive guide* (pp. 439–476). New York: Oxford University Press.

Satel, S. L., Becker, B. R., & Dan, E. (1993). Reducing obstacles to affiliation with Alcoholics Anonymous among veterans with PTSD and alcoholism. *Hospital and Community Psychiatry, 44*(11), 1061–1065.

Scott, J., Gilvarry, E., & Farrell, M. (1998). Managing anxiety and depression in alcohol and drug dependence. *Addictive Behaviors, 23*(6), 919–931.

Segal, B. (1988). *Drugs and behavior.* New York: Gardner Press.

Shaffer, D. (1988). The epidemiology of teen suicide: An examination of risk factors. *Journal of Clinical Psychiatry, 49*, 36–41.

Sowers, W., & Golden, S. (1999). Psychotropic medication management in persons with co-occurring psychiatric and substance use disorders. *Journal of Psychoactive Drugs, 31*(1), 59–70.

Steinglass, P. (1985). Family systems approaches to alcoholism. *Journal of Substance Abuse Treatment, 2*, 161–167.

Stoffelmayr, B. E., Benishek, L. A., Humphreys, K., et al. (1989). Substance abuse prognosis with additional psychiatric diagnosis: Understanding the relationship. *Journal of Psychoactive Drugs, 2*(2), 145–152.

Thomas, V., Melchert, T., & Banker, J. (1999). Substance dependence and personality disorders: Comorbidity and treatment outcome in an inpatient treatment population. *Journal of Studies of Alcohol, 60*, 271–277.

Wallen, M. C., & Weiner, H. D. (1989). Impediments to effective treatment of the dually diagnosed patient. *Journal of Psychoactive Drugs, 21*(2), 161–168.

Weiss, R. D., Marin, S. M., & Frances, R. J. (1992). The myth of the typical dual diagnosis patient. *Hospital and Community Psychiatry, 43*(2), 107–108.

Zweben, J. E. (1987). Can patients on medication be sent to 12-step programs? *Journal of Psychoactive Drugs, 19*(3), 299–300.

Zweben, J. E., & Smith, D. E. (1989). Considerations in using psychotropic medication with dual diagnosis patients in recovery. *Journal of Psychoactive Drugs, 2*(2), 221–228.

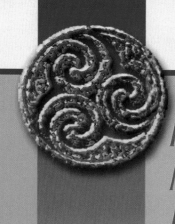

Psychosocial Aspects of Medically Compromised Persons

Gail L. Kongable-Beckman

PSYCHOLOGICAL ILLNESS RELATED TO SPECIFIC PHYSIOLOGIC DISORDERS

PSYCHOLOGICAL IMPACT OF PAIN
Biologic Basis of the Pain Response
Psychological Aspects of the Pain Response
Assessment of the Patient With Chronic Pain
Sensory and Pharmacologic Modulation of Pain

PSYCHOPATHOLOGIC COMPLICATIONS OF AIDS
Biologic Basis of Neurologic Manifestations of HIV
Psychological Aspects of AIDS
Assessment of the AIDS Patient
Biopsychosocial Treatment Interventions

PSYCHOLOGICAL ILLNESS RELATED TO TRAUMA
Biologic Basis of the Trauma Response
Psychological Aspects of the Trauma Response
Assessment of the Trauma Patient
Biopsychosocial Treatment Interventions

PSYCHOLOGICAL ILLNESS RELATED TO CENTRAL NERVOUS SYSTEM DISORDERS
Biologic Basis of Neurologic Impairment
Psychological Aspects of Neurologic Impairment
Assessment of the Neurologic Patient
Biopsychosocial Treatment Interventions

PSYCHOLOGICAL ILLNESS RELATED TO ACUTE AND CHRONIC MEDICAL ILLNESS
Biologic Aspects of Mental Illness Related to Medical Disease
Psychological Aspects of Medical Illness
Assessment of the Patient With Medical Illness
Clinical Features of Special Significance
Biopsychosocial Treatment Interventions

RECOGNITION OF MENTAL ILLNESS AND BIOPSYCHOSOCIAL INTERVENTIONS IN MEDICAL ILLNESS

LEARNING OBJECTIVES

After studying this chapter, you will be able to:

➤ Identify medically ill populations at risk for secondary mental illness.
➤ Analyze the impact on patients and their families of mental illness associated with medical illness.
➤ Discuss comorbid psychosocial and biologic disorders seen in psychiatric settings and their treatments.
➤ Discuss neurobiologic and psychological disturbances associated with specific medical illnesses and the medications used to treat them.
➤ Develop a plan of care for patients who are experiencing mental illness associated with medical illness.
➤ Discuss biopsychosocial interventions that promote patients' mental health in physical illness.

CHAPTER 34

KEY TERMS

allodynia
comorbidity
endorphins
gate-control model
HIV-1–associated
   cognitive-motor
   complex
hyperalgia
hyperesthesia
hypothalamic–
   pituitary–adrenal
   (HPA) axis

ischemic cascade
kindling
nociception
neurotransmitters
plasticity
self-efficacy
serotonin
substance P

KEY CONCEPTS

cognitive-biobehavioral model
neurochemical modulation

---

*P*sychiatric illness often accompanies medical illness and is a significant health care problem in the medically ill population. People who have chronic medical illnesses have a nearly 41% higher rate of psychiatric disorders than people without chronic medical illness. In addition, the chronically medically ill have a 28% higher lifetime prevalence of psychiatric disorders than other people (Cassem, 1990). Mood, anxiety, and substance use disorders are the most prevalent psychiatric conditions of patients with chronic or terminal illnesses, such as chronic pain, acquired immunodeficiency syndrome (AIDS), stroke, and cancer (Katon & Schulberg, 1992; Neese, 1991). Because most medically ill people are elderly, biologic, psychological, and social changes may place them at greater risk for mental illness and its potential complications.

PSYCHOLOGICAL ILLNESS RELATED TO SPECIFIC PHYSIOLOGIC DISORDERS

The biologic basis of mental disorders that are preceded by comorbid mental disorders is thought to be similar to the biologic basis of primary psychiatric disorders, in which neurochemical changes occur in the process of catecholamine metabolism (Arnsten, 1997). The neurochemicals (transmitters) that orchestrate thinking, learning, speaking, and motor responses also influence mood, perception, and emotional interpretation. Neurochemical modulation maintains a balance in the essential levels of these transmitters. When modulation is disrupted mechanically or chemically, biopsychosocial disorder occurs.

KEY CONCEPT Neurochemical Modulation. **Neurochemical modulation** maintains a balance in the essential levels of the neurotransmitters that influence mood, perceptions, and emotional interpretation.

    Unfortunately, mental illness is not commonly recognized or treated in general medical settings. Psychiatric symptoms may be masked by medical symptoms or misdiagnosed as somatoform disorders. The treatment regimen may contribute to psychosocial dysfunction because many medications prescribed for chronic illness alter affect (Neese, 1991). Generally, health care providers expect patients to exhibit depressed mood and anxiety as a normal response to illness. In fact, it is considered abnormal if a patient does not grieve over the loss of health or does not express discouragement or anxiety about treatment and the possibility of death.

When psychosocial dysfunction is not examined closely and is not treated, it can affect the course and outcome of associated medical illness. The presence of mental illness may weaken the motivation for self-care, impair symptom reporting, and delay the search for treatment (Katon & Schulberg, 1992). These symptoms may precede or occur during acute hospitalization and continue after discharge and apparent physical recovery. As a result, hospitalization may be prolonged and recovery delayed or impaired, at increased emotional and financial cost to the patient and the family (Levenson, 1992). In severe cases, mood disorders associated with medical illness increase morbidity and mortality (Hill et al., 1992). Careful assessment to identify and evaluate symptoms of concomitant mental illness separately from those of medical illness is required, together with appropriate treatment, to achieve the patient's best psychological and medical outcome.

A second aspect of psychiatric disorders and medical illness is the common **comorbidity** of physical disorders among people who require primary psychiatric care. Acute psychiatric settings, residential treatment settings, and psychiatric home health programs are reporting increasing numbers of patients with primary or secondary physical and medical problems (Katon, 1992). Factors associated with increased hospital stays of psychiatric patients include the presence of physical disability and concomitant medical illness (Cohen & Cosimer, 1989; Collins, 1991). Mental health care professionals must carefully evaluate and monitor changes in coexisting medical conditions to prevent their exacerbation or serious complications that would necessitate acute medical treatment or prolonged hospitalization.

This chapter reviews the prevalence of mental illness in the medically ill population and common comorbid medical disorders in the psychiatric population. The psychosocial disturbances associated with chronic pain, human immunodeficiency virus (HIV), trauma, neurologic disorders, stroke, and chronic medical illnesses such as heart disease and cancer are presented. Suggestions for diagnostic appraisal and appropriate intervention are given. These medical conditions were chosen because they are responsible for most hospitalizations and are frequently associated with psychiatric comorbidity. Psychiatric–mental health liaison clinicians are consulted to see patients with these conditions in all phases of their illness, from acute hospitalization and treatment to rehabilitation and return to the community.

PSYCHOLOGICAL IMPACT OF PAIN

Physiologic pain is a protective response to noxious stimuli that serves as a warning of injury. Clinical pain related to inflammation and pathologic processes is characterized by low-threshold sensitization. Despite major advances in treatments that lessen its force, pain remains one of the most powerful and complex human experiences. Assessing and treating pain is difficult because the pain response is subjective and a patient's degree of pain cannot be observed directly. A patient's complaints may be difficult to localize. In addition, the person's discomfort may seem out of proportion to the observed conditions or influenced by disordered emotions, personality, or abnormal environmental conditioning. Severe or chronic pain may affect mentally healthy people in adverse ways. The prevalence and impact of pain have led to numerous approaches to therapy, including the use of antipsychotic drugs, antidepressants, antianxiety agents, and stimulants. Considerable evidence suggests that psychiatric medications and interventions can be effective in treating both acute and chronic pain.

The **gate-control model** of pain response is based on physiologic evidence that pain perception (**nociception**) involves pathways in the dorsal horn of the spinal cord that relay noxious stimuli to the brain. In addition, certain other nerve fibers function as an antagonistic "gate" to augment or dampen the subjective experience of pain (Melzack, 1993; Melzack & Wall, 1965). The cognitive-biobehavioral model (Turk et al., 1983) considers not only the patient's emotive and cognitive perception of pain but also the interaction of environmental influences, physical factors, and pain perceptions over time. From this perspective, patients' interpretations of pain, their coping resources, and their emotive-psychological processes interact with the experience of pain and can influence the physiologic activities that characterize pain (Turk & Marcos, 1994). Some pain theorists believe that the gate-control theory has been largely discredited (McCaffery & Pasero, 1999); others are working to refine the theory as more knowledge of pain becomes available.

KEY CONCEPT Cognitive-Biobehavioral Model. The **cognitive-behavioral model** is the model of pain perception that includes emotion, cognition, environment, and physical and psychological factors.

Biologic Basis of the Pain Response

Pain is transmitted through specific neural pathways that carry information about touch and temperature (Fig. 34-1). Recent physiologic evidence obtained from magnetic resonance imaging and positron emission tomography has demonstrated that painful stimuli also

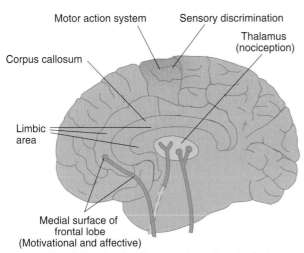

FIGURE 34.1 Pain stimuli activate regions of the brain that influence memory, emotion, and personality.

cause significant activation in areas of the brain responsible for memory, emotion, and personality (Talbot et al., 1991) (Fig. 34-2). Pain receptors may be activated by mechanical, thermal, or chemical stimuli. **Neurotransmitters** are chemicals circulating in the synaptic areas of neurons. They serve to initiate, block, or modulate nerve signal transmission and ultimately control neural function. Several neurotransmitters within primary pain pathways are involved in pain transmission (Text Box 34-1). When these neurochemicals are released, they initiate local inflammatory reactions and sensitize and stimulate central pain receptors. **Substance P** is the most common nociceptive transmitter that is released and transported along the central and peripheral pain synapses in the presence of noxious stimuli. **Endorphins,** neurotransmitters that have opiate-like behavior, produce an inhibitory effect at opiate receptor sites and are probably responsible for pain tolerance. The release of endorphins is centrally mediated by **serotonin** (Coderre et al., 1993; Kandel & Schwartz, 1987). Serotonin, histamine, and bradykinin sensitize and stimulate the pain receptors to generate experienced pain. Direct demonstrations of changes in endorphin levels during pain and relief from pain are being reported (Ren, 1994; Sosnowski, 1994). The role of endorphins may go beyond pain modulation to include mood enhancement, behavior modification, and influence on the development of tolerance or dependence on narcotics.

Acute pain is one of the most common symptoms of patients in emergency and acute care settings (Atkinson & Slater, 1989). It can result from a variety of physiologic abnormalities and trauma. It is characterized by sudden, severe onset and generally subsides as the injury heals. Postoperative incisional pain is an iatrogenic (physician-induced) tissue injury most often seen in medical settings. Careful assessment and treatment of

pain in these settings have a great impact on healing and recovery (Carpenter, 1996).

Chronic pain, defined as pain on a daily basis or pain that is constant for more than 6 months (Atkinson & Slater, 1989), can be related to a variety of pathologies and takes the form of syndromes such as headache, temporomandibular pain disorders, back pain, and arthritis. Clinical syndromes with chronic pain symptoms include neoplasia (cancer), thalamic stroke (central pain), neuropathies (diabetes), and reflex sympathetic dystrophy (Text Box 34-2). Nervous tissue injury leads to neuropathic pain that may be described as burning, aching, pricking, or lancinating. This central or neuropathic pain is the underlying mechanism for most chronic pain and leads to **hyperalgia** (increased sensation of pain), **allodynia** (lowered pain threshold), and **hyperesthesia** (increased nociceptor sensitivity). Permanent change in central pain interpretation frequently results in abnormal physiologic, biochemical, cellular, and molecular responses that misinterpret nonpainful sensations as painful (**plasticity**) (Coderre et al., 1993). This neural plasticity contributes to the development of errant firing and the pain syndromes of referred pain (pain felt in a part other than where it was produced) and phantom pain (pain that feels as though its source is a missing [amputated] limb).

Psychological Aspects of the Pain Response

Pain is not only a sensation but also a perceptual phenomenon with an important affective component. When a patient's pain persists for an extended period, a range of psychosocial influences, such as the patient's mood, fears, expectancies, coping efforts, and financial and social resources, and the responses of significant others begin to influence the patient's perception of the pain. Affective and anxiety disorders are prevalent among people with chronic pain. They may be a symptom of or a defense against psychological stress caused by continuous nociceptive input (Koob, 1999). Biopsychosocial stimuli and responses may cause the patient with chronic pain to become preoccupied with the pain and can contribute to depression. Also, the presence of persistent noxious sensations contributes to neurochemical and neurohormonal imbalances that lead to depressed mood and anxiety. Whether the psychological pain is primary or secondary may be difficult to determine because the neurovegetative symptoms of depression may resemble the patient's attempts to control the pain or the concomitant medical-physical conditions. Anorexia, sleep disturbance, and agitation or psychomotor retardation may be present. Also, affective disturbances, such as sadness, loss of interest in life, feelings of worthlessness, self-reproach, excessive guilt, indecisiveness, and suicidal ideation, are all symptoms re-

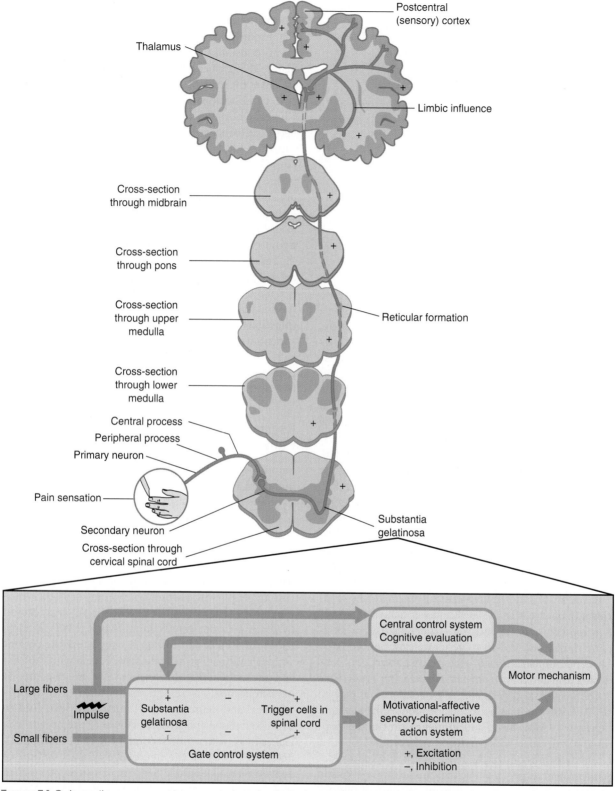

FIGURE 34.2 Ascending sensory pathways: anterior spinothalamic tract with a schematic diagram of the gate control theory of pain mechanism.

TEXT BOX 34.1

Neurotransmitters Active in Pain Sensation and Induced Plasticity

C-Fiber Neuropeptides Released by Noxious Stimulation Peripherally

Substance P

Neurokinin A

Somatostatin

Calcitonin gene-related peptide (CGRP)

Galanin

Vasoactive intestinal polypeptide (VIP)

Cholecystokinin

Excitatory Amino Acids That Have Widespread Activity in the Central Nervous System (Thalamus and Somatosensory Cortices)

L-glutamate

N-methyl-D-aspartate (NMDA)

Neurotransmitters Active as Pain Modulators

Endorphins

Enkephalin

Serotonin

Note: Many of these same neurotransmitters are released in large amounts during brain injury and contribute to neuronal cell death in a variety of neurologic and psychological disease processes.

---

ported by patients with chronic pain (Turk & Okifuji, 1994). Substance use disorder may arise from the patient's search for relief through overuse of drugs that lessen the pain sensation. A formal psychiatric assessment is essential when these symptoms exist.

Assessment of the Patient With Chronic Pain

Appropriate diagnosis and treatment of pain as a primary presenting symptom must begin with a comprehensive history and physical examination. In talking with the nurse about the pain, a patient will not only describe its characteristics, location, and severity but may also provide information about possible psychosocial and behavioral factors that are influencing the pain experience. No direct relationship may be evident between the severity or extent of detectable disease and the intensity of the patient's pain (Rudy & Turk, 1991). A number of assessment instruments have been developed to aid in evaluation (Bradley et al., 1992), but a fundamental approach is necessary to determine the impact of pain on the patient's life. All systems must be examined in the patient to determine the degree to which biomedical, psychosocial, and behavioral factors interact to influence the nature, severity, and persistence

of the patient's pain and disability. Text Box 34-3 presents a pain assessment tool.

Sensory and Pharmacologic Modulation of Pain

Chronic pain occurs with a wide variety of medical illnesses. Proper diagnosis of the underlying condition determines primary treatment, which could eliminate or significantly reduce the need for analgesic drugs. Unsuspected medical conditions, such as alcoholism, autoimmune disease, or cancer, must be considered if pain develops in the absence of a known cause. Caregivers must know the mechanisms of action of analgesic drugs to administer them safely and monitor their effects. Patients' responses to individual drugs vary, and many agents at different doses may be tried before pain relief is achieved. Table 34-1 presents treatment approaches to pain. The use of physical and psychological modulation techniques as well as pharmacotherapy or physical therapy is more successful than the latter therapies alone (Katz, 1994). Combination treatment often affects mood and anxiety levels as well. Patients trained to use cognitive strategies such as biofeedback, a positive emotional state, relaxation, physical therapy or exercise, meditation, guided imagery, suggestion, hypnosis, placebos, and positive self-talk are able to tolerate higher levels of pain than patients without specific coping strategies (Turk & Feldman, 1992). Most of these techniques involve redirecting the patient's attention away from the pain and helping the patient learn strategies of **self-efficacy** (self-effectiveness). Some of the biopsychosocial outcomes that can be measured to determine effectiveness of prescribed therapies include improvements in biologic, psychological, and sociocultural variables (Fig. 34-3). The biologic basis for the effectiveness of these strategies may be their ability to increase brain endorphin production (Bandura et al., 1987).

Many barriers exist to effective pain management (Text Box 34-4). Reluctance on the part of health professionals and the patient may contribute to persistent pain, which ultimately can adversely affect the patient's quality of life. Patients with chronic pain experience not only decreased functional capability but also diminished strength and endurance, nausea, poor appetite, and poor, interrupted sleep. The psychological impact includes diminished leisure and enjoyment, anxiety and fear, depression, somatic preoccupation, and difficulty concentrating. Social impairment may exist in the form of diminished social and sexual relationships, altered appearance, and increased dependence on others. All these contribute to the suffering caused by the pain experience.

(text continues on page 902)

TEXT BOX 34.2

Pain Syndromes Seen in the Primary Care Setting

Migraine headache: a cerebrovasomotor disorder in which a focal reduction of cerebral blood flow initiates an ischemic headache. May be preceded by a visual aura and followed by nausea, vomiting, and incapacitating head pain.

Low back pain: pain arising from the vertebral column or surrounding muscles, tendons, ligaments, or fascia. Causes range from simple muscle strain to arthritis, fracture, or nerve compression from a ruptured disk.

Chronic benign orofacial pain: temporomandibular joint pain.

Rheumatoid arthritis: more than 100 different types of joint disease produce inflammation of the joints. Associated with varying degrees of pain and stiffness and eventual loss of use of the affected joints.

Reflex sympathetic dystrophy: causalgia. A painful burning syndrome that occurs after peripheral nerve injury. Associated with hyperesthesia, vasomotor disturbances, and dystrophic changes due to sympathetic hyperactivity.

Cancer pain: pain from malignant tumors that is caused by local infiltration or metastatic spread involving specific organs, bones, or peripheral or cranial nerves, or the spinal cord. Pain therapy is aimed at providing sufficient relief to allow maximum possible daily functioning and a relatively pain-free death.

Neuropathic pain

  Polyneuropathy: neuropathy involving multiple peripheral nerves

  Diabetic neuropathy: neuropathy due to diabetes mellitus; marked by diminished sensation secondary to vascular changes

  Inflammatory neuropathy: neuropathy related to the presence of chemical or microorganic pathogens

  Traumatic neuropathy: neuropathy caused by avulsion or compression

  Plexopathy: neuropathy involving a peripheral nerve plexus

  Peripheral or central neuralgia: abrupt, intense, paroxysmal pain due to intrinsic nerve injury or extrinsic nerve compression

  Herpetic neuralgia: pain associated with the dermatomal rash of acute herpes zoster

  Radiculopathy: pain radiating along a peripheral nerve tract, such as sciatica

Vasoocclusive pain: thrombotic crisis of sickle cell anemia in joints and peripheral muscles that is caused by ischemia

Myofascial pain: pain in palpable bands (trigger points) of muscle. Associated with stiffness, limitation of motion, and weakness.

TEXT BOX 34.3

Assessment of Patients Who Report Pain

A. What is the extent of the patient's disease or injury (physical impairment)?

B. What is the magnitude of the illness? That is, to what extent is the patient suffering, disabled, and unable to enjoy usual activities?

C. Does the person's behavior seem appropriate to the disease or injury, or is there any evidence of amplification of symptoms for any of a variety of psychological or social reasons or purposes?

D. How often and for how long does the patient perform specific behaviors, such as reclining, sitting, standing, and walking?

E. How often does the patient seek health care and take analgesic medication (frequency and quantity)?

The Multiaxial Assessment of Pain (MAP) (Rudy & Turk, 1991) includes evaluation of three axes: biomedical, psychosocial, and behavioral.

Pain Behavior Checklist

Pain behaviors have been characterized as interpersonal communications of pain, distress, or suffering. Pain behavior may be a more accurate indication of intensity and toler-

ance than verbal reports. Check the box of each behavior you observe or infer from the patient's comments.

☐ Facial grimacing, clenched teeth

☐ Holding or supporting of affected body area

☐ Questions such as, "Why did this happen to me?"

☐ Distorted gait, limping

☐ Frequent shifting of posture or position

☐ Requests to be excused from tasks or activities; avoidance of physical activity

☐ Taking of medication as often as possible

☐ Moving extremely slowly

☐ Sitting with rigid posture

☐ Moving in a guarded or protective fashion

☐ Moaning or sighing

☐ Using a cane, cervical collar, or other prosthetic device

☐ Requesting help in ambulation; frequent stopping while walking

☐ Lying down during the day

☐ Irritability

TABLE 34.1 Treatment Approaches to Pain

Principles of Pain Treatment	Second Step	Third Step	Fourth Step

• Establish the correct diagnosis.
• Recognize that pain reduction, rather than complete pain control, is a reasonable goal.
• Control other symptoms besides pain. This includes treating the symptoms that were present before treatment (such as depression and anxiety) and the adverse effects associated with the pain therapy.
• Treat physical conditions that may initiate or exacerbate the pain.
 	
First Step
Analgesics for treatment of pain and:
Nonsteroidal antiinflammatory drugs (NSAIDs)
  Acetaminophen
  Acetylsalicylic acid
  Ibuprofen
Oral local anesthetics
  Flecainide
  Mexiletine
  Tocainide
Topical agents
  Capsaicin
  EMLA
  Lidocaine gel
Baclofen
Neuroleptics
  Pimozide
Corticosteroids
Calcitonin
Benzodiazepines
  Clonazepam
Drugs for sympathetically maintained pain
  Nifedipine
  Phenoxybenzamine
  Prazosin
  Propranolol
	Antidepressants, TENS, and psychosocial support, and/or:
	Tricyclic and tetracyclic antidepressants
	  Amitriptyline
	  Clomipramine
	  Desipramine
	  Doxepin
	  Imipramine
	  Maprotiline
	  Nortriptyline
	  Mirtazapine
	Selective and nonselective serotonin reuptake inhibitors
	  Buproprione
	  Fluoxetine
	  Fluvoxamine
	  Nefazodone
	  Olanzopine
	  Paroxetine
	  Sertraline
	  Trazodone
	  Venlafaxine
	Anticonvulsants
	  Carbamazepine
	  Neurontin
	  Phenytoin
	Opioid analgesics
	  Codeine
	  Meperidine
	  Morphine
	Monoamine oxidase inhibitors
	  Isocarboxazid
	  Phenelzine sulfate
	  Tranylcypromine
	Herbal and alternative medicine
	  SamE
	  Ginseng
	  Swedish massage
	  Acupressure
	  Acupuncture
	  Zero balancing
	  Reflexology
	  Meditation
	  Prayer
	Note: Treat the adverse effects of all the agents used.
		Adrenergic agents, TENS, and psychosocial support, and/or:
		Clonidine
		Naloxone infusion, and/or:
		Other agents (mexiletine, diphenhydramine)
		Note: Add the third-step agents to partially helpful agents used in first step, or use alone and treat the adverse effects of all the agents used.
			Psychiatric intervention Psychotherapy with pain patients:
			
			Cognitive
			• Explain the nature of the pain sensation.
			• Describe realistic expectations about the degree and course of pain.
			• Describe realistic expectations of treatment and side effects.
			• Use the placebo effect by supporting the treatment efficacy.
			• Relieve anxiety.
			
			Behavioral
			• Make the initial doses large rather than small, to effect some relief.
			• Reassure that medication will be available, not contingent on proof of need.
			• Reinforce healthy behavior/adaptation; do not reinforce obsession with pain.
			• Assure of regular evaluation not contingent on presence of pain.
			
			Ablative Procedure for Selected Patients
			
			Neuroblockade
			• Trigger point injection (TPI)
			• Epidural steroid injection (ESI)
			• Facet joint injection (FJI)
			• Nerve root blocks
			• Medical branch blocks
			• Peripheral nerve block
			• Sympathetic nerve block
			
			Spinal Cord Stimulation
			• Neurostimulator implants
			• TENS
			• Thalamic stimulation

TENS, transcutaneous electrical nerve stimulation
Note: If the patient has failed all standard pharmacologic treatments, psychiatric evaluation for underlying problems (such as severe depression and risk for suicide) should be emphasized.

Maladaptive coping by patients with chronic pain leads them to fear pain and to acquire a negative attitude about pain and how it affects their lives. These negative views can adversely influence biopsychological and physiologic processes, thereby sustaining or even exacerbating the pain. Noncompliance by these patients with sequential prescription changes and combined treatments can be problematic as well (Turk & Rudy, 1994). Strategies to assess compliance are regular self-report, assessment of behavioral change, biochemical assay, clinical improvement, and outcome assessment. The nurse can enhance compliance by closely monitoring the therapeutic efficacy and untoward effects of the treatments being used, involving the patient and family in treatment planning, educating the patient and family about self-care, and instructing the patient in noninvasive approaches to pain control.

PSYCHOPATHOLOGIC COMPLICATIONS OF AIDS

The medical syndrome of AIDS is characterized by multiple opportunistic infections and is associated with malignancy. People with AIDS are often overwhelmed by devastating disorders that cause profound fatigue, insomnia, anorexia, emaciation, pain, and disfigurement. The psychological impact of AIDS is considerably worsened by the social stigma associated with the infection and the special affinity of HIV for

brain and central nervous system (CNS) tissue (Lipton & Gendelman, 1995).

Biologic Basis of Neurologic Manifestations of HIV

In up to 60% of those who have AIDS, neurologic complications occur that are directly attributable to infection of the brain. Important clinical manifestations include impaired cognitive and motor function. This aspect of the syndrome is referred to as the **HIV-1–associated cognitive-motor complex.** Neuronal injury and frank nerve cell loss probably contribute to the neurologic deficits (Lipton & Gendelman, 1995). Evidence suggests that the presence of HIV stimulates brain cells to release neurotoxins and excitatory amino acids in excess. The resultant neurochemical changes and disrupted cell membrane integrity cause cell death similar to that which occurs with other types of brain injury. These neurochemical changes and eventual catecholamine depletion contribute to the cognitive, motor, and psychiatric manifestations of HIV infection.

Psychological Aspects of AIDS

The most common initial signs and symptoms of the AIDS dementia complex are changes in mentation and personality, followed by delirium, dementia, organic mood disorder, and organic delusional disorder. The

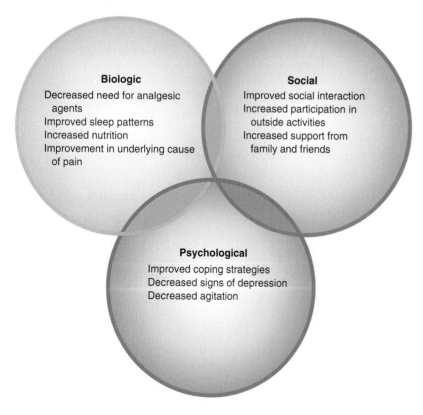

Biologic
Decreased need for analgesic agents
Improved sleep patterns
Increased nutrition
Improvement in underlying cause of pain

Social
Improved social interaction
Increased participation in outside activities
Increased support from family and friends

Psychological
Improved coping strategies
Decreased signs of depression
Decreased agitation

FIGURE 34.3 Biopsychosocial outcomes for patients with pain.

TEXT BOX 34.4

Barriers to Pain Management

Problems Related to Health Care Professionals
Inadequate knowledge of pain management

Poor assessment of pain

Concern about regulation of controlled substances

Fear of patient tolerance and addiction

Concern about side effects of analgesics

Problems Related to Patients
Reluctance to report pain

Concern about primary treatment of underlying disease

Fear that pain means the disease is worse

Concern about being a "good" patient, not a complainer

Reluctance to take pain medications

Fear of addiction, tolerance, and addict image

Fear of unmanageable side effects

Problems Related to the Health Care System
Low priority given to pain treatment

Cost or inadequate reimbursement

Restrictive regulation of controlled substances

Problems with availability of treatment or access to it

---

onset of major depression and uncomplicated bereavement soon after diagnosis is common. Comorbid neurologic infections such as encephalitis and meningitis can predispose the patient with AIDS to delirium. The clinical picture reflects the areas of the brain invaded by HIV; however, physiologic conditions such as addiction to alcohol or drugs, brain damage, chronic illness, hypoxia related to pneumonia, infections, space-occupying brain lesions, and systemic reactions to medications may contribute to the progression of mental changes. Loss of normal cortical function may lead to abnormal social behavior, depression, psychosis, and anxiety. The psychological influences of stress and sleep and sensory deprivation can further contribute to the altered perception and mentation. Figure 34-4 shows the possible pathologic progression of HIV neuronal injury.

Psychiatric disorders contribute to the course of AIDS in several ways. Mood disorder may be reflected in the patient who has an initial substance abuse disorder or an antisocial personality that predisposes him or her to a lifestyle that increases the patient's risk for exposure to HIV. The neuropathology associated with the presence of HIV then contributes to the progression of the disease and deterioration. AIDS-associated psychopathology is frequently unrecognized, misdiagnosed, and incorrectly treated. Diagnosis can be difficult when risk factors are not known or when cognitive or psychiatric symptoms precede the onset of other manifesta-

tions of HIV infection. Early CNS involvement is detected through neuropsychological testing and magnetic resonance imaging. The degree of cognitive dysfunction may not be a valid indication of the degree of organic involvement. Also, such diagnostic findings on computed tomography scanning as cerebral atrophy and prominent basal ganglia calcification may not correlate with the severity of the patient's dementia (Gabuzda & Hirsch, 1987).

Assessment of the AIDS Patient

Early recognition of psychiatric disorders associated with AIDS is important to enhance our understanding of the behavior of people with AIDS. Mental status changes and altered affect should be investigated through formal neurologic and psychological testing to determine the extent of impairment. Successful coping and cognitive adaptation are often further hindered by the presence of psychiatric disorders associated with HIV (Text Box 34-5). These mental illnesses include mood disorders, adjustment disorders, anxiety disorders, substance abuse disorders, and personality disorders. Organic mood disorder may be characterized by symptoms of a major depressive or manic episode. The depressed mood, feelings of guilt, anhedonia, and hopelessness can be accompanied by insomnia or hypersomnia, psychomotor retardation or agitation, and suicidal ideation. Low self-esteem, feelings of worthlessness and hopelessness, and impaired thinking or concentration are other likely findings. It is important to differentiate between major depression and complicated or uncomplicated grieving over the loss of health or of significant others to premature death due to HIV. When diagnosed with AIDS, the patient may face social isolation, severe life-threatening complications, unfamiliar and perhaps ineffective treatments, and the prospect of premature death. As with any life crisis, the patient and family members experience severe anxiety, fear, and depression. They may develop obsessive-compulsive rituals to allay anxiety related to the infection. In addition, panic disorders are frequently seen in these patients.

People who do not engage in high-risk behavior and who are unlikely to have been exposed to HIV may nevertheless report physical and psychological manifestations associated with HIV. Anxiety about the disease can produce symptoms not unlike those of HIV infection. Phobias, delusions, and factitious (Munchausen's) AIDS disorders have all been reported in uninfected people. In many of these cases, psychotherapy for the underlying psychological disorder is effective.

Biopsychosocial Treatment Interventions

Treatment of AIDS should be directed toward the underlying cause. In addition, treatment should attempt

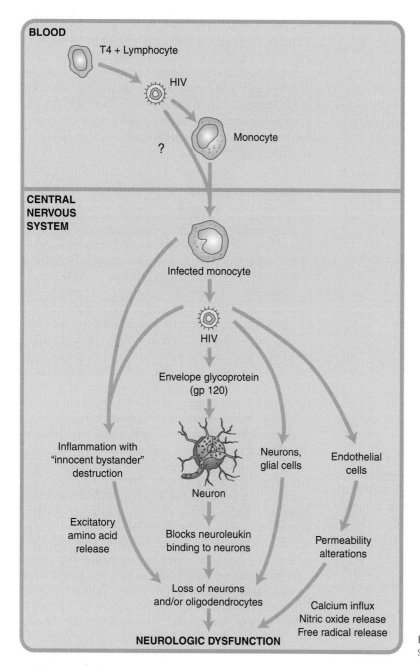

BLOOD

T4 + Lymphocyte

HIV

?

Monocyte

CENTRAL NERVOUS SYSTEM

Infected monocyte

HIV

Envelope glycoprotein (gp 120)

Inflammation with "innocent bystander" destruction

Neuron

Neurons, glial cells

Endothelial cells

Excitatory amino acid release

Blocks neuroleukin binding to neurons

Permeability alterations

Loss of neurons and/or oligodendrocytes

Calcium influx
Nitric oxide release
Free radical release

NEUROLOGIC DYSFUNCTION

FIGURE 34.4 Possible pathologic progression of HIV neuronal injury.

to maintain normal hydration, electrolyte balance, and nutrition as well as a safe, comfortable environment. Antiviral agents, such as zidovudine, ribavirin, and phosphonoformate, cross the blood–brain barrier and achieve adequate anti-HIV concentrations in cerebrospinal fluid after systemic administration. These agents have been administered with some success (Cohen, 1990). It is important to provide the patient and the patient's family, friends, and caregivers with emotional and educational support. Psychotherapy may be especially needed by those close to the patient if the patient is young. Treatment of psychiatric dis-

orders should include individual and family therapy as well as psychotropic medications, in a manner similar to the treatment of primary psychiatric disorders. Tricyclic antidepressants or serotonin reuptake inhibitors may be used in low doses for depressed mood. The administration of haloperidol (Haldol), 0.5 to 10 mg for sleep support, may be appropriate in some cases.

Early diagnosis and treatment are imperative to maximize the patient's adherence to risk reduction regimens and to prevent the transmission of infection. Treatment plans can often be tailored to meet the needs of the patient and family. The consultation-liaison psychiatric

TEXT BOX 34.5

Psychiatric Disorders Associated With HIV Infection

Organic Mental Disorder
Dementia
  HIV dementia or AIDS–dementia complex
  Dementia associated with opportunistic infection
    Fungal
      Cryptococcoma
      Cryptococcal meningitis
      Candidal abscesses
    Protozoal
      Toxoplasmosis
    Bacterial
      Mycobacterium avium–intracellulare
    Viral
      Cytomegalovirus
      Herpesvirus
      Papovavirus progressive multifocal leukoencephalopathy
  Dementia associated with cancer
    Primary cerebral lymphoma
    Disseminated Kaposi's sarcoma

Delirium
Organic delusional disorder
Organic mood disorder
  Depression
  Mania
  Mixed
Affective disorders
  Major depression
  Dysthymic disorder
Adjustment disorders
  Adjustment disorder with depressed mood
  Adjustment disorder with anxious mood
Substance abuse disorder
Borderline personality disorder
Antisocial personality disorder
Bereavement
Anxiety disorders
  Obsessive-compulsive disorder
  Panic

professional can recommend appropriate multidisciplinary interventions to meet the challenge of AIDS with compassion and dignity.

PSYCHOLOGICAL ILLNESS RELATED TO TRAUMA

Physiologic trauma activates the overall stress response of the autonomic nervous system (McEwen, 1994; Stratakis & Chrousos, 1995). Massive catecholamine release causes certain cardiovascular, muscular, gastrointestinal, and respiratory symptoms that release energy stores and support survival. Tissue destruction, musculoskeletal pain, physical disability, and body image changes all contribute to the physiologic and psychological stress response, which continues long after the injury is sustained. The overwhelming behavioral responses are hypervigilance, fear, and anxiety; psychological sequelae may include social isolation, agitation, personality disorders, posttraumatic stress disorder, and depression or, in extreme cases, dissociative identity disorders.

Biologic Basis of the Trauma Response

The neurotransmitters responsible for behavioral responses to fear and anxiety are usually held in balance to maintain a level of arousal appropriate for environmental threat. Information from the sensory processing areas in the thalamus and cortex alerts the amygdala (the lateral and central nucleus). Events that are interpreted

as threatening activate the **hypothalamic–pituitary–adrenal (HPA) axis,** initiating the stress response. Adrenal steroids are released and trigger the physiologic reactions just described. Complex neurochemical processes involving norepinephrine, γ-aminobutyric acid (GABA), and serotonin are overwhelmed by the catecholamine release. For example, norepinephrine receptors adjust to the increased level of hyperstimulation. Then, as the catecholamines are depleted, the norepinephrine receptors react to the relative catecholamine shortage. This response alters cognitive and affective function similar to the altered function that occurs in anxiety disorders. Persistent, severe distress leads to a general dysregulation of the HPA axis and inappropriate and prolonged secretion of high levels of catecholamines. This chronic stress disorder has been linked to increased susceptibility to immunosuppressive medical illness, such as certain cancers, as well as to infection, myocardial disease, and neurologic degenerative disorders (McEwen, 1994; Mastorakos et al., 1995).

Adaptation to trauma is related to such factors as the severity of the trauma, the person's maturity and age when the trauma occurs, available social support, and the person's ability to mobilize coping strategies (Heim, 2000). During adaptation to prolonged stress, the patient's cognitive thought processes and coping behaviors cause dopamine to be released in the prefrontal cortex of the brain. These dopaminergic systems are presumed to play a major role in physiologic and emotional coping responses, storage of the trauma experience into memory, and possibly the development of posttraumatic stress disorder (Charney et al., 1993). Serotonin is also thought to influence adaptation and mobilize coping strategies.

Psychological Aspects of the Trauma Response

Individual behavior and perception are essential components of the stress reaction. Response to the challenge depends on prior experience, developmental history, and physical status. Individual differences in the extent of endocrine and autonomic activity occur during stress as well. Psychological sequelae of sustained stress and trauma may be manifested as flashbacks, intrusive recurring thoughts, panic or anxiety attacks, paranoia, inappropriate startle reactions, nightmares, or the extreme of posttraumatic stress disorder. Catecholamine depletion and activation of the dopamine pathways may contribute to a deterioration in social and intellectual functioning after severe physical or emotional trauma. The patient may become so withdrawn and depressed that he or she stops participating in activities of daily living (ADLs). Toward the other extreme, the patient may become agitated and combative, perceiving any treatment as a continued threat.

Extreme forms of maladaptation are manifested in **kindling** and dissociative identity disorder. Kindling is thought to be responsible for the spontaneous recurrence of depressive illness that is associated with loss and trauma at an early age. Permanent biochemical changes from the early trauma response precipitate the sudden onset of affective disorder in the absence of any present stressor (Post, 1992). Dissociation disorders are rare but take the form of somatization (physical symptoms), agnosia, multiple personalities, or amnestic fugue states in which the patient escapes the stressor by subconscious loss of identity or adoption of a new identity. Although these disorders are not common, mood and anxiety disorders may occur after a trauma event. They are associated with slowed rehabilitation and deterioration in social functioning and ADLs after the trauma period has passed (Jorge et al., 1994) (see Chap. 37).

Assessment of the Trauma Patient

Complete physical assessment after physical traumatic injury is imperative in life-threatening circumstances. Multiple trauma and head injury are the major causes of death and disability in young adults. Emergency care and intensive care providers are highly trained to recognize signs and symptoms of physiologic injury and to intervene to stabilize primary and secondary trauma in the general medical setting. Trauma scales and triage models have been developed to assist in immediate assessment and to measure neurologic and physical condition (Fig. 34-5) (Burke, 1991). They have also been used to predict long-term outcome in patients in whom permanent cognitive and physical disability may limit recovery and challenge adaptive responses.

Psychological injury must be evaluated thoroughly through observation and interview to determine prevalent signs and symptoms of accompanying psychological disorders. This process includes evaluating the patient's adjustment and coping skills, personal way of dealing with the trauma, social circumstances, and environmental and life stressors. Assessment must be ongoing to help the patient deal with disfigurement, sudden disability, and changes in self-care. The evaluation should include assessment of the patient's perception of experienced stress, feelings related to the stress, predominant mood, cognitive functioning, defense and coping mechanisms, and available support systems. In addition, assessment of the risk for self-inflicted injury or suicide is critical.

Biopsychosocial Treatment Interventions

Psychiatric clinicians provide an important aspect of emergency care. Interventions that establish trust, reduce anxiety, promote adaptive coping, and cultivate a sense of control help the patient to begin recovery and maintain emotional health. Crisis intervention methods, stress management, cognitive-behavioral therapies, psychotherapy, and psychotropic medications, alone or in combination, may be useful in achieving the best possible outcome.

When trauma causes the patient's death, the family must be informed of the death and allowed to grieve, to prevent the development of a pathologic or prolonged grief response. Traumatic death is sudden and unexpected, and the victim is often young. Surviving family members usually have a severe emotional reaction to the death. Dysfunctional family dynamics may become evident during this period. The psychiatric–mental health liaison nurse can use family intervention strategies to enhance or improve relationships while the family's motivation to do all that is possible is high.

PSYCHOLOGICAL ILLNESS RELATED TO CENTRAL NERVOUS SYSTEM DISORDERS

Neurologic impairment is most often related to brain cell (neuron) destruction. The primary causes of neuronal damage are traumatic injury, ischemia, infarction (cerebrovascular accident), abnormal neuron growth (brain tumor), and metabolic poisoning associated with systemic disease. Brain cell loss may also be the result of

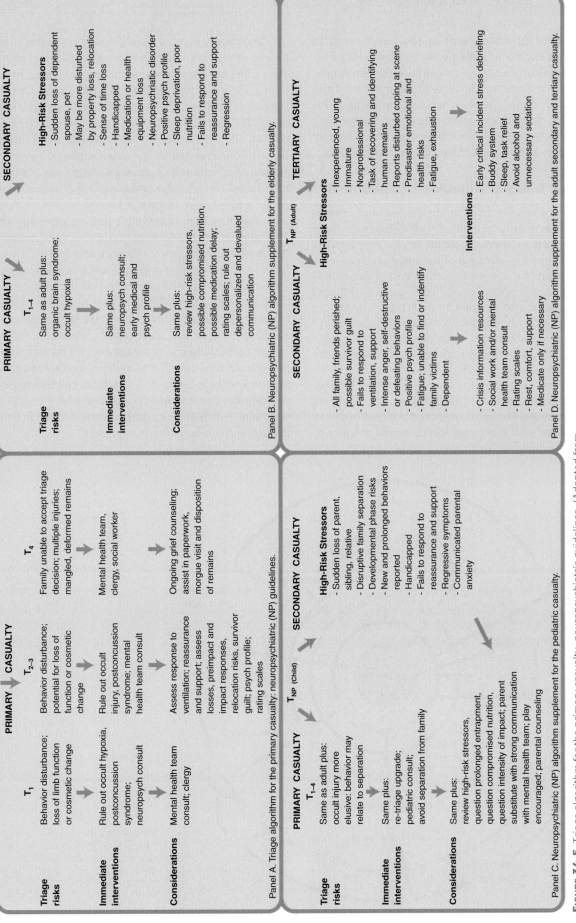

Figure 34.5 Triage algorithm for the primary casualty: neuropsychiatric guidelines. (Adapted from Burkle, F. G., Jr. [1991]. Triage of disaster-related neuropsychiatric casualties. *Psychiatric Aspects of Emergency Medicine, 9*[1], 87–104.)

SECONDARY CASUALTY

High-Risk Stressors

- Sudden loss of dependent spouse, pet
- May be more disturbed by property loss, relocation
- Sense of time loss
- Handicapped
- Medication or health equipment loss
- Neuropsychiatric disorder
- Positive psych profile
- Sleep deprivation, poor nutrition
- Fails to respond to reassurance and support
- Regression

PRIMARY CASUALTY

T₁₋₄

Triage risks — Same as adult plus: organic brain syndrome; occult hypoxia

Immediate interventions — Same plus: neuropsych consult; early medical and psych profile

Considerations — Same plus: review high-risk stressors, possible compromised nutrition, possible medication delay; rating scales; rule out depersonalized and devalued communication

Panel B. Neuropsychiatric (NP) algorithm supplement for the elderly casualty.

TERTIARY CASUALTY

T_NP (Adult)

High-Risk Stressors

- Inexperienced, young
- Immature
- Nonprofessional
- Task of recovering and identifying human remains
- Reports disturbed coping at scene
- Predisaster emotional and health risks
- Fatigue, exhaustion

SECONDARY CASUALTY

High-Risk Stressors

- All family, friends perished; possible survivor guilt
- Fails to respond to ventilation, support
- Intense anger, self-destructive or defeating behaviors
- Positive psych profile
- Fatigue; unable to find or indentify family victims
- Dependent

Interventions

- Early critical incident stress debriefing
- Buddy system
- Sleep, task relief
- Avoid alcohol and unnecessary sedation

- Crisis information resources
- Social work and/or mental health team consult
- Rating scales
- Rest, comfort, support
- Medicate only if necessary

Panel D. Neuropsychiatric (NP) algorithm supplement for the adult secondary and tertiary casualty.

PRIMARY CASUALTY

T₁

Triage risks — Behavior disturbance; loss of limb function or cosmetic change

Immediate interventions — Rule out occult hypoxia, postconcussion syndrome; neuropsych consult

Considerations — Mental health team consult; clergy

T₂₋₃

Behavior disturbance; potential for loss of function or cosmetic change

Rule out occult injury, postconcussion syndrome; mental health team consult

Assess response to ventilation; reassurance and support; assess losses, preimpact and impact responses, relocation risks, survivor guilt; psych profile; rating scales

T₄

Family unable to accept triage decision; multiple injuries; mangled, deformed remains

Mental health team, clergy, social worker

Ongoing grief counseling; assist in paperwork, morgue visit and disposition of remains

Panel A. Triage algorithm for the primary casualty: neuropsychiatric (NP) guidelines.

SECONDARY CASUALTY

High-Risk Stressors

- Sudden loss of parent, sibling, relative
- Disruptive family separation
- Developmental phase risks
- New and prolonged behaviors reported
- Handicapped
- Fails to respond to reassurance and support
- Regressive symptoms
- Communicated parental anxiety

PRIMARY CASUALTY

T_NP (Child)

T₁₋₄

Triage risks — Same as adult plus: occult injury more elusive; behavior may relate to separation

Immediate interventions — Same plus: re-triage upgrade; pediatric consult; avoid separation from family

Considerations — Same plus: review high-risk stressors, question prolonged entrapment, question compromised nutrition, question intensity of impact; parent substitute with strong communication with mental health team; play encouraged; parental counseling

Panel C. Neuropsychiatric (NP) algorithm supplement for the pediatric casualty.

degenerative processes, such as those that occur in Alzheimer's or Parkinson's disease (see Chap. 31). Psychological illness is often a complication of organic neurologic disease and may be difficult to distinguish from the neuropathology itself. Therefore, appropriate intervention depends on skilled assessment to discriminate and detect mental status changes related to organic brain injury as well as disorders of mood and thought.

Biologic Basis of Neurologic Impairment

All mechanisms of brain cell injury destroy brain cells directly or initiate a cascade of cell breakdown from ischemia. This **ischemic cascade** begins with hypoxia and is followed by paralysis of the ion exchange across the cell membrane, edema, calcium influx, free-radical production, and lipid peroxidation (Fig. 34-6) (Hickey, 1992). The severity of brain injury is related to the degree and duration of ischemia. Complete ischemia results in brain infarction, commonly known as stroke. The resulting neurologic impairment is related to the size and location of the affected brain area (Fig. 34-7). More eloquent areas of the brain, such as the internal capsule, are extremely sensitive to ischemia. They are typically injured first and contribute to more generalized impairment, such as memory loss or altered judgment.

The primary psychological disorder experienced by people with brain injury is depression (Astrom et al., 1993). Depressive symptoms related to organic brain injury are generated by altered biochemical neurotransmitter systems. Hyperactivity and dysregulation of the HPA axis probably contribute to the elevated cortisol and catecholamine levels after cerebral insult. In addition, changes in the metabolism of biogenic amines after brain cell death and ischemia may mediate both mood disturbances and cognitive dysfunction in patients with stroke (Brown & Gershon, 1993).

In cognitive brain function, dopamine is essential for normal neurotransmission of motor messages, motivation, and level of anxiety and mood; epinephrine establishes learning and memory; and serotonin regulates the level of alertness, the categorization of information, and the perception of well-being. These neurotransmitter pathways are temporarily interrupted or permanently disrupted during the acute injury. Secondary injury caused by swelling and compression may further compromise neurons in surrounding areas, causing marginal neurotransmitter function. In addition, circulating catecholamines can lead to oversecretion of dopamine or serotonin, which disrupts the necessary balance in production and uptake of the transmitters.

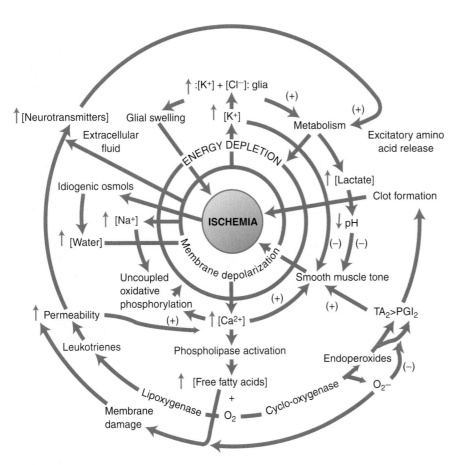

FIGURE 34.6 Ischemic cascade causes secondary brain injury and altered neurotransmitter function. (Adapted from Raichle, M. E. [1983]. The pathophysiology of brain ischemia. *Annals of Neurology, 13*[1], 2–10.)

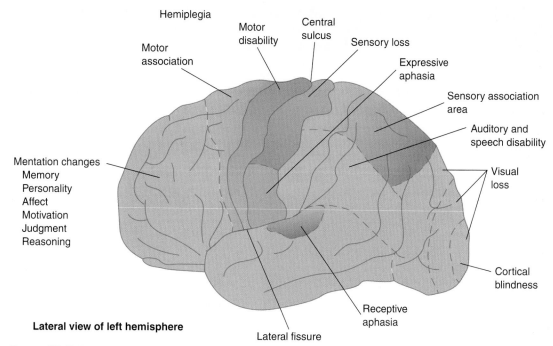

Hemiplegia

Motor disability

Central sulcus

Sensory loss

Motor association

Expressive aphasia

Sensory association area

Auditory and speech disability

Mentation changes
Memory
Personality
Affect
Motivation
Judgment
Reasoning

Visual loss

Cortical blindness

Lateral view of left hemisphere

Receptive aphasia

Lateral fissure

FIGURE 34.7 Functional cerebral anatomy and stroke.

Psychological Aspects of Neurologic Impairment

Depressive disorder is a frequent complication of brain injury, particularly ischemic stroke. This mood disorder occurs in 30% to 60% of stroke patients, depending on age, level of disability, and psychosocial factors such as family and social support (Morris & Raphael, 1990). About 20% of acute stroke patients have the symptom cluster of *DSM-IV-TR* criteria (American Psychiatric Association, 2000) for major depression (see Chap. 20). Other symptoms, such as sleep disturbances, cognitive dysfunction, poor concentration, difficulty making decisions, somatic discomfort, poor appetite, social withdrawal, and fatigue or agitation, often accompany the mood disturbance. The high-risk period extends for 2 years after the stroke, and left untreated, the depression generally lasts for at least 6 months (Sinyor et al., 1986). Table 34-2 compares *DSM-IV-TR* diagnostic criteria for depression and cerebrovascular accident–related emotional sequelae.

Minor and moderate depression may go unrecognized and undiagnosed when patients with stroke describe somatic symptoms and demonstrate lack of motivation in ADLs. Depression is more likely to develop in stroke patients if they have altered speech or aphasia, severe hemiparesis, or both. Stroke patients, however, experience depression more frequently than other disabled and chronically ill patients, even though the level of functional disability is the same (Morris & Raphael, 1990). This phenomenon is thought to be possibly related to the combination of permanent disability and altered neurotransmitter systems that persist after cerebral infarction.

Although the mechanism of neuronal injury is one of degeneration in Parkinson's disease and other neuromuscular diseases, the neurochemical changes in the brain after a stroke are similar with respect to the loss of dopamine secretion and receptor sites in the internal capsule motor pathways. In addition, the serotonergic system is disrupted as the neuronal synapses are destroyed or injured. This generalized loss of dopaminergic activity and decreasing functional ability probably contribute to depressed mood in stroke patients as well.

Mental illness related to organic brain injury is consistently dependent on the degree of functional impairment, particularly loss of the ability to communicate and administer self-care. Depressed mood may become evident in the acute recovery phase or during rehabilitation. Depression often negatively affects survival and recovery. It impedes progress throughout the rehabilitation process and ultimately prevents an optimal outcome. Early evaluation assists in the detection of mental illness after brain injury (Robinson, 1997).

Assessment of the Neurologic Patient

A thorough neurologic examination is important in determining the location and degree of disability but even more critical in establishing the locus of retained function. Many scales exist that accurately assess neurologic function and that are easy to administer and generally ac-

TABLE 34.2   Comparison of *DSM-IV-TR* Diagnostic Criteria for Depression and Stroke Related Affective Sequelae

Major Depression	Dysthymia*	Stroke Residual Sequelae†	Other Symptoms Associated With Depression
Depressed mood	Depressed mood	Depressed mood	Decreased sexual desire or sexual functioning
Anhedonia	Appetite change	Anhedonia	Loss of insight
Weight change	Sleep disturbance	Weight loss	Autonomic symptoms (eg, sweating, tachycardia)
Low energy or fatigue	Low energy or fatigue	Low energy or fatigue	Somatic anxiety symptoms
Motor disturbance	Low self-esteem	Paralysis or paresis	Psychic anxiety symptoms
Sleep disturbance	Decreased concentration	Sleep disturbance	Somatic preoccupation (hypochondriasis)
Feelings of worthlessness or guilt	Hopelessness	Feelings of guilt	Pain, especially chronic pain
Decreased concentration		Decreased concentration	Diminished self-care
Thoughts of death or suicide		No psychotic symptoms	Social incapacitation
No independent psychosis		Diminished self-care	
Some psychotic symptoms		Pain, usually chronic	
		Social withdrawal	
		Isolation	
		Hopelessness	
		Somatic preoccupation	

*Cameron, O. G. (1990). Guidelines for diagnosis and treatment of depression in patients with medical illness. *Journal of Clinical Psychiatry, 51,* 7(Suppl.), 49–54.
†Hickey, J. V. (1992). *The clinical practice of neurological and neurosurgical nursing* (3rd ed., pp. 529–530). Philadelphia: J. B. Lippincott.

cepted as reliable tools to detect the degree and limitations of disability. Cognition and mentation can be more discretely measured by the Folstein Mini-Mental State Examination (Folstein et al., 1975), and functional ability for self-care can be measured using the Barthel Index (Mahoney & Barthel, 1965). The evaluation of mood using the Center for Epidemiological Studies Depression Scale (CES-D) or the Beck Depression Inventory (Beck et al., 1961) provides important information for designing intervention strategies for the at-risk stroke patient. Findings of depressive symptoms indicate the need for a more definitive neuropsychological referral. The dexamethasone suppression test (DST) has also been used to diagnose clinical depression. However, it is not completely reliable, and frequent false-positive test results limit its clinical utility (Carroll et al., 1981).

Biopsychosocial Treatment Interventions

Isolation, lack of companionship, bereavement, and poverty are associated with depressive symptoms in the general population and compound the relative risk of depression developing after brain damage. In addition, a prior history or family history of major depression increases the risk for depressed mood. Prevention strategies should be used as early as possible for patients known to have these risks. These strategies include the assessment and provision of social support resources while the patient is hospitalized and as an important

component of discharge planning to rehabilitation services; the prescription of therapies to enhance competence in the performance of ADLs, with a focus on the use of retained function rather than on adaptation to disabilities only; formal psychosocial testing and psychopharmacologic treatment when appropriate (Palomaki, 1999; Robinson, 2000); and the education of the patient and family to increase their awareness of signs and symptoms of depressed mood, so that they will know when to seek medical attention and treatment to avert major depression, if possible. In addition, the presence of depressed mood and other symptoms of the depressive cluster indicate the need for cognitive, behavioral, biologic, and social interventions to support appropriate psychopharmacologic treatment.

PSYCHOLOGICAL ILLNESS RELATED TO ACUTE AND CHRONIC MEDICAL ILLNESS

Systemic medical illness is associated with a higher prevalence of concurrent psychiatric disorders. Disorders such as cancer, heart disease, endocrine abnormalities, and organ failure are often associated with more functional disability than most chronic medical illnesses and may be the basis of medically unexplained somatic symptoms. Among the psychiatric disorders, substance use disorder, anxiety, and depressive disorder occur most frequently in patients with chronic medical illnesses. Within the anxiety disorders, phobias are most common; panic disorder and obsessive-compulsive disorder are much less common (Cassem, 1990; Neese, 1991). Table 34-3 compares the prevalence rates of depressive and anxiety disorders in people who are medically ill with the rates in people who are not.

Biologic Aspects of Mental Illness Related to Medical Disease

The nervous, endocrine, and immune systems and their components are designed to communicate and interact through biochemical means. The cerebral cortex and limbic system initiate neuroendocrine HPA axis activity by thought processes in response to environmental stimuli. Various hormonal messengers travel between the hypothalamic, pituitary, and adrenal systems to initiate secondary peripheral responses. The immune system responds to signals from the HPA axis and returns messages as well. Its protective activities rely on neurochemicals to initiate the infection defense and stress response. At all levels, the circulating hormone levels serve as feedback messengers to inhibit HPA activity after sufficient response has occurred.

Dysregulation of the hypothalamic, pituitary, and adrenal systems at all levels leads to malfunction of the other systems. Abnormal nervous system firing in the hippocampus alerts the adrenal and immune systems unnecessarily, and vice versa. The principal neurochemical messengers in this regulation are thought to be norepinephrine, endorphins, cortisol, and dopamine. Metabolic and cellular disease processes that eventually cause signs and symptoms of medical diseases are de-

tected by this trio of systems, and body resources are initiated to stop these pathologic processes. Psychiatric conditions occur in the course of these medical illnesses and in some instances may contribute to the genesis of the physiologic disease.

A psychiatric disorder may be the first manifestation of a primary disease, such as depressive syndrome in Huntington's chorea, multiple sclerosis, Parkinson's disease, HIV, Cushing's disease, and systemic lupus erythematosus. Depressive symptoms are an intrinsic part of the primary pathophysiology of endocrine disorders, metabolic disturbances, malignancies, viral infections, inflammatory disorders, and cardiopulmonary conditions. Tables 34-4 and 34-5 list medical conditions associated with anxiety disorders and symptoms of depression, respectively.

Endocrine system pathologic processes involve abnormal HPA axis function, which affects neurotransmitter balance (Stratakis & Chrousos, 1995). Depression and anxiety are often present in patients with hyperthyroidism and hypothyroidism, Cushing's disease (hyperadrenalism), and Addison's disease (hypoadrenalism), complicating the clinical picture in up to 40% of cases (Gold et al., 1995).

Malignancies have also been associated with anxiety and depression. Depressive syndromes have been associated with cancer in up to 50% of cancer cases, and biologic relationships between the two disorders may exist such that the onset of depression may herald undetected carcinoma. Diagnoses range from major depression to adjustment disorder with depressed mood.

Systemic infections and generalized inflammatory disorders such as rheumatoid arthritis that acutely and

TABLE 34.3	Prevalence of Psychiatric Disorders in Medically Ill Compared With Nonmedically Ill People	
Prevalence of Psychiatric Disorders*	Medically Ill (%)	Nonmedically Ill (%)
Six-month prevalence	24.7	17.5
Substance abuse	8.5	
Anxiety	11.9	
Affective disorder	9.4	
Lifetime prevalence	42.4	33.0
Substance use	26.2	
Anxiety	18.2	
Phobias	12.1	
Panic disorder	1.5	
Obsessive-compulsive disorder	2.4	
Affective disorder	12.9	

*Prevalence rates are sex- and age-adjusted.
Adapted from National Institute of Mental Health Epidemiologic Catchment Area Program; Burkle, F. M., Jr. (1991). Triage of disaster-related neuropsychiatric casualties. *Psychiatric Aspects of Emergency Medicine, 9*(1), 87–104.

TABLE 34.4   Medical Conditions Associated With Anxiety Disorders

Psychiatric Disorder	Medical Illness	Incidence (%)
Panic disorder	Parkinson's disease	20
	Primary biliary cirrhosis	10
	Chronic obstructive pulmonary disease	24
	Cardiomyopathy	83
	Post–myocardial infarction	16
	Chronic pain	16
	Focal seizures	*
Social phobia	Parkinson's disease	17
Obsessive-compulsive disorder	Sydenham's chorea	13
Phobia	Multiple sclerosis	*
	Primary biliary cirrhosis	10
Generalized anxiety	Graves' disease	62

*Incidence not significant but reportable.

chronically stress the immune system or that may be the result of immune dysfunction are associated with up to 50% of psychological disorders (Chrousos & Gold, 1992). In addition, renal, pancreatic, and hepatic transplant recipients, who are artificially immunosuppressed because of treatment with prophylactic antiinfectious agents, experience primary neuropsychiatric symptoms, related metabolic imbalances, and neuropsychiatric side effects from treatment.

Cardiac disease deserves special attention because it has been associated with precipitated depressive syndromes in 20% to 50% of patients and anxiety disorders in up to 80%. The fact that more than 70% of patients who have an acute myocardial infarction remain depressed for up to a year after the event indicates that the mental illness may not be simply an adjustment disorder. The incidence of depression is similar in cardiac transplant recipients (54%) but is much lower in cardiac bypass surgery patients (6% to 15%). In a study by Hill and coworkers (1992), 75% of cardiac patients who received therapy for their depression responded to treatment.

In addition to the disease process contributing to psychological complications, the drugs used to treat chronic disease may induce mental illness as well. Psychotropic and nonpsychotropic medications can be potent generators of depression and anxiety (Cameron, 1990) (Table 34-6). The indications and pharmacologic activity of these medications often have biopsychosocial implications. In addition, medically ill elderly patients are particularly susceptible to medication effects at lower doses. Depressive and anxiety-related symptoms may in fact have an additive effect on patient function, well-being, and recovery when combined with medical illness. When a drug is suspected of causing mental changes, the recommended course of action is to withdraw the drug

and find an effective alternative. When an alternative is not available, the dosage should be decreased to an effective level at which symptoms resolve.

Psychological Aspects of Medical Illness

In all cases of medical illness, it is natural for patients to respond to the loss of health with hopelessness, particularly when the illness is demoralizing, life-threatening, and without a clear prognosis. People who are chronically ill are distressed by loss of function and limitations on their daily activities. They are often forced to comply with treatments that add discomfort but no apparent benefit. Medical patients commonly experience weight loss, insomnia, fatigue, and motor retardation, but perhaps not to the degree of "conspicuous" psychiatric illness. In addition, chronic life stress and mental illness may have set into motion a series of biologic processes, ultimately resulting in the medical disorder, which may be further exacerbated by the stress of hospitalization. A vicious cycle of medical and mental disorders may arise.

Mental illness in medically ill people is potentially lethal because normal affective and cognitive functioning may be essential to recovery and compliance with the medical treatment plan. In addition, the use of excessive analgesics and reluctance to perform self-care and rehabilitative activities hinder recovery and expose the person to other potential complications. The detection and diagnosis of any secondary mental illnesses in patients with medical illnesses is critical. The physiologic and pharmacologic factors that contribute to the mental illness must be explored and ruled out before effective intervention can begin.

TABLE 34.5	Medical Illnesses Associated With Symptoms of Depression
Endocrinopathies	Hypothyroidism and hyperthyroidism
	Hypoparathyroidism and hyperparathyroidism
	Cushing's syndrome (steroid excess)
	Adrenal insufficiency (Addison's disease)
	Hyperaldosteronism
Malignancies	Abdominal carcinomas, especially pancreatic
	Brain tumors (temporal lobe)
	Breast cancer
	Gastrointestinal cancer
	Lung cancer
	Prostate cancer
	Metastases
Neurologic disorders	Ischemic stroke
	Subarachnoid hemorrhage
	Parkinson's disease
	Normal-pressure hydrocephalus
	Multiple sclerosis
	Closed head injury
	Epilepsy
Metabolic imbalance	Serum sodium and potassium reductions
	Vitamin B_{12}, niacin, vitamin C deficiencies; iron deficiency (anemias)
	Metal intoxication (thallium and mercury)
	Uremia
Viral/bacterial infection	Infectious hepatitis
	Encephalitis
	Tuberculosis
	AIDS
Hormonal imbalance	Premenstrual, premenopausal, postpartum periods
Cardiopulmonary	Acute myocardial infarction
	Post–cardiac arrest
	Post–coronary artery bypass graft
	Post–heart transplantation
	Cardiomyopathy
Inflammatory disorders	Rheumatoid arthritis

TABLE 34.6	Medications Associated With Mental Illness in Medically Ill Patients
Analgesics and nonsteroidal antiinflammatory drugs (NSAIDs)	Ibuprofen
	Indomethacin
	Opiates
	Pentazocine
	Phenacetin
	Phenylbutazone
Antihypertensives	Clonidine
	Hydralazine
	Methyldopa
	Propranolol
	Reserpine
Antimicrobials	Ampicillin (gram-negative agents)
	Clotrimazole
	Cycloserine
	Griseofulvin
	Metronidazole
	Nitrofurantoin
	Streptomycin
	Sulfamethoxazole (sulfonamides)
Neurologic agents	L-Dopa
	Levodopa
Antiparkinsonian drugs	Amantadine
Anticonvulsants	Carbamazepine
	Phenytoin
Antispasmodics	Baclofen
	Bromocriptine
Cardiac drugs	Digitalis
	Guanethidine
	Lidocaine
	Oxprenolol
	Procainamide
Psychotropic drugs	Benzodiazepines
Stimulants/sedatives	Amphetamines
	Barbiturates
	Chloral hydrate
	Chlorazepate
	Diethylpropion
	Ethanol
	Fenfluramine
	Haloperidol
Steroids and hormones	Adrenocorticotropic hormone
	Corticosteroids
	Estrogen
	Oral contraceptives
	Prednisone
	Progesterone
	Triamcinolone
Antineoplastic drugs	Bleomycin
	C-Asparaginase
	Trimethoprim
	Vincristine
Other miscellaneous drugs	Anticholinesterases
	Cimetidine
	Diuretics
	Metoclopramide

Assessment of the Patient With Medical Illness

Unfortunately for the clinician who is evaluating a medically ill patient in whom psychiatric symptoms develop, it is almost impossible to ascertain whether these symptoms are the result of direct psychobiologic changes brought about by the illness. People at obvious risk have a family or personal history of mental illness or were experiencing psychological problems before symptoms of the medical illness were present. The main problem for the clinician is to determine which signs and symptoms are part of the medical illness and its treatment and which signify the presence of a psychological disorder. A complete health assessment and physical examination, including a psychological examination and a cognitive-affective assessment, will help determine the priority and severity of symptoms. In some instances, the primary diagnosis may be depression, although the symptoms may be similar to those of medical illness in the absence of diagnostic findings. Factors to be considered in diagnosing mental illness in medical patients are outlined in Text Box 34-6.

Several important cognitive-affective symptoms best differentiate the effects of depression from those of medical illness. These include feelings of failure, low self-esteem, guilt feelings, loss of interest in people, feelings of being punished, suicidal ideation, dissatisfaction, difficulty with decisions, and crying (Neese, 1991). The severity of the vegetative symptoms generally increases with the severity of the depressive disorder as well as the severity of the medical illness. Decreased appetite, sleep disturbances, and loss of energy are not considered indicators of depression in the medically ill patient because these symptoms are common in medical illness as well. The Beck Depression Inventory and the CES-D are easy to administer and will provide some indication of whether a psychiatric liaison referral is needed.

TEXT BOX 34.6

Factors to Consider in Diagnosing
Depression in Medical Patients

- Presence of one or more specific medical illnesses
- Presence of the defining criteria for one of the depressive syndromes
- Family psychiatric history of any affective disorder
- Past psychiatric history of the patient
- Patient's response to treatments, if any, for any prior depressive episodes
- Sex of the patient
- Patient's age at onset of depression
- Depression that preceded the medical illness
- Presence of psychosocial precipitants before onset of depression
- Duration of depressive illness
- Biologic markers of depression
- Relative frequency in the population of diagnoses under consideration
- Diagnosis by commission, not omission

Clinical Features of Special Significance

Two problems of special significance, psychosis and suicidal thoughts, are related in that patients with delusions or hallucinations tend to be at greater risk for suicide attempts or more likely to resist treatment (eg, to refuse to eat or take medication) for their medical condition. It is important to distinguish between a mentally competent patient's right to refuse life-saving medical treatment and a depressed patient's desire to die. A clinical evaluation of the effect of depression on the patient's capacity to make competent decisions is imperative. If optimal medical and psychiatric treatments have been provided and the patient has been found competent enough to make decisions about further medical care, it may be appropriate to honor the patient's desire to die.

Patients with chronic medical illness and patients with primary mental illness may pose similar problems in psychiatric hospitals when their medical condition fails. The use of advance directives helps in addressing these problems.

Biopsychosocial Treatment Interventions

It is essential to provide optimal treatment of patients' medical illnesses without neglecting their mental distress. Most reports suggest that clinicians should be more aggressive in the pharmacologic treatment of mental illness in the medically ill (Cameron, 1990; Stoudemire et al., 1990, 1991). The basic rules for medicating patients include using the minimum dose initially, advancing the dose slowly, and performing frequent blood level monitoring. The doses required to achieve therapeutic blood levels may be lower or even half the usual therapeutic dose and take longer to titrate. It is important to understand the pharmacokinetics (absorption, distribution, metabolism, and elimination) of the treatment of choice, to prevent further systemic insult. Tricyclic antidepressants and selective serotonin reuptake inhibitors (SSRIs) are used equally as the treatment for depression in the medically ill patient population. The safest and best-tolerated drugs have been found to be nortriptyline and desipramine. Because the side effects of psychopharmacologic agents can be especially troublesome in medically ill people, treatment must be changed or stopped if drug or illness interactions occur, or if treatment of the mental illness appears to be unsuccessful. SSRIs are increasingly popular in treating medically ill patients because their side-effect profile is more tolerable within a wider therapeutic range. Most patients respond to antidepressant therapy with a decrease in the severity of their vegetative symptoms in 4 to 8 days.

Both supportive individual psychotherapy and family therapy are helpful. Assisting the patient and family in understanding the nature and relationship of the medical and psychiatric diagnoses may strengthen the support system, alter the perception of caregiver burden, and identify appropriate coping strategies. Mutually agreed-on goals and therapy actively involve the patient in progress toward recovery. At some point, the clinician may need to help the patient identify psychodynamic conflicts and maladaptive coping strategies that may be contributing to his or her distress. Cognitive intervention should address those areas of the patient's life that can be controlled, despite major lifestyle changes, to reinforce a feeling of competence. Also, it is important to convey the fact that although medical and mental illness are difficult to prevent, they are often treatable.

RECOGNITION OF MENTAL ILLNESS AND BIOPSYCHOSOCIAL INTERVENTIONS IN MEDICAL ILLNESS

The relationship between stress and illness is becoming more apparent as studies increasingly disclose the effects of stress on the body. Chronic illness is viewed as a stressor and is associated with increased psychological distress, and interventions can minimize that distress. Nurses are committed to preventing illness and promoting healthy living. It is essential, therefore, that they be aware of the physiologic and psychological impact of chronic stress, understand the coping process, and know appropriate alternative strategies for coping with illness (see Chap. 35). In addition, nurses can evaluate the effectiveness of strategies being used and revise care plans to improve outcomes for the patient.

Patients with primary mental illness in need of medical care are at particular risk when somatic complaints are viewed as part of the primary process. Undiagnosed pathophysiologic processes may become advanced while being attributed to somatization. A thorough medical history and physical examination are standard practice for these patients in all settings.

Ideally, a multidisciplinary team of care providers that includes a psychiatric liaison nurse should work closely together to deliver optimum treatment of complex medical and mental illness. All patients with chronic medical illnesses are at risk for psychological distress and should be approached with this understanding. Clinicians should include a general cognitive-affective status evaluation in their assessment of all medically ill patients and make appropriate psychiatric liaison consultation to offset the negative impact of mental illness on recovery.

A psychosocial review of systems (Goldberg & Novack, 1992) is a useful tool to include in admission assessment, to detect psychosocial stress or risk. This review provides the minimum information needed for each patient—neglect of even one area could compromise patient care. Information on substance use, stressful life events, expectations, fears, meanings, social support, sexual concerns, work, finances, education, psychiatric history, mood, cognition, culture, and functional status is obtained from the review. This information is useful in determining relevant nursing diagnoses and developing the plan of care.

Stress management training, systematic relaxation, supportive education, and stress monitoring should be built into the plan of care, regardless of the medical diagnosis. Assessment of anxiety and depression are ongoing, and crisis intervention with psychotherapy may be necessary to reduce the severity of mental distress. Physiologic stress factors, such as increased heart rate, blood pressure, and respiration, and signs of restlessness and sadness can be measured to determine the effectiveness of the intervention. Secondary mental illness can be approached using the same strategies that are effective for primary mental dysfunction. Interventions overlap across criteria, and all interventions provide some element of supportive therapy or social support.

Mental health can and should be monitored in patients who have physical illnesses. Certain kinds of pathologic processes place patients at greater risk for mental illness. These processes can be identified and interventions prescribed to prevent psychiatric disorders from developing or to minimize their severity. Cognitive and behavioral strategies have a place in the treatment regimen and offer the practitioner an opportunity to expand the boundaries of traditional patient-oriented practice in effective ways.

Alternatives to traditional medical intervention are increasingly employed as adjunct therapy in patients with pain related to cancer, neuropathy, or degenerative disorders. Natural and herbal therapies, therapeutic massage, zero balancing, thought-field therapy, imaging, prayer, and meditation, have all been found to be useful in easing the mental and physical discomfort of the patient with medical illness. Also, these therapies are more satisfying to patients who otherwise must receive toxic medication as part of their conventional medical treatment (see Table 34-1).

Summary of Key Points

➤ Psychiatric disorders are more common in people with systemic or chronic medical illnesses than in other people. Comorbid depression is common in certain medical diseases, such as endocrine and metabolic disturbances, viral infections, inflammatory disorders, and cardiopulmonary diseases. Specific anxiety disorders are associated with other medical conditions, such as Parkinson's disease, focal seizures, primary biliary cirrhosis, and chronic pain.

➤ Psychiatric illness that accompanies medical illness is seldom recognized and treated. Psychiatric symptoms may precede the onset of disease symptoms, and it may be difficult to distinguish between the symptoms of the two conditions.

➤ The biologic basis of mental illness associated with medical illness (eg, catecholamine depletion, disorders in metabolism or production of neurotransmitters) is similar to that of primary psychiatric illness, and biopsychosocial treatment strategies are effective.

➤ Mental illness in medically ill people is potentially lethal because normal affective-cognitive function may be critical to recovery and compliance with the medical treatment plan. Therefore, it is imperative that mental health be included in the standard health assessment of all medically ill persons and that appropriate referrals be made.

Critical Thinking Challenge

1. You are caring for a stroke patient who refuses breakfast and a morning bath. Applying what you know about the neurologic damage caused by stroke and the frequency of depression in stroke patients, develop a care plan addressing the patient's biopsychosocial needs.

2. As you care for an AIDS patient, you notice that his partner is pacing and hyperventilating. Using your knowledge of relationships, systems, and the interconnectedness of physical and psychological illness, how would you approach him?

3. Discuss the pain syndromes you may see in the primary care setting.

4. A patient is being seen for chronic pain. Discuss how you would go about assessing barriers to pain management with this patient.

5. You are a psychiatric–mental health liaison nurse and have been asked to prepare a program for the medical-surgical nursing staff on psychiatric aspects of medical illnesses. What topics would you include, and what would be your rationale for including each?

REFERENCES

American Psychiatric Association. (2000). *Diagnostic and Statistical Manual of Mental Disorders* (4th edition, Text revision). Washington, DC: Author.

Arnsten, A. F. (1997). Catecholamine regulation of the prefrontal cortex. *Journal of Psychopharmacology, 11,* 151–162.

Astrom, M., Adolfsson, R., & Asplund, K., (1993). Major depression in stroke patients: A 3-year longitudinal study. *Stroke, 24,* 976–982.

Atkinson, J. H. Jr., & Slater, M. A. (1989). Psychiatric medications and pain management in emergency medicine. *Topics in Emergency Medicine, 11*(3), 1–10.

Bandura, A., O'Leary, A., & Taylor, C. B. (1987). Perceived self-efficacy and pain control-opioid and nonopioid mechanisms. *Journal of Personality and Social Psychology, 53,* 563–571.

Beck, A. T., Ward, C. H., Mendelson, M., et al. (1961). An inventory for measuring depression. *Archives of General Psychiatry, 4,* 561–656.

Bradley, L. A., Haile, J. M., & Jaworski, T. M. (1992). Assessment of psychological status using interviews and self-report instruments. In D. C. Turk & R. Melzack (Eds.), *Handbook of pain assessment* (pp. 193–213). New York: Guilford.

Brown, A. S., & Gershon, S., (1993). Dopamine and depression. *Journal of Neural Transmission, 91,* 75–109.

Burkle, F. M., Jr. (1991). Triage of disaster-related neuropsychiatric casualties. *Psychiatric Aspects of Emergency Medicine, 9*(1), 87–104.

Cameron, O. G. (1990). Guidelines for diagnosis and treatment of depression in patients with medical illness. *Journal of Clinical Psychiatry, 51*(7 Suppl.), 49–54.

Carpenter, R. L. (1996). Future directions for outcome research in acute pain management: Design of clinical trials. *Regional Anesthesia, 21*(6 Suppl.), 137–138.

Carroll, B. J., Feinberg, M., Greden, J. F., et al. (1981). A specific laboratory test for the diagnosis of melancholia: Standardization, validation and clinical utility. *Archives of Clinical Psychiatry, 38,* 15–22.

Cassem, E. H. (1990). Depression and anxiety secondary to medical illness. *Psychiatric Clinics of North America, 13*(4), 597–612.

Charney, D. S., Deutch, A. Y., Krystal, J. H., et al. (1993). Psychobiologic mechanisms of posttraumatic stress disorder. *Archives of General Psychiatry, 50*(4), 294–305.

Chrousos, G. P., & Gold, P. W. (1992). The concepts of stress and stress system disorders: Overview of physical and behavioral homeostasis. *JAMA, 267*(9), 1244–1252.

Coderre, T. J., Katz, J., Vaccarino, A. L., & Melzack, R. (1993). Contribution of central neuroplasticity to pathological pain: Review of clinical and experimental evidence. *Pain, 52*(3), 259–285.

Cohen, C., & Cosimer, G. (1989). Factors associated with increased hospital stay by elderly psychiatric patients. *Hospital and Community Psychiatry, 40*(7), 741–743.

Cohen, M. A. (1990). Biopsychosocial approaches to the human immunodeficiency virus epidemic: A clinician's primer. *General Hospital Psychiatry, 12*(2), 98–123.

Collins, J. G. (1991). Acute pain management. *International Anesthesiology Clinics, 29*(1), 23–36.

Folstein, M. F., Folstein, S. E., & McHugh, P. R. (1975). Mini-mental state: A practical method for grading the cognitive state of patients for the clinician. *Journal of Psychiatric Research, 12,* 189–198.

Gabuzda, D. H., & Hirsch, M. S. (1987). Neurologic manifestations of infection with human immunodeficiency virus: Clinical features and pathogenesis. *Annals of Internal Medicine, 107,* 383–391.

Gold, P. W., Licinio, J., Wong, M. L., & Chrousos, G. P. (1995). Corticotropin releasing hormone in the pathophysiology of melancholic and atypical depression and in the mechanism of action of antidepressant drugs. *Annals of the New York Academy of Sciences, 771,* 716–729.

Goldberg, R. J., & Novack, D. H. (1992). The psychosocial review of systems. *Social Science and Medicine, 35*(3), 261–269.

Heim, C., Newport, D. J., Heit, S., et al. (2000). Pituitary-adrenal and autonomic responses to stress in women after sexual and physical injury in childhood. *JAMA, 5,* 592–597.

Hickey, J. V. (1992). The clinical practice of neurological and neurosurgical nursing (3rd ed., pp. 529–530). Philadelphia: J. B. Lippincott.

Hill, D. R., Kelleher, K., & Shumaker, S. A. (1992). Psychosocial interventions in adult patients with coronary heart disease and cancer: A literature review. *General Hospital Psychiatry, 14*(6 Suppl.), 28S–42S.

Jorge, R. E., Robinson, R. G., Starkstien, S. E., & Arndt, S. V. (1994). Influence of major depression on 1-year outcome in patients with traumatic brain injury. *Journal of Neurosurgery, 81,* 726–733.

Kandel, E. R., & Schwartz, J. H. (1987). *Principles of neural science* (2nd ed.). New York: Elsevier.

Katon, W., & Schulberg, H. (1992). Epidemiology of depression in primary care. *General Hospital Psychiatry, 14,* 237–247.

Katz, N. (1994). Role of invasive procedures in chronic pain management. *Seminars in Neurology, 14*(3), 225–237.

Koob, G. F. (1999). Corticotrophin-releasing factor, norepinephrine and stress. *Biological Psychiatry, 46,* 1167–1180.

Levenson, J. L. (1992). Psychosocial interventions in chronic medical illness: An overview of outcome research. *General Hospital Psychiatry, 14*(6 Suppl.), 43S–49S.

Lipton, S. A., & Gendelman, H. E. (1995). Dementia associated with the acquired immunodeficiency syndrome. *New England Journal of Medicine, 332,* 934–940.

Mahoney, F. T., & Barthel, D. W., (1965). Functional evaluation: Barthel index. *Maryland Medical Journal, 14,* 61–65.

Mastorakos, G., Magiakou, M. A., & Chrousos, G. P. (1995). Effects of the immune/inflammatory reaction on the hypothalamic-pituitary-adrenal axis. *Annals of the New York Academy of Science, 771,* 438–448.

McCaffery, M., & Pasero, C. (1999). *Pain clinical manual* (2nd ed.). St. Louis: Mosby.

McEwen, B. (1994). Introduction: Stress and the nervous system. *Seminars in the Neurosciences, 6,* 195–196.

Melzack, R. (1993). Pain: Past, present and future. *Canadian Journal of Experimental Psychology, 47*(4), 615–629.

Melzack, R., & Wall, P. D. (1965). Pain mechanisms: A new theory. *Science, 150,* 971–980.

Morris, P. L. P., & Raphael, B. (1990). Prevalence and course of depressive disorders in hospitalized stroke patients. *International Journal of Psychiatry in Medicine, 20*(4), 349–364.

Neese, J. B., (1991). Depression in the general hospital. *Nursing Clinics of North America, 26*(3), 613–622.

Palomaki, H., Kaste, M., Berg, A., et al. (1999). Prevention of poststroke depression: 1 Year randomised placebo controlled double blind trial of mainserin with 6 month follow up after therapy. *Journal of Neurology, Neurosurgery and Psychiatry, 66,* 490–494.

Post, R. M. (1992). Transduction of psychosocial stress in the neurobiology of recurrent affective disorder. *American Journal of Psychiatry, 149*(8), 999–1010.

Ren, K. (1994). Wind-up and the NMDA receptor: From animal studies to human pain. *Pain, 59,* 157–158.

Robinson, R. G. (1997). Neuropsychiatric consequences of stroke. *Annual Review of Medicine, 48,* 217–229.

Robinson, R. G., Schultz, S. K., Castillo, C., et al. (2000). Nortriptyline versus fluoxetine in the treatment of depression and in short-term recovery after stroke: A placebo-controlled, double-blind study. *American Journal of Psychiatry, 157,* 351–359.

Rudy, T. E., & Turk, D. C. (1991). Psychological aspects of pain. *International Anesthesiology Clinics, 29*(1), 9–21.

Sinyor, D., Amato, P., Kaloupek, D. G., et al. (1986). Poststroke depression: Relationships to functional impairment, coping strategies, and rehabilitation outcome. *Stroke, 17,* 1102–1107.

Sosnowski, M. (1994). Pathophysiology of acute pain. *Pain Digest, 4,* 100–105.

Stoudemire, A., Moran, M. G., & Fogel, B. S. (1990). Psychotropic drug use in the medically ill: Part 1. *Psychosomatics, 31*(4), 377–390.

Stoudemire, A., Moran, M. G., & Fogel, B. S. (1991). Psychotropic drug use in the medically ill: Part 2. *Psychosomatics, 32*(1), 34–46.

Stratakis, C. A., & Chrousos, G. P. (1995). Neuroendocrinology and pathophysiology of the stress system. *Annals of New York Academy of Science, 771,* 1–18.

Talbot, J. D., Marrett, S., Evans, A. C., et al. (1991). Multiple representations of pain in human cerebral cortex. *Science, 251*(3), 1355–1358.

Turk, D. C., & Feldman, C. S. (1992). Facilitating the use of non-invasive pain management strategies with the terminally ill. *Hospice Journal, 8*(1–2), 193–214.

Turk, D. C., & Marcos, D. A. (1994). Assessment of chronic pain patients. *Seminars in Neurology, 14*(3), 206–212.

Turk, D. C., Meichenbaum, D., & Genest, M. (1983). *Pain and behavioral medicine: A cognitive-behavioral perspective.* New York: Guilford.

Turk, D. C., & Okifuji, A. (1994). Detecting depression in chronic pain patients: Adequacy of self-reports. *Behavioral Research and Therapy, 32*(1), 9–16.

Turk, D. C., & Rudy, T. E. (1994). Methods for evaluating treatment outcomes: Ways to overcome potential obstacles. *Spine, 19*(15), 1759–1763.

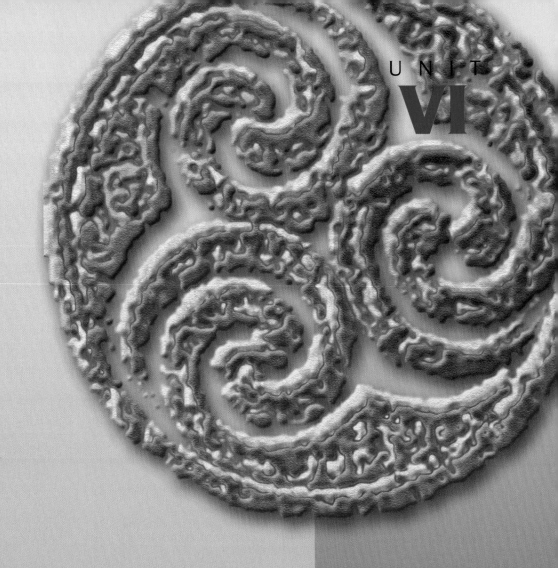

Care Challenges in Psychiatric Nursing

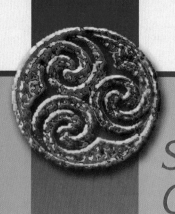

Stress Management and Crisis Intervention

Mary Ann Boyd

LEARNING OBJECTIVES

After studying this chapter, you will be able to:

➤ Examine person–environment factors that contribute to the stress experience.

➤ Relate the cognitive appraisal of the person–environment relationship to stress and coping.

➤ Determine when problem-focused and emotion-focused coping should be used.

➤ Define adaptation in terms of health, psychological well-being, and social function.

➤ Apply the nursing process to a person who is experiencing stress.

➤ Differentiate generalist and specialist psychiatric mental health nursing interventions that promote successful coping in stressful situations.

➤ Define a crisis as an example of severe stress.

➤ Differentiate between a crisis resulting from chronic stress and a psychiatric emergency.

➤ Delineate generalist and specialist interventions that promote positive resolution of crises.

CHAPTER 35

KEY TERMS

bereavement
cognitive appraisal
constraints
demands
dissupport
emotion-focused
    coping
emotions
life events

person–environment
    relationship
problem-focused
    coping
reappraisal
social functioning
social network
social support

KEY CONCEPTS

adaptation
coping
crisis
stress

*M*ost of this text has focused on developing an understanding of mental illness and the specialized care of people with mental health disorders. Now it is time to broaden the scope and focus on all people—those who have no diagnosis of or risk for a mental disorder as well as those who do. Stress and crises are inevitable in everyone's life. Sometimes, successfully coping with stress and surviving crises make the difference between being mentally healthy and mentally ill. This chapter explores the concepts of stress and crisis, describes which types of problems are appropriate for generalist psychiatric–mental health nurses to treat and which are appropriate for specialist psychiatric–mental health nurses, and explains generalist nursing interventions that promote successful coping in stressful situations and positive resolution of crises.

Stress and coping should be viewed as a natural part of life. If children are protected from experiencing stress and developing coping skills, they are likely to be vulnerable to stress in later life and unable to cope effectively with **life events** (eg, relocation, marriage, death). Even though being under stress is usually viewed as a negative experience, its outcomes can be positive. During severe stress or a severe crisis, some people draw on resources that they never realized they had. People can actually grow from stressful experiences.

The concept of stress seems deceptively simple yet has intrigued researchers for centuries. Stress is one of the most complex concepts in health and nursing. It is difficult to define, but its detrimental effects are well known. Stress is associated with manifestations of physical illness (eg, myocardial infarction), mental disorders (eg, posttraumatic stress disorder), and social disruption (eg, divorce). It can also interfere with the best treatment and rehabilitation efforts.

In his explanation of the general adaptation syndrome, Selye viewed stress as a nonspecific response to any demand or stressor (Selye, 1956, 1974). He believed that many diseases, including hypertension, peptic ulcer, and autoimmune illnesses, were products of excessive or "adaptive" reactions in which corticosteroids played a pathogenic role. The stressors stimulated neuroendocrine activity that in turn produced the illness. He differentiated stress (a nonspecific response) from a stressor, the external or internal event that initiates the response. He argued that stressors can be physical (eg, infection, intense heat or cold, surgical operations, debilitating illnesses), psychological (eg, psychological trauma, interpersonal problems), or social (eg, lack of social support).

Although ample evidence supports the notion of biologic responses to stress, some are questioning Selye's idea that there is a general physical reaction to diverse environmental stimuli. Many responses, such as those within the neuroendocrine system, are not general at all but very specific. Also, similar stressors do not necessarily produce similar results

(Lazarus & Folkman, 1984). In fact, a stressor for one person may not be a stressor for another. Furthermore, according to Selye's model, if adaptation responses are ineffective, "diseases of adaptation" will develop. Although many diseases (eg, essential hypertension) are related to stress, others are not (eg, rheumatoid arthritis) (McCain & Smith, 1994). Overall, Selye's view oversimplified the concept of stress and did not account for the individuality of stress responses.

In 1984, Richard Lazarus published his classic work, Stress, Appraisal and Coping. *Arguing that stress is much more complicated than a stimulus response, he offered a new approach to understanding stress. He focused on what happens inside a person's mind, defining stress as "a particular relationship between the person and the environment that is appraised by the person as taxing or exceeding his or her resources and endangering his or her well-being" (Lazarus & Folkman, 1984, p. 18). The experience of stress, the person's responses, and the effects of the stress are presented in the stress, coping, and adaptation model depicted in Figure 35-1. This systems model has four components: (1) antecedents to the stress, (2) stress, (3) coping, and (4) adaptation. This model, which is consistent with the biopsychosocial approach of psychiatric–mental health nursing practice, is used as a framework in this chapter for understanding stress and crisis.*

KEY CONCEPT   Stress. **Stress** is the relationship between the person and the environment that is appraised as exceeding the person's resources and endangering the person's well-being.

ANTECEDENTS TO STRESS

There are two important antecedents or precursors to the stress response. First is the person–environment relationship, which involves many factors. The second antecedent is the person's cognitive appraisal of the risks and benefits of the situation, which mediates or moderates the interpretation of its meaning. The appraisal of the relationship determines the manifestation of stress and the potential for coping.

Person–Environment Relationship

Let's first discuss the person–environment relationship. The **person–environment relationship** can be defined as the interaction between the individual and the environment that changes throughout the stress experience.

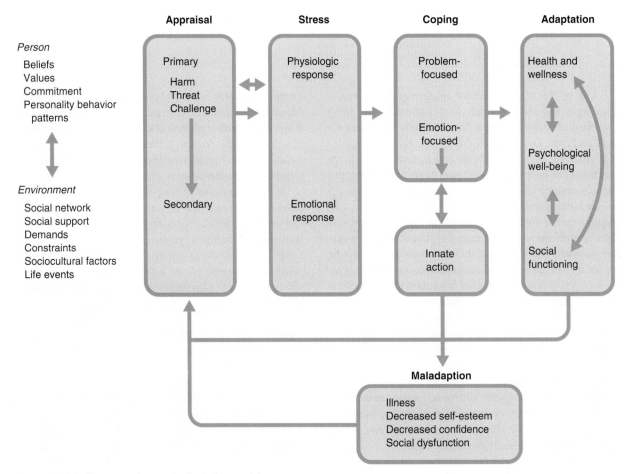

FIGURE 35.1 Stress, coping, and adaptation model.

The Person

A person brings to any interaction a set of values and beliefs that he or she has developed over a lifetime. These values are based on cultural, ethnic, family, and religious traditions that form the person's beliefs about the world. A person's underlying values and beliefs shape his or her decision about the significance of any particular situation. For one person, a college education may be important because of the underlying belief that it is the road to economic success. For another, living successfully with neighbors in a small, isolated community is much more important than formal education and economic success. Therefore, what is important to one person may not be to another.

Values and Commitment. When a person values a particular outcome such as a college education, the person is likely to be committed to activities directed toward that outcome. According to Lazarus, the commitment to a goal is an important factor in the stress response. The following example illustrates the relationship between values and commitment.

Students who earn mostly or all As are often more stressed and worried about examinations than students who earn Bs and Cs. Before they take a test, the former often express fear that they will flunk, a worry that is a source of great irritation to other students, who may remind them that they have never failed an examination. These high-achieving students are devastated if they earn a B or C, whereas other students are often relieved to receive a B or C. Although it seems illogical that students who consistently earn higher grades are more stressed than those who perform less well, the test-taking situation is actually more threatening to the better students, who place a higher value on the A grade than do the other students. The more committed students are to getting an A, the more likely they are to experience severe stress.

Personality Behavior Patterns. People bring not only their values, beliefs, and goals to any situation but also their own behavioral characteristics. Some people tend to avoid new experiences and situations, whereas others embrace them. Each person develops ways of interacting with the world from early childhood. These behaviors form patterns over a lifetime, so that people automatically respond to events with a particular behavior pattern. For example, the preschool-aged child who refuses to attend nursery school often fears going to kindergarten and may later have difficulty leaving home for college.

The importance of behavior patterns is demonstrated by type A and B personalities. In the mid-1970s, cardiologists Meyer Friedman and Ray Rosenman observed that their patients' personalities and lifestyles seemed to be related to the development of cardiovascular disease. They identified two distinct personality behavior patterns: type A and type B. They believed that the type A behavior pattern led to changes in the neuroendocrine system that resulted in cardiovascular problems. They also believed that the type B behavior pattern did not produce these changes. From their work, the widely known conceptualization of type A and B personality behavior patterns evolved (Friedman & Rosenman, 1974).

Type A people are competitive, aggressive, ambitious, and impatient. They speak rapidly, emphatically, and explosively. Alert, tense, and restless, they think and act at an accelerated pace. In their interactions with their environment, they reflect an aggressive, hostile, and time-urgent style of living that is often associated with increased psychophysiologic arousal. In contrast, type B people do not exhibit these chronic behaviors and are generally more relaxed, easy-going, and easily satisfied. They have an accepting attitude about trivial mistakes and a problem-solving approach to major problems. Rarely do type B people push themselves to obtain excesses from the environment or try to accomplish too much in too little time (Rosenman & Chesney, 1985).

These two behavior patterns have been studied extensively in relation to the development of cardiovascular illnesses. The initial studies supported a link between type A personality and atherosclerosis leading to coronary heart disease. More recent studies suggest that type A behavior and coronary disease are evident primarily in people with middle-class occupations and lifestyles, not in people with low-status occupations. Nevertheless, these concepts of type A and B personality behavior patterns demonstrate the significance of personal behavior patterns in everyday life.

The Environment

The external environment is conceptualized as everything outside a person, including physical surroundings and social interactions. Crowding, temperature, and noise are all physical aspects of the environment. Social aspects include living arrangements and personal contacts. Unique interactions occur daily between the person and physical and social aspects of the environment. The following section discusses environmental factors.

Social Networks. People live within a **social network** consisting of linkages among a defined set of people with whom there are personal contacts (Mitchell, 1969). A person develops and maintains his or her social identity within this social network (Walker et al., 1977). He or she acquires emotional support, material aid, services, information, and new social contracts within this framework. A social network can increase a person's resources, enhance the ability to cope with change, and influence the course of illnesses (Simmons, 1994).

A social network may be large, consisting of numerous family and community contacts, or small, consisting of few. Contacts can be categorized according to three different levels. Level I consists of 6 to 12 people with whom the person has close contact. Level II consists of a larger number of contacts, generally 30 to 40 people whom the person sees regularly. Level III consists of the large number of people with whom a person has direct contact, such as the grocer and mail carrier. Level III can represent several hundred people. Each person's social network is slightly different. These multiple contacts allow several networks to interact. Generally, the larger the network is, the more support that is available to the person. An ideal network structure is fairly dense and interconnected—people within the network are also in contact with one another. Dense networks are better able to respond in times of stress and crisis and to provide emotional support to a person in distress (Simmons, 1994).

Two concepts relate to social networks. Intensity is the degree of closeness of a relationship. Some relationships are naturally more intense than others. Ideally, a person's social network reflects a balance between intense and less intense relationships. Intense relationships can restrict a person's opportunity to interact with other network members, but without at least a few intense relationships, a person becomes isolated. Reciprocity is the extent to which there is give and take. Network members both provide and receive support, aid, services, and information. Sometimes, network members are on the giving side; at other times, they are on the receiving side. Reciprocity is particularly important because most friendships do not last without give and take of support and services. A person who is always on the receiving end eventually becomes isolated from other network members.

Social Support. One of the important functions of the social network is to provide **social support,** the positive and harmonious interpersonal interactions that occur within social relationships. Social support is a process, and the social network is the structure within which social support occurs. Social support serves three functions:

1. Emotional support contributes to a person's feelings of being cared for or loved.
2. Tangible support provides a person with additional resources.
3. Informational support helps a person view situations in a new light (Table 35-1).

Ample research evidence indicates that social support enhances health outcomes and reduces mortality. Social support helps people make needed behavior changes. Through social support, a person also feels helped, valued, and in personal control, which in turn may help reduce the "fight-or-flight" response and strengthen the immune system. Social support also either directly or indirectly buffers stressful life events. This buffering effect works in two ways. The first is that during stressful events, network members collect and analyze information, offer guidance, and help the person under stress interpret the world. Second, by treating the person under stress as a unique, special human being, members of the social network provide comfort and a sanctuary or place of refuge (Caplan, 1974).

The relationship between stressful life events and support is complicated. People who are relatively healthy are more likely to have a stronger support system and to be able to prevent undesirable life events than those who are physically or mentally ill. Also, some life events, such as marriage, divorce, and bereavement, actually change the level of social support by adding to or subtracting from a person's social network. For example, if a person loses a spouse and the spouse was the main source of support, the stress is greater because not only the spouse but also the support is lost. Therefore, social support should be viewed as a dynamic process that is in constant flux and varies with life events and health status (Beels et al., 1984; Thoits, 1982).

TABLE 35.1	Examples of Functions of Social Support
Function	**Example**
Emotional support	Attachment, reassurance, being able to rely on and confide in a person
Tangible support	Direct aid such as loans or gifts, services such as taking care of someone who is ill, doing a job or chore
Informational support	Providing information or advice, and giving feedback about how a person is doing

From Schaefer, C., Coyne, J., & Lazarus, R. (1982). The health-related functions of social support. *Journal of Behavioral Medicine, 44,* 381–406.

Not all interpersonal interactions within a network are supportive. A person can have a large, complex social network but little social support.

The concept of **dissupport** derives from the observation that many relationships are actually harmful, stressful, and damaging to a person's self-esteem. Social dissupport is the opposite of social support and refers to relationships that hinder growth, are emotionally destructive, and deplete resources. Social relationships can fluctuate between providing support at one end of a continuum and dissupport at the other (Malone, 1988). Some relationships can be both supportive and dissupportive, such as those that provide tangible support (eg, money) but that are emotionally destructive at the same time. The following behaviors are manifestations of social dissupport:

- Expressing negative emotions
- Disagreeing with or discounting the appropriateness of a person's opinions or values
- Discouraging a person from openly expressing his or her feelings
- Withholding advice or blocking a person's access to useful information
- Consuming a person's material resources
- Conveying information that makes a person feel isolated (Malone, 1988)

Only those interactions that a person perceives as being positive and harmonious are considered social support. If a person views a relationship as destructive or negative, the interactions are not considered supportive.

Demands and Constraints. Within the social network are external and internal demands and personal and environmental constraints. Internal **demands** are generated by physiologic and psychological needs. The physical environment imposes some external demands, such as crowding, crime, noise, and pollution; the social environment imposes others, such as behavioral and role expectations. In contrast to demands, **constraints** are limitations that are both personal and environmental. Personal constraints include internalized cultural values and beliefs that dictate actions or feelings and psychological deficits that are products of the person's unique development. Environmental constraints are finite resources, such as money and time, that are available to people.

These demands and constraints vary with the individual and contribute to or initiate a stress response (Lazarus & Folkman, 1984). They also interact with one another (Text Box 35-1). For instance, work demands, such as changing shifts, may interact with physical demands, such as a need for sleep, creating a high-risk situation in which stress is likely.

TEXT BOX 35.1

Clinical Vignette: Demands Are Not Equal

Two women lost their jobs at a local company. One was a single parent who was the sole supporter of two small children, and the other had no children but lived with a man who paid most of their expenses. Because the demands and constraints of the environment are different for the two women, the meaning of the job loss is different for each. The job loss significantly affects the single parent's ability to support her children, whereas it is merely an inconvenience for the other woman because her partner helps share expenses. The economic demands on the single parent are greater, and thus she is likely to experience greater stress.

Caregivers represent a group of people who are burdened by excessive demands and constraints. The care of a chronically ill person places additional stress on the caregiver and the patient's family. The caregiver is particularly vulnerable to stress because the patient's biopsychosocial demands take priority over the caregiver's own needs. In time, the caregiver becomes chronically stressed.

Sociocultural Factors. Cultural expectations and role strain serve as both demands and constraints in the experience of stress. If a person violates cultural group values to meet role expectations, stress occurs. For example, a person may stay in an abusive relationship to avoid the stress of violating a cultural norm that values lifelong marriage, no matter what the circumstances. The potential guilt associated with norm violation and the anticipated isolation from being ostracized are worse for that person than the physical and psychological pain caused by the abusive situation.

Employment is a highly valued cultural norm and provides social, psychological, and financial benefits. In all cultures, work is assigned significance beyond economic compensation. It is often the central focus of adulthood and, for many, a source of personal identity. Even if a person's employment brings little real happiness, being employed implies that a person's or family's financial needs are being met. Work offers status, regulates life activities, permits association with others, and provides a meaningful life experience. Even though work is demanding, unemployment can actually be more stressful because of the associated isolation and loss of social status.

Gender expectations often become a source of demands and constraints for women who assume multiple roles. In most cultures, women who work outside the home are expected to assume primary responsibility for care of the children and household duties. Most women are adept at separating these roles and can compartmentalize problems at work from those at home. Thus, problems do not usually spill over from one role to another. When problems occur or demands increase simultaneously within more than one role, however, women experience stress. Thus, women who have problems both at work and at home report psychological distress, but those who have difficulty in only one area, such as at work, do not experience distress at home (Barnett & Marshall, 1992).

Life Events. In 1967, Holmes and Rahe presented a psychosocial view of illness by pointing out the complex relationship between life changes and the development of illnesses (Holmes & Rahe, 1967). They hypothesized that people become ill after they experience life event changes. The more frequent the changes are, the greater is the possibility of becoming sick. The investigators cited the events that they believed partially accounted for the onset of illnesses and began testing whether these life changes were actual precursors to illness. It soon became clear that not all events have the same effects. For example, the death of a spouse is usually much more devastating and stressful than a change in residence. From their research, the investigators were able to assign relative weights to various life events according to the degree of associated stress. Rahe devised the Recent Life Changes Questionnaire (Table 35-2) to evaluate the frequency and significance of life change events (Rahe, 1994). Numerous research studies subsequently demonstrated the relationship between a recent life change and the severity of near-future illness (Rahe, 1994). If several life changes occur within a short period, the likelihood of an illness appearing is even greater. This line of research is important because it defines life event changes and provides a way of measuring their relationship with the development of illnesses.

Appraisal

Physiologic stress caused by tissue trauma is not the same as psychological stress, which involves thinking and feeling. The difference centers on the issue of personal meaning (Lazarus, 1993). All stress responses are affected by the personal meaning of the situation. For example, chest pain is stressful to a person not only because of the immediate pain and incapacitation it causes but also because it may mean that the person is having a heart attack. The fear of having a heart attack and dying is part of the stress of chest pain. Thus, the significance of the event actually determines the importance of the person–environment relationship.

A given event or situation may be extremely stressful to one person but not to another. Lazarus attributes this variation in response to stress to the significance of the outcome of the situation to the person involved.

The person who regards the outcome as important is naturally worried, concerned, or anxious. That person is also more likely to be stressed by the situation than another. The more important or meaningful the outcome is, the more vulnerable the person is to stress.

The meaning of the person–environment situation is evaluated or appraised for its risks and benefits. **Cognitive appraisal** is the term that Lazarus used to refer to the process of examining the demands, constraints, and resources of the environment and negotiating them with personal goals and beliefs. During this appraisal process, the person integrates his or her personality and environmental factors into a relational meaning based on the relevance of what is happening to the person's well-being (Lazarus, 1991). The Clinical Vignette demonstrates the relationship between personal meaning and stress (Text Box 35-2). An analysis of this scenario makes it clear that even though both students took the same test, Susan was less stressed than Joanne. A comparison of the two students reveals obvious differences. Susan was rested, had studied, and was interested in the content, whereas Joanne was sleep deprived and inadequately prepared. These differences, however, do not explain Joanne's severe stress reaction. The critical factor is the risk involved. For Susan, a failed test meant a retake; for Joanne, a failed test meant not returning to school.

The appraisal process has two levels: primary and secondary. During primary appraisal of a goal, the person determines whether (1) the goal is relevant, (2) the goal is consistent with his or her values and beliefs, and (3) a personal commitment is present. In the vignette, Susan's commitment to the goal of doing well on the test was consistent with her valuing the content, which in turn motivated her to study regularly and prepare carefully for the examination. She believed that the test would be difficult. Joanne had a commitment to pass the test but did not value the content. Unlike Susan, Joanne believed that the test would be relatively easy because she expected the questions to be the same as those on the previous examination.

The second level, secondary appraisal, involves making decisions about blame or credit, coping potential, and future expectations. In the example, Susan was nervous but took the test. Joanne's secondary appraisal of the test-taking situation began with the realization that she might not pass the test because the questions were different. She acted impulsively by blaming the teacher for giving a different examination and by storming out of the room. She clearly did not cope effectively with a difficult situation.

Therefore, stress is initiated not by a single stressor but by an unfavorable person–environment relationship that is meaningful in terms of the risks or benefits to that person's well-being. The person's commitment to the goal influences the stress response as well as the meaning of the situation. The more committed the person is

TABLE 35.2 Life Changing Event Questionnaire

Social Area	Life Changes	LCU Values*
Family	Death of spouse	105
	Marital separation	65
	Death of close family member	65
	Divorce	62
	Pregnancy	60
	Change in health of family member	52
	Marriage	50
	Gain of new family member	50
	Marital reconciliation	42
	Spouse begins or stops work	37
	Son or daughter leaving home	29
	In-law trouble	29
	Change in number of family get-togethers	26
Personal	Jail term	56
	Sex difficulties	49
	Death of a close friend	46
	Personal injury or illness	42
	Change in living conditions	39
	Outstanding personal achievement	33
	Change in residence	33
	Minor violations of the law	32
	Begin or end school	32
	Change in sleeping habits	31
	Revision of personal habits	31
	Change in eating habits	29
	Change in church activities	29
	Vacation	29
	Change in school	28
	Change in recreation	28
	Christmas	26
Work	Fired at work	64
	Retirement from work	49
	Trouble with boss	39
	Business readjustment	38
	Change to different line of work	38
	Change in work responsibilities	33
	Change in work hours or conditions	30
Financial	Foreclosure of mortgage or loan	57
	Change in financial state	43
	Mortgage (home, car, etc)	39
	Mortgage or loan less than $10,000 (stereo, etc)	26

Directions: Sum the LCUs for your life change events during the past 12 months.
  250 and 400 LCUs per year: Minor life crisis
  Over 400 LCUs per year: Major life crisis
*LCU, Life change unit. The number of LCUs reflects the average degree or intensity of the life change.
Adapted from Rahe, R. (1990). Psychosocial stressors and adjustment disorder: Van Gogh's life chart illustrates stress and disease. *Journal of Clinical Psychiatry, 51* (11, Suppl.), 15.

to a specific goal, the greater is his or her vulnerability to stress.

STRESS RESPONSES

Once a person–environment relationship is established and the person appraises it as threatening, harmful, or challenging, an internal stress response oc-

curs. The person has simultaneous physiologic and emotional responses. These responses are discussed in the next section.

Physiologic Responses

Physiologic changes are automatic and not under voluntary control. Their intensity will depend on the

TEXT BOX 35.2

Clinical Vignette: Stress and Students

Two students are preparing for the same examination. Susan is genuinely interested in the subject, prepares by studying throughout the semester, and reviews the content 2 days before test day. The night before the examination, she goes to bed early, gets a good night's sleep, and wakes refreshed but is slightly nervous about the test. She wants to do well and expects a difficult test but knows that she can retake it at a later date if she does poorly.

In contrast, Joanne is not interested in the subject matter and does not study throughout the semester. She "crams" 2 days before the test date and does an "all nighter" the night before. This is the last time that Joanne can take the examination, but she believes that she will pass because she has already taken it twice and is familiar with the questions. If she does not pass, she will not be able to return to school. On entering the room, Joanne is physically tired and somewhat fearful of not passing the test. As she looks at the test, she instantly realizes that it is not the examination she expected. The questions are new. She begins hyperventilating and tremoring. After yelling obscenities at the teacher, she storms out of the room. She is very distressed and describes herself as "being in a panic."

appraised risk of the situation. The riskier the situation, the more intense the response. Both the immune system and the sympathetic nervous system are implicated in the stress response.

The locus ceruleus in the brain initiates the stress response by responding to the appraisal by releasing norepinephrine, which in turn stimulates the sympathetic nervous system centers located in the hypothalamus (see Chap. 7). If the person experiences fear or pain, the sympathetic nervous system responds by discharging almost as a complete unit, causing excitatory effects in some organs and inhibitory effects in others (Table 35-3). This "mass discharge" activates large portions of the system and is called a *sympathetic alarm reaction* or the fight-or-flight response. The body is physically prepared to perform vigorous muscle activity because of the following sympathetic responses:

- Increased arterial pressure
- Increased blood flow to active muscle concurrent with decreased blood flow to organs that are not needed for rapid motor activity, such as the gastrointestinal tract and kidneys
- Increased rates of cellular metabolism throughout the body
- Increased blood glucose concentration
- Increased glycolysis in the liver and in muscle
- Increased muscle strength
- Increased mental activity
- Increased rate of blood coagulation

One structure that is stimulated during the sympathetic nervous system discharge is the adrenal gland through activation of the hypothalamic–pituitary–adrenal (HPA) axis. That is, the hypothalamus secretes corticotropin-releasing hormone (CRH), which causes a marked increase in adrenocorticotropic hormone (corticotropin) secretion by the pituitary gland, which in turn stimulates the adrenocortical secretion of cortisol (Rossen & Buschmann, 1995). The benefits of the increase in circulating cortisol to the human body are unclear. Speculation is that, because cortisol stimulates gluconeogenesis (formation of carbohydrate from proteins and some other substances), proteins then become available to needy cells for glucose synthesis to maintain life processes that are perceived to be threatened (Guyton & Hall, 2000).

Other neurobiologic reactions occur during a stress response. For example, CRH is secreted into the amygdala and hippocampus, a process important for memory retrieval and emotional analysis. The locus ceruleus has connections with the cerebrum, which has dopamine-producing neurons that project into the mesolimbic and mesocortical dopamine tracts, helping to control motivation, reward, and reinforcement.

Stress also adversely affects the functioning of the immune system. The hypothesized connection between the immune and sympathetic nervous systems is immune cells, which have receptors for cortisol and catecholamines that have the capacity to bind with lymphatic cells and suppress the immune system. Cortisol is primarily immunosuppressive, contributing to reductions in lymphocyte numbers and function (primarily T-lymphocyte and monocyte subsets) and natural killer activities. Therefore, during stress, when the production of both cortisol and norepinephrine increases, the immune system is negatively affected.

Not all appraisals provoke a severe fight-or-flight response. Chronically unfavorable person–environment relationships, however, also elicit both sympathetic and immune system responses. Academic examinations, job strain, caregiving for a family member with dementia, marital conflict, and daily hassles elevate white blood cell counts and lower those for T, B, and natural killer (NK) cells. Negative moods (chronic hostility, depression, and anxiety) also adversely affect the immune system. Antibody titers to Epstein-Barr and herpes simplex viruses are elevated in stressed populations. If the stress is long term, the immune alteration continues (Hayes, 1995; Herbert & Cohen, 1993). Social isolation also negatively affects immune functioning, especially in elderly people, poor people, and African Americans (House et al., 1988).

Over time, biologic responses to stress compromise a person's health status. The responses of the neurohormonal and immune systems can precipitate more severe stress responses. Ideally, through positive coping,

	TABLE 35.3 Effects of Sympathetic Nervous System Stimulation			

Organ	Effect of Sympathetic Stimulation	Organ	Effect of Sympathetic Stimulation
Eye		Kidney	Decreased output and renin secretion
Pupil	Dilated		
Ciliary muscle	Slight relaxation (far vision)	Bladder	
Glands	Vasoconstriction and slight secretion	Detrusor	Relaxed (slight)
Nasal		Trigone	Contracted
Lacrimal		Penis	Ejaculation
Parotid		Systemic arterioles	
Submandibular		Abdominal viscera	Constricted
Gastric		Muscle	Constricted (adrenergic α)
Pancreatic			Dilated (adrenergic β_2)
Sweat glands	Copious sweating		Dilated (cholinergic)
Apocrine glands	Thick, odoriferous secretions	Skin	Constricted
Heart		Blood	
Muscle	Increased rate	Coagulation	Increased
	Increased force of contraction	Glucose	Increased
		Lipids	Increased
Coronaries	Dilated (β_2); constricted (α)	Basal metabolism	Increased up to 100%
Lungs		Adrenal medullary secretion	Increased
Bronchi	Dilated	Mental activity	Increased
Blood vessels	Mildly constricted	Piloerector muscles	Contracted
Gut		Skeletal muscle	Increased glycogenolysis
Lumen	Decreased peristalsis and tone		Increased strength
Sphincter	Increased tone (most times)	Fat cells	Lipolysis
Liver	Glucose released		
Gallbladder and bile ducts	Relaxed		

From Guyton, A., & Hall, J. (2000). *Textbook of Medical Physiology* (10th ed.) (p. 775), Philadelphia: W. B. Saunders.

a person can counteract the stress and return to a healthy state. A person who does not cope with stress successfully is at higher risk for more serious physiologic changes.

Emotional Responses

After cognitively appraising a situation, a person experiences specific emotions along with physiologic changes. Lazarus defines **emotions** as organized psychophysiologic reactions. The emotion the person experiences depends on the significance of the person–environment event to his or her personal well-being. The person's mental state is one of excitement or distress, marked by strong feelings and usually accompanied by an impulse toward definite action. If the emotion is intense, a disturbance in intellectual functions occurs.

Dissociation can also occur and a strong impulse to act (Lazarus, 1991). In the previous example, the students experienced two very different emotions that were specific to the meaning to them of the test-taking experience. Susan experienced nervousness that most likely increased her ability to cope with a challenging

test, whereas Joanne experienced panic. One student was challenged and the other threatened.

Emotions are developed through a process: anticipation, provocation, unfolding, and outcome (Table 35-4). For an emotion to occur, an individual must subjectively evaluate a situation or person–environment relationship as having certain harms or benefits. The significance or meaning of the evaluation depends on the person's goals and beliefs and the environmental context (family conflict has a different meaning from stranger conflict). Some emotions are evaluated as being negative and others as positive. The person is more likely to experience positive emotions when he or she views the situation as a challenge. Conversely, negative emotions are elicited if the person evaluates the episode as threatening or harmful. According to Lazarus, emotions are categorized as follows:

- *Negative emotions* occur when there is a threat to, delay in, or thwarting of a goal or a conflict between goals: anger, fright, anxiety, guilt, shame, sadness, envy, jealousy, and disgust

TABLE 35.4   Stages of Emotion

Stages	Definition	Example
Anticipation	A change in the person–environment relationship, warning of an upcoming harm or benefit. Expectations are created about the outcome that can exacerbate the emotion. Positive expectations increase the likelihood of disappointment; negative expectations can make a negative outcome seem positive.	A person anticipates a promotion because of the boss's increased attention. Instead, the person is reprimanded for unsatisfactory work. He is extremely disappointed. *Or* a person buys a lottery ticket and does not expect to win. When the person does not win, she shrugs and says that buying the ticket was fun.
Provocation	Any occurrence in the environment or within a person that is judged as having changed the person–environment relationship in the direction of harm or benefit.	An unexpected relative arrives at an inopportune time.
Unfolding	Flow of emotion within an encounter. It usually involves an interaction with another, who in turn is provoked and reacts emotionally.	A jealous husband accuses his wife of infidelity. She in turn becomes angry at her husband.
Outcome	An emotional state that reflects an appraisal of what has happened as it relates to a person's well-being.	A wife is very sad after a violent argument with her husband.

Adapted from Lazarus, R. (1991). *Emotion and adaptation* (pp. 104–112). New York: Oxford University Press.

- *Positive emotions* occur when there is movement toward or attainment of a goal: happiness, pride, relief, and love
- *Borderline emotions* are somewhat ambiguous: hope, compassion, empathy, sympathy, and contentment
- *Nonemotions* connote emotional reactions but are too ambiguous to fit into any of the preceding categories: confidence, awe, confusion, and excitement

Each emotion is expressed as a theme that summarizes the personal harms and benefits of each person–environment relationship. This core relational theme is unique and specific to each emotion. For instance, physical danger stimulates fear in a person. A loss produces feelings of sadness (Table 35-5). Each emotion also has its own innate response that is automatic and unique to a particular person. For example, anger may automatically provoke tremors in one person but both tremors and perspiration in another. Sadness may provoke tears in one person but not in another.

Along with a theme and automatic response, each emotion provokes an impulse or innate action tendency. Emotions provoke an automatic tendency to act. Anger produces a tendency to attack the person who is blamed for the perceived offense. Compassion produces a tendency to reach out. Guilt produces an impulse to atone for the harm or seek punishment. Fear produces an impulse to escape to safety. For example, a young musician facing his first performance at Carnegie Hall experiences stage fright. His first impulse is to run home.

Therefore, the stress response is an automatic and sometimes intense biopsychological reaction in response to an appraised unfavorable person–environment situation. The physiologic responses involve the autonomic nervous and immune systems. Corresponding emotions occur that elicit an immediate, innate action to the appraised risks and benefits of the situations.

COPING

It is not usually in a person's best interest to act on his or her initial impulse. Fortunately, thinking usually takes over, and the person begins coping, a cognitive process followed by action. The person begins thinking and acting in ways to manage specific external or internal demands and conflicts that are taxing or exceeding personal resources (Lazarus, 1985). Coping is the process through which the person manages the demands and emotions generated by the appraised stress. The coping process, a deliberate, planned, and psychological activity, may inhibit or override the innate urge to act. Positive coping leads to adaptation, which is characterized by a balance between health and illness, a sense of well-being, and maximum social functioning. When a person does not cope positively, maladaptations occur that can shift the balance toward illness, a diminished self-concept, and deterioration in social functioning.

> **KEY CONCEPT** Coping. **Coping** is the process whereby a person manages the demands and emotions that are generated by the appraisal.

The process of coping alters the person–environment relationship and a person's emotional state; that is, the

TABLE 35.5 Core Relational Themes for Each Emotion

Emotion	Relational Meaning
Anger	A demeaning offense against me and mine
Anxiety	Facing an uncertain, existential threat
Fright	Facing an immediate, concrete, and overwhelming physical danger
Guilt	Having transgressed a moral imperative
Shame	Having failed to live up to an ego ideal
Sadness	Having experienced an irrevocable loss
Envy	Wanting what someone else has
Jealousy	Resenting a third party for the loss of or a threat to another's affection
Disgust	Taking in or being too close to an indigestible object or idea (metaphorically speaking)
Happiness	Making reasonable progress toward the realization of a goal
Pride	Enhancement of one's ego-identity by taking credit for a valued object or achievement, either our own or that of someone or a group with whom we identify
Relief	A distressing goal-incongruent condition that has changed for the better or gone away
Hope	Fearing the worst but yearning for better
Love	Desiring or participating in affection, usually but not necessarily reciprocated
Compassion	Being moved by another's suffering and wanting to help

Adapted from Lazarus, R. (1991). *Emotion and adaptation* (p. 122). New York: Oxford University Press.

person feels different after coping than during the stress. There are two types of coping: problem focused, which actually changes the person-environment relationship, and emotion focused, which changes the meaning of the situation. In **problem-focused coping**, the person attacks the source of stress by eliminating it or changing its effects. In **emotion-focused coping**, the person reinterprets the situation, reducing the stress and the need for further coping without changing the actual person–environment relationship (Table 35-6).

After a person has succeeded in coping, he or she reevaluates or reappraises the new situation. This reappraisal is important because of the changing nature of the person–environment relationship. **Reappraisal**, which is the same as appraisal except that it happens after coping, provides feedback about the outcomes and allows for continual adjustment to new information. Thus, the stress response becomes part of the dynamic relationship between the person and the environment.

No one coping strategy is best for all situations. Throughout their lives, people learn which coping strategies work best in particular situations. These strategies become automatic and develop into patterns for each person. In some instances, people use the coping mechanisms discussed in Chapter 6. Some situations require a combination of strategies and activities.

Ideally, a person can cope with an unfavorable person–environment situation by matching the resources that are needed with the events that are unfolding. Social support can be critical in helping people cope with difficult situations. We know that coping can influence the frequency, intensity, duration, and patterning of physiologic stress reactions (Lazarus, 1985). Successful coping with life stresses is linked to quality of life as well as to physical and mental health.

ADAPTATION

Adaptation can be conceptualized as a person's capacity to survive and flourish (Lazarus, 1985, p. 182). Adaptation or lack of it affects three important areas: health, psychological well-being, and social functioning. A period of stress may compromise any or all of these areas. If a person copes successfully with stress, he or she returns to a previous level of adaptation. Successful coping results in an improvement in health, well-being, and social functioning. Unfortunately, at times, maladaptation occurs.

KEY CONCEPT Adaptation. **Adaptation** is the person's capacity to survive and flourish. Adaptation affects three important areas: health, psychological well-being, and social functioning.

It is impossible to separate completely the adaptation areas of health, well-being, and social functioning. A

TABLE 35.6 Ways of Coping: Problem-Focused Coping Versus Emotion-Focused Coping	
Problem-Focused Coping	**Emotion-Focused Coping**
When noise from the television interrupts a student's studying and causes the student to be stressed, the student turns off the television and eliminates the noise.	A husband is adamantly opposed to visiting his wife's relatives because they keep dogs in their house. Even though the dogs are well cared for, their presence in the relative's home violates his need for an orderly, clean house and causes the husband sufficient stress that he copes by refusing to visit. This becomes a source of marital conflict. One holiday, the husband is given a puppy and immediately becomes attached to the dog, who soon becomes a valued family member. The husband then begins to view his wife's relatives differently and willingly visits their house more often.
An abused spouse is finally able to leave her husband because she realizes that the abuse will not stop, even though he promises never to hit her again.	A mother is afraid that her teenaged daughter has been in an accident because she did not come home after a party. Then the woman remembers that she gave her daughter permission to stay at a friend's house. She immediately feels better.

maladaptation in any one area can negatively affect the others. For instance, the appearance of psychiatric symptoms can cause problems in performance in the work environment that in turn elicit a negative self-concept. Even though each area will be discussed separately, the reader should realize that when one area is affected, most likely all three areas are affected (Fig. 35-2).

Health and Illness

A relationship between stress and illness has been implied throughout this chapter. Selye linked stressors to illnesses, Holmes and Rahe related life events to new illnesses, and Friedman and Rosenman linked personality behavior patterns to cardiovascular problems. Although

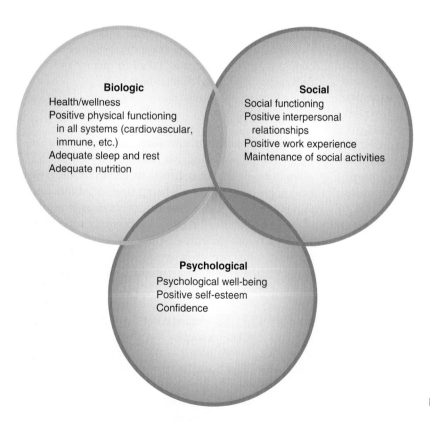

Biologic
Health/wellness
Positive physical functioning
in all systems (cardiovascular,
immune, etc.)
Adequate sleep and rest
Adequate nutrition

Social
Social functioning
Positive interpersonal
relationships
Positive work experience
Maintenance of social activities

Psychological
Psychological well-being
Positive self-esteem
Confidence

FIGURE 35.2 Biopsychosocial adaptation.

studies support this connection, the underlying mechanisms have not yet been elucidated. Abundant research, however, indicates that stress and coping are related to a person's health status. Extreme stress can produce deleterious effects on a person's health by exacerbating already existing health problems or contributing to the development of new ones. Once a health problem exists, it becomes part of the stress equation; that is, once a person has an illness or disorder, it can interfere with the ability to cope with other situations.

Health is negatively affected when coping is ineffective. When the damaging condition or situation is not ameliorated or the emotional distress is not regulated, stress occurs that in turn affects a person's health. The wrong coping strategy for a given situation will be ineffective. For instance, if emotion-focused coping is used when a problem-focused approach is appropriate, stress is not relieved. Also, if a coping strategy violates cultural norms and lifestyle, stress is often exaggerated. Some coping strategies actually increase the risk for mortality and morbidity, such as the excessive use of alcohol, drugs, or tobacco. Many people use overeating, smoking, or drinking to reduce stress. They may feel better temporarily but are actually increasing their risk for illness. For people whose behaviors exacerbate their illnesses, learning new behaviors becomes important. Healthy coping strategies such as exercising and obtaining adequate sleep and nutrition contribute to stress reduction and the promotion of long-term health.

Psychological Well-Being

If a person feels good about the end result of a stressful encounter, that is an ideal outcome. Whether a person has positive feelings about the results depends on whether he or she views the outcome as satisfactory. Appraising a situation as challenging, rather than harmful or threatening, is more likely to result in increased self-confidence and a sense of well-being. An encounter that a person accurately appraises as harmful or threatening is more likely to have a positive outcome if the person views it as manageable.

Outcome satisfaction for one person does not necessarily represent outcome satisfaction for another. For instance, suppose that two young men receive the same passing score on an examination. One man may feel a sense of relief, but the other may feel anxious because he appraises his score as too low. Understanding a person's emotional response to an outcome is essential to analyzing its personal meaning. People who consistently have positive outcomes from stressful experiences are more likely to have positive self-esteem and self-confidence. Unsatisfactory outcomes from stressful experiences are associated with negative mood states, such as depression, anger, guilt leading to decreased self-esteem, and feelings of helplessness.

Social Functioning

Social functioning, the performance of daily activities within the context of interpersonal relations and family and community roles, can be seriously impaired during stressful episodes. For instance, a person who is experiencing the stress of a divorce may not be able to carry out job responsibilities satisfactorily. If successful coping with a stressful encounter leads to a positive outcome, social functioning returns to normal or is improved. If the person views the outcome as unsuccessful and experiences negative emotions, social functioning will continue to be impaired.

NURSING MANAGEMENT: HUMAN RESPONSE TO DISORDER

Individuals experiencing stress may or may not have a diagnosis designated by the American Psychiatric Association (APA). If an existing Axis I or II disorder is present, the stress responses are usually conceptualized within the particular diagnosis. If there are significant emotional or behavioral symptoms in response to an identifiable stressful situation but the psychiatric disorder does not account for the response or there is no existing disorder, a diagnosis of adjustment disorder may be made. This residual category is used to describe responses to a stressful situation that do not meet criteria for an Axis I disorder. There are six subtypes: with depressed mood, with anxiety, with anxiety and depressed mood, with disturbance of conduct, with mixed disturbance of emotions and conduct, and unspecified. To be classified as an adjustment disorder, the onset of the emotional or behavioral response has to be within 3 months of the stressful situation and last for no more than 6 months after the stressor (APA, 2000) (Table 35-7).

Nurses provide service to individuals who are currently experiencing stress and those who are high risk for stress. The overall goals for those with active stress responses are to eliminate the unfavorable person–environment situations (when possible), reduce the stress response, and develop positive coping skills. The goals for those who are at high risk for stress (experiencing recent life changes, vulnerable to stress, or have limited coping mechanisms) are to recognize the potential for stressful situations and strengthen positive coping skills. These people benefit from education and practice of new coping skills. They often access the nurse through health promotion services. Those actually experiencing stress require a more intense level of intervention than those who are high risk for stress.

TABLE 35.7 Key Diagnostic Characteristics of Adjustment Disorder	
Diagnostic Criteria	**Target Symptoms and Associated Findings**
• Emotional or behavioral symptoms in response to an identifiable stressor occurring within 3 months of the onset of the stressors. • Clinically significant symptoms or behaviors (1) are characterized by distress that is in excess of what would be expected from exposure to the stressor, or (2) cause a significant impairment in social or occupational (academic) functioning. • Stress-related disturbance does not meet the criteria for another specific Axis I disorder and is not merely an exacerbation of a pre-existing Axis I or Axis II disorder. • Symptoms do not represent bereavement. • Symptoms do not persist for more than 6 months after the stressor has terminated. Acute: disturbance lasts more than 6 months Chronic: disturbance lasts for 6 months or longer 309.0 With depressed mood 309.24 With anxiety 309.28 With mixed anxiety and depressed mood 309.3 With disturbance of conduct 309.4 With mixed disturbance of emotions and conduct 309.9 Unspecified	• Subjective distress or impairment in functioning • Decreased performance at work or school • Temporary changes in relationships *Associated Physical Examination Findings* • Decreased compliance with recommended medical regimen

This section explains nursing management for those experiencing a stress response.

Assessing Human Responses to Stress

Stress responses vary from one person to another. Some people have primarily somatic responses, such as headaches, dermatitis, flushing, or stomach pains. Others experience fear and apprehension or withdraw from social situations. Usually, the person becomes emotionally upset and cannot think clearly for a short time. Nursing assessment in these situations is fairly complex because the nurse must consider many aspects: the situation, the biologic responses, the emotions, and the coping responses. From the assessment data, the nurse can determine any illnesses, the intensity of the stress response, and the effectiveness of coping strategies. Nurses typically identify stress responses in people or family members who are receiving treatment for other health problems.

Biologic Assessment

The nurse should include a careful health history, focusing on past and present illnesses in the assessment. An illness or a recent trauma may be either a result of or a contributing factor to stress. If a psychiatric disorder is present, psychiatric symptoms may spontaneously reappear even when no alteration has occurred in the patient's medication regimen. Nurses should also pay special attention to disorders of the neuroendocrine system, such as hypothyroidism. These illnesses can significantly affect the person's ability to deal with stress.

Review of Systems. A review of systems highlights the susceptibility of different biologic areas. Because physiologic responses to stress result from the activation of the sympathetic nervous system and the immune system, the person may experience symptoms from any of the body systems. A systems review can elicit the person's own unique response to stress (Table 35-8). A systems review can also provide important data on the effect of chronic illnesses. Thus, biologic data are useful for analyzing the person–environment situation and the person's stress reactions, coping responses, and adaptation.

Physical Functioning. Physical functioning usually changes during a stress response. Typically, sleep is disturbed, appetite either increases or decreases, body weight fluctuates, and sexual activity changes. Physical appearance may be uncharacteristically disheveled—a projection of the person's feelings. Body language expresses muscle tension, which conveys a state of anxiety not usually present. Because exercise is an important strategy in stress reduction, the nurse should assess the amount of physical activity, tolerance for exercise, and usual exercise patterns. Sometimes, a person was exercising regularly until changes in daily activities interrupted the routine. Determining the details of the person's exercise pattern can help in formulating reasonable interventions.

Pharmacologic Assessment. In assessing a person's coping strategies, the nurse needs to ask about the use of alcohol, tobacco, marijuana, and any other addic-

TABLE 35.8	Physiologic Stress-Related Symptoms
System	**Symptom**
Cardiovascular	Headache
	Chest pain
	Increased pulse
	Palpitations
	Fainting (blackouts, spells)
	Increased blood pressure
Respiratory	Shortness of breath
	Smoking history
	Increased rate and depth of breathing
	Chest discomfort (pain, tightness, ache)
Gastrointestinal	Nausea
	Vomiting
	Abdominal pain (cramps, stomach ache)
	Change in appetite
	Change in stool
	Obesity/frequent weight changes
Musculoskeletal	Pain
	Weakness
	Fatigue
Genitourinary	Menstrual changes
	Urinary discomforts (pain, burning, urgency, hesitancy)
	Sexual difficulty (pain, impotence, altered libido, anorgasmia)
Dermatologic	Itching
	Rash
	"Sweats"
	Eczema

Adapted from Carpenito, L. (2000). *Nursing diagnosis: Application to clinical practice* (8th ed.) (p. 265). Philadelphia: Lippincott Williams & Wilkins.

tive substances. Many people begin or increase the frequency of using these substances as a way of coping with stress. In turn, substance abuse contributes to the stress behavior. Knowing details about the person's use of these substances (number of times a day or week, amount, circumstances, side effects) helps in determining the role these substances play in overall stress reduction or management. The more important the substances are in the person's handling of stress, the more difficult it will be to change the addictive behavior.

Stress often prompts people to use anxiolytics without provider supervision. Use of over-the-counter sleep

medications for sleep disturbances is common. The nurse should carefully assess the use of any drugs to manage stress symptoms. If someone is using medication as a primary coping strategy, he or she may need further evaluation and referral to a mental health specialist. If the person is being treated for a psychiatric disorder, the nurse should assess him or her for medication compliance, especially if the psychiatric symptoms are reappearing.

Psychological Assessment

Unlike assessment for other health problems, psychological assessment of the person under stress does not ordinarily include a mental status examination. Instead, psychological assessment focuses on the person's emotions and their severity and his or her coping strategies. The assessment elicits the person's appraisal of risks and benefits, the personal meaning of the situation, and the person's commitment to a particular outcome. The nurse can then understand how vulnerable the person is to stress.

Using therapeutic communication techniques, the nurse assesses a person's emotional state in a nurse–patient interview. By beginning the interview with a statement such as, "Let's talk about what you have been feeling," the nurse can elicit the feelings that the person has been experiencing. Because emotions have different behavioral manifestations (tears for sadness, tenseness for anxiety), these responses can be indicators of specific emotions. Identifying the person's emotions can be helpful in assessing the intensity of the stress being experienced. Emotions often thought of as negative (anger, fright, anxiety, guilt, shame, sadness, envy, jealousy, and disgust) are usually associated with an inability to cope and severe stress.

After identifying the person's emotions, the nurse determines how the person reacts initially to them. For example, does the person who is angry respond by carrying out the innate urge to attack someone whom the person blames for the situation? Or does that person respond by thinking through the situation and overriding the initial innate urge to act? The person who tends to act impulsively has few real coping skills. The nurse should consider a nursing diagnosis of Ineffective Coping. For the person who can resist the innate urge to act and has developed coping skills, the focus of the assessment becomes determining their effectiveness.

According to the stress, coping, and adaptation model, there are two types of coping: problem-solving coping and emotion-focused coping (see Table 35-6). Each type can be effective in certain situations. In an assessment interview, the nurse can determine whether the person uses coping strategies effectively.

Problem-focused coping is effective when the person can accurately assess the situation. In this case, the person sets goals, seeks information, masters new skills, and seeks help as needed. Emotion-focused coping is effective when the person has inaccurately assessed the situation and coping corrects the false interpretation. Among the various emotion-focused coping strategies are minimizing the seriousness of the situation and projecting, displacing, or suppressing feelings (Table 35-9).

Social Assessment

Social assessment data are invaluable in determining the person's resources. The ability to make healthy lifestyle changes is strongly influenced by the person's health beliefs and family support system. Even the expression of stress is related to social factors, particularly cultural expectations and values. The assessment should include discovering the person's social network, social support, and underlying sociocultural attitudes and beliefs that relate to the current stress.

Recent Life Changes. Assessment should include use of the Life Change Event Questionnaire to determine the number and importance of life changes that the patient has experienced within the past year. If several recent life changes have occurred, the person–environment relationship has changed. The person is likely to be either at high risk for or already experiencing stress.

Social Network and Social Support. Social assessment includes identification of the person's social network. Because employment is the mainstay of adulthood and the source of many personal contacts, assessment of any recent changes in employment status is important. If a person is unemployed, the nurse should determine the significance of the unemployment and its effects on the person's social network. For children and adolescents, nurses should note any recent changes in their attendance at school. The nurse should elicit the following data:

- Size and extent of the network, both relatives and nonrelatives, professional and nonprofessional, and how long known
- Functions that the network serves (eg, intimacy, social integration, nurturance, reassurance of worth, guidance and advice, access to new contacts)
- Degree of reciprocity between the patient and other network members, that is, who provides support to the patient and who the patient supports
- Degree of interconnectedness, that is, how many of the network members know one another and are in contact (Simmons, 1994)

The nurse should assess both the supportive and non-supportive relationships within the patient's environment. The Malone Social Network Inventory (MSNI) is a scale that assesses a person's social relationships by using an open-ended interview format. The patient specifies who is helpful in his or her environment and who is not. The patient can use this inventory to assess the helpfulness of those who most and least affect his or her life and to determine those who are members of the patient's formal and informal groups (eg, work, clubs, religious organizations). The MSNI elicits the following information:

- Who is in the network
- The relationship (eg, spouse, child, minister)
- A brief description of what each relationship provides
- The degree of helpfulness
- The expected degree of helpfulness (Malone, 1988, p. 20)

On the inventory, the patient responds on a scale of 1 to 5 (highest) as to how helpful each person in the environment is. Next, the patient responds to how helpful they should be. A variation in scores between how helpful the person is and how helpful he or she should be gives a dissonance score—the discrepancy between the reality of the relationship and what the person would like the relationship to be. The higher the score, the higher the dissonance (Table 35-10).

Nursing Diagnosis and Outcome Identification

The nurse can generate several nursing diagnoses from the assessment data. The data may support any nursing diagnosis that involves the person–environment interaction related to a stress response (Anxiety, Powerlessness, Fear, Fatigue, Low Self-Esteem) or a coping process (Ineffective Coping, Disabled Family Coping, Ineffective Role Performance). The challenge of generating nursing diagnoses is to make sure that they are based on the person's appraisal of the situation. A response to stress is not a problem unless the person views it as one.

Outcomes should be individualized for each diagnosis. People who are experiencing stress are not usually hospitalized. They live in the community and seek services in community clinics, in private providers' offices, and at wellness centers. Stress in people who have an existing mental or physical disorder, however, may be detected while they are in the hospital. These people should receive follow-up care for the stress response after they are discharged. Caregivers of people with long-term or complicated illnesses should be considered at high risk for stress.

TABLE 35.9 Problem-Focused and Emotion-Focused Behaviors

Behavior	Problem or Emotion Focused	Definition	Effective	Ineffective
Goal setting	Problem focused	The conscious process of setting time limitations on behavior	When goals are attainable and manageable; eg, making an appointment with boss to discuss pay raise	When the appraisal of the situation is missed or inaccurately evaluated
Information seeking	Problem focused	Process of learning about all aspects of a problem that provides perspective and reinforces self-control	When situations are complex and additional information is needed; eg, attending a parent effectiveness class because of being unsure about discipline techniques	When the needed information is already obtained and the activity delays action
Mastery	Problem focused	Learning of new procedures or skills that facilitate self-esteem, reinforce self-control	When there are new procedures to learn; eg, self-care activities, insulin injection, catheter care	When the situation does not require learning new procedures, or they have nothing to do with the stressful situation
Help seeking	Problem focused	Reaching out to others for support; sharing feelings provides an emotional release, reassurance, and comfort	When similar problems are shared by others; eg, in Alcoholics Anonymous, weight loss programs, psychosocial programs	When using help seeking to avoid action in the current situation
Minimization	Emotion focused	The seriousness of the problem is minimized	Useful way of providing needed time for appraisal; eg, a person is told that her child is in an automobile accident and forces herself to think the accident is minor until additional information is received	When the appraisal of the situation is missed or inaccurately evaluated
Projection, displacement, and suppression of anger	Emotion focused	When anger is attributed to or expressed toward a less-threatening person or thing	When threat is reduced, the individual can deal with the situation; eg, the boss reprimands a worker for submitting a report late—the worker in turn hits his fist on the copying machine as he walks by	When reality is distorted and relationships disturbed, which further compounds the problem; suppression of anger may result in stress-related physical symptoms
Anticipatory preparation	Emotion focused	Mental rehearsal of possible consequences of behavior or outcomes of stressful situations	Provides the opportunity to develop perspective as well as to prepare for the worst; eg, when waiting for exam results, the patient develops a plan of action if the results are negative	When anticipation creates unmanageable stress as in anticipatory mourning
Attribution	Emotion focused	Finding personal meaning in the problem situation, which may be through religious faith or individual belief	May offer consolation; eg, fate, the will of the divine, luck	When all sense of self-responsibility is lost

Adapted from Carpenito, L. (2000). *Nursing diagnosis: Application to clinical practice* (8th ed.) (pp. 261–262). Philadelphia: Lippincott Williams & Wilkins.

TABLE 35.10   Malone Social Network Inventory

Initials	Relationship	What Relationship Provides	Level 1 (lowest)–5 (highest) Helpfulness Rating	
			Is	Should Be

From Malone, J. (1994). The social support dissupport continuum. *Journal of Psychosocial Nursing, 26*(12), 21.

Planning and Implementing Nursing Interventions

Biologic Interventions

People under stress can usually benefit from several biologic interventions. Their activities of daily living are usually interrupted, and they often feel that they have no time for themselves. The stressed patient who is normally fastidiously groomed and dressed may appear disheveled and unkempt. Simply reinstating the daily routine of shaving (for a man) or applying makeup (for a woman) can improve the person's outlook on life and ability to cope with the stress (see Chap. 14).

Stress is commonly manifested in the areas of nutrition and activity. During stressful periods, a person's eating patterns change. To cope with stress, a person may either overeat or become anorexic. Both are ineffective coping behaviors and actually contribute to stress. Educating the patient about the importance of maintaining an adequate diet during the period of stress will highlight its importance. It will also allow the nurse to help the person decide how eating behaviors can be changed.

Exercise can reduce the emotional and behavioral responses to stress. In addition to the physical benefits of exercise, a regular exercise routine can provide structure to a person's life, enhance self-confidence, and increase feelings of well-being. People who are stressed are often not receptive to the idea of exercise, particularly if it has not been a part of their routine. Exploring the patient's personal beliefs about the value of activity will help to determine whether exercise is a reasonable activity for that person.

The person under stress tends to be tense, nervous, and on edge. Simple relaxation techniques help the person relax and may improve coping skills. If these techniques do not help the patient relax, the nurse may teach distraction or guided imagery to the patient (see Chap. 14). Nurses should consider referral to a mental health specialist for hypnosis or biofeedback for patients who have severe stress responses.

Psychological Interventions

Numerous psychological interventions help reduce stress and support coping efforts. All the interventions are best carried out within the framework of a supportive nurse–patient relationship. The Nursing Interventions Classification (NIC) interventions in the behavioral domain support psychological functioning and facilitate lifestyle changes. The NIC includes six classes of useful generalist and specialist nursing interventions: behavior therapy, cognitive therapy, communication enhancement, coping assistance, patient education, and psychological comfort promotion. The interventions are listed in Table 35-11. Depending on the nursing diagnosis, the nurse may use any one of these interventions.

Social Interventions

Because the experience of stress and the ability to cope are a result of the appraisal of the person–environment relationship, interventions that affect the environment are important. People who are coping with stressful situations can often benefit from interventions that facilitate family unit functioning and promote the health and welfare of family members. For the nurse to intervene

TABLE 35.11 Interventions for Stress Reduction and Coping Enhancement

Behavior Therapy*	Cognitive Therapy	Communication Enhancement	Coping Assistance Interventions	Patient Education	Psychological Comfort Promotion
Reinforce or promote desirable behaviors or alter undesirable behaviors	Reinforce or promote desirable cognitive functioning or alter undesirable functioning	Facilitate interaction *or* receive or deliver verbal or nonverbal messages	Help another to build on own strengths, adapt to a change in function, or achieve a higher level of function	Facilitate learning	Promote comfort using psychological techniques
Generalist Interventions					
Assertiveness training	Anger control	Active listening	Anticipatory guidance	Learning facilitation	Anxiety reduction
Behavior management	Bibliotherapy	Communication enhancement	Body image enhancement	Learning readiness enhancement	Calming technique
Behavior modification	Reality orientation	Socialization enhancement	Counseling	Parent education	Distraction
Limit setting			Grief work facilitation	Teaching: disease process	Simple guided imagery
Mutual goal setting			Guilt work facilitation	Teaching: group, individual	Simple relaxation therapy
Patient contracting			Decision-making support	Teaching: activity, exercise, diet, medication, procedure/treatment, psychomotor skills, safe sex	
Self-modification assistance			Care of the dying		
Self-responsibility assistance			Emotional support		
Smoking cessation assistance			Hope instillation		
Substance use prevention			Humor		
Activity therapy			Role enhancement		
			Recreation therapy		
			Self-awareness enhancement		
			Self-esteem enhancement		
			Spiritual support		
			Support system enhancement		
			Values clarification		
Specialist (Advanced Practice) Interventions†					
Psychotherapy	Psychotherapy	Psychotherapy	Psychotherapy, individual and group	Same as generalist	Psychopharmacologic agents prescribed
Consultation	Consultation	Consultation	Consultation		Autogenic training
Animal-assisted therapy	Cognitive restructuring	Complex relationship building	Genetic counseling		Biofeedback
Substance use treatment	Cognitive stimulation	Music therapy	Grief therapy		Hypnosis
Art therapy	Memory training	Art therapy	Guilt work		Meditation
	Reminiscence therapy	Play therapy	Sexual counseling		
		Animal-assisted therapy	Touch therapy		

*Behavioral interventions: care that supports psychological functioning and facilitates lifestyle changes.
†Specialist interventions require additional training. Specialist interventions are in addition to those at the generalist level.
McCloskey, J., & Bulechek, G. (1996). *Nursing interventions classification (NIC)*. St. Louis: Mosby.

with the total family, the stressed person must agree for the family members to be involved. If the data gathered from the assessment of supportive and dissupportive relationships indicate that the family members are not supportive, the nurse should assist the patient to consider expanding his or her social network. If the family is the major source of support, the nurse should design interventions that support the functioning of the family unit.

Nurses can use many interventions to support the functioning of the family unit. The NIC includes the following generalist interventions in family care: caregiver support, family integrity promotion, family involvement, family mobilization, family process maintenance, family support, respite care, and home maintenance assistance. Parent education can also be effective in supporting family unit functioning. If family therapy is needed, the nurse should refer the family to an advanced practice specialist.

Evaluation and Treatment Outcomes

The treatment outcomes established in the initial plan of care guide the evaluation. Individual outcomes relate to improved health, well-being, and social function. Depending on the level of intervention, there can also be family and network outcomes. Family outcomes may be related to improved communication or social support. For instance, caregiver stress is reduced once other members of the family help in the care of the ill member. Social network outcomes focus on modifying the social network.

CRISIS

A crisis is a severely stressful experience for which coping mechanisms fail to provide any adaptation, whether the experience is positive or negative. Usually, a crisis occurs when the precipitating event is unusual or rare. For example, one woman coped with chronic physical abuse by her husband, who abused both drugs and alcohol. She managed to cope with her stressful living situation by maladaptive means—smoking and withdrawing from her husband with a chronic headache. When the woman discovered that her husband had been sexually abusing their 7-year-old daughter, she moved into a shelter. She had few economic resources and no social supports. When she left her husband, chronic stress became a crisis.

Either internal or external demands that are perceived as threats to a person's physical or emotional functioning can initiate a crisis. If a person has the biopsychosocial resources to cope with the threat, a crisis does not occur. If the person's coping methods are insufficient to deal with the threat, tension rises, and normal functioning (occupational, social, or familial) is disrupted.

KEY CONCEPT **Crisis.** **Crisis** is a severely stressful experience for which coping mechanisms fail to provide any adaptation, whether the experience is positive or negative.

The person's habits and coping patterns are suspended. Often, unexpected emotional (eg, depression) and biologic (eg, nausea, vomiting, diarrhea, headaches) responses occur. Even though a person may become extremely anxious, depressed, or elated, feeling states do not determine whether a person is in a crisis. If biopsychosocial functioning is severely impaired, then a crisis is occurring.

A state of crisis is generally regarded as time limited, lasting no more than 4 to 6 weeks. At the end of that time, the person in crisis has begun to come to grips with the event and to harness resources to cope with its long-term consequences. By definition, there is no such thing as a chronic crisis. People who live in constant turmoil are not in crisis but in chaos (Callahan, 1994). A crisis can also represent a turning point in a person's life, with either positive or negative outcomes. It can be an opportunity for growth and change because new ways of coping are learned.

A crisis should not be viewed as a psychiatric emergency, which requires immediate intervention. Psychiatric emergencies, including potential suicide, potential violence, and acute psychosis, require immediate response to prevent physical harm or serious biopsychosocial deterioration (Callahan, 1994). A patient in crisis needs to be seen soon but not immediately. Many people do not seek out help until several weeks after the event has occurred and difficulties in functioning are being noticed.

A person in crisis should not be viewed as having a mental disorder. If the person is significantly distressed or his or her social functioning is impaired, however, a diagnosis of acute stress disorder should be considered (APA, 2000). The person with an acute stress disorder has dissociative symptoms and persistently reexperiences the event (APA, 2000) (Table 35-12).

Many life events can evoke a crisis. Lindemann studied the bereavement of those who lost loved ones during a catastrophic community fire (Text Box 35-3). Other obvious crisis-evoking events include natural and man-made disasters (floods, fires, tornadoes, earthquakes, wars, bombings, and airplane crashes), trauma (rape, sexual abuse, assault), and interpersonal crises (divorce, marriage, birth of a child). The crisis response is similar in all these different situations. First, an event occurs that is perceived by the person as a threat and for which the usual coping methods do not work. Tension builds, and the person attempts to adapt to the situation by using new coping techniques that emerge naturally or are supported by helpers. If adaptation occurs, the person is able to cope with future threat-

TABLE 35.12 Key Diagnostic Characteristics of Acute Stress Disorder

Diagnostic Criteria	Target Symptoms and Associated Findings
• Experienced, witnessed, or was confronted with an event or events that involved actual or threatened death or serious injury, or threat to the physical integrity of self or others • Intense fear, helplessness, or horror • Dissociative symptoms (at least three), including a subjective sense of numbing, detachment, or absence of emotional responsiveness, reduction in awareness of surroundings ("being in a daze"), derealization, depersonalization, dissociative amnesia (inability to recall important aspects of trauma) • Traumatic event is persistently re-experienced—recurrent images, thoughts, dreams, flashbacks, illusions • Anxiety or increased arousal • Causes significant distress or impairment in social, occupational, or other important areas of functioning • Disturbance lasts for at least 2 days and no more than 4 weeks; occurs within 4 weeks of the traumatic event • Disturbance is not due to direct physiologic effects of substance abuse or other medical conditions.	• Despair and hopelessness • Guilt (especially if patient survived a trauma and others did not) about not providing enough help to others • Neglects basic health and safety needs • Impulsive and risk-taking behavior • Increased risk for posttraumatic stress disorder *Associated Physical Examination Findings* • General medical conditions may occur as a result of the trauma (eg, head injury, burns)

TEXT BOX 35.3

Historical Perspective on Understanding Crises

Our understanding of the biopsychosocial implications of a crisis began in the 1950s when Eric Lindemann studied bereavement reactions among the friends and relatives of the victims of the Coconut Grove nightclub fire in Boston in 1942. That fire, in which 493 people died, was the worst single building fire in the country's history at that time. Lindemann's goal was to develop prevention approaches at the community level that would maintain good health and prevent emotional disorganization. He described both grief and prolonged reactions as a result of loss of a significant person. From these results, he hypothesized that during the course of one's life, situations occur—such as the birth of a child, marriage, and death—that evoke adaptive mechanisms leading either to mastery of a new situation (psychological growth) or impairment in functioning.

In 1961, psychiatrist Gerald Caplan defined a crisis as occurring when a person faces a problem that cannot be solved by customary methods of problem solving. When the usual problem-solving methods no longer work, a person's life balance of equilibrium is upset. During the period of disequilibrium, there is a rise in inner tension and anxiety followed by emotional upset and an inability to function (Caplan, 1961). Caplan argued that during a crisis, a person is open to learning new ways of coping to survive the current crisis. The outcome of a crisis is governed by the kind of interaction that occurs between the person and his or her key social contacts. Research has focused on categorizing types of crisis events, understanding biopsychosocial responses to crisis, and developing intervention models that support people through crisis.

ening events. If the person cannot cope, overall functioning decreases, and the person does not return to the precrisis level of functioning.

Developmental Crisis

While Lindemann and Caplan were creating their crisis model, Erik Erikson was formulating his ideas about crisis and development. He proposed that maturational crises are a normal part of growth and development and that successfully resolving a crisis at one stage allows the child to move to the next. According to this model, the child develops positive characteristics if he or she resolves the crisis successfully, whereas he or she develops less desirable traits if the crisis is not resolved (see Chap. 6).

The concept of developmental crisis assumes that psychosocial development progresses by an easily identifiable, orderly process. The developmental models such as the ones proposed by Miller and Gilligan do not fit into a stage model (see Chap. 6). The concept of developmental crisis, however, continues to be used today to describe unfavorable person–environment relationships that relate to maturational events, such as leaving home for the first time, completing school, or accepting the responsibility of adulthood.

Situational Crisis

A situational crisis occurs whenever a stressful event threatens a person's biopsychosocial integrity and results in some degree of disequilibrium. The event can be an internal one, such as a disease process, or any number of external threats. A move to another city, a job promotion, or graduation from high school can initiate a crisis, even though they are positive events. For example, graduation from high school marks the end of an established routine of going to school, participating in school activities, and doing homework assignments. On starting a new job after graduation, the former student must learn an entirely different routine and acquire new knowledge and skills. If a person enters a new situation without adequate coping skills, a crisis can develop.

Anne Burgess, a psychiatric nurse and one of the foremost experts in crisis intervention, and her colleague Lynda Holmstrom have identified another category of situational crisis, *victim crisis.* They argue that in certain situations, people must face overwhelmingly hazardous events that may entail injury, trauma, destruction, or sacrifice. Such an event involves a physically aggressive and forced act by a person, a group, or an environment. National disasters (eg, racial persecutions, riots, war) and violent crimes (eg, rape, murder, and assault and battery) are examples (Burgess & Holmstrom, 1979).

Death of a Loved One: A Crisis Event

One of the most common crisis-provoking events is the loss of a loved one. Even though death is a certainty, much is unknown about the process of death. Fear of the unknown contributes to the mystique of death for the person who is dying as well as the loved one. **Bereavement,** the process of grieving, can last months or years, but it begins during a crisis.

Phases of Bereavement

Normally, the death of a loved one produces feelings of grief (Aguilera, 1993). Any subsequent loss can also reactivate these feelings. Bereavement is conceptualized in phases that are useful in describing the grieving process; however, these phases should not be considered universal. Individual differences and cultural practices influence the grieving process. Even though these phases are discussed as if progression from one to another is linear, in reality, they may be concurrent or vary from the proposed phase sequence. The nurse can use the following phases to understand the process but should not use them to determine whether a patient is experiencing normal grief (Text Box 35-4).

Shock and Disbelief. During the first phase, the person is in a state of shock and disbelief. This stage lasts from hours to weeks and is characterized by varying degrees of disbelief and denial of the loss (Zisook, 1987). The person experiences tightness in the throat, chok-

TEXT BOX 35.4

Stages of Grief

I. Shock: denial and disbelief

II. Acute mourning

   A. Intense feeling states: crying spells, guilt, shame, depression, anorexia, insomnia, irritability, emptiness, and fatigue

   B. Social withdrawal: preoccupation with health; inability to sustain usual work, family, and personal relationships

   C. Identification with the deceased: transient adoption of habits, mannerisms, and somatic symptoms of the deceased

III. Resolution: acceptance of loss, awareness of having grieved, return to well-being, and ability to recall the decreased without subjective pain

Reprinted from Zisook, S. (1987). Unresolved grief. In S. Zisook (Ed.), *Biopsychosocial aspects of bereavement* (p. 25). Washington, DC: American Psychiatric Press.

ing, shortness of breath, a need to sigh, an empty feeling in the abdomen, and a lack of muscular power. The person has a sense of unreality, feels increased emotional distance from others, and is intensely preoccupied with the image of the deceased. Also, the person may harbor exaggerated guilt feelings for minor negligence. Mourning rites, family, and friends facilitate the passage through this phase.

Acute Mourning. The acute mourning phase begins when the person becomes gradually aware of the loss. This phase, which may last several months, has three distinct periods:

> *Intense feeling:* The person becomes disorganized and experiences waves of intense pain. An insatiable yearning for the deceased person occurs. The person cries, feels helpless, and possibly identifies with or idealizes the deceased.
>
> *Social withdrawal:* In an attempt to avoid pain, the person avoids other people, including friends. The person feels irritable or angry, misses work, and emotionally distances himself or herself from others. The person spends time searching for evidence of failure in the relationship.
>
> *Identification with the deceased:* The person's thought content and affect become consumed by the deceased. Mourners may adopt mannerisms, habits, and somatic symptoms of the deceased (Zisook, 1987).

Resolution. Gradually, the person experiences the return of feelings of well-being and the ability to continue with life. He or she reviews the relationship with the deceased and realizes the sorrow and sense of loss.

The person recognizes that he or she has been grieving and now is ready to focus on the rest of the world. Finally, it is possible to reexperience pleasure and seek the companionship and love of others.

The bereavement process is often applied to other situations in which a loss occurs but not necessarily the death of a person. The "empty nest syndrome" is an example of bereavement for children who have grown up and left home. This bereavement experience is less intense than that triggered by a loss through death, but the bereaved person nevertheless has many of the same responses. Interventions may also be needed in this type of situation.

Dysfunctional Grieving

Grieving is a normal process of life. Dysfunctional grieving occurs when the grief response is either absent or exaggerated. Determining exactly what abnormal grieving is, however, is difficult. The absence of a grief reaction to a loss of a significant person is considered abnormal. If a person does not exhibit grief in response to a significant loss, he or she will eventually have a reaction.

Dysfunctional grieving occurs if a person fails to move from one bereavement phase to another (Table 35-13). When a person becomes stuck in one phase, he or she experiences exaggerated grief feelings associated with that phase. For example, depressive symptoms in a person who remains in the acute mourning phase become a full-blown depressive episode. In dysfunctional grieving, the bereaved becomes a chronic mourner, fixed on the deceased and events surrounding the person's death. Dysfunctional grieving often leads to depression.

NURSING MANAGEMENT: HUMAN RESPONSE TO DISORDER

The goal for people experiencing a crisis is to return to the precrisis level of adaptation. The nurse's role is to support the patient through the crisis and to facilitate the use of positive coping skills. For people who are experiencing a crisis, nursing management can easily serve as a framework for care.

Assessing Human Responses to Crises

Assessment of a person in crisis is similar to assessment of a person under stress. If a person is in crisis, however, he or she may be at high risk for suicide or homicide. The nurse should complete a careful assessment of suicidal or homicidal risk. If a person is at high risk for either, the nurse should consider hospitalization.

Biologic Assessment

Biologic assessment focuses on areas that usually undergo change during extreme stress. Eliciting information about changes in health practices provides important data that the nurse can use to ascertain the severity of the disruption in functioning. Biologic functioning is important because a crisis can be physically exhausting. Disturbances in sleep and eating patterns and the reappearance of physical or psychiatric symptoms are common. If the person's sleep patterns are disturbed or nutrition is inadequate, he or she will not have the physical resources to deal with the crisis. Pharmacologic interventions may be needed to help maintain a high level of physical functioning.

Psychological Assessment

Psychological assessment focuses on the person's emotions and coping strengths. In the beginning of the crisis, the person may report feeling numb and in shock. Later, as the reality of the crisis sinks in, he or she will be able to recognize the felt emotions. The nurse should expect those emotions to be intense and will need to provide some support during their expression. At the beginning of a crisis, coping by problem solving may be disrupted. By assessing the person's ability to solve prob-

TABLE 35.13 Syndromes Associated With Nonresolution of Grief		
Phase	**Resolution**	**Nonresolution**
I. Shock-denial	Acceptance	Psychotic denial
II. Acute mourning		
A. Intense feeling states	Equanimity	Depression
B. Withdrawal	Reinvolvement	Hypochondriasis
C. Identification	Individuation	Grief-related facsimile illness
III. Resolution	Work, love, play	Chronic mourning

Reprinted from Zisook, S. (1987). Unresolved grief. In S. Zisook (Ed.), *Biopsychosocial aspects of bereavement* (p. 25). Washington, DC: American Psychiatric Press.

lems, the nurse can judge whether the person can cognitively cope with the stressful situation and determine the amount of support needed.

Social Assessment

Assessment of the impact of the crisis on the person's social functioning is essential because a crisis usually severely disrupts social aspects. Shelter, money, and food may not be available. Basic human needs such as a place to live or immediate transportation can quickly become a priority.

Nursing Diagnosis and Outcome Identification

Many nursing diagnoses are appropriate for the person experiencing a crisis. Some were presented earlier in the chapter. Those that typically relate to crisis include Grieving, Post-Trauma Syndrome, or Relocation Stress Syndrome.

Planning and Implementing Nursing Interventions

Many nursing interventions previously discussed are useful for the person in crisis. The person's safety needs are of paramount importance, including protection from suicide or homicide. Addressing the person's need for shelter and food is also a priority. Approaches to crisis intervention and examples are presented in Table 35-14.

During a disaster that affects many people, such as a flood or hurricane, the nurse's interventions will be a part of the community's efforts to respond to the crisis. On the other hand, when a personal crisis occurs, the person in crisis may have only the nurse to respond to his or her needs. After the assessment, the generalist nurse must decide whether to provide the care needed or to refer the person to a mental health specialist. The decision tree in Text Box 35-5 offers guidance in making that decision.

Psychopharmacologic Interventions

Medication cannot resolve a crisis, but the judicious use of psychopharmacologic agents can help reduce its

---

TABLE 35.14 Guidelines for Crisis Intervention

Approach	Rationale	Example
Assist the person in confronting reality.	During the crisis experience, the person may use denial as a coping mechanism. Denial is ineffective in resolving the crisis. Emotional support will help the person face reality.	Accompany the husband to view the body of his deceased wife.
Encourage the expression of feelings (within limits).	Identification and expression of feelings about the crisis events help the person understand the significance of the crisis.	Encourage a woman who survived a house fire but lost her home to explore the meaning of the lost home.
Encourage the person to focus on one implication at a time.	Focusing on all the implications at once can be too overwhelming.	A woman left her husband because of abuse. At first, focus only on living arrangements and safety. At another time, discuss the other implications of the separation.
Avoid giving false reassurances, such as "It will be all right."	Giving false reassurances blocks communication. It may not be all right.	Patient: "My doctor told me that I have a terminal illness." Nurse: "What does that mean to you?"
Clarify fantasies with facts.	Accurate information is needed to problem solve.	A young mother believes that her comatose child will regain consciousness, although the medical evidence contradicts it. Gently clarify the meaning of the medical evidence.
Link the person and family with community resources, as needed.	Strengthening the person's social network so that social support can be obtained reduces the effect of the crisis.	Provide information about a meeting of a support group such as that of the American Cancer Society.

Adapted from Lazarus, R. (1991). *Emotion and adaptation* (p. 122). New York: Oxford University Press.

TEXT BOX 35.5

Decision Tree for Determining Referral

Situation: A 35-year-old woman is being seen in a clinic because of minor burns she received during a house fire. Her home was completely destroyed. She is tearful and withdrawn, and she complains of a great deal of pain from her minor burns. Biopsychosocial assessment is completed.

Patient has psychological distress but believes that her social support is adequate. She would like to talk to a nurse when she returns for her follow-up visit. ⟶ Provide counseling and support for the patient during her visit. Make an appointment for her return visit to the clinic for follow-up.

Patient is severely distressed. She has no social support. She does not know how she will survive. ⟶ Refer the patient to a mental health specialist. The patient will need crisis intervention strategies provided by a mental health specialist.

---

emotional intensity. For example, Mrs. Brown has just learned that both of her parents have perished in an airplane crash. When she arrives at the emergency department to identify their bodies, she is shaking, sobbing, and unable to answer questions. The emergency physician orders lorazepam (Ativan) (see Drug Profile: Lorazepam).

Initiation. Because Mrs. Brown is overcome by grief and severe anxiety from seeing her parents' bodies, 2 mg of lorazepam is administered intramuscularly. The nurse monitors the patient for onset of action and any side effects. If she does not have some relief within 20 to 30 minutes, another injection can be given.

Stabilization. Over the next half-hour, Mrs. Brown regains some of her composure. She is no longer shaking, and her crying is occasional. She is reluctant to identify her parents but can do so accompanied by the nurse. Once the paperwork is completed, Mrs. Brown is sent home with a prescription for lorazepam, 2 to 4 mg every 12 hours.

Maintenance. Mrs. Brown takes the medication over the next week as she plans and attends her parents' funeral and manages the affairs surrounding their deaths. The medication keeps her anxiety at a manageable level, enabling her to do the tasks required of her.

Medication Cessation. Two weeks after the death of her parents, Mrs. Brown is no longer taking lorazepam. She is grieving normally, has periods of teariness and sadness over her loss, but can cope. She visits with friends, reminisces with family members, and reads inspirational poems. All these activities help her get through the changes in her life brought about by her parents' sudden death.

This example demonstrates how a medication can be used to assist someone through a crisis. Once that crisis is past, the person can use his or her own coping mechanisms to adapt.

Biopsychosocial Interventions

Safety interventions to protect the person in crisis from harm should be used, such as preventing the person from committing suicide or homicide, arranging for food and shelter (if needed), and mobilizing social support. Once the person's safety needs are met, the nurse can address the psychosocial aspects of the crisis. Counseling reinforces healthy coping behaviors and interaction patterns. Counseling, which focuses on identifying the person's emotions and positive coping strategies for the corresponding nursing diagnosis, helps the person integrate the effects of the crisis into his or her life. At times, telephone counseling may provide the person with enough help that face-to-face counseling is not necessary. If counseling strategies do not work, other stress reduction and coping enhancement interventions can also be used (see Table 35-11). The nurse should refer anyone who cannot cope with a crisis to a mental health specialist for short-term therapy.

A crisis often disrupts the person's social network, leading to changes in available social support. Sometimes, the development of a new social support system can help the person more effectively cope with the crisis. Supporting the development of more contacts within the social network can be done by referring the person to support groups or religious groups.

Crisis Intervention in the Community

Telephone Hot Lines. Public and private funding and the efforts of trained volunteers permit most communities to provide crisis services to the public. For example, telephone hot lines for problems ranging from child abuse to suicide are a part of most communities' health delivery systems. Crisis services permit immediate access to the mental health system for people who are experiencing an emergency (such as threatened suicide) or for those who need help with stress or a crisis.

Residential Crisis Services. Many communities provide, as part of the health care network, residential

DRUG PROFILE: Lorazepam
Benzodiazepine
(Antianxiety Agent/Sedative and Hypnotic)
Trade Name: Ativan, Alzapam, Various Generic Formulations

Receptor affinity: Acts mainly at the subcortical levels of the central nervous system (CNS), leaving the cortex relatively unaffected. Main sites of action may be the limbic system and reticular formation. It potentiates the effects of α-aminobutyric acid, an inhibitory neurotransmitter. Exact mechanism of action is unknown.

Indications: Management of anxiety disorders or for short-term relief of symptoms of anxiety or anxiety associated with depression (oral forms). Also used as preanesthetic medication in adults to produce sedation, relieve anxiety, and decrease recall of events related to surgery (parenteral form). Unlabeled parenteral uses for management of acute alcohol withdrawal.

Route and dosage: Available in 0.5-, 1-, and 2-mg tablets; 2 mg/mL concentrated oral solution and 2 mg/mL and 4 mg/mL solutions for injection.

Adult dosage: Usually 2–6 mg/d orally, with a range of 1–10 mg/d in divided doses, with largest dose given at night. 0.05 mg/kg IM up to a maximum of 4 mg administered at least 2 h before surgery. Initially 2 mg total or 0.044 mg/kg IV (whichever is smaller). Doses as high as 0.05 mg/kg up to a total of 4 mg may be given 15–20 min before the procedure to those benefiting by a greater lack of recall.

Geriatric: Dosage not to exceed adult IV dose. Orally, 1–2 mg/d in divided doses initially, adjusted as needed and tolerated.

Children: Drug should not be used in children under 12 years of age.

Half-life (peak effect): 10–20 h (1–6 h [oral]); 60–90 min [IM]; 10–15 min [IV]).

Select adverse reactions: Transient mild drowsiness, sedation, depression, lethargy, apathy, fatigue, light-headedness, disorientation, anger hostility, restlessness, confusion, crying, headache, mild paradoxical excitatory reactions during first 2 weeks of treatment, constipation, dry mouth, diarrhea, nausea, bradycardia, hypotension, cardiovascular collapse, urinary retention, drug dependence with withdrawal symptoms.

Warning: Contraindicated in psychoses, acute narrow angle glaucoma, shock, acute alcoholic intoxication with depression of vital signs, and during pregnancy, labor and delivery, and while breast-feeding. Use cautiously in patients with impaired liver or kidney function or those who are debilitated. When given with theophylline, there is a decreased effect of lorazepam. When using the drug IV, it must be diluted immediately prior to use and administered by direct injection slowly or infused at a maximum rate of 2 mg/min. When giving narcotic analgesics, reduce its dose by at least half in patients who have received lorazepam.

Special patient/family education:

- Take the drug exactly as prescribed; do not stop taking the drug abruptly.
- Avoid alcohol and other CNS depressants.
- Avoid driving or other activities that require alertness.
- Notify prescriber before taking any other prescription or over-the-counter drug.
- Change your position slowly and sit at the edge of the bed for a few minutes before arising.
- Report any severe dizziness, weakness, drowsiness that persists, any rash or skin lesions, palpitations, edema of the extremities, visual changes, or difficulty urinating to the prescriber.

---

crisis services for people who need short-term housing. The specific residential crisis services available within a community reflect those problems that it judges as particularly important. For example, some communities provide shelter for teenaged runaways; others offer shelter for abused spouses. Still others provide shelter for people who would otherwise require acute psychiatric hospitalization. These settings provide residents with a place to stay in a supportive, homelike atmosphere. The people who use these services are linked to other community services, such as financial aid.

Evaluation and Treatment Outcomes

Outcomes established in the care plan will guide evaluation. The patient should come through the crisis well, with improved health, well-being, and social function.

Summary of Key Points

➤ Stress occurs when a person–environment relationship is appraised as being unfavorable. Stress responses are simultaneously emotional and physiologic, leading to an innate tendency to act.

➤ Many personal factors, such as personality patterns, beliefs, values, and commitment to an outcome, interact with environmental demands and constraints that produce a person–environment relationship.

➤ Within the social network, social support can help a person cope with stress.

➤ Effective coping can be either problem focused or emotion focused. The outcome of successful coping is enhanced health, psychological well-being, and social functioning.

➤ A crisis is a severely stressful situation that causes exaggerated stress responses. The nursing process is similar for the person experiencing a stress response except that increased attention is paid to safety issues.

Critical Thinking Challenges

1. Compare and contrast Selye's stress response to Lazarus' model of stress, coping, and adaptation.
2. Explain why one person may experience the stress of losing a job differently from another.
3. Explain the neuroendocrine response to stress.
4. A woman at the local shelter announced to her group that she was returning to her husband because it was partly her fault that her husband beat her. Is this an example of problem-focused or emotion-focused coping? Justify your answer.
5. After the death of his mother, a 24-year-old single man with schizophrenia moves into an apartment. He continues to take his medication but feels sad about his mother's death. He is not adjusting well to living alone and tells his nurse that he no longer wants to go to work. In tears, he admits that he is lonely and can no longer cope with the apartment. The nurse generates the following nursing diagnosis: Ineffective Coping related to inadequate support system. Develop a plan of care for this young man.
6. Distinguish among the terms crisis, stress, and psychiatric emergency.
7. Analyze factors that determine when the generalist nurse should refer a person under stress to a specialist.
8. Discuss the role of the generalist psychiatric–mental health nurse who is caring for a person in crisis.
9. Discuss the phases of medication use in crises.
10. List the phases of bereavement that can be considered a crisis and discuss the difference between normal and dysfunctional grief.

 WEB LINKS

www.tc.unl.edu/stress This site offers a review of the principles of stress management.

www.isma.org.uk This is the home page of the International Stress Management Association (ISMA) in the United Kingdom. ISMA is a leading professional body for stress management. Its website has articles from its journal.

www.stress-management-isma.org The International Stress Management Association seeks to advance the education of professionals and students and to facilitate methodically sound research in several professional interdisciplinary stress management fields.

www.ed.gov/databases/ERIC'Digests/ed405535. html This crisis intervention digest gives an overview of crisis intervention.

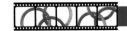 **MOVIES**

Schindler's List: 1993. The film presents the true story of Oskar Schindler, a member of the Nazi party, womanizer, and war profiteer, who saved the lives of more than 1,000 Jews during the Holocaust. The movie shows how during long periods of political turmoil and terror, life can become somewhat normalized. Yet, an underlying fear perpetuates daily lives. Crises erupt at different times during the very long period of chronic stress.

Viewing Points: Differentiate the periods of chronic stress from crisis in this film. Observe the reactions of different characters under stress. Is the behavior different from what you would expect? Observe your own feelings throughout the movie. Did you experience stress?

REFERENCES

Aguilera, D. (1993). *Crisis intervention: Theory and methodology.* St. Louis: Mosby.

American Psychiatric Association. (2000). *Diagnostic and statistical manual of mental disorders* (4th ed., Text revision). Washington, DC: Author.

Barnett, R., & Marshall, N. (1992). Worker and mother roles, spillover effects, and psychological distress. *Women and Health, 18*(2), 9–40.

Beels, C., Gutwirth, L, Berkeley, J., & Struening, E. (1984). Measurement of social support in schizophrenia. *Schizophrenia Bulletin, 10*(3), 399–411.

Burgess, A., & Holmstrom, L. (1979). *Rape, crisis, and recovery.* Bowie, MD: Robert J. Brady.

Callahan, J. (1994). Defining crisis and emergency. *Crisis, 15*(4), 164–171.

Caplan, G. (1961). *An approach to community mental health.* New York: Grune & Stratton.

Caplan, G. (1974). *Support systems and community mental health.* New York: Behavioral Publications.

Carpenito, L. (2000). *Nursing diagnosis: Application to clinical practice* (8th ed.). Philadelphia: Lippincott Williams & Wilkins.

Friedman, M., & Rosenman, R. (1974). *Type A and your heart.* New York: Knopf.

Guyton, A. C., & Hall, J. E. (2000). *Textbook of medical physiology* (10th ed.). Philadelphia: W.B. Saunders.

Hayes, A. (1995). Psychiatric nursing: What does biology have to do with it? *Archives of Psychiatric Nursing, 9*(4), 216–224.

Herbert, T., & Cohen, S. (1993). Stress and immunity in humans: A meta-analytic review. *Psychosomatic Medicine, 55*(4), 364–379.

Holmes, T., & Rahe, R. (1967). The social readjustment patient scale. *Journal of Psychosomatic Research, 11*(2), 213–218.

House, J., Landis, K., & Umberson, D. (1988). Social relationships and health. *Science, 241*, 540–545.

Lazarus, R. (1985). The costs and benefits of denial. In A. Monat & R. Lazarus (Eds.), *Stress and coping: An anthology* (2nd ed.). New York: Springer.

Lazarus, R. (1991). *Emotion and adaptation.* New York: Oxford University Press.

Lazarus, R. (1993). From psychological stress to the emotions: A history of changing outlooks. *Annual Review of Psychology, 44*, 1–21.

Lazarus, R., & Folkman, S. (1984). *Stress, appraisal and coping.* New York: Springer.

Malone, J. (1988). The social support dissupport continuum. *Journal of Psychosocial Nursing, 26*(12), 18–22.

McCain, N., & Smith, J. (1994). Stress and coping in the context of psychoneuroimmunology: A holistic framework for nursing practice and research. *Archives of Psychiatric Nursing, 8*(4), 221–227.

McCloskey, J., & Bulechek, G. (1996). *Nursing interventions classification.* St. Louis: Mosby–Year Book.

Mitchell, J. (1969). *Social networks in urban situations.* Manchester: Manchester University Press.

Rahe, R. (1994). The more things change. *Psychosomatic Medicine, 56*(4), 306–307.

Rosenman, R., & Chesney, M. (1985). Type A behavior pattern: Its relationship to coronary heart disease and its modification by behavioral and pharmacological approaches. In M. Zales (Ed.), *Stress in health and disease* (pp. 206–241). New York: Brunner/Mazel.

Rossen, E., & Buschmann, M. (1995). Mental illness in late life: The neurobiology of depression. *Archives of Psychiatric Nursing, 9*(3), 130–136.

Schaefer, C., Coyne, J., & Lazarus, R. (1982). The health-related functions of social support. *Journal of Behavioral Medicine, 4*(4), 381–406.

Selye, H. (1956). *The stress of life.* New York: McGraw-Hill.

Selye, H. (1974). *Stress without distress.* Philadelphia: J. B. Lippincott.

Simmons, S. (1994). Social networks: Their relevance to mental health nursing. *Journal of Advanced Nursing, 19*(2), 281–289.

Thoits, P. (1982). Conceptual, methodological, and theoretical problems in studying social support as a buffer against life stress. *Journal of Health and Social Behavior, 23*(2), 145–158.

Walker, K., MacBride, A., & Vachon, M. (1977). Social support networks and the crisis of bereavement. *Social Science and Medicine, 11*(1), 35–42.

Zisook, S. (1987). Unresolved grief. In S. Zisook (Ed.), *Biopsychosocial aspects of bereavement* (pp. 21–34). Washington, DC: American Psychiatric Press.

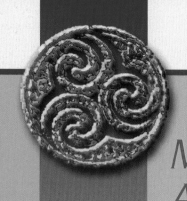

Management of Aggression

Sandy Harper-Jaques and Marlene Reimer

LEARNING OBJECTIVES

After studying this chapter, you will be able to:

➤ Explore feelings about the experience and expression of anger.

➤ Discuss the biopsychosocial factors that influence the expression of aggressive and violent behaviors.

➤ Discuss biopsychosocial theories used to explain anger, aggression, and violence.

➤ Identify behaviors or actions that escalate and de-escalate violent behavior.

➤ Recognize the risk for "nurse abuse" (attacks on nurses).

➤ Generate options for responding to the expression of anger and violent behaviors in clinical nursing practice.

➤ Apply the nursing process to the management of anger, aggression, and violence in patients.

catharsis
emotional circuit
restraint

seclusion
violence

aggression
anger
assertiveness

Definitions of anger, aggression, and violence vary and are influenced by experience, beliefs, culture, and gender. Individuals and groups develop their own views of acceptable and unacceptable words and actions. Theoretic distinctions can be made among anger, aggression, and violence, but clinically, their expression may be blurred. Each phenomenon may occur alone or in combination with one or both of the others.

All societies develop norms for acceptable and unacceptable behavior; some groups at some point in time have accepted all forms of aggression and violence (Megargee, 1993). Today, images and stories about aggressive and violent acts throughout the world are rampant. Like all other settings, health care settings are not immune to expressions of anger, aggression, and violence.

In any setting, aggression and violence are a reflection of the values of the individual, family, community, and society. Many people tend to minimize the frequency and severity of aggressive and violent acts. For example, couples who interact violently downplay the severity and effects of the episodes (Gortner et al., 1997).

The expression of anger, aggression, and violence by patients and, sometimes, their families is a tremendous challenge for nurses. This chapter discusses prominent theories about the nature and causes of these phenomena. It offers varying and sometimes controversial models, theories, and evidence, with each discussion attempting to explain the phenomena of anger, aggression, and violence. Clinicians can use each particular model as a basis for assessment, nursing diagnosis, planning, intervention, and evaluation. The chapter also explores how the nurse can apply the nursing process

in managing angry, aggressive, or violent patients and in preventing or de-escalating situations that may lead to aggression or violence.

ANGER

Anger can be defined as "a strong, uncomfortable emotional response to a provocation that is unwanted and incongruent with one's values, beliefs or rights" (Thomas, 1998b). Anger is usually described as a temporary state of emotional arousal, in contrast to hostility, which is associated with a more enduring negative attitude (Thomas, 1998b) (see Chap. 35). Anger is often portrayed as a bad emotion that always leads to aggression and violence. In fact, most episodes of anger do not progress to aggressive actions (Averill, 1982).

Language pertaining to anger is imprecise and confusing. The word anger is used to describe a wide range of feelings, from annoyance at having to wait at a red light when in a hurry to a severe emotional reaction to the news that a family member has been physically assaulted. Words used interchangeably with anger include (but are not limited to) annoyance, frustration, temper, resentment, hostility, hatred, and rage. Furthermore, the word anger is used to describe both a transient emotional state and a personality trait (Thomas, 1993). This imprecision is related to varying beliefs and theories, some of which include the following (Gerloff, 1997; Shannon, 2000; Thomas, 1998a, 1998b):

- Anger is a fixed quantity that is either dammed up or floods the system.
- Anger and aggression are linked. Anger is the feeling, and aggression is the behavior; both result from an innate instinct.
- Anger is the instinctive response to a threat or to the inability to meet goals or desires.
- If outward expression of anger is blocked, then it turns inward and develops into depression.
- Anger arises out of feelings of hurt or anxiety.

Text Box 36-1 invites the reader to explore variations in responses to anger through the use of an experiential exercise.

> **KEY CONCEPT**   **Anger.   Anger** is an affective state experienced as the motivation to act in ways that warn, intimidate, or attack those who are perceived as challenging or threatening. It occurs when there is a threat, delay, thwarting of a goal, or conflict between goals.

Experience of Anger

Anger offers a signal to those experiencing it that something is wrong in themselves, others, or their relationships with others (Lerner, 1986). Thomas (1998a, 1998b) suggests that the experience of anger can serve as a warning that demands are greater than available resources. If one accepts that human beings are rational and capable of appraising situations, then the subjective component of the experience of anger becomes an important area for study. With the exception of anger that arises from specific neurologic damage or biochemical imbalances, angry episodes can be viewed as social events (Thomas, 1998b). The meaning of angry episodes develops from the beliefs held about anger and the interpretation given to the episode (Shannon, 2000). According to Ellis (1977), people choose to experience anger, basing this choice on the related thinking processes. Following Ellis's model, the thinking process would be as follows:

- I wanted something.
- I didn't get what I wanted, and I feel frustrated.
- It's awful not to get what I want.
- Others should not frustrate me.
- Others are bad for frustrating me.
- Bad people should be frustrated.

The experience of anger is a normal human emotion; it is the inappropriate expression of anger that may be threatening to the self or others.

Expression of Anger

Difficulties in expressing anger have often been associated with psychiatric health problems. Anger turned inward has been implicated as a contributor to mood disorders, especially depression (Wolbert-Burgess, 1990). Several medical disorders have also been positively correlated with the suppression of anger. Among them are essential hypertension, migraine headaches, psoriasis, rheumatoid arthritis, and Raynaud's disease.

Behavioral expressions of anger vary. In the 19th century, anger was viewed as sinful, dangerous, and destructive—an emotion to be contained, controlled, and denied. This negatively viewed emotion was to be dominated and conquered, and the ideal family life was free of anger. Husbands and wives were discouraged from expressing anger toward each other; parenting manuals promoted the suppression of anger in children (Thomas, 1993). This view contributed to the development of a powerful taboo against feeling and expressing anger. People who have accepted this persistent taboo may have difficulty even knowing when they are angry (Shannon, 2000).

During the early 20th century, Freud and Lorenz advocated the use of **catharsis**, the release of ideas through talking and expressing appropriate emotion, in the expression of anger. Catharsis, however, has been shown empirically to promote, not reduce, anger (Thomas, 1998b).

As previously stated, anger is a normal and legitimate human emotion that should be expressed in a manner that is not harmful or hurtful. In recent years, interest has arisen in developing communication techniques that promote the expression of anger in nondestructive ways (Gerloff, 1997; Shannon, 2000). These varying beliefs have added to the confusion about anger. Differences in expectations about how men and women should express anger also contribute to the confusion.

TEXT BOX 36.1

Self-Awareness Exercise: Personal Experience of Anger

People's reactions differ when they experience anger. Some people report a sense of power, control, and calmness different from their usual experience; others report feeling shaky, tearful, and on the verge of collapse. Still others describe physical sensations of nausea and dizziness.

Think about the last time that you felt angry. List the body sensations and other emotions that you experienced. Now ask a friend, colleague, or family member to do the same. Compare lists. What are the similarities and differences between you? How will awareness of these differences help you in your clinical practice?

TABLE 36.1   Styles of Anger Expression

Style	Characteristic	Gender Socialization
Anger suppression	Emphasizing the need to keep angry feelings to oneself	In North America, girls are discouraged from expressing anger.
Anger expression	Expressing anger in an attacking or blaming way	In North America, boys are encouraged to express their anger, to not "lie down" or "give in" to others.
Anger discussion	Discussing the anger with a friend or family member Approaching a person with whom one is angry and discussing the concern directly	Popular and professional literature offers techniques in assertive expression.

Table 36-1 gives examples of different styles of anger expression.

Varying beliefs about appropriate ways to express anger become apparent when a patient and a nurse enter into a therapeutic relationship. Genetic predisposition, emotional development during infancy and childhood, and family environment influence the variations in expression for both the nurse and the patient (Thomas, 1993). Previous experiences in expressing anger and reactions from others will also be influential.

AGGRESSION AND VIOLENCE

In this chapter, aggression is defined as "verbal statements against someone that are intended to intimidate or threaten the recipient." **Violence** is defined as "a physical act of force intended to cause harm to a person or an object and to convey the message that the perpe-

trator's point of view is correct and not the victim's" (Harper-Jaques & Reimer, 1992, p. 312). Aggression and violent behavior reflect a continuum from suspicious behavior to extreme actions that threaten the safety of others or result in injury or death (see Table 36-2 for examples).

KEY CONCEPT   **Aggression.** **Aggression** is verbal statements that are intended to threaten. Aggression and violent behavior represent a continuum ranging from suspicious behavior to extreme actions that threaten the safety of others or result in injury or death.

Aggression does not occur in a vacuum. Both the patient and the context must be considered. Therefore, a multidimensional framework is essential for understanding and responding to these behaviors (Morrison, 1998) (Fig. 36-1).

TABLE 36.2   Examples of Behaviors on the Continuum of Aggression and Violence

Term	Description	Clinical Example
Suspicious behavior	Hypervigilance to external cues Attends more to cues that fit with current thinking patterns	A female patient with a long history of delusional disorder (including the belief that her family wants to "lock her away") questions the motives of a community mental health nurse when she asks the patient about her medication regimen. The patient misperceives the nurse's inquiry as evidence of a conspiracy against her.
Verbal hostility	Verbal comments that are sarcastic, coercive, or blaming and often expressed with the intent to hurt others May be used as a means of getting attention or inviting others to take action	When administration of PRN medication is delayed, a patient's mother comes to the nursing station and starts to yell. She states that the nurses don't care, are lazy, and should work harder. She also demands that someone give her daughter the analgesic. (Family members have been reported to use demanding behaviors to have needs met.)
Physical violence	Act of striking out, throwing an object, pushing, etc., that appears to be intended to cause harm to a person or object	A young man attending a mental health clinic has missed his appointment with the psychiatrist. When he finds out he cannot be scheduled to see her for another week, he yells at the receptionist, bangs his fist on the desk, and then picks up a chair and throws it at her.

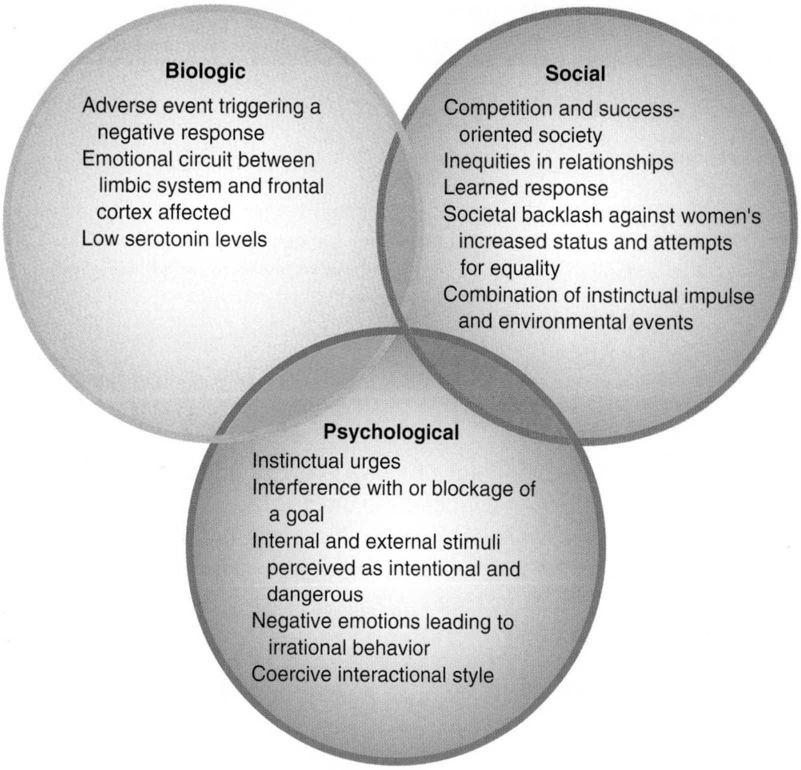

Biologic
Adverse event triggering a
negative response
Emotional circuit between
limbic system and frontal
cortex affected
Low serotonin levels

Social
Competition and success-
oriented society
Inequities in relationships
Learned response
Societal backlash against women's
increased status and attempts
for equality
Combination of instinctual impulse
and environmental events

Psychological
Instinctual urges
Interference with or blockage of
a goal
Internal and external stimuli
perceived as intentional and
dangerous
Negative emotions leading to
irrational behavior
Coercive interactional style

FIGURE 36.1 Biopsychosocial etiologies for patients with aggression.

MODELS OF ANGER, AGGRESSION, AND VIOLENCE

This section discusses some of the main theoretical explanations for anger, aggression, and violence. Most concepts will be familiar to the reader from earlier chapters and other sources. In our view, a single model or theory cannot fully explain anger, aggression, and violence; instead, the nurse must choose the most useful models for explaining a particular patient's experience and for planning interventions.

Biologic Theories

Evidence for a substantial biologic component to aggression will be considered first. From a biologic viewpoint, a tendency to have more frequent angry episodes may partially originate from developmental deficits, anoxia, malnutrition, toxins, tumors, or neurodegenerative diseases or trauma affecting the brain. Patients with a history of damage to the cerebral cortex are more likely to exhibit increased impulsivity, decreased inhibition, and decreased judgment than are those who have not experienced such damage. The interaction of neurocognitive impairment and social history of abuse or family violence increases the risk for violent behavior (Scarpa & Raine, 1997). The odds of violent behavior also increase when separate risk factors such as schizophrenia, substance abuse, and not taking prescribed medications coexist in the same person (Citrome & Volavka, 1999).

Before reading further research evidence, try the accompanying anger exercise in Text Box 36-2. What does daily experience suggest about biologically based aspects of the experience and expression of anger?

TEXT BOX 36.2

Self-Awareness Exercise: Intensity of Anger

Imagine this scene:

You are coming home late at night. You've been at the library studying for midterm examinations and are tired. As you come up the front walk, you trip over a skateboard, probably left by one of the neighborhood children. Before you know it, you are sprawled across the front step.

What emotions threaten to overwhelm you at that moment? What contributes to the intensity of the anger that you feel?

- The pain where you scraped your leg across the cement?

- Your general state of tiredness?

- The fact that you skipped supper?

- The five cups of coffee you had today?

- The careless children who left a toy in your way?

If the same thing had happened when you were well rested and feeling good, would the feeling and the intensity be the same?

Cognitive Neuroassociation Model

The cognitive neuroassociation model is one explanation for the interplay of biologic and other internal influences (Berkowitz, 1989). Initially, an averse event (like pain from tripping over the skateboard in Text Box 36-2) triggers a primitive negative response. Peripheral receptors communicate this response up the spinal cord through the spinothalamic tract to the hypothalamus (see Chap. 7). The hypothalamus, which synthesizes input from throughout the nervous system, is part of the limbic system. The limbic system mediates primitive emotion and basic drives to produce behaviors for survival, like the "fight-or-flight" response (Harper-Jaques & Reimer, 1992).

At first, cognitive appraisal is not involved in these rudimentary feelings of fear or anger other than identifying the stimulus as aversive; however, higher-order cognitive processing quickly begins to take over. The brain associates the current experience of physiologic sensations with memories, ideas, and previously experienced expressive-motor reactions. It then interprets and differentiates the experience. Depending on prior experience and associations, the response may be intensified or suppressed. It is this latter part of the process that is most amenable to modification through psychotherapy.

Neurostructural Model and the Emotional Circuit

The brain structures most frequently associated with aggressive behavior are the limbic system and the cerebral cortex, particularly the frontal and temporal lobes. Harper-Jaques and Reimer (1992) propose the phrase **emotional circuit** to describe the interrelationship between the emotional processes of the limbic system and the neurocognitive processes of the frontal lobe and other parts of the cortex. They hypothesize that the functioning of this system determines the meaning a person gives to a particular situation. Thus, meaning is influenced by physiologic capability to perceive incoming messages, prioritize among competing stimuli, and interpret these messages in relation to stored ideas, beliefs, and memories.

Neurochemical Model and Low Serotonin Syndrome

In recent decades, knowledge has exploded about the complex role of neurotransmitters in human behavior. As noted in Chapter 7, serotonin is one major neurotransmitter involved in mood, sleep, and appetite. Low serotonin levels are associated not only with depression but also with irritability, increased pain sensitivity, impulsiveness, and aggression (Kavoussi et al., 1997).

Serotonin is sensitive to fluctuations in dietary intake of its precursor, tryptophan, which is found in high-carbohydrate foods. Once it crosses the blood–brain barrier, tryptophan is synthesized into serotonin within the 5-hydroxytrytophan (5-HT) neurons by interaction with the enzyme tryptophan hydroxylase. Normally, the amount of tryptophan available in the plasma is below saturation (ie, below the amount that could be used if available). Tryptophan intake and the availability of binding sites on the plasma proteins affect synthesis of serotonin. Thus, assessing overall dietary intake is relevant, particularly of good tryptophan sources, such as wheat, flour, corn, milk, and eggs.

People with a history of aggressive behavior have been found to have a lower than average level of serotonin. Studies of humans with known aggressive tendencies, such as violent offenders, have repeatedly shown lower than average concentrations of 5-hydroxyindoleacetic acid (5-HIAA), the major metabolite for serotonin (Kavoussi et al., 1997). Similarly, plasma concentration of tryptophan is lower in alcoholic people with a history of aggressive behavior than in alcoholic people with no such history. Criminals whose acts of violence were committed impulsively have lower levels of 5-HIAA than criminals whose acts of violence were premeditated. Hyperarousal, as may occur through being constantly vigilant against possible attack (eg, in guerrilla warfare), may also contribute to aggressive behavior.

This evidence for a biologic component to aggressive behavior does not mean that only biologic means of treatment can be effective. Feedback between human behavior and biochemistry is continuous; verbal suggestions can affect biochemistry just as biochemistry affects behavior (Levine et al., 1992; Pardo et al., 1993). Environmental and learned behaviors influence the type and degree of aggression expressed, even by those for whom there is a biologic component (Kavoussi et al., 1997).

Psychological Theories

Several psychological explanations exist for aggressive and violent behaviors. This section discusses psychoanalytic, behavioral, and cognitive theories.

Psychoanalytic Theories

Psychoanalytic theorists view emotions as instinctual urges. They view suppression of these urges as unhealthy and possible contributors to the development of psychosomatic or psychological disorders (Thomas, 1998b). Freud struggled to understand the nature and expression of human aggressive behavior. In his early works, he linked aggression with libidinal factors; however, this association did not explain destructive actions during wars and armed conflict. In his later writings, Freud identified aggression as a separate instinct, like the sexual instinct. He viewed aggression as an innate human quality that could be expressed when a person was provoked or abused (Messner et al., 1975). In doing so, he challenged the commonly held belief that human beings are essentially good.

Freud explained aggressive or violent behavior as a combination of instinctual impulses and events in the environment that stimulated release of the instinctual urge. Freud's view fostered the use of catharsis. Therapeutic approaches, such as primal scream (Elkind, 1975), and nursing interventions that direct the patient to "let it out" by pounding a pillow find their origins in this theory (Tavris, 1989; Thomas, 1990). As previously stated, however, studies have not shown catharsis to be helpful in reducing anger. Venting can also have negative consequences when the action taken is hurtful to or blaming of others or damages property.

Erich Fromm (1900–1980), an American psychoanalyst best known for his application of psychoanalytic theory to social and cultural problems, held a different view. He believed that animals and humans shared one form of aggression he called benign. This genetically programmed response was designed as a defense to protect oneself against a threat. The distinction between humans and animals was that human beings could reason. This capability provided them with options that are not available to animals. Thus, unlike animals, human beings are capable of behaving aggressively for reasons other than self-preservation. Fromm defined aggression in humans as any behavior that causes or intends to cause damage to another person, animal, or object (1973). Humans may foresee both real and perceived threats. Perceived threats that are based on distorted perceptions may lead to aggressive and violent behaviors. For example, the cognitive and information-processing deficits of patients with psychosis or schizophrenia (see Chap. 18) are frequently implicated in episodes of aggression and violence.

Behavioral Theories

The goal of behaviorists is to predict and control behavior. Introspection has no role in these theories. Two behavioral theories, drive theory and social learning theory, are highlighted here.

Drive Theory. Drive theory suggests that violent behavior originates externally. A person experiences anger and acts violently in response to interference with or blocking of a goal. Laboratory experiments and the reality of everyday experience have proved the limitations of this theory (Thomas, 1990). Not all situations in which one's goal is blocked lead to anger or violence.

Social Learning Theory. In his research, Bandura (1973) drew attention to the role of learning and rewards in the expression of anger and violence (see Chap. 6). He studied interactions between mothers and children. The children learned that anger and aggressive behavior helped them get what they wanted from their mothers. Children's observation of aggressive behavior between family members and in their communities fosters a context for learning aggressive behavior. It may also lead to an assumption that aggressive behavior is appropriate. From this view, people learn to be aggressive by participating in an aggressive environment.

Cognitive Theories

Cognitive theorists are interested in how people transform internal and external stimuli into useful information. They emphasize understanding how a person takes new information and fits it into an already developed schema. Beck (1976) proposed that cognitive schema such as judgments, self-esteem, and expectations influence angry responses. In a situation perceived as intentional, dangerous, and unprovoked, the recipient's reaction will be intensified. The person's reaction will be further intensified if he or she views the offender as undesirable. In psychological disorders, cognitive processing may be compromised (Cheung & Schweitzer, 1998; Estroff et al., 1994).

Rational-emotive theory, one type of cognitive theory, considers cognition, affect, and behavior to be interrelated psychological processes (Ellis, 1977). This theory regards anger as an inappropriate negative emotion because it stems from irrational beliefs. Change is directed at altering irrational beliefs by identifying and working to change them and their associated psychological processes.

Sociocultural Theories

Western society is characterized by a competitive, success-oriented ideology that values the individual and individual accomplishments over collaboration and a sense of community. Self-esteem, particularly for men, may be based on social and economic status and influence over others and the environment (Jenkins, 1990). The pursuit of status produces inequities in relationships, whereby one person is superior and the other is subordinate. A hazard inherent in the pursuit of status is the view that a person is entitled to have influence and control, that the "entitled person" has the right to use whatever means necessary to obtain status (Jenkins, 1990). These means may include force or disregarding the rights and needs of others. The entitled person may also begin to consider other people responsible for his or her thoughts, feelings, or actions.

Violence against women is one example of the way in which men have used a belief in entitlement to justify such actions as threatening, hurting, or murdering women. The United Nations Children's Fund (UNICEF) (2000) has labeled violence against women as a worldwide epidemic. In recent decades, many societies have challenged men's position of entitlement. The challenge has evolved from an examination of the status quo and a call for society to view women as equal partners with men. Women now have greater access to education, increased economic independence, and opportunities to control the frequency and number of pregnancies. These changes have led some to suggest that the continuing prevalence of violence toward women (Tajaden & Thoennes, 2000) is a backlash against their increased efforts toward achieving equality.

Interactional Theory

E. F. Morrison (1989, 1990, 1992, 1993; Harris & Morrison, 1995) challenges research and theories suggesting that aggression and violence are biologically or psychologically based. She asserts that these views lead to excusing the person's behavior. She proposes that violence among people in psychiatric settings is the same as violence in other settings. Therefore, the patient's behavior should be considered a social problem and responded to on that basis. This challenge is grounded in several studies that examined the interactional style of the aggressive and violent individual. People with interactional styles that were argumentative or coercive were more likely to engage in aggressive or violent interchanges. Such people are often described as having a "chip on their shoulders." Morrison clearly states her view that the antecedent variables (ie, history of violence, psychiatric diagnosis, length of hospitalization) and the mediating variable of interactional style are the primary reasons for the behavior.

NURSING MANAGEMENT: HUMAN RESPONSE TO DISORDER

Aggression and violence often arise from one party's belief that his or her view of a situation is the only correct one. The first party considers other views wrong and in need of changing. A second party's refusal to give in to the view of the first may lead to violence (Capra, 1996). Text Box 36-3 illustrates such a scenario in the clinical setting. Paul dislikes the nurse's refusal to let him leave the unit. He believes it is time to leave, even though he continues to experience auditory and visual hallucinations. His view is that he is correct and that the nurse should change her mind.

Patients may use aggression and violence as ways to get what they want. They may resort to violence to force change or to regain or maintain control. Rewards from violence include attention from nursing staff and status and prestige among the patient group (Harris & Morrison, 1995). For example, the patient who behaves violently is observed more frequently

TEXT BOX 36.3

Clinical Vignette: Paul

Paul, a new patient on the unit, appears to be experiencing auditory hallucinations. The nurse approaches Paul, careful not to invade his personal space, and begins to walk with him. In an attempt to assess his current mental status, the nurse points out that he seems restless and asks if the voices have returned. Paul responds, "They are telling me this place isn't safe. The angel in the corner is signaling to me. She wants me to leave!" Paul starts to walk toward the door. In an attempt to offer an alternative point of view and orient him to the present, the nurse understands that what the patient is seeing and hearing are hallucinations. The nurse attempts to increase Paul's feeling of safety by identifying his perceptions as hallucinations and reassuring him of his safety. "No I won't stay and you can't make me." Paul pushes the nurse aside and runs to the door.

If you were the nurse in this situation, what would be your next response? How would you acknowledge Paul's concerns and encourage him to stay?

and has more opportunities to discuss concerns with nurses.

Nurses bring their own perceptions and reactions to clinical settings. They respond to the behaviors of the patients and families for whom they care. Patients and families, in turn, react to nurses (Leahey & Harper-Jaques, 1996). Nurses' beliefs about themselves as individuals and professionals will influence their responses to aggressive behaviors. For example, the nurse who considers any expression of anger or aggression inappropriate will approach an agitated patient differently than the nurse who considers agitated behavior to be meaningful.

The nurse's ability to maintain personal control is challenged when faced with angry, provoking patients. Some patients who are experiencing emotional problems have an uncanny ability to target verbally a nurse's vulnerable characteristics. It is a usual response to become defensive when one feels vulnerable. When nurses lose control of their own responses, however, the potential for punitive interventions or the use of threats or sarcasm is greater. The nurse who remains calm and detached will be more successful in preventing the escalation of potentially violent situations.

Contrary to popular belief, most patients who have mental health problems do not behave aggressively or violently (Kennedy, 1993). Nurses in all areas of clinical practice need to understand angry emotions, know how to prevent aggression and violence, and respond assertively (Duxbury, 1999). To better prepare themselves to respond to different types of behavior, many nurses take assertiveness training courses and workshops. Many nursing schools also teach assertiveness. Hopefully, nurses can understand the phenomena of anger, aggression, and violence as meaningful behaviors that warrant attention rather than as disruptive behaviors to control.

> **KEY CONCEPT** **Assertiveness.** **Assertiveness** is a set of behaviors and a communication style that is open, honest, direct, and confident. Assertiveness enables the expression of emotions, including anger, in a manner that assumes responsibility. It allows placement of boundaries and prevents acceptance of inappropriate aggression from others.

Assessing the Human Response to Anger, Aggression, and Violence

To develop a means of predicting aggressive and violent behaviors, some researchers have examined demographics, patient characteristics, and unit climate. Others have attempted to determine the relationship between medical diagnosis and violence. A third area of inquiry has been the role of the patient's history in predicting violence.

Several research reports have suggested that particular characteristics are predictive of violent behaviors. Low self-esteem that may be further eroded during hospitalization or treatment may influence a patient to use force to meet his or her needs or to experience some sense of empowerment. Many people who have chronic mental health problems "fight" the experience and refuse to accept medical treatment. When admitted to the hospital, they may experience turmoil from both the illness and the anger at the further loss of control that hospitalization mandates. Specific diagnoses have not been identified as predictive of violence, although some reports suggest that patients who have reduced impulse control (ie, diagnoses such as schizophrenia, bipolar disorder, organic brain syndrome, brain injury, attention deficit hyperactivity disorder) are at increased risk for violent episodes (Buckley, 1999; Kennedy, 1993; Tasman, 1997).

When assessing a patient, his or her history is probably the most important predictor of potential for violence. Important markers include previous episodes of rage and violent behavior, escalating irritability, intruding angry thoughts, and fear of losing control. Head injury, substance use or abuse, and temporal lobe epilepsy have also been discussed as possible predictors of violence (Harper-Jaques & Reimer, 1992; Mesulam, 2000). Whether a relationship exists between temporal lobe epilepsy and aggressive behavior is controversial (Citrome & Volavka, 1999). Aggressive behavior that occurs in the interictal period (ie, between seizures) may also be related to the intense frustration that people who have epilepsy often experience and could lead to violent behavior. Certain antiepileptic drugs, particularly barbiturates, may contribute to irritability and aggressive behavior. On the other hand, mood-stabilizing medications such as carbamazepine (Tegretol) and divalproex sodium (Depakote) have reduced aggressive behavior. The nurse should include any history of seizures, current medications, and compliance with pharmacotherapy in patient assessments. A qualitative study conducted by Morrison (1990) reported that all participants who exhibited violent behavior had been diagnosed with a chronic mental illness and had a history of previous hospitalization. Some physiologic and behavioral cues to anger are listed in Table 36-3.

Biologic Assessment

The nurse may encounter patients whose aggressive tendencies have been exacerbated by a biochemical imbalance. Nurses must recognize, however, that biologic alterations are neither necessary nor sufficient to account for most aggressive behaviors. In taking the patient's history, the nurse listens for evidence of industrial exposure to toxic chemicals (Carpenito, 2000), missed doses of medications (Simmons, 1996), alcohol

---

TABLE 36.3 **Physiologic and Behavioral Cues to Anger**

Internal Signs	External Signs
• Increased pulse, respirations, and blood pressure • Chills and shudders • Prickly sensations • Numbness • Choking sensations • Nausea • Vertigo	• Increased muscle tone • Changes in body posture; clenched fists; set jaw • Changes to the eyes: eyebrows lower and draw together, eyelids tense, eyes assume a "hard" appearance • Lips pressed together to form a thin line, or in a square shape • Flushing or pallor • Goose bumps • Twitching • Sweating

intoxication and withdrawal (Citrome & Valavka, 1999), or premenstrual dysphoric disorder (Megargee, 1993). Similarly, a history of even minor structural changes resulting in trauma, hemorrhage, or tumor may contribute to lowering a patient's anger threshold and thus requires investigation.

Aggressive episodes that are mainly biologic in origin share certain characteristics (Corrigan et al., 1993):

- The patient has a history or evidence of central nervous system (CNS) lesion or dysfunction.
- Onset of the episode is sudden and relatively unprovoked.
- The outburst is less controlled than those associated with external influences.
- The episode has a clear beginning and ending.
- The patient expresses remorse after the episode.

Psychological Assessment

Thought Processing. The nurse interested in working with patients to prevent and manage aggressive and violent behaviors should observe them for disturbances in thought processing. Patients may have disordered thoughts for various reasons, including associated psychiatric diagnoses (Buckley, 1999). Some common diagnostic categories that the nurse needs to look for in the patient's history are major depressive episode, bipolar disorder, delusional disorders, posttraumatic stress disorder, schizophrenia, and depersonalization. The nurse should also look for a current or past history of substance abuse because patients who abuse drugs, alcohol, or solvents may also exhibit disordered thought processing. Intoxication can trigger erratic thought processes and unpredicted violence. Some form of thought disorder may remain after a person is detoxified, becoming a permanent feature of the person's way of processing ideas. In addition, the nurse must look for acute and chronic medical conditions, such as brain tumor, encephalitis, electrolyte imbalance, and hepatic failure, which may also alter thought-processing (Citrome & Volavka, 1999).

The thought processes of greatest interest to the nurse in assessing a patient's potential for aggression and violence are perception and delusion.

Perception. Perception is awareness of events and sensations and the ability to make distinctions between them. Patients with disordered perceptions may misinterpret objects or events. Such misperception is called an illusion. For example, a patient may assume that a person walking toward him or her is going to strike out and thus take action to defend against this illusionary foe. The nurse can explore a patient's perception by asking such questions as, "I noticed you were looking very cautious as I approached you. I wonder what you are thinking?"

Delusion. Patients may maintain false or unreasonable beliefs, known as delusions, despite attempts to dissuade them from their point of view. The nurse may not notice any abnormalities in the patient's behavior or appearance until the patient begins to discuss delusional ideas. Discussion of the delusions may precipitate aggressive or violent behavior. To explore these false beliefs, the nurse could, with the patient's consent, ask questions respectfully. The nurse should match the pacing of such questions to the patient's responses. Attempts to dissuade the patient from his or her beliefs are usually ineffective.

Sensory Impairment. Sensory impairment and difficulties in communicating have been reported as one precipitant of agitation in older adults (Allen, 1999). The most common impairments are hearing loss and reduced visual acuity. A common component of nursing assessment documents is visual and hearing impairments. If a patient cannot provide information about his or her hearing and vision, the nurse should ask a family member or friend. If there are impairments, the nurse should ensure that hearing aids are working for patients who use them and assess patients for access to glasses or contact lenses.

Social Assessment

The nurse should evaluate factors related to the social domain that may be contributing to aggression or violence in a patient. For example, are conditions in the patient's home, family, or community leading to aggression or violent episodes? Are financial or legal troubles placing stress on the patient that places him or her at risk?

Nursing Diagnosis and Outcome Identification

The nurse analyzes assessment data to understand the dangers that the patient's behavior poses toward self or others. The most common nursing diagnoses for patients experiencing intense anger and aggression are Risk for Self-Directed Violence and Risk for Other-Directed Violence (North American Nursing Diagnosis Association [NANDA], 2001). Outcomes focus on aggression control (Johnson & Maas, 1999).

Planning and Implementing Nursing Interventions

Interventions are the treatment portion of nursing practice. A nursing intervention is any therapeutic response or action by the nurse that occurs within the context of the nurse–patient relationship and is designed to help the patient maintain or regain control over thoughts, feelings, and actions that are aggressive or potentially aggressive. This section emphasizes the development of a partnership between the nurse and patient, who work together to find solutions to prevent the recurrence of explosive episodes and to de-escalate volatile situations. Sometimes, however, the patient's condition (eg, advanced dementia) or the situation will prevent the development of a partnership. In such instances, the nurse must take charge. The nurse who intervenes from within the context of the therapeutic relationship must be cognizant of the fit of a particular intervention. The nurse's action is based on his or her response to the patient. The patient's affective, behavioral, and cognitive response to the intervention provides information about its effects and guides the nurse's next response (Wright & Leahey, 2000) (Fig. 36-2).

The following five assumptions are important to consider in planning interventions with this patient population (Harper-Jaques & Masters, 1994; McElheran & Harper-Jaques, 1994):

- The nurse and patient collaborate to find solutions and alternatives to aggressive and violent outbursts.
- Anger is a normal emotion. All people have the right to express their anger. All people have a responsibility to express their anger in a way that does not, emotionally or physically, threaten or harm others.

- In most instances, the person who behaves aggressively or violently can assume responsibility for the behavior.
- The nurse views the patient from the perspective of acknowledging that the patient has solved problems before and is only temporarily in need of help.
- The nurse understands that norms for behavior are created within the context of a particular environment and are influenced by the patient's history and culture.

Nurses who work collaboratively with potentially violent patients must also keep in mind that they can take certain actions to minimize personal risk:

- Using nonthreatening body language
- Respecting the patient's personal space and boundaries
- Positioning themselves so that they have immediate access to the door of the room in case they need to leave the room
- Choosing to leave open the door to an office while talking to a patient
- Knowing where colleagues are and making sure those colleagues know where they are
- Removing or not wearing clothing or accessories that could be used to harm them, such as scarves, necklaces, or dangling earrings

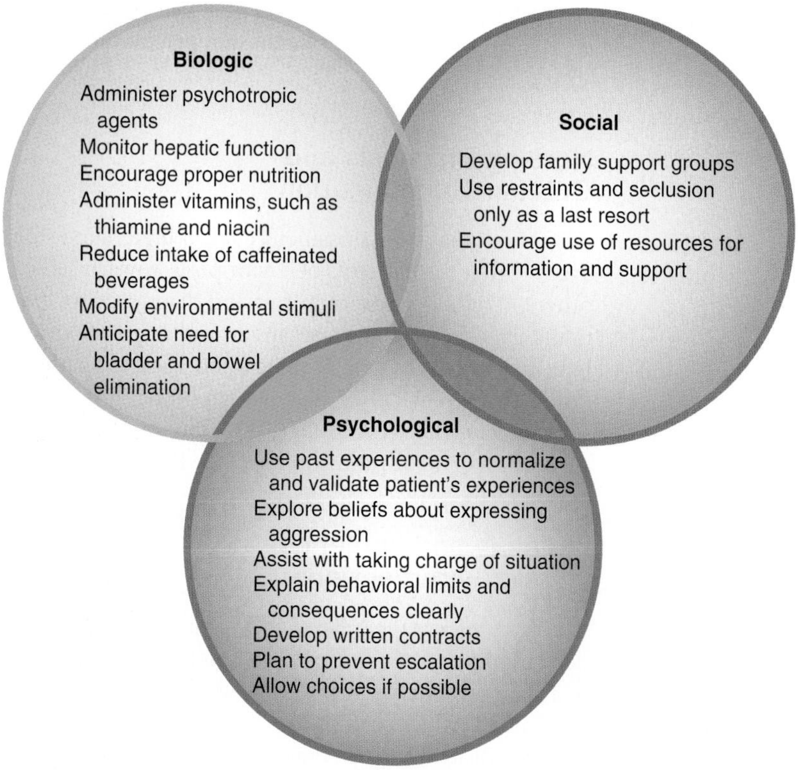

Biologic

Administer psychotropic agents
Monitor hepatic function
Encourage proper nutrition
Administer vitamins, such as thiamine and niacin
Reduce intake of caffeinated beverages
Modify environmental stimuli
Anticipate need for bladder and bowel elimination

Social

Develop family support groups
Use restraints and seclusion only as a last resort
Encourage use of resources for information and support

Psychological

Use past experiences to normalize and validate patient's experiences
Explore beliefs about expressing aggression
Assist with taking charge of situation
Explain behavioral limits and consequences clearly
Develop written contracts
Plan to prevent escalation
Allow choices if possible

FIGURE 36.2 Biopsychosocial interventions for patients with aggression.

TEXT BOX 36.4

Guidelines for Crisis Intervention

1. Call for assistance (eg, other nurses, security staff).

2. Brief all staff; plan intervention.

3. Assign staff to limbs should physical restraint or movement of the patient become necessary.

4. Remove other patients from the area. Also, remove any items that may impede the staff's movement.

5. Crisis intervention leader talks to the patient firmly and calmly. Other staff are present.

6. Leader gives patient choices (eg, go to room to calm down, talk with someone, lose privileges, take medication).

7. If patient continues to argue, leader tells the patient that staff will escort him or her to his or her room. If the patient refuses to walk, staff carry patient to the room.

When a violent outburst appears imminent or occurs, immediate intervention is required and should be directed by a designated leader (Text Box 36-4). Preassigning a crisis intervention leader at the change of shift or during a staff meeting can reduce confusion and time-consuming delays during a crisis. The crisis leader assumes responsibility for requesting additional staff, assigning staff duties, and designing and directing interventions (Brasic & Fogelman, 1999; Carpenito, 2000).

The nurse who works with potentially aggressive patients does so with respect and concern. The goal is to work with patients to find solutions other than violent outbursts. The nurse approaches these patients calmly, being mindful to use nonthreatening body language and to avoid violation of boundaries. In dealing with aggression, as in other aspects of nursing practice, the nurse will find that at times the best intervention is silence. It is easy to equate intervention with activity, the sense that "I must do something." But quiet calmness on the nurse's part may be enough to help a patient regain control of his or her behavior and perspective on the situation. Trying to clarify what has upset the patient is important. The nurse can use therapeutic communication techniques to prevent a crisis or defuse a critical situation (see Therapeutic Dialogue: The Potentially Aggressive Patient).

During daily interactions with patients, nurses intervene in many creative and useful ways. The intervention alone does not serve as the solution—it is the process or art of offering the intervention within the context of the nurse–patient relationship that is successful. These interventions will not be successful with all patients all the time. It is not the nurse's or patient's fault, however, when an intervention is ineffective. The intervention simply did not fit the situation at that particular time.

Biologic Interventions

Administering and Monitoring Medications. Several classes of drugs are used in the management of aggressive behavior. The rationale for their use is based on the, as yet, limited understanding of the interaction of neurotransmitter systems. Clinical trials on patients displaying aggressive behavior are difficult to conduct. Much current knowledge of effective medications is based on case studies (Buckley, 1999). Important points for the nurse to consider in making decisions about patient and family teaching, medication administration, and consultation with physicians and pharmacists are as follows:

- High-potency *typical antipsychotics* such as haloperidol (Haldol) are commonly used to manage

---

THERAPEUTIC DIALOGUE | **The Potentially Aggressive Patient**

Ineffective Approach

Nurse: I think you look angry. What is the problem?
Patient: Nothing!
Nurse: (Moves closer.) Let's talk about the problem.
Patient: (Backs up.) There is no problem!!
Nurse: You are raising your voice.
Patient: You are yelling at me. Get out of my face. . . .

Effective Approach

Nurse: You look upset. Are you OK? (Observation.)
Patient: I'm so angry. I feel like hitting someone.
Nurse: What happened? (Nonjudgmental question.)
Patient: I had to wait to see you! Everyone is out to get me!

Nurse: Oh. Did you get angry because of the waiting or have lots of things happened? (Clarification.)
Patient: Last night, my boyfriend dumped me, my roommate stole my money, and now I have no place to stay.
Nurse: A lot has happened to you. (Validation.) Let's talk about the most upsetting problem first.

Critical Thinking Challenge

- In the first scenario, how did the nurse escalate the situation?
- Compare the first scenario with the second. How are they different?

aggression. This class of drugs has sedative and antipsychotic effects. Typical antipsychotics are believed to act by depressing the CNS at the subcortical level of the brain, midbrain, and brain stem reticular formation. Haloperidol may reduce the seizure threshold (Citrome & Volavka, 1999).

- Evidence supports that *atypical antipsychotics*, such as risperidone (Risperdal) and olanzapine (Zyprexa), can be useful in reducing agitation (Buckley, 1999). Research on the use of these drugs in treating aggression has focused on people with schizophrenia; there have been isolated reports of the benefits of these medications for other conditions (Buckley, 1999). As with other psychotropic medications, the action of the atypical antipsychotics is not fully understood. It is thought that they block dopamine and serotonin receptors. Extrapyramidal side effects are few, which makes these drugs easier to tolerate than the typical antipsychotics (see Drug Profile: Risperidone).
- *Selective serotonin reuptake inhibitors* (SSRIs) are increasingly being used for their antiaggressive effects as well as for their antidepressant effects (eg, fluoxetine [Prozac], paroxetine [Paxil]). Their effects on aggressive behavior usually occur before their effects on depression.
- β-*Adrenergic receptor blockers*, such as propranolol (Inderal), may be used for their effect in decreasing the peripheral manifestations of rage that are associated with excitement of the sympathetic nervous system (Fava, 1997).

- *Lithium carbonate* has been effective in treating aggressive behavior associated with head injury.
- *Divalproex sodium* and *carbamazepine* have been shown to reduce aggressive behavior.
- Psychotropic drugs often interact with antiepileptic and antispasmodic agents, altering pharmacokinetics. For example, chlorpromazine may increase the risk for seizures in patients taking antiepileptic drugs (Fahs et al., 1997).
- The liver metabolizes most psychotropic drugs (except lithium). The nurse should be alert to possible hepatic dysfunction in patients with a history of alcohol or drug abuse.

Managing Nutrition. Patients with long-standing poor dietary habits (eg, indigent patients, patients with alcoholism) often have deficiencies of thiamine and niacin. Prolonged use of alcohol can block up to 70% of thiamine uptake. Increased irritability, disorientation, and paranoia may result. Encouraging patients to eat more whole grains, nuts, fruit, vegetables, organ meats, and milk instead of "junk" foods is important. The nurse may need to help patients with obtaining the resources needed to buy and prepare healthier food choices.

Caffeine is a potent stimulant (Simmons, 1996). Some inpatient psychiatric units have reduced patients' accessibility to coffee and other caffeinated beverages as a means of trying to reduce aggressive behavior. Results have been mixed.

Psychological Interventions

Psychological interventions help patients gain control over their expression of anger and aggressive behavior.

DRUG PROFILE: Risperidone
Antipsychotic Benzisoxazole
Trade Name: Risperdal

Receptor affinity: Dopamine, serotonin, blocks RAS; anticholinergic, antihistaminic and α-adrenergic

Mechanisms of action: Mechanism of action not fully understood; anticholinergic, antihistaminic, and α-adrenergic receptor blocking action may be reasons for its therapeutic action

Indications: In large doses, used for management of psychotic disorders and rapid control of aggressive or violent behavior; in small doses, can be used to stabilize mood and reduce irritability and hostility

Route and dosage: Low initial dosage, then work up; oral: tablets 1 mg, 2 mg, 3 mg, and 4 mg; suspension: 1 mg/1 mL

Initial dose: For management of psychosis or rapid control, 1 mg orally twice daily with an increase of 1 mg/d to a maximum daily dose of 3 mg twice daily; for mood stabilization or to reduce irritability, 0.5 mg orally HS to a maximum of 1 mg hs

Half-life (peak effect): Tablets, 1–3 h

Selected adverse reactions: Insomnia, anxiety, headache, nausea, unsteadiness, vomiting, tardive dyskinesias (refer to drug reference materials for a complete listing)

Warnings: Contraindicated in patients with a known allergy to risperidone and in women who are breastfeeding; use cautiously in cardiovascular disease, pregnancy, renal or hepatic impairment, or hypotension

Special Patient and Family Education

- Take drug exactly as prescribed.
- Do not make up missed dose.
- Do not stop taking the drug suddenly; gradual reduction is recommended.
- Take suspension with a liquid (but not with cola or tea).
- Report lethargy, weakness, fever, sore throat, malaise, mouth ulcers, or palpitations to nurse or physician.

In some instances, these interventions eliminate the need for chemical (medications) or mechanical restraints. De-escalating potential aggression is always preferable to challenging or provoking a patient. Anger control assistance, as set forth by the *Nursing Interventions Classification* (NIC) (McCloskey & Bulechek, 1996), is useful and can prevent deterioration of a patient's control of behavior (Text Box 36-5). For example, nurses at a psychiatric center in New York State (Visalli et al., 1997) developed an anger management assessment tool and a handout for use by patients. In a 1-year follow-up study, they reported a reduction in the use of seclusion and restraint and an increase in the successful use of alternative interventions to respond to aggression.

Affective Interventions. Affective interventions are designed to reduce or increase intense emotions that may hinder the patient from finding alternatives to the use of aggression or violence (Wright & Leahey, 2000). They include validating, listening to the patient's illness experience, and exploring beliefs.

Validating. Often, patients who experience intense anger and rage feel isolated and may view themselves as alone in having these feelings. The nurse can reduce the patient's feelings of isolation by acknowledging these intense feelings. By drawing on past experience with other patients, the nurse can also reassure the patient that others have felt the same way.

Listening to Patient's Illness Experience. Often, patients and their family members are invited to provide details about past medical treatments, medications, hospitalizations, and therapies. What is overlooked is the experience of the health problem or the experience of interactions with professionals. Inviting patients and families to talk about their previous experience with the health care system may highlight both their concerns and resources. See Text Box 36-6 for an example of how a nurse uses this intervention to improve a patient's care.

Exploring Beliefs. Exploring the patient's beliefs about the expression of angry feelings can be useful. Discussion of beliefs that prevent the patient from seeking alternate ways of handling distressing emotions and situations may help him or her to take charge of the situation.

Cognitive Interventions. Cognitive interventions are usually those that provide new ideas, opinions, information, or education about a particular problem. The

---

TEXT BOX 36.5

Anger Control Assistance

Definition: Facilitation of the expression of anger adaptively and nonviolently

Activities

- Establish basic trust and rapport with patient.
- Use a calm, reassuring approach.
- Determine appropriate behavior expectations for expression of anger, given patient's level of cognitive and physical functioning.
- Limit patient's access to frustrating situations until he or she can express anger adaptively.
- Encourage patient to seek assistance of nursing staff or responsible others during periods of increasing tension.
- Monitor patient's potential for inappropriate aggression and intervene before its expression.
- Prevent physical harm (eg, apply restraint, remove potential weapons) if patient directs anger at self or others.
- Provide reassurance to patient that nursing staff will intervene to prevent him or her from losing control.
- Use external controls (eg, physical or manual restraint, time-outs, seclusion) as needed to calm a patient who is expressing anger destructively.
- Provide feedback on behavior to help patient identify anger.

- Assist patient in identifying the source of anger.
- Identify the function that anger, frustration, and rage serves for the patient.
- Identify consequences of inappropriate expressions of anger.
- Assist patient in planning strategies to prevent the inappropriate expression of anger.
- Identify with patient the benefits of expressing anger adaptively and nonviolently.
- Establish expectation that patient can control his or her behavior.
- Instruct patient on use of calming measures (eg, time outs, deep breaths).
- Assist patient to develop appropriate methods of expressing anger to others (eg, assertiveness, use of statements).
- Provide role models who express anger appropriately.
- Support patient in implementing anger control strategies and appropriately expressing anger.
- Provide reinforcement for appropriate expression of anger.

Adapted from McCloskey, J., & Bulechek, G. (1996). *Nursing interventions classification (NIC)* (2nd ed.). St. Louis: Mosby.

TEXT BOX 36.6

Clinical Vignette: Mary

Mary, a 22-year-old single woman, was a regular patient at the crisis center. During previous visits, she came alone or with her mother and demanded immediate attention. This time she comes with her mother. The receptionist groans and rolls her eyes as she describes this family to the new intake nurse. "They are obnoxious. It is best to handle them fast and get them out of here!"

Before the interview, the nurse reviews Mary's extensive file. She notes that on many occasions Mary was aggressive and violent while in the center. The mother has complained to the local health authority about the center on at least two occasions.

During the interview, the nurse asks mother and daughter the following questions:

- What was the most useful thing that has happened during previous contacts at the center?
- What was the least useful thing about previous contacts at the center?

The family looks surprised to be asked these questions. They state that previous visits were useful only in providing them with written proof that Mary could not work. That information, required by the social service agency, ensured continuation of Mary's disability checks. Furthermore, Mary and her mother state that they often left the center feeling that the nurses were not interested in their concerns and believed that if Mary tried harder, her hallucinations would decrease. They add that they often waited 1 to 2 hours to be seen, whereas other patients were seen more quickly. Mary admits that she sometimes made a lot of noise in the waiting room to be seen sooner.

The nurse then asks: What would need to happen during your visit today to make you feel that coming here was worthwhile? The mother expresses interest in receiving information about hallucinations and how she could help Mary when she experiences them. Mary says she wants to know how to handle angry feelings.

nurse offers a cognitive intervention with the goal of inviting the patient to consider other possibilities (Wright & Leahey, 2000). Examples include giving commendations, offering information, providing education, and utilizing thought stopping and contracting.

Giving Commendations. Often, in clinical settings, the focus becomes "problem saturated" (White, 1988/89) and what the patient does well is overlooked. A commendation is a "statement of special praise that is specific to some aspect of patient and/or family functioning" (McElheran & Harper-Jaques, 1994, p. 7). A commendation focuses on the patient's behavior pattern over time and highlights his or her strengths and resources. For example, commending a patient's decision to request medication or to remove herself from an overstimulating environment highlights the woman's ability

to assume responsibility for thoughts and feelings that have previously invited aggressive behavior.

Offering Information. Nurses can offer information or arrange opportunities for patients to receive information from other professionals. Patients may sometimes become agitated and threaten to harm the nurse because they do not know what is expected of them or they do not remember why they need to be involved in treatment. The nurse can tell them about unit expectations or the reasons for hospitalization. The nurse can also determine the patient's information needs by asking questions. One option in providing information, education, and support is to develop a family support group, which can provide a forum for responding to general concerns and questions at the same time.

In the mental health setting, the nurse must make behavioral limits and consequences clear. Whenever possible, the nurse should match consequences to the patient's interests and desires. For example, Jane was slamming doors and banging down dishes in the kitchen of the group home. The nurse approached her to discuss other means of expressing her anger. During the conversation, the nurse reminded Jane that further agitated behavior would mean that Jane would not participate in a shopping trip planned that day. The trip was important to Jane, so she chose to discuss her concern with the nurse.

Providing Education. Nurses can offer education to patients and families about various topics. Greater understanding about mental health problems and altered mental status may help to prevent aggression by clarifying misunderstandings. Nurses can also teach patients and families about anger management.

Thought Stopping. In thought stopping, the nurse asks the patient to identify thoughts that heighten feelings of anger and invites the patient to "turn the thoughts off" by focusing on other thoughts or activities (Burns, 1980). Ideas of other activities include talking to someone, reading, baking, or thinking about a future event.

Contracting. A contract is a written document that the nurse and patient develop. The document clearly states acceptable and unacceptable behaviors, consequences and rewards, and the role of both the patient and nurse in preventing and managing aggressive behavior (Morrison, 1993).

Behavioral Interventions. Behavioral interventions are designed to assist the patient to behave differently (Wright & Leahey, 2000). Examples of such interventions include assigning behavioral tasks, using bibliotherapy, interrupting patterns, and providing choices.

Assigning Behavioral Tasks. Sometimes, the nurse may assign a behavioral task as a way to help the patient maintain or regain control over aggressive behaviors.

Behavioral tasks might include writing down a list of grievances that the patient will discuss with the nurse or observing how other people take charge of anger and aggression. For example, the nurse may ask the patient to observe patients or staff on the unit, people at a shopping mall, or particular movies or television shows to evaluate how other people in real or fictitious situations handle anger.

Using Bibliotherapy. In bibliotherapy, the nurse may ask the patient to read a particular pamphlet or article on anger management. The nurse and patient then discuss what the patient read to decide which, if any, of the ideas the patient can use when angry.

Interrupting Patterns. Although patients are not usually aware of it, escalation of feelings, thoughts, and behavior from calmness to violence usually follows a particular pattern. Disruption of the pattern can sometimes be a useful means of preventing escalation and can help the patient regain composure. Nurses can suggest several strategies to interrupt patterns:

- Counting to 10
- Removing oneself from interactions or stimuli that may contribute to increased distress
- Doing something different (eg, reading, exercising, watching television)

Providing Choices. Whenever possible, the nurse should provide the patient with choices, particularly those patients who have little control over their situation because of their condition. For example, the patient who is experiencing a manic episode and is confined to her room may have few options in her daily schedule. She may be allowed, however, to make choices about food, personal hygiene, and which pajamas to wear.

Social Interventions

Reducing Stimulation. Theorists have hypothesized that people differ as to the level of stimulation that they need or prefer (Kolanowski et al., 1994). Normally, people adjust their environments accordingly: some people like their music loud, whereas others want it soft; some people seek out the thrill of high-risk sports, whereas others prefer to be spectators. Within the context of a brain disorder or an unusually restrictive environment, such adjustments may not be within the patient's control. The patient with a brain injury, progressive dementia, or distorted vision may be experiencing intense and highly confusing stimulation, even though the environment, from the nurse or family's perspective, seems calm and orderly.

For people whose perceptions or thoughts are disordered from brain damage, degeneration, or other thought-processing difficulties, modification of the environment may be one of the main interventions. Like-

wise, introducing more structure into a chaotic environment can help decrease the risk for aggressive behavior (Citrome & Volavka, 1999). The nurse can make stimuli meaningful or can simplify and interpret the environment in many practical ways. Some examples are by identifying people or equipment that may be unfamiliar, providing cues as to what is expected (eg, posting signs with directions, putting toothbrush and toothpaste by the sink), and removing or silencing unnecessary stimuli (eg, turning off paging systems, which can be startling to patients). A good place to start is with the NIC environmental management interventions (Text Box 36-7).

Often, patients with cognitive impairment exhibit repetitive behaviors, such as wandering and making noises. These actions may be the patient's means of remaining connected to the environment, and attempts to interrupt them may lead the patient to strike out. Engaging the patient in a simple exercise, such as playing catch or moving to music, may help reduce such behavior. Other possible interventions include providing a safe, controlled environment for patients who need to pace and providing structured activities that use previously learned motor skills (eg, playing the piano).

Considering the environment from the patient's viewpoint is essential. For instance, if the surroundings are unfamiliar, the patient will need to process more information. Lack of a recognizable pattern or structure further taxes the patient's capacity to encode information. Appropriate interventions include clarifying the meaning and purpose of people and objects in the environment, enhancing the patient's sense of control and the predictability of the environment, and reducing other stimuli as much as possible (Stolley et al., 1999).

Anticipating Needs. The nurse can anticipate many needs of patients. In assuming responsibility for patients with cognitive impairment, the nurse needs to know when the patient last voided and the pattern of bowel movements. Regular toileting routines are not just interventions to prevent incontinence. Similarly, the anticipation of basic needs such as thirst and hunger is important, especially when working with adults or children who cannot readily express their needs. Other discomforts can arise from such conditions as ingrown toenails and adverse medication reactions.

The urge to void can be a powerful stimulus to agitated behavior. It is not uncommon in a neurologic observation unit to see a young man with a recent head injury become violent just before spontaneously voiding. From a biologic perspective, such a patient is probably normally sensitive or even hypersensitive to a full bladder. He probably also has sufficient cognitive function to recognize his need to void. Even some level of social inhibition may be operational in that he recognizes that

TEXT BOX 36.7

Environmental Management: Violence Prevention

Definition: Monitoring and manipulating the physical environment to decrease the potential of violent behavior directed toward self, others, or environment

Activities

- Remove potential weapons (eg, sharps, ropelike objects) from the environment.
- Search environment routinely to maintain it as hazard free.
- Search patient and belongings for weapons or potential weapons during inpatient admission procedures as appropriate.
- Monitor the safety of items that visitors bring to the environment.
- Instruct visitors and other caregivers about relevant patient safety issues.
- Limit patient use of potential weapons (eg, sharps, ropelike objects).
- Monitor patient during use of potential weapons (eg, razors).
- Place patient with potential for self-harm with a roommate to decrease isolation and opportunity to act on self-harm thoughts, as appropriate.
- Assign single room to patient with potential for violence toward others.
- Place patient in a bedroom located near a nursing station.
- Limit access to windows, unless locked and shatter-proof, as appropriate.
- Lock utility and storage rooms.
- Provide paper dishes and plastic utensils at meals.
- Place patient in the least restrictive environment that still allows for the necessary level of observation.
- Provide ongoing surveillance of all patient access areas to maintain patient safety and therapeutically intervene, as needed.
- Remove other individuals from the vicinity of a violent or potentially violent patient.
- Maintain a designated safe area (eg, seclusion room) for patient to be placed when violent.
- Provide plastic, rather than metal, clothes hangers, as appropriate.

Adapted from McCloskey, J., & Bulechek, G. (1996). *Nursing interventions classification (NIC)* (2nd ed.). St. Louis: Mosby.

voiding while lying on his back in bed, with strangers around, is inappropriate. But if he cannot speak or ask for help, he may become increasingly panic stricken. Thrashing around in bed, unable to communicate his need, he may strike out at staff. How might you manage this situation?

The following scenario is the true account of how one graduate student dealt with another common situation. A 75-year-old woman was pacing around the nursing station of a psychogeriatric unit in a nursing home, crying for her mother. Various people spoke kindly to her, trying to explain that her mother was not there. Donna, a graduate student, was studying the wandering behaviors of patients with Alzheimer's disease on the unit. Hypothesizing that there is purpose behind these actions, she walked alongside the woman. After talking a bit with her about the patient's mother, Donna asked the patient what she would like to do if her mother were there. Gradually the patient confided that she needed her mother to help her find the bathroom. Donna then offered to help the woman, walking her to the bathroom. After voiding copiously, the patient seemed greatly relieved and settled down.

Using Seclusion and Restraint. **Seclusion** and **restraint** are controversial interventions to use judiciously and only when other interventions have failed to control the patient's behavior. The availability of effective psychotropic medications since the 1950s has reduced the need for these interventions of last resort. Reasons usually cited for using them are to protect the patient from injury to self or others, to help the patient reestablish behavioral control, and to minimize disruption of unit treatment regimens. The controversy over these interventions and their potential to be applied punitively heightens the need for clear institutional standards for their use. The development and use of clear practice standards can reduce the likelihood that these interventions will be misused.

Evaluation is also important in tracking the use of seclusion and restraint. Morrison and colleagues (1997) evaluated the use of seclusion by examining its antecedents. Through the use of behavioral mapping, researchers could determine the location of incidents that resulted in seclusion. Most occurred in the day and dining rooms. This finding led to an examination of ward policies that restricted patient movement on the unit.

Interactional Processes

When the nurse develops a collaborative relationship with the patient, he or she can assist the patient to not exhibit aggressive behavior. Johnson and colleagues (1997) explored the experience of thought-disordered individuals preceding an aggressive incident. Three themes emerged from interviews with 12 patients who had a diagnosis of a thought disorder and a history of aggressive incidents:

- The strong influence of the external environment
- The use of aggressive behaviors to feel empowered briefly in a situation

- The occurrence of aggressive incidents despite knowledge of strategies to control anger

The skills the nurse uses in interactions with the patient may invite escalation or de-escalation of a tense situation (Morrison, 1998). When the nurse uses communication skills to draw out the patient's experience, together the nurse and patient coevolve an alternative view of the problem. Some nursing writers (Leahey & Harper-Jaques, 1996; Vosburgh & Simpson, 1993; Wright & Leahey, 2000) have highlighted the importance of attending to notions of reciprocity and circularity when providing nursing care. For example, the nurse explores the meaning of the expression of aggressive behaviors with the patient and the patient's beliefs about the ability to control aggressive impulses. Or the nurse and patient could discuss the effects of the nurse's behaviors on the patient and the effects of the patient's behaviors on the nurse. Such an approach facilitates the development of an accepting and equal nurse–patient relationship. The patient is a partner invited to assume responsibility for inappropriate actions. This approach is in contrast to a hierarchic nurse–patient relationship that emphasizes the nurse's role in controlling the patient's behaviors and defining changes the patient must make. In a collaborative approach, the nurse values the patient's experience and acknowledges his or her strengths. The nurse asks the patient to use those strengths to either maintain or resume control of behavior.

In Western cultures, events are typically thought of in a linear fashion (Wright & Leahey, 2000). The nurse who uses a linear causality frame of reference to think about patient aggression and violence will view the problem as follows:

PACING → leads to → THREATENING BEHAVIORS
(Event A)   (Event B)

From this linear perspective, the nurse labels the patient as the problem, and other factors assume secondary importance. The nurse might decide, first, to gain control over the patient's behavior. The nurse may base this decision on his or her affective response and previous experience (ie, that threatening behaviors frighten other patients and disrupt the unit routine). The nurse's response to a patient's behavior could be to ask the patient to stop yelling, to inform the patient that the behavior is inappropriate, or to suggest the use of medication if the patient does not calm down. When one thinks based on linear causality, he or she assumes that event A (pacing) causes event B (threatening behavior).

When one thinks using circular causality, he or she attempts to understand the link between behaviors and to determine how the threatening behavior will influ-

ence a continuation or cessation of pacing. The nurse who engages in circular thinking will also know that his or her responses to the patient will influence the situation. The nurse's responses will be in the domains of cognition (ideas, concepts, and beliefs), affect (emotional state), and behavior (Tomm, 1980). The nurse will be aware of the reciprocal influences of the nurse's and patient's behaviors (Wright & Leahey, 2000). In viewing the situation from a circular perspective, the nurse is interested in understanding how people are involved rather than in discovering who is to blame. This perspective does not ignore individual responsibility for aggressive or violent actions, nor does it blame the victim. It does invite the nurse to consider the multiple influences on the expression of aggressive and violent behavior (Robinson et al., 1994).

Responding to Assault

In recent years, compelling scientific evidence that violence portrayed in the media is harmful to children has fostered debate about violence and its effects. As a result, television networks have taken both voluntary and legislated actions to limit violent programming during hours when children are generally watching programs. These gains in limiting access to violence, however, have been countered by the growing availability of violent video games and websites.

Given today's societal context, it is not surprising that aggression and violence directed toward nurses is often ignored. Aggression and violence by patients can threaten the safety of nurses, other patients, other health care professionals, family members, and visitors. Of all health care professionals, nurses are the most frequent targets of patient violence (Arnetz et al., 1998). Family members may also direct aggression and violence toward nurses, especially when they disagree with staff about the patient's treatment plan or have been kept waiting for long periods (Duncan et al., 2000).

In health care settings, nurses assume an active role in preventing and managing aggressive and violent behaviors. Involuntary (as opposed to voluntary) admission to a psychiatric facility or altered mental status in any setting may constrain the development of a trusting relationship between nurse and patient. Nurses are more likely than physicians to be involved with patients who are aggressive or potentially violent because of the amount of time they are in close contact with patients. Nurses also have a major role in setting limits and defining boundaries (see Chap. 9).

Concern and investigation of assaults on nurses has been growing. In a survey of all registered nurses working in acute care institutions in one Canadian province, 17% reported one or more incidents of physical assault (defined as being spit on, bitten, hit, or pushed) in the last five shifts worked (Duncan et al., 2000). Assaults may occur in situations in which the patient perceives the nurse's actions as restricting, controlling, or aggressive (eg, the use of physical restraints) (Morrison, 1998).

The reported rates of assaults on nurses vary greatly. Reported incidence is higher in general hospitals and psychiatric facilities, but nurses who work in ambulatory care settings or community clinics are not immune to assault. Variations in statistics result from differences in definitions of violence, reporting practices, and data collection and analysis as well as underreporting.

Assaults on nurses by patients can have immediate and long-term consequences. Reported assaults range from verbal threats and minor altercations to severe injuries, rape, and murder. Any assault can produce severe consequences for the victim. In some instances, the response of nurse victims may correspond to the symptom profile for posttraumatic stress disorder (Caldwell, 1992).

Lanza's research (1992) has indicated that nurses experience a wide range of responses (Table 36-4) similar to those of victims of any other type of trauma. Because of their role as caregivers, however, nurses may suppress the normal range of feelings after an assault, believing that it is wrong to experience strong feelings of anger and fear in this situation. This belief may relate to the conflict nurses experience in having to care for patients who have hurt them.

Steps can be taken at a clinical and management level to reduce the risk for assaults on nurses by patients. Clinically, nurses must be provided with training programs in the prevention and management of aggressive behavior. These programs, like courses on cardiopulmonary resuscitation (CPR), impart both knowledge and skills. Like CPR training, these courses need to be made available to nurses regularly so that they have opportunities to reinforce and update what they have learned. Nurses who have participated in preventive training programs as students or as professionals are less likely to be involved in situations with aggressive or violent patients. Those with no training are at greater risk (Brasic & Fogelman, 1999). Less experienced staff with poor communication skills are at higher risk for assault (Brasic & Fogelman, 1999).

Evaluation and Treatment Outcomes

Treatment outcomes can be considered at both individual and aggregate levels. The desired outcome at the individual level is for the patient to regain or maintain control over aggressive or potentially aggressive thoughts, feelings, and actions. Aggression Control is the term used in the *Nursing Outcomes Classification* (NOC) (Johnson & Maas, 1997). The nurse may observe that the patient shows decreased psychomotor activity (eg, less pacing), has a more relaxed posture, speaks more directly about feelings of anger and personal needs, requires less sedating medication, shows increased tolerance for frustration and the ability to consider alternatives, and makes effective use of other coping strategies. Evidence of a reduction in risk factors may include decreased noise and confusion in the immediate environment, calmness on the part of nursing staff and others, and a climate of clear expectations and mutual acceptance and respect. In units, day hospitals, or group home settings, indicators of positive

TABLE 36.4 Nurses' Responses to Assault		
Response Type	**Personal**	**Professional**
Affective	• Irritability • Depression • Anger • Anxiety • Apathy	• Erosion of feelings of competence, leading to increased anxiety and fear • Feelings of guilt or self-blame • Fear of potentially violent patients
Cognitive	• Suppressed or intrusive thoughts of assault	• Reduced confidence in judgment • Consideration of job change
Behavioral	• Social withdrawal	• Possible hesitation in responding to other violent situations • Possible overcontrolling • Possible hesitation to report future assaults • Possible withdrawal from colleagues • Questioning of capabilities by coworkers
Physiologic	• Disturbed sleep • Headaches • Stomach aches • Tension	• Increased absenteeism from somatic complaints

RESEARCH BOX 36.1

Nurses' Experiences of Patient Aggression

Much previous research literature on aggression in health care settings has focused on the "aggressors" or the "victims" in a biomedical (internal) or environmental model. In the biomedical model, treatment focuses on containing aggression through a reactive approach. Research on environmental influences has identified contributing factors but has not sufficiently addressed the complexity of the problem. More recent literature has focused on interactional factors. Duxbury suggests that the way nurses choose to intervene in preventing or managing aggressive behavior may be shaped by which of these theoretic models dominates. She reports on an exploratory study to examine registered nurses' experiences of violent incidents with patients within both mental health and general nursing settings.

Duxbury collected data from 34 mental health nurses from acute inpatient settings and 32 nurses from acute medical-surgical units using the critical incident technique (CIT). Each participant received a blank sheet of paper with the question, "In your own words, please describe one or more incident(s) which has involved a patient being violent." Content analysis was done on this qualitative data to identify themes and explore differences between the two settings. The most common types of aggressive behaviors were verbal and physical. Most nurses were found to attribute aggressive behavior to internal factors, with noticeable emphasis on controlling interventions. Nurses identified environmental and interactional factors much less frequently, suggesting that the biomedical model predom-

inated. Experiences of the two groups of nurses were similar, but their patterns of response differed somewhat. Mental health nurses were more likely to manage the situation themselves, whereas general nurses were more likely to seek outside assistance (eg, medical staff, mental health teams, police). These findings should not be generalized to other environments, but they provide some insight into the experiences and behaviors of nurses in acute care settings. Unfortunately, in this study, the full set of questions needed for CIT was not used, so we do not know what was significant about these incidents from the nurses' point of view. The author also acknowledges that the wording of the one question may have influenced the lack of emphasis on prevention and de-escalation in the responses.

Utilization in the Clinical Setting. Research findings such as those reported here can remind nurses that how they think they practice may not be what they actually do and that the models held influence actions. These nurses recognized the importance of internal factors in contributing to aggressive behavior, a perspective that this chapter also emphasizes; however, they revealed less attention to environmental considerations. Of most significance was the lack of emphasis on interactional factors. Nurses must recognize that their behavior also greatly affects how patients feel and behave.

This research study is suitable for conceptual utilization, that is, expanding ways of thinking about nursing practice.

Duxbury, J. (1999). An exploratory account of registered nurses' experiences of patient aggression in both mental health and general nursing settings. *Journal of Psychiatric and Mental Health Nursing, 6*(2), 107–114.

treatment outcomes might be a reduction in the number and severity of assaults on staff and other patients, fewer incident reports, and increased staff competency in de-escalating potentially violent situations.

Continuum of Care

Anger and aggression occur in all settings. During periods of extreme aggression, in which people are a danger to themselves or others because of a mental disorder, they are admitted to an acute psychiatric unit. Removing individuals from their environment and hospitalizing them in a locked psychiatric unit provides enough safety that the aggressive behavior dissipates. Because uncontrolled anger and aggression interfere with their ability to function, people who have problems in these areas require referral to appropriate resources before these destructive behaviors erupt.

Further understanding of the phenomena of anger, aggression, and violence as they occur in the clinical set-

ting is needed. Research studies that have illuminated this problem from a nursing perspective need to be continued and expanded. Specific areas of study need to examine the link between biology, neurology, and psychology. Also, further explorations of the reciprocal influence of patient interactional style and treatment setting culture will assist in the development and management of humane treatment settings. Finally, and perhaps most importantly, nurses must research the effectiveness of particular nursing interventions (see Research Box 36-1).

Summary of Key Points

➤ Biopsychosocial theories used to explain anger, aggression, and violence include the following types:
  • Neurobiologic, including the cognitive neuroassociation model, neurostructural model (the emotional circuit), and neurochemical model (low serotonin syndrome)

- Psychological, including psychoanalytic theories, behavioral theories (eg, drive theory, social learning theory), and cognitive theories (eg, rational-emotive theory)
- Sociocultural theories
- Interactional theory

➤ Biologic factors to assess in patients who display aggressive and violent behaviors include exposure to toxic chemicals, use of medications, substance abuse, premenstrual dysphoric disorder, trauma, hemorrhage, and tumor.

➤ Psychological factors to assess in patients who display aggressive and violent behaviors include thought processing (eg, perception, delusion) and sensory impairment.

➤ Biologic intervention choices include administering medications and managing nutrition.

➤ Psychological intervention choices can be affective (eg, validating, listening, exploring beliefs), cognitive (eg, giving commendations, offering information, providing education, utilizing thought stopping or contracting), or behavioral (eg, assigning tasks, using bibliotherapy, interrupting patterns, providing choices).

➤ Social intervention choices include reducing stimulation, anticipating needs, and using seclusion or restraints.

➤ Patient aggression and violence are serious concerns for nurses in all areas of clinical practice. Training in and policies and procedures for the prevention and management of aggressive episodes should be available in all work settings.

Critical Thinking Challenges

1. Mr. K, a 32-year-old single man, is newly admitted to an inpatient psychiatric unit after threatening to kill himself. He seems extremely angry and agitated. The nurse initially approaches him and offers him an opportunity to talk or listen to music in a quiet area of the unit. He shakes his head "no" and walks away. Shortly after the nurse's offer, Mr. K walks to the nursing station, starts pounding on the desk, and demands that someone talk with him. What frameworks can the nurse use to understand Mr. K's behavior? At this point, what data does she have from which to develop a plan of care? What is the range of possible interventions that the nurse can use to assist Mr. K to behave in a manner that matches his context?

2. Discuss the influence of social expectations on the expression of anger. Identify how childhood experiences can influence expression of anger and aggression in adulthood.

3. Should perpetrators of aggressive and violent acts be held accountable for their behaviors? If so, under what circumstances?

4. Consider the following situation, and examine whether your responses differ according to the circumstances. Should legal charges be filed for: (1) a middle-aged man found drunk on admission to the emergency department, or (2) an elderly woman with dementia who is living in a nursing home?

5. When a nurse excuses verbally abusive behavior by a patient, family member, or health care colleague, what implicit message does he or she send?

6. In what ways do sociocultural theories influence the relationships between nurses and patients? Do these theories influence the relationships between nurses and their colleagues, patients, and family members?

7. Mr. J is sitting quietly and reading a magazine when Mr. T sits beside him and begins a conversation. Mr. J responds by pushing Mr. T onto the floor. How do you explain Mr. J's response? Could it have been prevented?

 WEB LINKS

www.journals.wiley.com/0096-140X This site provides a *Guide to the Literature on Aggressive Behavior* and information on the *Journal of the International Society for Research on Aggression*. The guide provides an extensive list of current publications on aggressive behavior.

www.helping.apa.org/warningsigns The American Psychological Association maintains this website. This section focuses on teen violence. It includes a personal risk evaluation for violent behavior, tips on helping when someone you know shows violence warning signs, and a free brochure.

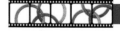 **MOVIES**

Caddyshack: 1980. Bill Murray plays a groundskeeper at a posh golf club. His determination and anger toward some gophers leads to interesting outcomes!
Viewing Points: How does the groundskeeper's thinking about the gophers change during the movie? How does his thinking influence his behavior? How does his thinking influence his ability to examine the consequences of his behavior?

The Insider: 1999. Russell Crowe plays a tobacco industry insider with scientific evidence that cigarettes are made to increase their addictive qualities. Al Pacino plays a news program producer who tries to get the story. Throughout the movie, many attempts are made to suppress the story.

Viewing Point: What is the goal of the people who use aggression and violence in this film?

Girl Interrupted: 2000. This movie tells the story of a young woman who is committed to a mental hospital after a suicide attempt.

Viewing Points: In what way do the behaviors of the staff encourage aggression and violence? How do nurses intervene to help the patients regain or maintain control of aggressive behaviors.

REFERENCES

Allen, L. A. (1999). Treating agitation without drugs. *American Journal of Nursing, 99*(4), 36–42.

Arnetz, J. E., Arnetz, B. B., & Soderman, E. (1998). Violence toward health care workers. *American Association of Occupational Health Nurses Journal, 46*(3), 107–114.

Averill, J. R. (1982). *Anger and aggression: An essay on emotion.* New York: Springer-Verlag.

Bandura, A. (1973). *Aggression: A social learning analysis.* New York: Prentice-Hall.

Beck, A. T. (1976). *Cognitive therapy and emotional disorders.* New York: International Universities Press.

Berkowitz, L. (1989). Frustration-aggression hypothesis: Examination and reformulation. *Psychological Bulletin, 106*(1), 59–73.

Brasic, J. R., & Fogelman, D. (1999). Clinician safety. *Psychiatric Clinics of North America, 22*(4), 923–940.

Buckley, P. F. (1999). The role of typical and atypical antipsychotic medications in the management of agitation and aggression. *Journal of Clinical Psychiatry, 60*(Suppl. 10), 52–60.

Burns, D. (1980). *Feeling good: The new mood therapy.* New York: Avon Books.

Caldwell, M. F. (1992). Incidence of PTSD among staff victims of patient violence. *Hospital and Community Psychiatry, 43*(8), 838–839.

Capra, F. (1996). *The web of life: A new scientific understanding of living systems.* New York: Anchor Books.

Carpenito, L. J. (2000). *Nursing diagnosis: Application to practice* (8th ed.). Philadelphia: Lippincott Williams & Wilkins.

Cheung, P., & Schweitzer, I. (1998). Correlates of aggressive behavior in schizophrenia: An overview. *Australian and New Zealand Journal of Psychiatry, 32*(2), 400–409.

Citrome, L., & Volavka, J. (1999). Violent patients in the emergency setting. *Psychiatric Clinics of North America, 22*(4), 789–801.

Corrigan, P. W., Yudofsky, S. C., & Silver, J. M. (1993). Pharmacological and behavioral treatment for aggressive psychiatric in-patients. *Hospital and Community Psychiatry, 44*(3), 125–133.

Duncan, S., Estabrookes, C. A., & Reimer, M. A. (2000). Violence against nurses. *Alberta RN, 56*(2), 13–14.

Duxbury, J. (1999). An exploratory account of registered nurses' experience of patient aggression in both mental health and general nursing settings. *Journal of Psychiatric and Mental Health Nursing, 6*(2), 107–114.

Elkind, D. (1975). Wilhelm Reich. In A. M. Freedman, H. I. Kaplan, & B. J. Sadock (Eds.), *Comprehensive textbook of psychiatry* (2nd ed., pp. 650–655). Baltimore: Williams & Wilkins.

Ellis, A. (1977). *Anger: How to live with and without it.* Secaucus, NJ: Citadel Press.

Estroff, S. E., Zimmer, C., Lachicotte, W. S., & Benoit, J. (1994). The influence of social networks and social support on violence by persons with serious mental illness. *Hospital and Community Psychiatry, 45*(7), 669–679.

Fahs, H., Potiron, G., Senon, J. L., & Perivier, E. (1997). Anticonvulsants in agitation and behavior disorders in demented subjects. *Encephale, 25*(2), 169–174.

Fava, M. (1997). Psychopharmacologic treatment of pathologic aggression. *Psychiatric Clinics of North America, 20*(2), 427–451.

Fromm, E. (1973). *The anatomy of human destructiveness.* New York: Holt, Rinehart and Winston.

Gerloff, L. (1997). Anger management. *Arkansas Nursing News, 14*(1), 5–7.

Gortner, E. T., Gollan, J. K., & Jacobson, N. S. (1997). Psychological aspects of perpetrators of domestic violence and their relationships with the victims. *Psychiatric Clinics of North America, 20*(2), 337–352.

Harper-Jaques, S., & Masters, A. (1994). Powerful words: The use of letters with sexual abuse survivors. *Journal of Psychosocial Nursing and Mental Health Services, 32*(8), 11–16.

Harper-Jaques, S., & Reimer, M. (1992). Aggressive behavior and the brain: A different perspective for the mental health nurse. *Archives of Psychiatric Nursing, 6*(5), 312–320.

Harris, D., & Morrison, E. F. (1995). Managing violence without coercion. *Archives of Psychiatric Nursing, 9*(4), 203–210.

Jenkins, A. (1990). *Invitations to responsibility.* Adelaide, NSW, Australia: Dulwich Centre Publications.

Johnson, B., Martin, M. L., Guha, M., & Montgomery, P. (1997). The experience of thought disordered individuals preceding an aggressive incident. *Journal of Psychiatric and Mental Health Nursing, 4*, 213–220.

Johnson, M., & Maas, M. (1999). *Nursing outcomes classification (NOC).* St. Louis: Mosby.

Kavoussi, R., Armstead, P., & Coccaro, E. (1997). The neurobiology of aggression. *Psychiatric Clinics of North America, 20*(2), 395–403.

Kennedy, M. G. (1993). Relationship between psychiatric diagnosis and patient aggression. *Issues in Mental Health Nursing, 14*(3), 263–273.

Kolanowski, A., Hurwitz, S., Taylor, L. A., et al. (1994). Contextual factors associated with disturbing behavior of institutionalized elders. *Nursing Research, 43*(2), 73–79.

Lanza, M. L. (1992). Nurses as patient assault victims: An update, synthesis, and recommendations. *Archives of Psychiatric Nursing, 6*(3), 163–171.

Leahey, M., & Harper-Jaques, S. (1996). Family-nurse relationship: Core assumptions and clinical implications. *Journal of Family Nursing, 2*(2), 133–151.

Lerner, H. (1986). *The dance of anger: A woman's guide to changing the patterns of intimate relationships.* New York: Harper & Row.

Levine, D. S., Leven, S. J., & Prueitt, P. S. (1992). Integration, disintegration and the frontal lobes. In D. S. Levine & S. J. Leven (Eds.), *Motivation, emotion, and goal direction in neural networks* (pp. 301–335). Hillsdale, NJ: Lawrence Erlbaum Associates.

McCloskey, J., & Bulechek, G. (1996). *Nursing interventions classification (NIC)* (2nd ed.). St. Louis: Mosby.

McElheran, N., & Harper-Jaques, S. (1994). Commendations: A resource intervention for clinical practice. *Clinical Nurse Specialist, 8*(1), 7–10.

Megargee, E. I. (1993). Aggression and violence. In P. B. Sutker & H. E. Adams (Eds.), *Comprehensive handbook of psychopathology* (2nd ed., pp. 617–644). New York: Plenum Press.

Messner, W. W., Mack, J. E., & Semrad, E. V. (1975). Psychoanalysis. In A. M. Freedman, H. I. Kaplan, & B. J. Sadock (Eds.), *Comprehensive textbook of psychiatry* (2nd ed., pp. 482–566). Baltimore: Williams & Wilkins.

Mesulam, M. (2000). *Principles of behavioral and cognitive neurology* (2nd ed.). Oxford: Oxford University Press.

Morrison, E. F. (1989). Theoretical modeling to predict violence in hospitalized psychiatric patients. *Research in Nursing and Health, 12,* 31–40.

Morrison, E. F. (1990). Violent psychiatric inpatients in a public hospital. *Scholarly Inquiry for Nursing Practice, 4*(1), 65–82.

Morrison, E. F. (1992). A coercive interactional style as an antecedent to aggression in psychiatric patients. *Research in Nursing and Health, 15,* 421–431.

Morrison, E. F. (1993). Toward a better understanding of violence in psychiatric settings: Debunking the myths. *Archives of Psychiatric Nursing, 7*(6), 328–335.

Morrison, E. F. (1998). The culture of caregiving and aggression in psychiatric settings. *Archives of Psychiatric Nursing, 12*(1), 21–31.

Morrison, P., Lehane, M., Palmer, C., & Meehan, T. (1997). The use of behavioral mapping in a study of seclusion. *Australian and New Zealand Journal of Mental Health Nursing, 6,* 11–18.

North American Nursing Diagnosis Association. (2001). *Nursing diagnoses: Definitions and classification 2001–2002.* Philadelphia: Author.

Pardo, J. V., Pardo, P. J., & Raichle, M. E. (1993). Neural correlates of self-induced dysphoria. *American Journal of Psychiatry, 150*(5), 713–719.

Robinson, C., Wright, L., & Watson, W. (1994). A nontraditional approach to family violence. *Archives of Psychiatric Nursing, 8*(1), 30–37.

Scarpa, A., & Raine, A. (1997). Psychophysiology of anger and violent behavior. *Psychiatric Clinics of North America, 20*(2), 375–394.

Shannon, J. W. (2000). *Understanding and managing anger: Diagnosis, treatment and prevention.* Presentation by Mind Matters Seminar, April, 2000, Calgary Alberta, Canada.

Simmons, D. H. (1996). Caffeine and its effect on persons with mental disorders. *Archives of Psychiatric Nursing, 10*(2), 116–122.

Stolley, J. M., Gerdner, L. A., & Buckwalter, K. C. (1999). Dementia management. In G. M. Bulechek & J. C. McCloskey (Eds.), *Nursing interventions: Effective nursing treatments* (3rd ed., pp. 533–548). Philadelphia: W. B. Saunders.

Tajaden, P., & Thoennes, N. (2000). *Findings from national violence against women survey.* Washington, DC: U.S. Department of Justice.

Tasman, A. (1997). *Psychiatry.* Philadelphia: W. B. Saunders.

Tavris, C. (1989). *Anger: The misunderstood emotion.* New York: Simon & Schuster.

Thomas, S. P. (1990). Theoretical and empirical perspectives on anger. *Issues in Mental Health Nursing, 11,* 203–216.

Thomas, S. P. (1993). *Women and anger.* New York: Springer.

Thomas, S. P. (1998a). Anger of African American women in the south. *Issues in Mental Health Nursing, 19*(4), 353–373.

Thomas, S. P. (1998b). Assessing and intervening with anger disorders. *Nursing Clinics of North America, 33*(1), 121–133.

Tomm, K. (1980). Towards a cybernetic systems approach to family therapy at the University of Calgary. In D. Freeman (Ed.), *Diagnosis and assessment in family therapy* (pp. 101–122). London: Aspen.

United Nations Children's Fund. (2000). *Domestic violence: An epidemic.* http://www.unicef.org/vaw.

Visalli, H., McNasser, G., Johnstone, L., & Lazzaro, C. A. (1997). Reducing high-risk interventions for managing aggression in psychiatric settings. *Journal of Nursing Care Quality, 11*(3), 54–61.

Vosburgh, D., & Simpson, P. (1993). Linking family theory and practice: A family nursing program. *Image—The Journal of Nursing Scholarship, 25*(3), 231–235.

White, M. (1988/89, Summer). The externalizing of the problem and the re-authoring of lives and relationships. *Dulwich Centre Newsletter,* 3–21.

Wolbert-Burgess, A. (1990). The combative patient. In A. Wolbert-Burgess (Ed.), *Psychiatric nursing in the hospital and the community* (5th ed., pp. 947–959). East Norwalk, CT: Appleton & Lange.

Wright, L. M., & Leahey, M. (2000). *Nurses and families: A guide to family assessment and intervention* (3rd ed.). Philadelphia: F. A. Davis.

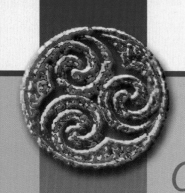

Caring for Abused Persons

Mary R. Boyd

After studying the chapter, you will be able to:

➤ Describe woman, child, and elder abuse.

➤ Describe biopsychosocial theories of abuse.

➤ Discuss theories explaining why some men become abusive and why some women remain in violent relationships.

➤ Describe biopsychosocial consequences of abuse.

➤ Describe the diagnostic criteria for posttraumatic stress disorder (PTSD).

➤ Discuss the three major symptom categories found in PTSD and their associated etiologic factors.

CHAPTER 37

➤ Describe the diagnostic criteria for dissociative identity disorder (DID).

➤ Integrate biopsychosocial theories into the analysis of human responses to survivors of abuse.

➤ Formulate nursing care plans for survivors of abuse.

KEY TERMS

acute stress disorder (ASD)

alexithymia

behavioral sensitization

cycle of violence

dissociation

dissociative identity disorder (DID)

emotional abuse

extinction

fear conditioning

intergenerational transmission

neglect

physical abuse

posttraumatic stress disorder (PTSD)

sexual abuse

traumatic bonding

KEY CONCEPTS

empowerment

self-esteem

Violence demonstrated in the abuse of women, children, and elders is a national health problem that causes significant impairment in survivors. Abuse of any type permanently changes the survivor's construction of reality and the meaning of his or her life. It wounds deeply, endangering core beliefs about self, others, and the world. It usually destroys the survivor's self-esteem.

Nurses encounter survivors of abuse in all health care settings. For this reason, they must be knowledgeable about abuse. They must understand its indicators, causes, assessment techniques, and effective nursing interventions. Unfortunately, few nurses ask about abuse because doing so is uncomfortable. It requires nurses to acknowledge evil in human nature and their own vulnerability to that evil. Protection and recovery from abuse, however, require survivors to remember and discuss terrible events. Secrecy and silence protect perpetrators and seriously endanger survivors. Nurses communicate a powerfully disturbing message with their silence: that the most traumatic event of a patient's life is too upsetting for others to hear. If nurses do not allow and encourage survivors to tell their stories, the
abuse experiences will continue to haunt patients as symptoms of mental disorders.

This chapter focuses on the nursing process with women, children, and elders who are survivors of abuse. It provides basic nursing information needed to address the multiple, complex problems that these patients present.

KEY CONCEPT **Self-esteem.** **Self-esteem** is how one feels about oneself. Its components are self-acceptance, self-worth, self-love, and self-nurturing.

TYPES OF ABUSE

Most abuse that women, children, and the elderly experience is intimate violence; that is, the perpetrator is a loved and trusted partner or family member. As a result, the world and home are no longer safe, people seem dangerous, and life may become a tortured existence of warding off ever-present threats. Empowerment is a foreign concept to those who are being abused.

KEY CONCEPT **Empowerment.** **Empowerment** is promotion of the continued growth and development of strength, power, and personal excellence.

Woman Abuse

Woman abuse, domestic violence, spouse abuse, partner abuse, wife abuse, and battered wives are all terms used interchangeably to denote violence directed toward women. Some of these terms, however, do not specifically refer to the abuse of a woman by an intimate partner. For example, the term domestic violence may be used in cases in which one person directs abuse against an entire family. The terms spouse abuse and partner abuse could indicate that the couple in whom abuse occurs, either heterosexual or homosexual, lives together but is unmarried. These terms, however, also imply that women abuse their male partners at the same frequency and with similar consequences as men direct violence against women (Ryan & King, 1998), which is simply not true. In most cases (90% to 95%), victims of battering are women, and the perpetrators are men (Sassetti, 1993; Sisley et al., 1999). When women use force against their male partners, they often do so in self-defense, and the injuries they receive are more severe than those they inflict (Flitcraft, 1997). For these reasons, woman abuse has been chosen as the most appropriate term to use in this chapter in designating violence, including rape, directed toward a woman by an intimate partner.

Woman abuse is a significant health problem that crosses all ethnic, racial, and socioeconomic lines. Estimates of its annual prevalence range from 2 million (Thompson et al., 1999) to 4.4 million cases (Campbell & Lewandowski, 1997). These figures may be low because underreporting contributes to conservative estimates. Many women are afraid or reluctant to identify their abusers. In some cases, they fear retaliation against themselves or their children. In other cases, they continue to hold strong feelings for their partners, despite the abuse.

Evidence suggests that single, divorced, and separated women may actually be at greater risk for abuse than married women (Flitcraft, 1997). Moreover, this group is at particularly high risk for severe violence. Danger assessments show that ex-partners exhibit obsessive threatening behavior after their relationships end and pose significant dangers to women (Flitcraft, 1997). Forty-three percent of women seen in emergency departments (EDs) attributed their abuse to a past partner (Flitcraft, 1997). These findings emphasize that ending a relationship often does not end violence (Flitcraft, 1997). This information is important for health care providers, who frequently pressure women to end abusive relationships.

The perpetuation of violence begins early in dating relationships. The prevalence of dating violence is unknown because, as with other forms of violence, it usually takes place in private and is not reported. A few studies provide some data on the extent of the problem. One study found that out of 1,870 cases of domestic assaults, 51.5% were classified as boyfriend or girlfriend violence (Barnett et al., 1997). About 20% to 50% of men and women in college-aged dating relationships have admitted physically abusing a dating partner (Barnett et al., 1997). These figures do not include date rape. One study found that behaviors that would qualify as date rape or sexual assault occurred at a rate of 15.4% or 38 per 1,000 women (Barnett et al., 1997).

To understand woman abuse, one must understand the dynamics of violent intimate relationships, especially gendered relationships (Flitcraft, 1995, 1997). Woman abuse is not just physical or sexual abuse. Rather, it is a chronic syndrome characterized by emotional abuse, degradation, restrictions on freedom, destruction of property, threatened or actual child abuse, threats against one's family, stalking, and isolation from family and friends (Flitcraft, 1995, 1997). Violence of this nature has at its core a pattern of coercive control and domination over all aspects of a woman's life (Flitcraft, 1995). Threats of violence against the woman and her loved ones are among the tactics that the batterer uses to enforce the woman's submission and secrecy (Sassetti, 1993). Many battered women report that physical violence is much less damaging than accompanying emotional abuse. Relentless emotional and psychological violence destroys and isolates women (Boyd & Mackey, 2000a).

Battering

Battering is the single greatest cause of serious injury to women. In a study performed in an urban ED, abuse accounted for 50% of all acute injuries and 21% of injuries that required emergency surgery to women (Sisley et al., 1999). Woman abuse contributes to a high rate of completed and attempted suicides in women; 81% of women reporting suicide attempts have experienced abuse by an intimate partner (Thompson et al., 1999). Moreover, many women who experience abuse develop posttraumatic stress disorder (PTSD). Individuals with PTSD are 15 times more likely to attempt suicide than the general population (Thompson et al., 1999).

Battered women are acutely aware that they are in danger of being killed by their abusers, especially when they take deliberate action to leave an abusive relationship. In 1996, 75% of 1,800 homicides perpetrated by intimate partners had female victims (Sisley et al., 1999). Indeed, the realistic fear of being killed is one factor that keeps many women from leaving abusive partners, even after years of severe abuse.

Battering also poses a significant danger to unborn children. Estimates of the prevalence of battering during pregnancy vary from 4% (Sisley et al., 1999) to as high as 22% (Parker et al., 1993). Differences in prevalence rates may be attributed to differences in definitions of abuse used by study authors. Abuse during pregnancy is a significant risk factor for several fetal and maternal complications, including low birth weight, low maternal weight gain, infections, and anemia. Moreover, abuse of women often results in their use of alcohol and other drugs, which, in turn, may harm unborn children (Parker et al., 1994; Sisley et al., 1999).

Rape and Sexual Assault

Rape and sexual assault are common in the United States. A sexual assault occurs once every 6.4 minutes (Petter & Whitehill, 1998). Expressed in another way, one in every three to four white women and one in every four African American women will be raped in their lifetime (Starling, 1998). Sexual assault includes any form of nonconsenting sexual activity, ranging from fondling to penetration. Most sexual assaults are underreported for the same reason that domestic violence is underreported—women are embarrassed and ashamed and fear being blamed for the assault. These reactions to sexual assault persist even though rape is a felony (Petter & Whitehill, 1998).

Rapists can be classified into three categories: the power rapist, the anger rapist, and the sadistic rapist (Petter & Whitehill, 1998). Power rapists account for 55% of sexual assaults. They often attack people their own age and use intimidation and minimal physical force to control their victims. Their assaults are generally premeditated. Anger rapists account for 40% of sexual assaults. These rapists tend to target either very young or elderly victims. They may use extreme force and restraint that results in physical injury to the victim. Sadistic rapists account for 5% of sexual assaults; however, they are the most dangerous. Their crimes are premeditated, and they often torture and kill their victims. Sadistic rapists derive erotic gratification from their victims' suffering (Petter & Whitehill, 1998).

Child Abuse

Child abuse can take several forms, and the definition of each type varies by state. All forms of child abuse rob children of rights that they should have. Those rights include the rights to be and behave like a child; to be safe and protected from harm; and to be fed, clothed, and nurtured so that the child can grow, develop, and fulfill his or her unique potential.

The prevalence of child abuse is unknown. In a 1996 survey, more than 3 million children were reported to Child Protective Services as suspected victims of child abuse (Wallace, 1999). That figure did not include cases that were unreported. Out of the total number of reported child abuse cases, estimates are that 62% rep-

resent neglect, 25% physical abuse, 7% sexual abuse, 3% emotional abuse, and 4% other types of abuse, including Münchausen's syndrome by proxy and witnessing abuse of a parent (Wallace, 1999).

Child Neglect

Child neglect is the most common form of child abuse reported (Wallace, 1999). There are several types of **neglect.** Failure to protect a child includes failure to prevent various kinds of accidental injury, such as ingestion of poison, electric shocks, falls, and burns (Barnett et al., 1997; Grant, 1995). Physical neglect includes failure to provide food, clothing, and shelter (Barnett et al., 1997; Grant, 1995). Indicators of physical neglect include diaper dermatitis, lice, scabies, dirty appearance, clothes inappropriate for the weather, and unclean and unsafe living environment. Medical neglect includes failure to provide for the child's medical needs, including failure to seek appropriate care or to comply with prescribed treatments (Grant, 1995; Wallace, 1999).

Physical Abuse

Physical abuse may include severe spanking, hitting, kicking, shoving, or any other type of physical action directed toward the child that results in nonaccidental injury. Injuries to children caused by physical abuse range from mild to severe and life-threatening. Types of injuries include skin and soft tissue injuries; internal injuries; dislocations and fractures; tooth loss; burns; abrasions or bruises made by fists or belts; hair loss from pulling the hair; wounds from guns, knives, razors, or other sharp objects; retinal hemorrhage; and conjunctival hemorrhage (Wallace, 1999). Often, clothing hides these injuries, and practitioners must look for other signs of abuse, such as fear, aggressive or withdrawn behavior, poor social relations, learning problems, delinquent behavior, and wearing clothing that is meant to cover injuries but is inappropriate for the weather (Wallace, 1999). In addition, when treating a child with such injuries, professionals should suspect abuse when explanations are implausible and inconsistent with injuries, involved parties give different versions of the incident, or treatment seeking is delayed (Wallace, 1999).

Sexual Abuse

Behaviors that constitute child **sexual abuse** range from mild, covert behaviors to overt sexual acts. Examples of sexual abuse include exhibitionism, voyeurism, touching the child's sexual organs, and oral, anal, and vaginal sex (Wallace, 1999). There are three categories of sexual abuse: incest, sexual abuse perpetrated by a nonfamily member, and pedophilia. Incest is defined as any form of sexual activity between a child younger than age 18 years and an immediate family member (parent, stepparent, sibling), extended family member (grandparent, uncle, aunt, cousin), or surrogate parent (Barnett et al., 1997; Wallace, 1999). Extrafamilial child sexual abuse is any form of sexual contact between a non-family member and a child younger than age 18 years. Pedophilia describes those who have a sexual fixation on young children that usually translates into sexual acts with the victims (Wallace, 1999). The following conditions qualify as pedophilia (Wallace, 1999):

- For at least 6 months, the person has recurrent intense sexual urges and sexually arousing fantasies involving sexual activity with a prepubescent child.
- The person has acted on or is extremely distressed by these urges.
- The person is at least 16-years-old and at least 5 years older than the child.

Research has shown that about 8% to 10% of child sexual abuse offenders are strangers, 47% are family members, and 40% are acquaintances (Wallace, 1999). High-risk years for child sexual abuse range between ages 4 and 9 (Wallace, 1999).

Several factors may mediate the effects of child sexual abuse. In general, younger children with a history of emotional difficulties may be more traumatized than will be older and more stable children. Repeated abuse over long periods with more violence and bodily penetration results in greater traumatization. Sexual abuse by someone that the child knows and trusts causes more severe trauma. The child abused by a family member experiences a devastating breach of trust, loss of a safe home, and threats to fundamental survival requirements (Boyd & Mackey, 2000a). Finally, negative reactions by significant others, health care professionals, or others may exacerbate the effects of trauma (Wallace, 1999).

Emotional Abuse

Emotional abuse includes acts or omissions that psychologically damage the child (Wallace, 1999). The emotionally abused child does not have visible injuries to alert others. Nevertheless, emotional abuse severely affects a child's self-esteem and often leaves permanent emotional scars (Wallace, 1999). Survivors of abuse frequently report that emotional abuse is worse than physical abuse.

There are several types of emotional abuse (Wallace, 1999). *Rejecting* involves refusing to acknowledge the child's worth and the legitimacy of his or her needs. The child receives the message that he or she is no good and is unwanted. *Isolating* involves cutting the child off from normal social experiences, preventing the child from forming friendships, and hindering the development of social skills. *Terrorizing* involves creating a climate of fear and making the child believe that the world is a capricious and hostile place. *Ignoring* means being

psychologically unavailable to the child and, therefore, starving him or her emotionally. Normal self-development depends on emotional connection to others. *Corrupting* involves mis-socializing the child to engage in destructive and antisocial behaviors and reinforcing deviance. This type of abuse makes the child unfit for normal social experience and sets him or her up for further rejection (Barnett et al., 1997; Wallace, 1999).

Münchausen's Syndrome by Proxy

Münchausen's syndrome by proxy is another form of child abuse. This disorder includes "the intentional production or feigning of physical or psychological signs or symptoms in another person who is under the individual's care for the purpose of indirectly assuming the sick role" (American Psychiatric Association [APA], 2000, p. 783). The signs of this disorder include repeated hospitalizations and medical evaluations of the child without definitive diagnosis; symptoms or medical signs that are inappropriate or inconsistent; symptoms that disappear when the child is away from the parent; a parent who encourages medical tests for the child; parental uneasiness as the child recovers; and a parent who is less concerned with the child's health than with spending time with caretakers (Wallace, 1999). One source estimates that about 10% of children who are victims of Münchausen's syndrome by proxy will die at the hands of their parents (Wallace, 1999).

Children of Battered Women

Children of battered women are often overlooked as abuse victims unless they demonstrate evidence of physical or sexual abuse themselves (Rhea et al., 1996). These children, however, often show signs of PTSD (Campbell & Lewandowski, 1997). Children may witness their mother being choked, threatened with a weapon, or threatened with death (Boyd & Mackey, 2000a; Campbell & Lewandowski, 1997). These children fear for both their own and their mother's safety (Boyd & Mackey, 2000a). In addition, children who grow up in violent families experience living with secrecy, relocations as the mother leaves home to seek safety, economic hardship, maternal depression that may reduce her ability to nurture, and frightening interactions with the police and court systems (Boyd & Mackey, 2000a; Campbell & Lewandowski, 1997). Moreover, many children who witness violence begin to accept it as a normal part of relationships and a way to deal with problems (Sisley et al., 1999).

Elder Abuse

Elder abuse is increasingly recognized as a serious problem in the United States and other countries. As the population continues to age, it is likely that the problem will worsen. As with other types of abuse, the prevalence of elder abuse is unknown; however, one report estimated 1.5 million cases of elder abuse each year in the United States (Wallace, 1999).

Types of elder abuse and their estimated prevalence rates are as follows: neglect (58.5%), physical abuse (15.7%), financial or material mistreatment (12.3%), emotional abuse (7.3%), and sexual abuse (.04%) (Comijs et al., 1998; Wallace, 1999). Neglect and physical, sexual, and emotional abuse are similar to that described for women and children. Financial or material mistreatment may include improper or illegal acts to obtain and use an elderly person's resources for personal benefit (Wallace, 1999).

Risk factors for elder abuse include older age, impairment in activities of daily living (ADLs), cognitive disability or other mental illness, dependency on the caretaker, isolation, stressful events, and a history of intergenerational conflict between the elder and the caregiver (Humphries-Lynch, 1997; Lichtenstein, 1997).

EXPLANATORY THEORIES OF ABUSE

Many theories have attempted to explain violence between intimate partners and in the family. The theories reviewed here have been categorized as biologic, psychological, and social. In all likelihood, family violence is truly a biopsychosocial phenomenon that no one of these theories can fully explain (Fig. 37-1). A separate section presents additional theories that are more specific to the phenomenon of woman abuse.

Biologic Theories

Neurologic Problems

Aggressive behavior may be associated with several neurologic conditions, including traumatic brain injury, seizure disorder, and dementia (see Chap. 36). Neurodevelopmental factors and traumatic brain injury can produce seizure disorders, attentional dysfunction, or focal neurobehavioral syndromes, all of which are associated with aggressive behavior. Moreover, neurodevelopmental disorders and traumatic brain injury are common antecedents of episodic dyscontrol syndrome. The most common association between seizures and aggressive behavior occurs during the postictal period (the period immediately after the seizure), during which the individual may be confused and react aggressively.

Damage to the orbitofrontal cortex often causes impulsive, labile, irritable, and socially inappropriate behavior. Individuals with such damage often respond aggressively to trivial stimuli (Rosenbaum et al., 1997). In addition, damage to the neocortex, limbic system, and hypothalamus may result in aggressive behavior. These systems have hierarchic control over one another.

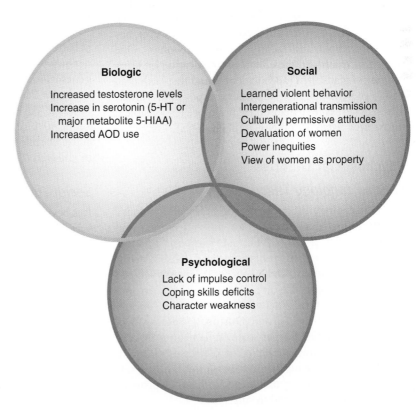

FIGURE 37.1 Biopsychosocial etiologies for patients with abuse.

Damage to higher centers may disinhibit aggression from lower centers.

Aggressive behavior also may be related to disruptions in neurotransmitter systems. Disruption in serotonin, dopamine, and γ-aminobutyric acid (GABA) systems has been linked with several psychiatric disorders, including depression, schizophrenia, impulsive behavior, suicide, and aggression (Rosenbaum et al., 1997).

Links With Substance Abuse

The use of alcohol and other drugs (AOD) is commonly associated with violent incidents; however, AOD use alone is rarely sufficient to account for violence. Other factors, such as low family income, stress, and abuse in the family of origin, are often more important (Collins & Messerschmidt, 1993; Wallace, 1999). The relationship of AOD to violence may result from three factors: (1) AOD-induced cognitive impairment, (2) the user's expectations that AOD increases the tendency toward aggression, and (3) socioculturally grounded beliefs that people are unaccountable for their behavior while intoxicated (Collins & Messerschmidt, 1993; Wallace, 1999).

Studies have demonstrated that drinking alcohol may change perceptions about accountability for behavior (Collins & Messerschmidt, 1993; Wallace, 1999). The belief that intoxicated behavior will be judged less harshly may encourage and provide an excuse for those who abuse substances to engage in normally unacceptable behavior. Research shows that people attempt to justify their criminal behavior by blaming alcohol after the fact (Collins & Messerschmidt, 1993; Wallace, 1999). The rules about AOD and accountability, however, appear to be applied differently to men and women. One study that examined the effects of intoxication on attributions of blame in a rape incident found that both men and women judged the rapist as less responsible if intoxicated, whereas they held the victim more responsible if intoxicated (Richardson & Campbell, 1982).

Psychosocial Theories

Psychopathology Theory

Psychopathology theory seeks to understand violence by examining characteristics of individual men and women (Wallace, 1999). Theorists from this perspective focus on personality traits, internal defense systems, and mental disorders. Older sources frequently labeled abusive men as infantile or lacking impulse control and gave them diagnoses of dependent, sociopathic, or borderline personality disorder (Dutton, 1995). An outdated theory that was particularly damaging labeled women masochistic, paranoid, or depressed (Bograd, 1999). One underlying assumption of this labeling was that some women enjoy abuse and deliberately provoke attacks because they need to suffer.

Although research has not consistently found one common mental disorder or set of characteristics in violent individuals, a recently identified typology of men who batter shows promise (Emery & Laumann-Billings, 1998). Type I batterers are violent in many situations, have many victims, and display antisocial characteristics. Type II batterers abuse only their family, commit less severe violence, are generally less aggressive, and demonstrate remorse. These men tend to be dependent, jealous, and unlikely to have personality or other disorders. Type III batterers display dysphoric-borderline or schizoid characteristics, such as emotional volatility, depression, feelings of inadequacy, and social isolation (Emery & Laumann-Billings, 1998). Type III batterers also tend to be violent, only within their families.

Social Learning Theory

Violent families create an atmosphere of tension, fear, intimidation, and tremendous confusion about intimate relationships (Boyd & Mackey, 2000a). Children in violent homes often learn violent behavior as an approved and legitimate way to solve problems, especially within intimate relationships. Social learning theory posits that men who witness violence in their homes often perpetuate violent behavior in their families as adults (Emery & Laumann-Billings, 1998; Wallace, 1999). Moreover, women who grow up in violent homes learn to accept violence and expect it in their own adult relationships (Boyd & Mackey, 2000a). These concepts are often referred to as the **intergenerational transmission** of violence.

Findings of extreme violence in the parental homes of battered individuals and individuals who grew up witnessing violence are common and support the intergenerational transmission of violence theory (Barnett et al., 1997). Not all those who batter or are abused, however, come from violent homes. Estimates are that about 40% of those who suffered abuse or witnessed abuse in childhood will consequently abuse their wives or children (Dutton, 1998).

Social Theories

It is beyond the scope of this chapter to cover the many sociologic theories of violence. Sociologic theories posit that abuse occurs because of cultural norms that permit and even glamorize violent behavior (Wallace, 1999). The permissive attitude toward violence in the United States is reflected in violence in the media, choice of heroes, spiraling rates of violent crimes, and lack of or inadequate response by the criminal justice system. For instance, some continue to view O. J. Simpson as a hero, and he was never arrested or prosecuted for battering his wife.

Acceptance of violence as normal appears widespread among young people. In one study, as many as

70% of a group of female college students listed at least one form of violence as acceptable in dating relationships (Girshick, 1993). Even more disturbing is that 80% of these women mentioned situations in which physical force between partners was tolerable (Girshick, 1993). Slapping was cited most often (49%), whereas punching was seen as acceptable by 21% of these women (Girshick, 1993). In addition, as many as 34% of women marry someone who abused them in a dating relationship (Barnett et al., 1997).

Family violence is also related to qualities of the community in which the family is embedded. Poverty, absence of family services, social isolation, lack of cohesion in the community, and stress contribute to family violence (Emery & Laumann-Billings, 1998). The relationship of poverty, social isolation, and child abuse has been well established (Emery & Laumann-Billings, 1998). Not all poor families, however, abuse their children. The main difference between poor families who do and do not abuse their children lies in the degree of social cohesion and mutual caring found in their communities (Emery & Laumann-Billings, 1998). Neighborhoods with high levels of child abuse frequently suffer from severe social disorganization and lack of community identity. In addition, they also have higher rates of juvenile delinquency, drug trafficking, and violent crime (Emery & Laumann-Billings, 1998).

One of the most accepted theories of elder abuse is the family stress theory (Wallace, 1999). This theory hypothesizes that providing care for an elder induces stress within the family. Family stress includes economic hardship, loss of sleep, and intrusions into family activities and routines. Moreover, caring for a dependent elder takes an enormous physical toll on the caregiver. If there is no relief, the caretaker may become overwhelmed, lose control, and abuse the elder (Wallace, 1999). Other characteristics of caretakers that may predispose them to abuse elderly parents include alcohol or drug abuse, dementia, restricted outside activities, unrealistic expectations, and a blaming, hypercritical personality.

Theoretic Dynamics Specific to Woman Abuse

Feminist Theories

Feminists contend that striving by men to perpetuate their control and dominance over women and their need to demonstrate power is at the heart of woman abuse (Sampselle et al., 1992; Wallace, 1999). According to the feminist perspective, woman abuse results from a patriarchal society that perpetuates attitudes that support violence against women (Wallace, 1999). Three major characteristics of such a patriarchal society are the devaluation of women, power inequities, and the view of women as property (Barnett et al., 1997; Wallace, 1999).

Feminists charge that patriarchal society is the product of a predominately white, male-dominated majority that believes that women are inherently inferior to men (Sampselle et al., 1992). Such societies value women primarily for their reproductive capacity and potential to please men (Sampselle et al., 1992; Wallace, 1999).

Feminists also point to a power inequity in society as a contributing factor to woman abuse. Women have made many advances in recent years; however, men continue to control most institutions (Sampselle et al., 1992; Stark & Flitcraft, 1996; Wallace, 1999). Women continue to earn less than men for paid work and are less likely to advance to positions of authority and power (Sampselle et al., 1992; Stark & Flitcraft, 1996; Wallace, 1999). Moreover, marriage often victimizes women in ways other than through violence. Although men now contribute to household work, most women who hold jobs outside the home continue to perform most household and child care tasks (Sampselle et al., 1992; Stark & Flitcraft, 1996; Wallace, 1999). This power inequity is reflected in higher depression rates for married women compared with married men (McGrath et al., 1990). In cases of divorce, most women become single parents with a standard of living significantly lower than that of their former spouse (Sampselle et al., 1992; Stark & Flitcraft, 1996; Wallace, 1999).

Until the early 1900s, women legally were the property of men in the United States (Sampselle et al., 1992). Ownership of women continues in many parts of the world and continues to influence attitudes toward women. The entertainment and advertising industries perpetuate the image of women as property by depicting them as objects and often portraying the dismembering of women's bodies (Kilbourne, 1987, 1999). The focus on women's body parts in advertising dehumanizes women, and that dehumanization is often the first step in making women acceptable targets of violence. Moreover, the explicit portrayal in the media of women in various states of undress and in seductive postures suggests that they are vulnerable and openly welcome sexual advances. Frequently, the message is, "Buy the product and get the woman" (Kilbourne, 1987). Just one example of this type of advertising was found in an advertisement for a popular red beer, which portrayed the beer bottle and a beautiful woman with red hair. The caption read, "Try a tall, cool red one" (Consumers for Socially Responsible Advertising, 1994).

Theory of Borderline Personality Organization and Violence

In a recent publication, Donald Dutton (1998) discusses the relationship of borderline personality organization (BPO) to the type of batterer who is chronically and intermittently abusive but abusive only within his family (see Chap. 37). Dutton's work combines aspects from several theoretic models, including social learning theory, reinforcement principles from learning theory, and evidence that early trauma can alter personality through changes that occur biologically or through learning. He bases his theory on his own research and that of others, such as Bandura (social learning theory) and van der Kolk (traumatic stress and its consequences).

Dutton (1998) describes three characteristics or cycles of BPO that shift over time and seem to coincide with the **cycle of violence** as first proposed by Walker (1979) and described later in this chapter. These characteristics can apply to men or women with BPO; however, because this discussion focuses on men's aggression toward their female partners, it addresses the individual with BPO as male. Phase I of the male borderline personality, or "cyclic personality," consists of an internal buildup of tensions, in which the man feels depressed and irritable but does not know how to verbalize his inner dysphoria. In fact, he may not even be able to recognize or label the painful feelings, a condition called **alexithymia** (Dutton, 1998). The inability to recognize or express painful feelings and ask for what he needs traps the man in a downward spiral of bad feelings, compounded by an inability to maintain his own self-integrity. He is dependent on his partner for his sense of self. Therefore, the loss of the partner carries the risk that he will lose himself. According to Dutton (1998), the reason that men with BPO become so abusive in their intimate relationships but not others is linked to their extreme dependency on their partners for sense of self and their inability to tolerate aloneness. This type of dependency is often called a "masked or hostile dependency." To maintain this relationship, the man with BPO must control his partner; therefore, his controlling behavior masks his dependency. The man with BPO expects his partner to do the impossible. When she fails, he erupts in extreme anger because his sense of self is threatened. Thus, the man with BPO converts dysphoria into abuse through (1) the belief that the partner should be able to soothe the bad feelings and (2) conversion of feelings of terror into rage (Dutton, 1998). His use of the defense mechanism of projection leads him to believe that it is her fault (Dutton, 1998). The explosive combination of ego needs, an inability to communicate them, chronic irritability, jealousy, and projective blaming combine to ensure a violent relationship (Dutton, 1998).

As this phase continues, the man with BPO becomes verbally abusive, and the partner withdraws. The man wants closeness, not withdrawal, but he does not have the skills to ask for it. In addition to increasing anger, the man with BPO becomes increasingly demanding. At this stage, the dichotomous thinking or splitting characteristic of BPO is evident, and the man sees the partner as "all bad"—unfaithful, unloving, and malev-

olent (Dutton, 1998). The unexpressed rage builds until the man with BPO erupts with violence. The violence drives the partner further away, increasing the man's feelings of abandonment. As a result, the abusive man promises anything to get the partner back. (This phase coincides with Walker's contrition phase in the cycle of violence.) The opposite side of splitting is now in evidence, as the man describes his partner as "all good"—"a Madonna" (Dutton, 1998, p. 96).

It is hypothesized that the abuser's BPO results from early physical abuse. Researchers suggest that early physical abuse causes long-term problems in modulating emotion and aggression and may lead to chronic anger (Dutton, 1998). The difficulty in modulating emotion often manifests first in affective numbing and constriction or alexithymia. Hyperarousal follows emotional numbing, a process that culminates in violence (Dutton, 1998). These symptoms are manifestations of PTSD, described later in this chapter. Abusive men also score higher than controls on other measures of trauma, such as depression, anxiety, sleep disturbances, and dissociation (Dutton, 1998). The form that the violence takes, however, appears to be learned. That is, boys tend to identify with the aggressor and act out, whereas girls often identify with the victim and turn to self-destructive acts, such as substance abuse and self-mutilation (Dutton, 1998).

One other aspect of this cycle appears to ensure its continuation, that of positive reinforcement. The type of violence perpetrated by men with BPO has been labeled "deindividuated violence," that is, the violence is responsive only to internal cues from the perpetrator and unresponsive to cues from the victim (Dutton, 1998, p. 54). The violence feeds on itself because it is rewarding; it reduces the perpetrator's aversive arousal and tension. As a result, batterers often continue the assault until they are exhausted. Expressing rage through violent acts is the only way they know how to reduce their tension or aversive arousal, and it becomes addictive (Dutton, 1998).

The cycle described by Dutton helps explain the descriptions of violent men provided by more than 200 women with whom he has worked. The following are examples of their descriptions of violent partners: "He's like Jekyll and Hyde," "He's completely different sometimes," and "His friends never see the other side of him; they think he's just a nice guy, just one of the boys" (Dutton, 1998, p. 53).

Theories of Why Women Stay in Violent Relationships

One important reason that battered women may stay in or return to abusive relationships is economic (Wallace, 1999). Despite years of progress, women still earn less than men for equal work. Many women lack the education or skills that would allow them to earn an adequate living outside the home. For these women, leaving their abusive partners means that they and their children would be homeless and without any source of support for even basic necessities. Furthermore, many shelters for battered women have long waiting lists and provide only temporary housing.

The socialization of women to assume major responsibility for their marriages and childrearing is often another barrier to leaving abusive relationships. Society teaches women that their proper place is at home and their primary responsibility is caring for their husbands and children (Chodorow, 1974; Gilligan, 1982; Wallace, 1999). Many women believe that making their marriage a success is their responsibility. Therefore, when they are abused, they assume that it is their fault and that their duty is to remain and try harder for their children's sakes (Boyd & Mackey, 2000a). Moreover, many women who were abused in childhood or witnessed abuse of their mothers think that abuse is part of a normal relationship (Boyd & Mackey, 2000a).

Women also face political and legal obstacles in leaving abusive partners. Although the legal response to wife battering is improving, police response remains inadequate in many areas of the United States (Boyd & Mackey, 2000a). If a man is arrested for assault and no action is taken to prevent future violence, he may be released shortly and retaliate against his partner. Fear for their lives and the lives of their children and other relatives often keeps women from attempting to leave abusive relationships (Boyd and Mackey, 2000a).

Even more difficult to understand is why some women stay in violent dating relationships. About 30% to 50% of dating couples continue their relationships despite violence (Barnett et al., 1997). One factor is that dating violence often does not occur until the relationship has been sustained for a long time. By then, many women feel that they have invested too much in the relationship to end it. Research has shown that the length of the relationship and the commitment level are positively correlated with physical and sexual abuse. Moreover, about 30% of those who stay in violent dating relationships interpret the violence as an act of love (Barnett et al., 1997). Another explanation is that abused women stay because they believe that they can change their partners and save their relationships.

Cycle of Violence. Many cases of woman abuse reflect a recognized cycle of violence (Walker, 1979; Wallace, 1999). The cycle consists of three recurring phases that often increase in frequency and severity (Walker, 1979). The cycle is fully described in Figure 37-2.

Traumatic Bonding. The formation of strong emotional bonds under conditions of intermittent maltreat-

ment has been reported in several studies with human and animal subjects (Dutton, 1995). For example, people taken hostage may show positive regard for their captors. Abused children often show strong attachment to their abusing parents. Cult members show strong loyalty to malevolent cult leaders (Dutton, 1995). Therefore, the relationship between battered women and their partners may be just one example of **traumatic bonding**—the development of strong emotional ties between two people, one of whom intermittently abuses the other (Dutton, 1995). Traumatic bonding suggests that a power imbalance and intermittent abuse help to form extremely strong emotional attachments. Traumatic bonding theory (Dutton & Painter, 1993) explains why the cycle of violence is so powerful in entrapping a woman in a violent relationship.

The woman in a power imbalance perceives herself to be in a powerless position in relation to her partner, whom she perceives as extremely powerful. As the power imbalance intensifies, she feels increasingly worthless, less capable of fending for herself, and therefore, more in need of her partner. This cycle of dependency and lowered self-esteem is continually repeated, eventually creating a strong affective bond to the partner (Dutton, 1995).

Intermittent reinforcement or punishment is one of the strongest learning paradigms in behavioral theory, especially in maintaining a particular behavior (Dutton, 1995). An example that is often used to illustrate this concept is the gambler who persistently puts coins in a slot machine. Despite substantial losses, the gambler persists because the next time just might be the big payoff. Therefore, the gambler is not rewarded every time, but intermittently. To apply this to battered women, women may stay because this time the man may actually mean what he says and stop the abuse. After all, he had been kind and loving intermittently.

Research suggests that traumatic bonding is especially important when a woman attempts to leave her abusive partner (Dutton, 1995). When a woman leaves an abusive relationship, especially after a battering incident, she is emotionally drained and vulnerable. As time passes, her fear of her abuser diminishes, and needs supplied by the partner become evident. At this time, she is particularly susceptible to the abuser's attempts to persuade her to return to the relationship (Dutton & Painter, 1993).

SURVIVORS OF ABUSE: HUMAN RESPONSES TO TRAUMA

The experience of violence and abuse is overwhelming for most survivors and often has devastating long-term consequences (Hendricks-Matthews, 1993; Herman, 1992). Victimization does not produce a single uniform

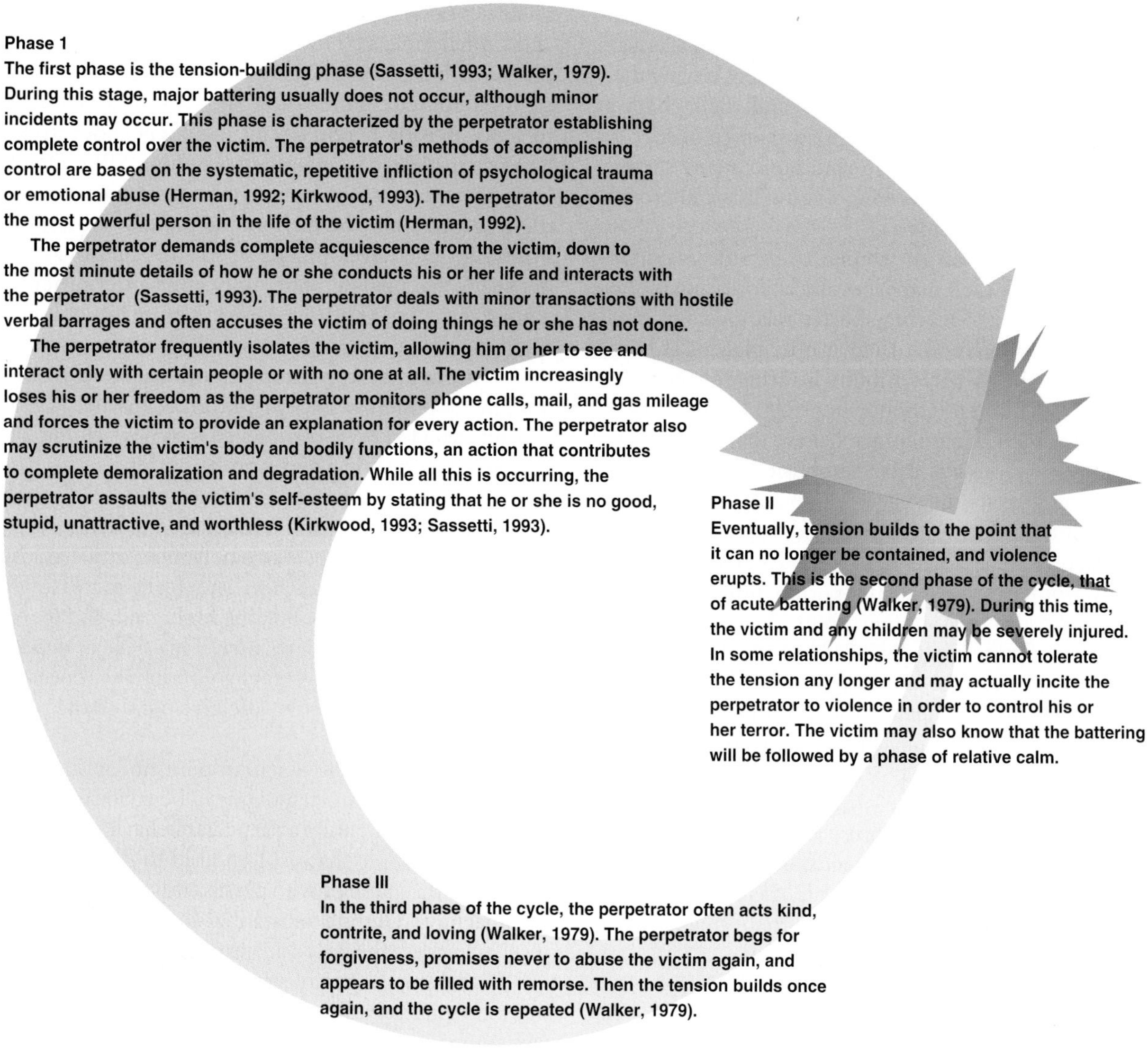

Phase 1

The first phase is the tension-building phase (Sassetti, 1993; Walker, 1979). During this stage, major battering usually does not occur, although minor incidents may occur. This phase is characterized by the perpetrator establishing complete control over the victim. The perpetrator's methods of accomplishing control are based on the systematic, repetitive infliction of psychological trauma or emotional abuse (Herman, 1992; Kirkwood, 1993). The perpetrator becomes the most powerful person in the life of the victim (Herman, 1992).

The perpetrator demands complete acquiescence from the victim, down to the most minute details of how he or she conducts his or her life and interacts with the perpetrator (Sassetti, 1993). The perpetrator deals with minor transactions with hostile verbal barrages and often accuses the victim of doing things he or she has not done.

The perpetrator frequently isolates the victim, allowing him or her to see and interact only with certain people or with no one at all. The victim increasingly loses his or her freedom as the perpetrator monitors phone calls, mail, and gas mileage and forces the victim to provide an explanation for every action. The perpetrator also may scrutinize the victim's body and bodily functions, an action that contributes to complete demoralization and degradation. While all this is occurring, the perpetrator assaults the victim's self-esteem by stating that he or she is no good, stupid, unattractive, and worthless (Kirkwood, 1993; Sassetti, 1993).

Phase II

Eventually, tension builds to the point that it can no longer be contained, and violence erupts. This is the second phase of the cycle, that of acute battering (Walker, 1979). During this time, the victim and any children may be severely injured. In some relationships, the victim cannot tolerate the tension any longer and may actually incite the perpetrator to violence in order to control his or her terror. The victim may also know that the battering will be followed by a phase of relative calm.

Phase III

In the third phase of the cycle, the perpetrator often acts kind, contrite, and loving (Walker, 1979). The perpetrator begs for forgiveness, promises never to abuse the victim again, and appears to be filled with remorse. Then the tension builds once again, and the cycle is repeated (Walker, 1979).

FIGURE 37.2 The cycle of violence.

syndrome or response. Research on the effects of victimization reflects considerable consistency in the biopsychosocial responses to overwhelming trauma, whether the victim is a child, adult, or elder (Hendricks-Matthews, 1993).

Biologic Responses

Victims of violence suffer several mild to severe physical consequences. Mild injuries may include bruises and abrasions of the head, neck, face, trunk, and extremities. Severe injuries include multiple traumas, major fractures, major lacerations, and internal injuries, including chest and abdominal injuries and subdural hematomas (Barnett et al., 1997; Wallace, 1999). Loss of vision and hearing can result from blows to the head.

Victims who have suffered sexual abuse may have vaginal and perineal trauma that is sufficient to require surgical repair (Barnett et al., 1997). Anorectal injuries may also be present, including disruption of anal sphincters, retained foreign bodies, and mucosal lacerations. Physical or sexual violence may result in head injuries that can produce changes in cognition, affect, motivation, and behavior (Barnett et al., 1997).

The following section covers the most common responses to violence and abuse:

- Depression (the dysregulated stress response theory of depression)
- Acute stress disorder (ASD)
- Posttraumatic stress disorder (PTSD)
- Dissociative identity disorder (DID)

therapeutic care of survivors. *Journal of Psychiatric and Mental Health Nursing, 5*, 129–136.

Lundberg-Love, P. K. (1997). Current treatment strategies of adult incest survivors and their partners. In R. Geffner, S. B. Sorenson, & P. K. Lundberg-Love (Eds.), *Violence and sexual abuse at home: Current issues in spousal battering and child maltreatment* (pp. 293–311). New York: Haworth Maltreatment & Trauma Press.

McGrath, M. E., Bettacchi, A., Duffy, S. J., et al. (1997). Violence against women: Provider barriers to intervention in emergency departments. *Academy Emergency Medicine, 4*, 297–300.

McGrath, E., Keita, G. P., Strickland, B. R., & Russo, N. F. (1990). *Women and depression: Risk factors and treatment issues.* Final report of the American Psychological Association National Task Force on Women and Depression. Washington, DC: American Psychological Association.

Ouimette, P. C., Wolfe, J., & Chrestman, K. R. (1996). Characteristics of posttraumatic stress disorder-alcohol abuse comorbidity in women. *Journal of Substance Abuse, 8*(3), 335–346.

Parker, B., McFarlane, J., & Soeken, K. (1994). Abuse during pregnancy: Effects on maternal complications and birth weight in adult and teenage women. *Obstetrics and Gynecology, 84*(3), 323–328.

Parker, B., McFarlane, J., Soeken, K., et al. (1993). Physical and emotional abuse in pregnancy: A comparison of adult and teenage women. *Nursing Research, 42*(3), 173–178.

Peled, E., Jaffe, P. G., & Edleson, J. L. (1995). *Ending the cycle of violence.* Thousand Oaks, CA: Sage.

Petter, M., & Whitehill, D. L. (1998). Management of female sexual assault. *American Family Physician, 58*(4), 920–929.

Putnam, F. W. (1994). Dissociative disorders in children and adolescents. In S. J. Lynn & J. W. Rhue (Eds.), *Dissociation: Clinical and theoretical perspectives* (pp. 175–189). New York: Guilford.

Resnick, H., Acierno, R., Holmes, M., et al. (1999). Prevention of post-rape psychology: Preliminary findings of a controlled acute rate treatment study. *Journal of Anxiety Disorders, 13*(4), 359–370.

Rhea, M. H., Chafey, K. H., Dohner, V. A., & Terragno, R. (1996). The silent victims of domestic violence-Who will speak? *Journal of Child and Adolescent Psychiatric Nursing, 9*(3), 7–15.

Richardson, D., & Campbell, J. L. (1982). Alcohol and rape: The effect of alcohol on attributions of blame for rape. *Personality and Social Psychology Bulletin, 8*(3), 468–476.

Roesler, T. A., & Dafler, C. A. (1993). Chemical dissociation in adults sexually victimized as children: Alcohol and drug use in adult survivors. *Journal of Substance Abuse Treatment, 10*, 537–543.

Root, M. P. P. (1989). Treatment failures: The role of sexual victimization in women's addictive behavior. *American Journal of Orthopsychiatry, 59*(4), 542–549.

Rosenbaum, A., Geffner, R., & Benjamin, S. (1977). A biopsychosocial model for understanding relationship aggression. In R. Geffner, S. B. Sorenson, & R. K.

Lundburg-Love (Eds.). *Violence and sexual abuse at home* (pp. 57–80), New York: Haworth Maltreatment & Trauma Press.

Rothbaum, B. O., & Foa, E. B. (1996). Cognitive-behavioral therapy for posttraumatic stress disorder. In B. A. van der Kolk, A. C. McFarlane, & L. Weisaeth (Eds.), *Traumatic stress: The effects of overwhelming experience on mind, body, and society* (pp. 491–509). New York: Guilford.

Rothschild, B. (1998). Post-traumatic stress disorder: Identification and diagnosis. *Swiss Journal of Social Work* [online], http://www.healing-arts.org

Ryan, J., & King, M. C. (1998). Scanning for violence: Educational strategies for helping abused women. *AWHONN Lifelines, 2*(3), 36–41.

Sampselle, C. M., Bernhard, L., Kerr, R. B., et al. (1992). Violence against women: The scope and significance of the problem. In C. M. Sampselle (Ed.), *Violence against women: Nursing research, education, and practice issues* (pp. 3–16). New York: Hemisphere.

Sassetti, M. R. (1993). Domestic violence. *Primary Care, 20*(2), 289–305.

Selzer, M. L. (1971). The Michigan Alcoholism Screening Test: The quest for a new diagnostic instrument. *American Journal of Psychiatry, 127*, 89–94.

Sisley, A., Jacobs, L. M., Poole, G., et al. (1999). Violence in America: A public health crisis-domestic violence. *Journal of Trauma, Injury, and Critical Care, 46*(6), 1105–1112.

Skinner, H. A. (1982). The Drug Abuse Screening Test. *Addictive Behavior, 7*, 363–371.

Southwick, S. M., Bremner, D., Krystal, J. H., & Charney, D. S. (1994). Psychobiologic research in post-traumatic stress disorder. *Psychiatric Clinics of North America, 17*(2), 251–264.

Spiegel, D., Koopman, C., & Classen, C. (1994). Acute stress disorder and dissociation. *Australian Journal of Clinical and Experimental Hypnosis, 22*(1), 11–23.

Stark, E., & Flitcraft, A. (1996). *Women at risk: Domestic violence and women's health.* Newbury Park, CA: Sage.

Starling, K. (1998). Black women and rape: The shocking secret no one talks about. *Ebony, 54*(1), 140–144.

Thompson, M. P., Kaslow, N. J., Kingree, J. B., et al. (1999). Partner abuse and posttraumatic stress disorder as risk factors for suicide attempts in a sample of low-income, inner-city women. *Journal of Traumatic Stress, 12*(1), 59–71.

Turnbull, G. J., & McFarlane, A. C. (1996). Acute treatments. In B. A. van der Kolk, A. C. McFarlane, & L. Weisaeth (Eds.), *Traumatic stress: The effects of overwhelming experience on mind, body, and society* (pp. 480–490). New York: Guilford.

Tyndall, C. I. (1997). Current treatment strategies for sexually abused children. In R. Geffner, S. B. Sorenson, & P. K. Lundberg-Love (Eds.), *Violence and sexual abuse at home: Current issues in spousal battering and child maltreatment* (pp. 277–293). New York: Haworth Maltreatment & Trauma Press.

van der Kolk, B. A., & Fisler, R. E. (1993). The biologic basis of posttraumatic stress. *Primary Care, 20*(2), 417–432.

van der Kolk, B. A., McFarlane, A. C., & Weisaeth, L. (Eds.). (1996). *Traumatic stress: The effects of overwhelming experience on mind, body, and society*. New York: Guilford.

Walker, L. (1979). *The battered woman*. New York: Harper & Row.

Walker, L. (1994). *The abused women: A survivor therapy approach* [Film]. Available from Newbridge Communications, Inc. 333 East Street, New York, NY 10016.

Wallace, H. (1999). *Family violence: Legal, medical, and social perspectives* (2nd ed.). Boston: Allyn & Bacon.

Wright, R. J., Wright, R. O., & Isaac, N. E. (1997). Response to battered mothers in the pediatric emergency department: A call for an interdisciplinary approach to family violence. *Pediatrics, 99*(2), 186–192.

Zust, B. L. (2000). Effect of cognitive therapy on depression in rural battered women. *Archives of Psychiatric Nursing, 14*(2), 51–63.

Case Finding and Care in Suicide: Children, Adolescents, and Adults

Emily J. Hauenstein

LEARNING OBJECTIVES

After studying this chapter, you will be able to:

➤ Define suicide, parasuicide, and suicide ideation.
➤ Describe population groups that have high rates of suicide.
➤ Discuss factors associated with rising rates of suicide in the young.
➤ Discuss the civil liberties of patients and other legal issues in care of suicidal patients.
➤ Determine factors that affect the nurse's responsibility in identifying suicidal patients.
➤ List screening measures for depression, suicide intent, and psychiatric diagnostic measures.
➤ Describe factors that increase the risk for suicide completion.
➤ Describe the no-suicide contract.
➤ Describe the nurse's responsibilities in promoting short and long-term recovery in suicidal adult inpatients.
➤ Discuss the patient's and nurse's responsibilities in discharging the patient to the community.

CHAPTER 38

KEY TERMS

case finding
confidentiality
informed consent
involuntary
    hospitalization
least restrictive
    environment
no-suicide contract
parasuicide
suicide
suicide ideation
voluntary
    hospitalization

KEY CONCEPTS

hopelessness
lethality

*S*uicide *is the voluntary act of killing oneself. It is sometimes called suicide completion. The behavioral definition of suicide is limited and does not consider the complexity of the underlying depressive illness, personal motivations, and situational and family factors that provoke the suicide act.*

Parasuicide is a voluntary, failed attempt to kill oneself. It is frequently called attempted suicide. Parasuicidal behavior varies by intent (Ferreira de Castro et al., 1998). For example, some people who attempt suicide truly wish to die, but others simply wish to feel nothing for awhile. Still others attempt suicide because they want to send a message to others about their emotional state.

Suicide ideation is thinking about and planning one's own death. It also includes excessive or unreasoned worrying about losing a significant other.

Although all mental illness is stigmatized in contemporary society, suicide is especially so. Speaking about or attempting suicide makes mental illness obvious to others. This is especially true if the person who attempted suicide requires medical intervention or psychiatric hospitalization. The subsequent visibility of the disorder discredits the person, leaving him or her open to stigmatization (Joachim & Acorn, 2000). The act of suicide stimulates others' fears of the mentally ill because of the common belief that the mentally ill are violent (Brunton, 1997; Steadman et al., 1998). Reports and portrayals of suicide in the popular press and television also con-

tribute to the stigmatization of those who consider or attempt suicide (Brunton, 1997; Wilson et al., 1999). Society's unwillingness to talk openly about suicide contributes to the common perception that firearms are used more often to commit murder than suicide. Firearm homicide deaths exceed the suicide rate in only 11 of the 50 states and the District of Columbia (Centers for Disease Control and Prevention, 2000). The fear of stigma plays a substantial role in suicide because it encourages the suicidal patient to avoid treatment.

Suicidal behaviors are direct consequences of certain mood disorders, especially recurrent major depressive disorder (MDD) (see Chap. 20). MDD is exceedingly common in both Western and developing nations. Data from the National Comorbidity Study show a 1-year prevalence rate of 11% for MDD (Kessler et al., 1994). This major epidemiologic study of mental disorders showed that MDD is most common among women, the poor, young people, and whites. Rates are also increased among people with comorbid physical illness (Hendin, 1999; Stevens et al., 1995) and among those who receive their health care in primary care settings (McQuaid et al., 1999). The concurrence of suicide and MDD is important because suicide prevention is based, in part, on understanding the nature and occurrence of MDD.

Suicide is highly preventable. People commit suicide because others do not recognize the signs, underlying MDD is not treated, or those with suicidal ideation fear the social stigma of discussing their problems. Because those at risk for suicide appear in most health care settings, nurses are in a unique position to prevent death by suicide. Nurses must be able to assess a patient's potential for suicide, determine its causes, and identify factors that enhance its risk. They must know what to do when working with a patient who is acutely suicidal. Nurses can do much to demystify suicide and destigmatize those at risk through individual and public education. This chapter contains tools nurses can use to reduce the broad effects of suicide and to provide appropriate care for suicidal patients.

EPIDEMIOLOGY OF SUICIDAL BEHAVIOR

More than 31,000 people die from suicide annually, making it the ninth leading cause of death in the United States (Anonymous, 1999; Anonymous, 2000a). Every 42 seconds, someone attempts suicide; every 17 minutes, someone completes it. There are 11 suicide attempts per 100,000 people annually.

Suicide occurs in all age groups, social classes, and cultures (Johansson, 1997). Its prevalence may be underestimated because suicide can be disguised as vehicular accidents or homicide, especially in young people (Ohberg & Lonnqvist, 1998). For this reason, the suicide rate may be as much as 10% higher than reported in national statistics. Parasuicide adds to the problem, placing significant demands on the health care system by increasing the use of emergency department and intensive care services and acute medical admissions. Failed suicide attempts often predate actual suicide completion.

The public health problem of suicidal behavior is so important that several goals of *Healthy People 2010* (Anonymous, 2000b), the nation's public health goals, directly target the reduction of deaths by suicide. Targeting suicide reduction as a national goal has somewhat reduced the rate of suicide overall and has dramatically reduced its incidence in elderly men.

Suicide

In 1997, 1.3% of all deaths were from suicide (Anonymous, 2000b). About 56% of people succeed in their first suicide attempt (Isometsa & Lonnqvist, 1998). About 25% of people hospitalized for a failed suicide attempt kill themselves within 3 months after discharge (Appleby et al., 1999a). Handguns are the most common method of suicide, accounting for 58% of all cases (Anonymous, 2000b). Suicides outnumber homicides by a ratio of 3:2. Suicide is more common among certain groups with specific risk factors (Text Box 38-1) and has been associated with loss, unemployment, transience, recent life events (eg, divorce, moving, prob-

TEXT BOX 38.1

Factors Enhancing Suicide Risk

Vulnerability
Primary family member who has completed suicide
Psychiatric disorder
Previous attempt by the patient
Loss (eg, death of significant other, divorce, job loss)
Unrelenting physical illness

Risk
White man
Older adulthood
Adolescence
Gay, lesbian, or bisexual orientation
Access to firearm

Intent
Suicide plan and means of executing it
Inability to enter into a no-suicide contract

Disinhibition
Impulsivity
Isolation
Psychotic thoughts
Drug or alcohol use

lems with children), interpersonal distress, and earlier attempts (Appleby et al., 1999b).

Age

KEY CONCEPT **Hopelessness. Hopelessness** is a state of despair characterized by feelings of inadequacy, isolation, and inability to act on one's own behalf. It is connected with the belief that one's situation is unlikely to improve.

Prepubertal Children. Suicide is rare among children younger than age 10 years, occurring at a rate of 0.02 per 100,000 (Anonymous, 1997a). Still, it is the sixth leading cause of death in this age group. White boys commit 75% of suicides deaths in this age group.

Preadolescents and Adolescents. Among children aged 10 to 14 years, suicide is the third leading cause of death. In this age group, suicide accounts for a death rate of 1.6 per 100,000. Boys in this age group commit 75% of successful suicides; 63.4% of these boys are white. In a study of 26 industrialized nations, the United States reported two suicides of children aged 10 to 14 years for every one committed in the remaining 25 nations combined (Anonymous, 1997b). The United States accounted for 54% of all suicide deaths reported by the 26 nations.

Suicide is the third leading cause of death among people aged 15 to 24 years. Among adolescents aged 15 to 19 years, the rate is 9.5 per 100,000, a total of 1,802 successful suicides (Anonymous, 2000a). Five boys commit suicide to every girl.

Among black male youth aged 15 to 19 years, suicide rates have increased rapidly. From 1980 to 1996, the suicide rate among black male teens more than doubled from 3.6 to 8.1 per 100,000 (Anonymous, 1999), an increase of 105% (Anonymous, 2000b). Homicides and "suicide by cop" (deliberately provoking a policeman to shoot) are prevalent among black male youth and may further contribute to the rates of suicide in black adolescents (Daugherty, 1999).

Death by firearm accounts for 63% of the increase in suicide among adolescents. Most of these teens (67%) obtain the guns at home (Shah et al., 2000). Alcohol also plays a role in suicide completion among adolescents. States that have set the minimum drinking age at 18 years have higher rates of suicide than those whose minimum drinking age is 21 years (Birckmayer & Hemenway, 1999).

Adults. Among adults aged 25 to 34 years, suicide is the second leading cause of death (Anonymous, 1997a). Childhood physical and sexual abuse has been linked to suicidal behavior in this age group (Santa Mina & Gallop, 1998). Other factors linked to suicidal behavior in young adults include unemployment and interpersonal distress (Appleby et al., 1999b; Foster et al., 1999; Gunnell et al., 1999). Suicide also is linked to mental illness in young adults; most young adults who commit suicide also have MDD, and many have personality disorders (Foster et al., 1999).

Older Adults. Older white men have the highest risk for completed suicide. They are more likely to be single, live in rural areas, and use a gun to commit suicide (Quan & Arboleda-Florez, 1999). Physical illness and financial difficulties also are important precipitants to suicide in elderly men (Uncapher et al., 1998). In contrast, elderly women who commit suicide are more likely to have a current psychiatric disorder (Agbayewa et al., 1998).

For both elderly men and women, suicide is associated with less education, previous attempts, depressive disorder, and substance abuse (Conwell et al., 2000). Elderly people who complete suicide are more likely to have severe depression, significant physical illness, decreased emotional and physical functioning, and increased functional impairment than other elderly people seen in primary care settings.

The ways that older adults approach their decision to commit suicide accounts for its lethality in this age group. Elderly people are more likely to have thought through the decision and the means to commit suicide (Marcus, 1996). Despite the impaired judgment that accompanies MDD, elderly people are more likely than younger people to have realistically assessed their life circumstances.

> **KEY CONCEPT**   Lethality. **Lethality** refers to the probability that a person will successfully complete suicide. Lethality is determined by the seriousness of the person's intent, the degree to which he or she has developed a viable plan, and the availability of the means to execute the plan.

Gender

Men have a suicide rate of 19.4 per 100,000, almost five times the rate of women (Anonymous, 2000a). The suicide rate in men peaks between ages 30 and 34 years (28 per 100,000) and slowly declines thereafter (Anonymous, 1997a). The rate then rapidly increases at age 65 years and continues upward; by age 85 years or older, the suicide rate in men is about 65 per 100,000. White men commit 72% of all suicides and 79% of all firearm suicides. In contrast, the suicide rate peaks in black men between ages 20 and 24 years (21 per 100,000) and then declines. The rate of suicide increases modestly in elderly black men.

The higher rate of suicide completion in men is related to their approach to decision making and interpersonal relationships (Murphy, 1998). Many men tend to be independent and decisive. They think vertically and linearly. These factors mean that men are more likely to think in absolutes and pay less attention to their interpersonal relationships. Men who commit suicide often have few or no significant others. Even when support is available, many suicidal men are reluctant to use it. MDD is often comorbid with substance abuse in men, and up to 33% of patients with alcoholism commit suicide (Angst et al., 1999; Berglund & Ojehagen, 1998). MDD also tends to be comorbid with other psychiatric disorders, which increases men's overall risk for suicide (Hall et al., 1999).

In women, the peak in the suicide rate is slightly older and longer, occurring between ages 35 and 44 years. Among white women, suicide rates peak between ages 45 and 54 years at less than 10 per 100,000 and decline thereafter. Like men, women who complete suicide often have several comorbid psychiatric disorders (Hall et al., 1999). Women who have MDD and comorbid schizophrenia or anxiety and those with bipolar disorder are at high risk for suicide (Rihmer & Pestality, 1999; Saarinen et al., 1999). Current or previous exposure to violence, sexual assault, or both also increases women's risk for suicide (see Chap. 37) (Davidson et al., 1996; Kaslow et al., 1998; Olson et al., 1999; Shrier et al., 1998).

Race

Black Americans commit suicide less often than whites (Kung et al., 1998). The major risk factor for suicide among blacks is a history of or current mental illness. Among blacks, men aged 15 to 29 years have the highest rates of suicide (Anonymous, 1997a). Historically, a major protective factor against suicide for many blacks was their fundamentalist Christian religious roots (Neeleman et al., 1998). Declining involvement of young blacks in religious activities is cited as one reason for the rapid increase in suicide in this age group. Involvement in gang activity and other homicidal deaths precipitated by the victim may also be means of committing suicide in young black men (Anonymous, 2000b). Suicides among black women in all age groups are less than 5 per 100,000 and are often precipitated by being a victim of violence from a known assailant (Kaslow et al., 1998).

Sexual Orientation

Gay, lesbian, and bisexual (GLB) youth have rates of attempted suicide between 20% and 42% (Remafedi, 1999). Research has shown that 28% of gay or bisexual male teens have attempted suicide, compared with 4.2% of heterosexual male teens (Remafedi, 1999). Similarly, 20.5% of lesbian teens reported attempting suicide, compared with 14.5% of heterosexual female teens. GLB youth aged 14 to 21 years were four times more likely to be depressed, five times more likely to think about suicide, and six times more likely to attempt suicide than heterosexual young people of the same ages (Fergusson et al., 1999). Findings were almost identical in a middle-aged group of GLB people (Herrell et al., 1999). GLB individuals who "came out" to their families reported more suicidal behavior than those who did not tell their families about their sexual orientation (D'Augelli et al., 1998).

Parasuicide and Suicide Ideation

Parasuicide and suicide ideation were evaluated as part of the National Comorbidity Study (Kessler et al., 1999). About 5% of people report a suicide attempt during their lifetime. Women are two to three times more likely to attempt suicide than men. Parasuicide occurs frequently in younger age groups and declines after age 44 years.

Parasuicide is among the best predictors of future suicide attempts and completions. As many as 20% of men and 40% of women attempt suicide and fail in the year preceding a completed suicide (Isometsa &

Lonnqvist, 1998). Most completed suicides occur in the first year after hospitalization for a failed suicide attempt. MDD, drug and alcohol abuse, schizophrenia, and borderline personality disorder are common among those who survive their attempt at suicide but have an ongoing wish to die (Ferreira de Castro et al., 1998). Polydrug use including alcohol, heroin, cocaine, and tobacco is associated with parasuicide (Tondo, et al., 1999).

Suicide ideation occurs in about 14% of people during their lifetimes (Kessler et al., 1999). Of those who experience suicide ideation, 34% form a plan; 72% of those who form a plan attempt suicide (Kessler et al., 1999). In addition to MDD, physical, cognitive, psychological, and social risk factors contribute to suicide ideation. Physical factors include medical illness and alcohol and drug use (Grant & Hasin, 1999; Hendin, 1999; Vilhjalmsson et al., 1998). Cognitive risk factors include problem-solving deficits and hopelessness (D'Zurilla et al., 1998). Psychological risk factors include internal distress and low self-esteem (Holden et al., 1998). Social risk factors include financial hardship, legal stress, family difficulties, and poor social support (Vilhjalmsson et al., 1998). As with parasuicide, childhood trauma (including physical and sexual abuse) has been linked to suicide ideation in adulthood (Boudewyn & Liem, 1995).

Parasuicide and suicide ideation are more common among adolescents than in other age groups. The estimated parasuicide rate among adolescents is 2.6% (Anonymous, 2000a). Suicide attempts are most common among teenage girls (3.3%) and Hispanics/Latinos (2.8%). About 25% of adolescents report suicidal ideation, and 15% report having a plan to commit suicide (Rey et al., 1998). Like adults, suicidal behavior in children and adolescents is associated with mental illness (Lee et al., 1999; McKeown et al., 1998). Adolescents who have panic attacks are particularly at risk (Gould et al., 1998; Pilowsky et al., 1999). Other causes of suicidal behavior in adolescents include family discord, neglect, physical abuse, adolescent unemployment, residential transience, chronic behavior problems, and recent interpersonal stress (Appleby et al., 1999b; Brent, 1997; Grilo et al., 1999; Groholt et al., 1998; Gunnell et al., 1999; McKeown et al., 1998). Substance abuse increases the likelihood that suicide ideation will result in parasuicide (Gould et al., 1998). Among children reporting neglect or physical or sexual abuse, 51% attempt suicide (Lipschitz et al., 1999).

Although adolescents make more attempts than do adults, they generally are less successful (Safer, 1997). Suicide attempts by adolescents also do not hold the same long-term risks for suicide completion as they do for adults.

ETIOLOGY OF SUICIDAL BEHAVIOR

Hauenstein (1996) described a stress-diathesis model designed to guide nursing practice for depressed women. In this model, vulnerable people exposed to stressors for which they have limited ability to cope respond with a host of biologic, psychological, and social responses called *stress responses*. If these stress responses continue over an extended period, the person develops one of many stress-related illnesses. MDD, a classic stress-related illness, and suicidal behavior are potential outcomes from this model.

Hauenstein's nursing practice paradigm (NPP) appears in Figure 38-1. The NPP is helpful in explaining suicidal behavior. First, it posits that some people are more likely to attempt or complete suicide than others because of certain genetic and biologic factors. Because certain people have specific vulnerability, not all depressed people need to be considered at risk for suicide. Second, the model permits variations in the factors or precipitants that lead to suicidal behavior. The model suggests that stressors can adversely affect those who are vulnerable to suicide but only under certain condi-

tions. Stressors become a catalyst to suicidal behavior only when they are novel and the affected person cannot readily meet them with an array of practiced coping strategies. When stressors are not novel but the person has few or maladaptive coping abilities, suicidal behavior might be an outcome. Finally, suicidal behavior can emerge when stressors simply exceed a person's psychological and other resources (Hauenstein, 1996). If these tenets are true, the nurse can target several behaviors for intervention to reduce suicide risk in those with specific vulnerability.

Biologic Theories

Suicide rarely occurs without psychopathology. Most people who attempt or complete suicide have severe MDD, either alone or in conjunction with another major acute psychiatric disturbance. Severe MDD tends to develop when a person who is vulnerable to it (because of genetic or other factors) is subjected to repeated or sustained stress.

Stress responsiveness in these people ultimately changes neurotransmitter and hormonal functioning

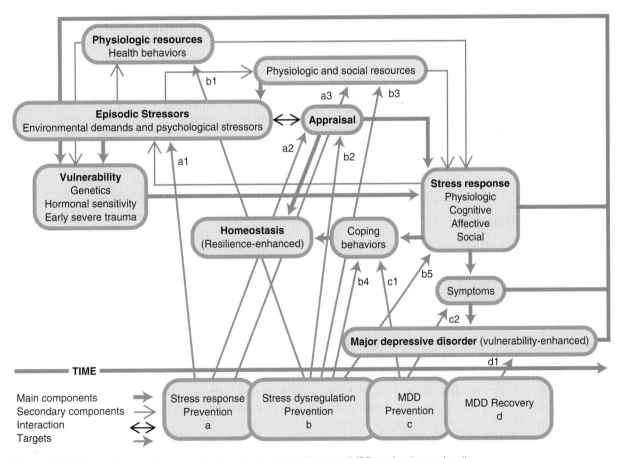

FIGURE 38.1 The nursing practice paradigm for depressed rural women. MDD, major depressive disorder. (Adapted from Hauenstein, E. [1996]. A nursing practice paradigm for depressed rural women: Theoretical basis. *Archives of Psychiatric Nursing, X*(5), 283–292.)

to affect a depressed state (Hauenstein, 1996). These neurochemical changes directly contribute to suicidal behavior. Those who complete suicide have extremely low levels of the neurotransmitter serotonin, or 5-hydroxytryptamine (5-HT). The cerebrospinal fluid of people who exhibit suicidal behavior contains extremely low levels of the 5-HT metabolite 5-hydroxyindoleacetic acid (5-HIAA) (Mann et al., 1999).

Evidence has shown that genetic factors may be involved in suicidal behavior. For example, suicide risk appears to be greater within families (Malone et al., 1995). Estimates are that the risk in first-degree relatives of psychiatric patients who have completed suicide is four times greater than that in first-degree relatives of psychiatric patients without a suicidal history. Suicide of a first-degree relative is highly predictive of a medically serious suicide attempt (Modai et al., 1999). Suicide rates are higher among families of adolescents who attempt suicide (Johnson et al., 1998). Depressed mothers with a history of suicide attempts are linked to higher rates of suicidal behavior in their children (Klimes-Dougan et al., 1999; Pfeffer et al., 1998). The genetic link to suicide is evident in studies of twins. One of these studies showed that when both members of a set of twins completed suicides, the pairs were always monozygotic (Roy et al., 1997). Another twin study showed that suicide attempts in one twin were the most powerful predictor of suicide attempts in the other twin (Statham et al., 1998). Adoption studies have shown that among adults who experience mood disorders and were adopted as children, the suicide rate among the biologic relatives of the adoptees is much higher than the rate among the adoptive relatives. These studies demonstrate that the biologic risk for suicide appears independent of environmental factors that might contribute to the depressive experience (Statham et al., 1998).

Psychological Theories

Psychodynamic theorists believe that suicide is anger and aggression turned inward. In a classic paper, Freud describes suicide as a sadomasochistic act that combines aggression toward oneself with punishment of a love object for real or imagined rejections (Freud, 1985). In other words, psychodynamic theorists believe that people who kill themselves sadistically punish themselves and the people who love them. When observing behavior of depressed people, it is easy to see why psychodynamic theorists describe suicide in this way. Their ideas were formulated long before the biologic basis of depression and suicide was understood; thus, their use in contemporary psychiatric nursing practice is limited.

Social learning theories of behavior are often more helpful in understanding and intervening successfully with suicidal behavior (Bandura, 1977). Stress-diathesis models of illness and outcome like Hauenstein's NPP

are direct outgrowths of the social learning perspective (Cohen et al., 1995; Hauenstein, 1996). According to social learning theory, environmental factors interact with individual biologic and psychological characteristics to cause certain behaviors. This perspective emphasizes that suicide results from an imbalance between a vulnerable individual's personal, physical, psychological, and social resources, and the nature and amount of personal and environmental stress he or she experiences. Using this theoretic perspective helps clinicians to target needed behavioral change.

Another psychological theory used to explain suicidal behavior is the cognitive model of depression (Abramson et al., 1985; Beck et al., 1979). According to this theory, negative dysfunctional thoughts and beliefs lead to feelings of hopelessness, helplessness, and worthlessness. Depressed people view themselves, their current situation, and their future negatively. They are pessimistic about themselves as people, their abilities (especially to effect change), the opinions of others about them, and the likelihood of improvement. People who engage in negative thinking believe that "No one is ever there for me," "Nothing I do makes any difference," and "My future is very bleak." These thoughts tend to be spontaneous, repetitive, and ultimately powerful motivators of suicidal behavior.

Social Theories

Suicide repeatedly is linked to lack of social support, loss, and interpersonal distress. Feeling connected to others is an important deterrent to suicide. Without such a connection, the risk for suicide, especially in those with existing MDD, is much higher. For these reasons, living alone and transience are major contributors to suicidal behavior (Appleby et al., 1999a; Johansson et al., 1997; Kung et al., 1998; Modai et al., 1999). Suicide is more common in unmarried people (Clark, 1995; Johansson, et al., 1997). Having little social support is especially difficult when experiencing loss, especially the loss of a loved one. For these reasons, interpersonal distress and divorce are linked to suicide. Job loss and unemployment figure prominently in suicide, especially for men (Modai et al., 1999; Statham et al., 1998). Social support is thought to reduce suicide because being connected with others reduces depressive symptoms (Hauenstein, 1996). Significant others also help the patient to manage the acute suicidal crisis and can summon help when needed. Figure 38-2 presents more information on causative factors in suicide.

EFFECTS OF SUICIDE

The financial costs of suicidal behavior are staggering. Estimated costs of medical and hospital care for a person who commits suicide are $5,700 (Clayton & Barcel,

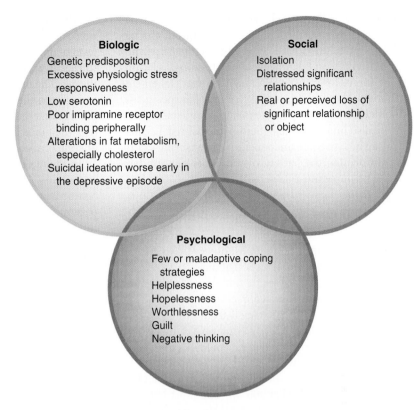

Biologic
Genetic predisposition
Excessive physiologic stress
  responsiveness
Low serotonin
Poor imipramine receptor
  binding peripherally
Alterations in fat metabolism,
  especially cholesterol
Suicidal ideation worse early in
  the depressive episode

Social
Isolation
Distressed significant
  relationships
Real or perceived loss of
  significant relationship
  or object

Psychological
Few or maladaptive coping
  strategies
Helplessness
Hopelessness
Worthlessness
Guilt
Negative thinking

FIGURE 38.2 Biopsychosocial etiologies of suicide.

1999). When considering the value of lost productivity for premature death, the estimated cost of suicide $844,184 per person. The total cost of one suicide is $849,877. Estimates of the costs of suicide attempts are much more difficult to obtain because record keeping of this behavior is less precise than that for completed suicide. In one study, however, estimates of the average hospital cost per suicide attempt were $2,639 (Waller et al., 1994), excluding ongoing outpatient pharmacologic costs and lost wages.

Beyond the financial implications, suicide has devastating effects on everyone it touches, but especially on the victim's family and close friends. Grief caused by a loved one's suicide is often severe and lengthy. Survivors often feel profoundly guilty and wonder if they could have done something to prevent the suicide. They feel guilty that they were unaware of how unhappy their loved one had become. Survivors also feel ambivalent and angry because of the strain of managing the chronic behavioral disturbance in their significant other who ultimately commits suicide (Van Dongen, 1988).

Survivors often have no experience with suicidal death and may not have the means to cope with this unnatural life event. Shneidman (1972) eloquently described the long-term effects of suicide on survivors:

> I believe that the person who commits suicide puts his psychological skeleton in the survivor's emotional closet—he sentences the survivor to deal with many negative feelings and, more, to be obsessed with thoughts regarding his own ac-

tual or possible role in having precipitated the suicidal act or having failed to abort it. It can be a heavy load. (p. ix)

LEGAL CONSIDERATIONS IN CARE FOR SUICIDAL PATIENTS

Patients have several legal rights that health care providers must consider during suicide prevention and treatment. Providers cannot deprive patients of their right to self-determination unless no other course is available to ensure a patient's safety. They must preserve the rights to privacy and anonymity unless they cannot protect a patient without disclosing his or her suicidal intent to others. Patients have the right of beneficence, which is the right to be free from harm. Physically restraining or hospitalizing a patient against his or her will has the potential for both physical and emotional harm. Providers should exercise such options only under the threat of imminent suicide or psychosis. The nurse must know the extent of the patient's legal rights and be prepared to inform patients of them in a way that they can understand.

Confidentiality

The nurse is responsible for explaining the patient's right to and the limits of **confidentiality**. The patient has a right to confidentiality unless he or she is in imminent danger of harming himself or herself. Only then can the nurse enlist the help of others to protect the patient's safety. Disclosing information without the patient's permission violates his or her rights to privacy and anonymity and damages the professional relationship. Patients lose trust when the nurse shares their suicidal intent with others unless the nurse has specifically explained the limits of confidentiality. Unwarranted disclosure also increases the patient's suicidal risk because he or she may become uncooperative in ensuring safety.

In informing the patient of the limits of confidentiality, the nurse must be very specific:

> Mr. Jones, when you tell me things that are very personal, I will not share that information with anyone else without your written permission. There are some specific times, however, when I may need to share information about you to provide you with proper care. If you ever tell me that you might want to hurt yourself and you do not think you can prevent yourself from doing so, I will be obligated to involve whomever I think necessary to preserve your safety. I would like for you to tell me if you do want to harm yourself because others and I can help you until you feel better and in more control of what you do. You must know ahead of time, though, that in this specific instance, I may need to tell others to keep you safe.

Protection of the patient's right to confidentiality is a special concern when a minor child has suicidal intent. As with adult patients, the nurse is required to describe the right to confidentiality and its limits. What differs is that the nurse must inform parents or legal guardians of a child who has suicidal intent. The parents of a minor child retain the privilege to determine the right care for their child, and they need sufficient information to make good decisions. Unfortunately, many suicidal children do not want their parents involved. Still, before beginning any suicide evaluation, nurses must let a child know that they could share anything that the child discloses with parents. They should emphasize that they will tell the parents of a child's intent to run away or to commit suicide or homicide. The child may become less cooperative, especially when he or she distrusts adults. Honesty about what the nurse can and cannot keep confidential, however, ultimately increases a child's trust and often results in a more therapeutic relationship. There may be times when the therapeutic relationship between the nurse and child or adolescent is best served by the parent suspending their privilege so that the relationship between patient and nurse can develop unimpeded. This is true especially when the child is an older adolescent or a young, but not emancipated, adult. When the minor child is actively suicidal, however, nurses must notify parents so that they can take action to protect their child.

After explaining the limits of confidentiality, the nurse must ask questions that will determine the patient's level of understanding. The nurse should ask the patient to repeat what he or she has heard and explain what it means. The nurse can then ask the patient how he or she feels about the limits imposed. The nurse should emphasize that the patient needs to trust the nurse, which is why the nurse is telling the patient about this limitation of confidentiality before they talk in depth.

In some settings, the patient signs confidentiality statements. Many settings also require health care professionals to sign statements that they will preserve the patient's confidentiality. When this is the case, the limits of confidentiality must appear in both the patient's statement and that to be signed by the health care professional.

Informed Consent

Obtaining fully **informed consent** from the patient protects his or her right to self-determination. The nurse ensures informed consent when he or she provides the patient with written and oral information about the proposed treatment. Consent is informed when it is presented in terms that the patient can readily understand. In non-English–speaking patients, informed consent requires the use of an interpreter to explain proposed treatments. Informed consent includes information about other treatment alternatives available to the patient and the risk and benefits of the proposed treatment. It requires that the patient is knowledgeable of who will be responsible for his or her care. It also includes information about what will be required of the patient.

Informed consent is especially important with the suicidal patient. Nurses must inform suicidal patients about limits to their self-determination and make efforts to obtain their cooperation. From the time that the nurse encounters a suicidal patient until a suitable placement is made, the nurse must share with the patient his or her right to be placed in the **least restrictive environment** that will ensure safety. The least restrictive environment is the setting that puts the fewest constraints on the patient's liberty while still ensuring the patient's safety. The patient has choices: a no-suicide contract or voluntary hospitalization, both of which preserve the patient's rights. By informing patients about their choices, the nurse gains the patient's trust and increases the likelihood that involuntary hospitalization will not be necessary.

Competence

To determine whether patients can make an agreement with the nurse that will keep them safe, the nurse needs to evaluate whether patients have sufficient judgment to enter into such agreements legally. The competent patient can reason and make decisions based on sound interpretations of the information available. The patient best demonstrates competence by asking knowledgeable questions about his or her rights and required treatment. Competence is task specific, which means that the nurse must judge the patient's competence with regard to the patient's ability to agree to the limits of confidentiality. He or she must consider the patient's competence when obtaining informed consent (see Chap. 4) and then again when discussing a no-suicide contract with the patient (discussed later in the chapter). With a psychiatric disorder such as depression, the patient is not necessarily incompetent to make decisions; the nurse and other mental health professionals must be able to demonstrate that the patient's judgment is impaired.

Beneficence

The ethical requirement of beneficence, doing no harm, is critical when considering restraining patients against their will. Touching patients in any way against their will is battery, and restraining patients without informing them that restraint may be imposed violates the legal requirement of informed consent. Managing patients who are suicidal and determined to get away is difficult without touching and actively restraining them. Still, nurses must do their best to disclose to patients the specifics of planned treatments, including restraints, and obtain their consent to proceed.

Documentation and Reporting

The nurse must document thoroughly encounters with suicidal patients. This action is for the patient's ongoing treatment and the nurse's protection. Lawsuits for malpractice in psychiatric settings often involve completed suicides. The medical record must reflect that the nurse took every reasonable action to provide for the patient's safety.

The record should describe the patient's history, methods used to determine a psychiatric disorder, and any diagnosis. The record should reflect all present risk factors for suicidal behavior, the level of the patient's intent, and any disinhibiting factors that might increase the patient's impulsivity. Documentation must include any use of drugs, alcohol, or prescription medications by the patient in the 6 hours before the assessment. It should include the use of antidepressants that are especially lethal (eg, tricyclics) as well as any medication that might impair the patient's judgment (eg, a sleep medication). Notes should reflect the level of the patient's judgment and ability to be a partner in treatment. If a no-suicide contract has been instituted, the record must contain specific aspects of the contract. It should include factors influencing the decision to use

the contract, including the patient's behaviors that led providers to believe that the patient could be safely managed as an outpatient. The documentation should reflect any medication and the amount prescribed. The record must also contain the provider's part in the contract, including information given to the patient about how to reenter the health care system during the term of the contract. Significant others who will care for the patient during the term of the no-suicide contract should also be mentioned.

Involuntary Hospitalization

Any patient who cannot be maintained safely in the community must be hospitalized. Health care professionals must make every effort to obtain the patient's permission to enter the hospital voluntarily, for both legal and therapeutic reasons. Legally, **voluntary hospitalization** protects the civil liberties of patients, permitting them some freedom in negotiating discharge from the hospital. Therapeutically, voluntary admission reinforces control of the situation for patients because they act as partners in their own care. Voluntary admission helps preserve the dignity and confidentiality of patients because it permits family members to take them to the hospital, and it does not necessitate additional outpatient evaluation.

When a patient will not or is not competent to agree to enter the hospital voluntarily, health care professionals must initiate **involuntary hospitalization**. Involuntary hospitalization is a lengthy process because the patient's civil liberties must be preserved. Two physicians must examine the patient and certify that he or she is a danger to self or others. These are the only legal reasons for detaining patients against their will. Typically, when the patient is considered in imminent danger of self-harm, providers must contact a judge who can issue a temporary detaining order (TDO). The TDO permits providers to contact the police, who then transport the patient to a community mental health center or hospital emergency department for evaluation or *preadmission screening*, as it is often called. If the mental health provider agrees with the initial evaluation, the patient can be admitted involuntarily for 60 days. The patient's next of kin must be notified of the admission in writing. The patient can ask for legal counsel and file a writ of habeas corpus with the court at any time. The writ asks the court to determine whether the patient's due process rights are being violated. The hospital is required to submit the writ immediately, and the court is obligated to hear the writ in a timely fashion.

Depriving patients of their civil liberties is serious and should be done only in life-threatening situations. Unfortunately, this drastic measure seriously impedes the patient's development of trust in the people whom they view as imprisoning them. Once a patient is hospitalized, every effort must be made to engage the person as a partner in his or her own care and to move the patient toward voluntary hospitalization. Special considerations in the hospitalization of children and adolescents are given in Text Box 38-2.

NURSING MANAGEMENT: HUMAN RESPONSE TO DISORDER

Suicidal behaviors are seriously underreported and often unrecognized by health care professionals. Estimates are that about 40% of people who commit suicide have visited a health care provider within 1 to 6 months of a suicide attempt (Foster et al., 1999; Purcell, Thrush, & Blanchette, 1999; Links et al., 1999). Nurses can play important roles in suicide prevention because they practice in diverse health care settings and thus work with many different kinds of patients.

Acutely suicidal behavior is a true psychiatric emergency. Nurses must act immediately and vigorously to prevent the patient's death. The NPP described earlier (see Fig. 38-1) is a useful guide for determining which people may be most at risk for suicide. By considering the patient's balance of stressors and resources, the

nurse can determine whether the patient has sufficient resources to manage his or her suicidal impulses. At this stage of suicide prevention, the nurse must identify people who may be suicidal, determine their risk for suicide, determine the presence of any psychiatric disorders, and provide for the patient's safety by initiating the least restrictive care possible.

As the initial suicidal crisis fades, the nurse's responsibility changes. The NPP provides structure for nursing action at this next stage of treatment. The nurse's focus should include reducing the patient's responsiveness to stress and strengthening existing resources. Nurses coach patients in self-care and coping skills, symptom management, identification of depressive symptoms, and relapse prevention. They identify and correct physical health problems as part of hospitalization for suicide or shortly after discharge. Social skills training may be an important part of relapse prevention. Nurses should encourage patients to identify sources of social support and, when appropriate, include these people in patient care.

Assessing the Suicidal Patient

Case Finding

Case finding refers to identifying people who are at risk for suicide to initiate proper treatment. Case finding for MDD and identifying risk factors associated with suicide are essential nursing roles that nurses must incorporate into the routine health care of patients. This is true for nurses working in primary care settings as well as for those who care for patients with psychiatric disorders.

Using the NPP, the nurse first identifies people who are experiencing extreme stress, have little social support, and have insufficient coping skills to manage the stressors that are affecting them. Case finding requires the nurse to inquire about emotional symptoms the patient may be having, specifically suicidal thoughts. Many nurses are concerned that asking patients about their suicidal thoughts will provoke a suicide attempt. This belief simply is not true. In most cases, the suicidal patient has been considering suicide for some time. Nurses who ask their patients about suicidal thoughts give them a chance to discuss what is troubling them, thereby reducing suicidal thoughts.

Asking about a patient's suicidal thoughts is difficult. Screening patients for depression is a good way to begin determining risk for suicidal behavior. Many useful screens for depressive symptoms are available. The Center for Epidemiological Studies Depression Scale (CES-D) (Radloff, 1977) is a 20-item self-report questionnaire that takes less than 10 minutes to complete. Each of the 20 items is a symptom of depression; the patient is asked to report how many days in the last week he or she has experienced the symptom. The

---

TEXT BOX 38.2

Child and Adolescent Hospitalization

Hospitalizing a child or adolescent is different from hospitalizing an adult. The decision to admit a child to the hospital rests with the parents and the mental health professional. The requirements for the least restrictive environment still pertain to children and adolescents, but minors do not have the same civil rights as do adults. Moreover, making decisions about the safety of children and adolescents is frequently difficult. Their competence to enter into contracts is often questionable, and their ability to manage their own behavior is hard to assess. For these reasons, many mental health professionals err on the side of hospitalization for young people with active suicidal ideation.

Hospitalization of suicidal children tends to be prolonged because as many as 60% have underlying mental illness (Shaffer et al., 1996). Mental disorders in children tend to be severe and require a family approach to treatment. Children who attempt suicide often have family members who also have attempted suicide, a factor that increases children's risk (McKeown et al., 1998; Pfeffer, Normandin, & Kakuma, 1998; Runeson, 1998). Childhood suicidal behavior often occurs in the context of extreme family discord, and children in these dysfunctional families may be the victims of abuse or neglect (Grilo et al., 1999; Lipschitz et al., 1999; Renaud et al., 1999). Nursing care is directed toward restoring the patient's functioning, decreasing the effects of the underlying illness, and establishing a stable environment to which the child or adolescent can return.

range of possible scores is 0 to 60. People with a score above 16 may have MDD; those with scores above 25 are probably clinically depressed. Other self-rating or clinician-rated scales include the Zung Self-Rating Depression Scale (Zung, 1965) and the Beck Depression Inventory (Beck et al., 1961). Nurses should ask patients who report moderate distress on at least five depressive symptoms from any of these scales if they are thinking about hurting or killing themselves.

Several scales are available to assess suicide risk. The best question to ask is, "Have you ever had a time where you felt so bad that you tried to kill or hurt yourself?" (Cloitre et al., 1997). Also useful are the questions, "During the last month, have you often been bothered by feeling down, depressed, or hopeless?" and "During the last month, have you often been bothered by little interest or pleasure in doing things?" (Whooley et al., 1997). People who answer yes to either question have a higher likelihood of being depressed.

Recently, Beck (1998) revised the Scale for Suicide Ideation (Beck et al., 1979) to include only eight items and renamed it the Suicide Intent Scale. This method is short and useful to determine whether a patient has a strong intent to die. Text Box 38-3 lists some questions that the nurse might ask in assessing the risk for suicide.

Determining Risk

The next stage of suicide risk assessment is determining the patient's actual risk for attempting or completing suicide. An important determinant of suicide risk is psychiatric disorders. The nurse or another experienced professional should assess the patient for other psychiatric disorders, especially those most commonly associated with suicidal behavior. Diagnoses especially associated with suicide completion are recurrent MDD, panic disorder, severe anxiety disorder, schizophrenia, substance abuse, borderline personality disorder, and antisocial personality disorder (Henriksson et al., 1996). Severity of MDD is associated with a greater likelihood of suicide completion (Alexopoulos et al., 1999; Grant & Hasin, 1999). For adolescents, a key question is whether any family member has attempted or completed suicide (Cerel et al., 1999; Klimes-Dougan et al., 1999; McKeown, et al., 1998). Alcoholism is another prominent factor in suicide. Patients with alcoholism account for 25% of completed suicides (Berglund & Ojehagen, 1998). Psychiatric diagnoses commonly associated with suicidal behavior are listed in Text Box 38-4.

Nurses in both general medical and psychiatric settings can use various methods of psychiatric diagnosis. The Quick Diagnostic Interview Schedule (QDIS) (Marcus et al., 1991) is a clinical diagnostic interview based on the National Institute of Mental Health's Diagnostic Interview Schedule (Robins et al., 1981). People who are not mental health providers can administer this computerized program. To qualify for a psychiatric diagnosis, the respondent must confirm one or more symptoms that qualify for the diagnosis and four or more symptoms that are associated with the disorder. The program provides the interviewer with a printout of each psychiatric condition found.

The QDIS takes between 30 to 60 minutes to complete, making its use in some clinical situations impractical. An alternative is the Primary Care Evaluation of Mental Disorders (PRIME-MD) (Spitzer et al., 1994).

TEXT BOX 38.3

Assessment of Suicidal Episode

Intent to Die
1. Have you been thinking about hurting or killing yourself?
2. How seriously do you want to die?
3. Have you attempted suicide before?
4. Are there people or things in your life who might keep you from killing yourself?

Severity of Ideation
1. How often do you have these thoughts?
2. How long do they last?
3. How much do the thoughts distress you?
4. Can you dismiss them or do they tend to return?
5. Are they increasing in intent and frequency?

Degree of Planning
1. Have you made any plans to kill yourself? If yes, what are they?
2. Do you have access to the materials (eg, gun, poison, pills) that you plan to use to kill yourself?
3. How likely is it that you could actually carry out the plan?
4. Have you done anything to put the plan into action?
5. Could you stop yourself from killing yourself?

TEXT BOX 38.4

Psychiatric Disorders Commonly Associated With Suicidal Behavior

Recurrent major depression

Substance abuse

Schizophrenia

Panic disorder

Dissociative disorders

Antisocial personality disorder

Borderline personality disorder

This program also is computer-based, generates diagnoses from the American Psychiatric Association's *Diagnostic and Statistic Manual of Mental Disorders*, 4th edition, and can be given by a trained lay interviewer (American Psychiatric Association, 1994). It is less precise than the QDIS but takes only 10 minutes to administer. For this reason, it is adaptable to various health care settings. The shorter interview may also be easier for highly distressed suicidal patients to tolerate.

What makes some patients more likely to kill themselves than others? A successful suicide requires intent, a plan, knowledge of how to carry out the act, and few obstacles to completing it. Patients who successfully complete suicide have made a clear decision and have developed a workable method of killing themselves. They are less likely to have young children or other immediate responsibilities and may not be concerned with religious prohibitions on the act. The relationship between the availability of a method of suicide and suicide completion is strong (Cantor & Baume, 1998). Firearms account for 59% of suicides (Anonymous, 2000b). White men account for 79% of all suicide deaths by firearms (Anonymous, 2000b). A person is 11 times more likely to use a firearm in the home for suicide than for self-defense (Kellerman et al., 1998). In Colorado, 67% of adolescents who complete suicide use a gun from their parents' home (Shah et al., 2000).

Many people who complete suicide have lowered inhibitions about death, either because of psychosis or substance abuse. In contrast to those who carefully prepare to take their own lives are those who decide impulsively to end their lives. These people are usually adolescents, people who abuse alcohol or drugs, or people with personality disorders. Patients with psychoses may act impulsively to "voices" that direct them to kill themselves. Patients with psychoses are at considerable risk because of their inability to separate psychotic thinking from reality.

Most victims of suicide are socially isolated. They generally cannot name anyone in their immediate environment with whom they can stay while they are acutely suicidal. They often wish to be alone or are unwilling to ask anyone for help. Patients at high risk for suicide may not subscribe to the rules and mores of any social group. Frequently, they can enter into a no-suicide agreement, but the lack of supportive people in their environment may indicate that they cannot safely remain in the community.

To determine how serious a patient is about dying, the nurse must ask about what thought the patient has put into the decision and why the patient views suicide as a solution. The nurse needs to determine whether the patient has considered other solutions to his or her difficulties, whether the patient has a specific plan for committing suicide, and the patient's means of completing the suicide. People who have developed a plan and the means to carry it out and who have executed some parts of the plan are serious about their intent to kill themselves. Inquiring about suicidal ideation and access to firearms has the potential to reduce successful suicides substantially.

Nursing Diagnosis and Outcome Identification

Several nursing diagnoses may be useful when dealing with a suicidal patient. They include but are not limited to Risk for Suicide, Interrupted Family Processes, Ineffective Health Maintenance, Risk for Self-Directed Violence, Impaired Social Interaction, Ineffective Coping, Chronic Low Self-Esteem, Disturbed Sleep Pattern, Social Isolation, and Spiritual Distress.

Planning and Implementing Nursing Interventions

If some or many of the risk factors for suicide (see Text Box 38-1) are present in a member of a high-risk group, the nurse must determine what is necessary to ensure the patient's ongoing safety, which is the nurse's first priority. Until the nurse has identified a patient's safety needs and implemented a plan to ensure the patient's safety, the nurse must not leave the acutely suicidal person alone for any reason, not even briefly.

The first thing the nurse should do if he or she decides that a patient may be suicidal is to get help. The nurse must not leave the patient alone but should call his or her supervisor or an experienced clinician immediately. Even if the nurse is an experienced mental health provider, he or she should not try to treat a potentially suicidal patient without help. Even the most experienced mental health professional may lose a patient in treatment because of suicide (Clark, 1995). The mental health provider is one person who must cope with the aftermath of a completed suicide and may experience some of the same feelings of guilt as family members of the victim. For this reason, even a highly experienced professional is better prepared to meet the challenges of a completed suicide when he or she works with another provider who is experienced in caring for suicidal patients. The reader is referred to **www.siec.ca/helpcard.htm** for a short checklist of things to do when a patient is suicidal.

Nursing interventions for the hospitalized suicidal patient can be derived from the NPP. The NPP prescribes stress response and symptom reduction and enhancement of psychological and social resources.

No-Suicide Contracts

One of the most important steps in determining the least restrictive environment that will ensure the patient's safety is engaging the patient in a no-suicide contract. In its simplest form, the **no-suicide contract** is a written or verbal agreement between the health care professional and the patient, stating that the patient will not engage in suicidal behavior for a specific period. Patients who can make such contracts may be at a lower risk for suicide than those who cannot. Moreover, they have a greater chance of being cared for in the community. Patients who make no-suicide contracts sometimes break them, but they do so infrequently.

The nurse should consider a no-suicide contract only after a thorough assessment of the patient (Simon, 1999). The nurse must consider several factors in making a no-suicide contract with a patient. The patient must be competent to enter into such a contract. Patients under the influence of drugs or alcohol or experiencing psychoses are not competent to make no-suicide contracts. Legal and professional scholars disagree on the ability of children and adolescents to make decisions of this gravity on their own behalf. Involving parents in the decision making about the appropriate mode of environment for their suicidal child is important. Patients who have made previous suicide attempts or are extremely isolated are not good risks for no-suicide contracts. Each of these types of patient can be characterized under the disinhibition category of risk in Text Box 38-1.

In making a no-suicide contract, the nurse must first help the patient dismantle the suicide plan. If the patient has a gun, it must be locked up in a room or cabinet to which the patient does not have access. If the patient's suicide plan involves taking medication, a family member must remove medications from the patient. If the plan involves the use of a motor vehicle, the patient must give the keys to that vehicle to someone for safekeeping. This facet of the no-suicide contract requires careful consideration because the determined patient may not disclose alternative methods. Isometsa & Lonnqvist (1998) showed that people completing suicide often have tried different methods in the past. A patient's cooperation in dismantling a suicide plan is an important indicator of his or her ability to maintain the no-suicide contract. Uncooperativeness at this stage may indicate that the patient cannot be maintained safely in his or her environment.

A second part of the no-suicide contract is assessing the patient's alcohol and drug use. Patients often have a strong propensity to use some kind of drug to escape their pain, or they may want drugs to help them sleep. The patient must refrain from using any mind-altering substances during the acute suicidal period because of their disinhibiting effects. Enlisting the help of the patient's family in removing mind-altering substances from the environment is essential. Asking the psychiatrist or primary care physician to provide a small amount of short-acting anxiety or sleeping medication may also be appropriate in managing the patient's emotional state.

Patients often cannot keep contracts if they are isolated from family or friends. They are much more likely to keep their part of the contract if they have support and some assistance in making their environment safe. It is critical, then, that patients identify someone who can stay with them or be nearby during the suicidal crisis. If they are unable or unwilling to do so, this may be sufficient reason for emergency hospitalization.

The mental health professional who makes a no-suicide contract agrees to participate in the patient's care in specific ways. For example, he or she agrees to be available personally or to ensure that another provider is available to the patient on a 24-hour basis until the suicidal crisis has passed. The provider must encourage the patient to make contact with him or her if resolve starts to wane. The suicidal patient must be able to reach the provider easily because the patient may lack sufficient motivation to connect with a professional who is difficult to reach. An inaccessible provider will make the patient feel abandoned and hopeless, perhaps fueling additional suicidal behavior.

Because the no-suicide contract is for a specific period, the mental health professional must be prepared to have contact with the patient before the contract period expires. A face-to-face meeting is preferable so that the nurse can assess nonverbal as well as verbal behavior. Face-to-face meetings also help patients to feel cared for, thereby decreasing suicidal risk. If the mental health professional finds the patient unimproved or improved but still actively suicidal, he or she must renew the contract with the patient for another specific period. It is often helpful to make the contract period somewhat longer the second time to help the patient re-establish a sense of personal control. Nurses must carefully reassess patients whose mental state has deteriorated since the last contract before these patients can be maintained in the community.

Careful initial and ongoing suicide assessment is vital to the success of the no-suicide contract. The entire basis of the contract is the patient's safety, something over which the nurse ultimately has no control. The contract is only as good as the therapeutic alliance on which it is formed (Simon, 1999). The no-suicide contract is not legally binding. Professionals who enter into these contracts are not protected from malpractice liability if the patient commits suicide. Thus, health care professionals must enter these contracts with considerable caution.

Inpatient Care and Acute Treatment

Suicidal patients were once hospitalized for extended periods to ensure that the suicidal crisis had passed and to provide sufficient time to establish a solid base of treatment for the underlying psychiatric disorder. This is no longer the case. Inpatient hospitalization is expensive, and insurance companies are reluctant to pay for extended inpatient care. Hospitals are overly restrictive environments that may inhibit the patient's development of the self-reliance needed to return to the community. Objectives of hospitalization are to maintain the patient's safety, reduce or eliminate the suicidal crisis, decrease the level of suicidal ideation, initiate treatment for the underlying disorder, evaluate for substance abuse, and reduce the patient's level of social isolation (Logue, & Parrish, 1998).

If the nurse and another professional determine that the patient is acutely suicidal and at considerable risk for completing suicide, he or she must decide whether to hospitalize the patient for the patient's safety. Safety in such cases is commonly determined by whether a patient may be a threat to self or others. Civil law requires the patient to be hospitalized only when he or she cannot make reasoned decisions to ensure his or her safety. Civil law also requires that the restriction of the patient occur only when it provides a therapeutic effect. The novice would argue that if a patient is suicidal, hospitalizing him or her makes sense because it will prevent completion of the act, which is clinically beneficial, but patients sometimes commit suicide in hospitals. In considering hospitalization of a patient, the nurse must consider how hospitalization will be useful in ensuring safety and relieving the patient's suicidal crisis.

Biologic Interventions

Ensuring Safety. During the early part of the hospitalization, the most important way to reduce stress is to help the patient feel more secure and hopeful. Nurses can do so by ensuring the patient's safety with as little intrusion as possible on the person's exercise of free will. Achieving this goal can be difficult. In a national study of all suicides reported during a 2-year period, the rate of suicide while hospitalized was 16% (Appleby et al., 1999a). The major deterrent to patients committing suicide in psychiatric hospitals is their continual observation by nurses. Each hospital has its own specific protocol for maintaining patients' safety. In addition to nursing standards of care, hospital staffing and other policies that affect the degree to which a suicidal patient can be restrained may influence the procedures mandated for maintaining patients.

Maintaining a safe environment includes observing the patient regularly for suicidal behavior, removing dangerous objects, and providing outlets for expression of the patient's feelings (Logue & Parrish, 1998; Robie et al., 1999). Part of ensuring patient safety is helping patients to re-establish personal control by including them in decisions about their care and restricting their behavior only as necessary. In this vein, the nurse must

reassure patients, inquire how they are feeling, and ask what they have been doing to manage their feelings and keep safe since the last observation period. Patients often feel shaky in the first hours of psychiatric hospitalization, and it is comforting to know that a caring person is nearby. Observational periods can be used to help the patient express a broad range of feelings and strengthen their belief in their own abilities to keep themselves safe. The nurse can help the patient who is not skilled in self-expression or self-management skills to describe feelings more effectively and cite ways of managing safety needs. Then, at the next observation time, the nurse may have the opportunity to reinforce the patient's own safety behavior. Thus, the observation period can be transformed from something negative ("The patient can't be trusted," "I am out of control") to something positive ("The patient is becoming safer," "Maybe I can keep myself safe after all") (Cardell & Pitula, 1999). As the patient becomes more confident of being able to control his or her behavior, the frequency of observation periods can be reduced.

Seclusion and restraint are two modalities sometimes used in the inpatient settings to maintain patient safety. These restrictive interventions, however, are extremely stressful for patients and may interfere with their recovery. Moreover, seclusion and restraint often are used to compensate for inadequate nursing staff. Unduly restraining patients to prevent their suicide interferes with the development of trusting relationships between patients and providers. The stress associated with restraints contributes to the biochemical disarray of their underlying psychiatric disorders. Restraints prevent patients from managing their own dysphoric and anxiety symptoms and reinforce their sense of hopelessness and helplessness. Restraints enhance patients' fears that they are "crazy" and incapable of controlling their impulses. These methods reinforce the patient's perception of being out of control and lessen their ability to form a partnership with mental health providers.

The no-suicide contract can also be used in the hospital to increase the length of time between observations and to provide opportunities for patients to have greater freedom (Drew, 1999). Use of the contract is another way to enhance the patient's perception of control and autonomy.

Assisting With Somatic Therapies. Often, suicidal patients are seriously depressed. During hospitalization, treatment of depression can begin, with observation of the patient's initial response to somatic therapies. The major somatic therapies used in the treatment of suicidal behavior are antidepressant medications and electroconvulsive therapy (ECT).

Patients with suicidal intent require an evaluation for medication. Because suicide is associated with low levels of serotonin, medication can increase serotonin levels and reduce suicide risk. Medication works faster than psychotherapy in decreasing the intensity and frequency of suicidal thoughts. It provides the added benefit of giving the patient hope. Because reducing suicidal impulses is a major objective of treatment, first-line treatment for suicidal ideation must always include consideration of medication.

First-generation, second-generation, and third-generation antidepressant medications all work equally well in the treatment of depression (Katon et al., 1995; Simon et al., 1996). The nurse must be aware of specific problems in the use of some of these medications. First-generation and second-generation antidepressants, including the tricyclics and monoamine oxidase inhibitors, are highly toxic medications that suicidal people can use to kill themselves. Resuscitation of a patient who has taken large amounts of one of these medications can be difficult because they are cardiotoxic. Medical sequelae may be long-term if the patient is saved. The side effects of early antidepressants may result in the patient stopping prescribed medication while still having suicidal thoughts. The need for laboratory assessment for therapeutic drug levels is another disadvantage of these drugs. Blood monitoring requires the patient's cooperation when his or her motivation may be at its lowest. These agents are inexpensive, however, and therefore may be the only medication option for some indigent patients. If this is the case, only small amounts of the medication should be provided to the patient at a time, until it is certain that the patient is mentally stable and no longer suicidal.

The third-generation and newer medications (fluoxetine [Prozac], sertraline [Zoloft], paroxetine [Paxil], nefazodone [Serzone], and bupropion [Wellbutrin]) are better choices for the suicidal patient. These drugs generally are not toxic and cause few side effects, especially after being taken for 1 to 2 weeks. They are often faster acting than the older drugs, but their onset of action varies. Especially useful are fluoxetine and paroxetine, which patients may take only once a day, requiring little manipulation in dose. Sertraline may be given once a day as well, but dosing varies. Patients who take overdoses of these medications have much better outcomes than those who abuse one of the early antidepressants. One drawback of these newer drugs is their relatively high cost. People without insurance coverage for prescription drugs can expect to pay between $60 and $100 or more each month for this type of medication.

ECT may be useful for selected inpatients with intractable suicidal ideation and severe depression. ECT often eliminates suicidal behavior in people who do not respond to medication. This treatment is also useful for people who do not tolerate antidepressant medications, such as elderly people and those with comorbid medical disorders. In those cases, ECT can stabilize the patient sufficiently to permit a return to the community.

Both patients and health care professionals often have distorted images of ECT. Movies like *One Flew Over the Cuckoos' Nest* have popularized the notion that ECT is a brutal procedure to avoid at all costs. Early in the history of its use, the procedure was extremely unpleasant. Contemporary ECT is conducted in an operating room or other specialized center. Patients are sedated, and ECT is given on one side of the brain only. This reduces the overall seizure and side effects of the procedure such as amnesia. ECT can be a life-saving procedure for the acutely suicidal patient. Nurses must understand this and not convey any personal biases that might affect the patient's decision to accept this treatment. It may be useful for the nurse to attend a few ECT sessions as an observer to get a better feel for the procedure and its effects.

Assisting With Treatment of Substance Abuse.   Suicidal behavior is often an outcome of substance abuse, especially among men. For men, substance abuse may be the primary psychiatric disorder and depression a side effect of it. For women, depression commonly is the primary psychiatric disorder, and substance abuse results from attempts to medicate the underlying depressive condition. Successful treatment of suicidal behavior in both men and women requires substance abuse treatment. Without this step, inpatient treatment of suicidal behavior is only palliative, and the danger of the patient's repeating a suicidal threat or attempt is high.

The nurse should work with the physician and patient to identify a suitable substance abuse treatment program. The nurse should also be sure that the patient understands the role that alcohol and drugs play in suicidal behavior.

Psychological Interventions.   Nurses need to use the brief hospitalization period to find out what may have precipitated or contributed to the suicidal crisis. Often, the precipitating factors and how the patient's coping process began to break down are evident. After identifying extreme stressors experienced by the patient, the nurse and patient can help determine ways for the patient to avoid those stressors in the future or, if they cannot be avoided, to manage them more effectively.

The hospitalization is a good time for the nurse to evaluate the patient's ways of thinking about problems and generating solutions. Some patients, by virtue of their depressive illness or social learning, have an unusually pessimistic view of life. They often think such thoughts as, "I am no good," "Everything I do is useless," "I have no future," or "Nobody has ever liked me, and nobody ever will." The nurse can point out negative thinking and invite the patient to begin to note instances in conversation when he or she is being pessimistic. Most patients can do so and are often surprised at the extent of their negativity. Once a patient is aware of this pessimistic outlook, the nurse can suggest that the patient "play detective" and try to figure out whether the negative views are true. For example, the nurse can ask the patient who feels that he or she is "no good" to write down on a piece of paper anything that the patient did that day that can be construed as "good." The nurse can help with that process by also keeping a list of "good" things that the patient does during that day. Then, if the patient says, "I did nothing good, I am no good," the nurse can counter with, "But I saw you helping Mrs. Barnes with her lunch. Why did you help her if you are no good?" The nurse and patient can then address these logical inconsistencies more straightforwardly (see Therapeutic Dialogue: Suicide).

The nurse and patient must also devise ways to prevent future suicidal behavior. Patients are likely to have periods of suicidal ideation throughout treatment. They must have a plan ready to manage these thoughts when they appear. The plan may include recalling that suicidal thoughts are caused by a biochemical imbalance and will go away. The plan may also include methods of distraction from suicidal thoughts. Exercise, such as taking

---

THERAPEUTIC DIALOGUE | Suicide

When the nurse asked Caroline about her family life, she once again began to cry softly. She said that she has been unhappy for a long time. Suddenly, the words tumbled out quickly. Caroline recalled that when she was very young, she was pretty happy. Things changed when her brother was born, 4 years after her. Her father began to abuse her sexually, starting when Caroline was 5 years old and continuing until he moved out of the house when she was 12 years old. Caroline suspects her mother knew of the abuse, although she did nothing about it.

Two years ago, Caroline's father committed suicide. Caroline feels relieved about his death but frustrated that she never got a chance to tell him how angry she was with him. Caroline's relationship with her mother has not improved. Caroline says that her mother favors her brother and is always telling her she won't amount to anything. Caroline begins to cry harder.

Ineffective Approach

Nurse: Clearly, many things are troubling you. Don't you think that things seem worse now because you have a cold?

Caroline: Well, that could be. What are you going to do to make me feel better?

Nurse: Give you some medicine to help you sleep and clear your nose. I think you should see a psychiatrist, too.

Caroline: I don't need a psychiatrist. I came here for my cold.

Nurse: I know you did, but you seem to be depressed.

Caroline: What are you, some kind of social worker? I am just tired.

Nurse: I am a nurse, and you seem down to me. Are you thinking about suicide?

Caroline: I don't think you know what you're talking about. I want to go now. Could you give me my medicine?

Effective Approach

Nurse: It seems as though many things have been piling up on you. Does it seem that way to you, too?

Caroline: It sure does. I've just been trying to get through one day at a time, but now with this cold and no sleep, I feel like I can't go on.

Nurse: When you say you can't go on, what does that mean to you?

Caroline: Lately, I have been thinking about running away to some place where I can't be found and maybe starting over. But then I think, where would I go? Where would I stay? Who would take care of me?

Nurse: When you think that your plan for escape won't work, what happens?

Caroline: (Starting to cry again.) Then I think that maybe it would be better if I just did what my father did. I really don't think anyone would miss me.

Nurse: So you think you might take your life, like your Dad did?

Caroline: Yeah, and what really scares me is lately I have been thinking about that a lot. I keep saying to myself, You're just tired, but I am so exhausted now that I can't chase the thoughts away.

Nurse: So, do you think about suicide every day?

Caroline: It seems like I never stop thinking about it.

Nurse: Is there anything you can do to make the thoughts go away?

Caroline: Nothing. (Silence.)

Nurse: What would you do?

Caroline: I think I would get as many pills as I could find, drink a lot of alcohol, and maybe smoke some pot and just go to sleep.

Nurse: Do you have enough pills at home to kill yourself?

Caroline (wan smile): I was hoping that the sleeping medicine you would give me might do the job.

Nurse: It sounds like you need some help getting through this time in your life. Would you like some?

Caroline: I honestly don't know—I just want to sleep for a long time.

Critical Thinking Challenge

- In the first interaction, the nurse made two key blunders. What were they? What effect did they have on the patient? How did they interfere with the patient's care?

- What did Caroline do that might have contributed to the nurse's behavior in the first interaction?

- In the second interaction, the nurse did several things that ensured reporting of Caroline's suicidal ideation. What were they? What differences in attitude might differentiate the nurse in the first interaction from the nurse in the second?

walks or engaging in some other pleasurable activities, should be part of the plan to help diminish the frequency and intensity of suicidal thoughts.

Social Interventions. Poor social skills may interfere with the patient's ability to engage others. The nurse should assess the patient's social capability early in the hospitalization and make necessary provisions for social skills training. The nurse must gently make the patient aware of any behaviors that may interfere with making friends and suggest alternative behaviors.

In many cases, although patients can identify family and friends who are willing to help, they are usually concerned about burdening these people or do not feel comfortable sharing their concerns with others. Helping the suicidal patient express these concerns and arrive at ways of reducing them is important. While hospitalized, the patient may be able to convey to the significant other how much he or she needs the other person's help and how difficult it is to ask for it. If patients can make that step, they and their significant others can develop a plan for managing those times when patients feel most isolated. Different friends and family members can use the plan at various times so that no one person is asked to assume too much of the patient's social care.

A final concern may be the patient's embarrassment about the hospitalization and his or her emotional state. Through education, the nurse can do much to destigmatize the situation for both the patient and significant others.

Before discharge, the patient should be able to name people who can act as a support. The nurse should encourage the patient to invite supportive others to visit the patient. When visitors are present, with the patient's permission, the nurse can work with them to begin to develop a network for the patient to rely on to remain safe. They also should have a plan to contact another person, either a confidante or mental health care provider, when they have distressing thoughts or feel unable to control their behavior.

Discharge Planning and Outpatient Care

The most desirable treatment outcome is the patient's return to the community. Because most hospitalizations for suicidal behavior are brief, discharge planning must begin immediately after the patient is admitted. The nurse needs to explain to the patient that hospitalization is likely to be short-term and immediately begin to form a partnership with the patient and family to ensure a smooth transition to the community. *Partnering* means empowering the patient to engage in self-care as soon as possible by helping to provide the tools he or she needs to manage behavior outside the security of the hospital.

Educating the Patient and Family. The objectives of patient and family education are to increase the patient's understanding of depressive illness and the biochemical origins of suicidal behavior; establish effective depressive treatment; provide for ongoing and seamless outpatient treatment; devise a plan for managing future suicidal ideation; identify a supportive other in the community; establish a plan for regularly using that person for support; and eliminate the patient's use of drugs and alcohol (see Psychoeducation Checklist). These objectives are demanding for both nurse and patient during brief hospitalization. Unfortunately, funding limits for inpatient care necessitate intensive nursing care to prevent future hospitalizations. Limits on mental health coverage have been associated with dramatically higher rates of completed suicide among those insured by managed care companies (Hall et al., 1999).

In addition to trying to reduce the stigma that the patient and family may associate with suicide, the nurse must educate them about depression, suicidal behavior, and treatments. Whenever possible, the nurse should schedule educational sessions to include significant others, so that they will better understand the patient's illness and also learn what is necessary in providing outpatient care (see Psychoeducation Checklist: Major Depression). The patient who is suicidal is likely to have low energy, weak motivation, and poor comprehension and retention because of the underlying depressive disorder. For this reason, nurses should keep instructions simple and educational sessions short. Whenever possible, written material that the patient can take home should supplement the educational sessions. Several sources of written material are listed in Text Box 38-5. The library, World Wide Web, and popular literature are all sources of supplementary information, but that information is not always accurate. Therefore, recommendations about written materials should be specific. The nurse should quiz the patient on his or her understanding of those materials, correcting any misinformation that might have been gleaned.

PSYCHOEDUCATION CHECKLIST
Major Depression

When teaching the patient and family about major depression, be sure to address the following topics:

- Symptoms of depression
- Suicidal behavior
- Identification of stressors
- Coping mechanisms
- Positive self-talk
- Information about medications and treatments

TEXT BOX 38.5

Educational Resources for Suicidal Clients

Aarons, L. (1996). *Prayers for Bobby: A mother's coming to terms with the suicide of her gay son*. San Francisco: Harper.

Fine, C. (1996). *No time to say goodbye: Surviving the suicide of a loved one*. New York: Doubleday.

Frankel, B., & Kranz, R. (1994). *Straight talk about teenage suicide*. New York: Facts on File.

Jamison, K. R. (1996). *An unquiet mind*. New York: Knopf.

Jamison, K. R. (1999). *Night falls fast: Understanding suicide*. New York: Knopf.

Marcus, E. (1996). *Why suicide?* San Francisco: Harper.

Nelson, R. E. (1994). *The power to prevent suicide: A guide for helping teens*. Minneapolis: Free Spirit Press.

Quinnett, P. G. (1995). *Suicide: The forever decision*. New York: Crossroad.

Slaby, A., & Garfinkel, L. F. (1994). *No one saw my pain: Why teens kill themselves*. New York: Norton.

Styron, W. (1990). *Darkness visible*. New York: Vintage Books.

Thompson, T. (1995). *The beast: A reckoning with depression*. New York: Putnam.

Identifying Continuing Sources of Social Support. Assisting the patient to make behavior changes is an immediate priority, and the nurse should make any patient's lack of social skills known to the community therapist. In addition to engaging family and friends in the patient's ongoing care, finding sources of help in the community, such as church groups, clubhouses, drop-in centers, or other social groups, is a necessary task. A patient's inability to name any significant others or social groups often means a poor outpatient course.

Establishing an Outpatient Care Plan. At the time of discharge, the patient is still considered very ill. Most suicides occur in the first week after discharge, and many happen within the first 24 hours (Appleby et al., 1999a). Before the patient's release, a specific, concrete plan for outpatient care must be in place. The care plan includes scheduling an appointment for outpatient care, providing for continuing medication until the first outpatient treatment visit, ensuring postrelease contact between the patient and significant other, providing for access to emergency psychiatric care, and arranging the patient's environment so that it provides both structure and safety.

At discharge, the patient should have enough medication on hand to last until the first outpatient provider visit. At that time, the community provider can assess the patient's level of stability and determine whether a full prescription can be given safely to the patient. At that visit, the patient and community provider can establish a plan of care that specifies the intensity of outpatient care. Very unstable patients may need two to three outpatient visits per week in the early days after hospitalization to maintain their safety in the community. In arranging outpatient care, the nurse must be certain to refer the patient to a community provider who can provide the intensity of care the patient may need.

The patient and significant other must have a plan for the patient's ongoing supervision. This plan must be established in such a way that the patient does not feel undermined in his or her ability to manage self-care but is reassured that help will be available when needed. The family members or friends involved must feel that they are resources for the patient but not responsible for the patient's life or death. In the end, it is the patient, not supporters, who must bear responsibility for his or her safety. The patient who feels connected to but not dependent on significant others will be most likely to maintain safety in the community.

The patient's outpatient environment should be made as safe as possible before discharge. The nurse must share the care plan with family members so that they can remove any objects in the patient's environment that could be of assistance in committing suicide. The nurse must explain this measure to the patient to reinforce his or her sense of self-control. It is important to be reasonable in deciding what to remove from the environment. Patients who are truly determined to kill themselves after discharge will succeed in doing so, using whatever means are available.

Finally, there should be some continuity between inpatient and outpatient care. The nurse must tell the patient specifically how to obtain emergency psychiatric care. He or she should place written instructions near the patient's telephone. It is helpful for the nurse to call periodically during the few first weeks after discharge to determine whether the patient is improving. These contacts will assist the patient to feel valued and connected to others. Once the nurse thinks that the patient is stabilized and moving forward in self-care, outpatient contact can be terminated. Lack of continuity is thought to contribute to significant suicide mortality after hospital discharge (Hulten & Wasserman, 1998).

Evaluation and Treatment Outcomes

Short-term outcomes for the suicidal patient include maintaining the patient's safety, averting suicide, and mobilizing the patient's resources. Whether the patient is hospitalized or maintained in the community, his or her emotional distress must be reduced. This often is accomplished in an environment that restricts suicidal behavior and provides sustained emotional support. The treatment during the suicidal crisis should also set the stage for meeting long-term objectives. Evidence has shown that many suicidal patients persist in their attempts to commit suicide and that 25% are successful within 3 months of discharge from hospitalization for a suicide attempt (Appleby et al., 1999a; Isometsa & Lonnqvist, 1998). Long-term outcomes must focus on maintaining the patient in psychiatric treatment, enabling the patient and family to identify and manage suicidal crises effectively, and widening the patient's support network.

Avoiding Secondary Trauma

Caring for suicidal patients is highly stressful and often leads to secondary trauma. Secondary trauma refers to the nurse's emotional reaction to certain circumstances of patients or to the repeated stress of coping with suicidal crises. Few other situations in nursing exist in which misinterpreting data that are often subjective can contribute to a preventable death. The nurse who experiences secondary trauma may begin to develop symptoms that reflect the early stage of posttraumatic stress disorder (PTSD) (see Chap. 37). These symptoms include fatigue, dysphoria, tearfulness without provocation, sleep disturbances or nightmares, preoccupation with the stressful situation or morbid thoughts, inability to be distracted from the stressor, anxiety, and cynicism. The nurse may begin to avoid the stress through absenteeism. These symptoms signal that a nurse's mental health is at risk. All nurses are vulnerable to this syndrome. Their vulnerability to secondary trauma increases when nurses manage crises similar to those in their own present or past. Caring for suicidal patients who are close to their own age or having a history of being abused or neglected in childhood enhances the risks. The suicidal behavior of a patient with whom the nurse can particularly identify can be especially upsetting.

To care successfully for suicidal patients or others prone to crises, the nurse must engage in an active program of self-care. Such a program begins with proper rest, exercise, and nutrition so that the nurse can better manage stress physiologically. Self-monitoring of symptoms is the next step. Nurses should be alert to fatigue, crying spells, and other symptoms of PTSD. Like their patients, nurses need to develop cognitive coping skills and engage in stress reduction exercises. An important component of developing these skills is debriefing. Nurses who care for suicidal patients must regularly share their experiences and feelings with one another. Talking about how the situations or actions of patients make them feel will help alleviate symptoms of stress. Some nurses find outpatient therapy helpful because it enhances their understanding of what situations are most likely to trigger secondary trauma. By demonstrating how to manage effectively stressors in their own lives, nurses can be powerful role models for their patients.

Summary of Key Points

➤ Suicide is a common and major public health problem that accompanies 15% of all cases of major depression.

➤ Suicide completion is more common in white men, especially elderly men.

➤ Rising rates of adolescent suicide correspond with the increasing availability of firearms and alcohol.

➤ More than half of all suicides are completed on the first attempt.

➤ Parasuicide is more common among women than men.

➤ People who attempt suicide most commonly do not seek medical or psychiatric assistance.

➤ People who attempt suicide and fail are likely to try again.

➤ Suicidal behavior is associated with genetic and biologic origins.

➤ People who threaten suicide have civil rights that must be preserved.

➤ The no-suicide contract is one means of increasing the suicidal patient's safety in the community.

➤ When a patient must be hospitalized, voluntary hospitalization is the method of choice.

➤ The major objectives of brief hospital care are to maintain the patient's safety, re-establish the patient's biologic equilibrium, strengthen the patient's cognitive coping skills, and develop an outpatient support system.

➤ The nurse who cares for suicidal patients is vulnerable to secondary trauma and must take steps to maintain personal mental health.

Critical Thinking Challenges

1. A religious black woman who lives with her three children, husband, and mother comes to her primary care provider. She is tearful and very depressed. What factors should be investigated to determine her risk for suicide and need for hospitalization?

2. A poor woman with no insurance is hospitalized after her third suicide attempt. Antidepressant medication is prescribed. What issues must be considered in providing medication for this woman?

3. A young man enters his workplace inebriated and carrying a gun. He does not threaten anyone but says that he must end it all. Assuming that he can be disarmed, what civil rights must be considered in taking further action in managing his suicidal risk?

4. You are a nurse in a large outpatient primary care setting responsible for a population that is 80% indigent. You want to implement a case-finding program for suicide prevention. Discuss how you would proceed and some potential problems you might face.

 WEB LINKS

www.save.org   Suicide Awareness\Voice of Education (SA\VE). The mission of SA\VE is to provide education about suicide prevention and to speak for suicide survivors. This site provides information about suicide and access to texts and books. It also gives information on what to do in the event that a loved one is suicidal.

www.nimh.nih.gov/research/suibib99.cfm   Sponsored by the National Institute of Mental Health, this site offers a selected bibliography on suicide research.

www.griefnet.org   GriefNet is an Internet community of people dealing with grief, death, and major loss. Their integrated approach to on-line grief support provides help to people working through loss and grief issues of all kinds. The site has a companion site, KIDSAID, for children and their parents to find information about grief and ask questions.

www.siec.ca

mailto:Suicide@rochford.org   The site has two different offerings. The Suicide Information & Education Centre (SIEC) is a special library and resource center providing information on suicide and suicidal behavior. This link contains a wealth of information and resources including information kits and pamphlets. The second link is to the Suicide Prevention Training Program (SPTP). The goal of these programs is to provide skills training that increases caregiver competence and confidence while improving community collaboration.

www.suicidology.org   The American Association of Suicidology, a nonprofit organization dedicated to the understanding and prevention of suicide, is designed as a resource for anyone concerned about suicide, including suicide researchers, therapists, prevention specialists, survivors of suicide, and people who are themselves in crisis. Links include resources, crisis centers, and support groups. The site also links to the latest national statistics about suicide.

www.cdc.gov/ncipc/factsheets/suifacts.htm   This site links to the home page of the Centers for Disease Control National Center for Injury Prevention and Control. It lists facts about suicide, including suicide national rates and distribution of suicides by gender, age, and ethnic origin.

www.afsp.org   The American Foundation for Suicide Prevention's home page provides information about suicide and its prevention. The site links to several of the foundation's activities, including giving information about research funding, providing information and education about depression and suicide, promoting professional education for the recognition and treatment of depressed and suicidal individuals, publicizing the magnitude of the problems of depression, and supporting programs for suicide survivor treatment, research, and education.

www.daretolive.org   The Dare to Live: Teen Suicide Prevention is designed for teenagers. It provides information about suicide that is written for and directed to helping teens who are considering suicide.

MOVIES

Night Mother: 1986. Sissy Spacek stars as Jessie Cates, who has decided to end her desperately unhappy life by shooting herself with her father's gun. While putting her house in order, she tries to explain her decision to her mother Thelma, played by Anne Bancroft. Thelma tries to talk Jessie out of suicide.
Viewing Points: What factors have contributed to Jessie's decision to end her life? What approach would you have taken to help Jessie?

Daughter of a Suicide: 1996 (Documentary). This personal documentary is the story of a woman whose mother committed suicide when the daughter was 18 years old. The daughter recounts the emotional struggle and depression left as the lifelong legacy of suicide and explores her efforts to heal. Combining digital video, 16-mm, and super-8 film, *Daughter of a Suicide* uses interviews with family and friends to tell the story of both mother and daughter.
Viewing Points: How does this movie show that the effects of suicide do not end with a person's death?

REFERENCES

Abramson, L. Y., Seligman, M. E. P., & Teasdale, J. D. (1985). Learned helplessness in humans: Critique and reformulation. In J. C. Coyne (Ed.), *Essential papers on depression* (pp. 259–301). New York: New York University Press.

Agbayewa, M. O., Marion, S. A., & Wiggins, S. (1998). Socioeconomic factors associated with suicide in elderly populations in British Columbia: An 11-year review. *Canadian Journal of Psychiatry, 43*(8), 829–836.

Alexopoulos, G. S., Bruce, M. L., Hull, J., et al. (1999). Clinical determinants of suicidal ideation and behavior in geriatric depression. *Archives of General Psychiatry, 56*(11), 1048–1053.

American Psychiatric Association. (1994). *Diagnostic and statistical manual of mental disorders* (4th ed.). Washington, DC: Author.

Angst, J., Angst, F., & Stassen, H. H. (1999). Suicide risk in patients with major depressive disorder. *Journal of Clinical Psychiatry, 60*(Suppl. 2), 57–62.

Anonymous. (1997b). Rates of homicide, suicide and firearm related death among children: 26 industrialized countries. *Morbidity and Mortality Weekly Report, 46,* 101–105.

Anonymous. (2000a). U.S. Department of Health and Human Services. *Healthy People 2010* (Conference Edition, in Two Volumes). Washington, DC: http://www.health.gov/healthypeople.

Anonymous. (1999). National Center for Health Statistics. http://www.cdc.gov/ncipc/factsheets/suifacts.htm.

Anonymous. (1997a). National Center for Health Statistics. http://www.cdc.gov./ncipc/data/us9704/Suic.htm.

Anonymous. (2000b). *The Surgeon General's call to action to prevent suicide.* http://www.surgeongeneral.gov/library/calltoaction/fact3.htm.

Appleby, L., Cooper, J., Amos, T., & Faragher, B. (1999b). Psychological autopsy study of suicides by people aged under 35. *British Journal of Psychiatry, 175,* 168–174.

Appleby, L., Shaw, J., Amos, T., et al. (1999a). Suicide within 12 months of contact with mental health services: National clinical survey. *British Medical Journal, 318*(7193), 1235–1239.

Bandura, A. (1977). Self-efficacy: Toward a unifying theory of behavior change. *Psychological Review, 84*(2), 191–215.

Beck, A. T. (1998). Suicidal Intent Scales—"selected items"—"adapted." *Journal of Clinical Psychology, 54*(8), 1063–1078.

Beck, A. T., Kovacs, M., & Weissman, A. (1979). Assessment of suicidal intention: The Scale for Suicidal Ideation. *Journal of Consulting and Clinical Psychology, 47*(2), 343–352.

Beck, A. T., Rush, A. J., Shaw, B. F., & Emery, G. (1979). *Cognitive therapy in depression.* New York: Guilford Press.

Beck, A. T., Ward, C. H., Mendelson, M., et al. (1961). An inventory for measuring depression. *Archives of General Psychiatry, 4,* 561—571.

Berglund, M., & Ojehagen, A. (1998). The influence of alcohol drinking and alcohol use disorders on psychiatric disorders and suicidal behavior. *Alcoholism: Clinical & Experimental Research, 22*(Suppl. 7), 3335–3455.

Birckmayer, J., & Hemenway, D. (1999). Minimum-age drinking laws and youth suicide, 1970–1990. *American Journal of Public Health, 89*(9), 1365–1368.

Boudewyn, A. C., & Liem, J. H. (1995). Childhood sexual abuse as a precursor to depression and self-destructive behavior in adulthood. *Journal of Traumatic Stress, 8*(3), 445–459.

Brent, D. A. (1997). The aftercare of adolescents with deliberate self-harm. *Journal of Child Psychology & Psychiatry & Allied Disciplines, 38*(3), 277–286.

Brunton, K. (1997). Stigma. *Journal of Advanced Nursing, 26*(5), 891–898.

Cantor, C. H., & Baume, P. J. (1998). Access to methods of suicide: What impact? *Australian & New Zealand Journal of Psychiatry, 32*(1), 8–14.

Cardell, R., & Pitula, C. R. (1999). Suicidal inpatients' perceptions of therapeutic and non-therapeutic aspects of constant observation. *Psychiatric Services, 50*(8), 1066–1070.

Centers for Disease Control. (2000). Deaths from 282 selected causes, by 5-year age groups, race, and sex: U.S. & each state. http://www.cdc.gov/nchs/data/96gm3'10.pdf.

Cerel, J., Fristad, M. A., Weller, E. B., & Weller, R. A. (1999). Suicide-bereaved children and adolescents: A controlled longitudinal examination. *Journal of the American Academy of Child and Adolescent Psychiatry, 38*(6), 672–679.

Clark, D. C. (1995). Epidemiology, assessment, and management of suicide in depressed patients. In E. E. Beckham & W. R. Leber (Eds.), *Handbook of depression* (pp. 526–538). New York: Guilford Press.

Clayton, D., & Barcel, A. (1999). The cost of suicide mortality in New Brunswick, 1996. *Chronic Diseases in Canada, 20*(2), 89–95.

Cloitre, M., Scarvalone, P., & Difede, J. (1997). Posttraumatic stress disorder, self- and interpersonal dysfunction among sexually retraumatized women. *Journal of Traumatic Stress, 10*(3), 437–452.

Cohen, S., Kessler, R. C., & Gordon, L. U. (1995). Strategies for measuring stress in studies of psychiatric and physical disorders. In S. Cohen, R. C. Kessler, & L. U. Gordon (Eds.), *Measuring stress: A guide for health and social scientists* (pp. 3–26). New York: Oxford University Press.

Conwell, Y., Lyness, J. M., Duberstein, P., et al. (2000). Completed suicide among older patients in primary care practices: A controlled study. *Journal of the American Geriatric Society, 48*(1), 23–29.

D'Augelli, A. R., Hershberger, S. L., & Pilkington, N. W. (1998). Lesbian, gay, and bisexual youth and their families: Disclosure of sexual orientation and its consequences. *American Journal of Orthopsychiatry, 68*(3), 361–371.

Daugherty, M. (1999). Suicide by cop. *Journal of the California Alliance for the Mentally Ill, 10*(2), 79–81.

Davidson, J. R. T., Hughes, D. C., George, L. K., & Blazer, D. G. (1996). The association of sexual assault and attempted suicide within the community. *Archives of General Psychiatry, 53*(6), 550–555.

Drew, B. L. (1999). No-suicide contracts to prevent suicidal behavior in inpatient psychiatric settings. *Journal of the American Psychiatric Nurses Association, 5*(1), 23–28.

D'Zurilla, T. J., Chang, E. C., Nottingham, E. J., & Faccini, L. (1998). Social problem-solving deficits and hopelessness, depression, and suicidal risk in college students and psychiatric inpatients. *Journal of Clinical Psychology, 54*(8), 1091–1107.

Fergusson, D. M., Horwood, L. J., & Beautrais, A. L. (1999). Is sexual orientation related to mental health problems and suicidality in young people? *Archives of General Psychiatry, 56*(10), 883–884.

Fierreira de Castro, E., Cunha, M. A., Pimenta, F., & Costa I. (1998). Parasuicide and mental disorders. *Acta Psychiatrica Scandinavica, 97*(1), 25–31.

Foster, T., Gillespie, K., McClelland, R., & Patterson, C. (1999). Risk factors for suicide independent of DSM-III-R Axis I disorder: Case-control psychological autopsy study in Northern Ireland. *British Journal of Psychiatry, 175*, 175–179.

Freud, S. (1985). Mourning and melancholia. In J. C. Coyne (Ed.), *Essential papers on depression* (pp. 48–63). New York: New York University Press.

Gould, M. S., King, R., Greenwald, S., et al. (1998). Psychopathology associated with suicide and attempts among children and adolescents. *Journal of the American Academy of Child & Adolescent Psychiatry, 37*(9), 915–923.

Grant, B. F., & Hasin, D. S. (1999). Suicidal ideation among the United States drinking population: Results from the National Longitudinal Alcohol Epidemiologic Survey. *Journal of Studies on Alcohol, 60*(3), 422–429.

Grilo, C. M., Sanislow, C. A., Fehon, D. C., et al. (1999). Correlates of suicide risk in adolescent inpatients who report a history of childhood abuse. *Comprehensive Psychiatry, 40*(6), 422–428.

Groholt, B., Ekeberg, O., Wichstrom, L., & Haldorsen, T. (1998). Suicide among children and younger and older adolescents in Norway: A comparative study. *Journal of the American Academy of Child & Adolescent Psychiatry, 37*(5), 473–481.

Gunnell, D., Lopatatzidis, A., Dorling, D., et al. (1999). Suicide and unemployment in young people: Analysis of trends in England and Wales, 1921–1995. *British Journal of Psychiatry, 175, 263–270.*

Hall, R. C., Platt, D. E., & Hall, R. C. (1999). Suicide risk assessment: A review of risk factors for suicide in 100 patients who have made severe suicide attempts: Evaluation of suicide risk in a time of managed care. *Psychosomatics, 40*(1), 18–27.

Hauenstein, E. (1996). A nursing practice paradigm for depressed rural women: Theoretical basis. *Archives of Psychiatric Nursing, X*(5), 283–292.

Hendin, H. (1999). Suicide, assisted suicide, and medical illness. *Journal of Clinical Psychiatry, 60*(Suppl. 2), 46–50.

Henriksson, M. M., Isometsa, E. T., Kuoppasalmi, K. I., et al. (1996). Panic disorder in completed suicide. *Journal of Clinical Psychiatry, 57*(7), 275–281.

Herrell, R., Goldberg, J., True, W. R., et al. (1999). Sexual orientation and suicidality: A co-twin control study in adult men. *Archives of General Psychiatry, 56*(10), 867–874.

Holden, R. R., Kerr, P. S., Mendonca, J. D., & Velamoor, V. R. (1998). Are some motives more linked to suicide proneness than others? *Journal of Clinical Psychology, 54*(5), 569–576.

Hulten, A., & Wasserman, D. (1998). Lack of continuity—a problem in the care of young suicides. *Acta Psychiatrica Scandinavica, 97*(5), 326–333.

Isometsa, E. T., & Lonnqvist, J. K. (1998). Suicide attempts preceding completed suicide. *British Journal of Psychiatry, 173*, 531–535.

Joachim, G., & Acorn, S. (2000). Stigma of visible and invisible chronic conditions. *Journal of Advanced Nursing, 32*(1), 243–248.

Johansson, L. M., Sundquist, J., Johansson, S. E., & Bergman, B. (1997). Ethnicity, social factors, illness and suicide: A follow-up study of a random sample of the Swedish population. *Acta Psychiatrica Scandinavica, 95*(2), 125–131.

Johansson, L. M., Sundquist, J., Johansson, S. E., et al. (1997). The influence of ethnicity and social and demographic factors on Swedish suicide rates. A four-year follow-up study. *Social Psychiatry & Psychiatric Epidemiology, 32*(3), 165–170.

Johnson, B. A., Brent, D. A., Bridge, J., & Connolly, J. (1998). The familial aggregation of adolescent suicide attempts. *Acta Psychiatrica Scandinavica, 97*(1), 18–24.

Kaslow, N. J., Thompson, M. P., Meadows, L. A., et al. (1998). Factors that mediate and moderate the link between partner abuse and suicidal behavior in African-American women. *Journal of Consulting & Clinical Psychology, 66*(3), 533–540.

Katon, W., Von Korff, M., Lin, E., et al. (1995). Collaborative management to achieve treatment guidelines. *Journal of the American Medical Association, 273*(13), 1026–1031.

Kellerman, A. L., Somes, G., Rivara, F. P., et al. (1998). Injuries and deaths due to firearms in the home. *Journal of Trauma Injury Infection and Critical Care, 45*(2), 263–267.

Kessler, R. C., Borges, G., & Walters, E. (1999). Prevalence of and risk factors for lifetime suicide attempts in the National Comorbidity Survey. *Archives of General Psychiatry, 56*(7), 617–626.

Kessler, R. C., McGonagle, K. A., Zhao, S., et al. (1994). Lifetime and 12-month prevalence of DSM-III-R psychiatric disorders in the United States: Results from the National Co-Morbidity Study. *Archives of General Psychiatry, 51*(1), 8–19.

Klimes-Dougan, B., Free, K., Rounsaville, D., et al. (1999). Suicidal ideation and attempts: A longitudinal investigation of children of depressed and well mothers. *Journal of the American Academy of Child & Adolescent Psychiatry, 38*(6), 651–659.

Kung, K. C., Liu, X., & Juon, H. S. (1998). Risk factors for suicide in Caucasians and in African-Americans: A matched case-control study. *Social Psychiatry & Psychiatric Epidemiology, 33*(4), 155–161.

Lee, C. J., Collins, K. A., & Burgess, S. E. (1999). Suicide under the age of eighteen: A 10-year retrospective study. *American Journal of Forensic Medicine & Pathology, 20*(1), 27–30.

Links, P. S., Balchand, K., Dawe, I., & Watson, W. J. (1999). Preventing recurrent suicidal behaviour. *Canadian Family Physician, 45*, 2656–2660.

Lipschitz, D. S., Winegar, R. K., Nicolaou, A. L., et al. (1999). Perceived abuse and neglect as risk factors for suicidal behavior in adolescent inpatients. *Journal of Nervous & Mental Disease, 187*(1), 32–39.

Logue, E. M., & Parrish, R. S. (1998). Suicide precautions in a medical/surgical unit. *Nurse Manager, 29*(10), 33–34.

Malone, K. M., Haas, G. L., Sweeny, J. A., & Mann, J. J. (1995). Major depression and the risk of attempted suicide. *Journal of Affective Disorders, 34*(3), 173–185.

Mann, J. J., Oquendo, M., Underwood, M. D., & Arango, V. (1999). The neurobiology of suicide risk: A review for the clinician. *Journal of Clinical Psychiatry, 60*(Suppl. 2), 7–11.

Marcus, E. (1996). *Why suicide?* San Francisco: Harper.

Marcus, S., Robins, L. N., & Bucholz, K. (1991). *The Quick Diagnostic Interview Schedule: Program manual.* St. Louis: Washington University Department of Psychiatry.

McKeown, R. E., Garrison, C. Z., Cuffe, S. P., et al. (1998). Incidence and predictors of suicidal behaviors in a longitudinal sample of young adolescents. *Journal of the American Academy of Child & Adolescent Psychiatry, 37*(6), 612–619.

McQuaid, J. R., Stein, M. B., Laffaye, C., & McCahille, M. E. (1999). Depression in a primary care clinic: The prevalence and impact of an unrecognized disorder. *Journal of Affective Disorders, 55*(1), 1–10.

Modai, I., Valevski, A., Solomish, A., et al. (1999). Neural network detection of files of suicidal patients and suicidal profiles. *Medical Informatics, 24*(4), 249–256.

Murphy, G. E. (1998). Why women are less likely than men to commit suicide. *Comprehensive Psychiatry, 39*(4), 165–175.

Neeleman, J., Wessely, S., & Lewis, G. (1998). Suicide acceptability in African and white Americans: The role of religion. *Journal of Nervous & Mental Disease, 186*(1), 12–16.

Ohberg, A., & Lonnqvist, J. (1998). Suicides hidden among undetermined deaths. *Acta Psychiatrica Scandinavica, 98*(3), 214–218.

Olson, L., Huyler, F., Lynch, A. W., et al. (1999). Guns, alcohol, and intimate partner violence: The epidemiology of female suicide in New Mexico. *Crisis, 20*(3), 121–126.

Pfeffer, C. R., Normandin, L., & Kakuma, T. (1998). Suicidal children grow up: Suicidal behavior and psychiatric disorders among relatives. *Journal of the Academy of Child and Adolescent Psychiatry, 33*(8), 1087–1097.

Pilowsky, D. J., Wu, L. T., & Anthony, J. C. (1999). Panic attacks and suicide attempts in mid-adolescence. *American Journal of Psychiatry, 156*(10), 1545–1549.

Pirkola, S. P., Isometsa, E. T., Henriksson, M. M., et al. (1999). The treatment received by substance-dependent male and female suicide victims. *Acta Psychiatrica Scandinavica, 99*(3), 207–213.

Purcell, D., Thrush, C. R., & Blanchette, P. L. (1999). Suicide among the elderly in Honolulu County: A multiethnic comparative study (1987–1992). *International Psychogeriatrics, 11*(1), 57–66.

Quan, H., & Arboleda-Florez, J. (1999). Elderly suicide in Alberta: Difference by gender. *Canadian Journal of Psychiatry, 44*(8), 762–768.

Radloff, L. (1977). The CES-D scale: A self-report depression scale for research in the general population. *Applied Psychological Measurement, 1*, 385–401.

Radomsky, E. D., Haas, G. L., Mann, J. J., & Sweeney, J. A. (1999). Suicidal behavior in patients with schizophrenia and other psychotic disorders. *American Journal of Psychiatry, 156*(10), 1590–1595.

Remafedi, G. (1999). Suicide and sexual orientation: Nearing the end of controversy? *Archives of General Psychiatry, 56*(10), 885–886.

Remafedi, G., French, S., Story, M., et al. (1998). The relationship between suicide risk and sexual orientation: Results of a population-based study. *American Journal of Public Health, 88*(1), 57–60.

Renaud, J., Brent, D. A., Birmaher, B., et al. (1999). Suicide in adolescents with disruptive disorder. *Journal of the American Academy of Child & Adolescent Psychiatry, 38*(7), 846–851.

Rey, G. C., Narring, F., Ferron, C., & Michaud, P. A. (1998). Suicide attempts among adolescents in Switzerland: Prevalence, associated factors and comorbidity. *Acta Psychiatrica Scandinavica, 98*(1), 28–33.

Rihmer, Z., & Pestality, P. (1999). Bipolar II disorder and suicidal behavior. *Psychiatric Clinics of North America, 22*(3), 667–673.

Robie, D., Edgemon-Hill, E. J., Phelps, B., et al. (1999). Suicide prevention protocol: One hospital's nursing protocol for identification and intervention. *American Journal of Nursing, 99*(12), 53, 55, 57.

Robins, L. N., Helzer, J. E., Croughan, C., & Ratcliff, K. S. (1981). National Institute of Mental Health Diagnostic Interview Schedule: Its history, characteristics, and validity. *Archives of General Psychiatry, 38*(4), 381–389.

Roy, A., Nielsen, D., Rylander, G., et al. (1999). Genetics of suicide in depression. *Journal of Clinical Psychiatry, 60*(Suppl. 2), 18–20.

Roy, A., Rylander, G., & Sarchiapone, M. (1997). Genetic studies of suicidal behavior. *Psychiatric Clinics of North America, 20*(3), 595–611.

Runenson, B. S. (1998). History of suicidal behavior in the families of young suicides. *Acta Psychiatrica Scandinavica, 98*(6), 497–501.

Saarinen, P. I., Lehtonen, J., & Lonnqvist, J. (1999). Suicide risk in schizophrenia: An analysis of 17 consecutive suicides. *Schizophrenia Bulletin, 25*(3), 533–542.

Safer, D. J. (1997). Self-reported suicide attempts by adolescents. *Annals of Clinical Psychiatry, 9*(4), 263–269.

Santa Mina, E. E., & Gallop, R. M. (1998). Childhood sexual and physical abuse and adult self-harm and suicidal behaviour: A literature review. *Canadian Journal of Psychiatry, 43*(8), 793–800.

Shaffer, D., Fisher, P., & Dulcan, M. K. (1996). The NIMH Diagnostic Interview Schedule for Children Version 2.3 (DISC–2.3): Description, acceptability, prevalence rates, and performance in the MECA study: Methods for the Epidemiology of Child and Adolescent Mental Disorders Study. *Journal of the American Academy of Child and Adolescent Psychiatry, 35*(7), 865–877.

Shah, S., Hoffman, R. E., Wake, L., & Marine, W. M. (2000). Adolescent suicide and household access to firearms in Colorado: Results of a case-control study. *Journal of Adolescent Health, 26*(3), 157–163.

Shneidman, E. S. (1972). Forward. In A. Cain (Ed.), *Survivors of suicide* (pp. ix–xi). Springfield, IL: Charles C. Thomas.

Shrier, L. A., Pierce, J. D., Emans, et al. (1998). Gender differences in risk behaviors associated with forced or pressured sex. *Archives of Pediatrics & Adolescent Medicine, 152*(1), 57–63.

Simon, G. E., Von Korff, M., Heiligenstein, J. H., et al. (1996). Initial antidepressant choice in primary care: Effectiveness and cost of fluoxetine vs. tricyclic antidepressants. *Journal of the American Medical Association, 275*(24), 1897–1902.

Simon, R. I. (1999). The suicide prevention contract: Clinical, legal and risk management issues. *Journal of the American Academy of Psychiatry & the Law, 27*(3), 445–450.

Spitzer, R. L., Williams, J. B., Kroenke, K., et al. (1994). Utility of a new procedure for diagnosing mental disorders in primary care: The PRIME-MD 1000 study.

Journal of the American Medical Association, 272(22), 1749–1756.

Statham, D. J., Heath, A. C., Madden, P. A., et al. (1998). Suicidal behavior: An epidemiological and genetic study. *Psychological Medicine, 28*(4), 839–855.

Steadman, H. J., Mulvey, E. P., Monahan, J., et al. (1998). Violence by people discharged from acute psychiatric inpatient facilities and by others in the same neighborhoods. *Archives of General Psychiatry, 55*(5), 393–401.

Stevens, D. E., Merikangas, K. R., & Merikangas, J. R. (1995). Comorbidity of depression and other medical conditions. In E. E. Beckham & W. R. Leber (Eds.), *Handbook of depression* (pp. 147–199). New York: Guilford Press.

Tondo, L., Baldessarini, R. J., Hennen, J., et al. (1999). Suicide attempts in major affective disorder patients with comorbid substance use disorders. *Journal of Clinical Psychiatry, 60*(Suppl. 2), 63–69.

Uncapher, H., Gallagher-Thompson, D., Osgood, N. J., & Bongar, B. (1998). Hopelessness and suicidal ideation in older adults. *Gerontologist, 38*(1), 62–70.

Van Dongen, C. J. (1988). The legacy of suicide. *Journal of Psychosocial Nursing, 26*(1), 8–13.

Vilhjalmsson, R., Kristjansdottir, G., & Sveinbjarnardottir, E. (1998). Factors associated with suicide ideation in adults. *Social Psychiatry and Psychiatric Epidemiology, 33*(3), 97–103.

Waller, J. A., Skelly, J. M., & Davis, J. H. (1994). Characteristics, costs, and effects of violence in Vermont. *Journal of Trauma, 37*(6), 921–927.

Whooley, M. A., Avins, A. L., Miranda, J., & Browner, W. S. (1997). Case-finding instruments for depression: Two questions are as good as many. *Journal of General Internal Medicine, 12*(7), 439–445.

Wilson, C., Nairn, R., Coverdale, J., & Panapa, A. (1999). Constructing mental illness as dangerous: A pilot study. *Australian & New Zealand Journal of Psychiatry, 33*(2), 240–247.

Zung, W. W. K. (1965). A self-rating depression scale. *Archives of General Psychiatry, 12*, 63–70.

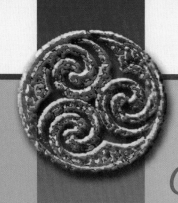

Glossary

absorption   Movement of drug from the site of administration into plasma.

abuse   Use of alcohol or drugs for the purpose of intoxication or, in the case of prescription drugs, for purposes beyond the intended use.

accommodation   Adjustment in cognitive organization that results from the demands of reality (Piaget).

accreditation   Process by which a mental health agency is judged by established standards to be providing acceptable quality of care.

acculturation   Act or process of assuming the beliefs, values, and practices of another, usually dominant culture.

acetylcholine (ACh)   An important neurotransmitter associated with cognitive functioning, and disruption of cholinergic mechanisms damages memory in animals and humans.

acetylcholinesterase (AChE)   Key enzyme that inactivates the neurotransmitter acetylcholine. AChE is found in high concentrations in the brain and is one of two cholinesterase enzymes capable of breaking down ACh.

acetylcholinesterase inhibitors (AChEI)   Mainstay of pharmacologic treatment of dementia; these drugs inhibit AChE, resulting in an enhancement of cholinergic activity. AChEIs have been shown to delay the decline in cognitive functioning but generally do not improve cognitive function once it has declined; therefore, it is important that this medication be started as soon as the diagnosis is made.

active listening   Focusing on what the patient is saying in order to interpret and respond to the message in an objective manner, while using techniques such as open-ended statements, reflection, and questions that elicit additional responses from the patient.

acute stress disorder (ASD)   A mental disorder characterized by persistent, distressing stress-related symptoms that last between 2 days and 1 month and that occur within 1 month after a traumatic experience.

adaptability   Capacity of a person to survive and flourish.

adaptive inflexibility   Rigidity in interactions with others, achievement of goals, and coping with stress.

addiction   Severe psychological and behavioral dependence on drugs or alcohol.

adherence   An individual's ability to follow directions for self-administration of medications and other biologic therapies; compliance.

advanced practice psychiatric–mental health nurse   A licensed registered nurse who is educationally prepared at the master's level and is nationally certified as a specialist by the American Nurses Credentialing Center (AANC).

advance care directives   Treatment directives (living wills) and appointment directives (power of attorney or health proxies) that apply only if the individual is unable to make his or her own decisions because the patient is incapacitated or, in the opinion of two physicians, is otherwise unable to make decisions for himself or herself.

adverse reactions   Unwanted medication effects that may have serious physiologic consequences.

affect   An expression of mood manifest in a pattern of observable behaviors.

affective blunting   Flat or blunted emotion.

affective instability   Rapid and extreme shifts in mood, erratic emotional responses to situations, and intense sensitivity to criticism or perceived slights; one of the core characteristics of borderline personality disorder.

affective lability   Abrupt, dramatic, unprovoked changes in the types of emotions expressed.

afferent   Toward the central nervous system or a particular structure.

affinity   Degree of attraction or strength of the bond between a drug and its receptor.

aggression   Behaviors or attitudes that reflect rage, hostility, and the potential for physical or verbal destructiveness; usually occurs if the person believes someone is going to do him or her harm.

agitation   Inability to sit still or attend to others, accompanied by heightened emotions and tension.

agnosia   Failure to recognize or identify objects despite intact sensory function, or a disturbance in executive functioning (ability to think abstractly, plan, initiate, sequence, monitor, and stop complex behavior).

agonists   Chemicals producing the same biologic action as the neurotransmitter.

agoraphobia   Anxiety about being in places from which escape might be difficult or embarrassing, or about being in places in which help may not be readily available if a panic attack should occur.

akathisia   An extrapyramidal side effect from phenothiazine, which includes restlessness that is easily mistaken for anxiety or increased psychotic symptoms.

alcohol-induced persisting amnestic disorder   Cognitive impairment deficits related to substance abuse.

alcohol tolerance   A phenomenon producing a more rapid metabolism of alcohol and a decreased response to its sedating, motor, and anxiolytic effects.

alcohol withdrawal syndrome   A syndrome that occurs after the reduction of alcohol consumption, or when abstaining from alcohol after prolonged use, causing changes in vital signs, diaphoresis, and other adverse gastrointestinal and central nervous system side effects.

alexithymia Inability to experience and communicate feelings consciously.

algorithms Systematic decision trees that depict the flow of decisions and outcomes.

allodynia Lowered pain threshold.

alogia Brief, empty verbal responses; often referred to as *poverty of speech.*

ambivalence Presence and expression of two opposing forces, leading to inaction.

amino acids Building blocks of proteins that have different roles. Amino acids function as neurotransmitters in as many as 60% to 70% of synaptic sites in the brain.

amygdala A bulb-like structure attached to the tail of the caudate and often considered part of the limbic system.

anger An affective state experienced as the motivation to act in ways that warn, intimidate, or attack those who are perceived as challenging or threatening.

anhedonia Inability to gain pleasure from activities.

animism A child's belief that inanimate objects are alive.

anorexia nervosa A life-threatening eating disorder characterized by refusal to maintain body weight appropriate for age, intense fear of gaining weight or becoming fat, a severely distorted body image, and refusal to acknowledge the seriousness of weight loss.

antagonists Chemicals blocking the biologic response at a given receptor site.

anticholinergic crisis A potentially life-threatening medical emergency that occurs as a result of overdose or sensitivity to drugs with anticholinergic properties.

antimotivational syndrome Attributed to long-term marijuana use, a syndrome marked by apathy, diminished interest in activities and goals, poor job performance, and reduced short-term memory.

anxiety Energy that arises when expectations that are present are not met (Peplau).

anxiogenic Anxiety provoking.

anxiolytics Drugs that reverse or diminish anxiety.

apathy Reactions to stimuli that are decreased, along with a diminished interest and desire.

aphasia Alterations in language ability.

apraxia Impaired ability to execute motor activities despite intact motor functioning.

arachnoid layer A thin, delicate sheet of collagenous tissue under the meningeal layer that follows the contours of the brain but does not dip down inside them.

area restriction Limitation of patient mobility to a specified area for purposes of safety or behavior management.

assertive community treatment Direct and individualized treatment and services provided by a selectively chosen interdisciplinary team that follows on a patient's progress during reintegration into the community.

assessment Deliberate and systematic collection of biopsychosocial information or data to determine current and past health and functional status and to evaluate present and past coping patterns.

association areas Areas of the cortex in which neighboring nerve fibers are related to the same sensory modality.

assortative mating Tendency for individuals to select mates who are similar in genetically linked traits such as intelligence and personality styles.

atropine flush Flushing of the face, neck, and upper arms due to a reflex blood vessel dilation that results from increased body temperature.

attachment Emotional bond between the infant and parental figure.

attention A complex mental process that involves concentrating on one activity to the exclusion of others, as well as sustaining interest over time.

autism A form of thinking or a style of relating that focuses subjectively on "me" to the exclusion of "not me."

autistic thinking Thinking restricted the literal and immediate so that the individual has private rules of logic and reasoning that make no sense to others.

automatic thinking Thinking that influences the person's actions or other thought; it is often subject to errors or tangible distortions of reality that contradicts objective appraisals.

autonomic nervous system Part of the nervous system that regulates involuntary vital functions including cardiac muscle, smooth muscles, and glands. It is composed of the sympathetic and parasympathetic systems.

autonomy Concept that each person has the fundamental right of self-determination.

avolition Inability to complete projects, assignments, or work.

axes A term used to describe domains of information. In a psychiatric diagnosis, there are five domains: Axis I, clinical domain that is the focus of treatment; Axis II, personality disorders or mental retardation, Axis III, general medical condition; Axis IV, psychosocial stress, and Axis V, level of functioning.

basal ganglia One set of structures in each hemisphere; areas of gray matter containing many cell bodies or nuclei.

basic level of practice According to the *Scope and Standards of Psychiatric–Mental Health Nursing*, this level includes two groups of nurses. The first group includes registered nurses who practice in psychiatric settings; the second includes those who have a baccalaureate degree in nursing and have worked in the field for 2 years.

behavior therapy Interventions that reinforce or promote desirable behaviors or alter undesirable ones.

behavioral sensitization A phenomenon by which a person has a magnified stress response to milder stressors after one or more exposures to a severe, uncontrollable stressor.

behaviorism A paradigm shift in understanding human behavior that was initiated by Watson, who theorized that human behavior is developed through a stimulus–response process rather than through unconscious drives or instincts.

beneficence The health care provider uses knowledge of science and incorporates the art of caring to develop an environment in which individuals achieve maximum health care potential.

bereavement A period of profound grieving following a loss.

bibliotherapy The use of books and other reading materials to help individuals cope with various life stressors.

binge eating Episodes of uncontrollable, ravenous eating of large amounts of food within discrete periods of time, usually followed by feelings of guilt that result in purging.

bioavailability Amount of a drug that reaches the systemic circulation for targeted treatment.

biogenic amines Small molecules manufactured in the neuron that contain an amine group. These include dopamine, norepinephrine, and epinephrine (all synthesized from the amino acid tyrosine), serotonin (from tryptophan), and histamine (from histidine).

biologic dimension Part of the biopsychosocial model that explains the biologic knowledge of mental health, including pathogenesis and treatment of mental illness.

biologic markers Physical indicators of disturbances within the central nervous system that differentiate one disease state from another.

biologic view A theoretic view or argument of the early 1900s that mental illness has a biologic cause and can be treated with physical interventions.

biopsychosocial model An organizational model consisting of three separate but interdependent dimensions: biologic, psychological, and social. Each dimension has an independent knowledge and treatment focus but can interact and be mutually interdependent with the other dimensions.

biosexual identity Anatomic and physiologic state of being male or female that results from genetic and hormonal influences.

bipolar type A subtype of schizophrenic disorder in which the patient exhibits manic symptoms alone or with a mix of manic and depressive symptoms.

board-and-care homes Facilities that provide 24-hour supervision and assistance with medications, meals, and some self-care skills, but in which individualized attention to self-care skills and other activities of daily living is generally not available.

body dysmorphic disorder Disorder in which there is a preoccupation with an imagined or slight defect in appearance, such as a large nose, thinning hair, or small genitals.

body image How each individual perceives his or her own body, separate from how the world or society views him or her.

body image disturbance Extreme discrepancy between one's perception of one's own body image and others' perceptions of one.

boundaries Limits in which a person may act or refrain from acting within a designated time or place.

bradykinesia An extrapyramidal condition characterized by a slowness of voluntary movement and speech.

brain stem Area of the brain containing the midbrain, pons, and medulla, which continues beneath the thalamus.

breach of confidentiality Release of patient information without the patient's consent in the absence of legal compulsion or authorization to release information.

Broca's area A section of the left frontal lobe of the brain thought to be responsible for the articulation of speech.

bulimia nervosa An eating disorder in which the individual engages in recurrent episodes of binge eating and compensatory behavior to avoid weight gain through purging methods such as self-induced vomiting, or use of laxatives, diuretics, enemas, or emetics, or through nonpurging methods such as fasting or excessive exercise.

butyrylcholinesterase (BuChE) A nonspecific cholinesterase found in the brain and especially in the glial cells. Both acetylcholinesterase and BuChE work in the gastrointestinal tract. If these enzymes are inhibited, the destruction of acetylcholine will be delayed, resulting in an increase in acetylcholine activity.

case management Problem solving and coordinating services for the patient to ensure continuity of services and overcome system rigidity, fragmentation of services, misuse of facilities, and inaccessibility.

cataplexy Bilateral loss of muscle tone triggered by a strong emotion such as laughter. This muscle atonia can range from subtle (drooping eyelids) to dramatic (buckling knees). Eye and respiratory muscles are not affected. Cataplexy usually lasts only seconds. Individuals are fully conscious, oriented, and alert during the episode. Prolonged episodes of cataplexy may lead to sleep episodes.

catatonic excitement Hyperactivity characterized by purposeless activity and abnormal movements like grimacing and posturing.

categoric diagnosis A subset of a given diagnosis that consists of criteria that include or exclude data for the purpose of giving a name to a set of symptoms.

central sulcus Posterior boundary of the frontal lobe that separates it from the parietal lobe.

cerebellum Part of the brain that is responsible for controlling movement and postural adjustments; it receives information from all parts of the body.

cerebrospinal fluid Cushioning fluid that circulates around the brain beneath the arachnoid layer in the subarachnoid space; it is colorless and contains sodium chloride and other salts.

chemical restraints Use of medication to control patients or manage behavior.

cholecystokinin A neuropeptide found in high levels in the cerebral cortex, hypothalamus, and amygdala; it is also excreted by the gastrointestinal system in response to food intake, which is believed to play a role in the control of eating and satiety by controlling the release of dopamine.

choroid plexus A collection of cells within the ventricles that produces cerebrospinal fluid.

chronic depression Depression that persists for months to years and that may be associated with some disability or distress.

chronic disaffiliation Lacking the love and support that come from being associated with a solid network of family and friends.

chronobiology Study and measure of time structures or biologic rhythms.

circadian rhythm (cycle) From the Latin *circa* and *dies*, meaning "about a day"; refers to a biologic system that fluctuates or oscillates in a pattern that repeats itself in about a day.

circumstantiality Extremely detailed and lengthy discourse about a topic.

clang association Repetition of word phrases that are similar in sound but in no other way, for example, "right, light, sight, might."

classical conditioning A learning situation in which an unconditioned stimulus initially produces an unconditioned response; over time, a conditioned response is elicited for a specific stimulus (Pavlov).

clearance Total amount of blood, serum, or plasma from which a drug is completely removed per unit of time.

clinical decision making A specific type of decision making that focuses on the decisions made in a clinical setting.

clinical domain outcome statements Statements that indicate a reduction in symptoms of illness or cure of a specific mental illness.

clinical path A plan of care for patients with a common problem represented by flow charts that usually contain assessment parameters, nursing diagnoses, nursing interventions, and outcomes.

closed group A group in which all the members begin at one time. New members are not admitted after the first meeting.

clubhouse model Psychosocial rehabilitation approach with the goal of integrating individuals with mental illness back into the community; these houses are run entirely by the patients or "clubhouse members."

codependence A maladaptive coping pattern in family members or others closely related to a substance abuser that results from prolonged exposure to the behaviors of the alcohol- or drug-dependent person; characterized by boundary distortions, poor relationship and friendship skills, compulsive and obsessive behaviors, inappropriate anger, sexual maladjustment, and resistance to change.

cognition A high level of intellectual processing in which perceptions and information are acquired, used, or manipulated.

cognitive appraisal The process of examining the demands, constraints, and resources of the environment and of negotiating them with personal goals and beliefs.

cognitive schema Patterns of thoughts that determine how a person interprets events. Each person's cognitive schema screen, code, and evaluate incoming stimuli.

cognitive therapy Interventions that reinforce and promote desirable cognitive functioning or alter undesirable cognitive functioning.

communication blocks interruptions in the content flow of communication that can be identified in process recordings as such changes in topic that either the nurse or patient makes.

communication disorders Disorders that involve speech or language impairments.

communication triad A technique used to provide a specific syntax and order for patients to identify and express their feelings and seek relief. The "sentence" consists of three parts: (1) an "I" statement to identify the prevailing feeling, (2) a nonjudgmental statement of the emotional trigger, and (3) a statement of what the person would like differently or what would restore comfort to the situation.

comorbidity (comorbid) Disease that coexists with the primary disease.

competence The degree to which the patient is able to understand and appreciate the information given during the consent process; the patient's cognitive ability to process information at a specific time; the patient's ability to gather and interpret information and make reasonable judgments based on that information to participate fully as a partner in treatment.

compliance The individual's ability to follow directions for self-administration of medications and other biologic therapies; adherence.

comprehensive assessment Collection of all relevant data to identify problems for which a nursing diagnosis is stated.

concrete thinking Lack of abstraction in thinking, in which people are unable to understand punch lines, metaphors, and analogies.

confidentiality An ethical duty of nondisclosure; the patient has the right to disclose personal information without fear of it being revealed to others.

conflict resolution A specific type of counseling in which the nurse helps the patient resolve a disagreement or dispute.

confused speech and thinking Symptoms of schizophrenia that render the patient unable to respond accurately to the ordinary signs and sounds of daily living.

connections Mutually responsive and enhancing relationships.

conservation The child's awareness that a quantity remains the same despite its shape.

constraints Limitations that are both personal (internalized cultural values and beliefs) and environmental (finite resources such as money and time).

content themes Repetition of concerns or feelings that occur within the therapeutic relationship. Themes may emerge as symbolic representations of fears.

continuum of care Providing care in an integrated system of settings, services (physical, psychological, and social), and care levels appropriate to the individual's specific needs in a continuous manner over time, with channels of communication among the service providers.

coordination of care Integration of the various components of the continuum of care, including the pre-entry, entry, pre-exit, and exit phases.

coping Thinking and acting in ways to manage specific external and internal demands and conflicts that are taxing or exceeding one's resources.

corpus callosum Functional link between the two hemispheres of the brain, made up of a thick band of fibers.

cortex Outer surface of the mature brain.

cortical dementia A type of dementia that is characterized by amnesia, aphasia, apraxia, and agnosia.

counseling interventions Specific time-limited interactions between a nurse and a patient, family, or group experiencing intermediate or ongoing difficulties related to their health or well-being.

countertransference The nurse's reactions to a patient that are based on the nurse's unconscious needs, conflicts, problems, and views of the world. It can significantly interfere with the nurse–patient relationship.

crisis A severely stressful experience for which coping mechanisms fail to provide any adaptation, whether the experience is positive or negative.

crisis intervention A specialized short-term (usually no longer than 6 hours) goal-directed therapy designed to assist patients in an immediate manner, after which they are usually transferred to an inpatient unit or to an intensive outpatient setting.

critical thinking An analytic and complex process that involves observing behaviors and responses; making purposeful, objective judgments; and constantly re-evaluating.

cultural brokering Act of bridging, linking, or mediating between groups or individuals of different cultural systems for the purpose of reducing conflict or producing change.

cultural competence A process (developed through cultural awareness, acquisition of cultural knowledge, development of cultural skills, and engagement in numerous cultural encounters) in which the nurse continually strives to achieve the ability to work effectively within the cultural context of an individual or community from a diverse cultural or ethnic background.

culture Any group of people who identify or associate with each other on the basis of some common purpose, need, or similarity of background; the set of learned, socially transmitted beliefs and behaviors that arise from interpersonal transactions among members of the cultural group.

cycle of violence A three-phase pattern of tension, abuse, and kindness in which the abuser engages first in abuse and then in seemingly sincere expressions of love, contrition, and remorse.

cyclothymic A term used to describe periods of hypomanic and depressive episodes that do not meet full criteria for a major depressive episode.

cytoarchitectonic analysis Study of the distribution and arrangement of cells within various parts of the brain using various staining procedures to identify differences throughout the brain.

de-escalation An interactive process of calming and redirecting a patient who has an immediate potential for violence directed at others or self.

defense levels Division of defense mechanisms that includes high adaptive, mental inhibitions (compromise formation), minor image-distorting, disavowal, major image-distorting, action level, and defense dysregulation.

defense mechanisms Coping styles; the automatic psychological process protecting the individual against anxiety and creating awareness of internal or external dangers or stressors.

defining characteristics Clues given by the signs and symptoms that join together in the nurse's mind to form a cluster that leads to a specific nursing diagnosis.

deinstitutionalization Release of patients with severe and persistent mental illness from state mental hospitals to community settings.

delirium tremens An acute withdrawal syndrome that occurs often in alcoholics after 10 or more years of heavy drinking and is characterized by tachycardia, sweating, hypertension, irregular tremor, delusions, vivid hallucinations, and wild, agitated behavior.

delusion Erroneous belief that usually involves a misinterpretation of perception or experience. These beliefs are false, fixed, and fall outside of the patient's social, cultural, or religious background.

delusional disorder A disorder in which there is the presence of nonbizarre delusions; includes several subtypes: ergotomania, grandiose, jealous, somatic, mixed, and specified.

demands External pulls (crowding, crime, noise, pollution) imposed by the physical environment, and internal pulls (behavior and role expectations) imposed by the social environment.

dementia From the Latin *de* (from or out of) and *mens* (mind); several cognitive deficits (one of which is impaired memory) that are due to the direct physiologic effects of a general medical condition, the persisting effects of a substance, or multiple biologic etiologies.

denial The patient's inability to accept loss of control over substance use or the severity of the consequences associated with substance abuse.

depersonalization A nonspecific experience in which the individual loses a sense of personal identity and feels strange or unreal.

depressive episode In a major depressive episode, either a depressed mood or a loss of interest or pleasure in nearly all activities must be present for at least 2 weeks. Four of seven additional symptoms must be present: disruption in sleep, appetite (or weight), concentration, energy; psychomotor agitation or retardation; excessive guilt or feelings of worthlessness; suicidal ideation.

depressive type A subtype of schizophrenic disorder in which the patient displays only symptoms of a major depressive episode during the illness.

desensitization A rapid decrease in drug effects that may develop within a few minutes or over a period of days, months, years, or lifetime of exposure to a drug.

detoxification Process of safely and effectively withdrawing a person from an addictive substance, usually under medical supervision.

developmental delay The impairment of normal growth and development that may not be reversible.

diagnosis-specific outcomes Outcomes based on nursing diagnoses.

Dialectical Behavior Therapy (DBT) An important biosocial approach to treatment that combines numerous cognitive and behavior therapy strategies. It requires patients to understand their disorder by actively participating in formulating treatment goals by collecting data about their own behavior, identifying treatment targets in individual therapy, and working with the therapists in changing these target behaviors.

dichotomous thinking Tendency to view things as absolute, either black or white, good or bad, with no perception of compromise.

differentiation of self An individual's resolution of attachment to his or her family's emotional chaos. It involves an intrapsychic separation of thinking from feelings and an interpersonal freeing of oneself from the chaos.

dimensional diagnoses A system of diagnosing patient problems by locating and describing them on a specified continuum; for example, aggression may be characterized as existing somewhere on a continuum from verbal anger to physical assault.

direct leadership behavior The leader controls the interaction of the group by giving directions and information and allowing little discussion.

discharge outcomes Those outcomes to be met before discharge.

discipline-specific outcomes Patient outcomes based on the standards of the discipline using them. These outcomes can be used to evaluate the individual practitioner's practice.

disconnections Lack of mutually responsive and enhancing relationships.

discrimination The differential treatment of others because they are members of a particular group.

disinhibition A concept borrowed from physics and biology and based on the idea of a dynamic, self-regulatory model of equilibrium in which equilibrium is defined (Piaget) as compensation for external disturbances; a mechanism for providing the self-regulation by which intelligence adapts to internal and external changes.

disordered water balance A state of chronic fluid imbalance, vacillating between normal and hyponatremic, that commonly occurs in psychiatric patients with chronic illnesses.

dissociation A disruption in the normally occurring linkages among subjective awareness, feelings, thoughts, behavior, and memories.

dissociative identity disorder (DID) A mental disorder characterized by the existence of two or more distinct identities with unique personality characteristics and the inability to recall important information about oneself or events.

dissupport The presence of relationships that are harmful, stressful, and damaging to a person's self-esteem.

distraction Consciously changing behaviors to take the focus off the physical sensations or unwanted thoughts, feelings, or behaviors.

distribution The amount of a drug that may be found in various tissues at the site of the drug action for which it is intended.

disturbances of executive functioning Problems in the ability to think abstractly, plan, initiate, sequence, monitor, and stop complex behavior.

diurnal weight gain Weight gain that occurs throughout a day that is caused by fluid and food intake that is regulated by the circadian rhythm.

domestic abuse Violence, including rape, directed toward a person by an intimate partner.

dosing Administration of medication over time so that therapeutic levels may be achieved or maintained without reaching toxic levels.

drug overdose A dose of a drug that causes an acute reaction such as agitation, delirium, coma, or death.

dual diagnosis Presence of both a psychoactive substance dependency and mental illness.

dura mater The tough layer of collagen fibers that forms a loose sac around the central nervous system (in Latin, "hard mother") and contains three layers: meningeal, arachnoid, and pia mater.

dyad A group of only two people who are usually related, such as a married couple, siblings, or parent and child.

dysfunctional family A family whose interactions, decisions, or behaviors interfere with the positive development of the family and its individual members.

dyslexia Significantly lower score for mental age on standardized test in reading that is not due to low intelligence or inadequate schooling.

dyspareunia A sexual pain disorder characterized by genital pain in men and women associated with sexual intercourse.

dysphagia Difficulty swallowing.

dysphoric (mood) Depressed, disquieted, and/or restless.

dyssomnia A disorder of initiating or maintaining sleep or of excessive sleepiness.

dysthymic disorder A milder but more chronic form of major depressive disorder.

dystonia An impairment in muscle tone that is generally the first extrapyramidal symptom to occur, usually within a few days of initiating an antipsychotic. Dystonia is characterized by involuntary muscle spasms, especially of the head and neck muscles.

early intervention programs Community outreach efforts designed to work with infants and preschool-aged children and their caretakers to foster healthy physical, psychological, social, and intellectual development.

echolalia Parrot-like repetition of another's words; inappropriate choice of topics.

echopraxia Involuntary imitation of another person's movements and gestures; regressed behavior that is child-like or immature.

efferent Away from the central nervous system or other particular structure.

efficacy Ability of a drug to produce a response as a result of the receptor or receptors being occupied.

egocentrism Tendency to view the world as revolving around oneself.

emotion Psychophysiologic reaction that define a person's mood and can be categorized as negative (anger, fright, anxiety, guilt, shame, sadness, envy, jealousy, and disgust), positive (happiness, pride, relief, and love), or somewhat ambiguous, or borderline (hope, compassion, empathy, sympathy, and contentment).

emotional abuse In reference to adults: degrading, threatening, stalking, or otherwise using psychological violence; in reference to children: rejecting, isolating, terrorizing, ignoring, or corrupting.

emotional dysregulation Inability to control emotion in social interactions.

emotional regulation A biosocial interaction between the innate emotional vulnerability of the individual and the ability to modulate that emotion in social interactions.

emotional vulnerability Sensitivity and reactivity to environmental stress.

emotion-focused coping A type of coping that changes the meaning of the situation.

empathetic linkage Ability to feel in oneself the feelings being expressed by another person or persons.

empathy A voluntary, nonprimordial experiencing of the situation of another within some form of interaction or relationship.

encopresis Soiling clothing with feces or depositing feces in inappropriate places.

endorphins Neurotransmitters that have opiate-like behavior and produce an inhibitory effect at opiate receptor sites; probably responsible for pain tolerance.

enuresis Involuntary excretion of urine after the age at which a child should have attained bladder control.

epidemiology The study of patterns of disease distribution in time and space that focuses on the health status of population groups or aggregates, rather than on individuals, and involves quantitative analysis of the occurrence of illnesses in population groups; basic science of public health.

epigenesis A concept borrowed from embryology: if a particular part does not manifest itself during the appropriate phase, it cannot reach full development because the moment for doing so has passed; each developmental stage must be completed at the appropriate time, or successful completion of the stage will not occur.

episode A period of a minimal duration of 2 weeks during which an individual experiences symptoms that meet the diagnostic criteria for that disorder.

epithalamus Area above and medial to the thalamus and adjacent to the roof of the third ventricle.

equilibration Compensation for external disturbances; a mechanism for providing the self-regulation by which intelligence adapts to external and internal changes (Piaget).

erectile dysfunction Inability of a male to achieve or maintain an erection sufficient for completion of sexual activity.

ergotomania Delusional belief that the person is loved intensely by the loved object, who is usually married and of a higher socioeconomic status, making him or her unattainable.

ethnic (ethnicity) People classified according to common traits, customs, thinking, and judgment.

euphoric (mood) An elated mood.

euthymic (mood) A normal mood.

exhibitionism A behavior associated with paraphilias involving exposing one's genitals to strangers, with occasional masturbation.

expansive (mood) A mood characterized by inappropriate lack of restraint in expressing one's feelings and frequently overvaluing one's own importance. Expansive qualities include an unceasing and indiscriminate enthusiasm for interpersonal, sexual, or occupational interactions.

exposure therapy The treatment of choice for agoraphobia that puts the patient into contact with the feared situations until the stimuli no longer produce anxiety.

expressed emotion Family members' responses that include one or more of the following dynamics: critical comments, hostility, or emotional overinvolvement.

extended family Several nuclear families who may or may not live together and function as one group.

external advocacy system Organizations that operate outside mental health agencies and serve as advocates for the treatment and rights of mental health patients.

externalizing disorders Disorders that are characterized by acting-out behavior.

extinction Elimination of a classically conditioned response by the repeated presentation of the conditioned stimulus without the unconditioned stimulus, or elimination of an operantly conditioned response by no longer presenting the reward after the response.

extrapyramidal motor system Collection of neuronal pathways that provides significant input in involuntary motor movements.

factitious disorder A type of psychiatric disorder characterized by somatization, in which the person intentionally causes an illness for the purpose of becoming a patient.

family development A broad term that refers to all the processes connected with the growth of a family, including changes associated with work, geographic location, migration, acculturation, and serious illness.

family dynamics The patterned interpersonal and social interactions that occur within the family structure over the life of a family.

family life cycle A process of expansion, contraction, and realignment of relationship systems to support the entry, exit, and development of family members.

family preservation Efforts made by professionals to preserve the family unit by preventing the removal of children from their homes through parental support and education and through work to facilitate a secure attachment between the child and parent.

family projection process The family projects its conflicts onto the child or spouse, and this member becomes the center of family conflicts.

family structure According to Minuchin, the organized pattern within which family members interact.

fear conditioning A type of classic conditioning in which a previously neutral stimulus (conditioned stimulus) elicits a fear response (conditioned response) after it has been paired with an aversive stimulus (unconditioned stimulus) that produces fear (unconditioned response).

fetal alcohol syndrome A syndrome that occurs in infants whose mothers ingested alcohol during pregnancy; includes symptoms such as permanent brain damage, often resulting in mental retardation.

fetishism A behavior associated with paraphilias, involving using an object for sexual arousal.

fissures The grooves of the cerebrum.

flight of ideas Repeated and rapid changes in the topic of conversation, generally with just one sentence or phrase.

flooding A type of therapy for agoraphobia in which highly anxiety-provoking stimuli are presented to the patient in vivo or with imagery, with no relaxation until the anxiety dissipates.

folk That which originates or is traditional to a group of people.

forensic commitment A special type of involuntary commitment of individuals with mental disorders who have been charged with a crime and are criminally committed to a mental hospital.

formal group roles The designated leader and members of a group.

formal operations The ability to use abstract reasoning to conceptualize and solve problems.

formal support system Large organizations that provide care to individuals, such as hospitals and nursing homes.

frontal, occipital, parietal, temporal Lobes of the brain located on the lateral surface of each hemisphere.

frotteurism A behavior associated with paraphilias, characterized by sexually arousing urges, fantasies, and behaviors resulting from touching or rubbing one's genitals on the breasts, genitals, or thighs of a nonconsenting person.

functional activities Activities of daily living necessary for self-care (ie, bathing, toileting, dressing, and transferring).

functional status Extent to which a person has the ability to carry out independent personal care, home management, and social functions in everyday life that has meaning and purpose.

gate-control theory Pain response based on the theory that pain perception involves pathways in the dorsal horn of the spinal column that relay noxious stimuli to the brain and that certain other nerve fibers function as an antagonistic "gate" to augment or dampen the subjective experience of pain.

gender identity A sense of self as being male or female.

gender identity disorder Disorder characterized by a strong and persistent identification with the opposite sex and the desire or perception that one is of that gender.

gender role How one functions and behave as a male or a female in relation to others in society, also referred to as *sex role identity*.

generic caring A phrase coined by Leininger to mean the foundational prototype included in local home remedies and folklore.

genogram A multigenerational schematic diagram that lists family members and their relationships.

gentrification The refurbishing of homes and buildings in rundown neighborhoods and the subsequent raising of rents.

glia (white matter) A fatty or lipid substance with a white appearance that surrounds the pathways of the cell body axons.

global risk factors Risk factors such as poverty, prejudice, and inadequate living situations that are associated with the risk for a mental disorder.

gray matter The cortex, with its gray-brown color because of the capillary blood vessels.

group Two or more people who are in an interdependent relationship with one another.

group cohesion Forces that act on the members to stay in a group.

group density effect An effect that accounts for the observed reality that individuals who live within their own cultural groups are protected from stressors that afflict people living as isolated minorities in a larger, incompatible culture or milieu.

group dynamics Interactions within groups.

group process The culmination of the session-to-session interactions of the members that move the group toward its goals.

groupthink The tendency of many groups to avoid conflict and adopt a normative pattern of thinking that is often consistent with the group leader's ideas.

gyri Bumps and convolutions in the brain.

half-life The time required for plasma concentrations of a drug to be reduced by 50%.

hallucinations Perceptual experiences that occur in the absence of actual external sensory stimuli and may be auditory, visual, tactile, gustatory, or olfactory.

hallucinogen A class of drug that produces euphoria or dysphoria, altered body image, distorted or sharpened visual and auditory perception, confusion, uncoordination, and impaired judgment and memory.

hallucinogen persisting perceptual disorder A transient and intermittent disorder associated with the long-term use of hallucinogens; includes depression, prolonged psychosis, and flashbacks.

hippocampus Subcortical gray matter embedded within each temporal lobe that may be involved in determining the best way to store information or memory; "time-dating" memory.

HIV-1–associated cognitive-motor complex Neurologic complications that occur with HIV-1 that are directly attributable to infection of the brain and include impaired cognitive and motor function.

homeless A description of a person who lives for a sustained period of time on the street, in a public shelter, or in other temporary living quarters.

homelessness State of being without a consistent dwelling place.

home visits Delivery of nursing care in a patient's living environment.

homophobia An intense fear of any contact whatsoever with gays or homosexuals and a dislike of homosexual lifestyles.

human sexual response cycle Usually viewed as consisting of four phases: excitement, plateau, orgasm, and resolution.

humanitarian domain outcome statements Statements that spell out behaviors or responses that show a sense of well-being of patients and personal fulfillment of patients and family members.

hyperactivity Excessive motor activity, movement, and/or utterances that may be either purposeless or aimless.

hyperalgia Increased nociceptor sensitivity.

hyperesthesia Increased sensation of pain.

hyperkinetic delirium A type of delirium in which the patient demonstrates behaviors most commonly recognized as delirium, including psychomotor hyperactivity, marked excitability, and a tendency toward hallucinations.

hypersexuality Inappropriate and socially unacceptable sexual behavior. The patient begins talking and behaving in ways that are uncharacteristic of the patient's behavior.

hypersomnia Oversleeping.

hypervigilance Sustained attention to external stimuli as if expecting something important or frightening to happen.

hypervocalization Screams, curse, moans, groans, and verbal repetitiveness that are common in the later stages of the cognitively impaired elders, often occurring during a hospitalization or nursing home placement.

hypnagogic hallucinations Intense dream-like images that occur when an individual is falling asleep and usually involve the immediate environment.

hypokinetic delirium A type of delirium in which the patient is lethargic, somnolent, and apathetic and exhibits reduced psychomotor activity.

hypomanic episode Mildly dysphoric mood that meets the same criterion as for a manic episode except that it lasts at least 4 days rather than 1 week and that no marked impairment in social or occupational functioning is present.

hyponatremia Decreased sodium concentration in the blood.

hyposthenuria Secretion of urine with a low specific gravity.

hypothalamus Immediately ventral and slightly anterior to the thalamus, forming the floor and part of the walls of the third ventricle.

hypothalamic–pituitary–adrenal (HPA) axis Neurotransmitters responsible for behavioral responses to fear and anxiety that are usually held in balance until information from the sensory processing areas in the thalamus and cortex alerts the amygdala. If events are interpreted as threatening, this axis is activated, initiating the stress response.

identity An integration of a person's social and occupational roles and affiliations, self-attributed personality traits, attitudes about gender roles, beliefs about sexuality and intimacy, long-term goals, political ideology, and religious beliefs.

identity diffusion Occurs when parts of a person's identity is absent or poorly developed; a lack of consistent sense of identity.

illusions Disorganized perceptions that create an oversensitivity to colors, shapes, and background activities that occur when the person misperceives or exaggerates stimuli in the external environment.

implosive therapy An imaginal technique useful in treating agoraphobia in which the therapist identifies individual phobic stimuli for the patient and then presents highly anxiety-provoking imagery in a dramatic fashion.

impulsiveness A sudden, irresistible urge or desire resulting from a particular feeling that can lead to an action.

impulsivity Acting without considering the consequences of the act or alternative actions.

incidence A rate that includes only new cases that have occurred within a clearly defined time period.

incompetent A person is legally determined not to be able to understand and appreciate the information given during the consent process.

indicated preventive interventions Preventive interventions that are targeted to high-risk individuals who are identified as having minimal but detectable signs and symptoms foreshadowing a disorder or as having biologic markers indicating a predisposition, but not the actual disorder.

indicators Representation of the dimension of outcome answering the question of how close the patient is coming toward an outcome.

indirect leader Leader who primarily reflects the group members' discussion and offers little guidance or information to the group.

individual roles Group roles that either enhance or detract from the group's functioning but have nothing to do with either the group task or maintenance.

individual treatment plan A plan of care that identifies the patient's problems, outcomes, interventions, the individuals assigned to implement interventions, and evaluation criteria.

informal group roles Positions in the group with rights and duties directed toward other group members. These positions are not formally sanctioned.

informal support systems Family members, friends, and neighbors who can provide care and support to the individual.

informed consent The right to determine what shall be done with one's own body and mind. To provide informed consent, the patient must be given adequate information on which to base decisions about care. The patient ultimately decides the course of treatment.

inhalants Organic solvents, also known as volatile substances, that are central nervous system depressants and when inhaled cause euphoria, sedation, emotional lability, and impaired judgment.

in-home mental health care The provision of skilled mental health nursing care under the direction of a psychiatrist or physician for individuals in their residences.

initial outcomes Those outcomes written after the patient interview and assessment.

insight The ability of the individual to be aware of his or her own thoughts and feelings and to compare them with the thoughts and feelings of others.

insomnia (initial) Difficulty falling asleep.

instrumental activities Activities that facilitate or enhance the performance of activities of daily living (eg, shopping, using the telephone, transportation). These aspects are critical to consider for any older adult living alone.

integration Incorporation of disparate ethnic or religious elements of the population into a unified society; the process by which networks communicate efficiently through cellular mechanisms that synthesize information from thousands of excitatory and inhibitory chemical signals before determining whether to respond.

intensive outpatient programs Programs focused on continued stabilization and prevention of relapse in vulnerable individuals who have returned to job or school, usually with sessions running 3 days per week and lasting 3 to 4 hours per day.

interdisciplinary approach Interventions from different disciplines integrated into the delivery of patient care.

interdisciplinary treatment plan   A plan of care that identifies the patient's problems, outcomes, interventions, and members of different disciplines assigned to implement interventions, and evaluation criteria.

internal rights protection system   Patient protective mechanisms developed by the United States mental health care system's organizations to help combat any violation of mental health patients' rights, including investigating any incidents of abuse or neglect.

internalizing disorders   Anxiety disorders and depression in which the symptoms tend to be within the individual.

interoceptive conditioning   Pairing a somatic discomfort, such as dizziness or palpitations, with an impending panic attack.

interpersonal relations   Characteristic interaction patterns that occur between human beings that are the basis of emotional and social connections.

intrinsic activity   The ability of a drug to produce a biologic response when it becomes attached to its receptor.

invalidating environment   A highly personal social situation that negates the individual's emotional responses and communication.

involuntary commitment   The confined hospitalization of a person without his or her consent, but with a court order (because the person has been judged to be a danger to self or others).

ischemic cascade   Cell breakdown resulting from brain cell injury.

judgment   The ability to reach a logical decision about a situation and to choose a course after looking at and analyzing various possibilities.

kindling   Repetitive stimulation of certain tracts may facilitate conduction of impulses in the future and lead to enhancement of intense behaviors after even mild stimulation.

kleptomania   A disorder in which the patient is unable to resist the urge to steal and independently steals items that he or she could easily afford. These items are not particularly useful or wanted. The underlying issue is the act of stealing.

Korsakoff's syndrome   An amnestic syndrome in which there is a profound deficit in the ability to form new memories; associated with a variable deficit in recall of old memories despite a clear sensorium.

lability of mood   Rapid alternations of mood, usually between euphoria and irritability.

language   A higher-order aspect of formulating and comprehending verbal communication.

lateral (sylvian) fissure   Separates the inferior aspects of the frontal and parietal lobes from the temporal lobe.

lateral ventricles   The horn-shaped first and second ventricles that are the largest of the brain's ventricles.

learning disorder   A discrepancy between actual achievement and expected achievement that is based on a person's age and intellectual ability.

least restrictive environment   The patient has the right to treatment in an environment that restricts the exercise of free will to the least extent; an individual cannot be restricted to an institution when he or she can be successfully treated in the community.

life review   A therapeutic intervention using recall and memory to conduct a critical analysis of one's life.

limbic system (limbic lobe)   Structures including the septum and the fornix, as well as the amygdala, hippocampus, cingulate, parahippocampal gyrus, epithalamus, portions of the basal ganglia, paraolfactory area, and the anterior nucleus of the thalamus.

longitudinal fissure   The longest and deepest groove of the cerebrum that separates the right and left hemispheres.

loose associations   Absence of the normal connectedness of thoughts and ideas; sudden shifts without apparent relationship to preceding topic.

maintenance function   A term used to describe the informal role of group members that encourages the group to stay together.

maintenance interventions   Supportive, educational, and pharmacologic interventions, aimed at decreasing the disability associated with a disorder, that are provided on a long-term basis to individuals who have been diagnosed with a disorder.

malingering   To produce intentionally illness symptoms with an obvious self-serving goal such as being classified as disabled or avoiding work.

managed care organizations   Large health care organizations whose goals are to increase access to care and to provide the most appropriate level of services in the least restrictive setting, which includes more outpatient and alternative treatment programs, while trying to avoid costly inpatient hospitalizations; in the long term, allowing patients better access to quality services while using health care dollars wisely.

manic episode   A distinct period during which there is an abnormally and persistently elevated, expansive, or irritable mood.

memory   One aspect of cognitive function; an information storage system composed of short-term memory (retention of information over a brief period of time) and long-term memory (retention of an unlimited amount of information over an indefinite period of time).

memory   The ability to recall or reproduce what has been learned or experienced.

meningeal layer   The inner layer of dura mater that becomes continuous with the spinal dura mater and sends extensions into the brain for support and protection of the different lobes or structures.

mental disorder   A disorder that is associated with the presence of psychological distress; impairment in psychological, social, or occupational functioning; or a significantly increased risk for death, pain, disability, or an important loss of freedom.

mental health problem   A term used when signs and symptoms of mental illnesses occur but do not meet specified criteria for a disorder.

mental illness   A term used to mean all diagnosable mental disorders.

mental retardation   Significantly below-average intelligence accompanied by impaired adaptive functioning.

mental status examination   An organized systematic approach to assessment of an individual's current psychiatric condition.

mesocortical   Medial aspects of the cortex.

metabolism   Biotransformation, or the process by which a drug is altered.

metonymic speech   Use of words with similar meanings interchangeably.

middle insomnia   Waking up during the night and having difficulty returning to sleep.

milieu therapy   An approach using the total environment to provide a therapeutic community; a therapeutic environment.

misidentification   Delusions in which the person believes that a familiar person is replaced by an imposter.

mixed episode Irritability or excitement and depression occurring at the same time.

modeling Pervasive imitation; one person trying to be like another person.

mood A pervasive and sustained emotion that colors a person's perception of the world.

mood disorder A clinically significant behavioral or psychological syndrome or pattern that occurs in an individual whereby the primary alteration is evident in mood rather than in thought or perception.

moral idealism To enjoy taking passionate philosophical positions on controversial issues such as abortion, sexism, legalization of drugs, gun use, and so forth.

moral treatment An approach to curing mental illness, popular in the 1800s, which was built on the principles of kindness, compassion, and a pleasant environment.

motivational interviewing Interviewing that helps the patient clarify personal goals and increases commitment to recovery; often used in treating people with substance abuse.

multiaxial diagnostic system A diagnostic structure that includes more than one domain of information, such as the psychiatric diagnoses of the *DSM-IV-TR*.

multidisciplinary approach Several disciplines providing services to a patient at one time.

multigenerational transmission process The transmission of emotional processes from one generation to the next.

multiple sleep latency test (MSLT) A standardized procedure that measures the amount of time a person takes to fall asleep during a 20-minute period.

music therapy The controlled use of music to promote physiologic or psychological well-being.

myoclonus Twitching or clonic spasms of a muscle group.

myoglobinuria The presence of myohemoglobin in the urine due to sustained muscular rigidity and necrosis.

negative outcome criteria Goals that direct interventions to prevent negative alterations in the patient such as complications, disabilities, or unwarranted death.

neglect Failure to protect from injury or to provide for the physical, psychological, and medical needs of a child or dependent elder.

neologisms Words that are made up that have no common meaning and are not recognized.

neuritic plaques Extracellular lesions consisting of β-amyloid protein and apolipoprotein A (apoA) cores that form in the nucleus basalis of Meynert, gradually increase in number, and are abnormally distributed throughout the cholinergic system.

neurofibrillary tangles Fibrous proteins, or *tau proteins*, that are chemically altered and twisted together and spread throughout the brain interfering with nerve functioning in cholinergic neurons. It is hypothesized that formation of these neurofibrillary tangles are related to the apolipoprotein E_4 (apoE_4).

neurohormones Hormones produced by cells within the nervous system, such as antidiuretic hormone (ADH).

neuroleptic malignant syndrome A syndrome caused by neuroleptic medications that are dopamine receptor blockers. The classic signs and symptoms include hyperthermia, lead-pipe rigidity, changes in mental status, and autonomic nervous system changes.

neuropeptide Y A recently discovered 36–amino-acid peptide that is a potent stimulator of feeding behavior especially selective for foods heavy in carbohydrates.

neuropeptides Short chains of amino acids that exist in the central nervous system and have a number of important roles, including as neurotransmitters, neuromodulators, or neurohormones.

neuropsychiatric disorders Those disease processes, toxic exposures, traumatic injuries, or other causes that change the structures in the central nervous system and produce psychiatric as well as neurologic symptoms.

neuropsychiatry A subspecialty of psychiatry that combines neurology and psychiatry.

neurotransmitters Small molecules that directly and indirectly control the opening or closing of ion channels.

nociceptive Pertaining to a neural receptor for painful stimuli.

nonbizarre delusions Beliefs that are characterized by adherence to possible situations that could appear in real life and are plausible in the context of the person's ethnic and cultural background.

non-REM (NREM) sleep A sleep cycle state of nonrapid eye movement.

nonverbal communication The gestures, expressions, and body language used in communications between the nurse and the patient.

no-suicide contract Written or verbal agreement between the health care professional and the patient that the patient will not engage in suicidal behavior for a specific period of time.

nuclear family Two or more people related by blood, marriage, or adoption.

nuclear family emotional process Patterns of emotional functioning in a family within single generations.

nurse–patient relationship A time-limited interpersonal process with definable phases during which the patient is able to consider alternative behaviors, try new health care strategies, and discuss complex health problems.

nursing diagnosis A clinical judgment about the individual, family, or community response to actual or potential health problems and life processes. It provides the basis for the selection of interventions and outcomes.

nursing intervention Nursing activities that promote and foster health, assess dysfunction, assist patients to regain or improve their coping abilities, or prevent further disabilities.

negative symptoms A lessening or loss of normal functions, such as restriction or flattening in the range of intensity of emotion; reduced fluency and productivity of thought and speech; withdrawal and inability to initiate and persist in goal-directed activity; and inability to experience pleasure.

nursing process The basis of clinical decision making and nursing actions.

object permanence The awareness that an object or person exists when not physically seen; behavior that results in a person attaining or retaining proximity to some other differentiated and preferred individual.

object relations The psychological attachment to another person or object.

observation Ongoing assessment of the patient's mental and health status to identify and subvert any potential problems.

obsessive-compulsive disorder (OCD) A disorder characterized by intrusive thoughts that are difficult to dislodge (obsessions) and ritualized behaviors that the person feels driven to perform (compulsions).

oculogyric crisis A medication side effect resulting from an imbalance of dopamine and acetylcholine, in which the muscles that control eye movements tense and pull the eyeball so that the patient is looking toward the ceiling; may be followed by torticollis or retrocollis.

ongoing assessments Shorter and more focused assessments made to monitor the progress and outcomes of the interventions implemented.

open group A group in which new members can join at any time.

operant behavior A type of learning that is a consequence of a particular behavioral response, not a specific stimulus.

opiate Any substance that binds to an opiate receptor in the brain to produce an agonist action, causing central nervous system depression, sleep or stupor, and analgesia.

orgasmic disorders Sexual dysfunction disorders characterized by the inability to reach an orgasm by any means, either alone or with a partner, or achieving orgasm only during masturbation or partner stimulation, but not during intercourse.

orientation phase The first phase of the nurse–patient relationship in which the nurse and the patient get to know each other. During this phase, the patient develops a sense of trust.

outcomes A patient's response to care received; the end result of the process of nursing.

outpatient detoxification A specialized form of partial hospitalization for patients requiring medical supervision during withdrawal from alcohol or other addictive substances, with or without use of a 23-hour bed during the initial withdrawal phase, including a requirement of attending a program 5 or 6 days per week for a period of 1 to 2 weeks.

panic A normal but extreme overwhelming form of anxiety often experienced when an individual is placed in a real or perceived life-threatening situation.

panic attacks Discrete periods of intense fear or discomfort that are accompanied by significant somatic or cognitive symptoms.

panic control treatment Systematic structured exposure to panic-invoking sensations such as dizziness, hyperventilation, tightness in chest, and sweating.

panicogenic Substances that produce panic attacks.

paranoia Suspiciousness and guardedness that is unrealistic and often accompanied by grandiosity.

paraphilias Recurrent, intense sexual urges, fantasies, or behaviors that involve unusual objects, activities, or situations and cause clinically significant distress or impairment in social, occupational, or other important areas of functioning.

parasomnia Disorders of abnormal physiologic or behavioral events that occur in relationship to sleep, specific sleep stages, or during transition from sleep to wakefulness.

parasuicide Deliberate self-injurious behavior accompanied by an intent to harm oneself.

parietal-occipital sulcus Separates the occipital lobe from the parietal lobe.

partial hospitalization A type of outpatient program that provides services to patients who spend only part of a 24-hour period in the facility but that does not provide overnight care; usually, the programs run 5 days per week for about 6 hours per day.

passive listening A nontherapeutic mode of interaction that involves sitting quietly and allowing the patient to talk without focusing on guiding the thought process; includes body language that communicates boredom, indifference, or hostility.

pedophilia A behavior associated with paraphilias involving sexual activity with a child (usually 13 years of age or younger) by an individual at least 15 years of age (or 5 years older than the child).

peer assistance programs Programs developed by state nurses' associations to assist nurses in securing evaluation, treatment, monitoring, and ongoing support.

peptide YY Related to neuropeptide Y, this peptide stimulates feeding behavior even more potently than neuropeptide Y.

perceptions The awareness reached as a result of sensory inputs of real stimuli that are usually altered.

persecutory delusions Delusions in which the person believes that he or she is being conspired against, cheated, spied on, followed, poisoned, drugged, maliciously maligned, harassed, or obstructed in the pursuit of long-term goals.

personal identity Knowing "who I am"; formed through the numerous biologic, psychological, and social challenges and demands faced throughout the stages of life.

personality A complex pattern of psychological characteristics, largely outside a person's awareness, that are not easily altered.

personality disorder An enduring pattern of inner experience and behavior that deviates markedly from the expectations of the individual's culture; is pervasive and inflexible; has an onset in adolescence or early adulthood; is stable over time; and leads to distress or impairment.

person–environment relationship The interaction between the individual and the environment that changes throughout the stress experience.

pet therapy The therapeutic use of animals as pets to promote physical, psychological, or social well-being.

pharmacodynamics The study of the biologic actions of drugs on living tissue and the human body in general.

pharmacokinetics The study of how the human body processes a drug, including absorption, distribution, metabolism, and elimination.

phenomena of concern Human responses to actual or potential health problems.

phobia Persistent, unrealistic fears of situations, objects, or activities that often lead to avoidance behaviors.

phonologic processing Thought to be the cause of reading disability; a process that involves the discrimination and interpretation of speech sounds. Reading disability is believed to be caused by some disturbance in the development of the left hemisphere.

phototherapy Also known as *light therapy;* involves exposing the patient to an artificial light source during winter months to relieve seasonal depression.

physical abuse Using physical force or a weapon against a person to do bodily injury.

physical restraints The application of wrist, leg, and body straps made of leather or cloth for the purpose of controlling or managing behavior.

pia mater The third layer of the central nervous system, in Latin, "soft mother."

pineal body Located in the epithalamus; contains secretory cells that emit the neurohormone melatonin (as well as other substances), which has been associated with sleep and emotional disorders and modulation of immune function.

plasticity Capability to change or adapt in form or physiology.

point prevalence Basic measure that refers to the proportion of individuals in a population who have a particular disorder at a specified point in time.

polydipsia Excessive thirst that can be chronic in patients with severe mental illness.

polypharmacy Use of several different medications at one time.

polysomnography   A special procedure that involves the recording of the electroencephalogram throughout the night. This procedure is usually conducted in a sleep laboratory.

polyuria   Excessive excretion of urine.

positive outcome criteria   Goals that direct interventions that provide the patient with improved health status, optimal levels of coping, maintenance of present optimal level of health, optimal adaptation to deterioration of health status, or collaboration and satisfaction with health care providers.

positive self-talk   Countering fearful or negative thoughts by using preplanned and rehearsed positive coping statements.

positive symptoms   An excess or distortion of normal functions, including delusions and hallucinations.

posttraumatic stress disorder   A mental disorder characterized by persistent, distressing symptoms lasting longer than 1 month after exposure to an extreme traumatic stressor.

prejudice   A hostile attitude toward others who belong to a particular group that is considered by some to have objectionable characteristics.

premature ejaculation   A male orgasmic disorder defined as the inability to control ejaculation before, during, or shortly after intromission; ejaculation before the individual desires it; or the inability to sustain erection long enough to satisfy the partner 50% of the time.

prevalence   The total number of people who have a particular disorder within a given population at a specific time.

prevention   Interventions used before the initial onset of a disorder that become distinct from the treatment.

priapism   A rare condition of prolonged and painful erection, usually without sexual desire; often the result of neurologic or vascular impairment.

privacy   That part of an individual's personal life that is not governed by society's laws and governmental intrusion.

problem-focused coping   A type of coping that actually changes the person–environment relationship.

process recording   A verbatim transcript of a verbal interaction usually organized according to the nurse–patient interaction. It often includes analysis of the interaction.

professional caring   Cognitively learned, practiced, and transmitted knowledge learned formally and informally through various schools of professional nursing education (Leininger).

projective identification   A psychoanalytic term used to describe behavior of people with borderline personality disorder when they falsely attribute to others their own unacceptable feelings, impulses, or thoughts.

provider domain outcome statements   Statements that describe behaviors and attitudes of nursing staff and responses to nurse–patient relationships.

pseudodementia   Memory difficulties in older adults with major depression (may be mistaken for early signs of dementia).

pseudoparkinsonism   Sometimes referred to as *drug-induced parkinsonism;* presents identically as Parkinson's disease without the same destruction of dopaminergic cells.

psychiatric pluralism   An integration of human biologic functions with the environment that was advocated by Meyer.

psychiatric rehabilitation programs   Programs that are focused on reintegrating people with psychiatric disabilities back into the community through work, educational, and social avenues while also addressing their medical and residential needs.

psychoanalytic movement   Freud's radical approach to psychiatric mental health care, which involved using a new technique called *psychoanalysis* based on unconscious motivations for behavior or drives.

psychodrama   A group role-playing technique used to encourage expression of emotion and exploration of problems.

psychoeducation   An educational approach used to enhance knowledge and shape behavior.

psychoeducational programs   A form of mental health intervention in which basic coping skills for dealing with various stressors are taught.

psychoendocrinology   The study of the relationships among the nervous system, endocrine system, and behavior.

psychoimmunology   The study of immunology as it relates to emotions and behavior.

psychopathy   Refers to individuals who behave impulsively and are interpersonally irresponsible, act hastily and spontaneously, are shortsighted, and fail to plan ahead or consider alternatives. Equated with antisocial personality disorder.

psychopharmacology   Subspecialty of pharmacology that includes medications used to affect the brain and behaviors related to psychiatric disorders.

psychosis   A state in which the individual is experiencing hallucinations, delusions, or disorganized thoughts, speech, or behavior.

psychosocial dimension   Part of the biopsychosocial model that explains the importance of the internal psychological processes of thoughts, feelings, and behavior (interpersonal dynamics) in influencing one's emotion, cognition, and behavior.

psychosocial theory   A theoretic argument or view from the early 1900s that mental disorders result from environmental and social deprivation.

psychosomatic   Conditions in which a psychological state contributes to the development of a physical illness.

public welfare domain outcome statements   Statements that show responses or behaviors that provide examples of preventing harm to self, family, and community.

purging   A compensatory behavior to rid oneself of food already eaten by means of self-induced vomiting or the use of laxatives, enemas, or diuretics.

pyromania   Irresistible impulses to start fires.

rapidly cycling bipolar disorder   The occurrence of four or more mood episodes during the past 12 months.

rapport   A series of interrelated thoughts and feelings that describe purposeful interactions between individuals; including empathy, compassion, sympathy, a nonjudgmental attitude, and respect for others.

rate   A proportion of the cases in the population when compared to the total population. It is expressed as a fraction in which the numerator is the number of cases, and the denominator is the total number in the population, including the cases and noncases.

reaction time   The lapse of time between stimulus and response.

receptor   Site to which a neurotransmitter substance can specifically adhere to produce a change in the cell membrane, serving a physiologic regulatory function.

recovery   A period of full remission for a minimum of 8 weeks.

referential thinking   Belief that neutral stimuli have special meaning to the individual, such as a television commentator speaking directly to the individual.

rehabilitative domain outcome statements Statements that provide examples of improvement or restoration of social and vocational functioning, leading to independent living.

reintegration A term used to describe the process of returning to the community through work, educational, and social avenues.

relapse Recurrence or marked increase in severity of the symptoms of the disease, especially following a period of apparent improvement or stability; the recurrence of alcohol- or drug-dependent behavior in an individual who has previously achieved and maintained abstinence for a significant time beyond the period of detoxification.

related factors Those factors (biologic, maturational, social, and treatment-related) that influence a health status change.

relaxation A mental health intervention that promotes comfort, reduces anxiety, alleviates stress, reduces pain, and prevents aggressive behavior.

religiosity A psychiatric symptom characterized by excessive or affected piety.

REM sleep A sleep cycle state of rapid eye movement.

reminiscence Thinking about or relating past experiences.

reminiscence therapy The process of looking back on specific times or events in one's life.

remission A restoration of baseline psychological functioning.

remotivation therapy The encouragement of interest and enthusiasm about events in one's life or the world.

residential treatment facility A facility that requires special accreditation and specialized licensing from the state that generally treats patients for 6 months or longer.

resolution phase The termination phase of the nurse–patient relationship that lasts from the time the problems are resolved to the close of the relationship.

restraint The use of any manual, physical, or mechanical device or material, which when attached to the patient's body (usually to the arms and legs) restricts the patient's movements.

retrocollis The neck muscles pull the head back.

revised outcomes Those outcomes written after each evaluation.

reward-seeking behavior A behavior that is initiated to gain a pleasurable outcome, such as feeling good, being rewarded, or gaining recognition or attention.

risk factors Characteristics that do not cause the disorder or problem and are not symptoms of the illness, but rather are factors that have been shown to influence the likelihood of developing a disorder.

role An individual's social position and function within an environment.

ruminations Repetitive thoughts that are forced into a patient's consciousness even when unwanted; when a person goes over and over the same ideas endlessly; part of an obsessive style of thinking.

safety Care that supports protection against harm.

satiety Internal signals that indicate one has had enough to eat.

schema A cognitive structure that screens, codes, and evaluates the incoming stimuli through which the individual interprets events.

schizoaffective disorder An interrupted period of illness during which at some point there is a major depressive, manic, or mixed episode, along with two of the following symptoms of schizophrenia: delusions, hallucinations, disorganized speech, disorganized or catatonic behavior, or negative symptoms (affective flattening, alogia, or avolition).

school phobia Anxiety in which the child refuses to attend school in order to stay at home and with the primary attachment figure. School phobia is a common presenting complaint in child psychiatric clinics and may be part of separation anxiety, general anxiety, social phobia, obsessive-compulsive disorder, depression, or conduct disorder.

screening assessments The collection of data with which to identify individuals who have not as yet recognized the presence of symptoms due to a psychiatric disorder; who have risk factors for development of a psychiatric disorder; or who may be experiencing emotional difficulties but have not yet formally sought treatment.

seclusion Solitary confinement in a full protective environment for the purpose of safety or behavior management.

sedative-hypnotics Medications that induce sleep and reduce anxiety.

segregation Separation of a cultural group from the majority through legally sanctioned societal practices.

selective preventive interventions Preventive interventions that are targeted to individuals or a subgroup of the population whose risk for a disorder is higher than average.

selectivity The ability of a drug to be specific for a particular receptor, interacting only with specific receptors in the areas of the body where the receptors occur and therefore not affecting tissues and organs where these receptors do not occur.

self-awareness Being cognizant of one's own beliefs, thought motivations, biases, physical and emotional limitations, and the impact one may have on others.

self-concept The sum of beliefs about oneself, which develops over time.

self-determinism The right to choose one's own health-related behaviors, which at times differ from those recommended by health professionals.

self-disclosure The act of revealing personal information about oneself.

self-efficacy Self-effectiveness.

self-esteem Attitude about oneself.

self-identity Formed through the integration of social and occupational roles and affiliations, self-attributed personality traits, attitudes about gender roles, beliefs about sexuality and intimacy, long-term goals, political ideology, and religious beliefs. Without an adequately formed identity, goal-directed behavior is impaired and interpersonal relationships are disrupted.

self-monitoring Observing and recording one's own information, usually behavior, thoughts, or feelings.

sensate focus A method for partners to learn what each finds sexually arousing and to learn to communicate those preferences. It begins with nongenital contact and gradually includes genital touch and.

separation-individuation A process during which the child develops a sense of self, a permanent sense of significant others (object constancy), and an integration of both bad and good as a component of the self-concept.

serotonin Centrally mediates the release of endorphin. Along with histamine and bradykinin, serotonin stimulates the pain receptors to generate experienced pain. Serotonin is involved in inhibiting gastric secretion, stimulating smooth muscle, and serving as a central neurotransmitter.

serotonin syndrome A toxic side effect that occurs as a result of the newer serotonergic drugs; this syndrome is thought to be caused by hyperstimulation of the 5-HT receptor in the brain stem and spinal cord.

severe and persistent mental illness Mental disorders that are long term and have recurring periods of exacerbation and remission.

sex role identity Outward expression of gender.

sexual abuse Sexual misconduct toward another person.

sexual addiction Out-of-control sexual behaviors that are somewhat tolerated by society (eg, compulsive masturbation, promiscuity).

sexual aversion (disorder) A sexual desire disorder characterized by a phobic reaction to real or anticipated sexual activity; occurs far more frequently in women than men.

sexual desire Ability, interest, or willingness to receive, or a motivational state to seek, sexual stimulation.

sexual orientation (sexual preference) An individual's feelings of sexual attraction and erotic potential.

sexuality Basic dimension of every individual's personality, undergoing periods of growth and development, and influenced by biologic and psychosocial factors.

side effects Unwanted or untoward effects of medications.

sleep architecture A predictable pattern during a night's sleep that includes the timing, amount, and distribution of REM and NREM stages.

sleep efficiency Expressed as a percentage of time in bed spent asleep.

sleep latency Amount of time it takes for an individual to fall asleep.

sleep paralysis Being unable to move or speak when falling asleep or waking.

social change The structural and cultural evolution of society, which is dependent on a complex interaction between economic and productivity factors as well as among political, religious, philosophical, and scientific ideas.

social dimension Part of the biopsychosocial model that accounts for the influence of social forces encompassing family, community, and cultural settings.

social distance Degree to which the values of a formal organization and its primary group members differ.

social functioning Performance of daily activities within the context of interpersonal relations and family and community roles.

social network Linkages among a defined set of people, among whom there are personal contacts.

social skills training A psychoeducational approach that involves instruction, feedback, support, and practice with learning behaviors that helps people interact more effectively with peers, and also children with adults.

social support Positive and harmonious interpersonal interactions that occur within social relationships.

somatization The manifestation of psychological distress as physical symptoms.

somatization disorder A polysymptomatic disorder that begins before age 30 years, extends over a period of years, and is characterized by a combination of pain, gastrointestinal, sexual, and psychoneurologic symptoms.

speech The motor aspects of speaking.

spinal cord A long, cylindrical collection of neural fibers continuous with the brain stem, housed within the vertebral column.

spirituality Beliefs and values related to hope and meaning in life.

stabilization Short-term care, lasting 7 to 14 days, with a primary focus on control of precipitating symptoms with medications, behavioral interventions, and coordination with other agencies for appropriate aftercare.

standards of care Standards that are organized around the nursing process and include assessment, diagnosis, outcome identification, planning, and implementation.

standards Authoritative statements established by professional organizations that describe the responsibilities for which nurses are accountable but that are not legally binding unless they are incorporated into a legal document, such as a nurse practice act or state board rules and regulations.

stereotypic behavior Repetitive, driven, nonfunctional, and potentially self-injurious behavior, such as head banging, rocking, and hand flapping, seen in autistic disorder, with an extraordinary insistence on sameness.

stereotyping Expecting individuals to behave in a manner that conforms to a negative perception of the cultural group to which they belong.

stereotypy Repetitive, purposeless movements that are idiosyncratic to the individual and to some degree outside of the individual's control.

stigmatization A process of assigning negative characteristics and identity to a person or group and causing that person or group to feel unaccepted, devalued, ostracized, and isolated from the larger society.

stranger anxiety Fear when approached by a person unknown to oneself.

stress (stressors) A pressure or force that puts strain on the system; can be either positive or negative but most often is used to mean a negative mental or physical tension or strain.

structured interaction Purposeful interaction that allows patients to interact with others in a way that is useful to them.

subcortical dementia Dementia that is caused by dysfunction or deterioration of deep gray- or white-matter structures inside the brain and brain stem.

subcortical Structures inside the hemispheres and beneath the cortex.

substance P The most common nociceptive transmitter that is released and transported along the central and peripheral pain synapses in the presence of noxious stimuli.

subsystems A systems term used by family theorists to describe subgroups of family members who join together for various activities.

suicidal ideation Thinking about and planning one's own death without actually engaging in self-harm.

suicide The act of killing oneself voluntarily.

surveillance The ongoing collection and analysis of information about patients and their environments for use in promoting and maintaining patient safety.

symbolism The use of a word or a phrase to represent an object, event, or feeling.

synapse The region across which nerve impulses are transmitted through the action of a neurotransmitter.

systematic desensitization A method used to desensitize patients to anxiety-provoking situations by exposing the patient to a hierarchy of feared situations. Patient is taught to use muscle relaxation as levels of anxiety increase through multisituational exposure.

tangentiality When the topic of conversation changes to an entirely different topic that is within a logical progression but causes a permanent detour from the original focus.

tardive dyskinesia A late-appearing extrapyramidal side effect of antipsychotic medication that includes abnormal involuntary movements in the mouth, tongue, and jaw such as lip smacking, sucking, puckering, tongue protrusion, the bon-bon sign, athetoid (worm-like) movements of the tongue, and chewing.

target risk factors Specific biopsychosocial stressors, such as genetic predisposition and traumatic situations, that are associated with mental disorders.

target symptoms Specific symptoms for which psychiatric medications are prescribed, such as hallucinations, delusions, paranoia, agitation, assaultive behavior, bizarre ideation, social withdrawal, disorientation, catatonia, blunted affect, thought blocking, insomnia, and anorexia.

task function   The group role that focuses on the task of the group.

temperament   A person's characteristic intensity, rhythmicity, adaptability, energy expenditure, and mood.

tenuous stability   Fragile personality patterns that lack resiliency under subjective stress.

terminal insomnia   Waking up too early and being unable to return to sleep.

thalamus   Thought to play a role in controlling electrical activity in the cortex; provides the relay mechanism for information to and from the cerebrum.

themes   Concerns or feelings expressed symbolically by the patient.

therapeutic communication   The ongoing process of interaction in which meaning emerges; may be verbal or nonverbal.

therapeutic foster care   The placement of patients in residences of families specially trained to handle individuals with mental illnesses.

therapeutic index   A ratio of the maximum nontoxic dose to the minimum effective dose.

thought stopping   A practice in which a person identifies negative feelings and thoughts that exist together, says "stop," and then engages in a distracting activity.

tolerance   A gradual decrease in the action of a drug at a given dose or concentration in the blood.

torticollis   The neck muscles pull the head to the side.

toxicity   The point at which concentrations of a drug in the blood stream become harmful or poisonous to the body.

transaction   Transfer of value between two or more individuals.

transfer   The formal shifting of responsibility for the care of an individual from one clinician to another or from one care unit to another.

transference   The unconscious assignment to others of feelings and attitudes that were originally associated with important figures such as parents or siblings.

transitional object   A symbolic attachment figure, such as a blanket or a stuffed animal, that a child may cling to when a parent is not available.

transition times   A term used to describe times of addition, subtraction, or change in status of family members.

transvestic fetishism   A fetish that applies generally to the heterosexual male who cross-dresses for the purpose of sexual excitement.

traumatic bonding   A strong emotional attachment between an abused person and his or her abuser, formed as a result of the cycle of violence.

triad   A group consisting of three people.

triangles   A three-person system and the smallest stable unit in human relations.

trichotillomania   Chronic, self-destructive hair pulling that results in noticeable hair loss, usually in the crown, occipital, or parietal areas, though sometimes of the eyebrows and eyelashes.

twelve-step programs   Anonymous self-help groups such as Alcoholics Anonymous that use 12 steps to recovery as part of their program.

twenty-three–hour beds   A specialized type of short-term treatment that is a relatively new trend for inpatient treatment (previously referred to as *observation units*); admits individuals to an inpatient setting, then discharges them before 24 hours.

unipolar   A term used to describe one abnormal mood state, usually depression.

universal preventive interventions   Preventive interventions that are targeted to everyone within a general public or whole population group.

urine specific gravity   A measure of the degree of concentration of solutes in urine.

use   The drinking of alcohol or the swallowing, smoking, sniffing, or injecting of a mind-altering substance.

vaginismus   A psychologically induced, spastic, involuntary constriction of the perineal and outer vaginal muscles due to imagined, anticipated, or actual attempts at vaginal penetration.

validation   An interactive process that affirms the patient's beliefs, no matter how bizarre.

ventricles   The four cavities of the brain.

verbal communication   The use of the spoken word, including its underlying emotion, context, and connotation.

verbigeration   Purposeless repetition of words or phrases.

vicious circles of behavior   A term used to describe the tendency to become trapped in rigid and inflexible patterns of behavior that are self-defeating.

violence (violent behavior)   A physical act of force intended to cause harm to a person or an object and to convey the message that the perpetrator's, and not the victim's, point of view is correct.

voluntary admission (committed)   The legal status of a patient who has consented to being admitted to the hospital for treatment, during which time he or she maintains all civil rights and is free to leave at any time, even if it is against medical advice.

voyeurism   A disorder that involves "peeping" at unsuspecting people who are nude, undressing, or engaged in sexual activity, for the purpose of sexual excitement.

water intoxication   A severe state of fluid overload; this disorder develops when large amounts of water are ingested and serum sodium levels rapidly fall to a level below 120 mEq/L. The specific etiology of this disorder is unknown.

waxy flexibility   Posture held in an odd or unusual fixed position for extended periods of time.

Wernicke's area   An area in the left superior temporal gyrus of the brain thought to be responsible for comprehension of speech.

Wernicke's syndrome   An alcohol-induced amnestic disorder caused by a thiamine-deficient diet and characterized by diplopia, hyperactivity, and delirium.

withdrawal   The adverse physical and psychological symptoms that occur when a person ceases to use a substance.

word salad   A string of words that are not connected in any way.

working phase   The second phase of the nurse–patient relationship, in which patients can examine specific problems and learn new ways of approaching them.

xerostomia   Dry mouth.

zeitgebers   specific events that function as time givers or synchronizers and that result in the setting of biologic rhythms.

DISORDERS USUALLY FIRST DIAGNOSED IN INFANCY, CHILDHOOD, OR ADOLESCENCE

Mental Retardation

Note: These are coded on Axis II.

317	Mild Mental Retardation
318.0	Moderate Mental Retardation
318.1	Severe Mental Retardation
318.2	Profound Mental Retardation
319	Mental Retardation, Severity Unspecified

Learning Disorders

315.00	Reading Disorders
315.1	Mathematics Disorders
315.2	Disorder of Written Expression
315.9	Learning Disorder NOS

Motor Skills Disorder

315.4	Developmental Coordination Disorder

Communication Disorders

315.31	Expressive Language Disorder
315.31	Mixed Receptive-Expressive Language Disorder
315.39	Phonological Disorder
307.0	Stuttering
307.9	Communication Disorder NOS

Pervasive Developmental Disorders

299.00	Autistic Disorder
299.80	Rett's Disorder

NOS = not otherwise specified.

An *x* appearing in a diagnostic code indicates that a specific code number is required.

An **ellipsis** (. . .) is used in the names of certain disorders to indicate that the name of a specific mental disorder or general medical condition should be inserted when recording the name (eg, 293 Delirium Due to Hypothyroidism).

*Indicate the General Medical Condition.

**Refer to Substance-Related Disorders for substance-specific codes.

***Indicate the Axis I or Axis II Disorder.

American Psychiatric Association. (2000). *Diagnostic and statistical manual of mental disorders.* (4th ed., Text revision). Washington, DC: Author.

299.10	Childhood Disintegrative Disorder
299.80	Asperger's Disorder
299.80	Pervasive Developmental Disorder NOS

Attention-Deficit and Disruptive Behavior Disorders

314.xx	Attention-Deficit/Hyperactivity Disorder
.01	Combined Type
.00	Predominantly Inattentive Type
.01	Predominantly Hyperactive-Impulsive Type
314.9	Attention-Deficit/Hyperactivity Disorder NOS
312.8	Conduct Disorder *Specify type:* Childhood-Onset/Adolescent-Onset
313.81	Oppositional Defiant Disorder
312.9	Disruptive Behavior Disorder NOS

Feeding and Eating Disorders of Infancy or Early Childhood

307.52	Pica
307.53	Rumination Disorder
307.59	Feeding Disorder of Infancy or Early Childhood

Tic Disorders

307.23	Tourette's Disorder
307.22	Chronic Motor or Vocal Tic Disorder
307.21	Transient Tic Disorder *Specify if:* Single Episode/Recurrent
307.20	Tic Disorder NOS

Elimination Disorders

—.-	Encopresis
787.6	With Constipation and Overflow Incontinence
307.7	Without Constipation and Overflow Incontinence
307.6	Enuresis (Not Due to a General Medical Condition) *Specify type:* Nocturnal Only/Diurnal Only/Nocturnal and Diurnal

Other Disorders of Infancy, Childhood, or Adolescence

309.21 Separation and Anxiety Disorder
        Specify if: Early Onset
313.23 Selective Mutism
313.89 Reactive Attachment Disorder of Infancy or Early Childhood
        Specify type: Inhibited/Disinhibited
307.3   Stereotypic Movement Disorder
        Specify if: With Self-Injurious Behavior
313.9   Disorder of Infancy, Childhood, or Adolescence NOS

DELIRIUM, DEMENTIA, AND AMNESTIC AND OTHER COGNITIVE DISORDERS

Delirium

293.0   Delirium Due to . . . *
—.-   Substance Intoxication Delirium**
—.-   Substance Withdrawal Delirium**
—.-   Delirium Due to Multiple Etiologies (code each of the specific etiologies)
780.09 Delirium NOS

Dementia

294.xx Dementia of the Alzheimer's Type, With Early Onset
  .10   Without Behavioral Disturbance
  .11   With Behavioral Disturbance
294.xx Dementia of the Alzheimer's Type, With Late Onset
  .10   Without Behavioral Disturbance
  .11   With Behavioral Disturbance
290.xx Vascular Dementia
  .40   Uncomplicated
  .41   With Delirium
  .42   With Delusions
  .43   With Depressed Mood
        Specify if: With Behavioral Disturbance
294.1x Dementia Due to HIV Disease
294.1x Dementia Due to Head Trauma
294.1x Dementia Due to Parkinson's Disease
294.1x Dementia Due to Huntington's Disease
294.10 Dementia Due to Pick's Disease
290.10 Dementia Due to Creutzfeldt-Jakob Disease
294.1   Dementia Due to . . . [Indicate the General Medical Condition not listed above]
—.-   Substance-Induced Persisting Dementia**
—.-   Dementia Due to Multiple Etiologies (code each of the specific etiologies)
294.8   Dementia NOS

Amnestic Disorders

294.0   Amnestic Disorder Due to . . . *
        Specify if: Transient/Chronic
—.-   Substance-Induced Persisting Amnestic Disorder**
294.8   Amnestic Disorder NOS

Other Cognitive Disorders

294.9   Cognitive Disorder NOS

MENTAL DISORDERS DUE TO A GENERAL MEDICAL CONDITION NOT ELSEWHERE CLASSIFIED

293.89 Catatonic Disorder Due to . . . *
310.0   Personality Change Due to . . . *
        Specify type: Labile/Disinhibited/Aggressive/Apathetic/Paranoid/Other/Combined/Unspecified
293.9   Mental Disorder NOS Due to . . . *

SUBSTANCE-RELATED DISORDERS

The following specifiers may be applied to Substance Dependence:

With Physiological Dependence/Without Physiological Dependence
Early Full Remission/Early Partial Remission
Sustained Full Remission/Sustained Partial Remission
On Agonist Therapy/In a Controlled Environment

The following specifiers apply to Substance-Induced Disorders as noted:

[I]With Onset During Intoxication/[W]With Onset During Withdrawal

Alcohol-Related Disorders

Alcohol Use Disorders

303.90 Alcohol Dependence
305.00 Alcohol Abuse

Alcohol-Induced Disorders

303.00 Alcohol Intoxications
291.8   Alcohol Withdrawal
        Specify if: With Perceptual Disturbances
291.0   Alcohol Intoxication Delirium
291.0   Alcohol Withdrawal Delirium
291.2   Alcohol-Induced Persisting Dementia
291.1   Alcohol-Induced Persisting Amnestic Disorder

291.x   Alcohol-Induced Psychotic Disorder
.5   With Delusions[I, W]
.3   With Hallucinations[I, W]
291.8   Alcohol-Induced Mood Disorder[I, W]
291.8   Alcohol-Induced Anxiety Disorder[I, W]
291.8   Alcohol-Induced Sexual Dysfunction[I]
291.   Alcohol-Induced Sleep Disorder[I, W]
291.9   Alcohol-Related Disorder NOS

Amphetamine (or Amphetamine-Like)-Related Disorders

Amphetamine Use Disorders

304.40 Amphetamine Dependence*
305.70 Amphetamine Abuse

Amphetamine-Induced Disorders

292.89 Amphetamine Intoxication
        Specify if: With Perceptual Disturbances
292.0   Amphetamine Withdrawal
292.81 Amphetamine Intoxication Delirium
292.xx Amphetamine-Induced Psychotic Disorder
.11   With Delusions[I]
.12   With Hallucinations[I]
292.84 Amphetamine-Induced Mood Disorder[I, W]
292.89 Amphetamine-Induced Anxiety Disorder[I]
292.89 Amphetamine-Induced Sexual Dysfunction[I]
292.89 Amphetamine-Induced Sleep Disorder[I, W]
292.9   Amphetamine-Related Disorder NOS

Caffeine-Related Disorders

Caffeine-Induced Disorders

305.90 Caffeine Intoxication
292.89 Caffeine-Induced Anxiety Disorder[I]
292.89 Caffeine-Induced Sleep Disorder[I]
292.9   Caffeine-Related Disorder NOS

Cannabis-Related Disorders

Cannabis Use Disorders

304.30 Cannabis Dependence*
305.20 Cannabis Abuse

Cannabis-Induced Disorders

292.89 Cannabis Intoxication
        Specify if: With Perceptual Disturbances
292.81 Cannabis Intoxication Delirium
292.xx Cannabis-Induced Psychotic Disorder
.11   With Delusions[I]
.12   With Hallucinations[I]

292.89 Cannabis-Induced Anxiety Disorder
292.9   Cannabis-Related Disorder NOS

Cocaine-Related Disorders

Cocaine Use Disorders

304.20 Cocaine Dependence*
305.60 Cocaine Abuse

Cocaine-Induced Disorders

292.89 Cocaine Intoxication
        Specify if: With Perceptual Disturbances
292.0   Cocaine Withdrawal
292.81 Cocaine Intoxication Delirium
292.xx Cocaine-Induced Psychotic Disorder
.11   With Delusions[I]
.12   With Hallucinations[I]
292.84 Cocaine-Induced Mood Disorder[I, W]
292.89 Cocaine-Induced Anxiety Disorder[I, W]
292.89 Cocaine-Induced Sexual Dysfunction[I]
292.89 Cocaine-Induced Sleep Disorder[I, W]
292.9   Cocaine-Related Disorder NOS

Hallucinogen-Related Disorders

Hallucinogen-Use Disorders

304.50 Hallucinogen Dependence*
305.30 Hallucinogen Abuse

Hallucinogen-Induced Disorders

292.89 Hallucinogen Intoxication
292.89 Hallucinogen Persisting Perception
        Disorder (Flashbacks)
292.81 Hallucinogen Intoxication Delirium
292.xx Hallucinogen-Induced Psychotic Disorder
.11   With Delusions[I]
.12   With Hallucinations[I]
292.84 Hallucinogen-Induced Mood Disorder[I]
292.89 Hallucinogen-Induced Anxiety Disorder[I]
292.9   Hallucinogen-Related Disorder NOS

Inhalant-Related Disorders

Inhalant Use Disorders

304.60 Inhalant Dependence*
305.90 Inhalant Abuse

Inhalant-Induced Disorders

292.89 Inhalant Intoxication
292.81 Inhalant Intoxication Delirium
292.82 Inhalant-Induced Persisting Dementia
292.xx Inhalant-Induced Psychotic Disorder
.11   With Delusions[I]

.12   With Hallucinations*
292.84 Inhalant-Induced Mood Disorder[I]
292.89 Inhalant-Induced Anxiety Disorder[I]
292.9   Inhalant-Related Disorder NOS

Nicotine-Related Disorders

Nicotine Use Disorder

305.10 Nicotine Dependence*

Nicotine-Induced Disorder

292.0   Nicotine Withdrawal
292.9   Nicotine-Related Disorder NOS

Opioid-Related Disorders

Opioid Use Disorders

304.00 Opioid Dependence*
305.50 Opioid Abuse

Opioid-Induced Disorders

292.89 Opioid Intoxication
          Specify if: With Perceptual Disturbances
292.0   Opioid Withdrawal
292.81 Opioid Intoxication Delirium
292.xx Opioid-Induced Psychotic Disorders
.11   With Delusions[I]
.12   With Hallucinations[I]
292.84 Opioid-Induced Mood Disorder[I]
292.89 Opioid-Induced Sexual Dysfunction[I]
292.89 Opioid-Induced Sleep Disorder[I, W]
292.9   Opioid-Related Disorder NOS

Phencyclidine (or Phencyclidine-Like)-Related Disorders

Phencyclidine Use Disorders

304.90 Phencyclidine Dependence*
305.90 Phencyclidine Abuse

Phencyclidine-Induced Disorders

292.89 Phencyclidine Intoxication
          Specify if: With Perceptual Disturbances
292.81 Phencyclidine Intoxication Delirium
292.xx Phencyclidine-Induced Psychotic Disorders
.11   With Delusions[I]
.12   With Hallucinations[I]
292.84 Phencyclidine-Induced Mood Disorder[I]
292.89 Phencyclidine-Induced Anxiety Disorder[I]
292.9   Phencyclidine-Related Disorder NOS

Sedative-Hypnotic- or Anxiolytic-Related Disorders

Sedative-Hypnotic- or Anxiolytic Use Disorders

304.10 Sedative, Hypnotic, or Anxiolytic Dependence*
305.40 Sedative, Hypnotic, or Anxiolytic Abuse

Sedative, Hypnotic, or Anxiolytic-Induced Disorders

292.89 Sedative, Hypnotic, or Anxiolytic Intoxication
292.0   Sedative, Hypnotic, or Anxiolytic Withdrawal
          Specify if: With Perceptual Disturbances
292.81 Sedative, Hypnotic, or Anxiolytic Intoxication Delirium
292.81 Sedative, Hypnotic, or Anxiolytic Withdrawal Delirium
292.82 Sedative-, Hypnotic-, or Anxiolytic-Induced Persisting Delirium
292.83 Sedative-, Hypnotic-, or Anxiolytic-Induced Persisting Amnestic disorder
292.xx Sedative-, Hypnotic-, or Anxiolytic-Induced Psychotic Disorder
.11   With Delusions[I, W]
.12   With Hallucinations[I, W]
292.84 Sedative-, Hypnotic-, or Anxiolytic-Induced Mood Disorder[I, W]
292.89 Sedative-, Hypnotic-, or Anxiolytic-Induced Anxiety Disorder[W]
292.89 Sedative-, Hypnotic-, or Anxiolytic-Induced Sexual Dysfunction[I]
292.89 Sedative-, Hypnotic-, or Anxiolytic-Induced Sleep Disorder[I, W]
292.9   Sedative-, Hypnotic-, or Anxiolytic-Induced Disorder NOS

Polysubstance-Related Disorder

304.80 Polysubstance Dependence*

Other (or Unknown) Substance-Related Disorders

Other (or Unknown) Substance Use Disorders

304.90 Other (or Unknown) Substance Dependence*
305.90 Other (or Unknown) Substance Abuse

Other (or Unknown) Substance-Induced Disorders

292.89 Other (or Unknown) Substance Intoxication
          Specify if: With Perceptual Disturbances

292.0   Other (or Unknown) Substance Withdrawal
      Specify if: With Perceptual Disturbances

292.81 Other (or Unknown) Substance-Induced
      Delirium

292.82 Other (or Unknown) Substance-Induced
      Persisting Dementia

292.83 Other (or Unknown) Substance-Induced
      Persisting Amnestic Disorder

292.xx Other (or Unknown) Substance-Induced
      Psychotic Disorder

  .11 With Delusions[I, W]

  .12 With Hallucinations[I, W]

292.84 Other (or Unknown) Substance-Induced
      Mood Disorder[I, W]

292.89 Other (or Unknown) Substance-Induced
      Anxiety Disorder[I, W]

292.89 Other (or Unknown) Substance-Induced
      Sexual Dysfunction[I]

292.89 Other (or Unknown) Substance-Induced
      Sleep Disorder[I, W]

292.9   Other (or Unknown) Substance-Induced
      Disorder NOS

SCHIZOPHRENIA AND OTHER PSYCHOTIC DISORDERS

295.xx Schizophrenia

The following Classification of Longitudinal Course applies to all subtypes of Schizophrenia:

Episodic With Interepisode Residual Symptoms
    (*Specify if:* With Prominent Negative Symptoms)/
      Episodic With No Interepisode Residual
      Symptoms/Continuous
    (*Specify if:* With Prominent Negative Symptoms)
Single Episode in Partial Remission
    (*Specify if:* With Prominent Negative Symptoms)
Single Episode in Full Remission
Other or Unspecified Pattern

  .30 Paranoid Type

  .10 Disorganized Type

  .20 Catatonic Type

  .90 Undifferentiated Type

  .60 Residual Type

295.40 Schizophreniform Disorder
      Specify if: Without Good Prognostic
      Features/With Good Prognostic Features

295.70 Schizoaffective Disorder
      Specify type: Bipolar/Depressive

297.1   Delusional Disorder
      Specify type: Erotomanic/Grandiose/
      Jealous/Persecutory Somatic/Mixed/
      Unspecified

298.8   Brief Psychotic Disorder
      Specify if: With Marked Stressor(s)

      Without Marked Stressor(s) With
      Postpartum Onset

297.3   Shared Psychotic Disorder

293.xx Psychotic Disorder Due to . . . *

  .81 With Delusions

  .82 With Hallucinations

—.- Substance-Induced Psychotic Disorder
      (refer to Substance-Related Disorders for
      substance-specific codes)
      Specify if: With Onset During
      Intoxication/With Onset During
      Withdrawal

298.9   Psychotic Disorder NOS

MOOD DISORDERS

Code current state of Major Depressive Disorder or Bipolar I Disorder in fifth digit

1 = Mild
2 = Moderate
3 = Severe Without Psychotic Features
4 = Severe With Psychotic Features
    Specify: Mood-Congruent Psychotic Features/
    Mood-Incongruent Psychotic Features
5 = In Partial Remission
6 = In Full Remission
0 = Unspecified

The following specifiers apply (for current or most recent episode) to Mood Disorders as noted:

[a]Severity/Psychotic/Remission
Specifiers/[b]Chronic/[c]With Catatonic
    Features/[d]With Melancholic Features/[e]With
    Atypical Features/[f]With Postpartum Onset
The following specifiers apply to Mood Disorders as noted:

[g]With or Without Full Interepisode Recovery/
    With Seasonal Pattern/[i]With Rapid Cycling

Depressive Disorders

296.xx Major Depressive Disorder,

  .2x Single Episode[a,b,c,d,e,f]

  .3x Recurrent[a,b,c,d,e,f,g,h]

300.4   Dysthymic Disorder
      Specify if: Early Onset/Late Onset
      Specify if: With Atypical Features

311   Depressive Disorder NOS

Bipolar Disorders

296.xx Bipolar I Disorder,

  .0x Single Manic Episode[a,c,f]
      Specify if: Mixed

.40   Most Recent Episode Hypomanic[a,h,j]
.4x   Most Recent Episode Manic[a,c,f,g,h,i]
.6x   Most Recent Episode Mixed[a,c,f,g,h,i]
.5x   Most Recent Episode Depressed[a,b,c,d,e,f,g,h,i]
.7   Most Recent Episode Unspecified[g,h,i]
296.89 Bipolar II Disorder[a,b,c,d,e,f,g,h,i]
       Specify (current or most recent episode):
       Hypomanic/Depressed
301.13 Cyclothymic Disorder
296.80 Bipolar Disorder NOS
293.83 Mood Disorder Due to . . . *
       Specify type: With Depressive Features/
       With Major Depressive-Like Episode/
       With Manic Features/With Mixed
       Features
—.-   Substance-Induced Mood Disorder**
       Specify type: With Depressive Features/
       With Manic Features/With Mixed
       Features
       Specify if: With Onset During
       Intoxication/With Onset during
       Withdrawal
296.90 Mood Disorder NOS

ANXIETY DISORDERS

300.01 Panic Disorder without Agoraphobia
300.21 Panic Disorder With Agoraphobia
300.22 Agoraphobia Without History of
       Panic Disorder
300.29 Specific Phobia
       Specify type: Animal Type/Natural Envi-
       ronment Type/Blood-Injection-Injury
       Type/Situational Type/Other Type
300.23 Social Phobia
       Specify if: Generalized
300.3   Obsessive-Compulsive Disorder
       Specify if: With Poor Insight
309.81 Posttraumatic Stress Disorder
       Specify if: Acute/Chronic
       Specify if: With Delayed Onset
308.3   Acute Stress Disorder
300.02 Generalized Anxiety Disorder
293.80 Anxiety Disorder Due to . . . *
       Specify if: With Generalized
       Anxiety/With Panic Attacks/
       With Obsessive Compulsive
       Symptoms . . . *
293.84 Substance-Induced Anxiety Disorder
       Specify if: With Generalized
       Anxiety/With Panic Attacks/
       With Obsessive-Compulsive
       Symptoms/With Phobic Symptoms
       Specify if: With Onset During

Intoxication/With Onset During
Withdrawal
300.00 Anxiety Disorder NOS

SOMATOFORM DISORDERS

300.81 Somatization Disorder
300.82 Undifferentiated Somatoform Disorder
300.11 Conversion Disorder
       Specify type: With Motor Symptom
       or Deficit/With Sensory Symptom or
       Deficit/With Seizures or Convulsions/
       With Mixed Presentation
307.xx Pain Disorder
.80   Associated With Psychological Factors
.89   Associated with Both Psychological Factors
       and a General Medical Condition
       Specify if: Acute/Chronic
300.7   Hypochondriasis
       Specify if: With Poor Insight
300.7   Body Dysmorphic Disorder
300.82 Somatoform Disorder NOS

FACTITIOUS DISORDERS

300.xx Factitious Disorder
.16   With Predominantly Psychological Signs
       and Symptoms
.19   With Predominantly Physical Signs and
       Symptoms
.19   With Combined Psychological and Physical
       Signs and Symptoms
300.19 Factitious Disorder NOS

DISSOCIATIVE DISORDERS

300.12 Dissociative Amnesia
300.13 Dissociative Fugue
300.14 Dissociative Identity Disorder
300.6   Depersonalized Disorder
300.15 Dissociative Disorder NOS

SEXUAL AND GENDER IDENTITY DISORDERS

Sexual Dysfunctions

*The following specifiers apply to all primary Sexual Dys-
functions:*

Lifelong Type/Acquired
Type Generalized Type/Situational Type
Due to Psychological Factors. Due to Combined
Factors

Sexual Desire Disorders

302.71 Hypoactive Sexual Desire Disorder
302.79 Sexual Aversion Disorder

Sexual Arousal Disorders

302.72 Female Sexual Arousal Disorder
302.72 Male Erectile Disorder

Orgasmic Disorders

302.73 Female Orgasmic Disorder
302.74 Male Orgasmic Disorder
302.75 Premature Ejaculation

Sexual Pain Disorders

302.76 Dyspareunia (Not Due to General Medical Condition)
306.51 Vaginismus (Not Due to a General Medical Condition)

Sexual Dysfunction Due to a General Medical Condition

625.8 Female Hypoactive Sexual Desire Disorder Due to . . . *
608.89 Male Hypoactive Sexual Desire Disorder Due to . . . *
607.84 Male Erectile Disorder Due to . . . *
625.0 Female Dyspareunia Due to . . . *
608.89 Male Dyspareunia Due to . . . *
625.8 Other Female Sexual Dysfunction Due to . . . *
608.89 Other Male Sexual Dysfunction Due to . . . *
—.- Substance-Induced Sexual Dysfunction**
Specify if: With Impaired Desire/With Impaired Arousal/With Impaired Orgasm/With Sexual Pain
Specify if: With Onset During Intoxication
302.70 Sexual Dysfunction NOS

Paraphilias

302.4 Exhibitionism
302.81 Fetishism
302.89 Frotteurism
302.2 Pedophilia
Specify if: Sexually Attracted to Males/Sexually Attracted to Females/Sexually Attracted to Both
Specify if: Limited to Incest
Specify type: Exclusive Type/Nonexclusive type
302.83 Sexual Masochism
302.84 Sexual Sadism

302.3 Transvestic Fetishism
Specify if: With Gender Dysphoria
302.82 Voyeurism
302.9 Paraphilia NOS

Gender Identity Disorders

302.xx Gender Identity Disorder
.6 in Children
.85 in Adolescents or Adults
Specify if: Sexually Attracted to Males/Sexually Attracted to Females/Sexually Attracted to Both/Sexually Attracted to Neither
302.6 Gender Identity Disorder NOS
302.9 Sexual Disorder NOS

EATING DISORDERS

307.1 Anorexia Nervosa
Specify type: Restricting, Binge-Eating/Purging
307.51 Bulimia Nervosa
Specify type: Purging/Nonpurging
307.50 Eating Disorder NOS

SLEEP DISORDERS

Primary Sleep Disorders

Dyssomnias

307.42 Primary Insomnia
307.44 Primary Hypersomnia
Specify if: Recurrent
347 Narcolepsy
380.59 Breathing-Related Sleep Disorder
307.45 Circadian Rhythm Sleep Disorder
Specify type: Delayed Sleep Phase/Jet Lag/Shift Work/Unspecified
307.47 Dyssomnia NOS

Parasomnias

307.47 Nightmare Disorder
307.46 Sleep Terror Disorder
307.46 Sleepwalking Disorder
307.47 Parasomnia NOS

Sleep Disorders Related to Another Mental Disorder

307.42 Insomnia Related to . . . ***
307.44 Hypersomnia Related to . . . ***

Other Sleep Disorders

780.xx   Sleep Disorder Due to . . . *
- .52   Insomnia Type
- .54   Hyposomnia Type
- .59   Parasomnia Type
- .59   Mixed Type
- —.-   Substance-Induced Sleep Disorder (refer to Substance-Related Disorders for substance-specific codes)
  Specify type: Insomnia/Hypersomnia/Parasomnia/Mixed
  Specify if: With Onset during Intoxication/With Onset During Withdrawal

IMPULSE-CONTROL DISORDERS NOT ELSEWHERE CLASSIFIED

- 312.34   Intermittent Explosive Disorder
- 312.32   Kleptomania
- 312.33   Pyromania
- 312.31   Pathological Gambling
- 312.39   Trichotillomania
- 312.30   Impulse-Control Disorder NOS

ADJUSTMENT DISORDERS

309.xx   Adjustment Disorder
- .0   With Depressed Mood
- .24   With Anxiety
- .28   With Mixed Anxiety and Depressed Mood
- .3   With Disturbance of Conduct
- .4   With Mixed Disturbance of Emotions and Conduct
- .9   Unspecified
  Specify if: Acute/Chronic

PERSONALITY DISORDERS

Note: These are coded on Axis II

- 301.0   Paranoid Personality Disorder
- 301.20   Schizoid Personality Disorder
- 301.22   Schizotypal Personality Disorder
- 301.7   Antisocial Personality Disorder
- 301.83   Borderline Personality Disorder
- 301.50   Histrionic Personality Disorder
- 301.81   Narcissistic Personality Disorder
- 301.82   Avoidant Personality Disorder
- 301.6   Dependent Personality Disorder
- 301.4   Obsessive-Compulsive Personality Disorder
- 301.9   Personality Disorder NOS

OTHER CONDITIONS THAT MAY BE A FOCUS OF CLINICAL ATTENTION

Psychological Factors Affecting Medical Condition

316 . . . [Specified Psychological Factor] Affecting . . . *

Choose name based on nature of factors:

Mental Disorder Affecting Medical Condition
Psychological Symptoms Affecting Medical Condition
Personality Traits or Coping Style Affecting Medical Condition
Maladaptive Health Behaviors Affecting Medical Condition
Stress-Related Physiological Response Affecting Medical Condition
Other or Unspecified Psychological Factors Affecting Medical Condition

Medication-Induced Movement Disorders

- 332.1   Neuroleptic-Induced Parkinsonism
- 333.92   Neuroleptic Malignant Syndrome
- 333.7   Neuroleptic-Induced Acute Dystonia
- 333.99   Neuroleptic-Induced Acute Akathisia
- 333.82   Neuroleptic-Induced Tardive Dyskinesia
- 333.1   Medication-Induced Postural Tumor
- 333.90   Medication-Induced Movement Disorder NOS

Other Medical-Induced Disorder

- 995.2   Adverse Effects of Medication NOS

Relational Problems

- V61.9   Relational Problem Related to a Mental Disorder or General Medical Condition
- V61.1   Partner Relational Problem
- V61.20   Parent-Child Relational Problem
- V61.8   Sibling Relational Problem
- V62.81   Relational Problem NOS

Problems Related to Abuse or Neglect

(code 995.5 if focus of attention is on victim)

- V61.21   Physical Abuse of Child
- V61.21   Sexual Abuse of Child
- V61.21   Neglect of Child
- V61.12   Physical Abuse of Adult
- V61.1   Sexual Abuse of Adult
- V62.83   Person Other Than Partner

Additional Conditions That May be Focus of Clinical Attention

V15.81 Noncompliance With Treatment
V65.2   Malingering
V71.01 Adult Antisocial Behavior
V71.02 Child or Adolescent Antisocial Behavior
V62.89 Borderline Intellectual Functioning
            Note: This is coded on Axis II.
780.9   Age-Related Cognitive Decline
V62.82 Bereavement
V62.3   Academic Problem
V62.2   Occupational Problem
313.82 Identify Problem

V62.89 Religious or Spiritual Problem
V62.4   Acculturation Problem
V62.89 Phase of Life Problem

ADDITIONAL CODES

300.9   Unspecified Mental Disorder
            (nonpsychotic)
V71.09 No Diagnosis or Condition on Axis I
799.9   Diagnosis or Condition Deferred on Axis I
V71.09 No Diagnosis on Axis II
799.9   Diagnosis Deferred on Axis II

BELIEFS ABOUT PSYCHIATRIC AND MENTAL HEALTH NURSING

Psychiatric and mental health nursing is a specialized area of nursing that has as its focus the promotion of mental health, the prevention of mental illness, and the care of clients experiencing mental health problems and mental disorders.

The psychiatric and mental health nurse works with clients in a variety of settings, including institutional facility and community settings. Clients may be unique in their vulnerability as, in this area of nursing practice, they can be involved involuntarily and can be committed to an institution under the law. Further, clients may receive treatment against their will. This fact affects the nature of the nurse-client relationship and often raises complex ethical dilemmas.

The centrality of PMHN practice is the therapeutic use of self; nurse-client interactions are purposeful and goal directed. The psychiatric and mental health nurse understands how the psychiatric disease process, the illness experience, the recuperative powers and the perceived degree of mental health are affected by contextual factors. Advances in knowledge (for instance, the current increase in understanding the biological basis of mental disorders, and the sociological determinants of behaviour) require that psychiatric and mental health nurses continually incorporate new research-based findings into their practice. PMH nurses acknowledge a responsibility to promote evidence-based, outcomes-oriented practice to enhance knowledge and skill development within the specialty. PMH nurses also acknowledge a responsibility to personal mental health promotion and maintenance.

PMHN knowledge is based on nursing theory, which is integrated with physical science theory, social science theory and human science theory. PMHN shares with other mental health disciplines a body of knowledge based on theories of human behaviour. As well, "reflection on practice" continues to develop the nurses habitual practices and skills of being truly present to the client situation at hand (Benner et al., 1996, p. 325). In some settings there may be an overlapping of professional roles and/or a sharing of competencies. PMH nurses recognize their accountability to society for both the discrete and shared functions of practice.

STANDARD I: PROVIDES COMPETENT PROFESSIONAL CARE THROUGH THE HELPING ROLE

The helping role is fundamental to all nursing practice. PMH nurses "enter into partnerships with clients, and through the use of the human sciences, and the art of caring, develop helping relationships" (CNA, 1997b, p. 43) and therapeutic alliances with clients. A primary goal of psychiatric and mental health nursing is the promotion of mental health and the prevention or diminution of mental disorder.

The Nurse:

1. Assesses and clarifies the influences of personal beliefs, values and life experiences on the therapeutic relationship.
2. Establishes and maintains a caring goal directed environment.
3. Uses a range of therapeutic communication skills, both verbal and nonverbal, including core communication skills (eg, empathy, listening, observing).
4. Makes distinctions between social and professional relationships.
5. Recognizes the influence of culture and ethnicity on the therapeutic process and negotiates care that is culturally sensitive.
6. Mobilizes resources that increase clients' access to mental health services.
7. Understands and responds to human responses to distress such as: anger, anxiety, fear, grief, helplessness, hopelessness and humour.
8. Guides the client through behavioral, developmental, emotional, or spiritual change while acknowledging and supporting the client's participation, responsibility and choices in own care.
9. Supports the client's sense of resiliency, for example self-esteem, power and hope.
10. Offers supportive and therapeutic care to the client's significant others.
11. Reflectively critiques therapeutic effectiveness of nurse-client relationships by evaluating

[1]Standards Committee of the Canadian Federation of Mental Health Nurses. (1998). *Canadian Standards of Psychiatric Mental Health Nursing Practice* (2nd ed.). Ottawa, Ontario: Canadian Nurses Association.

client responses to therapeutic processes, and by evaluating personal responses to client. Seeks clinical supervision with ongoing therapeutic skill development.

STANDARD II: PERFORMS/REFINES CLIENT ASSESSMENTS THROUGH THE DIAGNOSTIC AND MONITORING FUNCTION

Effective diagnosis and monitoring is central to the nurse's role and is dependent upon theory, as well as upon understanding the meaning of the health or illness experience from the perspective of the client. This knowledge, integrated with the nurse's conceptual model of nursing practice, provides a framework for processing client data and for developing client-focused plans of care. The nurse makes professional judgements regarding the relevance and importance of this data, and acknowledges the client as a valued and respected partner throughout the decision-making process.

The Nurse:

1. Collaborates with clients to gather holistic assessments through observation, examination, interview, and consultation, while being attentive to issues of confidentiality and pertinent legal statutes.
2. Documents and analyzes baseline data to identify health status, potential for wellness, health care deficits, potential for danger to self and others; alterations in thinking, perceiving, communicating and decision-making abilities; substance abuse and dependency; and history of abuse (emotional, physical, sexual or verbal).
3. Formulates and documents a plan of care in collaboration with the client and with the mental health team, recognizing variability in the client's ability to participate in the process.
4. Refines and extends client assessment information by assessing and documenting significant change in the client's status, and by comparing new data with the baseline assessment and intermediate client goals.
5. Anticipates problems in the future course of the client's functional status: eg, shifts in mood indicative of change in potential for self-harm; effects of "flashbacks."
6. Determines most appropriate and available therapeutic modality that will potentially best meet client's needs, and assists the client to access these resources.

STANDARD III: ADMINISTERS AND MONITORS THERAPEUTIC INTERVENTIONS

Due to the nature of mental health problems and mental disorders, there are unique practice issues confronting the psychiatric and mental health nurse in administering and monitoring therapeutic interventions. Safety in psychiatric and mental health nursing has unique meaning since many clients are at risk for self-harm and/or self-neglect. Clients may not be mentally competent to participate in decision-making. PMH nurse needs to be alert to adverse reactions as client's ability to self-report may be impaired. The PMH nurse uses evidence-based and experiential knowledge from nursing, health sciences and related mental health disciplines to both select and tailor nursing interventions. This is accomplished in collaboration with the client to the greatest possible extent.

The Nurse:

1. Assists and educates clients to select choices which will support positive changes in their affect, cognition, behavior and/or relationships (CNA, 1997b, p. 68).
2. Supports clients to draw on own assets and resources for self care and mental health promotion (CNA, 1997b, p. 68).
3. Makes discretionary clinical decisions, using knowledge of client's unique responses and paradigm cases as the basis for the decision, eg, frequency of client contact in the community.
4. Uses appropriate technology to perform safe, effective and efficient nursing intervention (CNA, 1997b, p. 68).
5. Administers medications accurately and safely, monitoring therapeutic responses, reactions, untoward effects, toxicity and potential incompatibilities with other medications or substances.
6. Assesses client responses to deficits in activities of daily living and mobilizes resources in response to client's capabilities.
7. Provides support and assists with protection for clients experiencing difficulty with self protection.
8. Utilizes therapeutic elements of group process.
9. Incorporates knowledge of family dynamics and cultural values and beliefs about families in the provision of care.
10. Collaborates with the client, health care providers and community to access and coordinate resources.

STANDARD IV: EFFECTIVELY MANAGES RAPIDLY CHANGING SITUATIONS

The effective management of rapidly changing situations is essential in critical circumstances which may be termed psychiatric emergencies. These situations include self harm and other assaultive behaviours and rapidly changing mental health states. This domain also includes screening for risk factors and referral related to psychiatric illnesses and social problems, ie, substance abuse, violence/abuse and suicide/homicide (SERPN, 1996, p. 41).

The Nurse:

1. Assesses clients for risk of substance use/abuse, victim violence/abuse, suicide or homicide.
2. Knows resources required to manage potential emergency situations and plans access to these resources.
3. Monitors client safety and utilizes continual assessment to detect early changes in client status, and intervenes in situations of acute agitation.
4. Implements crisis intervention as necessary.
5. Commences critical procedures: in an institutional setting, eg, suicide precautions, emergency restraint, elopement precautions, when necessary; in a community setting, uses appropriate community support systems, eg, police, ambulance services, crisis response resources.
6. Coordinates care to prevent errors and duplication of efforts where rapid response is imperative.
7. Considers the legal and ethical implications of responses to rapidly changing situations; invokes relevant provisions in mental health acts as necessary.
8. Evaluates the effectiveness of the rapid responses and modifies critical plans as necessary.
9. Explores with the client and/or family the precipitates of the emergency event and plans to minimize risk of recurrence.
10. Participates in "debriefing" process with team (including client and family) and other service providers, eg, reviews of critical event and/or emergency situation.
11. Incorporates knowledge of community needs or responses in the provision of care.
12. Encourages and assists clients to seek out support groups for mutual aid and support.
13. Assesses the client's response to, and perception of, nursing and other therapeutic interventions.

STANDARD V: INTERVENES THROUGH THE TEACHING-COACHING FUNCTION

All nurse-client interactions are potentially teaching/learning situations. The PMH nurse attempts to understand the life experience of the client and uses this understanding to support and promote learning related to health and personal development. The nurse provides mental health promotion information to individuals, families, groups, populations, and communities.

The Nurse:

1. In collaboration with the client, determines clients' learning needs.
2. Plans and implements, with the client, health education while considering the context of the client's life experiences on readiness to learn. Plans teaching times and strategies accordingly.
3. Provides anticipatory guidance regarding the client's situational needs, eg, assists the client in identifying living, learning or working needs and ways in which to access available community or other resources.
4. Facilitates the client's search for ways to integrate mental illness, chronic illness or improved functioning into lifestyle.
5. Considers a variety of learning models and utilizes clinical judgement when creating opportunities with clients regarding their learning needs.
6. Provides relevant information, guidance and support to the client's significant others within the bounds of any freedom of information legislation.
7. Documents the teaching/learning process (assessment, plan, implementation, client involvement and evaluation).
8. Evaluates and validates with the client the effectiveness of the educational process, and seeks clients input into developing other means of providing teaching opportunities.
9. Engages in learning/teaching opportunities as partners with consumer groups.

STANDARD VI: MONITORS AND ENSURES THE QUALITY OF HEALTH CARE PRACTICES

Clients may be particularly vulnerable as recipients of health care, because of the nature of mental health problems and mental disorders. Mental health care is conducted under the provisions of provincial/territorial Mental Health Acts and related legislation. It is essential for the PMH nurse to be informed regarding the interpretation of relevant legislation and its implications for nursing practice. The nurse has a responsibility to advocate for the client's right to receive the least restrictive form of care and to respect and affirm the client's right to pursue individual goals of equality and justice.

The Nurse:

1. Identifies limitations in the workplace or care setting that interfere with the nurse's ability to perform with skill, safety and compassion and takes appropriate action.
2. Identifies limitations at a community level that interfere with the entire health of the community, eg, poverty, malnutrition, unsafe housing.
3. Expands knowledge of innovations and changes in mental health and psychiatric nursing practice to ensure safe and effective care.
4. Critically evaluates current mental health and psychiatric research findings and uses research findings in practice.
5. Ensures and documents ongoing review and evaluation of psychiatric and mental health nursing care activities.
6. Understands and questions the interdependent functions of the team within the overall plan of care.
7. Advocates for the client within the context of institutional, professional, family and community interests.
8. Follows agency/institutional procedures when dissatisfied with the safety of a treatment plan and/or management interventions of other mental health care providers.
9. Uses sound judgement in advocating for safe, competent and ethical care for clients and colleagues even when there are system barriers to enacting an advocacy function.
10. Maintains and monitors confidentiality of client information.
11. Attends to changes in the mental health services system by recognizing changes that affect practice and client care, and by developing strategies to manage these changes (CNA, 1997b, p. 79).

STANDARD VII: PRACTICES WITHIN ORGANIZATIONAL AND WORK-ROLE STRUCTURES

The PMHN role is assumed within organizational structures, both community and institutional, particular to the provision of health care. In PMHN, the ethic of care is based on thoughtful and wise practice judgements within multiple, complex ??. As mental health care in Canada evolves into community based care, the psychiatric and mental health nurse needs to be skilled in collaborative partnering and decision-making, mental health promotion and community development.

The Nurse:

1. Collaborates in the formulation of mental health promotion, and in activities and overall treatment plans and decisions with the client and treatment team and, throughout the continuum of care (primary, secondary and tertiary).
2. Recognizes and addresses the impact of the dynamic of the treatment team on the therapeutic process.
3. Uses conflict resolution skills to facilitate interdisciplinary health team interactions and functioning.
4. Uses computerized and other mental health and nursing information systems in planning, documenting and evaluating client care.
5. Demonstrates knowledge of collaborative strategies in working with consumer/advocacy groups (SERPN, 1996, p. 50).
6. Actively participates in developing, implementing and critiquing mental health policy in the workplace.
7. Acts as a role model for nursing students and the beginning practitioner in the provision of psychiatric and mental health nursing care.
8. Practices independently within legislated scope of practice.
9. Supports professional efforts in psychiatric and mental health practice to achieve a more mentally healthy society.

DIRECTIONS: Place an X in the appropriate box to represent level of severity of each symptom.

	Not Present	Very Mild	Mild	Moderate	Mod. Severe	Severe	Extremely Severe
SOMATIC CONCERN—preoccupation with physical health, fear of physical illness, hypochondriasis.	☐	☐	☐	☐	☐	☐	☐
ANXIETY—worry, fear, overconcern for present or future, uneasiness.	☐	☐	☐	☐	☐	☐	☐
EMOTIONAL WITHDRAWAL—lack of spontaneous interaction, isolation deficiency in relating to others.	☐	☐	☐	☐	☐	☐	☐
CONCEPTUAL DISORGANIZATION—thought processes confused, disconnected, disorganized, disrupted.	☐	☐	☐	☐	☐	☐	☐
GUILT FEELINGS—self-blame, shame, remorse for past behavior.	☐	☐	☐	☐	☐	☐	☐
TENSION—physical and motor manifestations of nervousness, over-activation.	☐	☐	☐	☐	☐	☐	☐
MANNERISMS AND POSTURING—peculiar, bizarre unnatural motor behavior (not including tic).	☐	☐	☐	☐	☐	☐	☐
GRANDIOSITY—exaggerated self-opinion, arrogance, conviction of unusual power or abilities.	☐	☐	☐	☐	☐	☐	☐
DEPRESSIVE MOOD—sorrow, sadness, despondency, pessimism.	☐	☐	☐	☐	☐	☐	☐
HOSTILITY—animosity, contempt, belligerence, disdain for others.	☐	☐	☐	☐	☐	☐	☐
SUSPICIOUSNESS—mistrust, belief others harbour malicious or discriminatory intent.	☐	☐	☐	☐	☐	☐	☐
HALLUCINATORY BEHAVIOR—perceptions without normal external stimulus correspondence.	☐	☐	☐	☐	☐	☐	☐
MOTOR RETARDATION—slowed weakened movements or speech, reduced body tone.	☐	☐	☐	☐	☐	☐	☐
UNCOOPERATIVENESS—resistance, guardedness, rejection of authority.	☐	☐	☐	☐	☐	☐	☐
UNUSUAL THOUGHT CONTENT—unusual, odd, strange, bizarre thought content.	☐	☐	☐	☐	☐	☐	☐
BLUNTED AFFECT—reduced emotional tone, reduction in formal intensity of feelings, flatness.	☐	☐	☐	☐	☐	☐	☐
EXCITEMENT—heightened emotional tone, agitation, increased reactivity.	☐	☐	☐	☐	☐	☐	☐
DISORIENTATION—confusion or lack of proper association for person, place, or time.	☐	☐	☐	☐	☐	☐	☐

Global Assessment Scale (Range 1–100)

Reprinted with permission from Overall J. E. (1988). The Brief Psychiatric Rating Scale (BPRS): Recent developments in ascertainment and scaling. *Psychopharmacology Bulletin, 24*, 97–99.

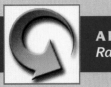
Patient's Name: **DOB:**   **Hospital no:**

Rater's Name: **Occupation:**

Patient's status at evaluation:
1. Inpatient.   2. Outpatient.   3. Day hospital/day centre patient.   4. Other (specify)

Scoring system:
U. Unable to evaluate.   0. Absent.   1. Mild or intermittent.   2. Moderate.   3. Severe.
Rating should be based on symptoms and signs occurring during two weeks prior to the interview.
No score should be given if symptoms result from physical disability or illness.
Total score is the sum of items 1 to 18. A score of 11 or more suggests significant clinical anxiety.

                                               Score

Worry	1. Worry about physical health.	
	2. Worry about cognitive performance (failing memory, getting lost when goes out, not able to follow conversation).	
	3. Worry over finances, family problems, physical health of relatives.	
	4. Worry associated with false belief and/or perception.	
	5. Worry over trifles (repeatedly calling for attention over trivial matters).	
Apprehension and vigilance	6. Frightened and anxious (keyed up and on the edge).	
	7. Sensitivity to noise (exaggerated startle response).	
	8. Sleep disturbance (trouble falling or staying asleep).	
	9. Irritability (more easily annoyed than usual, short tempered and angry outbursts).	
Motor tension	10. Trembling.	
	11. Motor tension (complain of headache, other body aches and pains).	
	12. Restlessness (fidgeting, cannot sit still, pacing, wringing hands, picking clothes).	
	13. Fatigueability, tiredness.	
Autonomic hypersensitivity	14. Palpitations (complains of heart racing or thumping).	
	15. Dry mouth (not due to medication), sinking feeling in the stomach.	
	16. Hyperventilating, shortness of breath (even when not exerting).	
	17. Dizziness or light-headedness (complains as if going to faint).	
	18. Sweating, flushes or chills, tingling or numbness of fingers and toes.	

Phobias: fears which are excessive, that do not make sense and tend to avoid—like afraid of crowds, going out alone, being in a small room, or being frightened by some kind of animals, heights, etc. *Describe.*

Panic attacks: feelings of anxiety or dread that are so strong that think they are going to die or have a heart attack and they simply have to do something to stop them, like immediately leaving the place, phoning relatives, etc. *Describe.*

PART I: SYMPTOMATOLOGY

Assessment Interval: Specify: _____ wks.

Total Score: _____

A. Paranoid and Delusional Ideation

  1. "People Are Stealing Things" Delusion

    (0) Not present

    (1) Delusion that people are hiding objects

    (2) Delusion that people are coming into the home and hiding objects or stealing objects

    (3) Talking and listening to people coming into the home

  2. "One's House Is Not One's Home" Delusion

    (0) Not present

    (1) Conviction that the place in which one is residing is not one's home (eg, packing to go home; complaints, while at home, of "take me home")

    (2) Attempt to leave domiciliary to go home

    (3) Violence in response to attempts to forcibly restrict exit

  3. "Spouse (or Other Caregiver) Is an Imposter" Delusion

    (0) Not present

    (1) Conviction that spouse (or other caregiver) is an imposter

    (2) Anger toward spouse (or other caregiver) for being an imposter

    (3) Violence towards spouse (or other caregiver) for being an imposter

  4. "Delusion of Abandonment" (eg, to an Institution)

    (0) Not present

    (1) Suspicion of caregiver plotting abandonment or institutionalization (eg, on telephone)

    (2) Accusation of a conspiracy to abandon or institutionalize

    (3) Accusation of impending or immediate desertion or institutionalization

  5. "Delusion of Infidelity"

    (0) Not present

    (1) Conviction that spouse and/or children and/or other caregivers are unfaithful

    (2) Anger toward spouse, relative, or other caregiver for infidelity

    (3) Violence toward spouse, relative, or other caregiver for supposed infidelity

  6. "Suspiciousness/Paranoia" (other than above)

    (0) Not present

    (1) Suspicious (eg, hiding objects that he/she later may be unable to locate)

    (2) Paranoid (ie, fixed conviction with respect to suspicions and/or anger as a result of suspicions)

    (3) Violence as a result of suspicions

    Unspecified? _____

    Describe _____

    _____

    _____

  7. Delusions (other than above)

    (0) Not present

    (1) Delusional

    (2) Verbal or emotional manifestations as a result of delusions

    (3) Physical actions or violence as a result of delusions

    Unspecified? _____

    Describe _____

    _____

    _____

B. Hallucinations

  8. Visual Hallucinations

    (0) Not present

    (1) Vague: not clearly defined

    (2) Clearly defined hallucinations of objects or persons (eg, sees other people at the table)

    (3) Verbal or physical actions or emotional responses to the hallucinations

  9. Auditory Hallucinations

    (0) Not present

    (1) Vague: not clearly defined

    (2) Clearly defined hallucinations of words or phrases

    (3) Verbal or physical actions or emotional response to the hallucinations

  10. Olfactory Hallucinations

    (0) Not present

    (1) Vague: not clearly defined

    (2) Clearly defined

    (3) Verbal or physical actions or emotional responses to the hallucinations

11. Haptic Hallucinations
    (0) Not present
    (1) Vague: not clearly defined
    (2) Clearly defined
    (3) Verbal or physical actions or emotional responses to the hallucinations
12. Other Hallucinations
    (0) Not present
    (1) Vague: not clearly defined
    (2) Clearly defined
    (3) Verbal or physical actions or emotional responses to the hallucinations
    Unspecified? _____
    Describe _____
    _____
    _____

C. Activity Disturbances
    13. Wandering: Away From Home or Caregiver
        (0) Not present
        (1) Somewhat, but not sufficient to necessitate restraint
        (2) Sufficient to require restraint
        (3) Verbal or physical actions or emotional responses to attempts to prevent wandering
    14. Purposeless Activity (Cognitive Abulia)
        (0) Not present
        (1) Repetitive, purposeless activity (eg, opening and closing pocketbook, packing and unpacking clothing, repeatedly putting on and removing clothing, opening and closing drawers, insistent repeating of demands or questions)
        (2) Pacing or other purposeless activity sufficient to require restraint
        (3) Abrasions or physical harm resulting from purposeless activity
    15. Inappropriate Activity
        (0) Not present
        (1) Inappropriate activities (eg, storing and hiding objects in inappropriate places, such as throwing clothing in wastebasket or putting empty plates in the oven; inappropriate sexual behavior, such as inappropriate exposure)
        (2) Present and sufficient to require restraint
        (3) Present, sufficient to require restraint, and accompanied by anger or violence when restraint is used

D. Aggressiveness
    16. Verbal Outbursts
        (0) Not present
        (1) Present (including unaccustomed use of foul or abusive language)
        (2) Present and accompanied by anger

(3) Present, accompanied by anger, and clearly directed at other persons
17. Physical Threats and/or Violence
    (0) Not present
    (1) Threatening behavior
    (2) Physical violence
    (3) Physical violence accompanied by vehemence
18. Agitation (other than above)
    (0) Not present
    (1) Present
    (2) Present with emotional component
    (3) Present with emotional and physical component
    Unspecified? _____
    Describe _____
    _____
    _____

E. Diurnal Rhythm Disturbances
    19. Day/Night Disturbance
        (0) Not present
        (1) Repetitive wakenings during night
        (2) 50% to 75% of former sleep cycle at night
        (3) Complete disturbance of diurnal rhythm (ie, less than 50% of former sleep cycle at night)

F. Affective Disturbance
    20. Tearfulness
        (0) Not present
        (1) Present
        (2) Present and accompanied by clear affective component
        (3) Present and accompanied by affective and physical component (eg, "wrings hands" or other gestures)
    21. Depressed Mood: Other
        (0) Present
        (1) Present (eg, occasional statement "I wish I were dead," without clear affective concomitants)
        (2) Present with clear concomitants (eg, thoughts of death)
        (3) Present with emotional and physical concomitants (eg, suicide gestures)
        Unspecified? _____
        Describe _____
        _____
        _____

G. Anxieties and Phobias
    22. Anxiety Regarding Upcoming Events (Godot Syndrome)
        (0) Not present
        (1) Present: Repeated queries and/or other activities regarding upcoming appointments and/or events

(2) Present and disturbing to caregivers

(3) Present and intolerable to caregivers

23. Other Anxieties

(0) Not present

(1) Present

(2) Present and disturbing to caregivers

(3) Present and intolerable to caregivers

Unspecified? _____

Describe _____

_____

_____

24. Fear of Being Left Alone

(0) Not present

(1) Present: Vocalized fear of being alone

(2) Vocalized and sufficient to require specific action on part of caregiver

(3) Vocalized and sufficient to require patient to be accompanied at all times

25. Other Phobias

(0) Not present

(1) Present

(2) Present and of sufficient magnitude to require specific action on part of caregiver

(3) Present and sufficient to prevent patient activities

Unspecified? _____

Describe _____

_____

_____

PART 2: GLOBAL RATING

With respect to the above symptoms, they are of sufficient magnitude as to be:

(0) Not at all troubling to the caregiver or dangerous to the patient

(1) Mildly troubling to the caregiver or dangerous to the patient

(2) Moderately troubling to the caregiver or dangerous to the patient

(3) Severely troubling or intolerable to the caregiver or dangerous to the patient

Cognitive Abilities Screening Instrument	Name_____ ID No. ⬚⬚⬚⬚⬚⬚ Date (mm/dd/yy) ⬚⬚ ⬚⬚ ⬚⬚ Examiner_____ ⬚⬚

SEX ☐ 1 = male ☐ 2 = female

EDUCATION (years of schooling completed) ⬚⬚
(code 99=Unk/Refused)

Testing start time (hr:min) _____:_____

1. WHERE WERE YOU BORN?

_____ [0   1]

City (Town/Village)

_____ [0   1]

State/Prefecture

add above 2 scores then circle the answer →

BPL
2
1
0

2. WHEN WERE YOU BORN?

_____ Accurate
Year Missed by 1–3 years
 Missed by > 3 years

BYR
2
1
0

_____ [0   1]
Month

_____ [0   1]
Date

add above 2 scores then circle the answer →

BDAY
2
1
0

3. HOW OLD ARE YOU?

_____ Accurate
 Missed by 1–3 years
 Missed by > 3 years

AGE
2
1
0

4. HOW MANY MINUTES ARE THERE IN AN HOUR? or HOW MANY DAYS ARE THERE IN A YEAR?

(score 2 if either question answered correctly)

_____

MNT
2
0

5. IN WHAT DIRECTION DOES THE SUN SET?
(If confused, may provide 4 choices)

SUN
2
0

Select version #, then circle corresponding words in Question 8 and Question 22.

VRS #
1
2
3

6. a. I AM GOING TO SAY 3 WORDS FOR YOU TO REMEMBER. REPEAT THEM AFTER I HAVE SAID ALL THREE.

☐ 1. SHIRT ___ BROWN ___ HONESTY ___
☐ 2. SHOES ___ BLACK ___ MODESTY ___
☐ 3. SOCKS ___ BLUE ___ CHARITY ___

RGS1
3
2
1
0

b. If participant can't answer the first time, elaborate and repeat up to a total of 3 times. Score last performance.

RGS2
3
2
1
0

7. I SHALL SAY SOME NUMBERS, AND YOU REPEAT WHAT I SAY BACKWARDS. FOR EXAMPLE, IF I SAY 1-2, YOU SAY 2-1. OK? REMEMBER: YOU REPEAT WHAT I SAY BACKWARDS.
(Rate: 1 digit/second)
1-2-3 (If unable, coach for 3-2-1, but score 0)

DBA
1
0

6-8-2

DBB
2
0

(If score is 0 in both DBA and DBB, score DBC 0)
3-5-2-9

DBC
2
0

8. WHAT THREE WORDS DID I ASK YOU TO REMEMBER EARLIER?

Spontaneous recall
After: "one word was something to wear"
After: "Was It SHOES, SHIRT, or SOCKS"?
Still Incorrect

RC1A
3
2
1
0

Spontaneous recall
After: "one word was a color"
After: "Was It BLUE, BLACK, or BROWN"?
Still Incorrect

RC1B
3
2
1
0

Spontaneous recall
After: "one word was a good personal quality"
After: "Was It HONESTY, CHARITY, or MODESTY"?
Still Incorrect

Unless recall is perfect, give another reminder of the 3 words.

RC1C
3
2
1
0

Cognitive Abilities Screening Instrument   CASI E-1.0   Record form page 2 of 4

(For the first error only: score 0, but provide the correct answer. If subject asks examiner to repeat answer from previous step, provide the answer but score 0 at that step.)	**SUB3A** 1 0	15. AN ORANGE AND A BANANA ARE BOTH FRUIT. *(pause for 2 sec. then ask:)* *(coach for correct answer if needed for "a." only)*	

9. a. FROM 100, TAKE AWAY 3, = HOW MANY? (97)

SUB3A 1 0

b. AND TAKE AWAY 3 FROM THAT EQUALS? (94)

SUB3B 1 0

(if a. and b. are both scored 0, score part c. 0)

c. Repeat "AND TAKE AWAY 3 AGAIN EQUALS?" three more times. 1 point each.
(91 88 85)

SUB3C 3 2 1 0

15. AN ORANGE AND A BANANA ARE BOTH FRUIT.
(pause for 2 sec. then ask:)

(coach for correct answer if needed for "a." only)

a. AN ARM AND A LEG ARE BOTH . . . ?

Body parts, limbs, extremities	2
Long, bend, muscles, bones, etc	1
Incorrect; DK; tells difference	0

b. LAUGHING AND CRYING ARE BOTH . . . ?

Expressions of <u>feelings/emotions</u>	2
other correct answer	1
incorrect; DK; tells difference	0

c. EATING AND SLEEPING ARE BOTH . . . ?

<u>Necessary</u> bodily functions	2
Other correct answer	1
Incorrect; DK; tells difference	0

add above 3 scores then circle the answer →

SIM
6
5
4
3
2
1
0

10. WHAT IS TODAY'S DATE? _____

Accurate	
[YEAR] Missed by 1 year	
Missed by 2–5 years	
Missed >= 6 years	

YR 4 2 1 0

Accurate or within 5 days	
[MONTH] Missed by 1 month	
Missed >= 2 months	

MO 2 1 0

(of the month) Accurate	
Missed 1 or 2 days	
[DATE] Missed 3–5 days	
Missed >=6 days	

DATE 3 2 1 0

11. WHAT DAY OF THE WEEK IS TODAY?   Accurate / Inaccurate

DAY 1 0

12. WHAT SEASON ARE WE IN?
   Accurate within 1 month
(may provide 4 choices   Missed by > 1 month if necessary)

SSN 1 0

13. a. WHAT _____ ARE WE IN?

State	[0	2]
City/Town/Village	[0	2]

add above 2 scores then circle the answer →

SPA 4 2 0

b. IS THIS PLACE A HOSPITAL (CLINIC). A STORE (   ), OR HOME?

SPB 1 0

14. WHAT ANIMALS HAVE 4 LEGS? TELL ME AS MANY AS YOU CAN. (30 sec.)

number of correct answers: 0 1 2 3 4 5 6 7 8 9 10

ANML

16. a. WHAT ACTIONS WOULD YOU TAKE IF YOU SAW YOUR NEIGHBOR'S HOUSE CATCHING FIRE?

(prompt "WHAT ELSE MIGHT YOU DO?" once only, if necessary)

No. of appropriate actions: 0   1   2

b. WHAT ACTIONS WOULD YOU TAKE IF YOU LOST A BORROWED UMBRELLA?

1 point for each category of actions:

* Inform/Apologize
* Replace/Compensate   0   1   2

c. WHAT WOULD YOU DO IF YOU FOUND AN ENVELOPE THAT WAS SEALED, ADDRESSED AND HAD A NEW STAMP?

Mail	2
Try to locate the owner	1
Inappropriate action	0

add above 3 scores then circle the answer →

JGMT
6
5
4
3
2
1
0

17. a. REPEAT EXACTLY WHAT I SAY: "HE WOULD LIKE TO GO HOME."

Correct	2
1 or 2 missed or wrong words	1
>= 3 missed or wrong words	0

RPTA
2
1
0

(for each part of 17b, score 1 only if repeated exactly as given)

b. NOW REPEAT . . .

"THIS YELLOW CIRCLE	[0	1]
IS HEAVIER THAN	[0	1]
BLUE SQUARE"	[0	1]

add above 3 scores then circle the answer →

RPTB
3
2
1
0

Cognitive Abilities Screening Instrument   CASI E-1.0   Record form page 3 of 4

---

18. PLEASE DO THIS:
(pause for 2 sec. then ask:)

	READ
(Point to statement "RAISE YOUR HAND")	
Raises hand without prompting	3
Raises hand after prompting	2
Reads correctly, but does not raise hand	1
Neither reads nor obeys	0

19. LET ME HAVE A SAMPLE OF YOUR HANDWRITING.
PLEASE WRITE:
(HE) WOULD LIKE TO GO HOME. (1 min.)
(may dictate 1 word at a time if necessary)   WRITE

0   1   2   3   4   5

20. PLEASE COPY THIS:
(show pentagons - 1 minute)

DRAW

	Left Pentagon	Right Pentagon	
			10
			9
5 approx. equal sides	4	4	8
5 but unequal (>2:1) sides	3	3	7
Any other enclosed figure	2	2	6
>=2 lines but without closure	1	1	5
Less than 2 lines	0	0	4
	Intersection:		3
4 cornered	2		2
Not 4-cornered enclosure	1		1
No enclosure	0		0

add above 3 scores then circle the answer →

(note: for question 21, do not repeat any part of the command)
(use non-dominant hand)

21. TAKE THIS PAPER WITH YOUR

			CMD
L(R) HAND	[0	1]	3
FOLD IT IN HALF, AND	[0	1]	2
HAND IT BACK TO ME.	[0	1]	1
			0

add above 3 scores then circle the answer →

---

22. WHAT THREE WORDS DID I ASK YOU TO REMEMBER EARLIER?

	RC2A
Spontaneous recall	3
After: "one word was something to wear"	2
After "Was it SHOES, SHIRT, or SOCKS"?	1
Still Incorrect	0

	RC2B
Spontaneous recall	3
After: "one word was a color"	2
After "Was it BLUE, BLACK, or BROWN"?	1
Still Incorrect	0

	RC2C
Spontaneous recall	3
After: "one word was a good personal quality"	2
After "Was it HONESTY, CHARITY, or MODESTY"?	1
Still Incorrect	0

---

23. WHAT DO WE CALL THIS PART OF THE FACE/BODY?
(2 sec. each)

			BODY
FOREHEAD	[0	1]	5
CHIN	[0	1]	4
SHOULDER	[0	1]	3
ELBOW	[0	1]	2
WRIST	[0	1]	1
add above 5 scores then circle the answer →			0

24. WHAT IS THIS? (show one at a time, any order OK)

			OBJA
SPOON	[0	1]	2
COIN	[0	1]	1
add above 2 scores then circle the answer →			0

			OBJB
TOOTHBRUSH	[0	1]	3
KEY	[0	1]	2
COMB	[0	1]	1
add above 3 scores then circle the answer →			0

	RPNM
(Total number of objects either named spontaneously or repeated correctly after coaching.) 0 1 2 3 4 5	

25. REMEMBER THESE 5 OBJECTS!
(Wait for 5 sec.; cover, then ask:)

RCOBJ

WHAT 5 OBJECTS DID I JUST SHOW YOU?
(Any order is OK, circle the correct ones.)

	5
	4
	3
SPOON COIN TOOTHBRUSH KEY COMB	2
	1
number of correct answers →	0

Finish time (hr:min) ___:___	Duration (minutes)	□□

VALIDITY OF SCORE	
Valid	1
Probably invalid: poor hearing	2
Probably invalid: poor eyesight	3
Probably invalid: impaired motor control	4
Probably invalid: language barrier	5
Probably invalid: impaired alertness or attentiveness	6
Probably invalid: significant physical or mental discomfort	7
Probably Invalid: other reasons (specify):	8

RAISE YOUR HAND

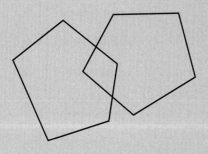

Activity intolerance
Risk for activity intolerance
Impaired adjustment
Ineffective airway clearance
Latex allergy response
Risk for latex allergy response
Anxiety
Death anxiety
Risk for aspiration
Risk for impaired parent/child/infant attachment
Autonomic dysreflexia
Risk for autonomic dysreflexia
Disturbed body image
Risk for imbalanced body temperature
Bowel incontinence
Effective breastfeeding
Ineffective breastfeeding
Interrupted breastfeeding
Ineffective breathing pattern
Decreased cardiac output
Caregiver role strain
Risk for caregiver role strain
Impaired verbal communication
Decisional conflict
Parental role conflict
Acute confusion
Chronic confusion
Constipation
Perceived constipation
Risk for constipation
Ineffective coping
Ineffective community coping
Readiness for enhanced community coping
Defensive coping
Compromised family coping
Disabled family coping
Readiness for enhanced family coping
Ineffective denial
Impaired dentition
Risk for delayed development
Diarrhea
Risk for disuse syndrome
Deficient diversional activity
Disturbed energy field
Impaired environmental interpretation syndrome
Adult failure to thrive
Risk for falls
Dysfunctional family processes: alcoholism
Interrupted family processes

Fatigue
Fear
Deficient fluid volume
Excess fluid volume
Risk for deficient fluid volume
Risk for imbalanced fluid volume
Impaired gas exchange
Anticipatory grieving
Dysfunctional grieving
Delayed growth and development
Risk for disproportionate growth
Ineffective health maintenance
Health-seeking behaviors (specify)
Impaired home maintenance
Hopelessness
Hyperthermia
Hypothermia
Disturbed personal identity
Functional urinary incontinence
Reflex urinary incontinence
Stress urinary incontinence
Total urinary incontinence
Urge urinary incontinence
Risk for urge urinary incontinence
Disorganized infant behavior
Risk for disorganized infant behavior
Readiness for enhanced organized infant behavior
Ineffective infant feeding pattern
Risk for infection
Risk for injury
Risk for perioperative-positioning injury
Decreased intracranial adaptive capacity
Deficient knowledge (specify)
Risk for loneliness
Impaired memory
Impaired bed mobility
Impaired physical mobility
Impaired wheelchair mobility
Nausea
Unilateral neglect
Noncompliance
Imbalanced nutrition: less than body requirements
Imbalanced nutrition: more than body
    requirements
Risk for imbalanced nutrition: more than body
    requirements
Impaired oral mucous membrane
Acute pain
Chronic pain

Impaired parenting
Risk for impaired parenting
Risk for peripheral neurovascular dysfunction
Risk for poisoning
Post-trauma syndrome
Risk for post-trauma syndrome
Powerlessness
Risk for powerlessness
Ineffective protection
Rape-trauma syndrome
Rape-trauma syndrome: compound reaction
Rape-trauma syndrome: silent reaction
Relocation stress syndrome
Risk for relocation stress syndrome
Ineffective role performance
Bathing/hygiene self-care deficit
Dressing/grooming self-care deficit
Feeding self-care deficit
Toileting self-care deficit
Chronic low self-esteem
Situational low self-esteem
Risk for situational low self-esteem
Self-mutilation
Risk for self-mutilation
Disturbed sensory perception (specify: visual, auditory, kinesthetic, gustatory, tactile, olfactory)
Sexual dysfunction
Ineffective sexuality patterns
Impaired skin integrity
Risk for impaired skin integrity
Sleep deprivation

Disturbed sleep pattern
Impaired social interaction
Social isolation
Chronic sorrow
Spiritual distress
Risk for spiritual distress
Readiness for enhanced spiritual well-being
Risk for suffocation
Risk for suicide
Delayed surgical recovery
Impaired swallowing
Effective therapeutic regimen management
Ineffective therapeutic regimen management
Ineffective family therapeutic regimen management
Ineffective thermoregulation
Disturbed thought processes
Impaired tissue integrity
Ineffective tissue perfusion (specify type: renal, cerebral, cardiopulmonary, gastrointestinal, peripheral)
Impaired transfer ability
Risk for trauma
Impaired urinary elimination
Urinary retention
Impaired spontaneous ventilation
Dysfunctional ventilatory weaning response
Risk for other-directed violence
Risk for self-directed violence
Impaired walking
Wandering

1. GAIT: The patient is examined as he walks into the examining room; his gait, the swing of his arms, his general posture, all form the basis for an overall score for this item. This is rated as follows:

   0 Normal
   1 Diminution in swing while the patient is walking.
   2 Marked diminution in swing with obvious rigidity in the arm.
   3 Stiff gait with arms held rigidly before the abdomen.
   4 Stooped shuffling gait with propulsion and retropulsion.

2. ARM DROPPING: The patient and the examiner both raise their arms to shoulder height and let them fall to their sides. In a normal subject, a stout slap is heard as the arms hit the sides. In the patient with extreme Parkinson's syndrome, the arms fall very slowly.

   0 Normal, free fall with loud slap and rebound.
   1 Fall slowed slightly with less audible contact and little rebound.
   2 Fall slowed, no rebound.
   3 Marked slowing, no slap at all.
   4 Arms fall as though against resistance; as though through glue.

3. SHOULDER SHAKING: The subject's arms are bent at a right angle at the elbow and are taken one at a time by the examiner who grasps one hand and also clasps the other around the patient's elbow. The subject's upper arm is pushed to and fro, and the humerus is externally rotated. The degree of resistance from normal to extreme rigidity is scored as follows:

   0 Normal
   1 Slight stiffness and resistance.
   2 Moderate stiffness and resistance.
   3 Marked rigidity with difficulty in passive movement.
   4 Extreme stiffness and rigidity with almost a frozen shoulder.

4. ELBOW RIGIDITY: The elbow joints are separately bent at right angles and passively extended and flexed, with the subject's biceps observed and simultaneously palpated. The resistance to this procedure is rated. (The presence of cogwheel rigidity is noted separately.) Scoring is from 0 to 4, as in the Shoulder Shaking test.

   0 Normal
   1 Slight stiffness and resistance.
   2 Moderate stiffness and resistance.
   3 Marked rigidity with difficulty in passive movement.
   4 Extreme stiffness and rigidity with almost a frozen shoulder.

5. FIXATION OF POSITION OR WRIST RIGIDITY: The wrist is held in one hand and the fingers held by the examiner's other hand, with the wrist moved to extension flexion and both ulnar and radial deviation. The resistance to this procedure is rated as in Items 3 and 4.

   0 Normal
   1 Slight stiffness and resistance.
   2 Moderate stiffness and resistance.
   3 Marked rigidity with difficulty in passive movement.
   4 Extreme stiffness and rigidity with almost a frozen shoulder.

6. LEG PENDULOUSNESS: The patient sits on a table with his legs hanging down and swinging free. The ankle is grasped by the examiner and raised until the knee is partially extended. It is then allowed to fall. The resistance to falling and the lack of swinging form the basis for the score on this item:

   0 The legs swing freely.
   1 Slight diminution in the swing of the legs.
   2 Moderate resistance to swing.
   3 Marked resistance and damping of swing.
   4 Complete absence of swing.

7. HEAD DROPPING: The patient lies on a well-padded examining table and his head is raised by the examiner's hand. The hand is then withdrawn, and the head allowed to drop. In the normal subject, the head will fall upon the table. The movement is delayed in extrapyramidal system disorder, and in extreme parkinsonism, it is absent. The neck muscles are rigid, and the head does not reach the examining table. Scoring is as follows:

0   The head falls completely, with a good thump as it hits the table.
1   Slight slowing in fall, mainly noted by lack of slap as head meets the table.
2   Moderate slowing in the fall, quite noticeable to the eye.
3   Head falls stiffly and slowly.
4   Head does not reach examining table.

8. GLABELLA TAP: Subject is told to open his eyes wide and not to blink. The glabella region is tapped at a steady, rapid speed. The number of times patient blinks in succession is noted:

0   0 to 5 blinks
1   6 to 10 blinks
2   11 to 15 blinks
3   16 to 20 blinks
4   21 or more blinks

9. TREMOR: Patient is observed walking into examining room and then is re-examined for this item:

0   Normal
1   Mild finger tremor, obvious to sight and touch.
2   Tremor of hand or arm occurring spasmodically.

3   Persistent tremor of one or more limbs.
4   Whole body tremor.

10. SALIVATION: Patient is observed while talking and then asked to open his mouth and elevate his tongue. The following ratings are given:

0   Normal
1   Excess salivation to the extent that pooling takes place if the mouth is open and the tongue raised.
2   When excess salivation is present and might occasionally result in difficulty in speaking.
3   Speaking with difficulty because of excess salivation.
4   Frank drooling.

Scoring: Each item is rated on a 5-point scale, with 0 meaning the complete absence of the condition, and 4 meaning the presence of the condition in extreme form. The score is obtained by adding the items and dividing by 10.

Reprinted with permission from Simpson G. M., Angus, J. W. S. (1970). A rating scale for extrapyramidal side effects. *Acta Psychiatrica Scandinavica, 212* (Suppl.), 11–19. Copyright 1970, Munksgaard International Publishers, Ltd.

		None	Minimal	Mild	Moderate	Severe
Facial and Oral Movements						
	1: Muscles of Facial Expression eg, movements of forehead, eyebrows, periorbital area, cheeks; include frowning, blinking, smiling, grimacing	0	1	2	3	4
	2: Lips and Perioral Area eg, puckering, pouting, smacking	0	1	2	3	4
	3: Jaw eg, biting, clenching, chewing, mouth opening, lateral movement	0	1	2	3	4
	4: Tongue Rate only increase in movement both in and out of mouth, NOT inability to sustain movement	0	1	2	3	4
Extremity Movements						
	5: Upper (arms, wrists, hands, fingers) Include choreic movements (ie, rapid, objectively purposeless, irregular, spontaneous), athetoid movements (ie, slow, irregular, complex, serpentine). Do NOT include tremor (ie, repetitive, regular, rhythmic).	0	1	2	3	4
	6: Lower (legs, knees, ankles, toes) eg, lateral knee movement, foot tapping, heel dropping, foot squirming, inversion and eversion of foot	0	1	2	3	4
Trunk Movements						
	7: Neck, shoulders, hips eg, rocking, twisting, squirming, pelvic gyrations	0	1	2	3	4
	8: Severity of abnormal movements	0	1	2	3	4
Global Judgment						
	9: Incapacitation due to abnormal movements	0	1	2	3	4
	10: Patient's awareness of abnormal movements Rate only patient's report	No awareness — 0 Aware, no distress — 1 Aware, mild distress — 2 Aware, moderate distress — 3 Aware, severe distress — 4				

		None	Minimal	Mild	Moderate	Severe

Global Judgment

11: Current problems with teeth and/or dentures — No 0 / Yes 1

12: Does patient usually wear dentures? — No 0 / Yes 1

Examination Procedures for AIMS

Either before or after completing the Examination Procedure, observe the patient unobtrusively, at rest (eg, in waiting room). The chair to be used in this examination should be a hard, firm one without arms.

1: Ask patient whether there is anything in his/her mouth (ie, gum, candy, etc.) and if there is, to remove it.

2: Ask patient about the *current* condition of his/her teeth. Ask patient if he/she wears dentures. Do teeth or dentures bother patient *now?*

3: Ask patient whether he/she notices any movements in mouth, face, hands, or feet. If yes, ask to describe and to what extent they *currently* bother patient or interfere with his/her activities.

4: Have patient sit in chair with hands on knees, legs slightly apart, and feet flat on floor. (Look at entire body for movements while in this position.)

5: Ask patient to sit with hands hanging unsupported. If male, between legs, if female and wearing a dress, hanging over knees. (Observe hands and other body areas.)

6: Ask patient to open mouth. (Observe tongue at rest within mouth.) Do this twice.

7: Ask patient to protrude tongue. (Observe tongue at rest within mouth.) Do this twice.

*8: Ask patient to tap thumb, with each finger, as rapidly as possible for 10–15 seconds; separately with right hand, then with left hand. (Observe facial and leg movements.)

9: Flex and extend patient's left and right arms (one at a time). (Note any rigidity and rate on NOTES.)

10: Ask patient to stand up. (Observe in profile. Observe all body areas again, hips included.)

*11: Ask patient to extend both arms outstretched in front with palms down. (Observe trunk, legs, and mouth.)

*12: Have patient walk a few paces, turn, and walk back to chair. (Observe hand and gait.) Do this twice.

---

*Activated movements.

Reprinted from Guy, W. (1976). ECDEU: Assessment manual for psychopharmacology (DHEW Publ No 76–338). Washington, DC: Department of Health, Education, and Welfare, Psychopharmacology Research Branch.

PREREQUISITES.—The three prerequisites are as follows. Exceptions may occur.

1. A history of at least 3 months' total cumulative neuroleptic exposure. Include amoxapine and metoclopramide in all categories below as well.

2. **SCORING/INTENSITY LEVEL.** The presence of a **TOTAL SCORE OF FIVE (5) OR ABOVE.** Also be alert for any change from baseline or scores below five which have at least a "moderate" (3) or "severe" (4) movement on any item or at least two "mild" (2) movements on two items located in different body areas.

3. Other conditions are not responsible for the abnormal involuntary movements.

DIAGNOSES.—The diagnosis is based upon the current exam and its relation to the last exam. The diagnosis can shift depending upon: (a) whether movements are present or not, (b) whether movements are present for 3 months or more (6 months if on a semiannual assessment schedule), and (c) whether neuroleptic dosage changes occur and effect movements.

- **NO TD.**—Movements **are not** present on this exam **or** movements are present, but some other condition is responsible for them. The last diagnosis must be NO TD, PROBABLE TD, or WITHDRAWAL TD.

- **PROBABLE TD.**—Movements **are** present on this exam. This is the first time they are present **or** they have never been present for 3 months or more. The last diagnosis must be NO TD or PROBABLE TD.

- **PERSISTENT TD.**—Movements **are** present on this exam **and** they have been present for 3 months **or** more with this exam or at some point in the past. The last diagnosis can be any except NO TD.

- **MASKED TD.**—Movements **are not** present on this exam **but** this is due to a neuroleptic dosage increase or reinstitution after a prior exam when movements were present. Also use this conclusion if movements are not present due to the addition of a non-neuroleptic medication to treat TD. The last diagnosis must be PROBABLE TD, PERSISTENT TD, WITHDRAWAL TD, or MASKED TD.

- **REMITTED TD.**—Movements **are not** present on this exam **but** PERSISTENT TD has been diagnosed **and** no neuroleptic dosage increase or reinstitution has occurred. The last diagnosis must be PERSISTENT TD or REMITTED TD. If movements re-emerge, the diagnosis shifts back to PERSISTENT TD.

- **WITHDRAWAL TD.**—Movements **are not seen while** receiving neuroleptics or at the last dosage level **but are seen within** 8 weeks following a neuroleptic reduction or discontinuation. The last diagnosis must be NO TD or WITHDRAWAL TD. If movements continue for 3 months or more after the neuroleptic dosage reduction or discontinuation, the diagnosis shifts to PERSISTENT TD. If movements do not continue for 3 months or more after the reduction or discontinuation, the diagnosis shifts to NO TD.

INSTRUCTIONS

1. The rater completes the Assessment according to the standardized exam procedure. If the rater also completes Evaluation items 1–4, he/she must also sign the preparer box. The form is given to the physician. Alternatively, the physician may perform the assessment.

2. The physician completes the Evaluation section. The physician is responsible for the entire Evaluation section and its accuracy.

3. IT IS RECOMMENDED THAT THE PHYSICIAN EXAMINE ANY INDIVIDUAL WHO MEETS THE THREE PREREQUISITES OR WHO HAS MOVEMENTS NOT EXPLAINED BY OTHER FACTORS. NEUROLOGICAL ASSESSMENTS OR DIFFERENTIAL DIAGNOSTIC TESTS WHICH MAY BE NECESSARY SHOULD BE OBTAINED.

4. File form according to policy or procedure.

OTHER CONDITIONS (partial list)

1. Age
2. Blind
3. Cerebral Palsy
4. Contact Lenses
5. Dentures/No Teeth
6. Down Syndrome
7. Drug Intoxication (specify)
8. Encephalitis
9. Extrapyramidal Side-Effects (specify)
10. Fahr's Syndrome
11. Heavy Metal Intoxication (specify)
12. Huntington's Chorea
13. Hyperthyroidism
14. Hypoglycemia
15. Hypoparathyroidism
16. Idiopathic Torsion Dystonia
17. Meige Syndrome
18. Parkinson's Disease
19. Stereotypies
20. Syndenham's Chorea
21. Tourette's Syndrome
22. Wilson's Disease
23. Other (specify)

Sprague, R. L., & Kalachnik, J. E. (1991). Reliability, validity, and a total score cutoff for the Dyskinesia Identification System, Condensed User Scale (DISCUS) with mentally ill and mentally retarded populations. *Psychopharmacology Bulletin, 27*(1), 51–58.

Clinic No. _____ Date _____ Rating No. _____ Code Number _____
Sex _____ Age _____ Patient's Name _____
Patient's Address _____ Tel _____

Item	Range	Score
1. Depressed mood	0–4	
2. Guilt	0–4	
3. Suicide	0–4	
4. Insomnia initial	0–2	
5. Insomnia middle	0–2	
6. Insomnia delayed	0–2	
7. Work and interest	0–4	
8. Retardation	0–4	
9. Agitation	0–4	
10. Anxiety (psychic)	0–4	
11. Anxiety (somatic)	0–4	
12. Somatic gastrointestinal	0–2	
13. Somatic general	0–2	
14. Genital	0–2	
15. Hypochondriasis	0–2	
16. Insight	0–4	
17. Loss of weight	0–2	
	Total Score	
Diurnal variation (M.A.E.)	0–2	
Depersonalization	0–4	
Paranoid symptoms	0–4	
Obsessional symptoms	0–4	

The scale is designed to measure the severity of illness of patients already diagnosed as suffering from depressive illness. It is obviously not a diagnostic instrument because that requires much more information (eg, previous history, family history, precipitating factors).

As far as possible, the scale should be used in the manner of a clinical interview. The first time the interview should be conducted in a relaxed, free, and easy manner, giving the patients time to unburden themselves and giving them the opportunity to speak of their problems and ask whatever questions they wish. It may then be necessary to obtain further information by asking them questions. At subsequent assessments, the interview can be briefer and more to the point.

An observer rating scale is not a checklist in which each item is strictly defined. The raters must have sufficient clinical experience and judgment to be able to interpret the patients' statements and reticences about some symptoms, and to compare them with other patients. They should use all sources of information (eg, from relatives and nurses).

The scale consists of 17 items, the scores on which are summed to give a total score. These are four other items, one of which (diurnal variation) is excluded on the grounds that it is not an additional burden on the patient. The last three are excluded from the total score because they occur infrequently, although information on them may be useful for other purposes.

The method of assessment is simple. For some symptoms it is difficult to elicit such information as will permit of full quantification. If present, score 2; if absent, score 0; and if doubtful or trivial, score 1. For those symptoms where more detailed information can be obtained, the score of 2 is expanded into 2 for mild, 3 for moderate, and 4 for severe. In case of difficulty, the raters should use their judgment as clinicians.

Hamilton, M. (1960). A rating scale for depression. *Journal of Neurology, Neurosurgery and Psychiatry, 23,* 56.

The CAGE is a very brief questionnaire for detection of alcoholism. Item responses on the CAGE are score 0 for *no* and 1 for *yes*, with a higher score an indication of alcohol problems. A total score of 2 or more is considered clinically significant and requires a more focused and detailed assessment. The following are the four questions that comprise the CAGE questionnaire.

Have you ever felt you should *Cut down* on your drinking?	Yes	No
Have people *Annoyed* you by criticizing your drinking?	Yes	No
Have you ever felt bad or *Guilty* about your drinking?	Yes	No
Have you ever had a drink first thing in the morning to steady your nerves to get rid of a hangover? *(Eyeopener)*	Yes	No

Ewing, J. A. (1984). Detecting alcoholism. *Journal of the American Medical Association. 252,* 1905–1907.
Additional readings:
Burge, S., & Schneider, F. (1999). Alcohol-related problems: Recognition and intervention. *American Family Physician,* American Academy of Family Physicians Home Page (www.aafp.org. 1/15/99).
Davis, M. (2000). Alcohol and drug addiction. *Medical Library* (www.medical-library.org. 9/30/00).
Wesson, D. (1995). *Detoxification from alcohol and other drugs.* Rockville, MD: Substance Abuse and Mental Health Services Administration, Center for Substance Abuse Treatment, Treatment Improvement Protocol # 19.

PATIENT CLINICAL PATHWAY FOR BIPOLAR AFFECTIVE DISORDER

Patient Name _____ Pt # _____ SOC Date: _____ Payor Source _____

Discharge Date: SN: _____ PT: _____ Actual Visits: SN: _____ PT: _____

Nursing Diagnosis:	1. Alteration in Thought Process 2. Ineffective Individual Coping 3. _____	Recommended frequency: 2–3 x/wk × 3 wks; 1–2 x/wk × 6 wks Recommended total visits: 21

KEY: Completed - Initial   To Be Completed in the Following Week = Circle/Initial   Not Applicable/Not Ordered = NA

Week/No. of Visits Key Functions	WEEK 1 2–3 Visits	Initial /Date	WEEK 2 2–3 Visits	Initial /Date	WEEK 3 2–3 Visits	Initial /Date	WEEK 4 1–2 Visits	Initial /Date	WEEK 5 1–2 Visits	Initial /Date
Patient Outcomes	Prevention of harm to self &/or others Daily adherence to med regimen Tolerating medication regimen Receptive to interventions Knowledge of >Disease process >Treatment >Identification of s/s >S/S's to report >Med. effects and SE's: _____ _____ _____ Psych. f/u appt. made Date _____		Daily adherence to med. regimen Tolerating medication regimen Receptive to interventions Knowledge of: >effects of decreased activity >reality testing >re-orientation skills >stress management skills >community programs >avoidance of caffeine >effects of poor diet Identification of stressors Able to maintain personal hygiene		Daily adherence to med. regimen Tolerating medication regimen Receptive to interventions Knowledge of: >need for socialization/ activity >effects of isolation and seclusion >psych. f/u		Daily adherence to med. regimen Tolerating medication regimen Receptive to interventions Knowledge of: >assertive communication skills >positive self talk >effects of negative thinking >medication effects and SE's: _____ _____ _____ _____		Daily adherence to med. regimen Tolerating medication regimen Receptive to interventions Able to express feelings Knowledge of: >_____ >_____ >_____ >_____	
Patient/ Family Education	I Disease process >Treatment >Identification of symptoms >s/s's to report Medication regimen Med. affects and SE's: _____ _____ _____ Psychiatric f/u		Effects of poor diet Effects of caffeine Effects of decreased activity Community programs Stress management skills Re-orientation skills Reality Testing		Effects of isolation & seclusion Need for socialization/ activities Short term goal setting		Med. effects and SE: _____ _____ _____ Effects of negative thinking Positive self talk Assertive communication skills		Re-instruct deficits in learning: _____ _____ _____ _____	

1085

PATIENT CLINICAL PATHWAY FOR BIPOLAR AFFECTIVE DISORDER (Continued)

Week No. of Visits	WEEK 1 2–3 Visits		WEEK 2 2–3 Visits		WEEK 3 2–3 Visits		WEEK 4 1–2 Visits		WEEK 5 1–2 Visits	
Key Functions		Initial /Date		Initial /Date		Initial /Date		Initial /Date		Initial /Date
Assessm't/ Treatment	Psychosocial assessment Medication effective- ness/ adverse SE's Therapeutic in- tervention/in struction Adherence to medication regimen		Psychosocial assessment Medication effective- ness/ adverse SE's Therapeutic intervention/ instruction Adherence to medication regimen		Psychosocial assessment Medication effective- ness/ad- verse SE's Therapeutic interven- tion/instruc- tion Adherence to medication regimen		Psychosocial assessment Medication ef- fectiveness/ adverse SE's Therapeutic intervention/ instruction Adherence to medication regimen		Psychosocial assessment Medication ef- fectiveness/ adverse SE's Therapeutic intervention/ instruction Adherence to medication regimen	
Referrals/ DME	Aide MSW PT OT RD						Community programs:			
Discharge Planning	Review pt pathway Explain goals of service/ expected LOS Initiate dis- charge planning				Review pt progress on pathway Discharge Planning				Review pt progress on pathway Discharge Planning	
Initial/ Signature Date	___ ___ ___ ___ ___ ___ ___ ___ ___ ___ ___ ___		___ ___ ___ ___ ___ ___ ___ ___ ___ ___ ___ ___		___ ___ ___ ___ ___ ___ ___ ___ ___ ___ ___ ___		___ ___ ___ ___ ___ ___ ___ ___ ___ ___ ___ ___		___ ___ ___ ___ ___ ___ ___ ___ ___ ___ ___ ___	

(Continued)

Patient Name _____ Pt # _____

KEY: Completed - Initial   To Be Completed in the Following Week = Circle/Initial   Not Applicable/Not Ordered = NA

Week/No. of Visits	WEEK 6 1-2 Visits		WEEK 7 1-2 Visits		WEEK 8 1-2 Visits		WEEK 9 1-2 Visits		WEEK 10 SN (1x/week)	
Key Functions		Initial /Date		Initial /Date		Initial /Date		Initial /Date		Initial /Date
Patient Outcomes	Daily adherence to med. regimen Tolerating medication regimen Receptive to interventions Knowledge of: >coping skills Decrease in identified problem behaviors		Daily adherence to med. regimen Tolerating medication regimen Receptive to interventions Enhanced coping skills Knowledge of: >problem solving skills Increased activity level and socialization		Daily adherence to med. regimen Tolerating medication regimen Receptive to interventions Knowledge of: >medication effects and SE's: _____ _____ _____		Daily adherence to med. regimen Tolerating med. regimen Receptive to interventions Prevention of rehospitalization Able to verbalize increase in life satisfaction Independent in med. preparation Knowledge of: >disease process & management >medication preparation >compliance issues >on-going psych. follow-up >community support services			
Patient/ Family Education	Coping skills		Problem solving skills		Medication Effects & SE's: _____ _____ Re-instruct deficits in learning: _____ _____		Long term management >Compliance issues >Psychiatric f/u >Community support services			
Assessm't/ Treatment	Psychosocial assessment Medication effectiveness/ adverse SE's Therapeutic intervention/ instruction Adherence to med. regimen		Psychosocial assessment Medication effectiveness/ adverse SE's Therapeutic intervention/ instruction Adherence to med. regimen Assess self-management skills		Psychosocial assessment Medication effectiveness/ adverse SE's Therapeutic intervention/ instruction Adherence to med. regimen		Psychosocial assessment Medication effectiveness/ adverse SE's Therapeutic intervention/ instruction Adherence to med. regimen			

(Continued)

Week No. of Visits	WEEK 6 1-2 Visits		WEEK 7 1-2 Visits		WEEK 8 1-2 Visits		WEEK 9 1-2 Visits		WEEK 10 SN (1x/week)	
Key Functions		Initial /Date		Initial /Date		Initial /Date		Initial /Date		Initial /Date
Referrals/ DME			Community programs: _____ _____ _____							
Discharge Planning	Review pt progress on pathway Discharge planning				Review pt progress on pathway Discharge planning		Discontinue services if outcomes are met/ pathway completed. Confirm psych. f/u Pathway completed/ outcomes not met/ continue with NCP			
Initial/ Signature Date	__ _____ __ __ _____ __ __ _____ __ __ _____ __		__ _____ __ __ _____ __ __ _____ __ __ _____ __		__ _____ __ __ _____ __ __ _____ __ __ _____ __		__ _____ __ __ _____ __ __ _____ __ __ _____ __		__ _____ __ __ _____ __ __ _____ __ __ _____ __

PATIENT CLINICAL PATHWAY FOR DEPRESSION

Patient Name _____ Pt # _____ SOC Date: _____ Payor Source _____

Discharge Date: SN: _____ PT: _____ Actual Visits: SN: _____ PT: _____

Nursing Diagnosis:	1. Alteration in Thought Process 4. _____ 2. Ineffective individual Coping 5. _____ 3. _____ 6. _____	Recommended frequency: 2–3 × wk × 1 wk; 1–2 × wk × 8 wks Recommended total visits: 15

KEY: Completed - Initial   To Be Completed in the Following Week = Circle/Initial   Not Applicable/Not Ordered = NA

Week/No. of Visits Key Functions	WEEK 1 2–3 Visits Initial /Date	WEEK 2 1–2 Visits Initial /Date	WEEK 3 1–2 Visits Initial /Date	WEEK 4 1–2 Visits Initial /Date	WEEK 5 1–2 Visits Initial /Date
Patient Outcomes	Prevention of harm to self &/or others Daily adherence to med. regimen Tolerating medication regimen Knowledge of >disease process >treatment >identification of s/s >s/s to report >med. effects and SE's	Receptive to interventions Daily adherence to med. regimen Tolerating medication regimen Psychiatric f/u appointment made. Knowledge of: >short term goal setting >effects of poor diet >effects of negative thinking >positive self-talk Able to maintain personal hygiene	Decrease in identified problem behaviors Daily adherence to med. regimen Tolerating medication regimen Receptive to interventions Knowledge of: >effects of isolation and seclusion >need for socialization and activity >community prog. >assertive communication skills	Daily adherence to med. regimen Tolerating med. regimen Receptive to interventions Able to express feelings Identification of stressors Knowledge of: >stress management skills >Med. effects and SE's: _____ _____	Daily adherence to med. regimen Tolerating med. regimen Enhanced coping skills Received psychiatric f/u Receptive to interventions Knowledge of: >problem solving skills >coping skills
Patient/ Family Education	I Disease process Treatment Identification of symptoms S/S's to report Medication regimen Med. effects and SE's: _____ _____ _____ Psychiatric f/u	Effects of poor diet Effects of decreased activity Effects of negative thinking Short term goal setting Positive self talk	Effects of isolation & seclusion Need for socialization/ activities Community programs Assertive communication skills	Med. effects and SE: _____ _____ _____ Stress management skills	Problem solving skills Coping skills
Assessm't/ Treatment	Psychosocial Assessment Medication effectiveness/ adverse SE's Therapeutic intervention/ instruction Adherence to medication regimen	Psychosocial Assessment Medication effectiveness/ adverse SE's Therapeutic intervention/ instruction Adherence to medication regimen	Psychosocial Assessment Medication effectiveness/ adverse SE's Therapeutic intervention/ instruction Adherence to medication regimen	Psychosocial Assessment Medication effectiveness/ adverse SE's Therapeutic intervention/ instruction Adherence to medication regimen	Psychosocial Assessment Medication effectiveness/ adverse SE's Therapeutic intervention/ instruction Adherence to medication regimen
Referrals/ DME	Aide MSW PT OT RD				

PATIENT CLINICAL PATHWAY FOR DEPRESSION (Continued)

Week/No. of Visits	WEEK 1 2–3 Visits	Initial /Date	WEEK 2 1–2 Visits	Initial /Date	WEEK 3 1–2 Visits	Initial /Date	WEEK 4 1–2 Visits	Initial /Date	WEEK 5 1–2 Visits	Initial /Date
Key Functions										
Discharge Planning	Review pt pathway Initiate discharge planning Explain goals of service/ expected LOS				Review pt progress on pathway Discharge Planning				Review pt progress on pathway Discharge Planning	
Initial/ Signature Date	__ __ __ __ __ __ __ __ __ __ __ __		__ __ __ __ __ __ __ __ __ __ __ __		__ __ __ __ __ __ __ __ __ __ __ __		__ __ __ __ __ __ __ __ __ __ __ __		__ __ __ __ __ __ __ __ __ __ __ __	

Patient Name _____ Pt # _____

KEY: Completed - Initial   To Be Completed in the Following Week = Circle/Initial   Not Applicable/Not Ordered = NA

Week/No. of Visits	WEEK 6 1–2 Visits	Initial /Date	WEEK 7 1–2 Visits	Initial /Date	WEEK 8 1–2 Visits	Initial /Date	WEEK 9 1–2 Visits	Initial /Date	WEEK 10 SN (1x/week)	Initial /Date
Key Functions										
Patient Outcomes	Daily adherence to med. regimen Tolerating medication regimen Clear communication of thoughts Receptive to interventions Enhanced coping skills Knowledge of: >reality testing >re-orientation skills		Daily adherence to med. regimen Tolerating medication regimen Receptive to interventions Knowledge of: _____ _____ _____ _____		Daily adherence to med. regimen Tolerating medication regimen Demonstrating self-management skills Receptive to interventions Knowledge of: >medication effects and SE's: _____ _____ _____		Daily adherence to med. regimen Tolerating medication regimen Receptive to interventions Prevention of rehospitalization Able to verbalize increase in life satisfaction Independent in med. preparation Knowledge of: >disease process & management >medication preparation >compliance issues >on-going psych. follow-up >community support services			
Patient/ Family Education	Reality testing Re-orientation skills		Re-instruct deficits in learning: _____ _____ _____		Medication Effects & SE's: _____ _____ _____		Long term management >Compliance issues >Psychiatric f/u >Community support services			

(Continued)

Week No. of Visits Key Functions	WEEK 6 1-2 Visits		WEEK 7 1-2 Visits		WEEK 8 1-2 Visits		WEEK 9 1-2 Visits		WEEK 10 SN (1x/week)	
		Initial /Date		Initial /Date		Initial /Date		Initial /Date		Initial /Date
Assessm't/ Treatment	Psychosocial assessment Medication effective- ness/ adverse SE's Therapeutic intervention/ instruction Adherence to med. regimen Assess self- manage- ment skills		Psychosocial assessment Medication effective- ness/ adverse SE's Therapeutic intervention/ instruction Adherence to med. regimen		Psychosocial assessment Medication effective- ness/ adverse SE's Therapeutic intervention/ instruction Adherence to med. regimen		Psychosocial Assessment Medication effective- ness/ Adverse SE's Therapeutic intervention/ instruction			
Referrals/ DME	Aide MSW PT OT		Community programs: _____ _____ _____ _____							
Discharge Planning	Review pt progress on pathway Discharge planning				Review pt progress on pathway Discharge planning		Discontinue services if outcomes are met. Confirm psych. f/u Pathway completed/ outcomes not met/ continue with NCP			
Initial/ Signature Date	__ _____ __ __ _____ __ __ _____ __ __ _____ __		__ _____ __ __ _____ __ __ _____ __ __ _____ __		__ _____ __ __ _____ __ __ _____ __ __ _____ __		__ _____ __ __ _____ __ __ _____ __ __ _____ __		__ _____ __ __ _____ __ __ _____ __ __ _____ __	

PATIENT CLINICAL PATHWAYS FOR SCHIZOPHRENIA

Patient Name _____ Pt # _____ SOC Date: _____ Payor Source _____

Discharge Date: SN: _____ PT: _____ Actual Visits: SN: _____ PT: _____

Nursing Diagnosis:	1. Alteration in Thought Process	Recommended frequency: 2–3 x/wk × 3 wks; 1–2 x/wk × 6 wks
	2. Ineffective individual Coping	Recommended total visits: 21

KEY: Completed - Initial   To Be Completed in the Following Week = Circle/Initial   Not Applicable/Not Ordered = NA

Week/No. of Visits	WEEK 1 2–3 Visits	Initial /Date	WEEK 2 2–3 Visits	Initial /Date	WEEK 3 2–3 Visits	Initial /Date	WEEK 4 1–2 Visits	Initial /Date	WEEK 5 1–2 Visits	Initial /Date
Key Functions										
Patient Outcomes	Daily adherence to med. regimen. Tolerating med. regimen Receptive to interventions Prevention of harm to self and/or others Knowledge of: >Disease proc. >Treatment >Identification of symptoms >S/S's to report >Effects and SE's of meds. Psychiatric f/u appt. made: Date: _____		Daily adherence to med. regimen. Tolerating med. regimen Ability to maintain personal hygiene Receptive to interventions Knowledge of: >Community programs >Re-orientation skills >Reality testing >Effects of poor diet >Avoidance of caffeine >Effects of decreased activity		Daily adherence to med. regimen. Tolerating med. regimen Receptive to interventions Knowledge of: >Short term goal setting >Need for socialization and activities. >Effects of isolation and seclusion >Psychiatric follow-up		Daily adherence to med. regimen. Tolerating med. regimen. Receptive to interventions Decrease in delusions & hallucinations. Knowledge of: >Effects of negative thinking >Positive self talk. >Assertive communication skills. >Community prog.'s >Med. effects and SE: _____		Daily adherence to med. regimen. Tolerating med. regimen. Receptive to interventions Able to express feelings Knowledge of: >_____ >_____ >_____ >_____	
Patient/ Family Education	Med. regimen. Disease proc. >Treatment >Identification of symptoms >S/S's to report. Psychiatric f/u Medication Effects and SE's: _____ _____		Community prog.'s Re-orientation skills. Reality testing. Effects of poor diet. Avoidance of caffeine Effects of decreased activity.		Short term goal setting. Need for socialization/ activities. Effects of isolation and seclusion.		Effects of negative thinking. Positive self talk. Assertive communication skills. Medication Effects and SE's: _____ _____ _____		Re-instruct deficits in learning: >_____ >_____ >_____ >_____	
Assessm't/ Treatment	Psychosocial assessment. Medication effectiveness/ Adverse SE's. Adherence to med. regimen Therapeutic interventions/ instructions.		Psychosocial assessment. Medication effectiveness/ Adverse SE's. Adherence to med. regimen Therapeutic interventions/ instructions.		Psychosocial assessment. Medication effectiveness/ Adverse SE's. Adherence to med. regimen Therapeutic interventions/ instructions.		Psychosocial assessment. Medication effectiveness/ Adverse SE's. Adherence to med. regimen Therapeutic interventions/ instructions.		Psychosocial assessment. Medication effectiveness/ Adverse SE's. Adherence to med. regimen Therapeutic interventions/ instructions.	
Referrals/ DME	Aide MSW PT RD OT						Community program(s): _____ _____			

PATIENT CLINICAL PATHWAYS FOR SCHIZOPHRENIA (Continued)

Week/No. of Visits	WEEK 1 2–3 Visits		WEEK 2 2–3 Visits		WEEK 3 2–3 Visits		WEEK 4 1–2 Visits		WEEK 5 1–2 Visits	
Key Functions		Initial /Date		Initial /Date		Initial /Date		Initial /Date		Initial /Date
Discharge Planning	Review pt pathway Explain goals of service/ expected LOS. Initiate D/C planning.				Review pt progress on pathway. D/C planning.				Review pt progress on pathway. D/D planning.	
Initial/ Signature Date	__ ____ __ __ ____ __ __ ____ __		__ ____ __ __ ____ __ __ ____ __		__ ____ __ __ ____ __ __ ____ __		__ ____ __ __ ____ __ __ ____ __		__ ____ __ __ ____ __ __ ____ __	

Patient Name _____ Pt # _____

KEY: Completed - Initial   To Be Completed in the Following Week = Circle/Initial   Not Applicable/Not Ordered = NA

Week/No. of Visits	WEEK 6 1-2 Visits		WEEK 7 1-2 Visits		WEEK 8 1-2 Visits		WEEK 9 1-2 Visits		WEEK 10 SN (1x/week)	
Key Functions		Initial /Date		Initial /Date		Initial /Date		Initial /Date		Initial /Date
Patient Outcomes	Tolerating med. regimen. Daily adherence to med. regimen Receptive to interventions Decrease in identified problem behaviors. Identification of stressors. Knowledge of: >Stress management skills. >Coping skills		Tolerating med. regimen. Daily adherence to med. regimen. Receptive to interventions Enhanced coping skills. Knowledge of: >problem solving skills >increased activity level/ socialization		Tolerating med. regimen. Daily adherence to med. regimen Receptive to interventions Clear verbalization of thoughts. Knowledge of: >Medication effects and SE's: _____ _____ _____		Tolerating med. regimen. Daily adherence to med. regimen Receptive to interventions Verbalizes increased life satisfaction Independent in medication preparation Knowledge of: >Ongoing psych. f/u >Compliance issues >Disease proc. and management. >Community support services Prevention of rehospitalization.			
Patient/ Family Education	Stress management skills Coping skills.		Problem solving skills.		Medication effects & SE's: _____ _____ Re-instruct deficits in learning: _____ _____		Long term management. >Compliance issues. >Psych. follow-up >Community support services.			

(Continued)

Week/No. of Visits	WEEK 6 1-2 Visits	Initial /Date	WEEK 7 1-2 Visits	Initial /Date	WEEK 8 1-2 Visits	Initial /Date	WEEK 9 1-2 Visits	Initial /Date	WEEK 10 SN (1x/week)	Initial /Date
Key Functions										
Assessm't/ Treatment	Psychosocial assessment. Medication effectiveness/ Adverse SE's. Adherence to med. regimen Therapeutic interventions/ instructions.		Psychosocial assessment Medication effectiveness/ Adverse SE's. Adherence to med. regimen Therapeutic interventions/ instructions.		Psychosocial assessment. Medication effectiveness/ Adverse SE's. Adherence to med. regimen Therapeutic interventions/ instructions.		Psychosocial assessment. Medication effectiveness/ Adverse SE's. Adherence to med. regimen Therapeutic interventions/ instructions.			
Referrals/ DME							Confirm f/u through community program(s): _____			
Discharge Planning			Review patient progress on pathway D/C planning.				Discontinue services if outcomes are met/ pathway completed. Confirm psych. f/u Pathway completed/ outcomes not met continue with NCP			
Initial/ Signature Date	__ ____ __ __ ____ __ __ ____ __ __ ____ __		__ ____ __ __ ____ __ __ ____ __ __ ____ __		__ ____ __ __ ____ __ __ ____ __ __ ____ __		__ ____ __ __ ____ __ __ ____ __ __ ____ __		__ ____ __ __ ____ __ __ ____ __ __ ____ __	

PATIENT CLINICAL PATHWAY FOR BIPOLAR AFFECTIVE DISORDER

Admission date _____ D/C date _____

Estimated LOS _____ Case manager _____

Case type & number (DRG - 430) Bipolar Affective Disorder

Date	Day 1/adm Loc ( )	Var n/s m u	Day 2–3 Loc ( )	Var n/s m u	Day 4–6 Loc ( )	Var n/s m u
Procedure/test	Organic workup (MD), EEG (MD), CT (MD), MRI (MD), EKG (MD), CXR (MD), electrolytes (MD), lithium level (MD), drug screen (MD), thyroid studies (MD), routine labs (MD), other (MD).		Lab results (ID abnormals)		——> Psych testing complete	
Consults	Medical (MD) Behavior Med. (MD) Psych Testing (MD) Other (MD)		ID additional consults		——>	
Meds/Tx	Meds ordered per MD including PRN to control behavior.		Monitor anti-depressant, lithium, tegretol, valproic acid, PRN meds. Other anti-psychotic meds; if mania DC anti-depressant ——>		——>	
	ECT (MD) —permits (Nsg) —teaching (Nsg) —team notified (Nsg)				——>	
Activity	Voluntary/involuntary SP/EP (MD, Nsg) Fall precautions (MS, Nsg)		Assess ADLs ——> ——> Integrate into milieu Partic. in groups Individual therapy		——> Assess pre-cautions ——> ——> ——>	
Nutrition	Assess appetite (MD, Nsg) Assess elimination patterns (MD, Nsg)		——> ——> Diet teach		——> ——> ——>	
Discharge planning	Legal guardian ID (Nsg)		SW acknowl. note Placement issues		Family mtg	
	Assess support system (Nsg, MD, SW, TR)					
	Initial plan (MD/Nsg)		MTP signed (MD/Nsg/SW)			
INTERVENTIONS: Assessment	H+P & psych orders (MD) Nsg assessment and ADB		Ongoing assess & treatment (MD, Nsg, SW, TR) BM initial assess, assess for dystonia		——>	
Functional assessment	Proper envir. assessed Mini mental (Nsg) Assess LOF (Nsg, SW) Assess methods to control behavior (Nsg) Remove ext. stimuli (Nsg)		If ADL assess needed OT referral		Assess: —thought patterns —orientation —cog. skills —task completion	
Patient teaching	Orient pt/family to unit (Nsg) Patient rights given (Nsg)		Ed. pt/family to various therapies Medication education Primary nurse ID		——> ——>	

Signatures & initials

_____   _____   _____   _____

_____   _____   _____   _____

Teaching (initial and date when complete):

1. Medication education_____
2. Education on illness_____
3. Social skills_____

Day 7–9 Loc ( )	Var n/s m u	Day 10–12 Loc ( )	Var n/s m u	Day 13–14 Loc ( )	Var n/s m u	Day 15 Loc ( )	Var n/s m u	Discharge expected outcome

Labs _____
Tests _____
Med. blood
  levels _____
		Labs _____
		Tests _____
		Med. blood
		  levels _____
				Labs _____
				Tests _____
				Chart copied
				  if appro-
				  priate
						DC orders
						  written		

——>		——>		F/u appts made		——>		
——>		——>		——>		Prescriptions written		Pt will verbalize/ demonstrate imp. or med- ication +/or other thera- pies in main- taining opti- mal level of fcn after DC as evidenced by _____

——>		——>
		Begin ECT
		  outpt
		  arrange-
		  ments
				——>
				——>				

——>
——>
——>
——>
——>
		——>
		——>
		——>
		——>
		——>
				DC teaching
				  r/t follow-
				  up therapy
						Plans finalized
						  r/t outpt
						  therapy		

——> ——>		——> ——>		DC teaching r/t nutrition		——>		
——>		——>						

Plan discussed
  with patient
  (MD)
				DC teaching
				  w/family
				  weekly
				  progress
				  note (MD,
				  SW, TR,
				  Nsg)
						MTP closed
						  or remains
						  ongoing
								Pt will return
								to least
								restrictive/
								most sup-
								portive envi-
								ronment
								after DC
								with im-

——>
Weekly
  progress
  note (MD,
  SW, Nsg,
  TR)
Complete SW
  assessment
Referrals
Resources
MTP
  developed
		——>		DC teaching
				  on utiliza-
				  tion of skills
				  learned
				  while in
				  hosp and
				  how to inte-
				  grate to
				  home.
				Written
				  info. r/t
				  resources
				  given.
						Final DC in-
						  structions
						  given to
						  pt/family
						
						F/U appt
						  finalized
								proved cop-
								ing skills and
								identified
								resources
								as demon-
								strated by
								_____

——>
Assess task
  completion
Encourage
  Incr. LOF
		——>
		——>
				——>
				——>
						Final assess-
						  ments & DC
						  summary
						  written		

——>
Assess
  lifestyle
  chgs
——>
		MMSE (Nsg)
		——>
		——>
		——>
				——>		——>		

——>
——>
		——>
		——>
				——>
				——>
				DC teaching
						Final DC
						  teaching to
						  Pt/Family
						Pt. response
						  to teaching
						  docu-
						  mented.		

4. Coping skills _____
5. ADLs _____
6. Self-esteem _____
7. Dealing with anger _____

8. Communication skills _____
9. Dealing with sadness _____
10. Decision making _____
11. Other _____

*Documented patient response in progress notes.
Refer to Nurses Notes for documentation regarding
  variances.
SW work week is M–F.
© G. Bufe 1994

PATIENT CLINICAL PATHWAY FOR DEPRESSION

Admission date _____ D/C date _____
Estimated LOS _____ Case manager _____

Case type & Number (DRG - 426) Depression

Date	Day 1/adm Loc ( )	Var n/s m u	Day 2–3/Phase I Loc ( )	Var n/s m u	Day 4–6/ Phase II Loc ( )	Var n/s m u
Procedure/test	Organic workup (MD), CT (MD), MRI (MD), EKG (MD), EEG (MD), CXR (MD), routine labs (MD), electrolytes (MD), thyroid studies (MD), DST (MD), other (MD).		Lab test results (MD/Nsg) Additional tests (MD)		Psych testing complete Monitor med levels (MD).	
Consults	Medical (MD) Psychology (Testing, MD) Dietary (if on MAOI) (MD) Other (MD)		Additional consults		——>	
Meds/Tx	Medications ordered: Antidepressants, MAOI, etc. (MD) ECT (MD) —permits (Nsg) —teaching (Nsg) —team notified (Nsg)		Monitor antidepressants, MAOI, and other meds ECT —preparations —staff informed —pt teaching/ response		——> ——>	
Activity	Voluntary/involuntary process started (MD, Nsg) Suicide/elopement precautions if indicated (MD, Nsg)		Assess ADLs Integrate into milieu Participate in pt/staff meeting Group therapy Individual therapy		Review/ update suicide/ Elopement precautions ——> ——> ——> ——>	
Nutrition	Assess appetite (Nsg, MD) Dietary teaching r/t MAOI		Assess appetite Assess compliance w/dietary restrictions		——> ——>	
Discharge planning	Legal guardian ID (Nsg) Plan discussed w/pt Assess support system (Nsg, MD, TR) Initial plan (MD, Nsg)		SW acknowledgement note Placement issues ID MTP signed (MD/Nsg/SW) SW initial plan TR initial plan		Family mtg (SW, MD) Resources ID (SW)	

INTERVENTIONS:

Assessment	H&P and psych orders written (MD) Nsg assessment, ADB (Nsg)		Ongoing assess and Tx (MD, Nsg, SW TR) BM—Initial assessment Assess sleep		——> ——>	
Functional assessment	Mini mental (Nsg) Assess LOF (Nsg) Baseline orthostatic BP Assess lethality (Nsg, MD)		If ADL assessment needed (OT referral) Assess cognitive ability and focusing on tasks (Nsg, SW).		Encourage/ promote LOF Assess lethality Assess coping	
Patient teaching	Orient Pt/family to unit (Nsg) Patient rights given (Nsg) Confidentiality disclosure Given (Nsg)		Medication education (Nsg) Educate pt/family on various therapies Primary nurse ID		——> ——>	

Signatures & initials

_____ _____ _____ _____

_____ _____ _____ _____

Teaching (initial and date when complete):
1. Medication education _____
2. Education on illness _____
3. Social skills _____

Day 7–8/ Phase III Loc ( )	Var. n/s m u	Day 9/ Phase IV Loc ( )	Var n/s m u	Day 10/ Phase V Loc ( )	Var n/s m u	Day 11/ Phase VI Loc ( )	Var n/s m u	Discharge expected outcome
Labs _____ ——>		Labs _____		Labs _____		DC orders written		
Tests _____ Monitor med blood levels		Tests _____		Tests _____				
——>		——>		Monitor med blood levels F/U appts made		——>		
——>		——>		——>		Prescript. written ——>		Pt will verbalize/ demonstrate imp of med- ication &/or other thera- pies in main- taining op- tional level of function as evidenced by _____
——>		——>		——>				
——>		Begin ECT. outpt arrange ID any changes in med/Tx		——>				
Encourage out-trips to integrate back to environ- ment						Pt informed of plans r/t activity after dis- charge		
——> ——> ——>		——> ——>		Milieu therapy Group therapy Individual therapy				
——> ——>		——> ——>		——> ——>		Dietary DC teaching		
DC plan reassessed, family informed Resource ID Weekly procedure (MD, Nsg, SW, TR) Complete SW assess in chart MTP developed		Help pt/family w/DC plans F/U plans ID		——> Outpt behav- ior therapy arranged ——> DC transport arranged: —complete —in chart —chart copied —release of info. —eval/ recomm. Weekly progress note (MD, Nsg, SW, TR) ——>		MTP closed or ID as ongoing Final DC in- structions given to pt/family F/U appt finalized		Pt will return to least restric- tive environ- ment after DC with im- proved copy- ing skills and identified resources as demon- strated by _____
——> Complete SW assessment in chart. ——>		——>		——>		Plans finalized r/t F/U therapy Final assess- ment & DC summary written		Pt will be able to state ap- propriate re- sources to utilize after DC
Encourage/ promote LOF BDI/HAM-D (Nsg) MMSE (Nsg) ——> ——> ——> ——> ——> ——>		——> ——> ——> ——> ——> Educ F/U & compliance ——> ——>		BDI/HAM-D (Nsg) MMSE (Nsg) ——> ——> ——> DC teaching to pt/family		Help pt ID phone #'s for commu- nity re- sources Final DC teaching done with pt/family Pt response to docu- mented		Pt will verbalize understand- ing of DC teaching

4. Coping skills_____
5. ADLs_____
6. Self-esteem_____
7. Dealing with anger_____

8. Communication skills_____
9. Dealing with sadness_____
10. Decision making_____
11. Other_____

*Documented patient response in progress notes.
Refer to Nurses Notes for documentation regarding
   variances.
SW work week is M–F.
© G. Bufe 1994

PATIENT CLINICAL PATHWAY FOR SCHIZOPHRENIA

Admission date _____ D/C date _____

Estimated LOS _____ Case manager _____

Case type & number (DRG - 430) Schizophrenia

Date	Day 1/adm Loc ( )	Var n/s m u	Day 2–3 Loc ( )	Var n/s m u	Day 4–6 Loc ( )	Var n/s m u
Procedure/test	Organic workup (MD), CT (MD), MRI (MD), EKG (MD), EEG (MD), CXR (MD), routine labs (MD), PET scan (MD), electrolytes (MD), drug screen (MD), thyroid studies (MD), Other (MD).		Lab/test results (MD/Nsg)		Labs Tests Monitor blood med levels if appropriate.	
Consults	Medical (MD) Behavior med. (MD) Psych testing (MD) Other (MD)		Additional consults		——>	
Meds/Tx	Meds ordered per MD including PRN for behavior		Monitor neuroleptics and other anti-psychotic drugs		——> ECT (MD) —permits (Nsg) —teaching (Nsg) —team notified (Nsg)	
Activity	Voluntary/involuntary Precautions if indicated		Assess ADLs Integrate into milieu Individual therapy Group therapy Encourage goal-oriented tasks		——> ——> ——> ——> Assess for task completion	
Nutrition	Assess appetite Assess elimination		——> ——>		——> ——> Nutrition education	
Discharge planning	Legal guardian ID (Nsg) Plan disc. w/pt Assess support system Initial plan (MD/Nsg)		SW acknowledge-ment note Placement issues Initial plan (SW, TR)		Family mtg	
INTERVENTIONS: Assessment	H+P & psych orders written (MD) Nsg assessment, ADB		Ongoing assess & treatment (MD, Nsg, SW, TR) Assess dystonia BM initial assess.		——> ——>	
Functional assessment	Assess for approp. environment Remove ext. stimuli (Nsg) Mini mental (Nsg) Assess LOF (Nsg. SW)		If ADL assessment needed (OT referral)		——> ——> Assess thought/ speech patterns	
Patient teaching	Orient pt/family to unit (Nsg) Patient rights given (Nsg)		Medication education Educate pt/family on various therapies Primary nurse ID		——> ——>	

Signatures & initials

_____ _____ _____ _____

_____ _____ _____ _____

Teaching (initial and date when complete):

1. Medication education_____
2. Education on illness_____
3. Social skills_____

Day 7–9 Loc ( )	Var n/s m u	Day 10–12 Loc ( )	Var n/s m u	Day 13–14 Loc ( )	Var n/s m u	Day 15 Loc ( )	Var n/s m u	Discharge expected outcome
⟶ ⟶		⟶ ⟶		Labs Tests Monitor blood med levels if appropriate		DC order written		
⟶		⟶		F/U appts made		⟶		
⟶		⟶		⟶		Prescriptions written		Pt will verbalize/ demonstrate imp. of medication +/or other therapies in maintaining optimal level of fcn after DC as evidenced by _____
ECT preparations, staff informed		ECT —teaching —response		⟶		⟶ Begin ECT outpt arrangements		
⟶ ⟶ ⟶ ⟶ ⟶		⟶ ⟶ ⟶ ⟶ ⟶		⟶ ⟶ ⟶ ⟶		Plans finalized r/t outpt therapy		
⟶ ⟶ ⟶		⟶ ⟶ ⟶		DC teaching r/t nutrition		⟶		
Plan discussed with patient (MD) Complete SW assessment MTP developed Weekly progress note (MD, Nsg, SW, TR) Assess for visit independence center or Day care Referrals Resources		⟶ DC teaching to pt/family F/U plans identified		⟶ ⟶ DC paperwork: —complete —chart copied —release of info —eval/ recommendations Transportation after DC arranged Outpt therapy arranged		MTP closed or remains ongoing Final DC instructions given to pt/family F/U appt finalized Weekly progress note (MD, SW, TR, Nsg)		Pt will return to least restrictive environment after DC with improved coping skills and identified resources as demonstrated by _____
⟶ ⟶ Encourage/ promote incr. LOF ⟶ ⟶ ⟶ ⟶		⟶ ⟶ Cognitive assessment Lifestyle changes assess ⟶ ⟶ ⟶ MMSE (Nsg)		⟶ ⟶ ⟶ MMSE-day 14 (Nsg)		Final assessments & DC summary written ⟶		
F/U on various therapies after DC		⟶ ⟶ D/C plan for therapies initialed		⟶ ⟶ ⟶		Final DC teaching with pt/ family A response to teaching documented.		

4. Coping skills_____
5. ADLs_____
6. Self-esteem_____
7. Dealing with anger_____

8. Communication skills_____
9. Dealing with sadness_____
10. Decision making_____
11. Other_____

*Documented patient response in progress notes. Refer to Nurses Notes for documentation regarding variances.
SW work week is M–F.
© G. Bufe 1994

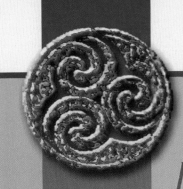

Index

Page numbers followed by "b" indicates boxed material; page numbers followed by "f" indicates figures; page numbers followed by "t" indicates tabular material.

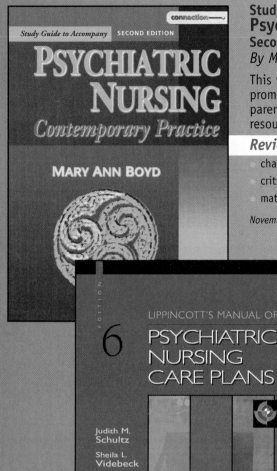
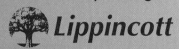

Get Connected!

http://connection.LWW.com

Connect into a one-of-a-kind resource for students!

connection

Access everything you need for your studies at connection

- **E-mail updates** notify you of recent changes on the site and of content updates to the texts.

- **Chat rooms** enable on-line discussions for you to efficiently discuss specific topics with your peers and professor.

- **Message boards** make communication a snap.

- **Create-your-own-website**, using **connection's** easy-to-use format, stores the syllabus, notes, and schedule.

And just for the student...

- **Detailed care plans** can be printed for use in the clinical setting.

- **Internet links** direct you to online resources for additional information on psychiatric nursing.

Register in 3 easy steps...

1. Simply log on to the **connection** website and access the Resource Center for Boyd: **Psychiatric Nursing, 2nd Edition**.

2. Enter your name and e-mail address, and set-up a user name and password.

3. Now you have immediate access to all the benefits of **connection**.

Connect today.
http://connection.LWW.com/go/boyd

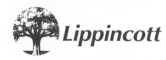 Lippincott

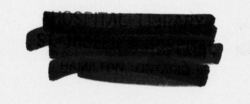